| Life stage group | Potassium (g/d) | Chloride (g/d) | Calcium (mg/d) | Phosphorus (mg/d) | Magnesium (mg/d) | Iron (mg/d) | Zinc (mg/d) | Selenium (µg/d) | Iodine (µg/d) | Copper (µg/d) | Manganese (mg/d) | Fluoride (mg/d) | Chromium (µg/d) | Molybdenum (µg/d) | Water (L/d)[8] |
|---|---|---|---|---|---|---|---|---|---|---|---|---|---|---|---|
| **Infants** | | | | | | | | | | | | | | | |
| 0-6 mo | 0.4* | 0.18* | 200* | 100* | 30* | 0.27* | 2* | 15* | 110* | 200* | 0.003* | 0.01* | 0.2* | 2* | 0.7* |
| 6-12 mo | 0.7* | 0.57* | 260* | 275* | 75* | 11 | 3* | 20* | 130* | 220* | 0.6* | 0.5* | 5.5* | 3* | 0.8* |
| **Children** | | | | | | | | | | | | | | | |
| 1-3 y | 3.0* | 1.5* | 700 | 460 | 80 | 7 | 3 | 20 | 90 | 340 | 1.2* | 0.7* | 11* | 17 | 1.3* |
| 4-8 y | 3.8* | 1.9* | 1,000 | 500 | 130 | 10 | 5 | 30 | 90 | 440 | 1.5* | 1* | 15* | 22 | 1.7* |
| **Males** | | | | | | | | | | | | | | | |
| 9-13 y | 4.5* | 2.3* | 1,300 | 1,250 | 240 | 8 | 8 | 40 | 120 | 700 | 1.9* | 2* | 25* | 34 | 2.4* |
| 14-18 y | 4.7* | 2.3* | 1,300 | 1,250 | 410 | 11 | 11 | 55 | 150 | 890 | 2.2* | 3* | 35* | 43 | 3.3* |
| 19-30 y | 4.7* | 2.3* | 1,000 | 700 | 400 | 8 | 11 | 55 | 150 | 900 | 2.3* | 4* | 35* | 45 | 3.7* |
| 31-50 y | 4.7* | 2.3* | 1,000 | 700 | 420 | 8 | 11 | 55 | 150 | 900 | 2.3* | 4* | 35* | 45 | 3.7* |
| 51-70 y | 4.7* | 2.0* | 1,000 | 700 | 420 | 8 | 11 | 55 | 150 | 900 | 2.3* | 4* | 30* | 45 | 3.7* |
| >70 y | 4.7* | 1.8* | 1,200 | 700 | 420 | 8 | 11 | 55 | 150 | 900 | 2.3* | 4* | 30* | 45 | 3.7* |
| **Females** | | | | | | | | | | | | | | | |
| 9-13 y | 4.5* | 2.3* | 1,300 | 1,250 | 240 | 8 | 8 | 40 | 120 | 700 | 1.6* | 2* | 21* | 34 | 2.1* |
| 14-18 y | 4.7* | 2.3* | 1,300 | 1,250 | 360 | 15 | 9 | 55 | 150 | 890 | 1.6* | 3* | 24* | 43 | 2.3* |
| 19-30 y | 4.7* | 2.3* | 1,000 | 700 | 310 | 18 | 8 | 55 | 150 | 900 | 1.8* | 3* | 25* | 45 | 2.7* |
| 31-50 y | 4.7* | 2.3* | 1,000 | 700 | 320 | 18 | 8 | 55 | 150 | 900 | 1.8* | 3* | 25* | 45 | 2.7* |
| 51-70 y | 4.7* | 2.0* | 1,200 | 700 | 320 | 8 | 8 | 55 | 150 | 900 | 1.8* | 3* | 20* | 45 | 2.7* |
| >70 y | 4.7* | 1.8* | 1,200 | 700 | 320 | 8 | 8 | 55 | 150 | 900 | 1.8* | 3* | 20* | 45 | 2.7* |
| **Pregnancy** | | | | | | | | | | | | | | | |
| ≤18 y | 4.7* | 2.3* | 1,300 | 1,250 | 400 | 27 | 12 | 60 | 220 | 1,000 | 2.0* | 3* | 29* | 50 | 3.0* |
| 19-30 y | 4.7* | 2.3* | 1,000 | 700 | 350 | 27 | 11 | 60 | 220 | 1,000 | 2.0* | 3* | 30* | 50 | 3.0* |
| 31-50 y | 4.7* | 2.3* | 1,000 | 700 | 360 | 27 | 11 | 60 | 220 | 1,000 | 2.0* | 3* | 30* | 50 | 3.0* |
| **Lactation** | | | | | | | | | | | | | | | |
| ≤18 y | 5.1* | 2.3 | 1,300 | 1,250 | 360 | 10 | 13 | 70 | 290 | 1,300 | 2.6* | 3* | 44* | 50 | 3.8* |
| 19-30 y | 5.1* | 2.3 | 1,000 | 700 | 310 | 9 | 12 | 70 | 290 | 1,300 | 2.6* | 3* | 45* | 50 | 3.8* |
| 31-50 y | 5.1* | 2.3 | 1,000 | 700 | 320 | 9 | 12 | 70 | 290 | 1,300 | 2.6* | 3* | 45* | 50 | 3.8* |

**Sources:** Data compiled from *Dietary Reference Intakes for Calcium, Phosphorus, Magnesium, Vitamin D, and Fluoride*. Washington, DC: National Academies Press; 1997. *Dietary Reference Intakes for Thiamin, Riboflavin, Niacin, Vitamin B6, Folate, Vitamin B12, Pantothenic Acid, Biotin, and Choline*. Washington, DC: National Academies Press; 1998. *Dietary Reference Intakes for Vitamin C, Vitamin E, Selenium, and Carotenoids*. Washington, DC: National Academies Press; 2000. *Dietary Reference Intakes for Vitamin A, Vitamin K, Arsenic, Boron, Chromium, Copper, Iron, Manganese, Molybdenum, Nickel, Silicon, Vanadium, and Zinc*. Washington, DC: National Academies Press; 2000. *Dietary Reference Intakes for Water, Potassium, Sodium, Chloride, and Sulfate*. Food and Nutrition Board. Washington, DC: National Academies Press; 2005. *Dietary Reference Intakes for Calcium and Vitamin D*. Washington, DC: National Academies Press; 2011. These reports may be accessed via http://nap.edu.

# Discovering
# Nutrition

## Fourth Edition

**Paul Insel**
Stanford University

**Don Ross**
California Institute of Human Nutrition

**Kimberley McMahon**
Benedictine University and Logan College

**Melissa Bernstein**
Rosalind Franklin University of Medicine and Science

JONES & BARTLETT
LEARNING

*World Headquarters*
Jones & Bartlett Learning
5 Wall Street
Burlington, MA 01803
978-443-5000
info@jblearning.com
www.jblearning.com

Jones & Bartlett Learning books and products are available through most bookstores and online booksellers. To contact Jones & Bartlett Learning directly, call 800-832-0034, fax 978-443-8000, or visit our website, www.jblearning.com.

Substantial discounts on bulk quantities of Jones & Bartlett Learning publications are available to corporations, professional associations, and other qualified organizations. For details and specific discount information, contact the special sales department at Jones & Bartlett Learning via the above contact information or send an email to specialsales@jblearning.com.

## Production Credits

Chief Executive Officer: Ty Field
President: James Homer
SVP, Editor-in-Chief: Michael Johnson
SVP, Chief Marketing Officer: Alison M. Pendergast
Publisher: Cathleen Sether
Executive Editor: Shoshanna Goldberg
Editorial Assistant: Agnes Burt
Production Manager: Julie Champagne Bolduc
Production Editor: Jessica Steele Newfell

Production Assistant: Emma Krosschell
Marketing Manager: Jody Yeskey
VP, Manufacturing and Inventory Control: Therese Connell
Composition: Publishers' Design and Production Services, Inc.
Cover and Title Page Design: Scott Moden
Permissions and Photo Research Assistant: Amy Rathburn
Cover and Title Page Image: © nuttakit/ShutterStock, Inc.
Printing and Binding: Courier Companies
Cover Printing: Courier Companies

**To order this product, use ISBN: 978-1-4496-6133-5**

## Library of Congress Cataloging-in-Publication Data

Discovering nutrition / by Paul Insel … [et al.]. — 4th ed.
    p. ; cm.
  Rev. ed. of: Discovering nutrition / Paul Insel, R. Elaine Turner, Don Ross. 3rd ed. c2010.
  Includes bibliographical references and index.
  ISBN 978-1-4496-3294-6 — ISBN 1-4496-3294-7
  I. Insel, Paul M. II. Insel, Paul M. Discovering nutrition.
  [DNLM: 1. Nutritional Physiological Phenomena. 2. Diet. QU 145]
  613.2—dc23
     2011046146

6048

Printed in the United States of America

16  15  14  13  12     10  9  8  7  6  5  4  3  2

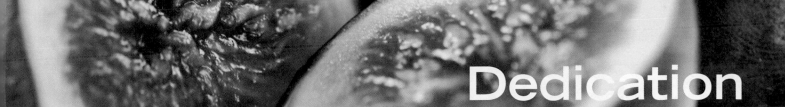

# Dedication

*To Michelle with love.*
*— Paul Insel*

*To Donna and Mackinnon for their sustenance of love, support, and patience.*
*— Don Ross*

*To Tom, Dawson, Emmett, and Quincy for your encouragement, patience, support, and love.*
*— Kimberley McMahon*

*To my family with all my love.*
*— Melissa Bernstein*

# Brief Contents

# Contents

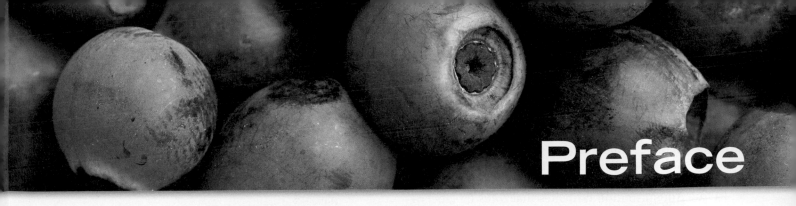

# Preface

Nutrition has never been more exciting or important than it is today. New discoveries about nutrition and its importance in overall health emerge daily. Because we are committed to providing comprehensive and accurate information on the most pressing current issues, we have prepared this fourth edition of *Discovering Nutrition*. The overall content, organization, and features remain, but, within this framework, key topics and issues are updated with the newest information available.

Learning nutrition can be exciting and engaging. *Discovering Nutrition* takes students on a fascinating journey beginning with curiosity and ending with a solid knowledge base and a healthy dose of skepticism for the endless ads and infomercials promoting "new" diets and food products. We want students to learn enough about their nutritional and health status to use this new knowledge in their everyday lives. Our mission is to give students the tools to logically interpret the nutrition information provided by the evening news, on food labels, in popular magazines, and by government agencies. Our goal is to help them become sophisticated consumers of both nutrients and nutrition information. Hopefully, students will come to understand that knowledge of nutrition allows them to personalize information rather than follow every guideline issued for an entire population.

*Discovering Nutrition* is unique in its behavioral approach. It challenges students to act, not just memorize the material. Familiar experiences and choices draw students into each chapter, and analogies illuminate difficult concepts. In addition, we address important topics that students are curious about, such as ethnic diets, functional foods, nutrient supplements, phytochemicals, vegetarianism, diets for athletes, food safety, and fad diets. We focus attention on alcohol, eating disorders, and complementary nutrition. Some instructors may wish to cover metabolism, so we include a Spotlight on Metabolism to provide a friendly tour of the metabolic pathways. Throughout the book, the relationship of diet and health is incorporated into appropriate chapters (e.g., lipids and cardiovascular disease; carbohydrates and diabetes).

*Discovering Nutrition* brings up-to-date nutritional research into your classroom. It features the latest standards: the Dietary Reference Intakes, *2010 Dietary Guidelines for Americans*, and the USDA MyPlate. *Discovering Nutrition* provides students with tools, such as the ancillary diet analy-sis software, to track and analyze their personal nutrient intakes. In addition, the book's website, **go.jblearning. com/inseldisco4e**, offers access to the constantly emerging developments in nutrition.

## Dietary Guidelines for Americans

The seventh edition of *Dietary Guidelines for Americans* places stronger emphasis on improving poor diets and increasing physical activity, two of the most important factors for combating the obesity epidemic. Eating a healthy balance of nutritious foods continues as a central point in the *Dietary Guidelines*, but simply balancing nutrients is not enough for health. Total calories also count, especially as more Americans are gaining weight. Because almost two-thirds of Americans are overweight or obese and more than half get too little physical activity, the *2010 Dietary Guidelines* place a stronger emphasis on calorie control and physical activity. The report identifies several key recommendations. As you read the chapters, look for these recommendations highlighted in the margins.

## USDA MyPlate

MyPlate, which replaces MyPyramid, is part of an overall food guidance system that emphasizes the need for a more individualized approach to improving diet and lifestyle. MyPlate incorporates recommendations from the *Dietary Guidelines for Americans* and uses interactive technology found at www.ChooseMyPlate.gov. These interactive activities allow individuals to obtain more personalized recommendations for daily calorie levels based on the *Dietary Guidelines for Americans* and to find general food guidance and suggestions for making smart choices from each food group. Concepts from MyPlate and the *Dietary Guidelines* are carried throughout the book and are fully integrated into the text.

## Trans Fat Labeling

*Discovering Nutrition* delivers the tools for students to understand food labels, including *trans* fat information, and to incorporate positive nutritional behaviors in their everyday lives. The *Dietary Guidelines for Americans* recommend reducing the intake of *trans* fats and saturated fats. The recent United States labeling requirement for *trans* fat provides a more complete picture of fat content in foods, allowing students and other consumers to choose foods low in *trans* fat, saturated fat, and cholesterol. The Food and Drug Administration estimates that *trans* fat labeling will prevent 600 to 1,200 cases of coronary heart disease and 250 to 500 deaths each year.

## Bioterrorism and the Food Supply

How safe is our food supply? In the aftermath of the terrorist attacks on the World Trade Center in September 2001 and the spread of anthrax through the mail, there is heightened concern over the vulnerability of our food supply to bioterrorism. *Discovering Nutrition* explores past attacks on U.S. and Canadian food supplies, points of vulnerability, and food safety strategies that students can use to help protect themselves.

## Updates to This Edition

Updates throughout this *Fourth Edition* include the latest DRIs, revised macronutrient chapters, the latest references, expanded coverage of diet and health, and much more. A chapter-by-chapter breakdown of updates can be downloaded from **go.jblearning.com/discovering4**. A few specific updates include:

- Position statements from the Academy of Nutrition of Dietetics (formerly the American Dietetic Association), the American Heart Association, the American College of Sports Medicine, and the Dietitians of Canada
- New section on dietary guidelines around the world, including the Japanese Food Guide
- Updated information on *Eating Well with Canada's Food Guide*
- New sections on diet and health, including in-depth coverage of obesity and physical activity

- Expanded discussion on preventing eating disorders, the impact of the college environment on eating disorders, and maladaptive coping patterns
- Updated discussion of Feeding America (formerly America's Second Harvest Food Bank)
- Revised discussion of overweight and obesity in childhood as well as pregnancy weight gain guidelines

## Accessible Science

*Discovering Nutrition* makes use of the latest in learning theory and balances the behavioral aspects of nutrition with an accessible approach to scientific concepts. This text is intended to be a comprehensive resource that communicates nutrition both graphically and personally.

We present technical concepts in an engaging, non-intimidating way with an appealing, stepwise, and parallel development of text and annotated illustrations. Illustrations in all chapters use consistent representations. Each type of nutrient, for example, has a distinct color and shape. Icons of an amino acid, a protein, a triglyceride, and a glucose molecule represent "characters" in the nutrition story and are instantly recognizable as they appear throughout the book.

This text is unique in the field of nutrition and leads the way in depicting important biological and physiological phenomena, such as emulsification, glucose regulation, digestion and absorption, and fetal development. Extensive graphic presentations make nutrition and physiological principles come alive. The illustrations use pictures to teach and are part of a multimedia package that coordinates the text with illustrations and software. The EatRight Analysis program is a fully integrated ancillary designed to help students track their diets, make choices, and hone their nutritional skills.

# The Pedagogy

*Discovering Nutrition* focuses on teaching behavioral change, personal decision making, and up-to-date scientific concepts in a number of novel ways. The interactive approach that addresses different learning styles makes it the ideal text to ensure a high likelihood of success by students. Beginning with Chapter 1, the material engages students in considering their own behavior in light of the knowledge they are gaining. The following pedagogical aids appear in most chapters.

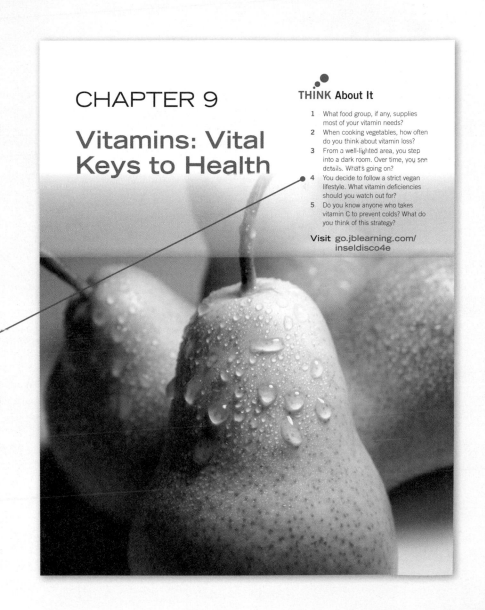

CHAPTER 9

## Vitamins: Vital Keys to Health

**THINK About It**

1  What food group, if any, supplies most of your vitamin needs?

2  When cooking vegetables, how often do you think about vitamin loss?

3  From a well-lighted area, you step into a dark room. Over time, you see details. What's going on?

4  You decide to follow a strict vegan lifestyle. What vitamin deficiencies should you watch out for?

5  Do you know anyone who takes vitamin C to prevent colds? What do you think of this strategy?

**Visit** go.jblearning.com/ inseldisco4e

**Think About It** questions present realistic nutrition-related situations and ask students to consider how they would behave in such circumstances.

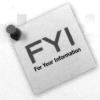

## Fresh, Frozen, or Canned? Raw, Dried, or Cooked?

**Selecting and Preparing Foods to Maximize Vitamin Content**

Wouldn't it be great if we could all shop daily for fresh fruits and vegetables? When picked at their peak ripeness, fresh fruits and vegetables contain many different vitamins. Remember that light, heat, air, acid, and alkali can destroy many vitamins, and cooking liquids can leach them out. Even if you can't buy fresh foods daily, you can still minimize nutrient loss after purchase. Start by choosing clean, undamaged produce on your regular shopping trips. Then store foods with minimal exposure to light and air. Many fruits, most vegetables, and all animal products require refrigeration. Get them cold right away, and keep them cold. Because vitamin content can decrease with time, plan on using fruits and vegetables soon after purchase. The vitamin C of fresh green beans, for example, drops by half after six days at home.

What about frozen and canned foods? Their vitamin content is much better than you might guess. When vegetables are frozen immediately after they are picked, they can be more healthful choices than fresh vegetables that lose nutrients during shipping and storage.[1] Although canning uses destructive heat, the processor typically uses fresh-picked produce, which is higher in vitamins than fresh food transported to faraway markets. When using canned vegetables, incorporate the liquid in soups and stews to get the benefit of any vitamins that end up in the liquid. Recipes prepared with canned foods have similar nutritional values to those prepared with fresh or frozen ingredients.[2]

Carotenoids are stable during the canning process. In fact, research suggests the lycopene in processed tomato products is better absorbed into the body than that from raw tomatoes.[3] Unfortunately, vitamin C is lost from fruits and vegetables during canning, but much of the lost vitamin remains in the canning liquid or juice. Ready-to-drink orange juice loses about 2 percent of its vitamin C content each day once opened.[4]

Dried fruits are also a good way to eat your daily fruit. The biggest concern is portion size because when fruits are dried their nutrient, calorie, and sugar content becomes concentrated, and it is easy to eat too much. Dried fruits have a low to moderate glycemic index and a glycemic response that's comparable to that of fresh fruits. They are a good source of nutrients such as potassium and fiber.[5] Data from the National Health and Nutrition Examination Survey (NHANES) showed that dried fruit consumption is associated with lower body mass index (BMI); reduced waist circumference; reduced abdominal obesity; improved nutrient intake (higher vitamin A, vitamin K, potassium, iron, magnesium, and fiber intake); more fruit servings per day; and healthier overall diets for both adults and children.[6]

What is the best way to cook vegetables? To maximize vitamin content, think minimal—minimal heat, minimal cooking water, and minimal exposure to air. A good rule of thumb: "minimize to maximize." Try to minimize handling the food before and during cooking. Dicing a food such as a potato reduces cooking time but also exposes more surface area to vitamin destruction. So, cut if you must, but not too small.

Because steaming, stir-frying, and microwaving minimize cooking time and water use, they are the best cooking methods for preserving vitamin content. If you boil foods, use the cooking water for sauces, stews, or soups to salvage lost water-soluble vitamins. And do not add baking soda to beans or vegetables (some folks do that to intensify color and tenderize). Baking soda destroys some vitamins.

Remember, to retain the most vitamins in your food, be gentle with storage, kind with cooking, and "minimize to maximize"!

1. Academy of Nutrition and Dietetics. Are fresh fruits and veggies better than frozen? http://www.eatright.org/Public/content.aspx?id=6442451896&terms=fresh+or+frozen. Accessed 7/12/11.
2. Fruit and Veggies—More Matters. Fresh, frozen canned, dried and 100% juice: all forms of fruits and vegetables matter! http://www.fruitsandveggiesmorematters.org/?page_id=47. Accessed 7/12/11.
3. Carlsen MH, Halvorsen BL, Holte K, et al. The total antioxidant content of more than 3,100 foods, beverages, spices, herbs, and supplements used worldwide. Nutr J. 2010;9:3.
4. Johnston CS, Bowling DL. Stability of ascorbic acid in commercially available orange juices. J Am Diet Assoc. 2002;102:525–529.
5. Fruit and Veggies—More Matters. About the buzz: fresh fruit is much healthier than dried fruit? Updated 7/6/11. http://www.fruitsandveggiesmatters.org/?page_id=18744. Accessed 7/12/11.
6. Fruit and Veggies—More Matters. About the buzz: fresh fruit is much healthier than dried fruit? Op. cit.; and Keast D, Jones J. Dried fruit consumption associated with reduced improved overweight or obesity in adults: NHANES, 1999–2004. Fed Am Soc Exp Bio J. 2009;23:LB511.

lost in milling. Moreover, the American diet contains lots of highly refined foods that are not fortified or enriched, foods that have calories but almost no micronutrients.

### Provitamins

Some vitamins in foods are in inactive forms, called **provitamins** or **vitamin precursors**. The body must change them to an active form. One familiar provitamin is beta-carotene, found in many fruits and vegetables. Your body

**provitamins** Inactive forms of vitamins that the body can convert into active usable forms. Also referred to as vitamin precursors.

**vitamin precursors** See *provitamins*.

The **For Your Information** feature offers more in-depth treatment of controversial and timely topics, such as unfounded claims about the effects of sugar, whether athletes need more protein, and the usefulness of the glycemic index.

**Key terms** are in boldface type the first time they are mentioned. Their definitions also appear in the margins near the relevant textual discussion, making it easy for students to review material and terms.

The **Label to Table** feature helps students apply their new decision-making skills at the supermarket. It walks students through the various types of information that appear on food labels, including government-mandated terminology, misleading advertising phrases, and amounts of ingredients.

**Key Concepts** summarize previous text and highlight important information.

**Quick Bites** are sprinkled throughout the book. They offer fun facts about nutrition-related topics such as exotic foods, social customs, origins of phrases, folk remedies, and medical history.

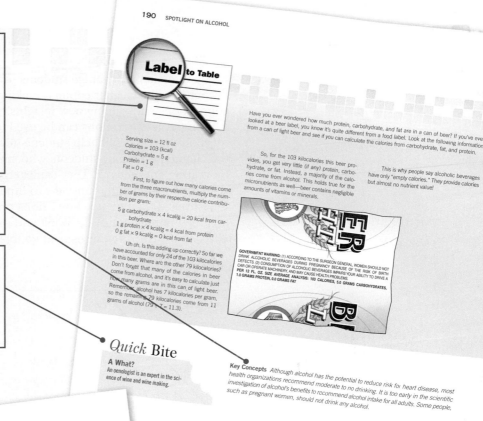

190 SPOTLIGHT ON ALCOHOL

**Label to Table**

Have you ever wondered how much protein, carbohydrate, and fat are in a can of beer? If you've ever looked at a beer label, you know it's quite different from a food label. Look at the following information from a can of light beer and see if you can calculate the calories from carbohydrate, fat, and protein.

Serving size = 12 fl oz
Calories = 103 (kcal)
Carbohydrate = 5 g
Protein = 1 g
Fat = 0 g

First, to figure out how many calories come from the three macronutrients, multiply the number of grams by their respective calorie contribution per gram:

5 g carbohydrate × 4 kcal/g = 20 kcal from carbohydrate
1 g protein × 4 kcal/g = 4 kcal from protein
0 g fat × 9 kcal/g = 0 kcal from fat

Uh oh. Is this adding up correctly? So far we have accounted for only 24 of the 103 kilocalories in this beer. Where are the other 79 kilocalories? Don't forget that many of the calories in beer come from alcohol, and it's easy to calculate just how many grams are in this can of light beer. Remember, alcohol has 7 kilocalories per gram, so the remaining 79 kilocalories come from 11 grams of alcohol (79 ÷ 7 = 11.3).

So, for the 103 kilocalories this beer provides, you get very little (if any) protein, carbohydrate, or fat. Instead, a majority of the calories come from alcohol. This holds true for the micronutrients as well—beer contains negligible amounts of vitamins or minerals.

This is why people say alcoholic beverages have only "empty calories." They provide calories but almost no nutrient value!

GOVERNMENT WARNING: (1) ACCORDING TO THE SURGEON GENERAL, WOMEN SHOULD NOT DRINK ALCOHOLIC BEVERAGES DURING PREGNANCY BECAUSE OF THE RISK OF BIRTH DEFECTS. (2) CONSUMPTION OF ALCOHOLIC BEVERAGES IMPAIRS YOUR ABILITY TO DRIVE A CAR OR OPERATE MACHINERY, AND MAY CAUSE HEALTH PROBLEMS. PER 12 FL. OZ. SIZE AVERAGE ANALYSIS: 103 CALORIES, 5.0 GRAMS CARBOHYDRATE, 1.0 GRAMS PROTEIN, 0.0 GRAMS FAT

*Quick* Bite

**A What?**
An oenologist is an expert in the science of wine and wine making.

**Key Concepts** Although alcohol has the potential to reduce risk for heart disease, most health organizations recommend moderate to no drinking. It is too early in the scientific investigation of alcohol's benefits to recommend alcohol intake for all adults. Some people, such as pregnant women, should not drink any alcohol.

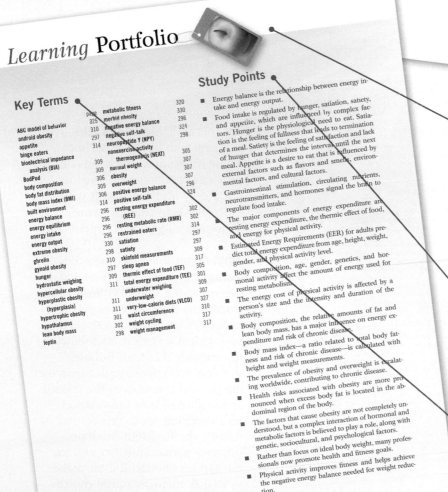

## *Learning* Portfolio

### Study Points

- Energy balance is the relationship between energy intake and energy output.
- Food intake is regulated by hunger, satiation, satiety, and appetite, which are influenced by complex factors. Hunger is the physiological need to eat. Satiation is the feeling of fullness that leads to termination of a meal. Satiety is the feeling of satisfaction and lack of hunger that determines the interval until the next meal. Appetite is a desire to eat that is influenced by external factors such as flavors and smells, environmental factors, and cultural factors.
- Gastrointestinal stimulation, circulating nutrients, neurotransmitters, and hormones signal the brain to regulate food intake.
- The major components of energy expenditure are resting energy expenditure, the thermic effect of food, and energy for physical activity.
- Estimated Energy Requirements (EER) for adults predict total energy expenditure from age, height, weight, gender, and physical activity level.
- Body composition, age, gender, genetics, and hormonal activity affect the amount of energy used for resting metabolism.
- The energy cost of physical activity is affected by a person's size and the intensity and duration of the activity.
- Body composition, the relative amounts of fat and lean body mass, has a major influence on energy expenditure and risk of chronic disease.
- Body mass index—a ratio related to total body fatness and risk of chronic disease—is calculated with height and weight measurements.
- The prevalence of obesity and overweight is escalating worldwide, contributing to chronic disease.
- Health risks associated with obesity are more pronounced when excess body fat is located in the abdominal region of the body.
- The factors that cause obesity are not completely understood, but a complex interaction of hormonal and metabolic factors is believed to play a role, along with genetic, sociocultural, and psychological factors.
- Rather than focus on ideal body weight, many professionals now promote health and fitness goals.
- Physical activity improves fitness and helps achieve the negative energy balance needed for weight reduction.

### Key Terms

The **Learning Portfolio** at the end of each chapter collects—in one place—all aspects of nutrition information students need to solidify their understanding of the material. The various formats will appeal to students according to their individual learning and studying styles.

**Study Points** is a bulleted list that summarizes the content of each chapter with a synopsis of each major topic. The points are in the order in which they appear in the chapter so related concepts flow together.

**Key Terms** lists all of the new vocabulary alphabetically with the page number of the first appearance. This arrangement allows students to review terms they do not recall and to turn immediately to the definition and discussion of it in the chapter. This approach promotes the acquisition of knowledge, not simply memorization.

**Study Questions** encourage students to probe deeper into the chapter content, making connections and gaining new insights. Although these questions can be used for pop quizzes, they also will help students review the chapter, especially students who study by writing out material. They can check their work by looking at the Answers to Study Questions (odd-numbered questions only) included in the back of the book and on the *Discovering Nutrition* website at **go.jblearning .com/inseldisco4e.**

---

- Abandoning unrealistic ideas of thinness and accepting body weight and shape are important elements in weight management.
- Long-term weight management includes a balanced diet of moderately restricted calorie intake, adequate exercise, cognitive-behavioral strategies for changing habits and behavior patterns, and attention to balancing self-acceptance and the desire for change.
- Surgical approaches to weight control should be considered only as a last resort for the morbidly obese.
- If the cause is not hereditary, being underweight can pose health problems.
- Gaining weight can be difficult for individuals who are underweight.

## Study Questions

1. Explain the concept of energy balance.
2. Define *hunger, satiation, satiety,* and *appetite.*
3. List and describe the three main components of energy expenditure.
4. Explain the three main factors that determine energy expenditure in activity.
5. What body mass index (BMI) values are associated with being underweight, overweight, and obese? Do these vary for men and women?
6. Obesity is seen as a complex disorder with multiple contributing factors. List the general types of factors involved in the development and maintenance of obesity.
7. What is the difference between hyperplastic and hypertrophic obesity?
8. Describe the concept of metabolic fitness.
9. What are the four components of a sound approach to weight management?
10. Explain how the ABCs of behavior modification can assist with weight control.
11. Define *underweight.*

## Try This

### A One-Week Energy Balance Check

The purpose of this exercise is to see if you're in energy balance by monitoring your body weight for one week. Measure your weight on a Monday morning soon after you wake up. Record your weight. Don't change your normal routine of exercise and food intake. One week later weigh yourself again (on a Monday morning just after waking). Did your weight change? If not, your energy intake closely matched your energy output. If so, did you gain or lose weight? What factors do you think contributed to your body weight change? Try repeating this exercise over a longer period of time. Measure and record your weight every Monday morning for six months. What happens?

### Increasing Your Energy Output

Physical activity is the part of your energy output that varies the most. The purpose of this exercise is to increase your energy expenditure by committing to daily exercise for one week. Make each exercise session about 30 minutes long, and remember that the longer the duration, the harder the intensity, and the larger the muscle groups involved, the greater the energy expenditure. Choose an exercise you enjoy—such as walking, jogging, cycling, swimming, or rollerblading. Once your week is complete, ask yourself these questions: How did this week's daily exercise affect my energy balance? Have I gained or lost weight during the week? Did I compensate for the extra energy expenditure by increasing my calorie intake?

### Changing Your Energy Input

Would you like to change your weight by a pound or two? The purpose of this exercise is to increase or decrease your energy input (calorie intake) so you gain or lose 1 pound by the end of a week. How? Make only minor adjustments in your usual diet but try to change the energy content for each of your meals by a small amount. Keep a food log and use the EatRight Analysis Software or Nutritionist Pro Software to estimate your calorie total for each of the days. Your goal is to change your calorie total by approximately 500 kilocalories per day. You should not consume fewer than 1,500 kilocalories (for women) or 1,800 kilocalories (for men) per day. Weigh yourself at the start of your week and at the end. What change, if any, do you see?

### What About Bobbie?

Remember, Bobbie is a 20-year-old college sophomore who weighs 155 pounds and is 5'4". She gained 10 pounds her freshman year and would like to lose it because she feels healthier when her weight is closer to 145 pounds. She exercises infrequently but likes to walk with her friends and occasionally goes to an aerobics class. How would you suggest she lose the extra 10 pounds? First, let's start by reducing her calorie intake slightly. Here is Bobbie's typical day of eating and some small changes in portion sizes that will save calories.

As you can see, small changes in Bobbie's diet can result in a 500-kilocalorie deficit, which will translate to approximately 1 pound per week of weight loss. This doesn't take into account any extra exercise she might do. If she starts to work out more regularly, she can make fewer changes in her calorie intake and still lose 1 pound per week.

---

**Try This** activities are for curious students who like to experiment. These suggestions for hands-on activities encourage students to put theory into practice. It will especially help students whose major learning style is experiential.

**What About Bobbie?** tracks the eating habits and health-related decisions of a typical college student so students can apply the material they learned in the chapter to a typical situation. By following the individual case of Bobbie, students move from understanding the general concepts to the specific application of new information. As a complement to this textual feature, the EatRight Analysis software allows students to track the various choices Bobbie makes as well as their own food choices.

## The Integrated Learning and Teaching Package

Integrating the text and ancillaries is crucial to deriving their full benefit. Based on feedback from instructors and students, Jones & Bartlett Learning offers the following supplements.

Dietary analysis software is an important component of the behavioral change and personal decision-making focus. **EatRight Analysis**, developed by ESHA Research and tailored by the authors, enables students to analyze their diets by calculating their nutrient intake and comparing it to recommended intake levels. It is available online (**eatright .jblearning.com**) and in CD format.

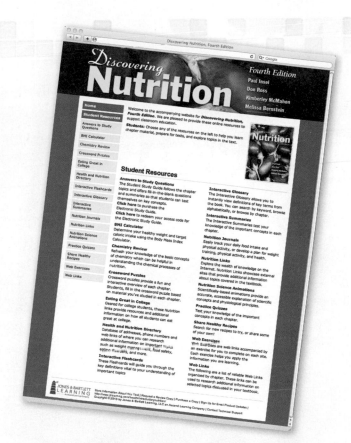

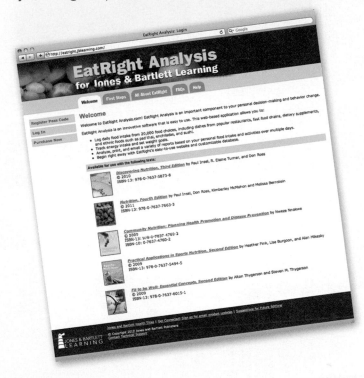

A downloadable Instructor's Manual and Test Bank also are available to adopters of this text. Contact your Nutrition Representative at **jblearning.com/nutrition**. The **website** for *Discovering Nutrition*, **go.jblearning.com/inseldisco4e**, offers students and instructors an unprecedented degree of integration between the text and the online world through many useful study tools, activities, and supplementary health information.

The **Instructor's Media CD** is a comprehensive teaching resource available to adopters of the book. It includes:

- PowerPoint Presentation Lecture Slides
- Image and Table Bank, which provides the art and tables from the text that can be imported into PowerPoints and tests or used to create transparencies

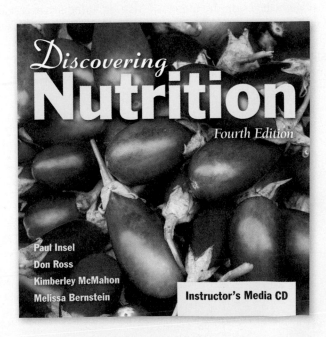

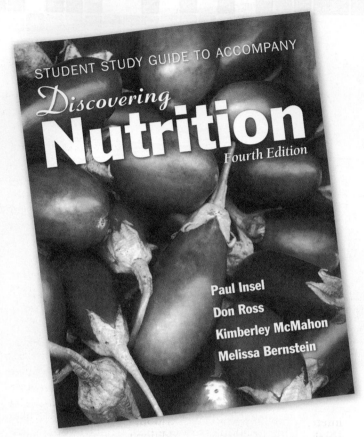

For the convenience of the student, the food composition tables and several additional appendices can now be found in the *Food Composition Tables and Appendices* supplement. This easy-to-use reference features the nutrient values found in a variety of foods. Additionally, students will have quick access to the USDA Food Intake Patterns, Vitamin and Mineral Summary Tables, Calculations and Conversions, and more. The supplement is available as a bundle item at no additional cost.

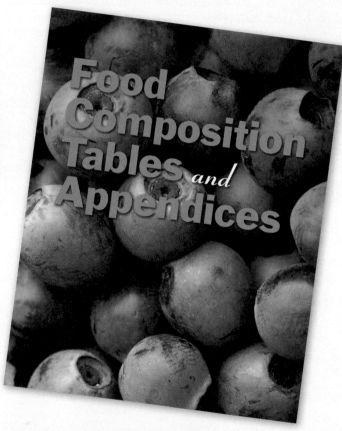

The online *Student Study Guide* provides a powerful learning tool for students using *Discovering Nutrition*. Available with every new text at no additional cost, the *Student Study Guide* follows the chapter topics and offers fill-in-the-blank questions and summaries so students can test themselves on the material. Also included are exercises for students to gain familiarity with the key terms in each chapter and ideas for making assessments of their own dietary habits. The *Student Study Guide* is accessible to students through the redeemable access code provided in every new text.

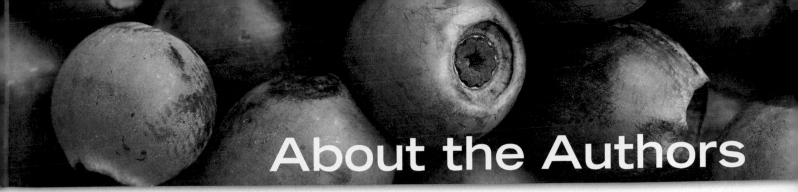

# About the Authors

The *Discovering Nutrition* author team represents a culmination of years of teaching and research in psychology and nutrition science. The combined experience of the authors yields a balanced presentation of both the science of nutrition and the components of behavioral change.

**Dr. Paul Insel** is Consulting Associate Professor of Psychiatry at Stanford University (Stanford, California). In addition to being the principal investigator on several nutrition projects for the National Institutes of Health (NIH), he is the senior author of the seminal text in health education and has co-authored several best-selling nutrition books.

**Don Ross** is Director of the California Institute of Human Nutrition (Redwood City, California). For more than 20 years, he has co-authored multiple textbooks and created educational materials about health and nutrition for consumers, professionals, and college students. He has special expertise in communicating complicated physiological processes with easily understood graphical presentations. The National Institutes of Health selected his *Travels with Cholesterol* for distribution to consumers. His multidisciplinary focus brings together the fields of psychology, nutrition, biochemistry, biology, and medicine.

**Kimberley McMahon** is a Registered Dietitian and Adjunct Instructor at both Benedictine University (Lisle, Illinois) and Logan College (St. Louis). She has taught basic nutrition, nutrition for exercise and sport, dietetics administration, and clinical nutrition courses. She co-authored *Eat Right! Healthy Eating in College and Beyond*. Her interests and experience are in the areas of wellness, weight management, sports nutrition, and eating disorders.

**Dr. Melissa Bernstein** is a Registered Dietitian, Licensed Dietitian, and Assistant Professor in the Department of Nutrition at Rosalind Franklin University of Medicine and Science (North Chicago, Illinois). She received her doctoral degree from the Gerald J. and Dorothy R. Friedman School of Nutrition Science and Policy at Tufts University. Dr. Bernstein has been teaching courses in nutrition for more than 15 years and is innovative in creating engaging and challenging online nutrition courses. Her interests include geriatric nutrition, physical activity, and nutritional biochemistry. In addition to co-authoring *Nutrition for the Older Adult*, Dr. Bernstein has contributed to and authored textbook chapters and peer-reviewed journal publications on the topics of nutrition and nutrition for older adults.

# Contributors

The following people contributed to the *Fourth Edition* of this text:

### R. Elaine Turner, PhD

Dr. R. Elaine Turner is a Registered Dietitian and Professor in the Food Science and Human Nutrition Department at the University of Florida (Gainesville, Florida), where she currently holds the position of Associate Dean in the College of Agricultural and Life Sciences. Dr. Turner has been teaching courses in introductory and life-cycle nutrition for more than 20 years. Her interests include nutrition labeling and dietary supplement regulations, computer applications in nutrition and education, maternal and infant nutrition, and consumer issues. Dr. Turner was named Undergraduate Teacher of the Year (2000–2001) for the College of Agricultural and Life Sciences, and, in 2004, she was recognized with a National Award for Excellence in College and University Teaching in the Food and Agricultural Sciences by the USDA.

### Hope McClusky Bilyk, MS, RD, LDN

*Chapter 1   Food Choices: Nutrients and Nourishment*

Hope Bilyk is an Assistant Professor at the Rosalind Franklin University of Medicine and Science, The Chicago Medical School. Her area of research includes healthcare communication and specializing in cultural competency and low literacy healthcare studies.

### Nancy Munoz, DCN, MHA, RD

*Chapter 13   Life Cycle: From Childhood Through Adulthood*

Nancy Munoz is the Clinical Nutrition Manager for Genesis Healthcare Corporation. She teaches courses on nutritional assessment and nutrition for a healthy lifestyle at the University of Massachusetts, Amherst, and is a University of Phoenix nursing instructor. Her areas of research include oral health and nutrition and wounds.

Contributors from past editions include the following:

Janine T. Baer, PhD, RD, University of Dayton (Chapters 11 and 12)

Katherine Beals, PhD, RD, FACSM, University of Utah (Chapter 8)

Toni Bloom, MS, RD, CDE, San Jose State University (pedagogy)

Boyce W. Burge, PhD, California Institute of Human Nutrition (Chapter 14)

Robert DiSilvestro, PhD, The Ohio State University (Chapter 7)

Eileen G. Ford, MS, RD, Drexel University (Chapter 12)

Ellen B. Fung, PhD, RD, University of Pennsylvania (Chapter 10)

Michael I. Goran, PhD, University of Southern California (Chapter 8)

Nancy J. Gustafson, MS, RD, FADA, Sawyer County (WI) Aging Unit (Chapters 5 and 7)

Rita H. Herskovitz, MS, University of Pennsylvania (Chapter 10)

Nancy I. Kemp, MD, University of California at San Francisco (Chapter 10)

Sarah Harding Laidlaw, MS, RD, MPA, Nutrition in Complementary Care DPG 18 (Chapter 13)

Rick D. Mattes, MPH, PhD, RD, Purdue University (Chapter 1)

Maye Musk, MS, RD, Past President of the Consulting Dietitians of Canada (Chapter 15)

Carla Miller, PhD, The Ohio State University (Chapter 5)

Joyce D. Nash, PhD (Chapter 8)

Rachel Stern, MS, RD, CNS, North Jersey Community Research Initiative (Chapters 6 and 15 and Spotlight on Alcohol)

Lisa Stollman, MA, RD, CDE, CDN, State University of New York at Stony Brook (Chapter 4)

Barbara Sutherland, PhD, University of California at Davis (Spotlight on Metabolism)

Debra M. Vinci, PhD, RD, CD, Appalachian State University (Chapter 11)

Stella L. Volpe, PhD, RD, FACSM, University of Massachusetts (Chapter 8)

Paula Kurtzweil Walter, MS, RD, Federal Trade Commission (Chapter 14)

The authors also would like to acknowledge the valuable contributions from the following people:

Pat Brown, MS, RD, Cuesta College

Alexandria Miller, PhD, RD/LD, Northeastern State University

Marcia Nelms, PhD, RD, Missouri State University

CJ Nieves, MS, University of Florida

Barbara Reynolds, MS, RD, College of the Sequoias

Elizabeth Quintana, MS, RD, LD, CDE, West Virginia University School (Chapter 6)

# Reviewers
## Reviewers of the *Third Edition*

Orville Bigelow, MS, RD, Mohave Community College

Deborah Cheater, MS, RN, Carl Albert State College

Laura Freeland Kull, MS, RD, Madonna University

Shelby Goldberg, RD, CDE, Pima Community College

Lisa P. Hall, MHA, MS, RD LD, CDE, Fayette County Memorial Hospital

Cathy Hix-Cunningham, PhD, RD, LDN, Tennessee Technological University

Colleen Kvaska, MA, RD, CDE, Fullerton College

David Lightsey, MS, Bakersfield College

Lourdes Lore, MS, Henry Ford Community College

Lisa Murray, MS, Pierce College, Fort Steilacoom

Karen Nguyen-Garcia, Community College of Denver

Stephanie Schroeder, PhD, Webster University

Annette R. Tommerdahl, PhD, University of Louisiana at Monroe

## Reviewers of the *Second Edition*

Helen C. Alexanderson-Lee, PhD, RD, California State University at Long Beach

Teresa Blair, MS, RD, LD, CDE, Eastern Kentucky University

Dr. Michele Brandenburger, BS, DC, MS, Presentation College

Lisa Burgoon, MS, RD, CSSD, LDN, University of Illinois at Urbana-Champaign

Alana D. Cline, PhD, RD, University of Northern Colorado

Jeanne Freeman, PhD, CHES, Butte-Glenn Community College

Bernard L. Frye, PhD, University of Texas at Arlington

Amy Gannon, MS, RD, LD, Marshall University

Shelby Goldberg, RD, CDE, Pima Community College

Michael I. Goran, PhD, University of Southern California

Donna Huisenga, MS, RD, LDN, Illinois Central College

Amy Kelly, MS, RD, LDN, Illinois Central College

Sarah Harding Laidlaw, MS, RD, MPA, CDE

Brett R. Merklet, MSN, RN, LDS Business College

Heather A. Minges Wols, PhD, Columbia College Chicago

Joyce D. Nash, PhD

Elizabeth Quintana, MS, RD, LD, CDE, West Virginia University School of Medicine

Lois A. Ritter, EdD, MS, California State University at East Bay

Lisa Sasson, MS, RD, New York University

Donal Scheidel, DDS, University of South Dakota

Shannon Seal, MS, RD, Front Range Community College

Rhoada Tanenbaum, EdD, Long Island University at CW Post

Norman R. Trezek, MS, Pima Community College

Amy A. Vaughn, MS, Radford University

Andrea M. Villarreal, MS, RD, Phoenix College

Debra M. Vinci, DrPh, RD, LDN, University of West Florida

Jennifer Weddig, MS, RD, Metropolitan State College of Denver

Maureen Zimmerman, EdD, MPH, RD, Mesa Community College

## Reviewers of the *First Edition*

Betty B. Alford, PhD, RD, LD, Texas Women's University

Nancy K. Amy, PhD, University of California at Berkeley

Susan I. Barr, PhD, RDN, University of British Columbia

Richard C. Baybutt, PhD, Kansas State University

Beverly A. Benes, PhD, RD, University of Nebraska at Lincoln

Virginia C. Bragg, MS, RD, CD, Utah State University

Katie Brown, BS, MS, Central Missouri State University

Melanie Tracy Burns, PhD, RD, Eastern Illinois University

N. Joanne Caid, PhD, California State University at Fresno

Sai Chidambaram, Canisius College

Janet Colson, PhD, RD, Middle Tennessee State University

Holly A. Dieken, PhD, MS, BS, RD, University of Tennessee at Chattanooga

Judy A. Driskell, PhD, RD, University of Nebraska

Liz Emery, MS, RD, CNSD, Drexel University

Joan Fischer, PhD, RD, LD, University of Georgia

Christine Goodner, MS, RD, Winthrop University

Margaret Gunther, PhD, Palomar Community College

Shelley R. Hancock, MS, RD, LD, University of Alabama

Nancy Gordon Harris, MS, RD, LDN, East Carolina University

Mary K. Head, PhD, RD, LD, University of West Virginia

Deloy G. Hendricks, PhD, CNS, Utah State University

Sharon Himmelstein, PhD, MNS, RD, LD, Albuquerque Technical Vocational Institute

Carolyn Holcroft-Burns, BSN, PhD, Foothill College

Claire B. Hollenbeck, PhD, San Jose State University

Kevin Huggins, PhD, Auburn University

Michael Jenkins, Kent State University

Zaheer Ali Kirmani, PhD, RD, LD, Sam Houston State University

Janet Levins, PhD, RD, LD, Pensacola Junior College

Samantha R. Logan, DrPH, RD, University of Massachusetts

Michael P. Maina, PhD, Valdosta State University

Patricia Z. Marincic, PhD, RD, LD, CLE, College of Saint Benedict/Saint John's University

Melissa J. Martilotta, MS, RD, Pennsylvania State University

Laura H. May, RD, Mesa Community College

Jennifer McLean, MSPH, Corning Community College

Mark S. Meskin, PhD, RD, California State Polytechnic University at Pomona

Stella Miller, BA, MA, Mount San Antonio College

Marilyn Mook, BS, MS, Michigan State University

Mary W. Murimi, PhD, Louisiana Technical University

Katherine O. Musgrave, MS, RD, CAS, University of Maine at Orono

J. Dirk Nelson, PhD, Missouri Southern State College

Nora Norback, MPH, RD, CDE, City College of San Francisco

Anne O'Donnell, MS, MPH, RD, Santa Rosa Junior College

Rebecca S. Pobocik, PhD, RD, Bowling Green State University

Roseanne L. Poole, MS, RD, LD/N, Tallahassee Community College

Amy F. Reeder, MS, RD, University of Utah

Robert D. Reynolds, PhD, University of Illinois at Chicago

Stephen W. Sansone, BS, EdM, Chemekata Community College

Susan T. Saylor, RD, EdD, Shelton State University

Brian Luke Seaward, PhD, University of Colorado at Boulder

Mohammad R. Shayesteh, PhD, RD, LD, Youngstown State University

Melissa Shock, PhD, RD, University of Central Arkansas

LuAnn Soliah, PhD, RD, Baylor University

Bernice Gales Spurlock, PhD, Hinds Community College

Christine Stapell, MS, RD, LDN, Tallahassee Community College

Barbara A. Stettler, MEd, Bluffton College

Beth Stewart, PhD, RD, University of Arizona

Kathy Timperman, MS, West Virginia University

Anna Sumabat Turner, Med, Bob Jones University

Karen M. Ulrich, BS, Paul Smith's College of Arts and Sciences

Janelle Walter, PhD, Baylor University

Beverly G. Webber, MS, RD, CD, University of Utah

Cynthia Wright, PhD, Southern Utah University

Shahla M. Wunderlich, PhD, Montclair State University

Erika M. Zablah, Louisiana State University at Baton Rouge

## Acknowledgments

We would like to thank the following people for their hard work and dedication. They have helped make this new edition a reality. Thank you to Jennifer Coker for a thorough and careful copyedit; to Jess Newfell of Jones & Bartlett Learning for shepherding the book through to completion; and to Mark Bergeron and the team at Publishers' Design and Production Services for making this book look so great. We also would like to thank Shoshanna Goldberg, Amy Bloom, Agnes Burt, and Jody Yeskey for giving us help and direction when we needed it. The authors would like to acknowledge Kimberley McMahon for her additional work updating the Study Guide, PowerPoints, Test Bank, Instructor's Manual, and web materials.

Finally, we would like to thank all of the instructors and students who were involved in the process of developing the majors edition of *Nutrition*, without whose involvement the creation of *Discovering Nutrition* would not have been possible. We are most grateful to Dr. Nancy Amy (University of California at Berkeley) and Dr. Sally Lederman (Columbia University), whose special nutrition expertise helped us strive for accuracy and precision. Special thanks also are owed to Helen Spremulli, RN, CP (Dr. Dario Del Rizzo Professional Medicine Corporation) and Sylvia Santosa, PhD (Department of Exercise Science, Concordia University) whose extensive knowledge of Canadian nutrition is especially valued by the authors, as well as the publisher, of this text.

# CHAPTER 1

# Food Choices: Nutrients and Nourishment

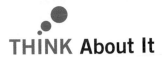

**THINK About It**

1   What, if anything, might induce you to change your food preferences?

2   Are there some foods you definitely avoid? If so, do you know why?

3   What do you think is driving the popularity of vitamins and other supplements?

4   Where do you get the majority of your information about nutrition?

Visit **go.jblearning.com/ inseldisco4e**

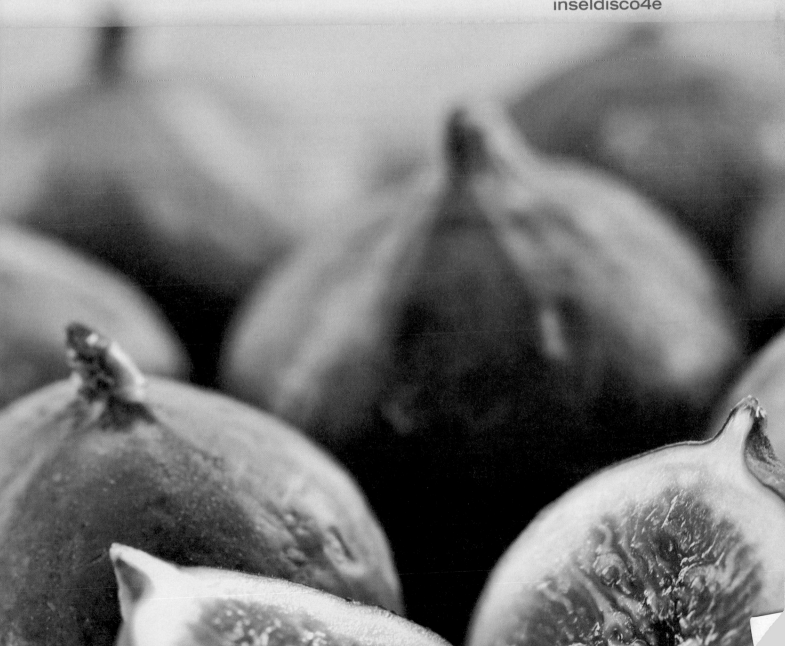

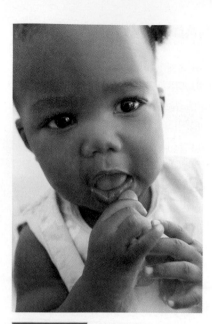

**Figure 1.1**    **Adventures in eating.** Babies and toddlers are generally willing to try new things.

nutrition    The science of foods and their components (nutrients and other substances), including the relationships to health and disease (actions, interactions, and balances); processes within the body (ingestion, digestion, absorption, transport, functions, and disposal of end products); and the social, economic, cultural, and psychological implications of eating.

neophobia    A dislike for anything new or unfamiliar.

A group of friends goes out for pizza every Thursday night. A college freshman greets his girlfriend with a box of chocolates. A 5-year-old imitates her parents after they salt their food. A firefighter who is asked to explain why hot dogs are his favorite food says it has something to do with going to baseball games with his father. A professor recently recruited from a Chinese university feels dissatisfied unless she eats a bowl of rice daily. A parent punishes a misbehaving child by withholding dessert. What do these people have in common? They are all using food for something other than its nutrient value. Can you think of a holiday that is not celebrated with food? For most of us, food is more than a collection of nutrients. Many factors affect what we choose to eat. Many of the foods people choose are nourishing and contribute to good health. The same, of course, may be true of the foods we reject.

The science of **nutrition** helps us improve our food choices by identifying the amounts of nutrients we need, the best food sources of those nutrients, and the other components in foods that may be helpful or harmful. Learning about nutrition will help us make better choices and not only improve our health but also reduce our risk of disease and increase our longevity. Keep in mind, though, that no matter how much you know about nutrition, you are still likely to choose some foods simply for their taste or just because they make you feel good.

## Why Do We Eat the Way We Do?

Do you "eat to live" or "live to eat"? For most of us, the first is certainly true—you must eat to live. But there may be times when our enjoyment of food is more important to us than the nourishment we get from it. Factors such as age, gender, genetic makeup, occupation, lifestyle, family, and cultural background affect our daily food choices. We use food to project a desired image, forge relationships, express friendship, show creativity, and disclose our feelings. We cope with anxiety or stress by eating or not eating; we reward ourselves with food for a good grade or a job well done; or, in extreme cases, we punish failures by denying ourselves the benefit and comfort of eating.

Food preferences begin early in life and then change as we interact with parents, friends, and peers. Further experiences with different people, places, and situations often—but not always—cause us to expand or change our preferences. Taste and other sensory factors such as texture are the most important things that influence our food choices; next are cost and convenience.[1] What we eat reveals much about who we are.

Age is a factor in food preferences. Young children prefer sweet or familiar foods; babies and toddlers are generally willing to try new things. (See **Figure 1.1**.) Experimental evidence suggests children repeatedly exposed to a variety of foods are more likely to accept these foods and have a healthier diet.[2]

Preschoolers typically go through a period of food **neophobia** (a dislike for anything new or unfamiliar), school-age children tend to accept a wider array of foods, and teenagers are strongly influenced by the preferences and habits of their peers. If you track the kinds of foods you have eaten in the past year, you might be surprised to discover how few basic foods your diet includes. By the time we reach adulthood, we have formed a core group of foods we prefer. Of this group, only about 100 basic items account for 75 percent of our food intake.

## Sensory Influences and Personal Preferences

Like many aspects of human behavior, food choices are influenced by both inborn (genetic) and environmental factors, and it's not always easy to sepa-

THINK
About It
1

**Environmental**
economic
environment
lifestyle
cultural beliefs and
    traditions
religious beliefs and
    traditions

**Sensory**
flavor (taste and smell)
texture
appearance

**Cognitive**
learned food habits
social factors
emotional needs
nutrition and
    health beliefs
advertising

**Health Status**
physical restrictions
    due to disease
declining taste
    sensitivity
age and gender

**Genetics**
taste sensitivity
preference for sweets
avoidance of bitter
possible "fat tooth"

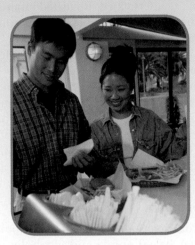

**Figure 1.2**    **Factors that affect food choices.** We often select a food to eat automatically without thought. But in fact, our choices are complex events involving the interactions of a multitude of factors.

rate them. However, we can look at food preferences in terms of the sensory properties of foods, cognitive factors that influence our choices, and environmental influences like culture. Exploring each of these areas may help you understand why you prefer certain foods. (See **Figure 1.2**.)

### Taste, Texture, and Smell

In making food choices, what appeals to our senses contributes to our personal preferences. People often refer to **flavor** as a collective experience that describes both taste and smell. Texture also plays a part. You may prefer foods that have a crisp, chewy, or smooth texture. You may reject foods that feel grainy, slimy, or rubbery. Other sensory characteristics that affect food choice are color, moisture, and temperature.

    We are familiar with the classic four tastes—sweet, sour, bitter, and salty—but studies show that there are more. One of these additional taste sensations is **umami**, which is a Japanese term for the taste produced by glutamate.[3] Glutamate is an amino acid (a building block of protein) that is found in monosodium glutamate (MSG), which gives food a distinctive meaty or savory taste.

### Habits

Your eating and cooking habits likely reflect what you learned from your parents. We typically learn to eat three meals a day, at about the same times each day. Quite often we eat the same foods, particularly for breakfast (e.g., cereal and milk) and lunch (e.g., sandwiches). This routine makes life convenient, and we don't have to think much about when or what to eat. But we don't have to follow this routine! How would you feel about eating mashed potatoes for breakfast and cereal for dinner? Some people might get a stomachache just thinking about it, while others may enjoy the prospect of doing things differently. Look at your eating habits and see how often you make the same choices every single day.

**flavor** The collective experience that describes both taste and smell.

**umami [ooh-MA-mee]** A Japanese term that describes a delicious meaty or savory sensation. Chemically, this taste detects the presence of glutamate.

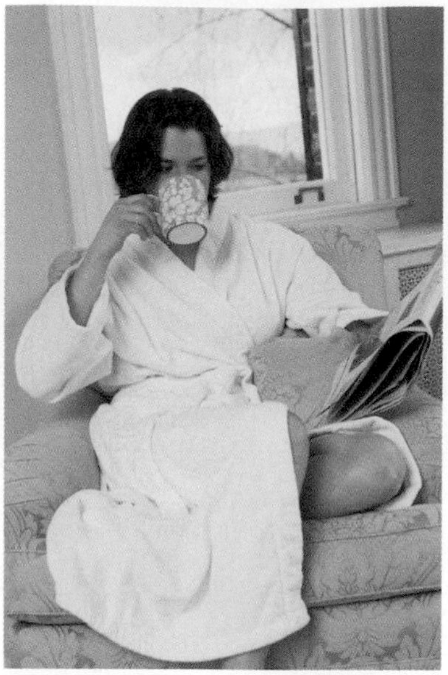

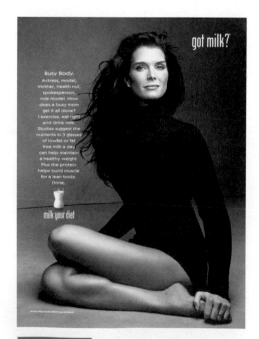

THINK
About It

2

### Comfort/Discomfort Foods

Our desire for particular foods often is based on behavioral motives, even though we may not be aware of them. For some people, food becomes an emotional security blanket. Consuming our favorite foods can make us feel better, relieve stress, and allay anxiety. (See **Figure 1.3**.) Starting with the first days of life, food and affection are intertwined. Breastfed infants, for example, experience physical, emotional, and psychological satisfaction when nursing. As we grow older, this experience is continually reinforced. For example, chicken soup and hot tea with honey are favorites when we feel under the weather because Mom and Dad fixed them especially for us. If we were rewarded for good behavior with a particular food (e.g., ice cream, candy, cookies), our positive feelings about that food may persist for a lifetime.

In contrast, children who have negative associations with certain foods are unlikely to choose those foods as adults. Maybe you avoid a certain food because you think it will make you sick. At some point in your childhood, you may have gotten sick soon after eating that food, and, consequently, the two events are linked forever.

**Figure 1.3**   **Comfort foods.** Depending on your childhood food experiences, a bowl of traditional soup, a remembered sweet, or a mug of hot chocolate can provide comfort in times of stress.

### Advertising and Promotion

It may not surprise you that some of the most popular food products are high-fat and high-sugar baked goods and alcoholic beverages. Aggressive and sometimes deceptive advertising programs can influence people to buy foods of poor nutritional quality. However, we are seeing more innovative and aggressive advertising from the commodity boards that promote milk, meat, cranberries, and other more nutrient-dense products.

According to the Federal Trade Commission (FTC), businesses spend $9.6 billion annually marketing food and beverages. More than $1.6 billion specifically targets children and adolescents, promoting items such as sugared breakfast cereals, fast food, and soft drinks.[4] Some advertising is positive. Ads like the one shown in **Figure 1.4**, for example, can be helpful, especially to consumers whose diets need improvement.

### Food and Diet Trends

The popularity of different diets can influence changes in food product consumption. Beginning in the late 1980s, low-fat diets became popular and were accompanied by an explosion of reduced-fat, low-fat, and fat-free products. When the "low-carb" diet became popular, so did the rise in low-carb or no-carb products. Diet and health-related products also compete for consumer dollars. For example, sales of gluten-free products in the United States are rising 15 to 25 percent a year due to the increased diagnosis of celiac disease and the belief that eliminating gluten from the diet will treat other conditions as well.[5]

### Social Factors

Social factors exert a powerful influence on food choice. Food is at the center of many social gatherings, parties, and events. Food often is the focus of family reunions, ice cream socials, and office holiday parties. When someone moves in, is sick, has a birthday, or has had a bad day at work—we bring food. Parents are influential models for infants and children. They learn which foods and combinations of foods are appropriate to consume and under what circumstances. Perhaps even more influential, though, are the messages from peers about what to eat or how to eat.

As **Figure 1.5** illustrates, eating is a social event that brings together different people for a variety of purposes (e.g., religious or cultural celebrations, business meetings, family dinners). Social pressures, however, also can restrict

**Figure 1.4**   **Healthy advertising.** Got milk? is an example of a successful healthy advertising campaign.

our food intake and selection. We might, for example, order nonmeat dishes when dining with a group of vegetarian friends.

### Nutrition and Health Beliefs

Many people select and emphasize certain foods they think are "good for them." (See **Figure 1.6**.) Consumer health beliefs, perceptions of disease susceptibility, and desires to take action to prevent or delay disease onset can have powerful influences on diet and food choices. For example, people who feel vulnerable to disease and believe that dietary change might lead to positive results are more likely to pay attention to information about links between dietary choices, dietary fat, and health risks. A desire to lose weight or alter one's physical appearance also can be a powerful force shaping decisions to accept or reject particular foods.

**Key Concepts** *Many factors influence our decisions about what to eat and when to eat. Some of the main factors include personal preferences such as taste, texture, and smell. Habits, experiences, social factors, advertising, and knowledge of relationships between food and health also influence our food decisions.*

## Environment

Your environment—where you live, how you live, who you live with—has a lot to do with what you choose to eat. People around us influence our food choices, and we prefer the foods we grew up eating. Other environmental factors include economics, lifestyle, culture, and religion. In America, our environment and the choices we make play a large role in the current obesity epidemic. The **obesogenic environment** in which many of us live promotes overconsumption of calories while at the same time discouraging physical activity.

### Economics

Where you live and the surrounding climate influence which foods are most accessible to you. Environmental factors such as location and climate also affect food costs, a major determinant of food choice. You may have "lobster taste" but a "hot dog budget." The types of foods purchased and the percentage of income used for food are affected by total income. Wealthier urban households tend to spend a larger portion of their food budget on food consumed away from home, ranging from approximately 44 percent for the wealthiest households to 30 percent for the poorest.[6] How much does it cost to follow dietary recommendations? For adults on a 2,000-calorie diet, the cost of meeting the *Dietary Guidelines for Americans* recommendations for fruit and vegetable consumption is $2.00 to $2.50 per day, according to an analysis by the U.S. Department of Agriculture (USDA).[7]

### Lifestyle

Another influential factor is lifestyle. Our fast-paced society has little time or patience for food preparation. Convenience foods, from frozen entrees to complete meals "in a box," saturate supermarket shelves. Americans spend almost half of their food budget on foods prepared away from home.[8] Many people, however, underestimate the amount of calories and fat contained in foods prepared away from home, which is likely contributing to overweight and obesity.[9] This trend has prompted an increase in interest for information on calories, fat, sodium, and other nutrients on menu labels.

Are people affected by menus that include calories? Yes! Studies have shown that people order foods with fewer calories when menus report calorie content.[10] In addition, when calories are shown

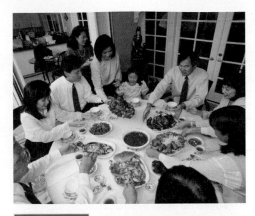

**Figure 1.5**    **Social facilitation.** Interactions with others can affect your eating behaviors.

**obesogenic environment**
Circumstances in which a person lives, works, and plays in a way that promotes the overconsumption of calories and discourages physical activity and calorie expenditure.

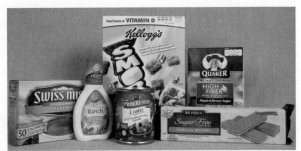

**Figure 1.6**    **Where do you get your nutrition information?** We are constantly bombarded by food messages. Which sources do you find most influential? Are they the most reliable?

## Quick Bite

### What Is an Ice Cream Headache?

After ingesting a cold substance quickly, such as when you take a big bite of ice cream, you may experience what is commonly known as an ice cream headache, or brain freeze. When cold substances touch the back part of the palate, blood vessels, including those that go to the brain, constrict (tighten), resulting in a sharp pain in the mid-frontal part of the brain. About one-third of the population experiences this phenomenon.

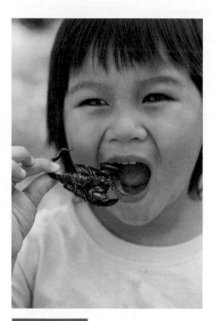

**Figure 1.7    Cultural influences.** If you were visiting China, would you sample the local delicacy—deep-fried scorpion?

## Quick Bite

### Nerve Poison for Dinner?

The puffer fish is a delicacy in Japan. Danger is part of its appeal; eating a puffer fish can be life threatening! The puffer fish contains a poison called tetrodotoxin (TTX), which blocks the transmission of nerve signals and can lead to death. Chefs who prepare the puffer fish must have special training and licenses to prepare the fish properly, so diners feel nothing more than a slight numbing feeling.

on a menu parents order foods with fewer calories for their children.[11] A number of cities and states have implemented legislation that will require restaurants to post nutritional information in an effort to aid consumers in making informed food choices.

### Availability

Poor access to healthy, nutritious foods can negatively affect health and well-being. Approximately 23.5 million Americans, including 6.5 million children, live in nutritional wastelands commonly referred to as *food deserts*. According to the Centers for Disease Control and Prevention (CDC), "Food deserts are areas that lack access to affordable fruits, vegetables, whole grains, low-fat milk, and other foods that make up the full range of a healthy diet."[12]

Not only do many people who live in food deserts lack the ability to get fresh, healthy, and affordable foods easily, but they often rely on "quick markets" that offer mostly highly processed, high-sugar, and high-fat foods. Their communities often lack healthy food providers, such as grocery stores and farmers' markets. Food needs typically are served by inexpensive restaurants and convenience stores that offer little fresh food. As part of its Let's Move! initiative, the Healthy Food Financing Initiative (HFFI) plans to help revitalize neighborhoods by eliminating food deserts that exist across urban and rural America.[13]

### Cultural Influences

One of the strongest influences on food preferences is tradition or cultural background. In all societies, no matter how simple or complex, eating is the primary way of initiating and maintaining human relationships.

Have you heard the saying "One man's food is another man's poison." To a large extent, culture defines our attitudes. Look at **Figure 1.7**. How does the photo make you feel? Insects, maggots, and entrails are delicacies to some, while just the thought of ingesting them is enough to make others retch. So powerful are cultural forces that if you were permitted only a single question to establish someone's food preferences, a good choice would be "What is your ethnic background?"[14] (See the FYI feature "Food and Culture.")

Knowledge, beliefs, customs, and habits all are defining elements of human culture.[15] Although genetic characteristics tie people of ethnic groups together, culture is a learned behavior and, consequently, can be modified through education, experience, and social and political trends.[16]

In many cultures, food has symbolic meanings related to family traditions, social status, and even health.[17] Indeed, many folk remedies rely on food. Some of these have gained wide acceptance, such as the use of spices and herbal teas for purposes ranging from allaying anxiety to preventing cancer and heart disease.[18] Just as cultural distinctions eventually blur when ethnic groups take part in the larger American culture, so do many of the unique expectations about the ability of certain foods to prevent disease, restore health among those with various afflictions, or enhance longevity. Food habits are among the last practices to change when an immigrant adapts to a new culture.[19]

### Religion

Food is an important part of religious rites, symbols, and customs. Some religious rules apply to everyday eating whereas others are concerned with special celebrations. Christianity, Judaism, Hinduism, Buddhism, and Islam, for example, all have distinct dietary laws, but within each religion different interpretations of these laws give rise to variations in dietary practices.

### Social-Ecological Model

The social-ecological model included in the *Dietary Guidelines for Americans* is designed to illustrate how individual factors, environmental settings, various sectors of influence, and social and cultural elements of society overlap to form the food and physical activity choices for an individual.[20] You can use the social-ecological model to think about how your current food and physical activity choices affect your calorie balance and risk for chronic diseases.

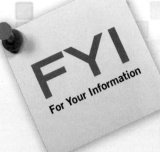

FYI
For Your Information

# Food and Culture

Ever wonder why people choose prickly pears over apples or pomegranates over blueberries? Food choices are a result of what people are accustomed to or what they have learned. Dietary habits are as diverse as individuals, and culture plays a key role in the food choices people make. Cultural influences often determine what roles various foods play in dietary habits, health beliefs, and everyday behaviors. Although beliefs and traditions may be modified through geography, economics, or experiences, core values and customs typically remain similar within a specific group.

Food plays a major role in most religions and religious customs. Religious beliefs usually are learned early and can define certain dietary habits. For example, Jewish dietary laws specify that foods must be *kosher*. To be kosher, meat must come from animals that chew their cud, have split hooves, and are free from blemishes to their internal organs. Fish must have fins and scales. Pork, crustaceans and shellfish, and birds of prey are not kosher. Kosher laws prohibit eating meat and milk at the same meal or even preparing or serving them with the same dishes and utensils. Islam identifies acceptable foods as halal and has rules similar to those of Judaism for the slaughtering of animals. Islam prohibits the consumption of pork, the flesh of clawed animals, alcohol, and other intoxicating drugs. The Church of Jesus Christ of Latter Day Saints disapproves of coffee, tea, and alcoholic beverages. Most Hindus are vegetarians and do not eat eggs, and some avoid onions and garlic. The Orthodox Jain religion in India forbids eating meat or animal products (e.g., milk, eggs) and any root vegetables (e.g., potatoes, carrots, garlic). In Buddhism, mind-altering substances or intoxicating beverages are prohibited, but dietary habits vary considerably based on the sect and geographic location. Some Buddhists follow strict forms of vegetarianism whereas others do not. In Christianity and many other religions, food plays a key role in religious ceremonies and various religious holidays, from what foods may or may not be eaten (e.g., no meat during Lent) to when foods can be consumed (e.g., only from sundown to sunrise during Islam's Ramadan). Food plays an important role not only in physical survival but also in many people's spiritualism.

Many cultures have traditional medical practices based on the belief that nature is composed of two opposing forces. In traditional Chinese medicine, for example, these forces, called *yin* and *yang*, must be in proper balance for good health. It is believed that excesses in either direction cause illness. The illness must then be treated by giving foods of the opposite force. This idea of balance or harmony, accompanied by terms describing illness and foods as either cold (e.g., banana, fish, juices) or hot (e.g., beef, nuts, ginger) or yin or yang, also is found in other Asian cultures, including India and the Philippines, and in Latin American cultures and ethnicities.

Numerous cultures view a variety of foods as having medicinal properties. Treatments commonly use assorted herbs, herbal teas, and special foods. From generation to generation, knowledge of such remedies is passed on. Remarkably, various cultures all over the world use remedies based on similar common substances, such as chamomile, garlic, and honey. These familiar substances often are more trusted and are considered safer than modern medicines. In addition to traditions and culture, the complete array of herbs and foods used daily and also as medicines is based on the geographic region, growing conditions, and climate.

The interplay of diet and culture helps to define a person's values, preferences, and practices. As a result, even in the face of changing world events and populations, neither is abandoned easily or quickly. Just as there is diversity in individuals and families, there is also diversity within cultures. One must be alert to avoid the assumption that all people of a specific culture eat, believe, or follow traditions in the exact same manner. Even so, the question arises: What impact will our increasing mobility and globalization have on food choice? Undoubtedly, cultural interactions and exposure to various cuisines will increase. Will this expand our appreciation and preservation of cultural culinary practices and result in the formation of new hybrid cuisines?

1　Welcome to food culture and tradition. http://www.food-links.com. Accessed 9/30/11.

2　Culture. http://ethnomed.org/culture. Accessed 9/30/11.

3　The meaning of food. http://www.pbs.org/opb/meaningoffood/food_and_culture. Accessed 9/30/11.

4　The meaning of food: you're going to eat that? http://www.pbs.org/opb/meaningoffood/food_and_culture/gonna_eat_that. Accessed 9/30/11.

5　Encyclopedia of food and culture. http://www.enotes.com/food-encyclopedia. Accessed 9/30/11.

6　Foods of world religions. http://www.interfaith-calendar.org/Foodsofreligions.htm. Accessed 9/30/11.

7　Top 20 herbs. http://www.herbmed.org/#param.wapp?sw_page=top20. Accessed 9/30/11.

8　Chinese medicinal cuisine. http://www.chinahighlights.com/travelguide/chinese-food/medicinal-cuisine.htm. Accessed 9/30/11.

## Quick Bite

**America's Favorite Vegetables**
When Americans eat vegetables, they are most likely to eat potatoes (especially french fries), tomatoes (usually part of tomato sauce or ketchup), onions, and iceberg lettuce.

**Key Concepts** *The cultural environments in which people grow up have a major influence on what foods they prefer, what foods they consider edible, and what foods they eat in combination and at what time of day. Many factors work to define a group's culture: environment, economics, access to food, lifestyle, traditions, and religious beliefs. As people from other cultures immigrate to new lands, they will adopt new behaviors consistent with their new homes. However, food habits are among the last to change. The social-ecological model of food and physical activity behavior shows how individual factors, environmental settings, sectors of influence, and cultural social values influence our food and physical activity behavior.*

## The American Diet

What, then, is a typical *American diet*? As a country influenced by the practices of so many cultures, religions, backgrounds, and lifestyles, there is no easy, single answer to this question. The U.S. diet is as diverse as Americans themselves, even though many people around the world imagine that the American diet consists mainly of hamburgers, french fries, and cola drinks! Our fondness for fast food and the marketability of such restaurants overseas make them seem like icons of American culture—and many of the stereotypes are true. The most commonly consumed grain product in the United States is white bread, the favorite meat is beef, and the most frequently eaten vegetable is the potato, usually as french fries. Despite the variety available to us, the American diet is still heavy on meat and potatoes and light on fruits, vegetables, low-fat dairy, and whole grains. Americans ages 2 and older consume, on average, 2,157 calories daily.[21] Grain-based desserts (e.g., cookies, cakes, pastries), soda, pizza, and alcohol are among the top 10 sources of daily calories (see Table 1.1).[22] Table 1.2 shows the usual U.S. intake from each food group based on a 2,000-calorie diet.

**Table 1.1    Top 10 Sources of Calories Among Americans Ages 2 Years and Older, NHANES 2005–2006[a]**

| Rank | Overall, Ages 2+ Years (Total Daily Calories = 2,157) |
|---|---|
| 1 | Grain-based desserts[b] (138 kcal) |
| 2 | Yeast breads[c] (129 kcal) |
| 3 | Chicken and chicken mixed dishes[d] (121 kcal) |
| 4 | Soda/energy/sports drinks[e] (114 kcal) |
| 5 | Pizza (98 kcal) |
| 6 | Alcoholic beverages (82 kcal) |
| 7 | Pasta and pasta dishes[f] (81 kcal) |
| 8 | Tortillas, burritos, and tacos[g] (80 kcal) |
| 9 | Beef and beef mixed dishes[h] (64 kcal) |
| 10 | Dairy desserts[i] (62 kcal) |

[a] Data are drawn from analyses of usual dietary intakes conducted by the National Cancer Institute. Foods and beverages consumed were divided into 97 categories and ranked according to calorie contribution to the diet. Table shows each food category and its mean calorie contribution for each age group. Additional information on calorie contribution by age, gender, and race/ethnicity is available at http://riskfactor.cancer.gov/diet/foodsources.

[b] Includes cake, cookies, pie, cobbler, sweet rolls, pastries, and donuts.

[c] Includes white bread or rolls, mixed-grain bread, flavored bread, whole-wheat bread, and bagels.

[d] Includes fried or baked chicken parts and chicken strips/patties, chicken stir-fries, chicken casseroles, chicken sandwiches, chicken salads, stewed chicken, and other chicken mixed dishes.

[e] Sodas, energy drinks, sports drinks, and sweetened bottled water, including vitamin water.

[f] Includes macaroni and cheese, spaghetti, other pasta with or without sauces, filled pasta (e.g., lasagna, ravioli), and noodles.

[g] Also includes nachos, quesadillas, and other Mexican mixed dishes.

[h] Includes steak, meatloaf, beef with noodles, and beef stew.

[i] Includes ice cream, frozen yogurt, sherbet, milk shakes, and pudding.

**Source:** US Department of Agriculture and US Department of Health and Human Services. *Dietary Guidelines for Americans, 2010.* 7th ed. Washington, DC: US Government Printing Office; December 2010.

| Table 1.2 | Usual U.S. Intake, Average Daily Intake at or Adjusted to a 2,000-Calorie Level |
| --- | --- |

| Pattern | Usual U.S. Intake Adults[a] |
| --- | --- |
| *Food Groups* | |
| **Vegetables: total (c)** | 1.6 |
| Dark-green (c) | 0.1 |
| Beans and pasta (c) | 0.1 |
| Red and orange (c) | 0.4 |
| Other (c) | 0.5 |
| Starchy (c) | 0.5 |
| **Fruit and juices (c)** | 1.0 |
| **Grains: total (oz)** | 6.4 |
| Whole grains (oz) | 0.6 |
| **Milk and milk products (dairy products) (c)** | 1.5 |
| *Protein Foods* | |
| Meat (oz) | 2.5 |
| Poultry (oz) | 1.2 |
| Eggs (oz) | 0.4 |
| Fish/seafood (oz) | 0.4 |
| Beans and pasta (oz) | See vegetables |
| Nuts, seeds, and soy products (oz) | 0.5 |
| **Oils (g)** | 18 |
| **Solid fats (g)** | 43 |
| **Added sugars (g)** | 79 |
| **Alcohol (g)** | 9.9 |

[a] **Source:** US Department of Agriculture, Agricultural Research Service, and US Department of Health and Human Services, Centers for Disease Control and Prevention. What We Eat in America, NHANES 2001–2004. 1 day mean intakes for adult males and females, adjusted to 2,000 calories and averaged.

**Source:** US Department of Agriculture and US Department of Health and Human Services. *Dietary Guidelines for Americans, 2010.* 7th ed. Washington, DC: US Government Printing Office; December 2010.

*Quick* Bite

"Poor diet and physical inactivity are the most important factors contributing to an epidemic of overweight and obesity affecting men, women, and children in all segments of our society."

**Source:** Reproduced from US Department of Agriculture and US Department of Health and Human Services. *Dietary Guidelines for Americans, 2010.* 7th ed. Washington, DC: US Government Printing Office; December 2010.

So, how healthful is the "American" diet? As shown in **Figure 1.8**, Americans are eating too little of the nutrient-dense food identified by nutrition experts as important for good health and too much of the foods known to be harmful! Together, solid fats and added sugars contribute nearly 800 calories per day while providing no important nutrients.[23] Soda, sugar-sweetened beverages, and grain-based desserts are the major sources of added sugars for many Americans. Regular cheese, grain-based desserts, and pizza are the top contributors of solid and saturated fat in the American diet. In addition, Americans of all age groups are eating more than the recommended amounts of sodium, mainly in the form of processed foods.[24]

Although we are bombarded with information about health and nutrition, this doesn't necessarily translate into better food choices. People are not "natural nutritionists"; that is, they don't know instinctively which foods to choose for good health. The majority of the population has never taken a course in nutrition. They probably will never take the time to become well-informed consumers—not just of food but also of information about food and nutrition. So it is probably not surprising when national surveys indicate that although Americans know that nutrition and food choices are important factors in health, few have made the recommended changes (e.g., eating less fat, sugar, and salt; eating more fruits and vegetables).

You are in a position to gather more information than the average consumer. By taking this course in nutrition, you will be getting the full story: the nutrients we need for good health, the science behind the health messages, and

**Figure 1.8**  How do typical American diets compare to the recommended intake levels or limits?

*a* SoFAS, solid fats and added sugars.

*Note:* Bars show average intake for all individuals (ages 1 or 2 years or older, depending on the data source) as a percentage of the recommended intake level or limit. Recommended intakes for food groups and limits for refined grains, solid fats, and added sugars are based on amounts in the USDA 2,000-calorie food pattern. Recommended intakes for fiber, potassium, vitamin D, and calcium are based on the highest average intake (AI) or recommended daily allowance (RDA) for ages 14 to 70 years. Limits for sodium are based on the UL and for saturated fat on 10 percent of calories. The protein foods group is not shown here because, on average, intake is close to recommended levels.

**Source:** US Department of Agriculture and US Department of Health and Human Services. *Dietary Guidelines for Americans, 2010.* 7th ed. Washington, DC: US Government Printing Office; December 2010.

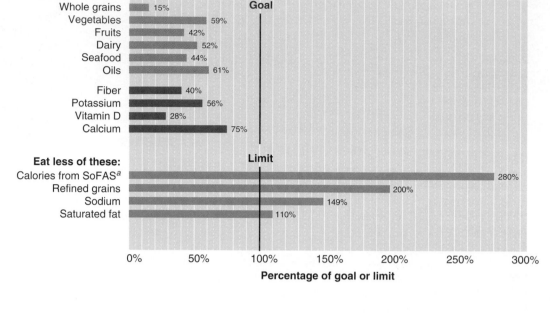

Usual intake as a percentage of goal or limit

Eat more of these:
- Whole grains — 15% — Goal
- Vegetables — 59%
- Fruits — 42%
- Dairy — 52%
- Seafood — 44%
- Oils — 61%
- Fiber — 40%
- Potassium — 56%
- Vitamin D — 28%
- Calcium — 75%

Eat less of these:    Limit
- Calories from SoFAS*a* — 280%
- Refined grains — 200%
- Sodium — 149%
- Saturated fat — 110%

Percentage of goal or limit

the food choices it will take to implement them. Whether you use this information is up to you, but at least you will be a well-informed consumer!

**Key Concepts**  *"American" cuisine is truly a melting pot of cultural contributions to foods and tastes. Although Americans receive and believe many messages about the role of diet in good health, these beliefs do not always translate into better food choices. The typical American diet contains too much sodium, solid fat, saturated fat, and sugar and not enough fruits, vegetables, low-fat diary, and whole-grain foods.*

## Introducing the Nutrients

Although we give food meaning through our culture and experience and make dietary decisions based on many factors, ultimately the reason for eating is to obtain nourishment—nutrition.

Just like your body, food is a mixture of chemicals, some of which are essential for normal body function. These essential chemicals are called **nutrients**. You need nutrients for normal growth and development, for maintaining cells and tissues, for fuel to do physical and metabolic work, and for regulating the hundreds of thousands of body processes that go on inside you every second of every day. Further, food must provide these nutrients; the body either cannot make these **essential nutrients** or cannot make enough of them. There are six classes of nutrients in food: carbohydrates, lipids (fats and oils), proteins, vitamins, minerals, and water. (See **Figure 1.9**.) The minimum diet for human growth, development, and maintenance must supply about 45 essential nutrients.

### Definition of Nutrients

In studying nutrition, we focus on the functions of nutrients in the body so that we can see why they are important in the diet. However, to define a nutrient in technical terms, we focus on what happens in its absence. A nutrient is a chemical whose absence from the diet for a long enough time results in a specific change in health; we say that a person has a deficiency of that nutrient. A lack of vitamin C, for example, will eventually lead to scurvy. A

**nutrients**  Any substances in food that the body can use to obtain energy, synthesize tissues, or regulate functions.

**essential nutrients**  Substances that must be obtained in the diet because the body either cannot make them or cannot make adequate amounts of them.

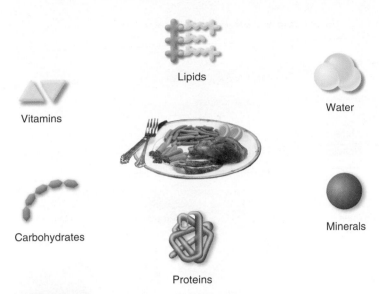

Lipids

Water

Vitamins

Minerals

Carbohydrates

Proteins

| Figure 1.9 | **The six classes of nutrients.** Water is the most important nutrient, and we cannot survive long without it. Because our bodies need large quantities of carbohydrate, protein, and fat, they are called macronutrients. Our bodies need comparatively small amounts of vitamins and minerals, so they are called micronutrients. |
|---|---|

diet with too little iron will result in iron-deficiency anemia. To complete the definition of a nutrient, it also must be true that putting the essential chemical back in the diet will reverse the change in health, if done before permanent damage occurs. If taken early enough, supplements of vitamin A can reverse the effects of deficiency on the eyes. If not, prolonged vitamin A deficiency can cause permanent blindness.

Nutrients are not the only chemicals in food. Other substances add flavor and color, some contribute to texture, and others like caffeine have physiological effects on the body. Some substances in food, like fiber, have important health benefits but do not fit the classical definition of a nutrient. One of the newest areas of research in nutrition is the area of **phytochemicals**. Although these "plant chemicals" are not nutrients, they have important health functions, such as **antioxidant** activity, which may reduce risk for heart disease or cancer.

The six classes of nutrients serve three general functions: They provide energy (fuel), regulate body processes, and contribute to body structures (see **Figure 1.10**). Although virtually all nutrients can be said to regulate body processes, and many contribute to body structures, only proteins, carbohydrates, and fats are sources of energy. Because the body needs large quantities of carbohydrates, proteins, and fats, they are called **macronutrients**; vitamins and minerals are called **micronutrients** because the body needs comparatively small amounts of these nutrients.

In addition to their functions, there are several other key differences among the classes of nutrients. First, the chemical composition of nutrients varies widely. One way to divide the nutrient groups is based on whether the compounds contain the element carbon. Substances that contain carbon are **organic** substances; those that do not are **inorganic**. Carbohydrates, lipids, proteins, and vitamins are all organic; minerals and water are not. Structurally, nutrients can be very simple—minerals such as sodium are single elements, although we often consume them as larger compounds (e.g., sodium chloride, which is table salt). Water also is very simple in structure. The organic nutrients

**phytochemicals** Substances in plants that may possess health-protective effects, even though they are not essential for life.

**antioxidant** A substance that combines with or otherwise neutralizes a free radical, thus preventing oxidative damage to cells and tissues.

**macronutrients** Nutrients, such as carbohydrate, fat, or protein, that are needed in relatively large amounts in the diet.

**micronutrients** Nutrients, such as vitamins and minerals, that are needed in relatively small amounts in the diet.

**organic** In chemistry, any compound that contains carbon, except carbon oxides (e.g., carbon dioxide) and sulfides and metal carbonates (e.g., potassium carbonate). The term *organic* also is used to denote crops that are grown without synthetic fertilizers or chemicals.

**inorganic** Any substance that does not contain carbon, excepting certain simple carbon compounds such as carbon dioxide and monoxide. Common examples include table salt (sodium chloride) and baking soda (sodium bicarbonate).

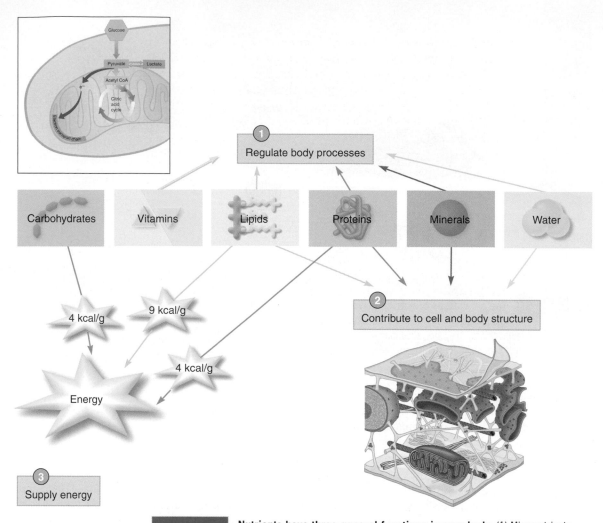

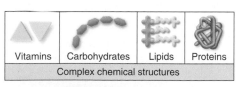

Organic – contains carbon

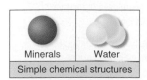

Inorganic – no carbon

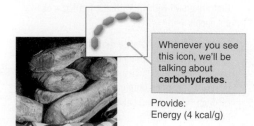

Whenever you see this icon, we'll be talking about **carbohydrates**.

Provide:
Energy (4 kcal/g)

**Figure 1.10**   **Nutrients have three general functions in your body.** (1) Micronutrients, some lipids and proteins, and water help regulate body processes such as blood pressure, energy production, and temperature. (2) Lipids, proteins, minerals, and water help provide structure to bone, muscle, and other cells. (3) Macronutrients supply energy to power muscle contractions and cellular functions.

have more complex structures—the carbohydrates, lipids, and proteins we eat are made of smaller building blocks whereas the vitamins are elaborately structured compounds.

It is rare for a food to contain just one nutrient. Meat is not just protein any more than bread is solely carbohydrate. Foods contain mixtures of nutrients, although in most cases protein, fat, or carbohydrate dominates. So while bread is certainly rich in carbohydrates, it also contains some protein, a little fat, and many vitamins and minerals. If it's whole-grain bread you're eating, you also get fiber, which is not technically a nutrient, but an important compound for good health nonetheless.

**Key Concepts** *Nutrients are the essential chemicals in food that the body needs for normal functioning and good health and that must come from the diet because they either cannot be made in the body or cannot be made in sufficient quantities. Six classes of nutrients—carbohydrates, proteins, lipids, vitamins, minerals, and water—can be described by their composition or by their function in the body.*

## Carbohydrates

If you think of water when you hear the word *hydrate*, then the word *carbohydrate*—or literally "hydrate of carbon"—tells you exactly what this nutrient is made of. **Carbohydrates** are made of carbon, hydrogen, and oxygen and are a major source of fuel for the body. Dietary carbohydrates are the starches and sugars found in grains, vegetables, legumes (dry beans and peas), and fruits. We also get carbohydrates from dairy products, but practically none from meats. Your body converts most dietary carbohydrates to glucose, a simple sugar compound. It is glucose that we find in **circulation**, providing a source of energy for cells and tissues.

## Lipids

The term *lipids* refers to substances we know as fats and oils but also to fatlike substances in foods, such as cholesterol and phospholipids. Lipids are organic compounds and, like carbohydrates, contain carbon, hydrogen, and oxygen. Fats and oils—or, more correctly, **triglycerides**—are another major fuel source for the body. In addition, triglycerides, cholesterol, and phospholipids have other important functions: providing structure for body cells, carrying the fat-soluble vitamins (A, D, E, and K), and providing the starting material (cholesterol) for making many **hormones**. Dietary sources of lipids include the fats and oils we cook with or add to foods, the naturally occurring fats in meats and dairy products, and less obvious plant sources, such as coconut, olives, and avocado.

## Proteins

**Proteins** are organic compounds made of smaller building blocks called **amino acids**. Unlike carbohydrates and lipids, amino acids contain nitrogen as well as carbon, hydrogen, and oxygen. Some amino acids also contain the mineral sulfur. The amino acids that we get from dietary protein combine with the amino acids made in the body to make hundreds of different body proteins. Body proteins help build and maintain body structures and regulate body processes. Protein also can be used for energy.

Proteins are found in a variety of foods, but meats and dairy products are among the most concentrated sources. Grains, **legumes**, and vegetables all contribute protein to the diet, while fruits contribute negligible amounts.

## Vitamins

**Vitamins** are organic compounds that contain carbon and hydrogen and perhaps nitrogen, oxygen, phosphorus, sulfur, or other elements. Vitamins regulate body processes such as energy production, blood clotting, and calcium balance. Vitamins help to keep organs and tissues functioning and healthy. Because vitamins have such diverse functions, a lack of a particular vitamin can have widespread effects. Although the body does not break down vitamins to yield energy, vitamins have vital roles in the extraction of energy from carbohydrate, fat, and protein.

Vitamins are usually divided into two groups: fat-soluble and water-soluble. The four fat-soluble vitamins—A, D, E, and K—have very diverse roles. What they have in common is the way they are absorbed and transported in the body and the fact that they are more likely to be stored in larger quantities than the water-soluble vitamins. The water-soluble vitamins include vitamin C and eight B vitamins: thiamin ($B_1$), riboflavin ($B_2$), niacin ($B_3$), pyridoxine ($B_6$), cobalamin ($B_{12}$), folate, pantothenic acid, and biotin. Most of the B vitamins are involved in some way with the pathways for energy metabolism.

**carbohydrates** Compounds, including sugars, starches, and dietary fibers, that usually have the general chemical formula $(CH_2O)_n$, where *n* represents the number of $CH_2O$ units in the molecule. Carbohydrates are a major source of energy for body functions.

**circulation** Movement of substances through the vessels of the cardiovascular or lymphatic system.

**lipids** A group of fat-soluble compounds that includes triglycerides, sterols, and phospholipids.

**triglycerides** Fats composed of three fatty acid chains linked to a glycerol molecule.

**hormones** Chemical messengers that are secreted into the blood by one tissue and act on cells in another part of the body.

**proteins** Large, complex compounds consisting of many amino acids connected in varying sequences and forming unique shapes.

**amino acids** Organic compounds that function as the building blocks of protein.

**legumes** A family of plants with edible seed pods, such as peas, beans, lentils, and soybeans; also called *pulses*.

**vitamins** Organic compounds necessary for reproduction, growth, and maintenance of the body. Vitamins are required in miniscule amounts.

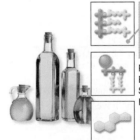

Whenever you see one of these three icons, we'll be talking about **lipids**.

Provide:
Energy (9 kcal/g)
Structure
Regulation (hormones)

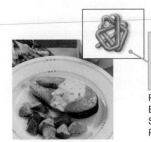

Whenever you see this icon, we'll be talking about **proteins**.

Provide:
Energy (4 kcal/g)
Structure
Regulation

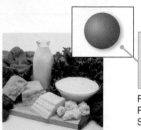

Whenever you see these icons, we'll be talking about **vitamins**.

Provide:
Regulation

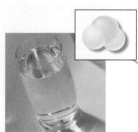

Whenever you see this icon, we'll be talking about **minerals**.

Provide:
Regulation
Structure

Whenever you see this icon, we'll be talking about **water**.

Provides:
Regulation
Structure

**minerals**  Inorganic compounds needed for growth and for regulation of body processes.

**macrominerals**  Major minerals required in the diet and present in the body in large amounts compared with trace minerals.

**microminerals**  See *trace minerals*.

**trace minerals**  Trace minerals are present in the body and required in the diet in relatively small amounts compared with major minerals; also known as *microminerals*.

**energy**  The capacity to do work. The energy in food is chemical energy, which the body converts to mechanical, electrical, or heat energy.

Vitamins are found in a wide variety of foods, not just fruits and vegetables—although these are important sources—but also meats, grains, legumes, dairy products, and even fats. Choosing a well-balanced diet usually makes vitamin supplements unnecessary. In fact, when taken in large doses, vitamin supplements (especially those containing vitamins A, D, $B_6$, or niacin) can be harmful.

THINK
About It

3

## Minerals

Structurally, **minerals** are simple, inorganic substances. At least 16 minerals are essential to health; among them are sodium, chloride, potassium, calcium, phosphorus, and magnesium. Because the body needs these minerals in relatively large quantities compared with other minerals, they are often called **macrominerals**. The body needs the remaining minerals only in very small amounts. These **microminerals**, or **trace minerals**, include iron, zinc, copper, manganese, molybdenum, selenium, iodine, and fluoride. As with vitamins, the functions of minerals are diverse. Minerals can be found in structural roles (e.g., calcium, phosphorus, and fluoride in bones and teeth) as well as regulatory roles (e.g., control of fluid balance, regulation of muscle contraction).

Food sources of minerals are just as diverse. Although we often associate minerals with animal foods, such as meats and milk, plant foods are important sources as well. Deficiencies of minerals, except iron and perhaps calcium, are uncommon. A balanced diet provides enough minerals for most people. However, individuals with iron-deficiency anemia may need iron supplements, and others may need calcium supplements if they cannot or will not drink milk or eat dairy products. As is true for vitamins, excessive intake of some minerals as supplements can be toxic.

## Water

Next to the mineral elements, water is chemically the simplest nutrient. Water also is the most important nutrient! We can survive far longer without any of the other nutrients in the diet, indeed without food at all, than we can without water. Water has many roles in the body, including temperature control, lubrication of joints, and transportation of nutrients and wastes.

Because your body is nearly 60 percent water, regular fluid intake to maintain adequate hydration is important. Water is found not only in beverages but also in most food products. Fruits and vegetables in particular are high in water content. Through many chemical reactions, the body makes some of its own water, but this is only a fraction of the amount needed for normal function.

**Key Concepts**  *The body needs larger amounts of carbohydrates, lipids, and proteins (macronutrients) than vitamins and minerals (micronutrients). Carbohydrates, lipids, and proteins provide energy; proteins, vitamins, minerals, water, and some fatty acids regulate body processes; and proteins, lipids, minerals, and water contribute to body structure.*

## Nutrients and Energy

One major reason we eat food, and the nutrients it contains, is for **energy**. Every cellular reaction, every muscle movement, every nerve impulse requires energy. Three of the nutrient classes—carbohydrates, lipids (triglycerides only), and proteins—are energy sources. When we speak of the energy in foods, we are really talking about the *potential* energy that foods contain. Energy itself is not a food component.

Different scientific disciplines use different measures of energy. In nutrition, we discuss the potential energy in food, or the body's use of energy, in units of heat called **kilocalories** (1,000 calories). One kilocalorie (or kcal) is the amount of energy (heat) it would take to raise the temperature of 1 kilogram (kg) of water by 1 degree Celsius. For now, this may be an abstract concept, but, as you learn more about nutrition, you will discover how much energy you likely need to fuel your daily activities. You also will learn about the amounts of potential energy in various foods.

## Energy in Foods

Energy is available from foods because foods contain carbohydrate, fat, and protein. These nutrients can be broken down completely (metabolized) to yield energy in a form that cells can use. When completely metabolized in the body, carbohydrate and protein yield 4 kilocalories of energy for every gram (g) consumed; fat yields 9 kilocalories per gram; and alcohol contributes 7 kilocalories per gram. (See **Figure 1.11**.) Therefore, the energy available from a given food or from a total diet is reflected by the amount of each of these substances consumed. Because fat is a concentrated source of energy, adding or removing fat from the diet can have a big effect on available energy.

### When Is a Kilocalorie a Calorie?

Many people inappropriately use the terms *calorie* and *kilocalorie* interchangeably. To clear up this confusing situation, you should use the term *calorie* as a general term for energy and *kilocalorie* as a specific measurement or unit of that energy. *Calories* is like referring to gas for a car, and *kilocalories* is like referring to gallons of fuel. When in doubt, substitute the word *energy* for calories. The following sentence illustrates the use of kilocalorie and calorie: Because fat contains 9 *kilocalories* per gram, more than double that of protein or carbohydrate, foods high in fat are rich in *calories* (energy).

You'll find that food labels, diet books, and other sources of nutrition information use the term *calorie*, not *kilocalorie*. Technically, the potential energy in foods is best measured in kilocalories; however, the term *calorie* has become familiar and commonplace.

### How Can We Calculate the Energy Available from Foods?

To calculate the energy available from food, multiply the number of grams of fat, carbohydrate, and protein by 9, 4, and 4, respectively; then add the results. For example, if we assume that one bagel with one and a half ounces of cream cheese contains 39 grams of carbohydrate, 10 grams of protein, and 16 grams of fat, we can determine the available energy from each component.

**39 g carbohydrate × 4 kcal/g = 156 kcal**

**10 g protein × 4 kcal/g = 40 kcal**

**16 g fat × 9 kcal/g = 144 kcal**

**Total = 340 kcal**

To calculate the *percentage* of calories each of these components contributes to the total, divide the individual results by the total, and then multiply by 100. For example, to determine the percentage of calories from fat in this example, divide the 144 fat kilocalories by the total of 340 kilocalories and then multiply by 100 (144 ÷ 340 × 100 = 42 percent).

### Be Food Smart: Calculate the Percentages of Calories in Food

Current health recommendations suggest limiting fat intake to about 20 to 35 percent of *total* energy intake. You can monitor this for yourself in two

**kilocalories (kcal) [KILL-oh-kal-oh-rees]** Units used to measure energy. Food energy is measured in kilocalories (1,000 calories = 1 kilocalorie).

**calorie** The general term for energy in food and used synonymously with the term *energy*. Often used instead of kilocalorie on food labels, in diet books, and in other sources of nutrition information.

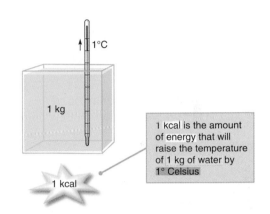

1°C

1 kg

1 kcal

1 kcal is the amount of energy that will raise the temperature of 1 kg of water by 1° Celsius

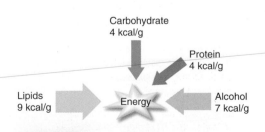

Carbohydrate
4 kcal/g

Protein
4 kcal/g

Lipids
9 kcal/g

Energy

Alcohol
7 kcal/g

**Figure 1.11**    **Energy sources.** Carbohydrate, fat, protein, and alcohol provide different amounts of energy per gram.

CALCULATING THE ENERGY
AVAILABLE FROM FOODS

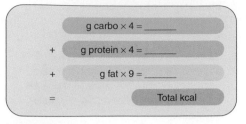

Example:
275 g carbohydrate × 4 kcal/g = 1,100 kcal

75 g protein × 4 kcal/g = 300 kcal

67 g fat × 9 kcal/g = 600 kcal (rounded
from 603 kcal)

Total = 2,000 kcal

CALCULATING THE PERCENTAGE OF
KILOCALORIES FROM NUTRIENTS

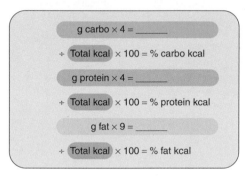

Example:
275 g carbohydrate × 4 = 1,100 kcal
1,100 kcal ÷ 2,000 kcal × 100 = 55% carbo. kcal

75 g protein × 4 = 300 kcal
300 kcal ÷ 2,000 kcal × 100 = 15% protein kcal

67 g fat × 9 = 600 kcal (rounded
from 603 kcal)
600 kcal ÷ 2,000 kcal × 100 = 30% fat kcal

ways. If you like counting fat grams, you can first determine your suggested maximum fat intake. For example, if you need to eat 2,000 kilocalories each day to maintain your current weight, at most 35 percent of those calories can come from fat:

$$2{,}000 \text{ kcal} \times 0.35 = 700 \text{ kcal from fat}$$

$$700 \text{ kcal from fat} \div 9 \text{ kcal/g} = 77.8 \text{ g of fat}$$

Therefore, your maximum fat intake should be about 78 grams. You can check food labels to see how many fat grams you typically eat.

Another way to monitor your fat intake is to know the percentage of calories that come from fat in various foods. If the proportion of fat in each food choice throughout the day exceeds 35 percent of calories, then the day's total of fat will be too high as well. Some foods contain virtually no fat calories (e.g., fruits, vegetables) whereas others are nearly 100 percent fat calories (e.g., margarine, salad dressing). Being aware that a snack like the bagel with cream cheese provides 42 percent of its calories from fat can help you select lower-fat foods at other times of the day.

## Diet and Health

What does it mean to be healthy? The World Health Organization (WHO) defines health as "a state of complete physical, mental, and social well-being and not merely the absence of disease or infirmity."[25] Although we often focus on the last part of that definition, "the absence of disease or infirmity," the first part is equally important. As you have learned, nutrition is an important part of physical, mental, and social well-being. It also is important for preventing disease.

*Disease* can be defined as "an impairment of the normal state of the living animal or plant body or one of its parts that interrupts or modifies the performance of the vital functions" and can arise from environmental factors or specific infectious agents, such as bacteria or viruses.[26] Diseases can be *acute* (short-lived illnesses that arise and resolve quickly) or *chronic* (diseases with a slow onset and long duration). Although nutrition can affect our susceptibility to acute diseases—and contaminated food is certainly a source of acute disease—our food choices are more likely to affect our risk for developing chronic diseases such as heart disease or cancer. Other lifestyle factors, such as smoking and exercise, in addition to genetic factors, also may determine who gets sick and who remains healthy. The 10 leading causes of death are listed in Table 1.3. Nutrition plays a role in the prevention or treatment of more than half of the conditions listed. Heart disease and cancer, together, account for almost half of all deaths.[27]

### *Obesity*

Once considered merely an aesthetic issue, obesity is now widely recognized as a major public health problem. The prevalence of obesity has steadily increased among men, women, and children of all ages, racial/ethnic groups, and educational levels. Currently, more than two-thirds of U.S. adults are overweight or obese. Among children, approximately 12.4 percent of those ages 2 to 5, 17 percent of those ages 6 to 11, and 17.6 percent of those ages 12 to 19 are overweight or obese.[28]

Overweight and obesity are risk factors for the major chronic diseases of public health significance in the United States and Canada: coronary heart disease, cancer, diabetes, hypertension, and metabolic syndrome as well as conditions like those shown in Table 1.4. Individuals who are obese have a significantly increased risk of death from all causes, but most often cardio-

**Table 1.3** Leading Causes of Death: United States

| Rank | Cause of Death |
|------|----------------|
| 1 | Heart disease[a] |
| 2 | Cancer[a] |
| 3 | Chronic lower respiratory diseases |
| 4 | Stroke |
| 5 | Accidents (unintentional injuries) |
| 6 | Alzheimer's disease |
| 7 | Diabetes mellitus[a] |
| 8 | Influenza and pneumonia |
| 9 | Kidney disease[a] |
| 10 | Intentional self-harm (suicide) |

[a] Causes for which nutrition is thought to be important in the prevention or treatment of the condition.

**Source:** Kochanek KD, Xu J, Murphy SL, Miniño AM, Kung H-C. Deaths: preliminary data for 2009. *National Vital Statistics Report.* 59(4):2011. http://www.cdc.gov/nchs/data/nvsr/nvsr59/nvsr59_04.pdf. Accessed 9/10/11.

vascular causes, compared with individuals at a healthy weight. Obesity is associated with over 112,000 excess deaths due to cardiovascular disease, over 15,000 excess deaths due to cancer, and over 35,000 excess deaths due to noncancer, noncardiovascular disease causes per year in the U.S. population, relative to healthy-weight individuals.[29]

A number of factors influence overweight or obesity, including the following:

- *Behavior:* Eating too many calories while not getting enough physical activity.
- *Environment:* Home, work, school, or community can provide barriers to or opportunities for an active lifestyle.
- *Genetics:* Heredity plays a large role in determining how susceptible people are to overweight and obesity. Genes also influence how the body burns calories for energy or stores fat.

**Table 1.4** Health Risks from Overweight and Obesity

Type 2 diabetes
Coronary heart disease
High LDL ("bad") cholesterol
Stroke
Hypertension
Nonalcoholic fatty liver disease
Gallbladder disease
Osteoarthritis (degeneration of cartilage and bone of joints)
Sleep apnea and other breathing problems
Some forms of cancer (breast, colorectal, endometrial, and kidney)
Complications of pregnancy
Menstrual irregularities

**Source:** Weight-Control Information Network (WIN). Overweight and obesity statistics. http://win.niddk.nih.gov/statistics/#overweight. Accessed 9/10/11.

Behavioral and environmental factors are the main contributors to overweight and obesity and provide the greatest opportunity for prevention and treatment.

The foods we choose do more than provide us with an adequate diet. The balance of energy sources can affect our risk of chronic disease. For example, high-fat diets have been linked to heart disease and cancer. Excess calories contribute to obesity, which also increases disease risk. Other nutrients, such as the minerals sodium, chloride, calcium, and magnesium, affect blood pressure while a lack of the vitamin folate prior to conception and in early pregnancy can cause serious birth defects. Non-nutrient components in the diet (e.g., phytochemicals) may have antioxidant or immune-enhancing properties that also can keep us healthy. The choices we make can reduce our disease risk, as well as provide energy and essential nutrients.

### Physical Activity

A sedentary lifestyle is a significant risk factor for chronic disease. Physically active people generally outlive those who are inactive, and, as a risk factor for heart disease, inactivity can be almost as significant as high blood pressure, smoking, or high blood cholesterol. Physical activity also plays a significant role in long-term weight management. The 2008 Physical Activity Guidelines states, "Physical activity is safe for almost everyone and the health benefits of physical activity far outweigh the risks. … For all individuals, some activity is better than none."[30] At least 30 minutes per day of moderate physical activity such as brisk walking or cycling helps reduce chronic disease risk, and higher amounts of exercise—at least 60 minutes per day—have a positive impact on weight-management efforts.

**Key Concepts**  *All cells and tissues need energy to keep the body functioning. Energy in foods and in the body is measured in kilocalories. The carbohydrates, lipids, and proteins in food are potential sources of energy, meaning that the body can extract energy from them. Triglycerides (fats) are the most concentrated source of energy, with 9 kilocalories per gram. Carbohydrates and proteins provide 4 kilocalories per gram, while alcohol has 7 kilocalories per gram. Excess energy intake is a contributing factor to obesity, a major public health issue. All individuals should aim to be physically active for at least 30 minutes daily to reduce risk of chronic disease and manage body weight.*

## Applying the Scientific Process to Nutrition

Whether it's identifying essential nutrients, establishing recommended intake levels, or exploring the effects of vitamins on cancer risk, scientific studies are the cornerstone of nutrition. Although we may use creative, artistic talents to choose and serve a pleasing array of healthful foods, the fundamentals of nutrition are developed through the scientific process of observation and inquiry.

The scientific process enables researchers to test the validity of **hypotheses** that arise from observations of natural phenomena. For example, it was common knowledge in the eighteenth century that sailors on long voyages would likely develop scurvy (which we now know results from a deficiency of vitamin C). Scurvy had been recognized since ancient times, and its common symptoms—pinpoint skin hemorrhages, swollen and bleeding gums, joint pain, fatigue and lethargy, and psychological changes such as depression and hysteria—were well known. Native populations discovered plant foods that would cure this illness; among Native Americans these included cranberries in the Northeast and many tree extracts in other parts of the country. From observations such as these come questions that lead to hypotheses, or "educated guesses," about factors that might be responsible for the observed phe-

**hypotheses** Scientists' "educated guesses" to explain phenomena.

| Table 1.5 | Common Study Designs Used in Nutrition Research |
|---|---|

**Epidemiological Studies**

An epidemiological study compares disease rates among population groups and attempts to identify related conditions or behaviors such as diet and smoking habits. Epidemiological studies can provide useful information about relationships but often do not clarify cause and effect. The results of these studies show **correlations**—relationships between two or more factors, however. Epidemiological studies can provide important clues and insights that lead to animal and human studies that can further clarify diet and disease relationships. The relationship between inadequate vitamin C intake and scurvy is one example of this.

**Animal Studies**

Animal studies can provide preliminary data that often lead to human studies. Although animal studies can provide scientists with important information that furthers nutrition knowledge, the results of animal studies cannot be assumed to transfer directly to humans. Animal studies need to be followed with cell culture studies and ultimately human clinical studies to determine specific effects on humans.

**Cell Culture Studies**

Another way to study nutrition is to isolate specific types of cells and grow them in the laboratory. Scientists then can use those cells to study the effects of nutrients or other components on metabolic processes in the cell. An important area of nutrition research, called **nutrigenomics**, explores the effect of specific nutrients and other chemical compounds on gene expression. This area of molecular biology will help us explain individual differences in chronic disease risk factors and may lead to designing diets based on an individual's genetic profile.

**Case Control Studies**

**Case control studies** are small-scale epidemiological studies in which individuals who have a condition (e.g., breast cancer) are compared with similar individuals who do not have the condition. Researchers then identify factors other than the disease in question that differ between the two groups. These factors provide researchers with clues about the cause, progression, and prevention of the disease.

**Clinical Trials**

**Clinical trials**, also called **intervention studies**, are controlled studies where some type of intervention (e.g., a nutrient supplement, controlled diet, exercise program) is used to determine its impact along certain health parameters. These studies include an **experimental group** (the people experience the intervention) and a **control group** (similar people who are not treated). Scientists measure aspects of health or disease in each group and compare the results.

nomenon. Scientists then test hypotheses using appropriate research designs. Poorly designed research can produce useless results or false conclusions.

Nutrition research is exciting and always changing. Scientists ask questions to be answered and define problems to be solved. Investigators choose a study design that will best answer their research question or hypothesis. Throughout the research process researchers must follow rigorous ethical procedures in all areas of the study design. Common study designs used in nutrition research are defined in Table 1.5.

James Lind's experiments with sailors aboard the *Salisbury* in 1747 are considered to be the first dietary clinical trial. (See **Figure 1.12**.) His observation that oranges and lemons were the only dietary elements that seemed to cure scurvy was an important finding. However, it took more than 40 years before the British Navy began routinely giving all sailors citrus juice or fruit, such as lemons or limes—a practice that led to the nickname "limeys" when referring to British sailors. It took nearly 200 years (until the 1930s) for scientists to isolate the compound we call vitamin C and show that it had antiscurvy activity.[31] The chemical name for vitamin C, ascorbic acid, comes from its role as an antiscorbutic (antiscurvy) compound.

There are several important elements in a modern clinical trial: random assignment to groups, use of placebos, and the double-blind method. Subjects are assigned randomly—as by the flip of a coin—to the experimental group or the control group. This reduces the risk of introducing bias into either group. People in the experimental group receive the treatment or specific protocol (e.g., consuming a certain nutrient at a specific level). People in the control group do not receive the treatment but usually receive a placebo.

**correlations** Connections co-occurring more frequently than can be explained by chance or coincidence but without a proven cause.

**nutrigenomics** The study of how nutrition interacts with specific genes to influence a person's health.

**case control studies** Investigations that use a group of people with a particular condition rather than a randomly selected population. These cases are compared with a control group of people who do not have the condition.

**clinical trials** Studies that collect large amounts of data to evaluate the effectiveness of a treatment.

**intervention studies** See *clinical trials*.

**experimental group** A set of people being studied to evaluate the effect of an event, substance, or technique.

**control group** A set of people used as a standard of comparison to the experimental group. The people in the control group have characteristics similar to those in the experimental group and are selected at random.

1. **Observation**
   Sailors on long voyages all became ill with scurvy.
2. **Hypothesis**
   Lack of certain foods causes scurvy.
3. **Experimentation**
   Experiment to test hypothesis.
   Predicts that some dietary element will cure scurvy.

**Key**

| Controlled variables |
| Experimental variables |
| Results |
| Conclusions |

James Lind: A Treatise of the Scurvy in Three Parts.
Containing an inquiry into the Nature, Causes and Cure of that Disease,
together with a Critical and Chronological View of what has been
published on the subject. A. Millar, London, 1753.

On the 20th May, 1747, I took twelve patients in the scurvy on board, the Salisbury at sea. Their cases were as similar as I could have them. They all in general had putrid gums, the spots and lassitude, with weakness of their knees. They lay together in one place, being a proper apartment for the sick in the fore-hold; and had one diet in common to all, viz., water gruel sweetened with sugar in the morning; fresh mutton broth often times for dinner; at other times puddings, boiled biscuit with sugar etc.; and for supper barley, raisins, rice and currants, sago and wine, or the like. Two of these were ordered each a quart of cyder a day. Two others took twenty five gutts of elixir vitriol three times a day upon an empty stomach, using a gargle strongly acidulated with it for their mouths. Two others took two spoonfuls of vinegar three times a day upon an empty stomach, having their gruels and their other food well acidulated with it, as also the gargle for the mouth. Two of the worst patients, with the tendons in the ham rigid (a symptom none the rest had) were put under a course of sea water. Of this they drank half a pint every day and sometimes more or less as it operated by way of gentle physic. Two others had each two oranges and one lemon given them every day. These they eat with greediness at different times upon an empty stomach. They continued but six days under this course, having consumed the quantity that could be spared. The two remaining patients took the bigness of a nutmeg three times a day of an electuary recommended by an hospital surgeon made of garlic, mustard seed, rad. raphan, balsam of Peru and gum myrrh, using for common drink narley water well acidulated with tamarinds, by a decoction of wich, with the addition of cremor tartar, they were gently purged three or four times during the course.

The consequence was that the most sudden and visible good effects were perceived from the use of the oranges and lemons; one of those who had taken them being at the end of six days fit four duty. The spots were not indeed at that time quite off his body, nor his gums sound; but without any other medicine than a gargarism or elixir of vitriol he became quite healthy before we came into Plymouth, which was on the 16th June. The other was the best recovered of any in his condition, and being now deemed pretty well was appointed nurse to the rest of the sick ...

As I shall have occasion elsewhere to take notice of the effects of other medicines in this disease, I shall here only observe that the result of all my experiments was that oranges and lemons were the most effectual remedies for this distemper at sea. I am apt to think oranges preferable to lemons...

4. **Publication**
   Publication subjects the findings to peer review by fellow scientists.
5. **More experiments**
   Further experiments replicate the findings and extend knowledge.
6. **Theory**
   Scientists consolidate acquired knowledge into a theory that explains the observed phenomenon.

**Figure 1.12**   **The first clinical trial.** In 1758, physician James Lind reported the careful process of his clinical trial among British sailors afflicted with scurvy.

A **placebo** is an imitation treatment (such as a sugar pill) that looks the same as the experimental treatment but has no effect. The placebo also is important for reducing bias because subjects do not know if they are r eceiving the intervention and are less inclined to alter their responses or reported symptoms based on what they think should happen. The *expectation* that a medication will be effective can be nearly as effective as the medication itself—a phenomenon called the **placebo effect**. Because the placebo effect can exert a powerful influence, research studies must take it into account.

When the members of neither the experimental nor the control groups know what treatment they are receiving, we say the subjects are "blinded" to the treatment. If a clinical trial is designed so neither the subjects nor the researchers collecting data are aware of the subjects' group assignments (experimental or control), the study is called a **double-blind study**. This reduces the possibility that researchers will see the results they want to see even if these results do not occur. In this case, another member of the research team holds the code for subject assignments and does not participate in the data collection. Double-blind, placebo-controlled clinical trials are considered the "gold standard" of nutrition studies. These studies can show clear cause-and-effect relationships but often require large numbers of subjects and are expensive and time consuming to conduct.

**Key Concepts** *The scientific method is used to expand our nutrition knowledge. Hypotheses are formed from observations and are then tested by experiments. Epidemiological studies observe patterns in populations. Animal and cell culture studies can test effects of various treatments. For human studies, randomized, double-blind, placebo-controlled clinical trials are the best research tools for determining cause-and-effect relationships.*

## Headlines Can Be Confusing

THINK
About It

4

What about the nutrition and health headlines we see in the newspapers, hear on television, or read on the Internet daily? Consumers often are confused by what they see as the "wishy-washiness" of scientists—for example, coffee is good, then coffee is bad. Margarine is better than butter … No wait, maybe butter is better after all. These contradictions, despite the confusion they cause, show us that nutrition is truly a science: dynamic, changing, and growing with each new finding.

**placebo** An inactive substance that is outwardly indistinguishable from the active substance whose effects are being studied.

**placebo effect** A physical or emotional change that is not due to properties of an administered substance. The change reflects participants' expectations.

**double-blind study** A research study set up so neither the subjects nor the investigators know which study group is receiving the placebo and which is receiving the active substance.

## *Quick* Bite

**Controlling the Pesky Placebo**
When researchers tested the effectiveness of a medication in reducing binge eating among people with bulimia, they used a double-blind, placebo-controlled study to eliminate the placebo effect. After a baseline number of binge-eating episodes was determined, 22 women with bulimia were given the medication or a placebo. After a period of time, the number of binge-eating episodes was reassessed. The group taking the medication had a 78 percent reduction in binge-eating episodes. Sounds good, right? But, the placebo group had a similar reduction of 70 percent. The placebo effect was nearly as powerful as the medication.

**SCIENTISTS DISPUTE CLAIMS OF GINKGO BILOBA EFFECTIVENESS**

Schwabe Co. of Karlsruhe, Germa producer of the proprietary extra EGb 761. Ginkgo extract is a goo exa mu deli scie the for

There have been over four hundred scientific studies conducted on proprietary standardi

**Researchers Link Caffeine and Cancer**

**Some Say Ginkgo Biloba Improves Memory**

**Cancer and Vitamin E Link Disputed**

Besides causing a multitude of other offenses against human health, free radicals are the main culprits underlying cardiovascular disease. Growing edical literature suggests that terol)

hardening of the arteries. Briefly, here's how it works: Excess free radicals in the bloodstream oxidize particles of LDL. Immune system cells in the arterial walls recognize the oxidized LDLs as toxic to the body and gobble them up. When the immune cells become overloaded with LDLs, they break down logical cells called foam cells. The foam

**Vitamin E Reduces Risk of Cancer**

The walls recognize the risk of oxidized LDLs as toxic to the body and gobble them up. This vitamin has been shown to be instumental in reducing some forms of cancer in certain patient. When the immune

Vitamin E reduces the risk of LDL cholesterol being oxidized and therefore attaching to the cell wall. Because it is fat soluble, Vitamin E can get inside the LDL chol

logical cells called foam cells. The foam cells attach readily to the vessel wall and start the of bardening at

| Figure 1.13 | **Sifting facts and fallacies.**
From original research to the evening news, each step along the way introduces biases as information is summarized and restated. Whether on television, radio, the Internet, or in print, the best consumer information cites sources for reported facts.

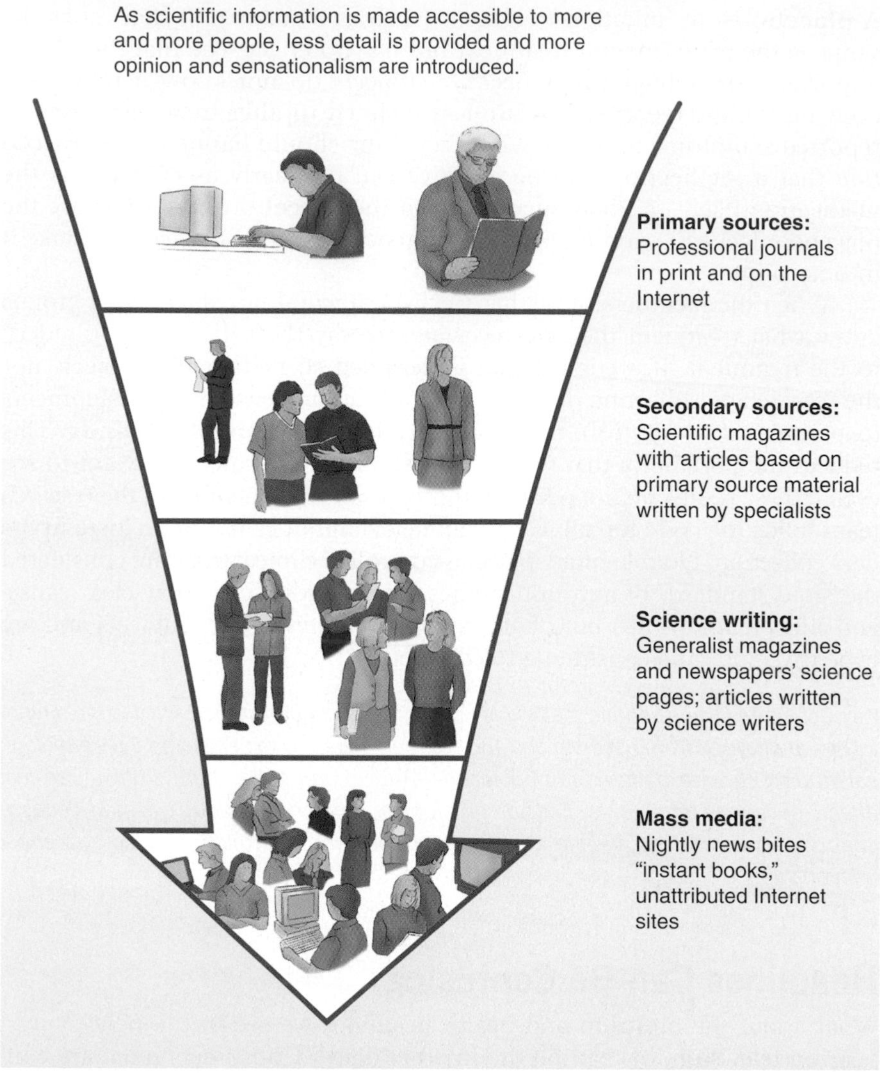

As scientific information is made accessible to more and more people, less detail is provided and more opinion and sensationalism are introduced.

**Primary sources:** Professional journals in print and on the Internet

**Secondary sources:** Scientific magazines with articles based on primary source material written by specialists

**Science writing:** Generalist magazines and newspapers' science pages; articles written by science writers

**Mass media:** Nightly news bites "instant books," unattributed Internet sites

**peer review** An appraisal of research against accepted standards by professionals in the field.

## Publishing Experimental Results

Once an experiment is complete, scientists publish the results in a scientific journal to communicate new information to other scientists. Generally, before articles are published in scientific journals, other scientists who have expert knowledge of the subject critically review them. **Peer review** ensures that only high-quality research findings are published. Unfortunately, peer-reviewed journals such as the *American Journal of Clinical Nutrition* and the *Journal of the American Dietetic Association* are not the main sources of information presented in the popular media.

A news article becomes a 30-second sound bite that often fails to reflect the original data. In some cases, the study may be distorted, with its results misstated or overstated. (See **Figure 1.13**.)

## Sorting Facts and Fallacies in the Media

People tend to believe what they hear repeatedly. Even when it has no basis in fact, a claim can seem credible if heard often enough. For example, do you believe that sugar makes kids hyperactive? There is no scientific evidence to support this claim! Although news stories may be based on reports in the

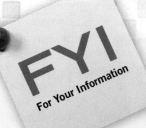

# Evaluating Information on the Internet

Surfing the Web has made life easier in many ways. You can buy a car, check stock prices, search out sources for a paper you're writing, chat with like-minded people, and stay up-to-date on news or sports scores. Hundreds of websites are devoted to nutrition and health topics, and you may be asked to visit such sites as part of your course requirements. So, how do you evaluate the quality of information on the Web? Can you trust what you see?

First, it's important to remember that there are no rules for posting on the Internet. Anyone who has the equipment can set up a website and post any content he or she likes. Although the Health on the Net Foundation has set up a Code of Conduct for medical and health websites, following their eight principles is completely voluntary.[1]

Second, consider the source, if you can tell what it is! Many websites do not specify where the content came from, who is responsible for it, or how often it is updated. If the site lists the authors, what are their credentials? Who sponsors the site itself? Educational institutions (.edu), government agencies (.gov), and organizations (.org) generally have more credibility than commercial (.com) sites, where selling rather than educating may be the primary motive.[2] Identifying the purpose for a site can give you more clues about the validity of its content.

Third, when you see claims for nutrients, dietary supplements, or other products and results of studies or other information, keep in mind the scientific method and the basics of sound science. Who did the study? What type of study was it? How many subjects? Was it double-blind? Were the results published in a peer-reviewed journal? Think critically about the content, look at other sources, and ask questions of experts before you accept information as truth. What is true of books, magazines, and newspapers also applies to the Internet: Just because it is in print or online doesn't mean it's true.

Finally, be on the lookout for "junk science"—sloppy methods, interpretations, and claims that lead to public misinformation. The Food and Nutrition Science Alliance (FANSA) is a coalition of several health organizations, including the Academy of Nutrition and Dietetics. FANSA has developed the "10 Red Flags of Junk Science" to help consumers identify potential misinformation.[3] Use these red flags to evaluate websites.

## The 10 Red Flags of Junk Science

1. Recommendations that promise a quick fix
2. Dire warnings of danger from a single product or regimen
3. Claims that sound too good to be true
4. Simplistic conclusions drawn from a complex study
5. Recommendations based on a single study
6. Statements refuted by reputable scientific organizations
7. Lists of "good" and "bad" foods
8. Recommendations made to help sell a product
9. Recommendations based on studies not peer reviewed
10. Recommendations from studies that ignore differences among individuals or groups

Use the Internet; it's fun and can be educational. Don't forget about the library, though; many scientific journals are not available online. Treat claims as "guilty until proven innocent"—in other words, don't accept what you read at face value until you have evaluated the science behind it. If it sounds too good to be true, it probably is!

1  Health on the Net Foundation. http://www.hon.ch/HONcode/Conduct.html. Accessed 9/9/11.

2  The wheat from the chaff: sorting out nutrition information on the Internet. *J Am Diet Assoc.* 1998;98:1270–1272.

3  Academy of Nutrition and Dietetics Media Guide, 2010–2011. http://www.eatright.org/media. Accessed 9/9/11.

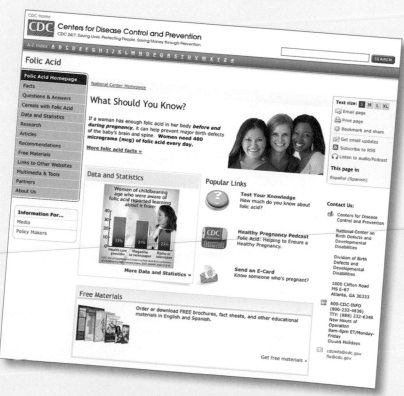

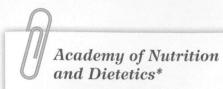

## Academy of Nutrition and Dietetics*

### Food and Nutrition Misinformation

It is the position of the American Dietetic Association that food and nutrition misinformation can have harmful effects on the health and economic status of consumers. Nationally credentialed dietetics professionals working in health care, academia, public health, nutrition communications, media, and the food industry and serving in policy-making/regulatory roles are uniquely qualified to advocate for and promote sound, science-based nutrition information to the public, function as primary nutrition educators to health professionals, and actively counter and correct food and nutrition misinformation.

**Source:** Reproduced from Warsink B. Position of the Academy of Nutrition and Dietetics: food and nutrition misinformation. *J Am Diet Assoc.* 2006;106(4):601–607.

\* Formerly the American Dietetic Association

scientific literature, the media may distort the facts through omission of details. (See the FYI feature "Evaluating Information on the Internet.")

As you learn about nutrition, you will undoubtedly be more aware not only of your eating and shopping habits but also of nutrition-related information in the media. As you see and hear reports, stop to think carefully about what you are hearing. Headlines and news reports often overstate the findings of a study. Two other things to keep in mind: One study does not provide all the answers to our nutrition questions; and if it sounds too good to be true, it probably is!

Your study of nutrition is just beginning. As you learn about the essential nutrients, their functions, and food sources, be alert to your food choices and the factors that influence them. When the discussion turns to the role of diet in health, think about your preconceived ideas and evaluate your beliefs in the light of current scientific evidence. Keep an open mind, but also think critically. Most of all, remember that food is more than the nutrients it provides; it is part of the way we enjoy and celebrate life!

# Learning Portfolio

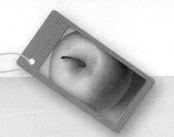

## Key Terms

## Study Points

- Most people make food choices for reasons other than nutrient value.

- Taste and texture are the two most important factors that influence food choices.

- In all cultures, eating is the primary way of maintaining social relationships.

- Although most North Americans know about healthful food choices, their eating habits do not always reflect this knowledge.

- Food is a mixture of chemicals. Essential chemicals in food are called nutrients.

- Carbohydrates, lipids, proteins, vitamins, minerals, and water are the six classes of nutrients found in food.

- Nutrients have three general functions in the body: They serve as energy sources, structural components, and regulators of metabolic processes.

- Vitamins regulate body processes such as energy metabolism, blood clotting, and calcium balance.

- Minerals contribute to body structures and to regulating processes such as fluid balance.

- Water is the most important nutrient in the body. We can survive much longer without the other nutrients than we can without water.

- Energy in foods and the body is measured in kilocalories. Carbohydrates, fats, and proteins are sources of energy.

- Carbohydrate and protein have a potential energy value of 4 kilocalories per gram, and fat provides 9 kilocalories per gram.

- Scientific studies are the cornerstone of nutrition. The scientific method uses observation and inquiry to test hypotheses.

- Double-blind, placebo-controlled clinical trials are considered the "gold standard" of nutrition studies.

- Research designs used to test hypotheses include epidemiological, animal, cell culture, and human studies.

- Information in the public media is not always an accurate or complete representation of the current state of the science on a particular topic.

## Study Questions

1. Name three sensory aspects of food that influence our food choices.
2. How do our health beliefs affect our food choices?
3. List the six classes of nutrients.
4. List the 13 vitamins.
5. What determines whether a mineral is a macromineral or a micro- (trace) mineral?
6. How many kilocalories are in 1 gram of carbohydrate, of protein, and of fat?
7. What is an epidemiological study?
8. What is the difference between an experimental and control group?
9. What is a placebo?

## Try This

### Try a New Cuisine Challenge

Expand your culinary taste buds and try a new cuisine. Take your local phone book and see how many ethnic restaurants are near campus. Choose a cuisine you are not very familiar with and take some friends along for dinner so you can order and share several dishes. While you're there, don't be afraid to ask questions about the menu, so you can gain a better understanding of the foods, preparation techniques, spices, and even the cultural meaning attached to some of the dishes.

## Food Label Puzzle

The purpose of this exercise is to put the individual pieces of the food label together to determine how many kilocalories are in a serving. Pick six foods in your dorm room or apartment that have complete food labels. Ask a friend to write down the value for calories on each label and then black out these numbers on the labels. Remember that the term *calories* on a food label is really referring to kilocalories. Your job is to determine how many kilocalories are in a serving of each of these foods. You can do this by putting together the individual pieces (carbohydrate, protein, and fat). If you need help, review this chapter and pay close attention to the section on the energy-yielding nutrients. How many kilocalories does each have per gram? You may find that the results of your calculations don't exactly match the numbers on the label. Within labeling guidelines, food manufacturers can round values.

# What About Bobbie?

The "What About Bobbie?" feature appears in most chapters of this text. Bobbie is a college student whom you'll follow to learn the strengths and weaknesses of her diet. Look for this feature to see how the information you learn in each chapter can be applied to real life.

Bobbie is a 20-year-old college sophomore. She lives on campus and has one roommate. She has the standard meal plan with her university, so she eats most of her meals in the cafeteria. Sometimes she'll get a snack from the local coffee shop or a vending machine. Her schedule is fairly typical, with classes spread out in both the morning and afternoon. Occasionally at night, she and her friends will order pizza or go out for ice cream.

Bobbie weighs 155 pounds and is 5 feet, 4 inches tall. She gained 10 pounds her freshman year in college and would like to lose it because she feels that her ideal weight is more like 145 pounds. She exercises infrequently but likes to walk with her friends and take an occasional aerobics class. Here is a typical day of eating for Bobbie:

**Sample one-day menu from Bobbie's diet**

**7:45 A.M.**
1 raisin bagel, toasted
3 tablespoons light cream cheese
10 fluid ounces regular coffee
   2 packets of sugar
   2 tablespoons of 2% milk

**10:15 A.M.**
1 banana

**12:15 P.M.**
Turkey and cheese sandwich
2 slices sourdough bread
2 ounces sliced turkey lunch meat
2 teaspoons regular mayonnaise
2 teaspoons mustard
2 slices tomato
2 slices dill pickle
Shredded lettuce
Salad from cafeteria salad bar
   2 cups shredded iceberg lettuce
   2 tablespoons each:
      Shredded carrot
      Chopped egg
      Croutons
      Kidney beans
      Italian salad dressing
12 fluid ounces diet soda
1 small chocolate chip cookie

**3:30 P.M.**
16 fluid ounces water
1.5 ounces regular tortilla chips
½ cup salsa

**6:00 P.M.**
Spaghetti with meatballs
   1.5 cups pasta
   3 ounces ground beef (meatballs)
   3 ounces spaghetti sauce
   2 tablespoons Parmesan cheese
1 piece garlic bread
½ cup green beans
   1 teaspoon butter
12 fluid ounces diet soda

**10:15 P.M.**
1 slice cheese pizza

# References

1   Kittler PG, Sucher KP, Nelms M. *Food and Culture*. 6th ed. Belmont, CA: Wadsworth; 2011.

2   Cooke L. The importance of exposure for healthy eating in childhood: a review. *J Hum Nutr Diet*. 2007;20(4):294–301.

3   Yamaguchi S, Ninomiya K. Unami and food palatability. *J Nutr*. 2000:284(3): 32–39.

4   Federal Trade Commission. Marketing food to children and adolescents: a review of industry expenditures, activities, and self-regulation. July 2008. http://www.ftc.gov/os/2008/07/P064504foodmktingreport.pdf. Accessed 8/30/11.

5   Business booming for gluten-free products: growing awareness of celiac disease sparks new foods free of gluten. MSNBC.com. http://www.msnbc.msn.com/id/28437360/ns/business-small_business/t/business-booming-gluten-free-products. Accessed 8/31/11.

6   Blisard N, Stewart H. Food spending in America 2003–2004. Economic Information Bulletin (EIB-23). US Department of Agriculture (USDA), Economic Research Service, March 2007. http://www.ers.usda.gov/Publications/EIB23. Accessed 8/8/11.

7   Hayden S, Hyman J, Buzby JC, Frazão E, Carlson A. How much do fruits and vegetables cost? Economic Information Bulletin (EIB-71), USDA, Economic Research Service, February 2011. http://www.ers.usda.gov/Publications/EIB71/EIB71.pdf. Accessed 8/8/11.

8   Larsen N, Story M. Menu labeling: does providing nutrition information at the point of purchase affect consumer behavior? A research synthesis. June 2009, Healthy Eating Research, a National Program of the Robert Wood Johnson Foundation. http://www.rwjf.org/files/research/20090630hermenulabeling.pdf. Accessed 10/1/11.

9   Burton S, Creyer E, Kees J, et al. Attacking the obesity epidemic: the 27 potential health benefits of providing nutrition information in restaurants. *Am J Pub Health*. 2006;96(9):1669–1675.

10   Roberto CA, Larsen PD, Agnew H, Baik J, Brownell KD. Evaluating the impact of menu labeling on food choices and intake. *Am J Public Health*. 2010;100(2):312–318.

11   Tandon PS, Wright J, Zhou C, Rogers CB, Christakis DA. Nutrition menu labeling may lead to lower-caloric restaurant meal choices for children. *Pediatrics*. 2010;125(2):244–248.

12   Centers for Disease Control and Prevention. Food deserts. http://www.cdc.gov/features/fooddeserts. Accessed 9/11/11.

13   Let's Move! Taking on "food deserts." http://www.letsmove.gov/blog/2010/02/24/taking-food-deserts. Accessed 9/11/11.

14   Fieldhouse P. *Food and Nutrition: Customs and Culture*. UK: Chapman and Hall; 1996.

15   Kittler PG, Sucher KP. Op. cit.

16   Bryant CA, DeWalt KM, Courtney A, Schwartz J. *The Cultural Feast: An Introduction to Food and Society*. 2nd ed. Belmont, CA: Wadsworth; 2004.

17   Ibid.

18   Sloan AE. Top 10 food trends. *Food Tech*. 2007;61(4):22–38.

19   Kittler PG, Sucher KP. Op. cit.

20   US Department of Agriculture and US Department of Health and Human Services. *Dietary Guidelines for Americans, 2010*. 7th ed. Washington, DC: US Government Printing Office; December 2010.

21   Ibid.

22   Ibid.

23   Ibid.

24   Ibid.

25   World Health Organization. WHO definition of health. https://apps.who.int/aboutwho/en/definition.html. Accessed 9/11/11.

26   MedlinePlus Medical Dictionary. http://www.merriam-webster.com/medlineplus/disease. Accessed 9/11/11.

27   Centers for Disease Control and Prevention, National Center for Health Statistics. Stroke drops to fourth leading cause of death in 2008; life expectancy declines slightly according to latest CDC deaths report. December 9, 2010. http://www.cdc.gov/media/pressrel/2010/r101209.html. Accessed 9/10/11.

28   US Department of Health and Human Services, Weight-Control Information Network (WIN). Overweight and obesity statistics. Updated 2/10. http://win.niddk.nih.gov/statistics/#overweight. Accessed 9/10/11.

29   Ibid.

30   US Department of Health and Human Services. 2008 Physical Activity Guidelines for Americans. http://www.health.gov/Paguidelines/pdf/paguide.pdf. Accessed 9/9/11.

31   Levine M, Katz A, Padayatty SJ. Vitamin C. In: Shills ME, Shike M, Ross AC, Cabellero B, Cousins RJ, eds. *Modern Nutrition in Health and Disease*. 10th ed. Philadelphia: Lippincott, Williams & Wilkins; 2006.

# CHAPTER 2

# Nutrition Guidelines: Tools for a Healthful Diet

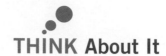

## THINK About It

1 Do you and your friends discuss food and diet?

2 Have you ever taken a large dose of a vitamin or mineral supplement?

3 Do you eat the same foods most days, or do you prefer a variety of choices?

4 What food group makes up the biggest part of your diet?

Visit go.jblearning.com/ inseldisco4e

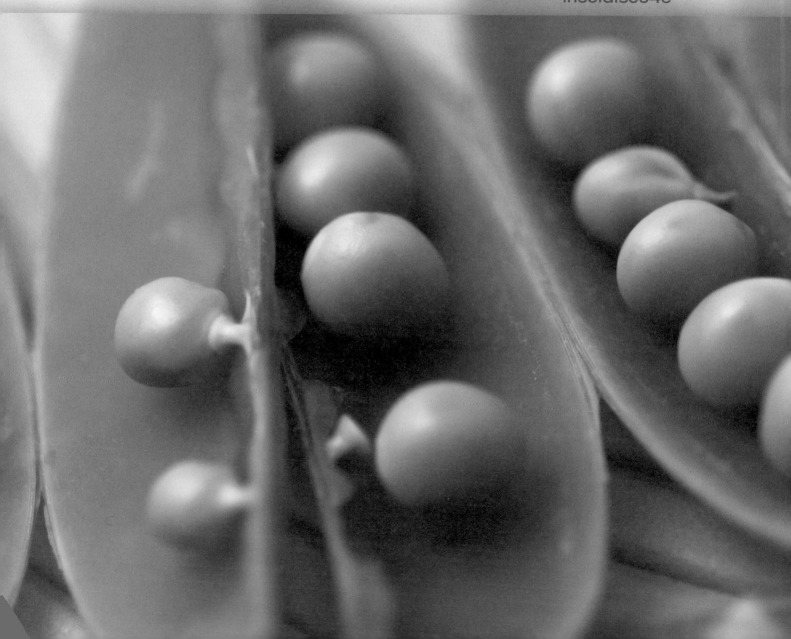

So, you want to be healthier—maybe that's why you are taking this course! You probably already know that a well-planned diet is a prerequisite of being healthy. Although most of us know that the foods we choose have a major impact on our health, we aren't always certain about what to choose. Selecting the right foods isn't any easier when we are bombarded by headlines and advertisements: Eat less fat! Get more fiber! Build strong bones with calcium!

For many Americans, nutrition is simply a lot of hearsay . . . or maybe the latest slogan coined from last week's news headline. Conversations about nutrition start off with "*They* say you should . . ." or "Now *they* think that . . ." Have you ever wondered who "they" are and why "they" are telling you what to eat or what not to eat?

It's no secret that a healthy population is a more productive population, so many of our nutrition guidelines come from the federal government's efforts to improve our overall health; thus the government is one "they." Many important elements of nutrition policy focus on relieving undernutrition in some population groups. To prevent widespread deficiencies, the government requires food manufacturers to add nutrients to certain foods: iodine to salt; vitamin D to milk; and thiamin, riboflavin, niacin, iron, and folic acid to grains. Dietary standards, such as the Dietary Reference Intakes, make it easier to define adequate diets for large groups of people.

Overnutrition has led to changes in public policy as well. Health researchers have discovered links between diet and obesity, high blood pressure, cancer, and heart disease. As a result, nutritionists suggest that we make informed food choices by reducing our intake of excess calories, sodium, saturated fats, and *trans* fats while being physically active. The public's desire to know about food items and the larger food supply has led to increased information on food labels. In addition, public education efforts have developed teaching tools such as MyPlate.

New information about diet and health will continue to drive public policy. This chapter explores current dietary standards, guidelines, and diet-planning tools. While you read, think about your diet and how it measures up to current guidelines and standards.

## Linking Nutrients, Foods, and Health

**THINK**
**About It**
**1**

We all know that what we eat affects our health. Nutrition science has made significant advancements in identifying essential nutrients and the foods in which they are found. Eating foods with all the essential nutrients prevents nutritional deficiencies such as scurvy (vitamin C deficiency) or pellagra (deficiency of the B vitamin niacin). Many people in the United States are malnourished, but fewer people suffer nutritional deficiencies from dietary inadequacies than from chronic diseases (such as heart disease, cancer, hypertension, and diabetes) that develop from overconsumption, nutrition imbalance, and poor lifestyle choices. Your future health depends on today's lifestyle choices, which includes what you eat.

### Planning How You Will Eat

Living in a high-tech world, we expect immediate solutions to long-term problems. Wouldn't it be nice if we could avoid the consequences of overeating by taking a pill, drinking a beverage, or getting a shot? As you know, no magic food, nutrient, or drug exists. Instead, we have to rely on healthful foods, exercise, and lifestyle choices to reduce our risk of chronic disease—a task that challenges many Americans.

Many tools are available to help us select healthful foods to eat. The U.S. Department of Agriculture's MyPlate food guidance system and the Diabetic Exchange Lists are two common and comprehensive tools. Although different, these tools rely on the same core nutrition concepts: adequacy, balance, calorie (energy) control, nutrient density, moderation, and variety. These underlying concepts help to keep the focus of healthy eating on the total diet approach. Let's look at how each concept can shape our eating patterns.

## Adequacy

Having an adequate diet means that the foods you choose to eat provide all the essential nutrients, fiber, and energy in amounts sufficient to support growth and maintain health.[1] Many Americans consume more calories than they need while not getting 100 percent of the recommended intake for a number of nutrients. Take, for example, a meal of soda pop, two hard-shell beef tacos, and cinnamon twists. Although this meal provides foods from different food groups, it is high in sugar and fat and is low in many vitamins and minerals that are found in fruit and vegetables. Occasionally skipping fruits and vegetables at a meal will not create a vitamin or mineral deficiency; however, dietary habits that skimp on fruit and vegetables most of the time will provide an overall inadequate diet. Most people could improve their diet adequacy by choosing meals and snacks that are high in vitamins and minerals but low to moderate in energy (calorie) content. Doing so offers important benefits: normal growth and development of children, health promotion for people of all ages, and reduced risk for a number of chronic diseases.[2]

## Balance

A healthful diet requires a balance of food groups (grains, vegetables, fruits, oil, milk, and meat and beans), energy sources (carbohydrates, protein, and fat), and other nutrients (vitamins and minerals). Your diet is balanced if the amount of energy (calories) you eat equals the amount of energy you expend in daily activities and exercise. Your diet also is balanced when the foods you choose to eat provide you with adequate nutrients. The trick is to consume enough, but not too much, from all of the different food groups.

## Calorie Control

The challenge is to figure out how to maintain a healthy weight while balancing your optimally healthful diet. This entails identifying the amount of calories you need to maintain or achieve a healthy weight and then choosing an adequate diet that balances the calories you eat with the amount of calories your body uses. The formula for weight maintenance seems simple: if you eat the same amount of calories that you use each day, your weight will stay the same. If you cat more than you use, you will gain weight, and, if you eat less than you use, you will lose weight. In this chapter, we focus on how to control the amount of calories you eat by making food choices that provide the most nutrients per calorie. This is like a lesson on budgeting money: you should demand value for your expenditures. Let's put the concept of calorie control together with nutrient density to see how it works.

## Nutrient Density

The Dietary Guidelines Advisory Committee report and the *Dietary Guidelines for Americans, 2010* confirm that many Americans are overweight or obese, yet many of these same people are also undernourished.[3] Understanding nutrient density can help explain how overeating can nevertheless result in undernutrition, and it also can help people make informed food choices.

How does this condition relate to the previously mentioned budget? Just as each of us has a monetary budget—a certain amount of money to spend on things such as food, rent, books, and transportation—in a sense we all have a calorie budget, too. Once you determine how many calories your body uses each day and how to manipulate your calorie expenditure to reach certain health goals, you will be making food choices to match your calorie needs. Every time you eat, you are choosing to spend some of your calorie budget for that day. Those who spend their budget wisely tend to be healthier than those who do not.

The **nutrient density** of food provides a clue to how "healthy" a food is. Nutrient-dense foods are those foods that provide substantial amounts of vitamins and minerals in proportion to relatively few calories.[4] Foods that are low in nutrient density are foods that supply calories but relatively small amounts of vitamins and minerals, sometimes none at all.[5] If a food is high in calories but low in vitamins and minerals, we say that food is less nutrient dense than one that has a high vitamin and mineral content compared with its overall calories.

Take, for example, a potato. We can prepare a potato many different ways. We eat baked potatoes, mashed potatoes with toppings, or french fries. Regardless of how it is cooked, the potato is still a potato, but, depending on how it is cooked and what is added to it before we eat it, the nutrient density of that potato changes. The most nutrient-dense form of this potato would be a plain baked potato, which provides the highest amount of vitamins and minerals with relatively few calories. The least nutrient-dense version of this potato is french fries because frying adds a lot more calories without adding more vitamins and minerals. In this case, the proportion of vitamins and minerals is low compared to the overall higher calorie content. French fries are not nutrient dense.

Foods with little or no added sugar or fat are usually nutrient dense. For example, you might decide to eat a pear instead of a handful of jelly beans. Both provide about the same amount of calories. But, by choosing to eat the nutrient-dense pear instead of the jelly beans, you are working toward meeting your daily nutrient needs on a lower energy budget. These choices over time will create a diet that is healthier overall.

## Moderation

Not too much or too little—that's what moderation means. Moderation does not mean that you have to eliminate low nutrient–dense foods from your diet but rather that you can include them occasionally. Moderation also means not taking anything to extremes. Here is an example: You probably have heard that vitamin C has positive health effects, but that doesn't mean huge doses of this essential nutrient are appropriate for you. It's also important to remember that substances that are healthful in small amounts can sometimes be dangerous in large quantities. For example, the body needs zinc for hundreds of chemical reactions, including those that support normal growth, development, and immune function. Too much zinc, however, can cause deficiency of another essential mineral, copper, which can lead to impaired immune function. Being moderate in your diet means that you do not restrict or completely eliminate any one type of food, but rather that you fit all types of food into a healthful diet.

Food guides and their graphics convey the message of moderation by showing suggested amounts of different food groups. Appearing in diverse

THINK
About It
2

**nutrient density** A description of the healthfulness of foods. Foods high in nutrient density are those that provide substantial amounts of vitamins and minerals and relatively few calories; foods low in nutrient density are those that supply calories but relatively small amounts of vitamins and minerals (or none at all).

## *Quick* Bite

### How Much Do Doctors and Dentists Know About Nutrition?

Nutrition training in medical schools and residency programs has been identified as an essential component of medical education by numerous organizations, including the American Society for Clinical Nutrition, the American Medical Student Association, the National Academy of Sciences, and the U.S. Congress, which passed the National Nutritional Monitoring and Related Research Act of 1990 mandating nutrition as a part of the medical school curriculum. Findings indicate, however, that significant variation in nutrition knowledge of U.S. medical students exists and that the amount of time medical schools spend on nutrition education varies significantly, ranging from a mandatory course in nutrition to nutrition education relegated to just a component of another required course.

# Japanese Food Guide Spinning Top
Do you have a well-balanced diet?

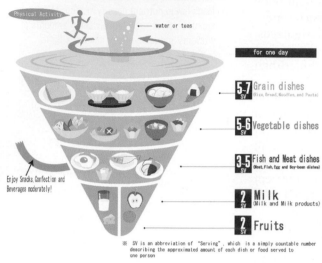

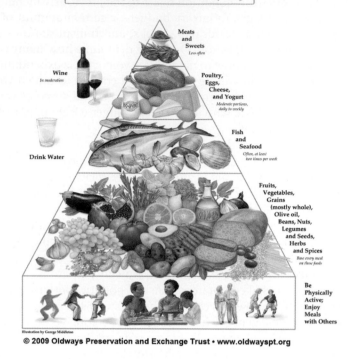

(a) The Japanese food guide spinning top.
**Source:** Courtesy of the Japanese Ministry of Health, Labor and Welfare/USDA.

(b) The Mediterranean diet pyramid.
**Source:** © 2009 Oldways Preservation & Exchange Trust

**Figure 2.1**  **Dietary guidelines around the world.** Global differences in environment, culture, socioeconomics, and behavior create significant differences in the foods that make up our diets. Despite this, dietary guidelines from one country to the next show surprising similarities. Whether a country has only 3 guidelines or as many as 23, all share similar basic recommendations.

shapes, food guides from other countries reflect their cultural contexts. Japan, for example, uses the shape of a spinning top. (See **Figure 2.1**.)

## Variety

How many *different* foods do you eat on a daily basis? Ten? Fifteen? Would it surprise you that one of Japan's dietary guidelines suggests eating 30 different foods each day?[6] Now *that's* variety!

Variety means including a lot of different foods in the diet: not just different food groups, such as fruits, vegetables, and grains but also different foods from within each group. Eating two bananas and three carrots each and every day may give you the minimum number of recommended daily servings for fruits and vegetables, but it doesn't add much variety.

THINK
About It
3

Variety is important for a number of reasons. Eating a variety of fruits, for example, will provide a broader mix of vitamins, minerals, and phytochemicals than just including one or two fruits. Choosing a variety of protein sources will give you a different balance of fats and other nutrients. Variety can add interest and excitement to your meals over and above merely preventing boredom with your diet. Perhaps most important, variety in your diet helps ensure that you get all the nutrients you need. Studies have shown that people who have varied diets are more likely to meet their overall nutrient needs.[7]

Remember, there are no magic diets, foods, or supplements. Instead, your overall, long-term food choices can bring you the benefits of a healthful diet.

A healthful diet is something you create over time; it is not the way you eat on any given day. Using the principles of adequacy, balance, calorie (energy) control, nutrient density, moderation, and variety will help you attain and achieve healthy eating habits, which, in turn, will contribute to your overall healthy lifestyle. Let's take a look at some general guidance for making those food choices.

**Key Concepts** *Food and nutrient intake play a major role in health and risk of disease. For most Americans, overnutrition is more of a problem than undernutrition. The diet-planning principles of adequacy, balance, calorie (energy) control, nutrient density, moderation, and variety are important concepts in choosing a healthful diet.*

## Dietary Guidelines

To help citizens improve overall health, many countries develop dietary guidelines—simple, easy-to-understand statements about food choices. Dietary guidelines are used to develop educational materials and aid policymakers in designing and carrying out nutrition-related programs.

### A Brief History of the *Dietary Guidelines for Americans*

In 1980 the **U.S. Department of Agriculture (USDA)** and the **U.S. Department of Health and Human Services (DHHS)** jointly released the first edition of the *Dietary Guidelines for Americans*. Revised guidelines have been released every 5 years as scientific information about links between diet and chronic disease is updated. The ultimate goal of the *Dietary Guidelines for Americans* is to improve the health of our nation's current and future generations by facilitating and promoting healthy eating and physical activity choices so that these behaviors become a way of life for all individuals.[8]

### The *Dietary Guidelines for Americans, 2010*

The *Dietary Guidelines for Americans, 2010* offers a roadmap intended to guide personal choices and help individuals make informed food and activity decisions. The result of a systematic, evidence-based review of the scientific literature, the *Dietary Guidelines for Americans, 2010* is based on what experts have determined to be the best advice for Americans to reduce their risk for chronic diseases and reduce the prevalence of overweight and obesity through improved nutrition and physical activity. The *Guidelines* are the cornerstone of federal nutrition policy and education. They are used to develop educational materials and to aid in the design and implementation of nutrition-related programs, such as the National School Lunch Program and Meals on Wheels. The *Dietary Guidelines for Americans* serves as the basis for nutrition messages and consumer materials developed by nutrition educators and health professionals for the general public.[9]

Lifestyle choices, including a poor diet and lack of physical activity, are the most important contributors to the overweight and obesity epidemic that is currently affecting men, women, and children throughout the United States. Even in individuals who are not overweight, a poor diet and physical inactivity are well-known to be associated with the major causes of morbidity and mortality. Currently, the number of Americans who are overweight or obese is at an all-time high, and, as a consequence, the risk for various chronic diseases also is on the rise. In an effort to address this growing problem, the *Dietary Guidelines for Americans, 2010* focuses on the integration of government, agriculture, health care, business, educators, and communities working together to encourage individuals to make healthy lifestyle changes.[10]

**U.S. Department of Agriculture (USDA)** The government agency that monitors the production of eggs, poultry, and meat for adherence to standards of quality and wholesomeness. The USDA also provides public nutrition education, performs nutrition research, and administers the WIC program.

**U.S. Department of Health and Human Services (DHHS)** The principal federal agency responsible for protecting the health of all Americans and providing essential human services. The agency is especially concerned with those Americans who are least able to help themselves.

***Dietary Guidelines for Americans, 2010*** The *Guidelines* are the foundation of federal nutrition policy and is jointly developed by the U.S. Department of Agriculture (USDA) and the Department of Health and Human Services (DHHS). These science-based guidelines are intended to reduce the number of Americans who develop chronic diseases such as hypertension, diabetes, cardiovascular disease, obesity, and alcoholism.

The main objective of the *Guidelines* is to encourage Americans to balance calorie intake with physical activity to manage weight. This means helping Americans make the choices they need to eat a healthier diet by promoting the consumption of more vegetables, fruits, whole grains, fat-free and low-fat dairy products, and seafood and foods with less sodium, saturated and *trans* fats, added sugars, and refined grains and emphasizing the importance of daily physical activity.

The two overarching concepts in the *Dietary Guidelines for Americans, 2010* are:

- *Maintain calorie balance over time to achieve and sustain a healthy weight.* To decrease the number of overweight and obese children and adults, many Americans would benefit from a decrease in calorie consumption and an increase in calorie expenditure each day.
- *Focus on consuming nutrient-dense foods and beverages.* An eating pattern that frequently includes foods that are low in nutrients and high in calories (unhealthy) will often take the place of more nutrient-dense (healthier) foods in one's diet. In a healthy eating pattern, the majority of foods should be those foods and beverages that have a high nutrient content; foods with a low nutrient density should be limited.

These two overarching concepts form the basis of the *Dietary Guidelines for Americans, 2010.* The chapters include 23 Key Recommendations for the general population as well as additional Key Recommendations for specific population groups, such as women who are pregnant. The following is a review of the concepts and recommendations from each chapter of the *Dietary Guidelines for Americans, 2010.* You can access the full report at http://www.dietaryguidelines.gov.

## Balancing Calories to Manage Weight

Being successful at maintaining a healthy body weight requires a balance between the amount of calories you eat and the amount of calories you expend every day. Participating in physical activity on a regular basis also helps make it easier for you to maintain a healthy weight. The *2008 Physical Activity Guidelines for Americans* suggests that adults should do the equivalent of 150 minutes of moderate-intensity aerobic activity each week—that's an average of only 30 minutes a day, 5 days a week. For children and adolescents age 6 years or older, the recommendation is 60 minutes or more of physical activity per day.[11]

The environment in which many Americans now live, work, learn, and play may also be a roadblock for many people trying to achieve or maintain a healthy body weight. An **obesogenic environment** is a significant contributor to America's obesity epidemic because it affects both sides of the calorie balance equation.[12] In our modern lifestyle, the availability of high-calorie, palatable, inexpensive food is coupled with many mechanized labor-saving devices. The result is that we live in an environment that often promotes overeating while at the same time discouraging physical activity.

### *Key Recommendations*

The following Key Recommendations are intended to help each of us balance calories to manage weight:

- Prevent and/or reduce overweight and obesity through improved eating and physical activity behaviors.

**obesogenic environment**
According to the *Dietary Guidelines for Americans, 2010,* an environment that promotes overconsumption of calories and discourages physical activity.

- Control total calorie intake to manage body weight. For people who are overweight or obese, this will mean consuming fewer calories from foods and beverages.
- Increase physical activity and reduce time spent in sedentary behaviors.
- Maintain appropriate calorie balance during each stage of life—childhood, adolescence, adulthood, pregnancy and breastfeeding, and older age.

## Foods and Food Components to Reduce

This chapter of the *Dietary Guidelines for Americans, 2010* focuses on several foods and food components that Americans typically consume in excess. These foods/food components include sodium, solid fats, added sugars, and refined grains. Consistently eating too much of these foods/food components may increase the risk of certain chronic diseases, such as cardiovascular disease, diabetes, and certain types of cancer. In addition, when these foods/food components are a regular part of a person's diet, they tend to replace more nutrient-dense foods in the diet, making it even more difficult to meet recommended nutrient and calorie levels.

### *Key Recommendations*

The following Key Recommendations are intended to help each of us reduce our intake of certain foods and food components:

- Reduce daily sodium intake to less than 2,300 milligrams (approximately 1 teaspoon) and further reduce intake to 1,500 milligrams among persons who are 51 or older and those of any age who are African American or have hypertension, diabetes, or chronic kidney disease. The 1,500-milligram recommendation applies to about half of the U.S. population, including children and the majority of adults.
- Consume less than 10 percent of calories from saturated fatty acids by replacing them with monounsaturated and polyunsaturated fatty acids.
- Consume less than 300 milligrams per day of dietary cholesterol.
- Keep *trans* fatty acid consumption as low as possible by limiting foods that contain synthetic sources of *trans* fats, such as partially hydrogenated oils, and by limiting other solid fats.
- Reduce the intake of calories from solid fats and added sugars.
- Limit the consumption of foods that contain refined grains, especially refined-grain foods that contain solid fats, added sugars, and sodium.
- If alcohol is consumed, it should be consumed in moderation—up to one drink per day for women and two drinks per day for men—and only by adults of legal drinking age.

## Foods and Nutrients to Increase

In this chapter of the *Dietary Guidelines for Americans, 2010*, the focus is on food choices that many Americans should adopt to move toward more healthful eating. In the United States, intakes of vegetables, fruits, whole grains, milk and milk products, and oils are lower than recommended. As a result, dietary intakes of several nutrients, such as potassium, dietary fiber, calcium, and vitamin D, are low enough to be of public concern for both adults and children. Choosing healthful foods that provide these nutrients has been found to aid in preventing disease and be beneficial for overall well-being.

Keep in mind that recommendations for a healthy eating pattern will generally group foods based on commonalities in nutrients provided, their effects on health, and how the foods are viewed and used by consumers. When trying to adopt the following recommendations as part of a healthy eating pattern, it is important that you also consider the recommendations from the previous section to help ensure you are staying within your calorie needs. Examples of the health benefits from adopting the Key Recommendations, as well as tips for implementing them, can be found in Table 2.1.

### Key Recommendations

The following Key Recommendations are intended to help each of us increase consumption of particular foods and nutrients:

- Increase vegetable and fruit intake.
- Eat a variety of vegetables, especially dark-green and red and orange vegetables and beans and peas.
- Consume at least half of all grains as whole grains. Increase whole-grain intake by replacing refined grains with whole grains.
- Increase intake of fat-free or low-fat milk and milk products, such as milk, yogurt, cheese, or fortified soy beverages.
- Choose a variety of protein foods, which include seafood, lean meat and poultry, eggs, beans and peas, soy products, and unsalted nuts and seeds.
- Increase the amount and variety of seafood consumed by choosing seafood in place of some meat and poultry.

**Table 2.1** *2010 Dietary Guidelines for Americans:* **Benefits, Behaviors, and Tips**

| Dietary Guideline Recommendation | Benefits to Your Health | Goals or Behaviors That Could Make You Healthier | How-to Tips |
|---|---|---|---|
| **Control total calorie intake to manage body weight.** | • Helps you to achieve and sustain a healthy weight.<br>• Benefits your physical health by improving blood pressure.<br>• Benefits your physical health by improving your blood cholesterol levels.<br>• Benefits your physical health by improving your blood sugar levels.<br>• Improves your energy level.<br>• Improves your physical mobility.<br>• Improves your overall general mood and self-confidence. | • Consume foods and drinks to meet, not exceed, calorie needs.<br>• Plan ahead to make better food choices.<br>• Track food and calorie intake.<br>• Reduce portion sizes, especially of high-calorie foods.<br>• Cook and eat more meals at home, instead of eating out.<br>• Choose healthy options when eating out. | • Know your calorie needs.<br>• Prepare and pack healthy snacks at home to be eaten at school or work.<br>• Track and evaluate what you eat using a food journal or an online food planner.<br>• Pay attention to feelings of hunger. Eat only until you are satisfied, not full.<br>• Limit eating while watching television, which often leads to overeating.<br>• Choose smaller plates and smaller portions.<br>• To feel satisfied with fewer calories, replace large portions of high-calorie foods with lower-calorie foods, like vegetables and fruits.<br>• Cook and eat at home more often.<br>• When eating out, choose a smaller size option or take home part of your meal.<br>• Choose dishes that include vegetables, fruits, and/or whole grains, and avoid choosing foods with the following words: creamy, fried, breaded, battered, or buttered. |

| Table 2.1 | *2010 Dietary Guidelines for Americans:* Benefits, Behaviors, and Tips *(Continued)* |

| Dietary Guideline Recommendation | Benefits to Your Health | Goals or Behaviors That Could Make You Healthier | How-to Tips |
|---|---|---|---|
| **Increase physical activity and reduce time spent in sedentary behaviors.** | • Helps to control your weight.<br><br>• Promotes psychological well-being.<br><br>• Reduces feelings of pressure and anxiety.<br><br>• Helps reduce your risk for chronic diseases such as diabetes, metabolic syndrome, high blood pressure, and some cancers.<br><br>• Helps build and maintain healthy bones, muscles, and joints.<br><br>• Improves your ability to do daily activities.<br><br>• Helps older adults become stronger and better able to move about without falling.<br><br>• Increases your chances of living longer. | • Limit screen time.<br><br>• Be more active daily.<br><br>• Avoid couch time. Some physical activity is better than none.<br><br>• Slowly build up the amount of physical activity you choose. | • Limit the amount of time you spend watching television or using other media such as computers and video games.<br><br>• Pick activities you like and that fit into your life.<br><br>• Be active with family and friends. Having a support network can help you stay active.<br><br>• Keep track of your physical activity and gradually increase it to meet the recommendations of the *2008 Physical Activity Guidelines for Americans.*<br><br>• Start by being active for longer each time you exercise, and then do more by exercising more often.<br><br>• Adults should do the equivalent of 150 minutes of moderate-intensity aerobic activity each week. |
| **Increase vegetable and fruit intake.** | • Eating vegetables and fruits as part of a reduced-calorie diet can be of benefit to your body weight.<br><br>• Is associated with a decreased risk for many chronic diseases such as cardiovascular disease and many cancers.<br><br>• Contributes to healthy aging. | • Eat five or more servings of vegetables and fruit daily, made up of a variety of choices. | • Add dark-green, red, and orange vegetables to soups, stews, casseroles, and stir-fries and other main and side dishes.<br><br>• Add beans or peas to salad, soups, and side dishes, or serve as a main dish.<br><br>• Have raw, cut-up vegetables and fruit handy for a quick side dish, snacks, salad, or desserts.<br><br>• When eating out, choose a vegetable as a side dish. |
| **Increase intake of fat-free or low-fat milk and milk products, such as milk, yogurt, cheese, or fortified soy beverages.** | • Milk and milk products contribute many nutrients to the diet, including calcium and vitamin D, which help to build and maintain strong bones and teeth.<br><br>• Adequate milk intake is associated with decreased chance of developing metabolic syndrome and high blood pressure. | • Choose two to three servings of low-fat dairy products every day.<br><br>• Replace higher-fat milk and milk products with lower-fat options. | • Drink fat-free (skim) or low-fat (1%) milk.<br><br>• When drinking beverages such as cappuccino or latte, request fat-free or low-fat milk.<br><br>• When recipes call for sour cream, substitute plain fat-free or low-fat yogurt. |

*(Continues)*

**Table 2.1**    *2010 Dietary Guidelines for Americans:* **Benefits, Behaviors, and Tips** *(Continued)*

| Dietary Guideline Recommendation | Benefits to Your Health | Goals or Behaviors That Could Make You Healthier | How-to Tips |
|---|---|---|---|
| **Limit the consumption of foods that contain refined grains and added sugars.** | • Eating foods that contain whole grains offers a good source of antioxidants such as vitamin E, magnesium, iron, and fiber to your diet.<br><br>• Eating foods that contain fiber helps lower blood cholesterol levels, control blood glucose levels for people with diabetes, and causes a feeling of satiety.<br><br>• A diet high in sugar is associated with being overweight/obese. | • Increase whole-grain intake.<br><br>• Consume at least half of all grains as whole grains.<br><br>• Whenever possible, replace refined grains with whole grains.<br><br>• Choose foods and drinks with added sugars or caloric sweeteners (sugar-sweetened beverages) less frequently.<br><br>• Drink more water. | • Choose 100 percent whole-grain breads, crackers, rice, and pasta.<br><br>• Use the Nutrition Facts label to choose whole grains that are a good or excellent source of dietary fiber.<br><br>• Eat fewer refined grain products, such as cakes, cookies, other desserts, and pizza.<br><br>• Replace white bread, rolls, bagels, muffins, pasta, and rice with whole-grain versions.<br><br>• To increase fiber in your diet, choose foods such as oat bran, barley, kidney beans, fruits, vegetables, wheat bran, and whole grains.<br><br>• To increase insoluble fiber in your diet, choose foods such as wheat bran, vegetables, and whole grains.<br><br>• Drink few or no regular sodas, sports drinks, energy drinks, and fruit drinks.<br><br>• Eat less cake, cookies, ice cream, other desserts, and candy.<br><br>• Choose water, fat-free milk, 100 percent fruit juice, or unsweetened tea or coffee as drinks rather than sugar-sweetened drinks. |
| **Keep trans fatty acid consumption as low as possible.** | • Eating a diet that includes saturated fat, *trans* fat, and dietary cholesterol raises low-density lipoprotein (LDL), or "bad" cholesterol, levels, which increases the risk of coronary heart disease (CHD). | • Be aware of the most likely sources of *trans* fat in your diet, such as many pastry items and donuts, deep-fried foods, many types of snack chips, cookies, and crackers.<br><br>• Choose foods and drinks with added sugars or caloric sweeteners (sugar-sweetened beverages) less frequently.<br><br>• Drink more water. | • When using spreads, choose soft margarines with zero *trans* fats made from liquid vegetable oil, rather than stick margarine or butter.<br><br>• Use vegetable oils such as olive, canola, corn, or sunflower oil rather than solid fats (butter, stick margarine, shortening, lard).<br><br>• Check the Nutrition Facts label to choose foods with little or no saturated fat and no *trans* fat.<br><br>• Limit foods that contain partially hydrogenated oils and other solid fats. |
| **If alcohol is consumed, it should be consumed in moderation.** | • Excessive drinking has no benefits, and the health and social hazards of heavy alcohol intake are numerous and well known. | • If you are of legal drinking age you should drink alcoholic beverages in moderation.<br><br>• Avoid alcohol in situations that can put you at risk. | • Limit alcohol to no more than one drink per day for women and two drinks per day for men.<br><br>• Avoid excessive (heavy or binge) drinking.<br><br>• Avoid alcohol if you are pregnant or may become pregnant. |

| Table 2.1 | *2010 Dietary Guidelines for Americans:* **Benefits, Behaviors, and Tips** *(Continued)* |
|---|---|

| Dietary Guideline Recommendation | Benefits to Your Health | Goals or Behaviors That Could Make You Healthier | How-to Tips |
|---|---|---|---|
| **Follow food safety recommendations when preparing and eating foods to reduce the risk of foodborne illnesses.** | • Prevents foodborne illness. | • Learn proper food handling techniques.<br>• When in doubt, throw it out.<br>• Cook food to a safe temperature.<br>• Store food safely. | • Clean: Wash hands, utensils, and cutting boards before and after contact with raw meat, poultry, seafood, and eggs.<br>• Separate: Keep raw meat and poultry apart from foods that won't be cooked.<br>• Cook: Use a food thermometer.<br>• Chill: Chill leftovers and takeout foods within 2 hours and keep the refrigerator at 40 degrees Fahrenheit or below. |

**Source:** Modified from US Department of Health and Human Services, US Department of Agriculture. *Dietary Guidelines for Americans, 2010.* 7th ed, page 63. Washington, DC: US Government Printing Office, 2010.

- Replace protein foods that are higher in solid fat with choices that are lower in solid fats and calories and/or are sources of oils.
- Use oils to replace solid fats where possible.
- Choose foods that provide more potassium, dietary fiber, calcium, and vitamin D, which are nutrients of concern in American diets. These foods include vegetables, fruits, whole grains, and milk and milk products.

## Recommendations for Specific Population Groups

Within the "Foods and Nutrients to Increase" chapter, unique recommendations for specific population groups are described. These recommendations are designed to improve the food choices and health outcomes of certain individuals, such as pregnant and lactating women and older adults who have specific nutritional needs. The recommendations are as follows:

- Women capable of becoming pregnant
  - Choose foods that supply heme iron, which is more readily absorbed by the body; additional iron sources; and enhancers of iron absorption, such as vitamin C–rich foods.
  - Consume 400 micrograms per day of synthetic folic acid (from fortified foods and/or supplements) in addition to food forms of folate from a varied diet.
- Women who are pregnant or breastfeeding
  - Consume 8 to 12 ounces of seafood per week from a variety of seafood types.
  - Due to their methyl mercury content, limit white (albacore) tuna to 6 ounces per week, and do not eat the following four types of fish: tilefish, shark, swordfish, and king mackerel.
  - If pregnant, take an iron supplement as recommended by an obstetrician or other healthcare provider.
- Individuals age 50 years or older
  - Consume foods fortified with vitamin $B_{12}$, such as fortified cereals, or dietary supplements.

## Building Healthy Eating Patterns

The *Dietary Guidelines for Americans, 2010* also shows you how the recommendations and principles described in the previous chapters can be combined into a healthy overall eating pattern. Culture, ethnicity, tradition, personal preferences, food cost, and food availability are all factors people consider when creating the way they choose to eat. Americans have flexibility in the choices they make when forming their own healthy eating patterns. Americans also have access to established eating plans, such as the USDA Food Patterns and DASH Eating Plan, to help assist in such efforts.

In addition, this chapter focuses on eating patterns that prevent foodborne illness and identifies how the four basic food safety principles—*clean*, *separate*, *cook*, and *chill*—work together to reduce the risk of foodborne illnesses.

### Key Recommendations

The following Key Recommendations are intended to help each of us build healthy eating patterns:

- Select an eating pattern that meets nutrient needs over time at an appropriate calorie level.
- Account for all foods and beverages consumed and assess how they fit within a total healthy eating pattern.
- Follow food safety recommendations when preparing and eating foods to reduce the risk of foodborne illnesses.

## Helping Americans Make Healthy Choices

This chapter focuses on two important factors. The first is that people make choices about what to eat and how physically active they will be every day. Second, all elements of society, including individuals and families, communi-

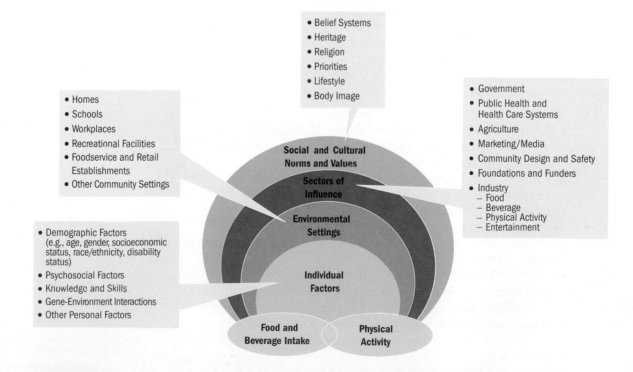

| Figure 2.2 | **A social ecological framework for nutrition and physical activity decisions.** |

**Sources:** US Department of Health and Human Services and US Department of Agriculture. *Dietary Guidelines for Americans, 2010.* 7th ed, page 56. Washington, DC: US Government Printing Office; 2010; Adapted from Centers for Disease Control and Prevention, Division of Nutrition, Physical Activity, and Obesity. *State Nutrition, Physical Activity and Obesity (NPAO) Program: Technical Assistance Manual.* January 2008, page 36. Accessed 4/21/10. http://www.cdc.gov/obesity/downloads/TA_Manual_1_31_08.pdf; Institute of Medicine. *Preventing Childhood Obesity: Health in the Balance.* Page 85. Washington, DC: National Academies Press; 2005; and Story M, Kaphingst KM, Robinson-O'Brien R, Glanz K. Creating healthy food and eating environments: policy and environmental approaches. *Annu Rev Public Health.* 2008;29:253–272.

ties, business and industry, and various levels of government, should have a positive and productive role in the efforts to make America healthy.[13] The *Dietary Guidelines for Americans, 2010* employs the social ecological model (see **Figure 2.2**) as a tool to illustrate how all elements of society combine to shape an individual's food and physical activity choices. As a result, they ultimately influence the choices people make every day about what they will eat and drink and what their daily activity will be.[14]

This chapter also includes the *2010 Dietary Guidelines'* Call to Action, which includes three guiding principles:

1.  Ensure all Americans have access to nutritious foods and opportunities for physical activity.
2.  Facilitate individual behavior change through environmental strategies.
3.  Set the stage for lifelong healthy eating, physical activity, and weight management behaviors.

The *Dietary Guidelines for Americans, 2010* (see **Figure 2.3**) also provides resources that can be used in developing policies, programs, and educational materials. These include:

- Guidelines for Specific Population Groups
- Key Consumer Behaviors and Potential Strategies for Professionals to Use
- Food Safety Principles and Guidance for Consumers
- Using the Food Label to Track Calories, Nutrients, and Ingredients

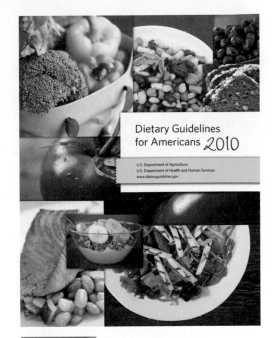

**Figure 2.3**    *Dietary Guidelines for Americans, 2010.* A revised *Dietary Guidelines for Americans* was released in 2010.

**Source:** US Department of Health and Human Services, US Department of Agriculture. *Dietary Guidelines for Americans, 2010.* 7th ed. Washington, DC: US Government Printing Office; 2010.

## How to Incorporate the Dietary Guidelines into Your Daily Life

Think about your diet and consider your overall food intake to determine whether it is consistent with the *Dietary Guidelines for Americans, 2010*. Choose more fruits, vegetables, and whole grains to make sure you are getting all the nutrients you need while lowering your intake of saturated fat, *trans* fat, and cholesterol. Eat fewer high-fat toppings and fried foods to balance your energy intake and expenditure. Exercise regularly. Use the extra things—sugar, salt, and alcohol—in moderation. Drink water more often than soft drinks, and, if you choose to drink alcohol at all, use caution. By using the *Dietary Guidelines* as your roadmap for finding a healthier way of eating, you may not only find it easier to meet your nutrition needs, but you also will be protecting your health and achieving or maintaining a healthy weight along the way. Table 2.1 offers suggestions of changes you can make in your own diet or lifestyle. Pick one or two of these suggestions, or come up with some simple changes of your own, to try to incorporate the *Dietary Guidelines for Americans, 2010* into your daily life. Table 2.2 gives a summary of daily limits or targets for a number of nutrients addressed in the *Dietary Guidelines*.

## Canada's Guidelines for Healthy Eating

Promoting healthy eating habits among Canadians has been a priority of Health Canada for many years. Health Canada is the federal department responsible for helping the people of Canada maintain and improve their health. In the 1980s, a high priority was given to developing a single set of dietary guidelines. The result of this effort was the 1990 *Nutrition Recommendations for Canadians* and *Canada's Guidelines for Healthy Eating*, Canada's first set of positive, action-oriented messages for healthy Canadians over the age of 2.

*Quick* Bite

**How Well Do School Cafeterias Follow Nutrition Guidelines?**

About one in three kids and teenagers is obese, and high-fat school lunches may be part of the problem. Until recently, the UDSA's nutritional standards for school meals had not been updated in more than 15 years. With the majority of school-age kids and teens getting 30 to 50 percent of their total calories from cafeteria meals each day, it's important that these meals be as healthy as possible. The Healthy, Hunger-Free Kids Act is a plan that will (1) boost the nutrition quality of school lunch by requiring fewer calories and sodium and more fresh fruits, vegetables, and whole grains; (2) expand the number of students enrolled in free- and reduced-cost meals; and (3) put into place a plan to eliminate things like unhealthy vending machines from school cafeterias.

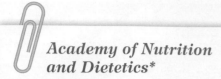

## Academy of Nutrition and Dietetics*

**Total Diet Approach to Communicating Food and Nutrition Information**

It is the position of the American Dietetic Association that the total diet or overall pattern of food eaten is the most important focus of a healthful eating style. All foods can fit within this pattern, if consumed in moderation with appropriate portion size and combined with regular physical activity. The Academy of Nutrition and Dietetics strives to communicate healthful eating messages to the public that emphasize a balance of foods, rather than any one food or meal.

**Source:** Reproduced from Nitzke S, Freeland-Graves J. Position of the Academy of Nutrition and Dietetics: total diet approach to communicating food and nutrition information. *J Am Diet Assoc.* 2007;107:1224–1232.

* Formerly the American Dietetic Association

## Quick Bite

**Pass Up the Salt**
Our bodies require only a few hundred milligrams of sodium each day, but this minimal amount would be difficult to achieve given our current food supply and would be unpalatable, given our acquired taste—so the guideline is to eat less sodium (not more than a teaspoon total) but to not cut down to the level of actual body requirements.

| Table 2.2 | Daily Targets for Nutrients as Addressed in the *Dietary Guidelines for Americans, 2010* |
|---|---|

| Nutrient or Food Group | Target for Adults Ages 19–50 |
|---|---|
| Total fat (percent of calories) | 20–35 |
| Saturated fat (percent of calories) | < 10 |
| Cholesterol (mg) | < 300 |
| Calcium (mg) | 1,000 |
| Potassium (mg) | 4,700 |
| Sodium (mg) | < 2,300 |
| Vitamin D (mcg)[a] | 15 |
| Fiber (g) | 14 g per 1,000 calories (28–34 g/day) |
| Vegetables and fruit (cups per day) | At least 4–5 |
| Refined grains (oz per day) | > 3 |
| Physical activity | 150 minutes of moderate-intensity aerobic activity each week |

[a] 1 mcg of vitamin D is equivalent to 40 IU.

**Source:** Data from US Department of Agriculture and US Department of Health and Human Services. *Dietary Guidelines for Americans, 2010.* 7th ed. Washington, DC: US Government Printing Office; December 2010.

The 2007 revision, *Eating Well with Canada's Food Guide*, recommends that Canadians do the following:[15]

- Eat at least one dark-green and one orange vegetable each day.
- Enjoy vegetables and fruits prepared with little or no added fat, sugar, or salt.
- Have vegetables and fruits more often than juice.
- Select whole grains for at least half of their grain products.
- Choose grain products that are low in fat, sugar, or salt.
- Drink skim, 1%, or 2% milk each day.
- Select lower-fat milk alternatives.
- Consume meat alternatives, such as beans, lentils, and tofu, often.
- Eat at least two *Food Guide* servings of fish each week.
- Select lean meat and alternatives prepared with little or no added fat or salt.
- Include a small amount of unsaturated fat each day.
- Satisfy thirst with water.
- Limit foods and beverages high in calories, fat, sugar, or salt.
- Be active every day.

Canada's Physical Activity Guide, released in January 2011 by the Canadian Society for Exercise Physiology, recommends that children ages 5 to 11 and youth ages 12 to 17 should get at least 60 minutes of moderate- to vigorous-intensity physical activity daily. Adults ages 18 to 64 and older adults age 65 and older should get at least 150 minutes of moderate- to vigorous-intensity aerobic physical activity per week, in bouts of 10 minutes or more (see http://www.csep.ca/english/view.asp?x=804 for detailed information).

Dietary guidelines in the United States and Canada address similar issues—less fat; more fruits, vegetables, and grains; less salt; and achieving healthy weights. In addition, both countries have developed graphic depictions of a healthful diet by showing the balance of food groups to be consumed each day.

**Key Concepts** *Dietary guidelines are statements based on current science that "guide" people toward more healthful choices. The Dietary Guidelines for Americans, 2010 pro-*

*vides two overarching themes and 23 Key Recommendations for making food choices that promote good health, a healthy weight, and prevention of disease for healthy Americans age 2 or older. Six additional key recommendations target specific population groups. Behavioral strategies and creating a healthy environment are important for adopting the recommendations in the Dietary Guidelines for Americans, 2010. Both the United States and Canada have guidelines that embody the basic principles of balance, variety, and moderation.*

# From Dietary Guidelines to Planning: What Will You Eat?

For many years, nutritionists and teachers have used **food groups** to illustrate the proper combination of foods in a healthful diet. The foods within each group are apparently similar because of their origins—fruits, for example, all come from the same part of different plants. But from a nutritional perspective, what fruits have in common are the balance of macronutrients and similarities in micronutrient composition. Even so, the foods in one group may differ significantly in their vitamin and mineral profiles. Some fruits (e.g., citrus, strawberries, kiwi) are rich in vitamin C, whereas others (e.g., apples, bananas) have very little. Here again, we can see the importance of variety, of choosing a variety of foods *within* each group, not simply including different food groups.

**food groups** Categories of similar foods, such as fruits or vegetables.

## A Brief History of Food Group Plans

When the U.S. Department of Agriculture published its first dietary recommendations in 1894, specific vitamins and minerals had not even been discovered.[16] The initial guide stressed the importance of consuming enough fat and sugar and energy-rich foods to support daily activity. Because people performed more manual labor in those days, many people were simply not getting enough calories! Canada's Official Food Rules (1942) recommended a weekly serving of liver, heart, or kidney and regular doses of fish liver oils— good sources of vitamins A and D. Later food group plans, including the Basic Four that was popular from the 1950s through the 1970s, focused on fruits, vegetables, grains, dairy products, and meats and their substitutes. The Basic Four was usually illustrated as either a circle or a square with each group having an equal share. The implication was that people should consume equal amounts of food from each group. Nutrition science now tells us that those proportions give us a diet too high in fat and protein for our modern lifestyle and not high enough in carbohydrates and fiber. After the development of the *Dietary Guidelines for Americans* in 1980, the USDA developed a new food guide that would promote overall health and be consistent with the *Dietary Guidelines*. To bring this new food guide and its key messages to the attention of consumers, the colorful Food Guide Pyramid was developed.[17] By law, the *Dietary Guidelines for Americans* is reviewed, updated if necessary, and published every 5 years; thus the current version, the *Dietary Guidelines for Americans, 2010* and MyPlate (see **Figure 2.4**) were created.

## MyPlate

MyPlate is the USDA's current icon and the primary food group symbol to accompany the *Dietary Guidelines for Americans, 2010*. As part of the federal government's healthy eating initiative, My Plate is designed to convey the seven key messages from the *Dietary Guidelines for Americans, 2010*: Enjoy food, but eat less; avoid oversized portions; make half your plate fruits and vegetables; drink water instead of sugary drinks; switch to fat-free or low-fat (1%) milk; compare sodium in foods; and make at least half your grains whole grains.

*Quick* **Bite**

**SuperTracker: My Foods, My Fitness, My Health**
MyPlate includes the SuperTracker. Get your personalized nutrition and physical activity plan. Track your foods and physical activities to see how they stack up. Get tips and support to help you make healthier choices and plan ahead. Visit https://www.choosemyplate.gov/SuperTracker/default.aspx.

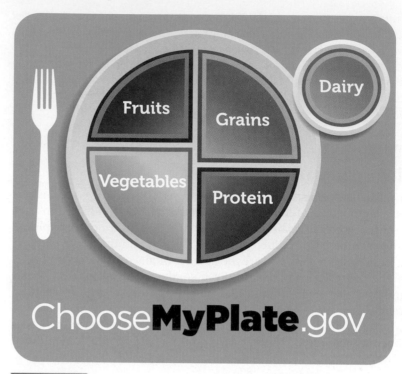

**Figure 2.4**    **MyPlate.** Released in 2011, MyPlate is an Internet-based educational tool that helps consumers implement the principles of the *Dietary Guidelines for Americans, 2010* and other nutritional standards.
**Source:** Courtesy of USDA.

MyPlate is an easy-to-understand visual image intended to empower people with the information they need to make healthy food choices and create eating habits consistent with the *Dietary Guidelines for Americans, 2010*. Experts suggest that, because we eat on plates, the design of the MyPlate icon is able to visually convey how much room on a plate each food group should occupy. The goal is for the MyPlate icon to remind people to think about and make better, more balanced food choices.[18] MyPlate uses the image of a dinner plate divided into four sections representing fruits, vegetables, grains, and proteins with a smaller plate (or glass) representing a serving of dairy.

THINK
About It
4

MyPlate is accompanied by a supporting website (http://www.Choose MyPlate.gov). The website provides tools, resources, and practical information on dietary assessment, nutrition education, and other user-friendly nutrition information.[19] Unlike the USDA's former food guide systems, MyPlate does not suggest particular foods or specific serving sizes and does not even mention desserts or sweets. The purpose behind these changes is clear—this food guide is different! It is not intended to tell people what to eat but to empower them to make their own healthy choices and to use the icon as a sensible guide.

## Eating Well with Canada's Food Guide

As science advanced and nutritional concerns changed, Canada's Official Food Rules evolved into *Eating Well with Canada's Food Guide*. (See **Figure 2.5**.) The amounts and types of foods recommended in the *Food Guide* are based on the nutrient reference values of the Dietary Reference Intakes (DRIs). The foods pictured in the *Food Guide* reflect the diversity of foods available in Canada. The *Food Guide* document essentially incorporates both the recommended eating pattern and associated dietary guidance.

*Eating Well with Canada's Food Guide* Recommendations to help Canadians select foods to meet energy and nutrient needs while reducing the risk of chronic disease. The *Food Guide* is based on the *Nutrition Recommendations for Canadians* and Canada's Guidelines for Healthy Eating and is a key nutrition education tool for Canadians aged 2 to 3 years and older.

The "rainbow" of the *Food Guide* places foods into four groups: Vegetables and Fruit, Grain Products, Milk and Alternates, and Meat and Alternatives. The *Food Guide* describes the kinds of foods to choose from each group. For example, under the Milk and Alternates group, the *Food Guide* suggests, "Drink fortified soy beverages if you do not drink milk." *Canada's Food Guide* illustrates that vegetables, fruits, and grains should be the major part of the diet with milk products and meats consumed in smaller amounts.

The *Food Guide* provides a "bar" that shows how many daily servings are recommended from each group for each age group and gives examples of serving sizes. The *Food Guide* also provides specific advice for different ages and stages. Limiting foods and beverages high in calories, fat, sugar, or salt is recommended. Label-reading is recommended, and a list of steps to healthy living is provided. The Health Canada website (http://www.healthcanada.gc.ca/foodguide) includes a link to "My Food Guide," an interactive tool for personalizing the information in the Food Guide.

## Using MyPlate or *Canada's Food Guide* in Diet Planning

The first step in using MyPlate or *Canada's Food Guide* for diet planning is to determine the amount of calories you should eat each day. Table 2.3 shows the recommended amounts of food for three calorie-intake levels. It also will give you an idea of how MyPlate varies with different energy needs. Next, become familiar with the types of food in each group, the number of recommended servings, and the appropriate serving sizes. (For an intuitive guide to serving sizes, see Table 2.4.) Finally, plan your meals and snacks using the suggested serving sizes for your appropriate calorie level.

Let's start to plan a 2,000-calorie diet. Beginning with breakfast, you could plan to have: 1 cup (1 ounce) of ready-to-eat cereal, ½ cup of skim milk, one slice of whole wheat toast with 1 teaspoon of butter, and 1 cup of orange juice.

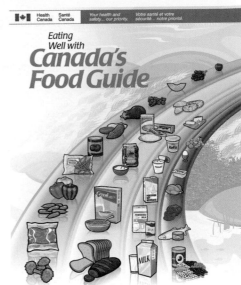

**Figure 2.5** *Eating Well with Canada's Food Guide.* The rainbow portion of *Canada's Food Guide* sorts foods into groups from which people can make wise food choices.

**Source:** *Eating Well With Canada's Food Guide*, Health Canada, 2007. © Reproduced with the permission of the Minister of Public Works and Government Services Canada, 2009.

**Table 2.3**  **MyPlate Suggested Daily Amounts for Three Levels of Energy Intake**

| Food Group | Energy Intake Level | | |
|---|---|---|---|
| | Low (1,400 kcal)[a] | Moderate (2,000 kcal)[b] | High (2,800 kcal)[c] |
| Grains | 5 oz eq | 6 oz eq | 10 oz eq |
| Vegetables | 1½ cups | 2½ cups | 3½ cups |
| Fruits | 1½ cups | 2 cups | 2½ cups |
| Milk | 2 cups | 3 cups | 3 cups |
| Meat and beans | 4 oz eq | 5½ oz eq | 7 oz eq |
| Oils | 4 teaspoons | 6 teaspoons | 8 teaspoons |
| Empty calories allowed[d] | 117 kilocalories | 267 kilocalories | 426 kilocalories |

[a] 1,400 kilocalories is about right for many young children.

[b] 2,000 kilocalories is about right for teenaged girls, active women, and many sedentary men.

[c] 2,800 kilocalories is about right for teenaged boys and many active men.

[d] Empty calorie allowance is the remaining amount of calories needed for all food groups, assuming that those choices are fat-free or low-fat and with no added sugars.

**Note:** Your calorie needs may be higher or lower than those shown. Women may need more calories when they are pregnant or breastfeeding.

**Source:** US Department of Agriculture. Adapted from MyPlate. http://www.choosemyplate.gov. Accessed 6/12/11.

**Table 2.4**    **Playing with MyPlate Portions**

Your favorite sports and games can help you visualize MyPlate portion sizes.

| GRAINS | 1 cup dry cereal | 2 ounce bagel | ½ cup cooked cereal, rice, or pasta |
|---|---|---|---|
| | 4 golf balls | 1 hockey puck | tennis ball |

| VEGETABLES | 1 cup of vegetables |
|---|---|
| | 1 baseball or 1 Rubik's cube |

| FRUITS | 1 medium fruit (equivalent of 1 cup of fruit) |
|---|---|
| | 1 baseball |

| OILS | 1 teaspoon vegetable oil | 1 tablespoon salad dressing |
|---|---|---|
| | 1 die (¹¹⁄₁₆″ size) | 1 jacks ball |

| MILK | 1½ ounces of hard cheese | ⅓ cup of shredded cheese |
|---|---|---|
| | 6 dice (¹¹⁄₁₆″ size) | 1 billiard ball or racquetball |

| MEAT AND BEANS | 3 ounces cooked meat | 2 tablespoons hummus |
|---|---|---|
| | 1 deck of playing cards | 1 ping pong ball |

Continue to plan your meals and snack for the rest of the day with the amount of servings you have remaining for each food group. In this case it would be:

| Food Group | Total Recommended for 2,000-Calorie Diet | Amount Used at Breakfast | Amount Left for Remainder of the Day |
|---|---|---|---|
| Grains | 6 oz eq | 2 oz eq | 4 oz eq |
| Vegetables | 2½ cups | 0 | 2½ cups |
| Fruits | 2 cups | 1 cup | 1 cup |
| Milk | 3 cups | ½ cup | 2½ cups |
| Meat and beans | 5½ oz eq | 0 | 5½ oz |
| Oils | 6 teaspoons | 1 teaspoons | 5 teaspoons |
| Discretionary calorie allowance | 267 calories | 0 calories | 267 calories |

Keep in mind that what you consider a serving may differ from the sizes defined in MyPlate. Research shows that Americans' serving sizes for common foods such as pasta, cookies, cereal, soft drinks, and french fries have increased significantly.[20] Do large portions promote overeating and obesity? (See the FYI feature "Portion Distortion" for a scientific exploration related to this question.)

Sometimes it's difficult to figure out how to account for foods that are mixtures of different groups—lasagna, casseroles, or pizza, for example. Try separating such foods into their ingredients (e.g., pizza contains crust, tomato sauce, cheese, and toppings, which might be meats or vegetables) to estimate the amounts. You should be able to come up with a reasonable approximation. All in all, MyPlate and *Canada's Food Guide* are easy-to-use guidelines that can help you select a variety of foods.

Watch the empty calories, too. Note in Table 2.3 that for a 2,000-calorie food plan 267 calories are unused even when all the other food groups are accounted for. However, this accounting with leftover calories assumes that all food choices are fat-free or low-fat and do not have added sugars. What does this all mean? If you are already in the habit of choosing low-fat and low-sugar options, you have a few calories to play with each day. These calories can be used for a higher-fat choice or for some sugar in your iced tea. But watch out! Those calories get used up quickly. One regular 12-ounce soft drink would take up 150 discretionary calories; an extra tablespoon of dressing on your salad would be 100 calories.

Using the http://www.ChooseMyPlate.gov website is easy and informative. You can use it to create a personalized plan, learn healthy eating tips, get weight loss information, plan a healthy menu, and analyze your diet. The website is an excellent tool to help guide you through the necessary steps of putting the *Dietary Guidelines* into practice. You can use it to learn about good nutrition and appropriate physical activity.

**Key Concepts** *MyPlate is a complete food guidance system based on the Dietary Guidelines for Americans, 2010 and Dietary Reference Intakes to help Americans make healthy food choices and remind them to be active every day. The interactive tools on the http://www.ChooseMyPlate.gov website can help you monitor your food choices. Eating Well with Canada's Food Guide illustrates the dietary guidelines for Canadians and the Dietary Reference Intakes. These graphic tools show the appropriate balance of food groups in a healthful diet: more whole grains, vegetables, and fruits and less dairy, meat, and added fats and sugars.*

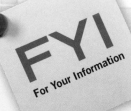

# Portion Distortion

The prevalence of obesity is of increasing concern in the United States. A notable increase in obesity has occurred over the past 20 years. In 2010, no state had an obesity rate less than 20 percent. Thirty-six states had obesity rates greater or equal to 25 percent; 12 of these states (Alabama, Arkansas, Kentucky, Louisiana, Michigan, Mississippi, Missouri, Oklahoma, South Carolina, Tennessee, Texas, and West Virginia) had obesity rates greater than 30 percent.[1]

Many factors are contributing to Americans' growing waistlines, but one observation in particular cannot be overlooked: the incidence of obesity has increased in parallel with increasing portion sizes.[2] In almost every eating situation, we are now confronted by huge portions, which are perceived as "normal" or "a great value." This perception that large portion sizes are appropriate has created an environment of *portion distortion.*[3] We find portion distortion in supermarkets, where the number

of larger sizes has increased 10-fold between 1970 and 2000. We find portion distortions in restaurants, where the jumbo-sized portions are consistently 250 percent larger than the regular portions.[4] We even find portion distortions in our homes, where the sizes of our bowls and glasses have steadily increased and where the surface area of the average dinner plate has increased 36 percent since 1960.[5] Research shows that people unintentionally consume more calories when faced with larger portions. In addition, research also shows that portion distortion seems to affect the portion sizes selected by young adults and children for some foods.[6] Consuming larger portion sizes can contribute to positive energy balance, which, over time, leads to weight gain and ultimately may result in obesity.

The phenomenon of portion distortion has the potential to hinder weight loss, weight maintenance, and health improvement efforts. Food and nutrition professionals must develop ways to "undistort" what people perceive to be typical portion sizes and help individuals recognize what is an appropriate amount to eat at a single eating occasion.[7]

To see whether you know how today's portions compare to the portions available 20 years ago, take the interactive portion distortion quizzes on the National Heart, Lung and Blood Institute's Portion Distortion website (http://hp2010.nhlbi-hin.net/portion). You can also learn about the amount of physical activity required to burn off the extra calories provided by today's portions.

1   Centers for Disease Control and Prevention. U.S. obesity trends: trends by state, 1985–2010. http://www.cdc.gov/obesity/data/trends.html. Accessed 11/24/11.

2   Schwartz J, Byrd-Bredbenner C. Portion distortion: typical portion sizes selected by young adults. *J Am Diet Assoc.* 2006;106(9):1412–1418.

3   Wansink B, van Ittersum K. Portion size me: downsizing our consumption norms. *J Am Diet Assoc.* 2007;7(7):1103–1106.

4   Ibid.

5   Ibid.

6   Schwartz J, Byrd-Bredbenner C. Op. cit.; and Lawhun SA, Starkoff B, Sundararajan S, et al. Influence of larger portion sizes on the diet of overweight children and adolescents. *J Am Diet Assoc.* 2008;108(9):A38.

7   Schwartz J, Byrd-Bredbenner C. Op. cit.

45 kcals    350 kcals

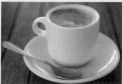

8 oz with milk and sugar    16 oz mocha coffee

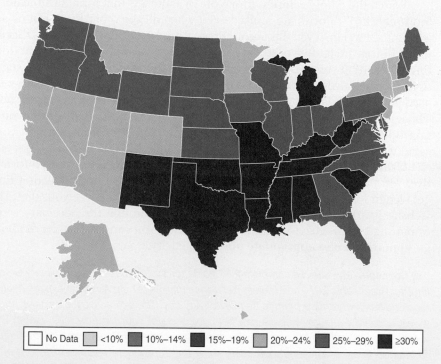

| | No Data | | <10% | | 10%–14% | | 15%–19% | | 20%–24% | | 25%–29% | | ≥30% |

Prevalence of obesity.

**Source:** Centers for Disease Control and Prevention. U.S. obesity trends: trends by state, 1985–2010. http://www.cdc.gov/obesity/data/trends.html. Accessed 11/24/11.

# Exchange Lists

Another tool for diet planning that uses food groups is the **Exchange Lists**. Like MyPlate, the Exchange Lists divide foods into groups. Diets can be planned by choosing a certain number of servings, or exchanges, from each group each day. The original purpose of the Exchange Lists was to help people with diabetes plan diets that would provide consistent levels of energy and carbohydrates—both of which are essential for dietary management of diabetes. For this reason, foods are organized into groups or lists not only by the type of food (e.g., fruits, vegetables) but also by the amount of macronutrients (carbohydrate, protein, and fat) in each portion. The portions are defined so that each "exchange" has a similar composition. For example, 1 fruit exchange is ½ cup of orange juice, 17 small grapes, 1 medium apple, or ½ cup of applesauce. All these exchanges have approximately 60 kilocalories, 15 grams of carbohydrate, 0 grams of protein, and 0 grams of fat. In the Exchange Lists, starchy vegetables such as potatoes, corn, and peas are grouped with breads and cereals instead of with other vegetables because their balance of macronutrients is more like bread or pasta than carrots or tomatoes.

**Figure 2.6** shows the amounts of carbohydrate, protein, fat, and kilocalories in one exchange from each group, along with a sample serving size. For a complete set of the Exchange Lists, go to **go.jblearning.com/inseldisco4e**.

> **Exchange Lists** Lists of foods that in specified portions provide equivalent amounts of carbohydrate, fat, protein, and energy. Any food in an Exchange List can be substituted for any other without markedly affecting macronutrient intake.

## Using the Exchange Lists in Diet Planning

In addition to their use by people with diabetes, Exchange Lists are used in many weight-control programs. Planning a diet using the Exchange Lists is done in much the same manner as using MyPlate. The first step is to become very familiar with the components of each group, the variations in fat content for the dairy and meat lists, and the ways other foods may be included. Then, select the specific meals and snacks to eat throughout the day. A diet plan based on Exchange Lists specifies the number of exchanges to be consumed from each group at each meal. For example, a 1,500-kilocalorie weight-reduction diet plan might have the following meal pattern:

| | |
|---|---|
| **Breakfast:** | 2 starch, 1 fruit, 1 milk, 1 fat |
| **Lunch:** | 3 meat, 2 starch, 1 fruit, 1 vegetable, 1 fat |
| **Snack:** | 1 milk, 1 starch, 1 fat |
| **Dinner:** | 2 meat, 1 starch, 2 vegetable, 2 fat |
| **Snack:** | 2 starch, 1 fruit |

Using this pattern and a complete set of the Exchange Lists, you could then plan out a day or week of menus. Here's one sample:

| | |
|---|---|
| **Breakfast:** | ½ cup orange juice, ¾ cup corn flakes, 1 cup 2% milk, 1 slice toast, 1 teaspoon margarine |
| **Lunch:** | 3 ounces cooked hamburger on bun, 1 teaspoon mayonnaise, ½ cup baby carrots, 1 medium apple |
| **Snack:** | ¾ cup low-fat yogurt, ½ bagel with 1 tablespoon cream cheese |
| **Dinner:** | 2 ounces cooked pork chop, ½ cup rice with 1 teaspoon margarine, ½ cup yellow squash, ½ cup zucchini stir-fried in 1 teaspoon vegetable oil |
| **Snack:** | 1 toasted English muffin, 1 medium pear |

**Key Concepts** *The Exchange Lists are diet-planning tools that work on the basis of food groups, but define groups specifically in terms of macronutrient (carbohydrate, fat, and protein) content. Individual diet plans can be developed for people who need to control energy or carbohydrate intake, such as for weight control or management of diabetes mellitus.*

**Key**

- Energy kilocalories
- Carbohydrate grams
- Protein grams
- Fat grams

**CARBOHYDRATES & MILK**

| Group | Energy (kcal) | Carbohydrate (g) | Protein (g) | Fat (g) | Examples |
|---|---|---|---|---|---|
| Starch | 80 | 15 | 3 | <1 | 1 slice bread = $\frac{1}{2}$ English muffin = $\frac{1}{2}$ c. corn or peas = $\frac{1}{3}$ c. pasta |
| Fruits | 60 | 15 | 0 | 0 | 1 small apple = 17 small grapes = $\frac{1}{2}$ c. orange juice = $\frac{1}{2}$ c. applesauce |
| Fat-free and low-fat milk | 90 | 12 | 8 | 0-3 | 1 cup fat-free or 1% milk = $\frac{2}{3}$ c. plain fat-free yogurt |
| Reduced fat milk | 120 | 12 | 8 | 5 | 1 cup 2% milk = $\frac{3}{4}$ c. plain low-fat yogurt |
| Whole milk | 150 | 12 | 8 | 8 | 1 cup whole milk |
| Other | Varies | 15 | Varies | Varies | 3 sm. sugar-free cookies = 2 Tbsp light syrup = $\frac{1}{2}$ c. gelatin |
| Vegetables | 25 | 5 | 2 | 0 | 1 c. raw salad greens = $\frac{1}{2}$ c. cooked carrots = 1 lg. tomato |

**MEAT & MEAT SUBSTITUTES**

| Group | Energy (kcal) | Carbohydrate (g) | Protein (g) | Fat (g) | Examples |
|---|---|---|---|---|---|
| Very lean | 35 | 0 | 7 | 0-1 | 1 oz chicken = 1 oz canned (water packed) tuna = $\frac{1}{2}$ c. cooked beans = $\frac{1}{4}$ c. low-fat cottage cheese |
| Lean | 55 | 0 | 7 | 3 | 1 oz beef tenderloin = 1 oz salmon = 1 oz roast pork |
| Medium fat | 75 | 0 | 7 | 5 | 1 oz ground beef = 4 oz tofu = 1 egg |
| High fat | 100 | 0 | 7 | 8 | 1 oz sausage = 1 oz cheese = 1 turkey hot dog |

**FAT**

| Group | Energy (kcal) | Carbohydrate (g) | Protein (g) | Fat (g) | Examples |
|---|---|---|---|---|---|
| Fats | 45 | 0 | 0 | 5 | 1 tsp butter = 8 large black olives = 1 slice bacon = 10 peanuts |

**Figure 2.6** **Exchange Lists.** The Exchange Lists are a widely used system for meal planning for people with diabetes. They also are helpful for people interested in healthy eating and weight control.

**Source:** Data from *Exchange Lists for Meal Planning*. Alexandria, VA: Academy of Nutrition and Dietetics; 2003.

# Recommendations for Nutrient Intake: The DRIs

So far, the tools we have described (*Dietary Guidelines for Americans, Eating Well with Canada's Food Guide*, MyPlate, and Exchange Lists) have dealt with whole foods and food groups rather than individual nutrient values; foods—rather than nutrients—are the units that we think about in planning our daily meals and shopping lists. Sometimes, though, we need more specific information about our nutritional needs—a healthful diet is healthful because of the balance of nutrients it contains. Before we can choose foods that meet our needs for specific nutrients, we need to know how much of each nutrient we require daily. This is what dietary standards do—they define healthful diets in terms of specific amounts of the nutrients.

## Understanding Dietary Standards

**Dietary standards** are sets of recommended intake values for nutrients. These standards tell us how much of each nutrient we should have in our diets. In the United States and Canada, the **Dietary Reference Intakes (DRIs)** are the current dietary standards.

Consider the following scenario. You are running a North Pole research center staffed by 60 people. Because they will not be able to leave the site to get meals, you must provide all their food. You must keep the group adequately nourished; you certainly don't want anyone to become ill as a result of a nutrient deficiency. How would you (or the nutritionist you hire) start planning? How can you be sure to provide adequate amounts of the essential nutrients? The most important tool would be a set of dietary standards! Essentially the same scenario faces those who plan and provide food for groups of people in more routine circumstances—the military, prisons, and even schools. To assess nutritional adequacy, diet planners can compare the nutrient composition of their food plans to recommended intake values.

## A Brief History of Dietary Standards

Beginning in 1938, Health Canada published dietary standards called Recommended Nutrient Intakes (RNIs). In the United States, the Recommended Dietary Allowances (RDAs) were first published in 1941. By the 1940s, nutrition scientists had been able to isolate and identify many of the nutrients in food. They were able to measure the amounts of these nutrients in foods

**All DRI values refer to intakes averaged over time**

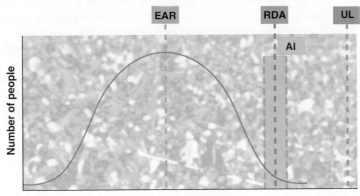

Figure 2.7 **Dietary Reference Intakes.**
The DRIs are a set of dietary standards that include Estimated Average Requirement (EAR), Recommended Dietary Allowance (RDA), Adequate Intake (AI), and Tolerable Upper Intake Level (UL).

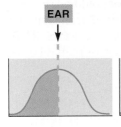 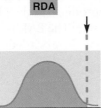 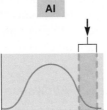 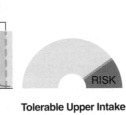

The **Estimated Average Requirement** is the nutrient intake level estimated to meet the needs of 50% of the individuals in a life-stage and gender group.

The **Recommended Dietary Allowance** is the nutrient intake level that is sufficient to meet the needs of 97–98% of the individuals in a life-stage and gender group. The RDA is calculated from the EAR.

**Adequate Intake** is based upon expert estimates of nutrient intake by a defined group of healthy people. These estimates are used when there is insufficient scientific evidence to establish an EAR. AI is not equivalent to RDA.

**Tolerable Upper Intake Level** is the maximum level of daily nutrient intake that poses little risk of adverse health effects to almost all of the individuals in a defined group. In most cases, supplements must be consumed to reach a UL.

and to recommend daily intake levels. These levels then became the first RNI and RDA values. Committees of scientists regularly reviewed and published revised editions; for example the tenth (and final) edition of the RDAs was published in 1989.

In the mid-1990s, the **Food and Nutrition Board** of the National Academy of Sciences began a partnership with Health Canada to make fundamental changes in the approach to setting dietary standards and to replace the RDAs and RNIs. In 1997, the first set of DRIs was published for calcium, phosphorus, magnesium, vitamin D, and fluoride—nutrients that are important for bone health.

## Dietary Reference Intakes

Since the inception of the RDAs and RNIs, we have learned more about the relationships between diet and chronic disease, and nutrient-deficiency diseases have become rare in the United States and Canada. The new DRIs reflect not just intake levels for dietary adequacy but also for optimal nutrition.

The DRIs are reference values for nutrient intakes to be used in assessing and planning diets for healthy people. (See **Figure 2.7**.) The DRIs include four basic elements: Estimated Average Requirement (EAR), Recommended

**dietary standards** Set of values for recommend intake of nutrients.

**Dietary Reference Intakes (DRIs)** A framework of dietary standards that include Estimated Average Requirement (EAR), Recommended Dietary Allowance (RDA), Adequate Intake (AI), and Tolerable Upper Intake Level (UL).

**Food and Nutrition Board** A board within the Institute of Medicine of the National Academy of Sciences. It is responsible for assembling the group of nutrition scientists who review available scientific data to determine appropriate intake levels of the known essential nutrients.

Dietary Allowance (RDA), Adequate Intake (AI), and Tolerable Upper Intake Level (UL). Underlying each value is the definition of a *requirement* as the "lowest continuing intake level of a nutrient that, for a specific indicator of adequacy, will maintain a defined level of nutriture in an individual."[21] *Nutriture* refers to the nutritional status of the body, especially with regard to a specific nutrient. In other words, a requirement is the smallest amount of a nutrient you should take in on a regular basis to remain healthy. In the DRI report on macronutrients, two other concepts were introduced: the Estimated Energy Requirement (EER) and the Acceptable Macronutrient Distribution Ranges (AMDRs).[22]

### Estimated Average Requirement

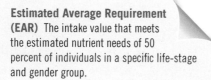

**Estimated Average Requirement (EAR)** The intake value that meets the estimated nutrient needs of 50 percent of individuals in a specific life-stage and gender group.

The **Estimated Average Requirement (EAR)** reflects the amount of a nutrient that would meet the needs of 50 percent of the people in a particular life-stage (age) and gender group. For each nutrient, this requirement is defined using a specific indicator of dietary adequacy. This indicator could be the level of the nutrient or one of its breakdown products in the blood, or the amount of an enzyme associated with that nutrient.[23] The EAR is used to set the RDA, and EAR values also can be used to assess dietary adequacy or plan diets for groups of people.

### Recommended Dietary Allowance

The Recommended Dietary Allowance (RDA) is the daily intake level that meets the needs of most people (97 to 98 percent) in a life-stage and gender group. The RDA is mathematically determined based on the EAR. A nutrient will not have an RDA value if there are not enough scientific data available to set an EAR value.

People can use the RDA value as a target or goal for dietary intake and make comparisons between actual intake and RDA values. It is important to remember, however, that the RDAs do not define an *individual's* nutrient

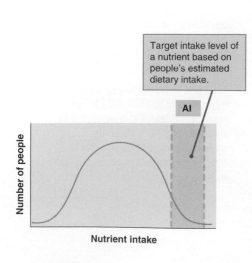

Target intake level of a nutrient based on people's estimated dietary intake.

AI

Number of people

Nutrient intake

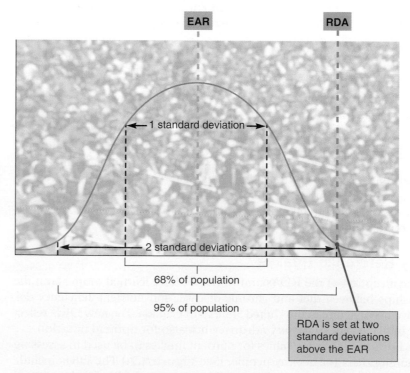

EAR

RDA

1 standard deviation

2 standard deviations

68% of population

95% of population

RDA is set at two standard deviations above the EAR

The RDA takes into account about 98 percent of the population.

requirements. Your actual nutrient needs may be much lower than average, and, therefore, the RDA would be much more than you need. An analysis of your diet might show, for example, that you consume 45 percent of the RDA for a certain vitamin, but that might be adequate for your needs. Only specific laboratory or other tests can determine a person's true nutrient requirements and actual nutritional status. An intake that is consistently at or near the RDA level is highly likely to be meeting your needs.

### Adequate Intake

If not enough scientific data are available to set an EAR level, a value called an **Adequate Intake (AI)** is determined instead. AI values are determined, in part, by observing healthy groups of people and estimating their dietary intake. All the current DRI values for infants are AI levels because there have been too few scientific studies to determine specific requirements in infants. Instead, AI values for infants are usually based on nutrient levels in human breast milk, a complete food for newborns and young infants. Values for older infants and children are extrapolated from human milk and from data on adults. For nutrients with AI instead of RDA values for all life-stage groups (e.g., calcium, vitamin D), more scientific research is needed to better define nutrient requirements of population groups. AI values can be considered target intake levels for individuals.

### Tolerable Upper Intake Level

**Tolerable Upper Intake Levels (ULs)** have been defined for many nutrients. Consumption of a nutrient in amounts higher than the UL could be harmful. The ULs have been developed partly in response to the growing interest in dietary supplements that contain large amounts of essential nutrients. The UL is not to be used as a target for intake, but rather should be a cautionary level for people who regularly take nutrient supplements.

### Estimated Energy Requirement

The **Estimated Energy Requirement (EER)** is defined as the energy intake that is estimated to maintain energy balance in healthy, normal-weight individuals. It is determined using an equation that considers weight, height, age, and physical activity. Different equations are used for males and females and for different age groups.

### Acceptable Macronutrient Distribution Ranges

**Acceptable Macronutrient Distribution Ranges (AMDRs)** indicate the recommended balance of energy sources in a healthful diet. These values consider the amounts of macronutrients needed to provide adequate intake of essential nutrients while reducing the risk for chronic disease. The AMDRs are shown in Table 2.5.

## Use of Dietary Standards

The most appropriate use of DRIs is for planning and evaluating diets for large groups of people. Remember the North Pole scenario at the beginning of this section? If you had planned menus and evaluated the nutrient composition of foods that would be included and if the average nutrient levels of those daily menus met or exceeded the RDA/AI levels, you could be confident that your group would be adequately nourished. If you had a very large group—thousands of soldiers, for instance—the EAR would be a more appropriate guide.

Dietary standards are also used to make decisions about nutrition policy. The Special Supplemental Food Program for Women, Infants, and Children

**Adequate Intake (AI)** The nutrient intake that appears to sustain a defined nutritional state or some other indicator of health (e.g., growth rate, normal circulating nutrient values) in a specific population or subgroup. AI is used when there is insufficient scientific evidence to establish an EAR.

**Tolerable Upper Intake Levels (ULs)** The maximum levels of daily nutrient intakes that are unlikely to pose health risks to almost all of the individuals in the group for whom they are designed.

**Estimated Energy Requirement (EER)** Dietary energy intake that is predicted to maintain energy balance in a healthy adult of a defined age, gender, weight, height, and level of physical activity consistent with good health.

**Acceptable Macronutrient Distribution Ranges (AMDRs)** Range of intakes for a particular energy source that are associated with reduced risk of chronic disease while providing adequate intakes of essential nutrients.

| Table 2.5 | Acceptable Macronutrient Distribution Ranges for Adults |

| | |
|---|---|
| Fat | 20–35 percent |
| Carbohydrate | 45–65 percent |
| Protein | 10–35 percent |
| *n*-6 polyunsaturated fatty acids | 5–10 percent |
| *α*-linolenic acid | 0.6–1.2 percent |

**Note:** All values are the percentage of total calorie intake.

**Source:** Data from Institute of Medicine, Food and Nutrition Board. *Dietary Reference Intakes for Energy, Carbohydrate, Fiber, Fat, Fatty Acids, Cholesterol, Protein, and Amino Acids.* Washington, DC: National Academies Press; 2002.

(WIC), for example, takes into account the DRIs as it provides food or vouchers for food. The goal of this federally funded supplemental feeding program is to improve the nutrient intake of low-income pregnant and breastfeeding women, their infants, and young children. The guidelines for school lunch and breakfast programs also are based on DRI values.

Often, we use dietary standards as comparison values for individual diets, something you may be doing in class. It can be informative to see how your daily intake of a nutrient compares to the RDA or AI. However, an intake that is less than the RDA/AI doesn't necessarily mean deficiency; your individual requirement for a nutrient may be less than the RDA/AI value. You can use the RDA/AI values as targets for dietary intake, while avoiding nutrient intake that exceeds the UL.

**Key Concepts**  *Dietary standards are levels of nutrient intake recommended for healthy people. These standards help the government set nutrition policy and also can be used to guide the planning and evaluation of diets for groups and individuals. Dietary Reference Intakes are the dietary standards for the United States and Canada. These standards focus on optimal health and lowering the risks of chronic disease, rather than simply on dietary adequacy.*

## Food Labels

Now that you understand diet-planning tools and dietary standards, let's focus on your use of these tools—for example, when making decisions at the grocery store. One of the most useful tools in planning a healthful diet is the **food label**.

**food label**  Labels required by law on virtually all packaged foods and having five requirements: (1) a statement of identity; (2) the net contents (by weight, volume, or measure) of the package; (3) the name and address of the manufacturer, packer, or distributor; (4) a list of ingredients; and (5) nutrition information.

Specific federal regulations control what can and cannot appear on a food label and what must appear on it. The Food and Drug Administration (FDA) is responsible for assuring that foods sold in the United States are safe, wholesome, and properly labeled. Only a small category of foods is not required by the FDA to have a particular food label. Examples of these foods are things like spices and flavorings. Such foods are exempted because they do not provide a significant amount of nutrients. Deli items and ready-to-eat foods that are prepared and sold in retail establishments also do not require a food label.[24] Raw fruits and vegetables and fresh fish generally do not carry food labels either; however, these foods fall under the FDA's voluntary, point-of-purchase nutrition information program, which establishes that the nutrition information for grocery stores' most commonly purchased items be posted somewhere near where that food is sold.[25] The FDA's jurisdiction does not include meat, meat products, poultry, or poultry products; the USDA regulates these foods.

Health Products and Food Branch of Health Canada is responsible for the regulation of health products and food. The Canadian Food Inspection Agency (CFIA) provides all federal inspection services related to food and enforces the food safety and nutritional quality standards.[26]

## Brief History of Food Labels

As information about the role of diet in chronic disease grew during the 1970s and 1980s, so did the demand for nutrition labels on all food products. As a result, in 1990 Congress passed the **Nutrition Labeling and Education Act (NLEA)**. Once the necessary regulations had been developed, "Nutrition Facts" labels began appearing on foods in 1994. Voluntary nutrition labeling was introduced in Canada in 1988, and a "Nutrition Facts" label was introduced in 2003. This label became mandatory for most prepackaged food products on December 12, 2007. Canadian nutrition labels now are similar in format to U.S. nutrition labels.

## Ingredients and Other Basic Information

The label on a food you buy today has been shaped by many sets of regulations. As **Figure 2.8** shows, food labels have five mandatory components:

1. A statement of identity/name of the food
2. The net weight of the food contained inside of the package, not including the weight of the package
3. The name and address of the manufacturer, packer, or distributor
4. A list of ingredients in descending order by weight
5. Nutrition information

Ingredients must be listed by common or usual name, in descending order by weight, so the first ingredient listed is the primary ingredient in that food product. Let's compare two cereals:

- *Cereal A ingredients:* Milled corn, sugar, salt, malt flavoring, high-fructose corn syrup
- *Cereal B ingredients:* Sugar, yellow corn flour, rice flour, wheat flour, whole oat flour, partially hydrogenated vegetable oil (contains one or more of the following oils: canola, soybean, cottonseed), salt, cocoa, artificial flavor, corn syrup

**Nutrition Labeling and Education Act (NLEA)** An amendment to the Food, Drug, and Cosmetic of 1938. The NLEA made major changes to the content and scope of the nutrition label and to other elements of the food labels. Final regulations were published in 1993 and went into effect in 1994.

## Quick Bite

**Truth in Tuna**
Due to an old regulation still in the law books, tuna companies can get away with skimping on canned tuna. Legally, a 6-ounce can of solid tuna has to contain only 3.75 ounces of actual tuna. Although the Tuna Foundation has set a voluntary minimum of 4 ounces, not all manufacturers subscribe to the minimum. The FDA is considering making companies use the drained weight on tuna cans so future labels may be more precise.

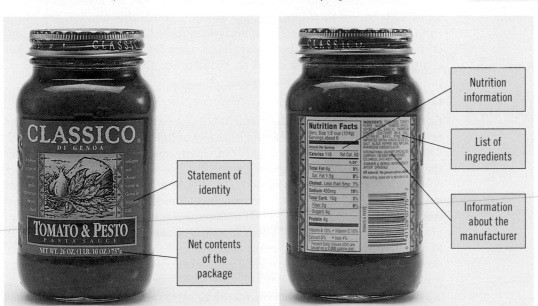

**Figure 2.8** **The five mandatory requirements for food labels.** Federal regulations determine what can and cannot appear on food labels.

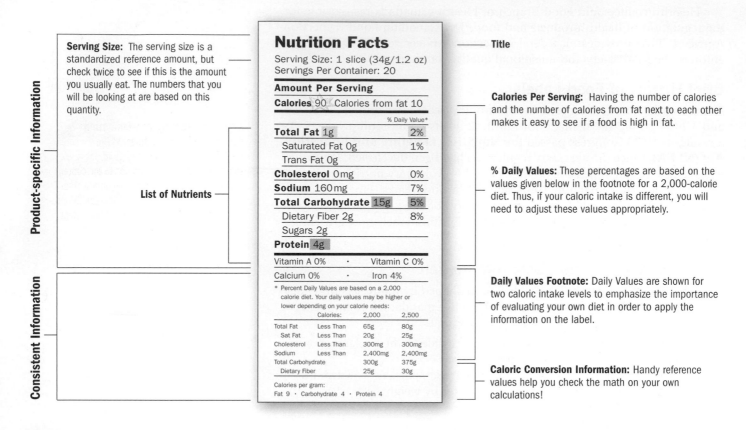

**Serving Size:** The serving size is a standardized reference amount, but check twice to see if this is the amount you usually eat. The numbers that you will be looking at are based on this quantity.

**Product-specific Information**

**List of Nutrients**

**Consistent Information**

**Nutrition Facts**
Serving Size: 1 slice (34g/1.2 oz)
Servings Per Container: 20

**Amount Per Serving**

**Calories** 90    Calories from fat 10

% Daily Value*

**Total Fat** 1g    2%

Saturated Fat 0g    1%

Trans Fat 0g

**Cholesterol** 0mg    0%

**Sodium** 160mg    7%

**Total Carbohydrate** 15g    5%

Dietary Fiber 2g    8%

Sugars 2g

**Protein** 4g

Vitamin A 0%    •    Vitamin C 0%

Calcium 0%    •    Iron 4%

\* Percent Daily Values are based on a 2,000 calorie diet. Your daily values may be higher or lower depending on your calorie needs:

| | | Calories: | 2,000 | 2,500 |
|---|---|---|---|---|
| Total Fat | Less Than | | 65g | 80g |
| Sat Fat | Less Than | | 20g | 25g |
| Cholesterol | Less Than | | 300mg | 300mg |
| Sodium | Less Than | | 2,400mg | 2,400mg |
| Total Carbohydrate | | | 300g | 375g |
| Dietary Fiber | | | 25g | 30g |

Calories per gram:
Fat 9 • Carbohydrate 4 • Protein 4

**Title**

**Calories Per Serving:** Having the number of calories and the number of calories from fat next to each other makes it easy to see if a food is high in fat.

**% Daily Values:** These percentages are based on the values given below in the footnote for a 2,000-calorie diet. Thus, if your caloric intake is different, you will need to adjust these values appropriately.

**Daily Values Footnote:** Daily Values are shown for two caloric intake levels to emphasize the importance of evaluating your own diet in order to apply the information on the label.

**Caloric Conversion Information:** Handy reference values help you check the math on your own calculations!

**Figure 2.9** **The Nutrition Facts panel.** Consumers can use the Nutrition Facts panel to compare the nutritional value of different products.

In Cereal B, the first ingredient listed is sugar, which means this cereal contains more sugar by weight than any other ingredient. Cereal A's primary ingredient is milled corn. If we were to read the nutrition information, we would find that a 1-cup serving of Cereal A contains 2 grams of sugars while a similar amount of Cereal B contains 12 grams of sugars. Quite a difference! Preservatives and other additives in foods must be listed, along with an explanation of their function. The labels of foods that contain any of the eight major food allergens (egg, wheat, peanuts, milk, tree nuts, soy, fish, and crustaceans) must include common names when listing these ingredients. For example, an ingredient list might show "albumen (egg)."

## Nutrition Facts Panel

Let's take a closer look at the elements of the Nutrition Facts panel. It was designed so that the nutrition information would be easy to find on the label. The heading *Nutrition Facts* stands out clearly. (See **Figure 2.9**.) Just under the heading is information about the serving size and number of servings per container. It is important to note the serving size, because all of the nutrient information that follows is based on that amount of food, and the listed serving size may be different from what you usually eat. An 8-ounce bag of potato chips may be a "small" snack to a hungry college student, but according to the manufacturer the bag really contains eight servings! Serving sizes are standardized according to reference amounts developed by the FDA. Similar products (cereals, for instance) will have similar serving sizes (1 ounce).

The next part of the label shows the calories per serving and the calories that come from fat. Following this is a list of the amounts of total fat, saturated fat, *trans* fat, cholesterol, sodium, total carbohydrate, dietary fiber, sugars, and protein in one serving. This information is given both in quantity (grams or milligrams per serving) and as a percentage of the Daily Value—a comparison standard specifically for food labels (this standard is described in the next section). Listed next are percentages of Daily Values for vitamins A and C, calcium, and iron, which are the only micronutrients that must appear on all standard labels. Manufacturers may choose to include information about other nutrients, such as potassium, polyunsaturated fat, additional vitamins, or other minerals, in the Nutrition Facts. However, if they make a claim about an optional component (e.g., "good source of vitamin E") or **enrich** or **fortify** the food, the manufacturers must include specific nutrition information for these added nutrients such as the fortification of milk with vitamin D to prevent rickets (a bone disease in children that results from vitamin D deficiency) or the fortification of enriched grain products with folic acid to reduce risk of birth defects. Food products that come in small packages (e.g., gum, candy, tuna) or that have little nutritional value (e.g., diet soft drinks) can have abbreviated versions of the Nutrition Facts on the label, as **Figure 2.10** shows.

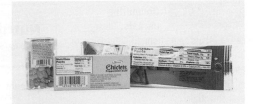

**Figure 2.10** **Nutrition Facts on small packages.** When a product package has insufficient space to display a full Nutrition Facts panel, manufacturers may use an abbreviated version.

## Daily Values

Let's come back to the Daily Values part of the label. The **Daily Values (DVs)** are a set of dietary standards used to compare the amount of a nutrient (or other component) in a serving of food to the amount recommended for daily consumption. The Percent Daily Values (%DV) are based on a 2,000-calorie diet. Your estimated needs may not be 2,000 calories per day, but you can still use the %DV as a guide whether or not you consume more than or less than 2,000 calories. The %DV helps you determine if a serving of a food is high or low in a nutrient. In other words, you can see if this food contributes a lot or a little to your daily recommended allowance. Let's say you rely on your breakfast cereal as a major source of dietary fiber intake. Comparing two packages, as in **Figure 2.11**, you find that a serving of cornflakes cereal has 4 percent of the DV for dietary fiber, but a bran flakes cereal has 20 percent. By eating one serving of the cornflakes (left label), you will get 4 percent of an estimated 100 percent of your fiber needs for the day. If you choose to eat the bran flakes (right label), you will get 20 percent of the 100 percent estimated needs of fiber for the day. You don't have to know anything about grams to see which food is higher in fiber!

## Claims That Can Be Made for Foods and Dietary Supplements

The U.S. Food and Drug Administration enforces numerous laws and regulations that dictate how food and dietary supplement labels are required to look and what language or claims are allowed to be printed on the label. Companies selling foods and dietary supplements can make three types of claims: nutrient content claims, health claims, and structure/function claims. The responsibility for ensuring that claims are accurate and follow appropriate laws rests with the manufacturer, the FDA, or, in the case of advertising, with the Federal Trade Commission.[27]

## Nutrient Content Claims

The NLEA and the associated FDA regulations allow food manufacturers to make **nutrient content claims** using a variety of descriptive terms on labels, such as low fat and high fiber. The FYI feature "Definitions for Nutrient

**enrich** To add vitamins and minerals lost or diminished during food processing, particularly the addition of thiamin, riboflavin, niacin, folic acid, and iron to grain products.

**fortify** Refers to the addition of vitamins or minerals that were not originally present in a good.

**Daily Values (DVs)** A single set of nutrient intake standards developed by the Food and Drug Administration to represent the needs of the "typical" consumer; used as standards for expressing nutrient content on food labels.

**nutrient content claims** These claims describe the level of a nutrient or dietary substance in the product, using terms such as *good source*, *high*, or *free*.

**Figure 2.11** **Comparing cereals.** These cereal labels come from different types of breakfast cereal: cornflakes cereal (left) and bran flakes cereal (right). What might influence your decision to buy one over the other?

## Nutrition Facts

Serving Size: 1 Cup (28g/1.0 oz.)
Servings Per Container: About 18

| Amount Per Serving | Cereal | with 1/2 cup Skim Milk |
|---|---|---|
| Calories | 100 | 140 |
| Fat Calories | 0 | 0 |
| | % Daily Value | |
| **Total Fat** 0g | 0% | 0% |
| Saturated Fat 0g | 0% | 0% |
| **Trans** Fat 0g | | |
| **Cholesterol** 0mg | 0% | 0% |
| **Sodium** 300mg | 13% | 15% |
| **Potassium** 25mg | 1% | 7% |
| **Total Carbohydrate** 24g | 8% | 10% |
| Dietary Fiber 1g | 4% | 4% |
| Sugars 2g | | |
| Other Carbohydrates 21g | | |
| **Protein** 2g | | |
| Vitamin A | 15% | 20% |
| Vitamin C | 25% | 25% |
| Calcium | 0% | 15% |
| Iron | 45% | 45% |
| Vitamin D | 10% | 25% |
| Thiamin | 25% | 30% |
| Riboflavin | 25% | 35% |
| Niacin | 25% | 25% |
| Vitamin B6 | 25% | 25% |
| Folate | 25% | 25% |
| Vitamin B12 | 25% | 35% |

## Nutrition Facts

Serving Size: 3/4 Cup (30g)
Servings Per Container: About 15

| Amount Per Serving | Cereal | with 1/2 cup Skim Milk |
|---|---|---|
| Calories | 100 | 140 |
| Calories from fat | 5 | 5 |
| | % Daily Value | |
| **Total Fat** 0.5g | 1% | 1% |
| Saturated Fat 0g | 0% | 0% |
| **Trans** Fat 0g | | |
| **Cholesterol** 0mg | 0% | 0% |
| **Sodium** 210mg | 9% | 12% |
| **Potassium** 200mg | 6% | 11% |
| **Total Carbohydrate** 24g | 8% | 10% |
| Dietary Fiber 5g | 20% | 20% |
| Sugars 5g | | |
| Other Carbohydrates 14g | | |
| **Protein** 3g | | |
| Vitamin A | 15% | 20% |
| Vitamin C | 0% | 2% |
| Calcium | 0% | 15% |
| Iron | 45% | 45% |
| Vitamin D | 10% | 25% |
| Thiamin | 25% | 30% |
| Riboflavin | 25% | 35% |
| Niacin | 25% | 25% |
| Vitamin B6 | 25% | 25% |
| Folate | 25% | 25% |
| Vitamin B12 | 25% | 35% |

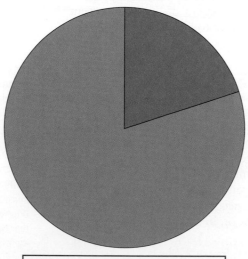

**Branflakes contribute fiber to your %DV allowance.**

- Amount of fiber allowance met by eating 1 serving of branflakes
- Amount of fiber allowance remaining for the day

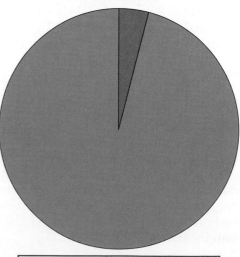

**Cornflakes contribute fiber to your %DV allowance.**

- Amount of fiber allowance met by eating 1 serving of cornflakes
- Amount of fiber allowance remaining for the day

Content Claims on Food Labels" shows a list of terms that may be used. The FDA has made an effort to make the terms meaningful, and the regulations have reduced the number of potentially misleading label statements. It would be misleading, for example, to print "cholesterol free" on a can of vegetable shortening—a food that is 100 percent fat and high in saturated and *trans* fatty acids (types of fats that raise blood cholesterol levels). This type of statement misleads consumers who associate "cholesterol free" with "heart healthy." Remember that only animal products have cholesterol in them. Under the NLEA regulations, statements about low cholesterol content can be used only when the product also is low in saturated fat (less than 2 grams per serving). In addition to the content claims defined in the regulations, companies may submit to the FDA a notification of a new nutrient content claim based on "an authoritative statement from an appropriate scientific body of the United States Government or the National Academy of Sciences."[28]

## Health Claims

With the passage of the NLEA, manufacturers also were allowed to add health claims to food labels. A **health claim** is a statement that links one or more dietary components to reduced risk of disease. A health claim must be supported by scientifically valid evidence for it to be approved for use on a food label.

> **health claim** Any statement that associates a food or a substance in a food with a disease or health related condition. The FDA authorizes health claims.

So far, the FDA has authorized the following health claims:

- *Calcium, vitamin D, and osteoporosis.* Adequate calcium and vitamin D along with regular exercise may reduce the risk of osteoporosis.
- *Dietary fat and cancer.* Low-fat diets may reduce the risk for some types of cancer.
- *Dietary fiber, such as that found in whole oats, barley, and psyllium seed husk, and coronary heart disease (CHD).* Diets low in fat and rich in these types of fiber can help reduce the risk of heart disease.
- *Dietary noncarcinogenic carbohydrate sweeteners and dental caries (tooth decay).* Foods sweetened with sugar alcohols do not promote tooth decay.
- *Dietary saturated fat and cholesterol and CHD.* Diets high in saturated fat and cholesterol increase risk for heart disease.
- *Dietary saturated fat, cholesterol, and* trans *fat and heart disease.* Diets low in saturated fat and cholesterol and as low as possible in *trans* fat may reduce the risk of heart disease.
- *Fiber-containing grain products, fruits, and vegetables and cancer.* Diets low in fat and rich in high-fiber foods may reduce the risk of certain cancers.
- *Fluoridated water and dental caries.* Drinking fluoridated water may reduce the risk of dental caries.
- *Folate and neural tube defects.* Adequate folate intake prior to and early in pregnancy may reduce the risk of neural tube defects (a birth defect).
- *Fruits and vegetables and cancer.* Diets low in fat and rich in fruits and vegetables may reduce the risk of certain cancers.
- *Fruits, vegetables, and grain products that contain fiber, particularly pectins, gums, and mucilages, and CHD.* Diets low in fat and rich in these types of fiber may reduce the risk of heart disease.
- *Plant sterol/stanol esters and CHD.* Diets low in saturated fat and cholesterol that contain significant amounts of these additives may reduce the risk of heart disease.

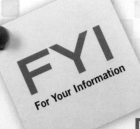

# Definitions for Nutrient Content Claims on Food Labels

- *Free:* Food contains no amount (or trivial or "physiologically inconsequential" amounts). May be used with one or more of the following: fat, saturated fat, cholesterol, sodium, sugar, and calories. Synonyms include *without*, *no*, and *zero*.
  - *Fat-free:* Less than 0.5 grams of fat per serving
  - *Saturated fat-free:* Less than 0.5 grams of saturated fat per serving, and less than 0.5 grams of *trans* fatty acids per serving
  - *Cholesterol-free:* Less than 2 milligrams of cholesterol and 2 grams or less of saturated fat per serving
  - *Sodium-free:* Less than 5 milligrams of sodium per serving
  - *Sugar-free:* Less than 0.5 grams of sugar per serving
  - *Calorie-free:* Fewer than 5 calories per serving
- *Low:* Food can be eaten frequently without exceeding dietary guidelines for one or more of these components: fat, saturated fat, cholesterol, sodium, and calories. Synonyms include little, few, and low source of.
  - *Low-fat:* 3 grams or less per serving

- *Low-saturated fat:* 1 gram or less of saturated fat per serving; no more than 15 percent of calories from saturated fat
- *Low-cholesterol:* 20 milligrams or less and 2 grams or less of saturated fat per serving
- *Low-sodium:* 140 milligrams or less per serving
- *Very low-sodium:* 35 milligrams or less per serving
- *Low-calorie:* 40 calories or less per serving
- *High:* Food contains 20 percent or more of the Daily Value for a particular nutrient in a serving.
- *Good source:* Food contains 10 to 19 percent of the Daily Value for a particular nutrient in one serving.
- *Lean and extra lean:* Describe the fat content of meat and main dish products, seafood, and game meat products.
  - *Lean:* Less than 10 grams of fat, 4.5 grams or less of saturated fat, and less than 95 milligrams of cholesterol per serving and per 100 grams
  - *Extra lean:* Less than 5 grams of fat,

less than 2 grams of saturated fat, and less than 95 milligrams of cholesterol per serving and per 100 grams
- *Reduced:* Nutritionally altered product containing at least 25 percent less of a nutrient or of calories than the regular or reference product. (Note: A "reduced" claim can't be used if the reference product already meets the requirement for "low.")
- *Less:* Food, whether altered or not, contains 25 percent less of a nutrient or of calories than the reference food. *Fewer* is an acceptable synonym.
- *Light:* This descriptor can have two meanings:
  1. A nutritionally altered product contains one-third fewer calories or half the fat of the reference food. If the reference food derives 50 percent or more of its calories from fat, the reduction must be 50 percent of the fat.
  2. The sodium content of a low-calorie, low-fat food has been reduced by 50 percent. Also, *light in sodium* may be used on a food in which the sodium content has been reduced by at least 50 percent.

- *Potassium and high blood pressure/stroke.* Diets that contain good sources of potassium may reduce the risk of high blood pressure and stroke.
- *Sodium and hypertension (high blood pressure).* Low-sodium diets may help lower blood pressure.
- *Soy protein and CHD.* Foods rich in soy protein as part of a low-fat diet may help reduce the risk of heart disease.
- *Whole-grain foods and CHD or cancer.* Diets high in whole-grain foods and other plant foods and low in total fat, saturated fat, and cholesterol may help reduce the risk of heart disease and certain cancers.

A new health claim may be proposed at any time, so this list will expand. The most current information on label statements and claims can be found on the FDA website (http://www.inspection.gc.ca/english/fssa/labeti/guide/tab7e.shtml).

**Note:** The term *light* can still be used to describe such properties as texture and color as long as the label clearly explains its meaning (e.g., light brown sugar or light and fluffy).

- *More:* A serving of food, whether altered or not, contains a nutrient that is at least 10 percent of the Daily Value more than the reference food. This also applies to fortified, enriched, and added claims, but, in those cases, the food must be altered.

- *Healthy:* A healthy food must be low in fat and saturated fat and contain limited amounts of cholesterol (less than 60 milligrams) and sodium (less than 360 milligrams for individual foods and less than 480 milligrams for meal-type products). In addition, a single-item food must provide at least 10 percent or more of one of the following: vitamins A or C, iron, calcium, protein, or fiber. A meal-type product, such as a frozen entrée or dinner, must provide 10 percent of two or more of these vitamins or minerals, or protein, or fiber, in addition to meeting the other criteria. Additional regulations allow the term *healthy* to be applied to raw, canned, or frozen fruits and vegetables and enriched grains even if the 10 percent nutrient content rule is not met. However, frozen or canned fruits or vegetables cannot contain ingredients that would change the nutrient profile.

- *Fresh:* Food is raw, has never been frozen or heated, and contains no preservatives. *Fresh frozen*, *frozen fresh*, and *freshly fro-*

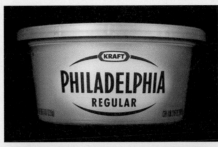
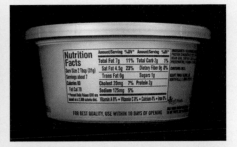
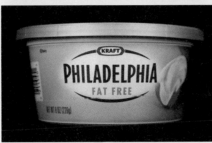
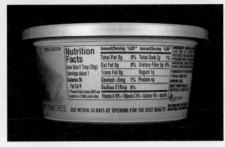

zen can be used for foods that are quickly frozen while still fresh. Blanched foods also can be called fresh.

- *Percent fat-free:* Food must be a low-fat or a fat-free product. In addition, the claim must reflect accurately the amount of nonfat ingredients in 100 grams of food.

- *Implied claims:* These are prohibited when they wrongfully imply that a food contains or does not contain a meaningful level of a nutrient. For example, a product cannot claim to be made with an ingredient known to be

a source of fiber (such as "made with oat bran") unless the product contains enough of that ingredient (e.g., oat bran) to meet the definition for "good source" of fiber. As another example, a claim that a product contains "no tropical oils" is allowed, but only on foods that are "low" in saturated fat, because consumers have come to equate tropical oils with high levels of saturated fat.

**Source:** Data from Food Labeling Guide, 2009. US Department of Health and Human Services, Food and Drug Administration.

## Structure/Function Claims

Food labels also may contain **structure/function claims** that describe potential effects of a food, food component, or dietary supplement component on body structures or functions, such as bone health, muscle strength, and digestion. As long as the label does not claim to diagnose, cure, mitigate, treat, or prevent a disease, a manufacturer can claim that a product "helps promote immune health" or is an "energizer" if *some* evidence can be provided to support the claim. Currently, structure/function claims on foods must be related to the food's nutritive value. Many scientists are concerned about the lack of a consistent scientific standard for both health claims and structure/function claims.

## Using Labels to Make Healthful Food Choices

What's the best way to start using the information on food labels to make food choices? Let's look at a couple of examples. Perhaps one of your goals is to add more iron to your diet. Compare the cereal labels in Figure 2.11.

**structure/function claims** These statements may claim a benefit related to a nutrient-deficiency disease (e.g., *vitamin C prevents scurvy*) or describe the role of a nutrient or dietary ingredient intended to affect a structure or function in humans (e.g., *calcium helps build strong bones*).

### Nutrition Facts

Serving Size: 1 Entree (240g)
Servings Per Container: 1

**Amount Per Serving**

**Calories** 400    Calories from fat 150

|  | % Daily Value* |
|---|---|
| **Total Fat** 16g | 25% |
| Saturated Fat 2.5g | 13% |
| Trans Fat 1g | |
| **Cholesterol** 10mg | 3% |
| **Sodium** 780mg | 33% |
| **Total Carbohydrate** 56g | 19% |
| Dietary Fiber 2g | 8% |
| Sugars 2g | |
| **Protein** 8g | |

| Vitamin A 2% | · | Vitamin C 4% |
|---|---|---|
| Calcium 6% | · | Iron 4% |

### Product A

### Nutrition Facts

Serving Size: 1 package (269g)
Servings Per Container: 1

**Amount Per Serving**

**Calories** 400    Calories from fat 140

|  | % Daily Value* |
|---|---|
| **Total Fat** 16g | 24% |
| Saturated Fat 6g | 30% |
| Trans Fat 2g | |
| **Cholesterol** 40mg | 14% |
| **Sodium** 690mg | 29% |
| **Total Carbohydrate** 48g | 16% |
| Dietary Fiber 2g | 9% |
| Sugars 5g | |
| **Protein** 15g | |

| Vitamin A 10% | · | Vitamin C 8% |
|---|---|---|
| Calcium 20% | · | Iron 15% |

### Product B

**Figure 2.12**    **Comparing product labels.** Labels may look similar, but appearances can be deceptive. Compare the amounts of saturated fat and sodium in these two products

Which cereal contains a higher percentage of the Daily Value for iron? How do they compare in terms of sugar content? What about vitamins and other minerals?

Maybe it's a frozen entrée you're after. Look at the two examples in **Figure 2.12**. Which is the best choice nutritionally? Are you sure? Sometimes the answer is not clear-cut. Product A is higher in sodium while Product B has more saturated and *trans* fat. It would be important to know about the rest of your dietary intake before making a decision. Do you already have quite a bit of sodium in your diet, or are you likely to add salt at the table? Maybe you never salt your food, so a bit extra in your entrée is okay. If you know that your saturated fat intake is already a bit high, however, Product A might be a better choice. To make the best choice, you should know which substances are most important in terms of your own health risks. The label is there to help you make these types of food decisions.

**Key Concepts**   *Making food choices at the grocery store is your opportunity to implement the Dietary Guidelines for Americans and your MyPlate-planned diet. The Nutrition Facts panel on most packaged foods contains not only specific amounts of nutrients shown in grams or milligrams, but also comparisons between the amounts of nutrients in a food and the recommended intake values. These comparisons are reported as %DV (Daily Values). The %DV information can be used to compare two products or to see how individual foods contribute to the total diet.*

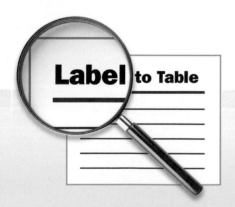

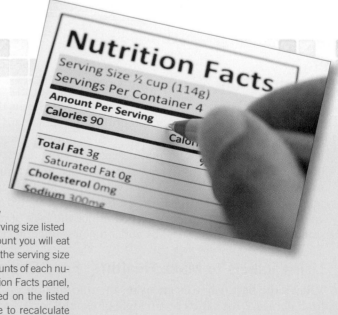

Many of us use food labels to determine such things as how many calories are in a food, how many grams of carbohydrate it provides, or how much saturated fat it contains. Sometimes we overlook the serving size that these numbers are based on, assuming that the amount we eat is considered one serving. But is the amount of food you eat equal to the serving size listed on the package? Consider a bowl of cereal or a box of snack crackers. About how much of either of these foods would you eat at one time? Not sure? Pour your typical serving into a bowl. Now, use a measuring cup to measure how much you have. Look at the serving size listed on that food's label. Is the amount you will eat smaller, larger, or the same as the serving size listed? Remember that the amounts of each nutrient listed on the food's Nutrition Facts panel, as well as the %DVs, are based on the listed serving size, so you may have to recalculate those numbers to get more accurate values.

# Learning Portfolio

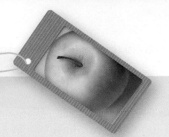

## Key Terms

## Study Points

- Moderation, balance, and variety are general guiding principles for healthful diets.

- The *Dietary Guidelines for Americans* advise consumers regarding general components of the diet.

- Dietary recommendations for Canadians are described in *Eating Well with Canada's Food Guide*. Intake recommendations are based on the Dietary Reference Intakes and depicted graphically in the *Food Guide*.

- MyPlate is a graphic representation of a food guidance system that supports the principles of the *Dietary Guidelines for Americans*.

- The Exchange Lists are a diet-planning tool most often used for diabetic or weight-control diets.

- Servings for each food in the Exchange Lists are grouped so that equal amounts of carbohydrate, fat, and protein are provided by each choice.

- Dietary standards are values for individual nutrients that reflect recommended intake levels. These values are used for planning and evaluating diets for groups and individuals.

- The Dietary Reference Intakes are the current dietary standards in Canada and the United States. The DRIs consist of several types of values: EAR, RDA, AI, UL, EER, and AMDR.

- Nutrition information on food labels can be used to select a more healthful diet.

- Label information not only provides the gram or milligram amounts of the nutrients present but also gives a percentage of Daily Values so the consumer can compare the amount in the food and the amount recommended for consumption each day.

- Nutrition information, label statements, and health claims are specifically defined by the regulations that were developed after passage of the Nutrition Labeling and Education Act of 1990.

## Study Questions

1. Define *undernutrition* and *overnutrition*.

2. What is the purpose of the *Dietary Guidelines for Americans*? List the two overarching concepts from the *Dietary Guidelines for Americans, 2010*.

3. What are the recommended MyPlate amounts for each food group for a 2,000-calorie diet?

4. Describe how the Exchange List system works and why people with diabetes might use it.

5. List and define the four main Dietary Reference Intake categories.

6. List the five mandatory components found on all food labels.

7. The standard Nutrition Facts panel shows information on which nutrients?

8. What is the purpose of the Percent Daily Value (%DV) listed next to most nutrients on the label?

9. Define the three types of claims that may be found on food labels.

## Try This

### Are You a MyPlate Pleaser?

Keep a detailed food diary for three days. Make sure to include the things you drink along with the amounts (e.g., cups, ounces, tablespoons) of each food or beverage. How well do you think your intake matches the Dietary Guidelines and MyPlate recommendations? To find out, go to http://www.ChooseMyPlate.gov. This feature allows you to complete an online assessment of your food intake. Follow the directions to register, and set up your Personal

Profile. Next, within the "Food-A-Pedia" box, select the "Food Tracker." Search for each food that you have eaten. Choose the appropriate food, serving size, and the meal or snack from which you ate it. As you are entering your meals and snacks, watch as your "Daily Food Group Targets" and "Daily Calorie Limits" add up. See how your intake compares to the Dietary Guidelines and MyPlate. How did you do? From which groups did you tend to eat more than is recommended? Were there any groups for which you did not meet the recommendations? Use the results of this activity to plan ways you can improve your diet. You may want to visit this site frequently to monitor changes you are making in your food intake.

## Grocery Store Scavenger Hunt

On your next trip to the grocery store, find a food item that has any number other than "0" listed for the two vitamins and two minerals required to be listed on the food label %DV. It doesn't matter if you choose a cereal, soup, cracker, or snack item, as long as it has numbers other than "0" for all four items. Once you're home, review the Daily Values and calculate the number of milligrams of calcium, iron, and vitamin C found in each serving of your food. Next, take a look at vitamin A: How many International Units

(IUs) does each serving of your product have? If you can calculate these, you should have a better understanding of %DVs.

## What About Bobbie?

Now that you have learned something about the recommendations for a healthful diet, how do you think Bobbie did? Review her one-day food record (see the "Food Choices: Nutrients and Nourishment" chapter). How closely does Bobbie's intake compare to the USDA-established Nutrition Targets? She can use the SuperTracker from the ChooseMyPlate website (https://www.choosemyplate.gov/SuperTracker/foodtracker.aspx) to find out. Was her diet balanced enough to meet most of the Dietary Guidelines recommendations?

How do you think Bobbie's food choices fit with the *Dietary Guidelines for Americans, 2010* and MyPlate? Can you classify all Bobbie's foods into one of the MyPlate groups? Some items, like the cheese pizza, have elements of more than one group. Others, like the dill pickle, don't seem to fit anywhere.

When Bobbie analyzed her food intake using the SuperTracker she got the following results:

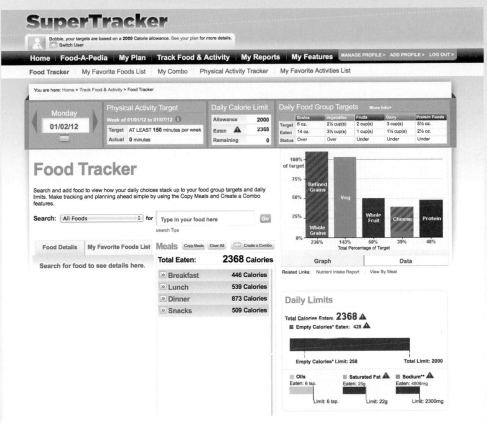

## Bobbie's Food Groups and Calories Report

Your plan is based on a **2000 Calorie** allowance.

| Food Groups | Target | Average Eaten | Status |
|---|---|---|---|
| ⊞ Grains | 6 ounce(s) | 14 ounce(s) | Over |
| ⊞ Whole Grains | ≥ 3 ounce(s) | 1 ounce(s) | Under |
| ⊞ Refined Grains | ≤ 3 ounce(s) | 13 ounce(s) | Over |
| ⊞ Vegetables | 2½ cup(s) | 3½ cup(s) | Over |
| ⊞ Dark Green | 1½ cup(s)/week | 0 cup(s) | Under |
| ⊞ Red & Orange | 5½ cup(s)/week | 1¾ cup(s) | Under |
| ⊞ Beans & Peas | 1½ cup(s)/week | ¼ cup(s) | Under |
| ⊞ Starchy | 5 cup(s)/week | 0 cup(s) | Under |
| ⊞ Other | 4 cup(s)/week | 1¾ cup(s) | Under |
| ⊞ Fruits | 2 cup(s) | 1 cup(s) | Under |
| ⊞ Whole Fruit | No Specific Target | 1 cup(s) | No Specific Target |
| ⊞ Fruit Juice | No Specific Target | 0 cup(s) | No Specific Target |
| ⊞ Dairy | 3 cup(s) | 1¼ cup(s) | Under |
| ⊞ Milk & Yogurt | No Specific Target | ¼ cup(s) | No Specific Target |
| ⊞ Cheese | No Specific Target | 1 cup(s) | No Specific Target |
| ⊞ Protein Foods | 5½ ounce(s) | 2½ ounce(s) | Under |
| ⊞ Seafood | 8 ounce(s)/week | 0 ounce(s) | Under |
| ⊞ Meat, Poultry & Eggs | No Specific Target | 2½ ounce(s) | No Specific Target |
| ⊞ Nuts, Seeds & Soy | No Specific Target | 0 ounce(s) | No Specific Target |
| ⊞ Oils | 6 teaspoon | 6 teaspoon | OK |

| Limits | Allowance | Average Eaten | Status |
|---|---|---|---|
| ⊞ Total Calories | 2000 Calories | 2368 Calories | Over |
| ⊞ Empty Calories* | ≤ 258 Calories | 428 Calories | Over |
| ⊞ Solid Fats | * | 375 Calories | * |
| ⊞ Added Sugars | * | 53 Calories | * |

*Calories from food components such as added sugars and solid fats that provide little nutritional value. Empty Calories are part of Total Calories.

**Note:** If you ate Beans & Peas and chose "Count as Protein Foods instead," they will be included in the Nuts, Seeds & Soy subgroup.

**Source:** Courtesy of USDA

As you can see, Bobbie's diet was low in Milk, Fruits, and Meat and Beans. She was high in the Grains group but without much whole grain. Her fat intake was also a little high, as was sodium. It's probably not fair to evaluate just this single day of eating, though. We would need to know much more about Bobbie's usual diet and lifestyle before making specific recommendations.

# References

1    Liu A, Berhane Z, Tseng M. Improved dietary variety and adequacy but lower dietary moderation with acculturation in Chinese women in the United States. *J Am Diet Assoc*. 2010;110(3):457–462.

2    Schwartz C, Scholtens PA, Lalanne A, et al. Development of healthy eating habits early in life. Review of recent evidence and selected guidelines. *Appetite*. 2011; May 27.

3    US Department of Health and Human Services, US Department of Agriculture. *Dietary Guidelines for Americans, 2010*. 7th ed. Washington, DC: US Government Printing Office, 2010.

4    Pennington J, Kandiah J, Nicklas T, et al. Practice paper of the Academy of Nutrition and Dietetics: nutrient density: meeting nutrient goals within calorie needs. *J Am Diet Assoc*. 2007;107(5):860–869.

5    Ibid.

6    Uauy R, Hertrampf E, Dangour AD. Food-based dietary guidelines for healthier populations: international considerations. In: Shils ME, Shike M, Ross AC, et al., eds. *Modern Nutrition in Health and Disease*. 10th ed. Baltimore, MD: Lippincott Williams & Wilkins, 2006.

7    Wengreen HJ, Neilso C, Munger R, Corcoran C. Diet quality is associated with better cognitive test performance among aging men and women. *J Nutr*. 2009;139(10):1944–1949.

8    US Department of Health and Human Services, US Department of Agriculture. Op. cit.

9    Ibid.

10    Ibid.

11    US Department of Health and Human Services. *2008 Physical Activity Guidelines for Americans*. Washington, DC: DHHS; 2008. Office of Disease Prevention and Health Promotion publication U0036.

12    US Department of Health and Human Services, US Department of Agriculture, p. 10.

13    Ibid, p. 4.

14    Ibid, p. 55.

15    Health Canada Office of Nutrition Policy and Promotion. *Eating Well with Canada's Food Guide*. http://www.hc-sc.gc.ca/fn-an/food-guide-aliment/index-eng.php. Accessed 1/3/12.

16    Davis C, Saltos E. Dietary recommendations and how they have changed over time. http://www.ers.usda.gov/publications/aib750/aib750b.pdf. Accessed 6/26/11.

17    US Department of Agriculture, Human Nutrition Information Service. *USDA's Food Guide: Background and Development*. Washington, DC: USDA; 1993. Miscellaneous publication 1514.

18    US Department of Agriculture. First Lady, Agriculture Secretary launch MyPlate icon as a new reminder to help consumers to make healthier food choices. Press release. 6/2/11.

19    US Department of Agriculture. http://www.ChooseMyPlate.gov. Accessed 10/16/11.

20    Burger KS, Kern M, Coleman KJ. Characteristics of self-selected portion size in young adults. *J Am Diet Assoc*. 2007;107(4):611–618.

21    Institute of Medicine, Food and Nutrition Board. *Dietary Reference Intakes: The Essential Guide to Nutrient Requirements*. Washington, DC: National Academies Press; 2006.

22    Ibid.

23    Academy of Nutrition and Dietetics. Practice paper of the Academy of Nutrition and Dietetics: using the Dietary Reference Intakes. *J Am Diet Assoc*. 2011;111(5):762–770.

24    US Food and Drug Administration. Food labeling and nutrition. 2007. http://www.cfsan.fda.gov/label.html. Accessed 4/11/11.

25    Ibid.

26    Canadian Food Inspection Agency. Acts and regulations. http://www.inspection.gc.ca/about-the-cfia/acts-and-regulations/eng/1299846777345/1299847442232. Accessed 1/23/12.

27    US Food and Drug Administration. Claims that can be made for conventional foods and dietary supplements. September 2003. http://www.fda.gov/Food/LabelingNutrition/LabelClaims/ucm111447.htm. Accessed 6/26/11.

28    US Food and Drug Administration. Guidance for industry: notification of a health claim or nutrient content claim based on an authoritative statement of a scientific body. http://www.cfsan.fda.gov/guidance.html. Accessed 4/11/11.

# CHAPTER 3

# Complementary Nutrition: Functional Foods and Dietary Supplements

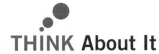

## THINK About It

1 When choosing food, what health benefits do you consider beyond basic nutrition?

2 How do you feel about the safety of high doses of nutrient supplements?

3 Would you ask your physician before taking an herbal supplement?

4 If a friend told you about a new herbal extract that is guaranteed to tone muscles, would you try it?

**Visit go.jblearning.com/ inseldisco4e**

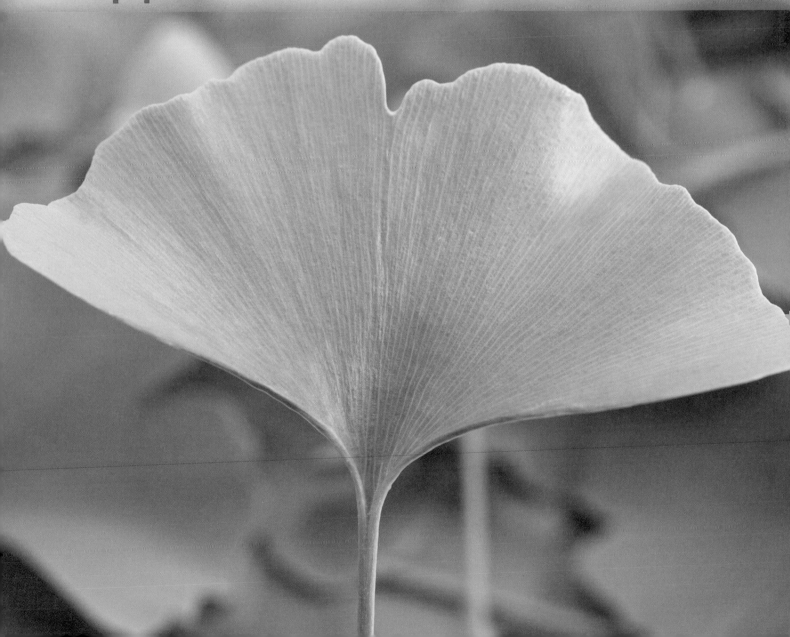

## Quick Bite

**isoflavones** Plant chemicals that include genistein and daidzein and may have positive effects against cancer and heart disease. Also called *phytoestrogens*.

**dietary supplements** Products taken by mouth in tablet, capsule, powder, gelcap, or other nonfood form that contain one or more of the following: vitamins, minerals, amino acids, herbs, enzymes, metabolites, or concentrates.

**complementary and alternative medicine (CAM)** A broad range of healing philosophies, approaches, and therapies that include treatments and health care practices not taught widely in medical schools, not generally used in hospitals, and not usually reimbursed by medical insurance companies.

**functional food** A food that may provide a health benefit beyond basic nutrition.

**lycopene** One of a family of plant chemicals, the carotenoids. Others in this big family include alpha-carotene and beta-carotene.

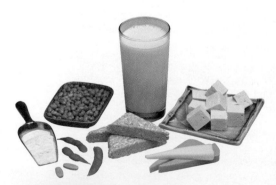

**Figure 3.1**    **Soy is rich in phytochemicals.** Soybeans contain phytochemicals called isoflavones. High intake of soy products such as tofu is linked to a lower incidence of heart disease and cancer.

W hen she feels down, Jana takes the herbal St. John's wort to give her a lift. Whenever she has the option, Sherina chooses calcium-fortified foods. Carlos swears by creatine in his muscle-building regime. Jason tries a new energy bar with added ginkgo biloba, hoping it will improve his memory. Others in search of better health turn to massage therapy, magnets, macrobiotic diets, homeopathy, acupuncture, and many other practices.

Any trip to the grocery store will tell you that a new era in product development is here—one in which food products are more often touted for what they contain (e.g., soy **isoflavones**, vitamins and minerals, herbal ingredients) than for what they lack (e.g., fat, cholesterol). Beverages, energy bars, and teas marketed as foods sit side by side on the shelf with similar products labeled as dietary supplements. The market for **dietary supplements**—which are much more than the simple vitamins and minerals our parents knew—continues to grow.

This chapter looks at functional foods, dietary supplements, and the role of nutrition in **complementary and alternative medicine (CAM)**. We will discuss not only the claims made for products and therapies in terms of current scientific knowledge but also the regulatory and safety issues. Making decisions about nutrition and health requires both consumers and professionals to stay informed and consult reliable sources before trying a new product or embarking on a new health regimen.

## Functional Foods

What do garlic, tomato sauce, tofu, and oatmeal all have in common? They aren't in the same food group, nor do they have the same nutrient composition. Instead, all of these foods could be considered "functional foods." Although there is not yet a legal definition for the term, a **functional food** is widely considered to be a food or food component that provides a health benefit beyond basic nutrition.[1] Garlic contains sulfur compounds that may reduce heart disease risk, and tomato sauce is rich in **lycopene**, a compound that may reduce prostate cancer risk. The soy protein in tofu and the fiber in oatmeal can help reduce the risk of heart disease. (See **Figure 3.1**.) The functional food industry has grown rapidly since its birth in Japan in the late 1980s. In the United States, functional foods comprise about 5 percent of the overall U.S. food market, with annual sales of $20 billion to $30 billion.

THINK About It

1

All the functional foods just mentioned get their health-promoting properties from naturally occurring compounds that are not considered nutrients but are called phytochemicals. While the word *phytochemical* itself may sound futuristic, its meaning is simple: "plant chemical." It seems you can't pick up a health magazine these days without seeing an article about phytochemicals. But, what do we really mean when we talk about phytochemicals, and why is there so much interest in these compounds?

### Phytochemicals Make Foods Functional

A vitamin is a food substance essential for life. Phytochemicals, in contrast, are substances in plants that may affect health, even though they are not essential for life. Phytochemicals are complex chemicals that vary from plant to plant. They include pigments, antioxidants, and thousands of other compounds, many of which have been associated with protection from heart disease, vision loss, hypertension, cancer, and diabetes. Table 3.1 lists many examples of phytochemicals and their potential benefits.

| Table 3.1 | Examples of Functional Components |

| Class/Components | Source[a] | Potential Benefit | Tips for Including Healthful Components in the Diet |
|---|---|---|---|
| **Carotenoids** | | | |
| Beta-carotene | Carrots, pumpkin, sweet potato, cantaloupe | Neutralizes free radicals, which may damage cells; bolsters cellular antioxidant defenses; can be made into vitamin A in the body | For beta-carotene–rich french fries: thinly slice sweet potatoes and coat with olive oil or fat-free cooking spray, add spices to taste (pepper, rosemary, thyme), bake in 425° oven until golden brown on both sides (10–15 minutes). Time-saver: buy precut sweet potatoes in the frozen foods section. |
| Lutein, zeaxanthin | Kale, collards, spinach, corn, eggs, citrus | May contribute to maintenance of healthy vision | Freezing kale can bring out a sweeter, more flavorful taste. For an easy sautéed side dish, try this simple recipe: add kale to skillet with oil and garlic, slivered almonds, and red pepper flakes. If kale doesn't top your list of food preferences, spinach, which provides the same health benefits, can be an easy substitute. Did you know that many multivitamin and mineral dietary supplements include lutein? |
| Lycopene | Tomatoes and processed tomato products, watermelon, red/pink grapefruit | May contribute to maintenance of prostate health | Research shows lycopene is best absorbed by the body when consumed from tomatoes that have been cooked using a small amount of oil. This includes products such as tomato sauce and tomato paste. Try adding 1 cup tomato sauce to sautéed zucchini for a fun and colorful side dish!<br>Don't like the bitter taste of grapefruit? Try sprinkling on a little sugar or a low-calorie sweetener before eating one to bring out the rich natural sweetness within. |
| **Dietary (Functional and Total) Fiber** | | | |
| Insoluble fiber | Wheat bran, corn bran, fruit skins | May contribute to maintenance of a healthy digestive tract; may reduce the risk of some types of cancer | Try adding a little dry wheat bran when making smoothies or muffins to bulk up the fiber content; this may help keep you full longer. |
| Beta-glucan[b] | Oat bran, oatmeal, oat flour, barley, rye | May reduce risk of coronary heart disease (CHD) | Jazz up your oatmeal with these tasty extras: 2 Tbsp peanut butter and jelly; cinnamon and pumpkin puree; or slivered almonds and ½ cup frozen berries.<br>Instant oatmeal packets are easily stored in your desk drawer to have on hand when you missed breakfast at home or need a hearty afternoon snack to tide you over until dinner. |
| Soluble fiber[b] | Psyllium seed husk, peas, beans, apples, citrus fruit | May reduce risk of CHD and some types of cancer | Try adding canned beans (black, pinto, or garbanzo) to your regular cuisine: layer them in a quesadilla, add to an omelet, or enjoy them cold in a mixed green salad. |
| Whole grains[b] | Cereal grains, whole wheat bread, oatmeal, brown rice | May reduce risk of CHD and some types of cancer; may contribute to maintenance of healthy blood glucose levels | Did you know that popcorn is a great source of whole grains? Keep a few mini-bags in your desk drawer to heat up for a quick, low-calorie snack at the office. Also, try spicing up your popcorn with garlic powder and cinnamon or rosemary and parmesan cheese. Yum!<br>Are your kids picky eaters? Try making their next sandwich visually appealing: use 1 slice of white bread and 1 slice of whole grain bread, cut the sandwich into 4 pieces, and turn two sections to create a checker board effect. |
| **Fatty Acids** | | | |
| Monounsaturated fatty acids (MUFAs)[b] | Tree nuts, olive oil, canola oil | May reduce risk of CHD | Fill the cradle of your cupped hand to make portion-controlled snack-bags of mixed nuts of your choosing (e.g., almonds, pecans). Throw in some dried fruit for an extra helping of fruit. Keep the bags on hand to grab on your way out the door for a quick and easy mid-morning or afternoon snack with healthful fats for your heart. |
| Polyunsaturated fatty acids (PUFAs)—omega-3 fatty acids—ALA | Walnuts, flax | May contribute to maintenance of heart health; may contribute to maintenance of mental and visual function | When cooking, try substituting flax seed oil in a recipe that calls for canola or olive oil 1 to 2 times a week. |

*(Continues)*

**Table 3.1    Examples of Functional Components (Continued)**

| Class/Components | Source[a] | Potential Benefit | Tips for Including Healthful Components in the Diet |
|---|---|---|---|
| PUFAs—*omega*-3 fatty acids—DHA/EPA[b] | Salmon, tuna, marine, and other fish oils | May reduce risk of CHD; may contribute to maintenance of mental and visual function | Salmon or tuna that is canned in water or in a shelf-stable pouch can make easy and affordable meals; add a few tablespoons of olive oil, and season with pepper and thyme to enjoy on top of whole grain crackers or wrapped with tomatoes in a lettuce leaf. |
| Conjugated linoleic acid (CLA) | Beef and lamb; some cheese | May contribute to maintenance of desirable body composition and healthy immune function | Bring Hawaii to your next cookout by preparing these kebabs for the grill: alternate pineapple, beef, onions, and bell peppers on wooden skewers and season for your grilling pleasure with garlic powder, pepper, paprika, oil, and lime. |
| **Flavonoids** | | | |
| Anthocyanins—cyanidin, delphinidin, malvidin | Berries, cherries, red grapes | Bolsters cellular antioxidant defenses; may contribute to maintenance of brain function | For a cold treat, try frozen berries. They are also tasty additions to any yogurt and can help to cool and flavor your oatmeal in the morning! |
| Flavanols—catechins, epicatechins, epigallocatechin, procyanidins | Tea, cocoa, chocolate, apples, grapes | May contribute to maintenance of heart health | Make your own iced tea by pouring boiling water over 3 to 4 bags of your favorite tea; let the tea sit for 5 minutes, and then pour over a pitcher of ice and fill to the brim with water. Stir and refrigerate to chill. Enjoy with freshly squeezed lemon as desired. |
| Flavanones—hesperetin, naringenin | Citrus fruits | Neutralize free radicals, which may damage cells; bolster cellular antioxidant defenses | Squeeze half an orange and half a lemon into a small dish; add olive or flax oil, dashes of salt, pepper, and basil for a perfectly refreshing salad dressing. Rushed for time? You can get the same benefits from fresh orange or grapefruit juice. |
| Flavonols—quercetin, kaempferol, isorhamnetin, myricetin | Onions, apples, tea, broccoli | Neutralize free radicals, which may damage cells; bolster cellular antioxidant defenses | Caramelized onions make a sweet and tasty garnish to many main dishes. Sautee onions over low heat in oil until a deep gold color; add on top of prepared steak, chicken, or fish. |
| Proanthocyanidins | Cranberries, cocoa, apples, strawberries, grapes, wine, peanuts, cinnamon | May contribute to maintenance of urinary tract health and heart health | Dice apples and simmer in water until soft, add to blender with dashes of cinnamon, and then puree. Enjoy as a spread on whole-wheat toast or crackers! |
| **Isothiocyanates** | | | |
| Sulforaphane | Cauliflower, broccoli, broccoli sprouts, cabbage, kale, horseradish | May enhance detoxification of undesirable compounds; bolsters cellular antioxidant defenses | Keep frozen broccoli and cauliflower on hand for an easy dinner side dish: in a microwaveable bowl, cover frozen vegetables with paper towel and cook 1 to 1.5 minutes. Add slivered almonds and cover with parmesan cheese, cook 30 to 60 seconds more or until the cheese melts and it's ready for the table! |
| **Minerals** | | | |
| Calcium[b] | Sardines, spinach, yogurt, low-fat dairy products, fortified foods and beverages | May reduce the risk of osteoporosis | Add cooked spinach (1 minute in boiling water), canned artichokes, and plain yogurt to blender or food processor; puree for a quality cracker spread or dip. Season to taste; try black pepper, basil, and garlic powder. |
| Magnesium | Spinach, pumpkin seeds, whole grain breads and cereals, halibut, brazil nuts | May contribute to maintenance of normal muscle and nerve function, healthy immune function, and bone health | Add pumpkin seeds to a stir-fry or sauté. You can also sprinkle a fish filet with seeds before baking to add extra flavor. |
| Potassium[b] | Potatoes, low-fat dairy products, whole grain breads and cereals, citrus juices, beans, banana | May reduce the risk of high blood pressure and stroke, in combination with a low sodium diet | Puree ripe bananas with crushed peanuts, portion into freezer cups to enjoy as a frozen "ice cream" treat! For extra indulgence, add some shavings of fresh chocolate as a topping. |

| Table 3.1 | Examples of Functional Components *(Continued)* |

| Class/Components | Source[a] | Potential Benefit | Tips for Including Healthful Components in the Diet |
|---|---|---|---|
| Selenium | Fish, red meat, grains, garlic, liver, eggs | Neutralizes free radicals, which may damage cells; may contribute to healthy immune function | LOVE garlic? Perhaps you need some convincing. Roasting garlic gives it a rich, buttery flavor. Cut a full bulb of garlic crosswise to expose wrapped cloves; drizzle with olive/flax oil, season with salt/pepper, cover with aluminum foil to bake in 400° oven for 30 minutes or microwave on high (NO foil) for 1 minute, turn bulb upside down, and cook 1 minute more. Delicious! |
| **_Phenolic Acids_** | | | |
| Caffeic acid, ferulic acid | Apples, pears, citrus fruits, some vegetables, coffee | May bolster cellular antioxidant defenses; may contribute to maintenance of healthy vision and heart health | Love your morning coffee? Good news—coffee is a powerful source of antioxidants. Pair it with apples and peanut butter for a powerful breakfast on the go. |
| **_Plant Stanols/Sterols_** | | | |
| Free stanols/sterols[b] | Corn, soy, wheat, wood oils, fortified foods and beverages | May reduce risk of CHD | Get your free stanols/sterols from fortified foods such as bread containing "whole-wheat flour," low-fat yogurt, and some cereals. Dietary supplements in soft-gel form that contain free stanols and sterols also are available and can provide similar benefits when used as part of a low-fat, low-cholesterol diet. |
| Stanol/sterol esters[b] | Stanol ester dietary supplements, fortified foods and beverages, including table spreads | May reduce risk of CHD | Many table spreads (butter or margarine alternatives) are now fortified with stanol and/or sterol esters. Other commercial products fortifying with stanols and sterols include some orange juices, yogurt beverages, chocolate, and granola bars. Be sure to check the product label and ingredient list to confirm the presence and amount of stanols and sterols. |
| **_Polyols_** | | | |
| Sugar alcohols[b]— xylitol, sorbitol, mannitol, lactitol | Some chewing gums and other food applications | May reduce risk of dental caries | Reduce your risk for dental caries and curb your appetite by chewing gum containing xylitol after eating. |
| **_Prebiotics_** | | | |
| Inulin, fructo-oligosaccharides (FOS), polydextrose | Whole grains, onions, some fruits, garlic, honey, leeks, fortified foods and beverages | May improve gastrointestinal health; may improve calcium absorption | Several new food products are beginning to appear fortified with prebiotics, but did you know that you can also get prebiotics by simply adding honey to some of your routine meals? Try honey in your oatmeal or yogurt, drizzle it over a banana, spread it on your morning toast, or treat yourself to half a peanut butter and honey sandwich as a snack. |
| **_Probiotics_** | | | |
| Yeast, _Lactobacilli_, _Bifidobacteria_, and other specific strains of beneficial bacteria | Certain yogurts and other cultured dairy and nondairy applications | May improve gastrointestinal health and systemic immunity; benefits are strain-specific | Add probiotics into your diet by choosing low-fat yogurt: choose from a variety of flavored yogurts with probiotics for a quick and tasty snack, 30-second smoothie-to-go: 6 to 8 oz yogurt, 6 oz orange juice, 1 Tbsp honey, half a banana, and ice. Blend gently and pour into a container for the person on the go. For a healthy breakfast snack, try topping pancakes with flavored yogurt and fresh fruit like strawberries and bananas. |
| **_Phytoestrogens_** | | | |
| Isoflavones— daidzein, genistein | Soy beans and soy-based foods | May contribute to maintenance of bone health, healthy brain and immune function; for women, may contribute to maintenance of menopausal health | Not a fan of tofu? Try "hiding" it in some of your favorite recipes. Get your isoflavones by getting soft, silken tofu and adding it to the cheese sauce mixture used to make lasagna. Other recipes that work well with tofu additions include quiches, veggie dips, quesadillas, chili, chocolate mousse, and even baked goods! |

*(Continues)*

| Table 3.1 | **Examples of Functional Components** *(Continued)* |

| Class/Components | Source[a] | Potential Benefit | Tips for Including Healthful Components in the Diet |
|---|---|---|---|
| Lignans | Flax, rye, some vegetables | May contribute to maintenance of heart health and healthy immune function | Add flax seeds—whole or ground—to a smoothie or a recipe for baked goods that can pack a lignan punch! You can also try substituting rye bread for your usual bread of choice at home once in a while. Or, when eating at a restaurant and offered a choice of bread, opt for rye. Did you know that most Reuben sandwiches are made with rye bread? |
| *Soy Protein* | | | |
| Soy protein[b] | Soy beans and soy-based foods | May reduce risk of CHD | Soy beans are also called "edamame" in many Asian cuisine restaurants; try ordering a plate to share before your meal arrives. When cooking at home, look for edamame in the frozen section to easily prepare as a healthy snack or party sampler; experiment with seasonings for additional taste—red pepper flakes add the perfect amount of heat! If you like your foods cold, edamame that has been cooked and removed from the pod adds great flavor and extra protein to any salad. |
| *Sulfides/Thiols* | | | |
| Diallyl sulfide, Allyl methyl trisulfide | Garlic, onions, leeks, scallions | May enhance detoxification of undesirable compounds; may contribute to maintenance of heart health and healthy immune function | Scallions, or "green onions," are milder than traditional onions and are commonly added at the last minute to salads or cooked sauces as a garnish. Try incorporating scallions into your diet by thinly chopping the green stalks and adding them to mashed potatoes, cold pasta salad, tuna salad, or canned soups! Leeks can also be an easy substitute, but more commonly used in soups. |
| Dithiolthiones | Cruciferous vegetables | May enhance detoxification of undesirable compounds; may contribute to maintenance of healthy immune function | Broccoli and cauliflower are the more commonly known cruciferous, or crossed-shaped, vegetables that we can eat, but did you also know that varieties of cabbage, bok choy, brussel sprouts, kale, and wasabi are also sources of dithiolthiones? Bok choy is great in any stir-fry or by itself. To cook, separate the white stem from the leaves and chop into 1-in. thick pieces. Add to oil in skillet on medium-high heat, sauté 3 minutes, add the leaves and ½ cup of water or vegetable stock, and stir until the leaves are wilted and cooked (about 5 to 10 minutes). Season to taste and enjoy! |
| *Vitamins* | | | |
| A[c] | Organ meats, milk, eggs, carrots, sweet potato, spinach | May contribute to maintenance of healthy vision, immune function, and bone health; may contribute to cell integrity | If you are not a fan of boiled or raw carrots, try buying the larger carrots and slice them lengthwise into wide strips: add them to the grill after lightly brushing with oil and season with fajita seasoning or other spices to give them a unique BBQ flavor. |
| $B_1$ (thiamin) | Lentils, peas, long-grain brown rice, brazil nuts, and certain fortified breakfast cereals | May contribute to maintenance of mental function; helps regulate metabolism | If you are still unsure about making the transition to long-grain brown rice, start slow and create a half white rice and half brown rice mixture. Think about adding dried cranberries and slivered almonds to the rice mix as well for appealing color and a little sweet flavor to complement the dense rice. |
| $B_2$ (riboflavin) | Lean meats, eggs, green leafy vegetables and certain fortified breakfast cereals | Helps support cell growth; helps regulate metabolism | Get lots of vitamin $B_2$ by bulking up a homemade sandwich made on a whole-wheat bread with lean-cut deli meat and double-stacked green and red leaf lettuce or spinach. The extra greens will give your sandwich that mouthwatering crunch in every bite—also adding fiber to keep you satisfied longer! |
| $B_3$ (niacin) | Dairy products, poultry, fish, nuts, eggs, and certain fortified breakfast cereals | Helps support cell growth; helps regulate metabolism | For a spicy twist on chicken, grill chicken breasts, cut into strips, toss in your favorite hot sauce, and serve with celery—healthful "chicken wings" for the next football party! |

**Table 3.1**    **Examples of Functional Components** *(Continued)*

| Class/Components | Source[a] | Potential Benefit | Tips for Including Healthful Components in the Diet |
|---|---|---|---|
| B$_5$ (pantothenic acid) | Organ meats, lobster, soybeans, lentils, and certain fortified breakfast cereals | Helps regulate metabolism and hormone synthesis | Looking for a healthful crunch? Try dried soy nuts with dried fruit for a fiber-rich, vitamin B$_5$-friendly snack. Soy nuts are easily added to yogurts, oatmeal, salads, stir-fries, chicken bakes, and much more. |
| B$_6$ (pyridoxine) | Beans, nuts, legumes, fish, meat, whole grains, and certain fortified breakfast cereals | May contribute to maintenance of healthy immune function; helps regulate metabolism | Legumes come in all shapes and varieties; to add more vitamin B$_6$ to your diet, try snacking on sugar snap peas to change up the routine of baby carrots once or twice a week. Keep frozen green beans on hand for a quick side dish or snack: boil beans 2 to 3 minutes until tender but firm. Season with oil, soy nuts or sunflower seeds, basil, salt, and pepper. |
| B$_9$ (folate)[b] | Beans, legumes, citrus foods, green leafy vegetables and fortified breads, cereals, pasta and rice | May reduce a woman's risk of having a child with a brain or spinal cord defect | Many breads and cereals are fortified with folate; check the nutrition facts panel to be sure. To get folate in your diet, think about buying canned or raw beans; not only are they affordable, but they can also be easy to prepare. Try this culturally charged take on lentils: sauté chopped onions until a deep golden brown, add drained, canned or cooked lentils, curry powder, salt, and pepper; stir in ½ cup water, and let simmer for 10 minutes. Serve over long-grain brown rice (or rice of your choice). |
| B$_{12}$ (cobalamin) | Eggs, meat, poultry, milk, and certain fortified breakfast cereals | May contribute to maintenance of mental function; helps regulate metabolism and supports blood cell formation | Hard-boiled eggs can be healthful, easy meal additions for the person on the go. Boil 6 to 8 eggs over the weekend to store as a time-saver in the mornings during the week. For an easy fail-proof method: add water over eggs placed on the bottom of a stove pot, add 1 to 2 tsp vinegar (to prevent cracking), and place on high heat. When water is at a rolling boil (big bubbles), cover and turn off the heat. Let sit for 30 minutes. Remove the eggs from the water, and store in the refrigerator until ready to enjoy! |
| Biotin | Liver, salmon, dairy, eggs, oysters, and certain fortified breakfast cereals | Helps regulate metabolism and hormone synthesis | Do you buy your lunches out? Instead of the grilled chicken or steak on a salad, try the salmon at least once a week. Think about keeping a can or pouch of salmon in your desk drawer to have on hand the next time someone brings bagels and cream cheese to the office. WOW—your coworkers will fancy your more healthful take on breakfast! |
| C | Guava, sweet red/green pepper, kiwi, citrus fruit, strawberries, fortified foods and beverages | Neutralizes free radicals, which may damage cells; may contribute to maintenance of bone health and immune function | A great way to boost your vitamin C is through a fruit smoothie. Save money and preparation time by using frozen fruit. Canned fruit in lite syrup can also be cost-friendly and nutritious—try adding canned fruit to low-fat or fat-free cottage cheese or yogurt. |
| D | Sunlight, fish, fortified foods and beverages, including milk, juices, and cereals | Helps regulate calcium and phosphorus; helps contribute to bone health; may contribute to healthy immune function; helps support cell growth | If choosing to get your vitamin C from a morning glass of orange juice, did you know you could also be getting calcium and vitamin D? Now, more milk and juice products around the supermarket are fortified with vitamin D and calcium. Make sure to check the label before making your next purchase. Dietary supplements of vitamin D are also a great way to add vitamin D to your diet. |
| E | Sunflower seeds, almonds, hazelnuts, turnip greens, fortified foods and beverages | Neutralizes free radicals, which may damage cells; may contribute to healthy immune function and maintenance of heart health | Raw and chopped hazelnuts can make excellent additions to vegetable sautés, pancake batter, and frozen yogurt. Sunflower seeds in the shell can be a good alternative or addition to taking peanuts to sporting events. Unshelled sunflower seeds are great as salad toppers; look for them at the end of the salad bar line the next time you go. |

[a] Examples are not an all-inclusive list.

[b] FDA approved health claim established for component.

[c] Preformed vitamin A is found in foods that come from animals. Provitamin A carotenoids are found in many darkly colored fruits and vegetables and are a major source of vitamin A for vegetarians.

**Source:** Reproduced with permission from the International Food Information Council Foundation, 2009.

## *Quick* Bite

### Functional Food Decisions

Are you a health-conscious consumer who seeks out functional foods? A 2009 survey found that 53 percent of consumers surveyed "strongly" agreed that functional foods offer health benefits. The top functional foods named by consumers included fruits and vegetables, fish and seafood, dairy, meat and poultry, herbs/spices, fiber, tea/green tea, nuts, whole grains, water, cereal, and oat products. The top three food components people look for when choosing foods and beverages for themselves and their children are fiber, whole grains, and protein.

**phytoestrogens**  Plant compounds that have weak estrogen activity in the body.

**free radicals**  Short-lived, highly reactive chemicals often derived from oxygen-containing compounds, which can have detrimental effects on cells, especially DNA and cell membranes.

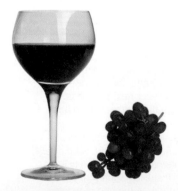

| Figure 3.2 | **Grapes, red wine, and heart disease.** Grapes and red wine |

contain phytochemicals that appear to reduce the risk of heart disease. Studies show that moderate consumption of alcohol independently reduces heart disease risk.

Plants contain phytochemicals in abundance because these substances are of benefit to the plant itself. For example, an orange has at least 170 distinct phytochemicals. Singly and together, these compounds help plants resist the attacks of bacteria and fungi, the ravages of free radicals, and high levels of ultraviolet light from the sun. When we eat these plants, the phytochemicals end up in our tissues and provide many of the same protections that plants enjoy.

Phytochemicals are part of the reason why the *Dietary Guidelines for Americans* recommends that we increase our consumption of fruits and vegetables each day and eat a variety of vegetables, especially dark-green and red and orange vegetables and beans and peas.[2] The emphasis also can literally be seen in the MyPlate food plan, which encourages you to make half your plate fruits and vegetables.[3] Fruits and vegetables are also naturally low in fat and calories and tend to be rich in fiber, potassium, and vitamins. In addition, studies show that groups of people who consume more fruits and vegetables tend to have lower rates of common chronic diseases.

### Benefits of Phytochemicals

What are some of the specific benefits of phytochemicals? People who eat tomatoes and processed tomato products take in lycopene, which is associated with a decreased risk of chronic diseases, such as cancer and cardiovascular diseases.[4] Scientists believe that the large consumption of soy products in Asian countries contributes to lower rates of colon, prostate, uterus, and breast cancers.[5] Depending on the source of the isoflavones, the kind of cancer, and the study population, the outcomes of these studies are occasionally conflicting.[6] The foods and herbs with the highest anticancer activity include garlic, soybeans, cabbage, ginger, and licorice as well as the family of vegetables that includes celery, carrots, and parsley.

How do phytochemicals work to prevent chronic disease? A number of phytochemicals, including those from soybeans and from the cabbage family, are able to modify estrogen metabolism or block the effect of estrogen on cell growth. Such compounds are known as **phytoestrogens**. Because levels of estrogen and other hormones are closely linked to the development of breast, ovarian, and prostate tumors, it is clear how phytochemicals might inhibit development of such cancers. However, because compounds in soy activate estrogen, which increases breast cancer risk and tumor growth, the safety of soy has been questioned. Evidence suggests that the protective effects from soy, specifically, the lower risk of breast cancer, may benefit women who consume moderate amounts of soy throughout their life.[7]

Other phytochemicals neutralize **free radicals**. Free radicals (active oxidants) are continually produced in our cells and over time can result in damage to DNA and important cell structures. Eventually, this damage can promote both cancer and cell aging. Free radical oxidation of lipids contributes to heart disease risk. Many different plant chemicals, such as the pigments in grapes and red wine (see **Figure 3.2**), are able to neutralize or reduce concentrations of free radicals, thus protecting us against the development of both cancer and heart disease.

Phytochemicals in fruits and vegetables have a number of other potential benefits. Lutein and zeaxanthin are carotenoids (plant pigments) found in dark-green leafy vegetables, corn, and egg yolks. Increased consumption of these compounds is associated with a lower incidence and slower progression of age-related macular degeneration, the leading cause of blindness in older people.[8] The phytochemicals in whole grains are generally similar to those found in fruits and vegetables and also are important in the prevention of both cancer and heart disease. One class of grain phytochemicals, the terpenoids, produces a significant reduction in total and LDL cholesterol levels, thus reducing the risk of heart disease. Before you reach for your next slice of bread, it is worth remembering that refined wheat, the source of white flour, has lost more than 99 percent of its phytochemical content, and only four vitamins and one mineral are added back when refined grains are enriched.

### Adding Phytochemicals to Your Diet

Since phytochemicals are so beneficial, why can't we just purify the important ones and add them to our diet as supplements, the way we put vitamins back into white flour after processing? The short answer is that we don't know enough about how phytochemicals function.

Many phytochemicals appear to act synergistically, both fighting free radicals and blocking the negative effects of hormones. It is not surprising, then, that when a single pure phytochemical, such as beta-carotene, is given as a long-term supplement, only minor benefits are seen. In fact, some studies have shown no health benefits from such purified supplements and have even found higher lung cancer rates in smokers taking beta-carotene supplements. Yet there is no doubt that consumption of plant foods containing multiple antioxidants is strongly associated with health benefits. The weight of evidence and experience strongly favors finding a place for more fruits and vegetables in the diet. (See **Figure 3.3**.) The FDA allows the dietary guidance message "Diets rich in fruits and vegetables may reduce the risk of some types of cancer and other chronic diseases" on food labels. The new MyPlate graphic and the Fruits & Veggies—More Matters® logo both encourage fruit and vegetable consumption. In addition, MyPlate's advice to "Make at least half your grains whole grains" helps promote intake of disease-fighting phytochemicals found in whole grains.

Changing your diet to include more functional foods and fewer empty calories needn't be painful if you use your imagination. Sometimes you can have your pizza and eat it too. The next time you indulge, ask for a pizza with minimum cheese and maximum vegetables. Whole-wheat crust would be a plus. The combination of lycopene from tomato sauce, quercetin from onions, glucarates from green peppers, and carotenoids from basil and spinach can turn a potential nutritional train wreck into a phytochemical cornucopia.

## Foods Enhanced with Functional Ingredients

Another type of functional food is one that gets its health-promoting properties from what has been added during processing. Calcium-fortified orange juice, breakfast cereals fortified with folic acid, yogurt with live active cultures, and margarines with added plant sterol and plant stanol esters are examples. Health properties come from added nutrients, bacteria, fiber, or other substances. Some are foods and beverages that contain added herbal compounds, such as those sold in pill form as dietary supplements. The result is a wide variety of products making an often confusing array of label statements and health claims.

## Regulatory Issues for Functional Foods

Food labeling is required for most prepared foods, such as breads, cereals, canned and frozen foods, snacks, desserts, drinks, and so on. Nutrition labeling for raw produce such as fruits and vegetables and fish is voluntary. The FDA refers to these products as *conventional* foods. The terms *functional foods* and *nutraceuticals* are widely used in the marketplace and media. Such foods are regulated by the FDA under the authority of the Federal Food, Drug, and Cosmetic Act, even though they are not specifically defined by law.[9] Although

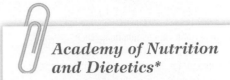

### Academy of Nutrition and Dietetics*

**Functional Foods**
All foods are functional at some physiological level, but it is the position of the American Dietetic Association that functional foods that include whole foods and fortified, enriched, or enhanced foods have a potentially beneficial effect on health when consumed as part of a varied diet on a regular basis, at effective levels. The Academy of Nutrition and Dietetics supports research to further define the health benefits and risks of individual functional foods and their physiologically active components. Health claims on food products, including functional foods, should be based on the significant scientific agreement standard of evidence, and the Academy of Nutrition and Dietetics supports label claims based on such strong scientific substantiation. Food and nutrition professionals will continue to work with the food industry, allied health professionals, the government, the scientific community, and the media to ensure the public has accurate information regarding functional foods and thus should continue to educate themselves on this emerging area of food and nutrition science.

**Source:** Reproduced from Hasler CM et al. Position of the Academy of Nutrition and Dietetics: functional foods. *J Am Diet Assoc.* 2009;109:735–746.

* Formerly the American Dietetic Association

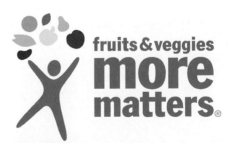

**Figure 3.3** **The National Fruit and Vegetable Program.** This program encourages Americans to increase their consumption of fruits and vegetables for better health. It is a public–private partnership, consisting of government agencies, nonprofit groups, and industry. For more information, visit http://www.fruitsandveggiesmorematters.gov.

**Source:** Courtesy of FruitsandVeggiesMatter.gov

**additives**  Substances added to food to perform various functions, such as adding color or flavor, replacing sugar or fat, improving nutritional content, or improving texture or shelf life.

**direct additives**  Substances added to foods for a specific purpose.

**indirect additives**  Substances that become part of the food in trace amounts due to its packaging, storage, or other handling.

this may sound a little confusing, a *food* is a product that we eat or drink as well as all the components of that product. This definition distinguishes a food from a *drug*, which is a substance intended to diagnose, cure, mitigate, treat, or prevent disease. Foods also are distinct from *dietary supplements*, which are products intended to supplement the diet but that do not represent themselves as a conventional food, meal, or diet. You will learn more about dietary supplements later in this chapter.

Although some manufacturers have tried to market functional products as dietary supplements rather than foods to take advantage of broader allowances for label claims, the FDA's position is that products that are conventional foods and beverages are subject to the regulations for food and not for dietary supplements. A substance added to a food for health benefits must still conform to FDA regulations for food **additives**.

**Key Concepts**  *Functional foods provide health benefits beyond basic nutrition. They get their health-promoting properties from naturally occurring compounds called phytochemicals. Phytochemicals are "plant chemicals" that include thousands of compounds, pigments, and natural antioxidants, many of which are associated with protection from heart disease, hypertension, cancer, and diabetes. Just like conventional foods, functional foods are subject to FDA regulations for claims and safety.*

## Food Additives

Food additives work in many different ways to give us a safe, plentiful, varied, and relatively inexpensive food supply. Food additives can be either direct or indirect. **Direct additives** are added to a food for a specific reason. Aspartame, saccharin, and sucralose are direct food additives, used instead of sugar to sweeten. Direct additives are identified in the ingredient list on the food label. **Indirect additives** are substances that unintentionally become part of the food in trace amounts—for example, chemicals from a food's packaging can become part of the food. The FDA evaluates both direct and indirect additives for safety.

Direct additives are used in foods for five main reasons:

1. *To maintain product consistency.* Emulsifiers give products such as peanut butter a consistent texture and prevent them from separating. Stabilizers and thickeners give ice cream a smooth, uniform texture. Anticaking agents help substances such as salt to flow freely.
2. *To improve or maintain nutritional value.* Vitamins and minerals are added to many common foods such as milk, flour, cereal, and margarine to make up for elements likely to be lacking in a person's diet, replace those lost in processing, or improve shelf life.
3. *To keep the food appetizing and wholesome.* Preservatives help protect against mold, air, bacteria, fungi, or yeast, which all can cause food to spoil.
4. *To provide leavening or control acidity and alkalinity.* Leavening agents help cakes, biscuits, and other baked goods to rise during baking. Other additives modify the acidity and alkalinity of foods for flavor, taste, and color.
5. *To enhance flavor or give a desired color.* Many spices and added flavors enhance the taste of foods. Colors, likewise, enhance the appearance of certain foods to make them more appealing or meet consumer expectations.

Although most people think additives are complex chemicals with unfamiliar names, three of the most common additives are sugar, salt, and corn

*Quick* Bite

**Early Food Laws**
In 1202, King John of England proclaimed the first English food law, the Assize of Bread, which prohibited adulteration of bread with such ingredients as ground peas or beans.

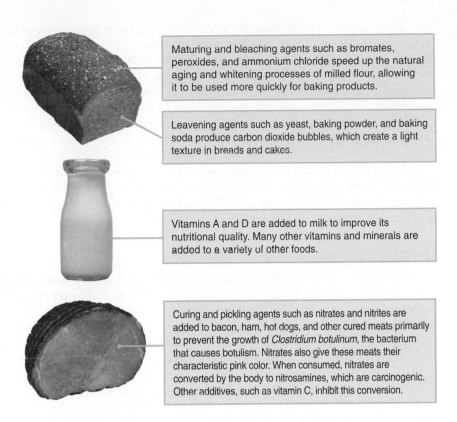

**Figure 3.4** **Common foods that contain additives.** Substances may be added to foods to improve texture, shelf life, nutritional quality, and safety.

Maturing and bleaching agents such as bromates, peroxides, and ammonium chloride speed up the natural aging and whitening processes of milled flour, allowing it to be used more quickly for baking products.

Leavening agents such as yeast, baking powder, and baking soda produce carbon dioxide bubbles, which create a light texture in breads and cakes.

Vitamins A and D are added to milk to improve its nutritional quality. Many other vitamins and minerals are added to a variety of other foods.

Curing and pickling agents such as nitrates and nitrites are added to bacon, ham, hot dogs, and other cured meats primarily to prevent the growth of *Clostridium botulinum*, the bacterium that causes botulism. Nitrates also give these meats their characteristic pink color. When consumed, nitrates are converted by the body to nitrosamines, which are carcinogenic. Other additives, such as vitamin C, inhibit this conversion.

syrup. These three, plus citric acid (found naturally in oranges and lemons), baking soda, vegetable colors, mustard, and pepper account for more than 98 percent by weight of all food additives used in the United States and Canada.

## Regulation by the FDA

Although additives serve important functions (see **Figure 3.4**), you might be skeptical about their safety. Additives fall into four regulatory categories: food additives, color additives, Generally Recognized as Safe (GRAS) substances, and prior-sanctioned substances. The FDA must approve a new food additive before it can be put on the market. The manufacturer must provide convincing research evidence that the additive not only performs its intended function but also is not harmful at expected consumption levels. Based on this and other scientific information, the FDA decides whether to approve the additive and determines the types of foods that may contain the additive, the quantities that can be used, and the way the substance will be identified on labels.

A **color additive** is any dye, pigment, or substance that can give color when added to a food, drug, or cosmetic or to the human body. Colors allowed for use in food are classified as either certified or exempt from certification. Certified colors are synthetic. The manufacturer and the FDA test each batch to ensure their purity. Certified colors added to a food must be listed on the food's ingredient list by common name. Colors exempt from certification include natural substances derived from vegetables, minerals, or animals. These colors also must be produced according to specifications that ensure purity.

A third type of additive falls under the category **Generally Recognized as Safe (GRAS)**. Congress first defined GRAS substances in 1958 when it passed the Food Additives Amendment to the Food, Drug, and Cosmetic

**color additive** Any dye, pigment, or other substance that can impart color when added or applied to a food, drug, or cosmetic or to the human body.

**Generally Recognized as Safe (GRAS)** Refers to substances that are "generally recognized as safe" for consumption and can be added to foods by manufacturers without establishing their safety by rigorous experimental studies. Congress established the GRAS list in 1958.

**prior-sanctioned substance** All substances that the FDA or the U.S. Department of Agriculture (USDA) had determined were safe for use in specific foods before passage of the 1958 Food Additives amendment are designated as prior-sanctioned substances. These substances are exempt from the food additive regulation process.

**Delaney Clause** The part of the 1960 Color Additives Amendment to the Federal Food, Drug, and Cosmetic Act that bars the FDA from approving any additives shown in laboratory tests to cause cancer.

Act. If a substance is classified as GRAS, experts generally consider it safe to use, either because it was safely used in food before 1958 or because there is published scientific evidence for its safety. Salt, sugar, spices, vitamins, and monosodium glutamate (MSG), along with several hundred other substances, are considered GRAS. Manufacturers themselves may assert that a food has GRAS status or petition the FDA to have a new additive be considered GRAS. In either case, the manufacturer must have evidence of safety and a basis for concluding that this evidence is known and accepted by qualified experts.

If the FDA or USDA had determined that an additive was safe for use in a specific food before the 1958 legislation, then it is a **prior-sanctioned substance**, the fourth category of additives. Examples include sodium nitrite and potassium nitrite to preserve luncheon meats.

## Delaney Clause

Food additives and color additives cannot be approved if they cause cancer in humans or animals. This provision of the law is often referred to as the **Delaney Clause**, named for the congressman who sponsored it.

Although the Delaney Clause sounds good in principle, it has become one of the most controversial food laws on the books. To determine a chemical's safety, researchers often administer massive doses to rodents. Many experts question whether an additive that causes cancer in laboratory animals at extremely high levels should be banned from use in foods at low levels. They argue that feeding animals large doses of a substance over their entire lifetimes may have little relevance to human consumption of trace amounts of that same substance.

For now, the Delaney Clause remains part of our food safety laws. Future scientific techniques might decrease reliance on animal testing and improve accuracy in predicting the effects of food additives on human health.

## Additives in Functional Foods

Using additives to create functional foods raises questions of how much should be used and how much is safe. In addition, while there are guidelines for the use of vitamins and minerals in the fortification of food and for the use of approved food additives, little is known about what happens to many novel ingredients, such as botanical extracts, when they are put into a food.[10]

Because so many products with added herbal and other novel ingredients have appeared on the market, the FDA has been reminding manufacturers that food additives not GRAS require approval before being sold. Any food containing an unapproved food additive is considered adulterated and cannot legally be marketed in the United States. Companies that have marketed foods containing novel or "new" ingredients, including botanicals that were not considered GRAS, have received warning letters from the FDA.[11] These companies were warned that, as formulated, the FDA considered the products to be adulterated.

**Key Concepts** *Direct additives are used for specific purposes. Indirect additives become part of the food in trace amounts when the food comes in contact with the substance. Additives are used for many reasons; these include improving product quality, maintaining freshness, and improving nutritional value. Unless a new additive meets the requirements to be considered GRAS or is a prior-sanctioned ingredient, the FDA demands that it undergo extensive testing to be proved safe and effective. The FDA is responsible for approving and regulating additives. The Delaney Clause prohibits the approval of an additive if it is found to cause cancer in humans or animals.*

*Quick* Bite

**Old Concept, New Frontier**
Functional foods are a new frontier of nutrition and food science, but the idea has been around for centuries. Hippocrates, the father of modern medicine, proclaimed, "Let food be your medicine, and medicine be your food."

## Claims for Functional Foods

When a functional food meets the appropriate FDA guidelines, it may make a nutrient content claim or health claim on the label. For example, tofu containing at least 6.25 grams of soy protein per serving may make a health claim about the role of soy protein in reducing the risk of heart disease. Oatmeal with an adequate amount of beta-glucan fiber can highlight its benefit in reducing risk of heart disease. Another health claim applies to a functional food created through the addition of plant sterol or plant stanol esters to a vegetable-oil-based spread. The Benecol and Take Control product lines (spreads and salad dressings) contain these plant esters, which have been shown to reduce cholesterol levels when consumed daily in adequate amounts.[12] (See **Figure 3.5**.)

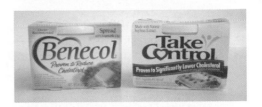

**Figure 3.5** **Some functional foods can make health claims.**
Manufacturers have obtained approval from the FDA to make health claims for these margarine products.

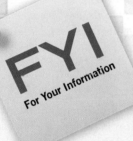

FYI
For Your Information

# The Saccharin Story

The granddaddy of all sugar substitutes is saccharin. Discovered in 1879, it was used during both world wars to sweeten foods, helping to compensate for sugar shortages and rationing. It is 300 times sweeter than sugar.

In 1907, an early attempt to ban saccharin was thwarted when President Theodore Roosevelt proclaimed the top safety official behind the effort to be "an idiot." Safety questions resurfaced in 1911 when a board of federal scientists called the artificial sweetener "an adulterant" that should not be used in foods. This same board later decided to limit saccharin just to products "intended for invalids," a restriction that was lifted after sugar shortages developed during World War I.

In 1958, when Congress passed the Food Additives Amendment to the Food, Drug, and Cosmetic Act, saccharin was one of the ingredients Generally Recognized as Safe (GRAS). That same year the saccharin-based product Sweet 'N Low took the public by storm. Food and beverage companies scrambled to offer saccharin-sweetened products, which came to include the diet soda Tab and a plethora of gelatins, candies, and baked goods.

By the early 1970s, studies of rats that had been fed saccharin raised concerns about the sweetener's role in causing bladder cancer, but scientists later suggested that impurities, not saccharin, may have caused the tumors. Then, in 1977, a Canadian study looked specifically at the role of saccharin in test animals. Researchers fed rats high doses of saccharin equivalent to 5 percent of their diet. The results again showed that saccharin caused bladder cancer in rats.

Because the Delaney Clause prohibits the use of any additive shown to cause cancer in animals or humans, the FDA proposed an immediate ban on saccharin. The FDA proposal prompted a public outcry, fueled in part by media reports that the test rats were fed the equivalent of as many as 800 diet sodas a day.[1] Congress responded by passing the Saccharin Study and Labeling Act, which placed a two-year moratorium on any ban of the sweetener while additional safety studies were conducted. Congress extended the moratorium several times over the years. The law also required that any foods containing saccharin must carry a label that reads "Use of this product may be hazardous to your health. This product contains saccharin, which has been determined to cause cancer in laboratory animals."

In May 2000, the National Toxicology Program (NTP) removed saccharin from its list of possible human carcinogens. The NTP concluded that the types of tumors caused by saccharin in rats arose from a mechanism that is not relevant to humans. This ruling is in keeping with the opinion of other scientific bodies. The National Cancer Institute (NCI) states that:

. . . questions about artificial sweeteners and cancer arose when early studies showed that cyclamate in combination with saccharin caused bladder cancer in laboratory animals. However, results from subsequent carcinogenicity studies of these sweeteners have not provided clear evidence of an association with cancer in humans. Similarly, studies of other FDA-approved sweeteners have not demonstrated clear evidence of an association with cancer in humans.[2]

Specifically regarding saccharin, the NCI states that "human epidemiology studies have shown no consistent evidence that saccharin is associated with bladder cancer incidence."[3] Other health groups, including the American Medical Association, the American Cancer Society, and the Academy of Nutrition and Dietetics, agree that saccharin use is acceptable. And, in 2000, Congress repealed the warning label requirements for saccharin-containing foods.

Saccharin remains on the market and continues to have a fairly large appeal as a tabletop sweetener, particularly in restaurants, where it is available in single-serving packets under trade names such as Sweet 'N Low.

1    Henkel J. Sugar substitutes: Americans opt for sweetness and lite. *FDA Consumer*, Nov/Dec 1999.

2    The National Cancer Institute (NCI). FactSheet: artificial sweeteners and cancer. http://www.cancer.gov/cancertopics/factsheet/Risk/artificial-sweeteners. Accessed 6/17/11.

3    Ibid.

**Table 3.2    Questions to Ask to Assess the Credibility of Websites**

- What is the background, credibility, and affiliation of the researchers or sources?
- Does the website identify the publisher and any sponsors?
- Does the website say who wrote it or how it was approved?
- Is the information up-to-date?
- Does the information include credible references such as peer-reviewed journals?
- Does the information present both perspectives of the issue?
- Is the information balanced and state any caveats?
- Is the website designed to sell products?
- Are there links that provide support or more detail?

Source: Reproduced from Position of the American Dietetic Association: food and nutrition misinformation. *J Am Diet Assoc.* 2006;106:601–607.

**Table 3.3    Red Flags of Junk Science**

1. Recommendations that promise a quick fix.
2. Dire warnings of danger from a single product or regimen.
3. Claims that sound too good to be true.
4. Simplistic conclusions drawn from a complex study.
5. Recommendations based on a single study.
6. Dramatic statements that are refuted by reputable scientific organizations.
7. Lists of "good" and "bad" foods.
8. Recommendations made to help sell a product.
9. Recommendations based on studies published without peer review.
10. Recommendations from studies that ignore individual or group differences.

Source: Reproduced from Position of the American Dietetic Association: food and nutrition misinformation. *J Am Diet Assoc.* 2006;106:601–607.

## Structure/Function Claims for Functional Foods

Structure/function claims on conventional or functional foods must be based on the food's nutritive value. An example is orange juice with added vitamin C, vitamin E, and zinc to "support your natural defenses." However, structure/function claims are not as stringently regulated by the FDA as health claims. So, at present, many manufacturers are making claims about non-nutrients in foods and their effects on body structure or function. For example, a cereal with added St. John's wort and kava extract is "accented with herbs to support emotional and mental balance," and a bottled tea is "infused with mind-enhancing ginkgo biloba and Panax ginseng." Consumers should beware; many companies continue to deliberately confuse consumers by exaggerating the health effects or ingredients of their products despite the FDA sending more warning letters to food manufacturers about misleading labeling.[13]

**Key Concepts**  *Under FDA guidelines, a functional food's label may have a nutrient content claim, health claim, or structure/function claim. A structure/function claim promotes a substance's effect on the structure or function of the body. For foods, the claimed effect must be based on the food's "nutritive value." Currently, many manufacturers make structure/function claims about non-nutrients in foods.*

## Strategies for Functional Food Use

So, should you go all out and fill your shopping cart with functional foods? Which ones would you buy? The best course of action is to stick with what scientists have agreed upon so far. First, fruits and vegetables promote health and reduce disease risk through a whole host of natural phytochemicals. Use the list of foods and phytochemicals in Table 3.1 to enhance your shopping list with nature's functional foods. Second, consider nutrient-fortified products when a particular nutrient is lacking in your diet and you either don't like or can't eat good food sources of that nutrient. For example, if you are allergic to milk and dairy products, consider calcium-fortified orange juice as a nutritious way to get the calcium that you need. Third, *read, read, read* about functional foods, and be skeptical when you evaluate what's on the Internet. Table 3.2 lists some questions to ask when assessing the credibility of websites. For more tips on how to evaluate health information on the Internet, visit the Office of Dietary Supplements website.[14] Do your homework by looking at scientific articles—your instructor can help you find and interpret studies of functional food components. Finally, be critical of advertising and hype—if it sounds too good to be true, it probably is! Table 3.3 lists some of the red flags of junk science.

## Dietary Supplements: Vitamins and Minerals

Dietary supplements come in various forms—vitamins, minerals, amino acids, herbs, glandular extracts, enzymes, and many others. The marketplace includes a wide variety of products claiming to do everything from enhancing immune function to improving mood. Table 3.4 lists many popular supplements, claims, and important cautions. Despite the enticing claims made for many non-nutrient supplements, scientific evidence of efficacy and long-term safety often is lacking.

"Should I take a vitamin (or mineral) supplement?" Apparently many people already have answered that question for themselves: Multivitamin/mineral supplements and other single vitamin or mineral supplements are popular supplements and are taken by a substantial percentage of Americans.[15] (See **Figure 3.6**.) We will look at two levels of vitamin and mineral

**Table 3.4    Examples of Dietary Supplements and Their Claims**

| Supplement | Claimed Benefits | Current Research Caveats |
|---|---|---|
| Beta-carotene | Prevents cancer and heart disease; boosts immunity; improves eye health | Diets rich in beta-carotene-containing fruits and vegetables reduce heart disease and cancer risk. Supplements have not been shown to be beneficial. Taking supplements may increase lung cancer risk in smokers. In combination with vitamin C, vitamin E, and zinc, may slow progression of age-related macular degeneration. |
| Chromium picolinate | Builds muscle, helps with blood glucose control in diabetes, promotes weight loss, reduces cholesterol | No solid evidence that chromium picolinate supplements perform as claimed or benefit healthy people. Some evidence that they may harm cells. |
| Coenzyme $Q_{10}$ | Prevents heart disease, improves health of people with heart disease and hypertension, cure-all | May have value in preexisting heart disease, but benefits for healthy people are unproved. |
| Cranberry | Prevents and treats urinary tract infections (UTIs) | Regular consumption of juice may reduce UTI incidence; limited evidence for supplements. |
| Creatine | Increases muscle strength and size, improves athletic performance | May enhance power and strength for some athletes, but is meaningless for casual exercisers and distance athletes. |
| Echinacea | Protects against and cures colds, boosts immunity | Inconsistent evidence of benefit. Many varieties exist; products on the market are unstandardized. |
| Ephedra | Weight control, herbal "high," decongestant | Ephedra raises heart rate and blood pressure and is dangerous for people with diabetes, hypertension, or heart disease. The FDA has prohibited sales of ephedra-containing supplements. |
| Feverfew | Prevents migraines | Some evidence of reduced severity and frequency of migraines, but high drop-out rates in studies. |
| Garlic | Lowers blood pressure and blood cholesterol, reduces cancer risk | Some evidence that garlic reduces cholesterol and blood pressure. Conflicting results related to cancer risk reduction. |
| Ginkgo biloba | Improves blood flow and circulatory disorders; prevents or cures absentmindedness, memory loss, dementia | Limited benefits for some Alzheimer's patients. No proven benefit for others. |
| Ginseng | Improves athletic performance, fights fatigue, helps control blood glucose in people with diabetes, reduces cancer risk | No evidence that ginseng has any beneficial effects. Many products on the market contain no ginseng. |
| Glucosamine and chondroiton sulfate | Relieves arthritis pain, slows progression of arthritis | Some evidence of reduced pain and improved symptoms, although more studies are needed. Does not reverse arthritis. Variable amounts in products. |
| Kava | Promotes relaxation and relieves anxiety | May cause liver damage. Banned in Switzerland, Germany, and Canada. |
| Melatonin | Promotes sleep, counters jet lag, improves sex life, prevents migraine | May be effective for jet lag, studies are contradictory relative to sleep. No evidence for anti-aging or sex-drive claims. No data on long-term safety. |
| Milk thistle | Reduces liver damage in alcoholic liver disease, promotes general liver health | No evidence of general liver health benefit, some evidence of benefit in those with alcoholic liver cirrhosis. |
| Saw palmetto | Shrinks prostate, reduces symptoms of benign prostatic hyperplasia, prevents prostate cancer | May improve urinary tract symptoms associated with prostate enlargement. No evidence for prevention of prostate cancer. May affect PSA test and diagnosis of prostate cancer. |
| St. John's wort | Alleviates depression, promotes emotional well-being | Studies in Europe suggest efficacy for mild depression. Clinical studies in the United States show no effect on major depression of moderate severity. Should not be taken with prescription antidepressants. |
| Valerian | Enhances sleep, reduces stress and anxiety | Inconclusive results to date, much more research is needed. |

Source: Adapted from Sarubin Fragakis A. *The Health Professional's Guide to Popular Dietary Supplements.* 3rd ed. Chicago, IL: Academy of Nutrition and Dietetics; 2006; Hendler S, Rorvik R. *Physician's Desk Reference for Nutritional Supplements.* 2nd ed. New York: Thomson Healthcare; 2008; and NIH Office of Dietary Supplements. Dietary supplement fact sheets. http://ods.od.nih.gov/factsheets/list-all. Accessed 6/20/11.

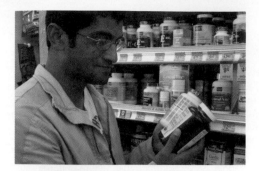

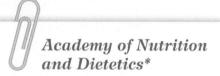

*Academy of Nutrition and Dietetics**

**Nutrient Supplementation**

It is the position of the American Dietetic Association that the best nutrition-based strategy for promoting optimal health and reducing the risk of chronic disease is to wisely choose a wide variety of foods. Additional nutrients from supplements can help some people meet their nutrition needs as specified by science-based nutrition standards such as the Dietary Reference Intakes.

**Source:** Reproduced from Marra MV, Boyar AP. Position of the Academy of Nutrition and Dietetics: nutrient supplementation. *J Am Diet Assoc.* 2009:109(12):2073–2085.

* Formerly the American Dietetic Association

**megadoses** Doses of a nutrient that are 10 or more times the recommended amount.

supplementation: (1) moderate doses that are in the range of the Daily Values (DVs) or levels you might eat in a nutrient-rich diet and (2) **megadoses**, or high levels that are typically multiples of the DVs and much greater amounts than diet alone could supply.

## Moderate Supplementation

Health care practitioners often recommend moderate nutrient supplementation for people with elevated nutrient needs and for people who may not always eat well enough.[16] Some examples include the following:

- *Women of childbearing age who may become pregnant as well as pregnant and breastfeeding women.* Taking supplemental folic acid prior to and during pregnancy can reduce the incidence of birth defects. During pregnancy, it's hard to meet the increased needs for iron and other nutrients through diet alone. "Morning sickness" makes it even harder. When a woman breastfeeds, some of her nutrient needs are even higher than they were in pregnancy.
- *Women with heavy menstrual bleeding.* Women with high iron losses may need a supplement, but they should not take high doses of iron without a doctor's recommendation. Lab tests can show whether a woman gets enough blood-building nutrients or whether she needs supplements.
- *Children.* A supplement can help balance the diets of picky eaters or children on a food jag (eating only a few specific foods), and it can ease parental worries. Children who do not consume the recommended amounts of vitamin D–fortified milk may need supplemental vitamin D.
- *Infants.* If their access to sunlight is restricted, infants may need supplemental vitamin D. Doctors also may prescribe fluoride in areas where water is not fluoridated.
- *People with severe food restrictions, either self-imposed or prescribed.* Supplements may help people on a strict weight-loss diet, those who have eating disorders, those who have mental illnesses, and those who limit their eating because of social or emotional situations.
- *Strict vegetarians who abstain from animal foods and dairy products.* People who don't eat meat or dairy products may need supplemental vitamin $B_{12}$, vitamin D, and perhaps calcium, zinc, iron, and other minerals.
- *Older adults.* Because inadequate stomach acid (which is needed for normal absorption of vitamin $B_{12}$) is common among older people, older adults may need extra vitamin $B_{12}$. When older adults have limited exposure to the sun and their diets lack dairy products, they should take supplements of vitamin D, calcium, and possibly other nutrients to help maintain bone health.

Other groups may also be vulnerable to nutrient inadequacies, such as individuals who are food insecure, alcohol/drug dependent, or those who have altered nutritional needs due to an illness or medication use. Many people take nutrient supplements to ensure they meet their nutritional needs. However, taking supplements to "fix" a poor diet is a bad idea. Foods provide not only nutrients but also fiber and other health-promoting phytochemicals. Whenever possible, meet your nutritional needs with food.

Many supplements contain multiple vitamins and minerals. If you are one of those who should take multivitamin/mineral supplements, look for brands that contain at least 20 vitamins and minerals, each no more than 100 percent of its Daily Value unless otherwise instructed by your doctor. (See **Figure 3.7.**). Although most products have appropriate nutrient levels, some formulas are irrational and unbalanced, with less than 10 percent of the Daily Value of some nutrients and more than 1,000 percent of others.

**Key Concepts** *Vitamin and mineral supplements are popular; however, it is better to obtain nutrients from food. Some conditions and circumstances make it difficult to meet nutritional needs through food alone or to consume enough food to accommodate increases in nutrient needs. Multivitamin/mineral supplements should be well balanced, with doses no greater than about 100 percent of the Daily Value of each nutrient.*

## Megadoses in Conventional Medical Management

High doses of vitamins and minerals have become so much a part of treating certain illnesses that when physicians prescribe these nutrients, many see themselves as following "standard medical practice" rather than as "practicing nutrition." Here are some situations in which physicians prescribe megadoses:

- When a medication dramatically depletes or destroys the stores or blocks the functions of vitamins or minerals, megadosing can overcome these effects. For example, folic acid and vitamin $B_6$ are used during long-term treatment with some tuberculosis drugs. B vitamins also may be prescribed along with seizure medications or medicines that block the metabolism of **nucleic acids**.[17]
- People with **malabsorption syndromes** often take large nutrient doses to compensate for nutritive losses and to override intestinal barriers to absorption. Megadoses routinely are given to patients with colitis or cystic fibrosis, for example.
- Megadoses of vitamin $B_{12}$ can overcome the malabsorption seen in pernicious anemia, a condition in which a key substance needed for vitamin $B_{12}$ absorption is lacking. Ordinarily, an intricate series of steps during digestion prepares $B_{12}$ for normal intestinal absorption; if there is a malfunction during any of these steps, the vitamin is lost. Megadoses allow a small amount of the vitamin to diffuse across the intestine, thus overriding the normal mechanism and preventing deficiency.[18]

A vitamin at megadose levels can have "pharmacological activity"—that is, it acts as a drug. Nicotinic acid (niacin) is the best example. At usual levels (around 10 or 20 milligrams), it functions as a vitamin, but at levels 50 or 100 times higher it acts as a drug to lower blood lipid levels. Like any drug, though, it can have serious side effects.[19] For example, a recent medical trial from the National Institutes of Health studying a combination of niacin (nicotinic acid) and another medication was stopped earlier than planned because the researchers found that in patients with heart and vascular disease who received the combination treatment there was a small and unexplained increase in ischemic stroke rates.[20]

Benefits from high doses of other vitamins are not clear-cut. Researchers have tried prescribing B vitamins, including niacin, for emotional disturbances and mental illnesses; they work well when there is an underlying deficiency, but otherwise results have been mixed and often disappointing. Vitamin E has been tried for some neurological illnesses, to minimize complications of diabetes mellitus, and to reduce the risk of coronary artery disease. A combination supplement of vitamin C, vitamin E, beta-carotene, and zinc with copper

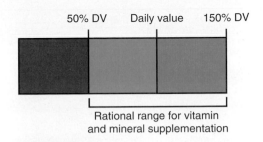

**Figure 3.7**   **Moderate supplementation.** Health care practitioners often recommend moderate nutrient supplementation for people with elevated nutrient needs and for people who have consistently poor diets.

**nucleic acids**  A family of more than 25,000 molecules found in chromosomes, nucleoli, mitochondria, and the cytoplasm of cells.

**malabsorption syndromes**  Conditions that result in imperfect, inadequate, or otherwise disordered gastrointestinal absorption.

called the AREDS formula has been shown to slow the progression of age-related macular degeneration.[21] Supplementation with vitamins $B_6$, $B_{12}$, and folic acid has been linked to reduced heart disease risk. However, experts have concluded that evidence is insufficient to recommend the use of antioxidant vitamin supplements to reduce the risk of cardiovascular disease.[22]

## Megadosing Beyond Conventional Medicine: Orthomolecular Nutrition

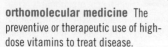

**orthomolecular medicine** The preventive or therapeutic use of high-dose vitamins to treat disease.

In 1968, Linus Pauling, the best-known advocate of megadosing, coined the term **orthomolecular medicine**. To him, *orthomolecular* meant achieving the optimal nutrient levels in the body.[23] Few nutritionists argue with the importance of optimum nutrition. In fact, some nutritionists share Pauling's concerns that the typical diet is too refined to provide adequate nutrients and that intake equal to RDA values may not be high enough to achieve optimal body levels.

Most nutritionists would argue, however, with the high doses Pauling recommended to attain those optimal body levels and with the therapeutic value he and his followers attributed to those doses. Most notably, Pauling suggested in the early 1970s that an optimal daily intake of vitamin C was 2,000 milligrams—more than 30 times the current Daily Value. (See **Figure 3.8**.) Some advocates of vitamin C recommend even higher doses, relying on intravenous administration to avoid causing diarrhea. Dr. Pauling claimed megadoses of vitamin C prevented or cured the common cold. Although many researchers have attempted to confirm this theory, studies do not support the idea that vitamin C prevents colds. A few studies found that colds were slightly less severe or less frequent in certain people, but most studies found no beneficial effect.[24]

## *American Heart Association*

**Vitamin and Mineral Supplements**

The American Heart Association recommends that healthy people get adequate nutrients by eating a variety of foods in moderation, rather than by taking supplements. The exception is *omega*-3 fatty acid supplements for people with documented heart disease.

"The Dietary Recommended Intakes (DRIs) published by the Institute of Medicine are the best available estimates of safe and adequate dietary intakes," says the AHA. "There aren't sufficient data to suggest that healthy people benefit by taking certain vitamin or mineral supplements in excess of the DRIs." Moreover, "vitamin or mineral supplements aren't a substitute for a balanced, nutritious diet that limits excess calories, saturated fat, trans fat, sodium and dietary cholesterol. This dietary approach has been shown to reduce coronary heart disease risk in both healthy people and those with coronary disease."

*What about antioxidant vitamins?*

Many people are interested in antioxidant vitamins (A, C, and E). This is due to suggestions from large observational studies comparing healthy adults consuming large amounts of these vitamins with those who didn't. However, these observations are subject to bias and don't prove a cause-and-effect relationship. *Scientific evidence does not suggest that consuming antioxidant vitamins can eliminate the need to reduce blood pressure, lower blood cholesterol, or stop smoking cigarettes.* Clinical trials are under way to find out whether increased vitamin antioxidant intake may have an overall benefit. However, a recent large, placebo-controlled, randomized study failed to show any benefit from vitamin E on heart disease. Although antioxidant supplements are not recommended, antioxidant food sources—especially plant-derived foods such as fruits, vegetables, whole-grain foods, and vegetable oils—are recommended.

*What about omega-3 fatty acid supplements?*

Fish intake has been associated with decreased risk of heart disease. On the basis of available data, the AHA recommends that patients without documented heart disease eat a variety of fish—preferably *omega*-3-containing fish—at least twice a week. Examples of these types of fish include salmon, herring, and trout. Patients with documented heart disease are advised to consume about 1 gram of EPA + DHA (types of *omega*-3 fatty acids), preferably from fish, although EPA + DHA supplements could be considered, but consult with a physician first. For people with high triglycerides (blood fats), 2 to 4 grams of EPA + DHA per day, in the form of capsules and under a physician's care, are recommended.

**Source:** Reproduced with permission, www.heart.org, © 2011 American Heart Association, Inc.

## Drawbacks of Megadoses

Megadose vitamins and minerals remain popular. But when taken without recommendation or prescription from a qualified health professional, they can cause problems. Because high doses of a nutrient can act as a drug, with a drug's risk of adverse side effects, people who choose to take megadoses should always check first with their doctors.

Excesses of some nutrients can create deficits of other nutrients. High doses of supplemental minerals, especially calcium, iron, zinc, and copper, can interfere with absorption of the others.[25] In general, it's riskier to megadose with minerals than with vitamins.

It's easy to reach toxic levels if you use high doses of the fat-soluble vitamins A and D. Vitamins E and K appear relatively safe, although at high doses vitamin E can interfere with normal use of vitamin K and blood clotting. Megadosing with water-soluble vitamin $B_6$ at 50 to 100 times the DV can cause nerve damage. You may want to review the DRI tables for tolerable upper intake levels (UL) for vitamins and minerals.

Megadoses often are recommended for sick people, but sick people may be least able to tolerate them. Supplemental iron, for example, is very hard on a sensitive digestive system, often causing constipation while high doses of vitamin C can cause diarrhea. Megadoses also can interfere with medications and treatments. Although some people who take antiseizure medications also may need folic acid supplementation, too much folic acid can allow "breakthrough seizures." Vitamin K interferes with medication to control blood clotting and should be taken only under a doctor's direction. People undergoing surgery should describe their nutritional supplements to their doctor because high-dose vitamin E, especially if accompanied by blood thinners such as ginkgo biloba, aspirin, or fish oil, can cause bleeding problems in the operating room. Antioxidant nutrients may counteract chemotherapy or radiation aimed at oxidative destruction of cancer cells.

**Key Concepts**  *High doses (megadoses) of vitamins or minerals turn nutrients into drugs—chemicals with pharmacological activity. Although there may be medical reasons for prescribing high-dose supplements, they should be taken under a physician's supervision. Many claims for high-dose supplements are not supported by clinical studies.*

## Dietary Supplements: Natural Health Products

Supplementation with herbal and other "natural" products is a popular form of complementary medicine. (See **Figure 3.9**.) The 1990s saw a dramatic rise in the popularity of dietary supplements. In the United States, more than 150 million people use dietary supplements, accounting for $26.9 billion in annual sales.[26] Health Canada estimates that 71 percent of Canadians have consumed natural health products: herbs, vitamins and minerals, and homeopathic products.[27] **Herbal therapy (phytotherapy)** is nothing new, however. Most cultures have long traditions of using plants (and some animal products) to treat illness or sustain health. For centuries there were no other medicines. Even now, most of the world's people depend primarily on plants for medications; in some remote areas, modern medicines are just not obtainable.

In the Western world, the feeling that "natural" is better than "chemical" or "synthetic" has launched the market for "natural" foods to a $12.9 billion industry, with "all natural" becoming the second most common claim to be found on new food labels in 2008.[28] Consumers interpret claims such as "100% natural" to mean the product is more wholesome, nutritious, and healthy.

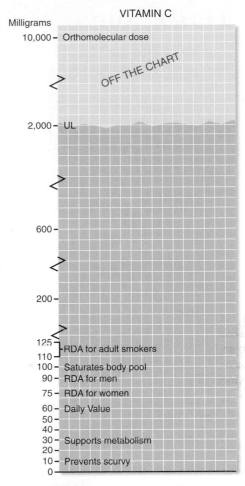

**Figure 3.8**  **Vitamin C megadoses.** Megadoses of vitamin C are much higher intakes than currently recommended.

**herbal therapy (phytotherapy)**  The therapeutic use of herbs and other plants to promote health and treat disease. Also called *phytotherapy*.

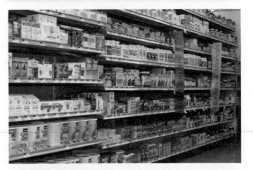

**Figure 3.9**  **Use of herbal supplements is growing in popularity.** Use of herbal supplements grew nearly eightfold during the last decade.

## *Quick* Bite

### Culinary Herbs Are Not Medicinal Herbs—Or Are They?

Herbs used in cooking are called *culinary herbs* to distinguish them from medicinal herbs. But culinary herbs are also rich in phytochemicals. Some examples are beta-carotene in paprika, the antioxidants in rosemary, the mild antibiotic allicin in garlic, and the mild antiviral curcumin in turmeric.

**National Center for Complementary and Alternative Medicine (NCCAM)** An NIH organization established to stimulate, develop, and support objective scientific research on complementary and alternative medicine for the benefit of the public.

**National Institutes of Health (NIH)** A Department of Health and Human Services agency composed of 27 separate institutes and centers with a mission to advance knowledge and improve human health.

THINK
About It

3

People who decide to use herbs instead of conventional medicines must choose their practitioners carefully. Herbalists must know their herbs, but they also must know when to tell patients to seek conventional care. People who use both an herbalist and a conventional doctor should tell both practitioners about the other and disclose all treatments.

Herbalists reason that natural products are likely to contain a complex of healing ingredients, whereas a purified pharmaceutical product contains only one or two. They believe that when active ingredients are combined with many other plant components their side effects may be blunted or neutralized. Using herbal medicine sounds simple and easy, but, in fact, herbalism calls for a great deal of skill. Traditional healers typically serve long apprenticeships and acquire a subjective "feel" for their therapies after much experience. They must learn to judge the safety and potency of individual plants, which vary from season to season, location to location, part of the plant, and age of the plant. They must know how to prepare the plant—whether to extract it and with what, or how to make it into a salve or an oral preparation. They must know how to blend it with other herbs and with other therapies. In traditional Chinese medicine, for example, a blend of herbs, sometimes 30 or more, can be used at once; the mixture usually is simmered in water and taken as a tea or "soup." Other herbal traditions use only one or two carefully chosen herbs at a time.

Traditional herbalists know their patients and individualize their herbal remedies accordingly. In the United States, that includes knowing results of diagnostic testing; in other cultures it includes recognizing and understanding symptoms. But those who turn to the mass market for herbal supplements rarely receive such attention and are likely to be confused by nutrition and health-related claims that surround foods and supplements.

## Helpful Herbs, Harmful Herbs

Until recently, most research on herbs had been published in obscure or foreign-language journals that were hard to locate or read. Traditional herbal medical practices are difficult to study in a controlled manner because they use plants to make teas or soups, a far cry from the purified extracts and herbal blends sold in a supermarket. Nevertheless, for some herbs, researchers have enough data to plan carefully controlled studies.

The mission of the **National Center for Complementary and Alternative Medicine (NCCAM)** within the **National Institutes of Health (NIH)** is to "define the usefulness and safety of CAM interventions and their roles in improving health and health care" through rigorous scientific investigation.[29] Some examples include:

- Scientific evidence suggests that St. John's wort may be useful for short-term treatment of mild to moderate depression.[30]
- Milk thistle may be helpful for liver disease, but more research is needed.[31]
- Studies on Ginkgo biloba have found it to be ineffective in lowering the overall incidence of dementia and Alzheimer's disease in older adults, improving memory, slowing cognitive decline, lowering blood pressure, or reducing the incidence of hypertension.[32]
- Several small studies indicate that saw palmetto extract may improve symptoms in men with benign prostate enlargement, but a recent review of the research found no difference between saw palmetto and the placebo.[33]

- Drinking cranberry juice may discourage urinary tract infections by inhibiting harmful bacteria from sticking to the lining of the urinary tract.[34] However, recent evidence from an NCCAM-supported study suggests that cranberry juice is not more effective in preventing the reoccurrence of urinary tract infections than a placebo.[35]

The suggested benefits of other herbs are based not on scientific study but on years of informal observation: Mint helps indigestion; ginger helps nausea and motion sickness; lemon perks appetite; chamomile helps insomnia.

If you're considering using an herb, remember this important rule of thumb: Any herb that is strong enough to help you can be strong enough to hurt you. Like any medicine, herbs can have side effects, and herbs can be contraindicated. Ginkgo biloba is a blood thinner and can cause harmful bleeding in some people.[36] Just like any other new, unusual substance, herbs can cause sudden allergic reactions.

Herbs can interfere with standard medicines,[37] and they can make people with underlying health problems quite sick. For example, licorice extract—even as a flavoring in chewing tobacco—flushes potassium from the body, raises blood pressure, and can interfere with blood pressure medication.[38] (Most licorice candy is now flavored synthetically; naturally flavored licorice has little effect unless routinely eaten in large amounts.) St. John's wort interacts with many commonly used medications, including oral contraceptives, blood thinners, and antidepressants, as well as drugs used in the treatment of HIV/AIDS, and could lead to serious clinical consequences.[39] Table 3.5 lists some possible interactions of herbs and drugs.

Some herbs and herbalist treatments are downright dangerous. (See Table 3.6.) Some hazardous therapies even use lead or arsenic, known poisons. St. John's wort, ginseng, ginkgo biloba, garlic, grapefruit juice, hawthorn, saw palmetto, danshen, echinacea, yohimbe, licorice, and black cohosh are just some common herbal remedies known to be potentially dangerous for people taking medications for cardiovascular disease.[40] Other herbs, such as ephedra (ma huang), chaparral, and comfrey, have also been shown to be dangerous. Senna, cascara, and rhubarb are powerful laxatives used in products described as "colon cleansers," "colon purifiers," or even "blood purifiers"; their overuse is

THINK
About It
**4**

## Table 3.5    Selected Herb–Drug Interactions

| Herb | Drug | Interaction |
|------|------|-------------|
| Feverfew, garlic, ginger, ginkgo biloba, guarana, and pau d'Arco | Warafin, aspirin | Increases anticoagulant effect by inhibiting platelet aggregation. |
| Hawthorn and horse chestnut | Digoxin, diuretics | Affects cardiac function and blood pressure; should not be taken with digoxin and diuretics. |
| Aloe, senna (laxative), cascara, and licorice | Digoxin, diuretics | Causes electrolyte imbalance; true licorice increases blood pressure. Do not take with digoxin and diuretics. |
| Kava and valerian | Anxiolytics, narcotics, alcohol | Increases sedative effects. |
| St. John's wort | Antidepressants, crixivan (indinavir) and other protease inhibitors, cyclosporine | Should not be taken with prescription antidepressants; risk of hypertensive crisis if taken with antidepressants. St. John's wort makes several prescription medications used in the treatment of AIDS less effective. The herb speeds up activity in a key pathway responsible for breaking down these drugs in the body. When the medications are taken with St. John's wort, blood levels of the drugs decrease because the body breaks them down faster. |

Table 3.6  **Potential Adverse Effects of Selected Herbs**

| Herb | Adverse Effects |
| --- | --- |
| Chamomile (tea) | Allergic reaction; digestive upset |
| Chaparral | Liver toxicity |
| Comfrey | Liver and kidney disease |
| Echinacea | Allergic reaction; stimulation of immune system; not for use by those with systemic/autoimmune diseases |
| Ephedra | Insomnia; headaches; nervousness; seizures; increased blood pressure; stroke; death |
| Ginkgo biloba | Inhibits blood clotting; do not take with aspirin, anticoagulants, or vitamin E; mild gastrointestinal upset; headaches; dizziness |
| Ginseng | Headaches; insomnia; diarrhea; heart palpitations; increased bleeding time |
| Kava | Slowed reaction time; scaly dermatitis; liver damage |
| Licorice | Headaches; fluid retention; increased blood pressure; electrolyte imbalance; heart failure |
| Pau d'Arco | Severe nausea and vomiting; anemia; bleeding tendencies |
| Pennyroyal | Liver damage; convulsions; abortions; coma; death; oil is very toxic |
| St. John's wort | Adverse interactions with antidepressants and HIV/AIDS medications; possible photosensitivity; gastrointestinal symptoms; headaches; dizziness |
| Senna | Laxative dependency; diarrhea; cramps; electrolyte disturbances |
| Valerian | Drowsiness; withdrawal symptoms if abruptly discontinued |

**Source:** Adapted from McGuffin M, Hobbs C, Upton R, Goldberg A. *American Herbal Products Association Botanical Safety Handbook.* Boca Raton, FL: CRC Press; 1997; Sarubin Fragakis A. *The Health Professional's Guide to Popular Dietary Supplements.* 3rd ed. Chicago: Academy of Nutrition and Dietetics; 2007; and Foster S, Tyler VE. *Tyler's Honest Herbal: A Sensible Guide to the Use of Herbs and Related Remedies.* Binghamton, NY: Haworth Herbal Press; 1999.

as damaging as overuse of conventional laxatives. In fact, in November 2002 the FDA ruled that aloe and cascara sagrada are not GRAS and therefore cannot be used in over-the-counter laxatives. In February 2004, the FDA issued a final rule prohibiting the sale of dietary supplements containing ephedra. Health Canada requested a recall of similar products in 2002. Also in 2002, both Health Canada and the FDA issued advisories warning consumers not to use products containing kava due to European reports of liver toxicity. In the United States, the ban on ephedra was overturned in a federal court in 2005, a ruling that the FDA subsequently appealed. In 2007, the FDA was granted a summary judgment in its favor.

Herbal blends marketed for specific conditions, such as "healthy bone formula" or "female blend," do not always make sense in light of current scientific knowledge. For example, pennyroyal and St. John's wort—herbs that should not be used during pregnancy—have shown up in some "prenatal formulas." Also, a popular blend used to treat prostate cancer actually had hormonal (estrogenic) activity, which promotes the growth of cancer cells.[41] Herbal preparations and teas marketed and sold specifically for infants were given to almost 1 out of 10 infants by their mothers for conditions such as teething, colic, and digestion problems as well as to help the infant relax and reduce fussiness; however, these products could contain potentially harmful contaminants or heavy metals and could cause serious adverse effects or interactions with medications.[42] Recently, products marketed as "male enhancers" containing ginseng, ginkgo biloba, l-arginine, and *Tribulus terrestris* extract, in addition to niacin, zinc, and copper, were found to cause changes in heart function in healthy men.[43]

Although many dietary supplements are probably safe, some, however, contain active ingredients or contaminants that have the potential to cause serious harm.[44] Quality control is a big issue in herbal medicines. The Government Accounting Office found that 92 percent of herbal supplements sampled contained trace amounts of lead and 80 percent contained one other contaminant, such as mercury.[45] Other contaminants have caused acute illness and death. A common problem is poorly standardized strength, or potency.[46] For example, red yeast rice, a common dietary supplement used by millions as a treatment for high cholesterol, was found to have a high variability in the active compound (called monacolin) that prevents the liver from synthesizing cholesterol, and one-third of the products were contaminated with a potentially harmful compound.[47] In 2007, the FDA issued final regulations requiring current good manufacturing practices (cGMPs) for the manufacturing, packaging, labeling, and storage of dietary supplements. Under the regulations, manufacturers are required to evaluate the identity, purity, strength, and composition of their products and ensure proper labeling.[48]

The use of traditional Chinese medicines are gaining popularity throughout the world. However, only recently have scientists begun to investigate techniques to improve the quality control to ensure the safety, efficacy, and consistency of these products, which contain hundreds of different chemically active compounds.[49]

To guarantee quality, each step from field to market must be monitored carefully. However, monitoring the production of herbal supplements poses special challenges. Herbs are grown and harvested in far-flung, sometimes remote areas of the world. Extraction or preparation of the herbs may take place somewhere else. Mixing the herbs and putting them in capsules, tonics, or teas typically takes place in yet another location.

## Other Dietary Supplements

The supplement market used to include only vitamins, minerals, and a handful of other products, such as brewer's yeast and sea salt. Today there are hundreds more products, with new ones continuously popping up. Although some are useful, many are of dubious benefit.

Supplement categories now include protein powders, amino acids, carotenoids, **bioflavonoids**, digestive aids, fatty acid formulas and special fats, lecithin and phospholipids, probiotics, products from sharks and other sea animals, algae, metabolites such as coenzyme Q10 and nucleic acids, glandular extracts, garlic products, and fibers such as guar gum. Supplement producers also blend these products with herbs and nutrients, resulting in the countless array of individual and combination supplements sold today. In many cases, labeling and advertising claims go beyond current knowledge about these products.

**Key Concepts** *Herbal products are among the many dietary supplements available today. Herbal medicine has a long history in many cultures. Although there is anecdotal support for the use of many herbal products, there is little scientific evidence to back it up. The FDA has set standards for production and sale of herbal supplements. It is important to remember that any herb that is strong enough to help you can also be strong enough to hurt you. Before taking any supplements, it's a good idea to consult your health care practitioner.*

## Dietary Supplements in the Marketplace

Although some dietary supplements have druglike actions (e.g., reducing cholesterol levels), government agencies regulate supplements differently

*Quick* Bite

**Office of Dietary Supplements**
The Office of Dietary Supplements (ODS) is a Congressionally mandated office in the National Institutes of Health (NIH). The Mission of ODS is to strengthen knowledge and understanding of dietary supplements by evaluating scientific information, stimulating and supporting research, disseminating research results, and educating the public to foster an enhanced quality of life and health for the U.S. population.

**bioflavonoids** Naturally occurring plant chemicals, especially from citrus fruits, that reduce the permeability and fragility of capillaries.

Maintains a healthy circulatory system
Maintains a healthy immune system

Helps you relax
Enhances libido
For muscle
enhancement

• For common symptoms of PMS
• For hot flashes
• For morning sickness

!

Beware the
exclamation point

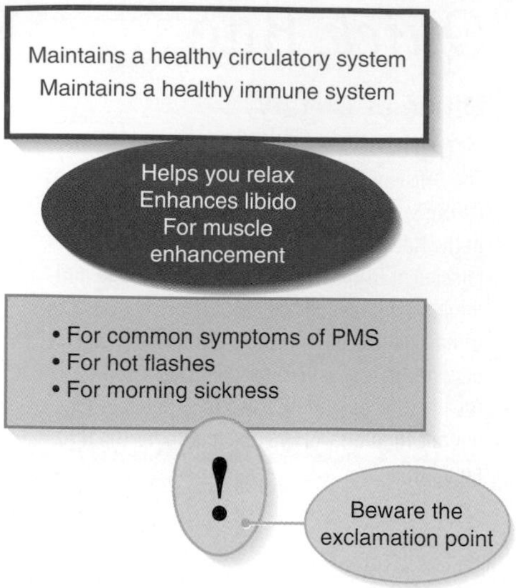

**Figure 3.10** **Dietary supplement label claims.** Although claims such as these appear on dietary supplement labels, they do not have to be approved by the FDA. All should be viewed with skepticism.

**Dietary Supplement Health and Education Act (DSHEA)** Legislation that regulates dietary supplements.

**Supplement Facts panel** Content label that must appear on all dietary supplements.

*Quick* Bite

**Pronouncing the Acronym**
The Dietary Supplement Health and Education Act of 1994 is better known by its acronym DSHEA, pronounced "da-shay."

from drugs. Manufacturers are allowed to make a wide variety of claims for product effects without having to provide scientific evidence to support those claims. The freedoms of speech and press prevail; in practical terms, almost anything goes. Promotional books, magazine articles, audio- and videotapes, lectures, staged interviews, and messages posted on Internet chat rooms—all are protected by the First Amendment, and their authors have the freedom to inform or to deceive. It's up to the listener or reader to distinguish fact from fiction. (See **Figure 3.10**.)

## The FTC and Supplement Advertising

The Federal Trade Commission (FTC) in the U.S. Department of Commerce is responsible for ensuring that advertisements and commercials are truthful and do not mislead. The agency depends on and encourages self-monitoring by the supplement industry. In pursuing companies that skirt the regulations, the FTC gives priority to cases that seriously put people's health and safety at risk or that affect sick and vulnerable consumers. The FTC's Operation Cure All targets false and unsubstantiated claims on the Internet.[50]

## The FDA and Supplement Regulation

The Food and Drug Administration has primary responsibility for regulating labeling and content of dietary supplements under the Federal Food, Drug, and Cosmetic Act, as amended by the 1994 **Dietary Supplement Health and Education Act (DSHEA)**.[51] How do you know a product is a "dietary supplement"? Simple. The law defines *dietary supplements*, in part, as products that are taken by mouth that contain a "dietary ingredient."[52] Dietary supplements include vitamins, minerals, herbs or botanicals, and amino acids as well as other substances, such as enzymes, organ tissues, metabolites, extracts, or concentrates, used to supplement the diet.

Dietary supplements are *not* drugs. A drug is intended to diagnose, cure, mitigate, treat, or prevent disease. Before marketing, drugs must undergo extensive studies of effectiveness, safety, interactions with other substances, and dosing. The FDA gives formal premarket approval to a drug and monitors its safety after the drug is on the market. If a drug is subsequently shown to be dangerous, the FDA can act quickly to have it removed from the market. None of this is true for dietary supplements.

Dietary supplements and their ingredients are *not* food additives, which also are subject to premarket approval. For new ingredients in dietary supplements, the manufacturer finds information (usually not scientific proof) to show the substance is safe if used as directed and submits this information to the FDA 75 days before the supplement is first marketed. However, formal approval by the FDA is not required. A new dietary supplement that contains ingredients already in use does not require such advance notification. Unlike pharmaceutical manufacturers, who must prove the safety and efficacy of their products before they sell them, supplement manufacturers can market their products without the FDA's approval. To restrict the sale and use of a dietary supplement, the FDA must prove that it isn't safe after it is on the market, a process that can take years.

## Supplement Labels

Like food labels, supplement labels have mandatory and optional information. All labels on dietary supplements must include ingredient information and a **Supplement Facts panel**.[53] You'll notice in **Figure 3.11** that the format is similar to the Nutrition Facts panel on food labels. However, a Supplement

Facts panel can include substances for which no Daily Value has been established. In combination products, any nutrients with Daily Values are listed first, followed by other dietary ingredients. Herbal ingredients must list the plant part, such as the root or leaf.

**Serving Size** is the manufacturer's suggested serving expressed in the appropriate unit (tablet, capsule, softgel, packet, teaspoonful).

**Each Tablet Contains** heads the listing of dietary ingredients contained in the supplement.

Each dietary ingredient is followed by the quantity in a serving. For proprietary blends, total weight of the blend is listed, with components listed in descending order by weight.

Dietary ingredients that have no Daily Value are listed below this line.

Botanical supplements must list the part of plant present and its common name (Latin name if common name not listed in *Herbs of Commerce*).

**List of Ingredients** shows the nutrients and other ingredients used to formulate the supplement, in decreasing order by weight.

**Contact Information** shows the manufacturer's or distributor's name, address, and zip code.

# Supplement Facts

Serving Size 1 Tablet

| Each Tablet Contains | | %DV |
|---|---|---|
| Vitamin A  5,000 IU | | 100% |
| 50% as Beta-Carotene | | |
| Vitamin C | 90 mg | 150% |
| Vitamin D | 400 IU | 100% |
| Vitamin E | 45 IU | 150% |
| Thiamin | 1.5 mg | 100% |
| Riboflavin | 1.7 mg | 100% |
| Niacin | 20 mg | 100% |
| Vitamin B$_6$ | 2 mg | 100% |
| Folate | 400 mcg | 100% |
| Vitamin B$_{12}$ | 6 mcg | 100% |
| Calcium | 100 mg | 10% |
| Iron | 18 mg | 100% |
| Iodine | 150 mcg | 100% |
| Magnesium | 100 mg | 25% |
| Zinc | 15 mg | 100% |
| Ginseng Root | | |
| (*Panax ginseng*)  25 mg | | * |
| Ginkgo Biloba Leaf | | |
| (*Ginkgo biloba*)  25 mg | | * |
| Citrus Bioflavonoids | | |
| Complex  10 mg | | * |
| Lecithin (*Glycine max*) | | |
| (bean)  10 mg | | * |
| Nickel | 5 mcg | * |
| Silicon | 2 mcg | * |
| Boron | 60 mcg | * |

* Daily Value (%DV) not established

**%DV** indicates the percentage of the Daily Value of each nutrient that a serving provides.

An **asterisk** under %DV indicates that a Daily Value is not established for that ingredient.

**INGREDIENTS:** Dicalcium Phosphate, Magnesium Oxide, Ascorbic Acid, Cellulose, Vitamin A Acetate, Beta-Carotene, Vitamin D, dl-Alpha Tocopherol Acetate, Ginseng Root (*Panax ginseng*), Gelatin, Ginkgo Biloba Leaf (*Ginkgo biloba*), Ferrous Fumarate, Niacinamide, Zinc Oxide, Silicon Dioxide, Lecithin, Citrus Bioflavonoids Complex, Pyridoxine Hydrochloride, Riboflavin, Thiamin Mononitrate, Folic Acid, Potassium Iodine, Boron, Cyanocobalamin, Nickelous Sulfate

DISTRIBUTED BY COMPANY NAME
P.O. BOX XXX
CITY, STATE 00000-0000

**Figure 3.11  Supplement Facts panel.** Similar to the Nutrition Facts panel on food labels, the Supplement Facts panel required on dietary supplement labels shows the product composition.

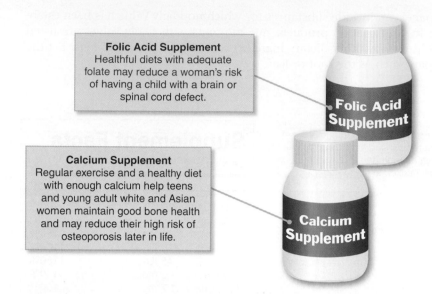

**Folic Acid Supplement**
Healthful diets with adequate folate may reduce a woman's risk of having a child with a brain or spinal cord defect.

**Calcium Supplement**
Regular exercise and a healthy diet with enough calcium help teens and young adult white and Asian women maintain good bone health and may reduce their high risk of osteoporosis later in life.

**Figure 3.12** **Health claims for supplements.** Calcium and folic acid supplements may carry health claims similar to these model statements.
**Source:** Data from U.S. Food and Drug Administration.

Supplement labels, like food labels, may contain health claims, structure/function claims, and nutrient content claims. However, only a few of the health claims approved for foods are appropriate for dietary supplements. "Adequate calcium may reduce risk of osteoporosis" and "adequate folate intake by women reduces risk of neural tube defects in newborns" are examples of health claims that could appear on supplement labels. (See **Figure 3.12**.) Qualified health claims may also apply to dietary supplements.

"Antioxidants maintain cell integrity," "fiber maintains bowel regularity," and "St. John's wort enhances mood" are examples of structure/function claims that might appear on supplement labels. Structure/function claims also may describe the link between a nutrient and a deficiency disease (like vitamin C and scurvy), as long as the statement also mentions the prevalence of the disease in the United States. Manufacturers can use structure/function claims without FDA authorization and can base their claims on their own review and interpretation of the scientific literature.

Structure/function claims are easy to spot because they are accompanied by the disclaimer "This statement has not been evaluated by the Food and Drug Administration. This product is not intended to diagnose, treat, cure, or prevent any disease."[54] There is often a fine line between structure/function claims and claims that would make the product an unauthorized drug. For example, the claim "promotes urinary tract health" on a bottle of cranberry extract capsules would be allowable, whereas "prevents urinary tract infections" would not. A dietary supplement with a label claiming to cure or treat a specific condition is considered an unapproved drug.[55]

Nutrient content claims must be consistent with definitions approved for foods. With few exceptions, nutrient content claims can be made only for a nutrient or dietary substance that has an established Daily Value.

For dietary ingredients without a Daily Value, manufacturers may describe the amount of the ingredient. Examples include simple percentage statements, such as "40% *omega*-3 fatty acids, 10 mg per capsule," and comparative percentage claims, such as "twice the *omega*-3 fatty acids per capsule (80 mg) as in 100 mg of menhaden oil (40 mg)."[56]

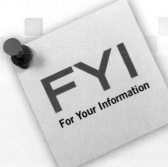

# Shopping for Supplements

Thinking about buying a dietary supplement? Before you do, ask yourself, "Why do I need this supplement?" and "Is it suitable for me?" Think about your typical diet and what it may be lacking. Remember, the word *supplement* means just that—a product meant to supplement your food. A well-chosen supplement can be beneficial under some circumstances, especially if your diet is limited. However, if you're healthy and eat a good balance of healthful foods, supplements won't help you much.

It's a good idea to let your doctor know your supplement plans. Some supplements are contraindicated during pregnancy or lactation; others should not be used with certain chronic illnesses. Supplements sometimes interfere with the action of medicines. Some slow blood clotting, which is a concern if surgery is planned.

To a great extent, you will need to rely on your own understanding of diet and nutrition to make your selection. And, you must rely on the supplement manufacturer for the product's safety, its purity and cleanliness, and the label's accuracy. If you are concerned about potential side effects or contraindications, you will probably need to contact the manufacturer or distributor.

## Choose Quality

In 2010, the FDA finalized guidelines for current good manufacturing practices by supplement manufacturers.[1] Additionally, you should also use tip-offs to judge a quality company—the kind you would expect to have good quality control procedures and to manufacture, store, and transport products safely and carefully.

A quality company will not promise miracles on its website, in catalogues, in commercials or advertisements, or in in-store promotions. Promises to make you smarter or thinner (unless you cut calories along with taking the supplement), to keep you young, to increase or decrease the size of various body parts, and so forth, should raise a red flag. A quality company will not manipulate statistics or distort research findings in an attempt to mislead you.

A quality company will take care with its labels, print materials, and web information. Misspelling of terms; confusion of milligrams, grams, and micrograms; and omission on labels of important or required information are indicators of the manufacturer's carelessness or ignorance.

## Confirm Supplement Ingredients

Use resources that analyze and confirm supplement content, dose, and purity. ConsumerLab.com (http://www.consumerlab.com) is one such service. Pharmaceutical researchers also report findings on supplement label accuracy; a search on PubMed (http://www.nlm.nih.gov) can lead you to this information.

Look for the U.S. Pharmacopeia (USP) logo (USP verification mark) on supplement labels.

The mark certifies that the USP has found the ingredients consistent with those stated on the label; that the supplement has been manufactured in a safe, sanitary, controlled facility; and that the product dissolves or disintegrates to release nutrients in the body. (However, the USP does not test the supplement's efficacy.)

## Choose Freshness

Finding the freshest supplement is often easier if you shop in a retail store. Avoid dust-covered containers. Choose a store where turnover is likely to be quick. Supplements should be displayed away from direct sunlight, bright lights, or nearby heat sources, because heat ages many supplements. Expiration dates also can give you a clue regarding freshness.

## Expect Accountability

How easily can you obtain information about the product? Look for a phone number on the label so you can call with questions or to report side effects. On websites, look for a domestic address and phone number, in addition to an email contact. Does a knowledgeable company representative respond to your questions, or is the only person available one who reads a scripted response?

If you're shopping online but are uncertain the supplement is right for you, check the web retailer's return policy. A web retailer that also has a brick-and-mortar outlet near your locale may be preferable.

1. Food and Drug Administration. Guidance for industry: current good manufacturing practice in manufacturing, packaging, labeling, or holding operations for dietary supplements; small entity compliance guide, December 2010. http://www.fda.gov/Food/GuidanceComplianceRegulatoryInformation/GuidanceDocuments/SmallBusinessesSmallEntityComplianceGuides/ucm238182.htm. Accessed 6/23/11.

### Be a Safe and Informed Consumer

When buying supplements, follow this advice from the Food and Drug Administration:

- Let your health care professional advise you on sorting reliable information from questionable information.
- Contact the manufacturer for information about the product you intend to use.
- Be aware that some supplement ingredients, including nutrients and plant components, can be toxic. Also, some ingredients and products can be harmful when consumed in high amounts, when taken for a long time, or when used in combination with certain other drugs, substances, or foods.
- Do not self-diagnose any health condition. Work with health care professionals to determine how best to achieve optimal health.
- Do not substitute a dietary supplement for a prescription medicine or therapy, or for the variety of foods important to a healthful diet.
- Do not assume that the term *natural* in relation to a product ensures that the product is wholesome or safe.
- Be wary of hype and headlines. Sound health advice is generally based upon research over time, not a single study.
- Learn to spot false claims. If something sounds too good to be true, it probably is.

**Source:** Food and Drug Administration. FDA 101: dietary supplements. http://www.fda.gov/Forconsumers/ConsumerUpdates/ucm050803.htm. Accessed 10/4/11.

## Canadian Regulations

Beginning January 1, 2004, all natural health products sold in Canada are subject to Health Canada's *Natural Health Products Regulations*.[57] By definition, natural health products include vitamins, minerals, herbal remedies, and homeopathic medicines. Health Canada has developed a product approval system whereby each product must meet the requirements of the *Natural Health Products Regulations* to acquire a license and be legally sold in Canada. Authorization requires evidence of safety and efficacy. The regulations also include provisions on site licensing, good manufacturing practices, labeling and packaging requirements, and adverse reaction reporting. The Canadian regulations go much further than DSHEA in terms of assuring the safety and efficacy of supplements.

**Key Concepts**  *Dietary supplements are neither foods nor drugs, and the government regulates their manufacture and sale differently than it does for foods, additives, and drugs. The FTC and FDA monitor advertising and labeling of dietary supplements. A Supplement Facts panel is now required on labels. Canada's regulations for natural health products require premarket approval and product licensing.*

## Choosing Dietary Supplements

DSHEA has made many improvements, such as the Supplement Facts panel, to help consumers choose dietary supplements wisely. By loosening previous restrictions, DSHEA also has made many more products available to consumers. However, with the resulting array of supplements, it is a challenge for the FDA to effectively monitor claims, quality, and safety. Because manufacturers can market their products without prior approval, you need to be wary. (For tips on choosing supplements, see the FYI feature "Shopping for Supplements.") Knowledge of nutrition science is your most valuable tool for evaluating a supplement. Read each label and judge each implied claim in light of what you know. Ask the following questions:

- *Is the quantity enough to have an effect or is it trivial?* Consider amino acids, for example. A product contains 25 milligrams of glycine. How does this compare to the amount of glycine you would obtain from a diet with 70 grams of protein? Has glycine been added to the product, or is it a component of the gelatin capsule? Is glycine an essential or a nonessential amino acid? What will happen if you take more than you need?
- *Is the product new to you?* Learn about it from the many reliable resources available. Evaluate the product in light of scientific research. Has it been studied in humans, rodents, or other animals, or only in cell cultures or *in vitro*? If in humans, was the study controlled to eliminate a placebo effect? For case report studies, could the placebo effect influence the results? Consider the type of preparation and the route of administration. An injected herbal extract may have a very different effect than the same herb in a pill.
- *Can the supplement cross the intestine and travel to its presumed site of action in the body?* The body digests enzyme preparations, for example, along with other proteins. There are little data on the absorption and **bioavailability** of herbal preparations and other types of non-nutrient supplements.
- *Can this supplement interact with any prescription or over-the-counter medications?* Some combinations of supplements or using some supplements together with either prescription or OTC medications could produce potentially harmful adverse effects.

**bioavailability** A measure of the extent to which a nutrient becomes available to the body after ingestion and thus is available to the tissues.

Consumers should check for advisories about these products, whether taken alone or in combination with other supplements or medications.

- *Does the product promise too much?* A product touted to control high blood cholesterol, hangnails, psoriasis, and insomnia is unlikely to do much of anything. Neither will a "low-calorie, high-energy" drink. It is possible that the same results can be achieved more cheaply and more enjoyably by eating regular foods. Why take lycopene capsules when you can eat tomatoes, even ketchup? Why take bilberry extract when blueberries (the American equivalent to European bilberries) are delicious and low in calories?
- *Who is selling the product?* Alternative practitioners, dietitians, and even physicians sometimes sell the supplements they recommend— which is a possible conflict of interest that could compromise their objectivity. The Academy of Nutrition and Dietetics has issued guidelines for practitioners' recommendations and sales of supplements.[58] In **multilevel marketing**, someone at each level in the system takes a commission on the supplements you buy, so expect to pay extra. When you buy a supplement over the phone, by catalogue, or over the web, you lose the chance to examine it before you buy it.

**multilevel marketing** A system of selling in which each salesperson recruits assistants who then recruit others to help them. The person at each level collects a commission on sales made by the later recruits.

**U.S. Pharmacopeia (USP)** Established in 1820, the USP is a nonprofit health care organization that sets quality standards for a range of health care products.

A good indicator of quality is the **U.S. Pharmacopeia (USP)** verification mark (see **Figure 3.13**), which verifies that the product meets the U.S. Pharmacopeia's standards for product purity, accuracy of ingredient labeling, and proper manufacturing practices.[59] Established in 1820, the USP is a voluntary, nonprofit organization that sets quality standards for a range of health care products, including prescription and nonprescription medicines, biotechnology drugs, vitamins and minerals, and other dietary supplements. The USP verification mark helps assure consumers, health care professionals, and supplement retailers that a product has passed USP's rigorous program and:

- Contains the ingredients declared on the product label
- Contains the amount or strength of ingredients declared on the product label
- Meets requirements for limits on potential contaminants
- Has been manufactured properly by complying with USP and FDA standards for current good manufacturing practices (cGMPs)

Many nationally known food and drug manufacturers have established their own standards, quality control, and manufacturing practices that they are likely to apply to their dietary supplements as well. Contact the company with your questions; you'll learn a lot, although maybe not what you expected. The "technical representative" may be unable to give you any more information than a brief readout from a computer database. Some companies respond to queries by sending a long printout of journal citations, most of them inappropriate, without text or even abstracts; many references are in a foreign language. However, some dietary supplement companies have on-site quality control and on-site nutritionists who are knowledgeable and happy to supply helpful information. Even the best-intentioned, most carefully considered supplement can prove ineffective or even risky. Take the example of beta-carotene supplements. Even though diets rich in beta-carotene are linked with reduced cancer risk, several large well-controlled studies found that beta-carotene supplements had no protective effect. For some groups of people, such as smokers, these supplements actually increased risk.[60] The

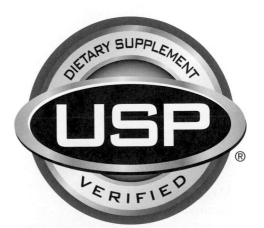

**Figure 3.13**  **U.S. Pharmacopeia verification mark.** Dietary supplements can earn the USP-Verified mark through a comprehensive product testing and evaluation process and manufacturing site audit.

**Source:** Reprinted with permission from The United States Pharmacopeial Convention, 12601 Twinbrook Parkway, Rockville, Maryland 20852.

## Quick Bite

**Jell-O and Your Nails**
You may have heard that taking gelatin can make your nails stronger. Not true. Fingernails get their strength from sulfur in amino acids. Gelatin has no sulfur-containing amino acids.

## Quick Bite

**Mayonnaise Protects Against Strokes**
Is this claim science or snake oil? Studies show that foods rich in vitamin E help protect against heart disease and stroke. In one study of stroke reduction in postmenopausal women, mayonnaise was the most concentrated food source of vitamin E. But to claim that mayonnaise prevents strokes is unwarranted and overstates the evidence.

results disappointed advocates of beta-carotene, but these studies demonstrate the value of carefully controlled studies and the risk of unproved assumptions about dietary supplements.

## Fraudulent Products

Some health advocates consider the burgeoning market of dietary supplements an unwelcome return to the "snake oil" era of the late nineteenth and early twentieth centuries, when "magic" potions and cures were sold door to door and at county fairs and markets. Most manufacturers work hard to ensure the quality of their products, yet some supplements on the market are nothing more than a mixture of ineffective ingredients.

The Food and Drug Administration (FDA) has found nearly 300 fraudulent products that contain hidden or deceptively labeled ingredients.[61] Most frequently recalled products with potentially harmful ingredients are those that are promoted for weight loss, sexual enhancement, and bodybuilding. The FDA has advice for consumers using or considering the use of dietary supplements.[62] Consumers should look for potential warning signs of tainted products marketed as dietary supplements, such as:

- Products claiming to be alternatives to FDA-approved drugs or to have effects similar to prescription drugs
- Products claiming to be a legal alternative to anabolic steroids
- Products that are marketed primarily in a foreign language or those that are marketed through mass e-mails
- Sexual enhancement products promising rapid effects, such as working in minutes to hours, or long-lasting effects, such as working for 24 to 72 hours
- Product labels warning that you may test positive in performance enhancement drug tests

Generally, if you are using or considering using any product marketed as a dietary supplement, the FDA suggests that you:

- Check with your health care professional or a registered dietician about any nutrients you may need in addition to your regular diet.
- Ask your health care professional for help distinguishing between reliable and questionable information.
- Ask yourself if it sounds too good to be true:
  - Be cautious if the claims for the product seem exaggerated or unrealistic.
  - Watch out for extreme claims—for example, "quick and effective," "cure-all," "can treat or cure diseases," or "totally safe."
  - Be skeptical about anecdotal information from personal "testimonials" about incredible benefits or results obtained from using a product.
  - See the FDA's website to help recognize fraudulent weight-loss products and claims.

Supplement users who suffer a serious harmful effect or illness that they think is related to supplement use should call a doctor or other health care provider. Practitioners and consumers can report problems and adverse reactions to the FDA's MedWatch by calling 1-800-FDA-1088 or by going to the MedWatch website.

**Key Concepts** *When considering a dietary supplement, it is important to consider the product and its claims carefully. Be aware that some products may promise more than they can deliver. A good indicator of quality is the USP verification mark, but even this does not guarantee that a product will fulfill its claims.*

# Complementary and Alternative Medicine

Complementary and alternative medicines (CAM) are therapies and treatments outside the medical mainstream. Historically they tended to be based mainly or solely on observation or anecdotal evidence rather than controlled research. According to the National Center for Complementary and Alternative Medicine:

> Defining CAM is difficult because the field is very broad and constantly changing. NCCAM defines CAM as a group of diverse medical and health care systems, practices, and products that are not generally considered part of conventional medicine. Conventional medicine (also called Western or allopathic medicine) is medicine as practiced by holders of M.D. (medical doctor) and D.O. (doctor of osteopathic medicine) degrees and by allied health professionals, such as physical therapists, psychologists, and registered nurses. The boundaries between CAM and conventional medicine are not absolute, and specific CAM practices may, over time, become widely accepted.[63]

The term *alternative* suggests practices that replace conventional ones. *Complementary* implies practices that are used *in addition to* conventional ones. A practice that combines both conventional and CAM treatments for which there is evidence of safety and effectiveness is referred to as *integrative*. For example, using only herbs and megavitamins to treat AIDS would be "alternative," whereas using herbs to combat diarrhea caused by conventional AIDS medications and taking supplements to replace lost vitamins would be "complementary." Many people find the terms *complementary* and *integrative* more acceptable than *alternative*, although all these terms often are used interchangeably. CAM includes a broad range of healing therapies and philosophies. Several among them involve nutrition, including special diet therapies, phytotherapy (herbalism), orthomolecular medicine, and other biologic interventions.

Almost 40 percent of adults and 12 percent of children in America use some form of CAM therapy.[64] Commonly used CAM therapies other than prayer are natural products, deep breathing exercises, meditation, chiropractic care, yoga, massage, and diet-based therapies. People seek out CAM for numerous reasons, including fear of aging, personal beliefs, and distrust of institutional medicine.

## Where Does Nutrition Fit In?

A number of alternative therapies involve nutrition, and sometimes the line between standard and alternative nutrition is not clear. A variety of health conditions, such as diabetes, gastrointestinal disorders, and kidney disease, require special diets. Alternative nutrition practices include diets to prevent and treat diseases not shown to be diet-related. (See **Figure 3.14**.) What often makes these practices "alternative" is the limited nature of the diet, the lack of rigorous scientific evidence showing effectiveness, and the divergence from science-based healthy eating patterns such as the DASH diet or MyPlate. Other practices outside the nutritional mainstream include reliance on only raw foods and the extensive use of herbal and botanical supplements as well as megadoses of vitamin/mineral supplements, which we have already discussed.

### *Vegetarian Diets*

Most nutritionists consider vegetarianism a routine variation of a normal diet, particularly if the vegetarian's motivation is religious or

*Quick* Bite

**The Yin and Yang of Food**
The early theory of yin and yang had its genesis during the Yin and Zhou dynasties (1766 B.C.E.–256 B.C.E.). The yin force is passive, downward flowing, and cold. Conversely, the yang force is aggressive, upward rising, and hot. The concept of balance and harmony between these life forces is the basis upon which food and herbs are used as medicine. In traditional Chinese healing methods, disease is viewed as the result of an imbalance of these energies in the body. To balance these energies, according to this view, your diet should balance yin foods and yang foods. Yin (cold) foods include milk, honey, fruit, and vegetables; yang (hot) foods include beef, poultry, seafood, eggs, and cheese. Foods are also classified as sweet (earth), bitter (fire), sour (wood), pungent (metal), and salty (water). Each class supposedly has specific effects on different parts of the body.

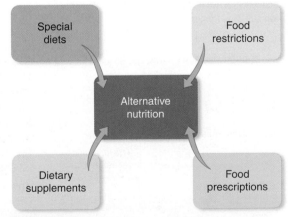

**Figure 3.14** **Alternative nutrition practices.** Although many mainstream medical practices may involve special dietary regimens, alternative nutrition practices often are overly restrictive, depart from established dietary guidelines, and lack rigorous scientific evidence.

philosophical, the result of a concern for animals, or an aversion to animal products. When a meat eater goes vegetarian in an attempt to prevent or cure disease, that's "alternative."

### Macrobiotic Diet

**macrobiotic diet** A highly restrictive dietary approach applied as a therapy for risk factors or chronic disease in general.

Aside from vegetarianism, the **macrobiotic diet** probably is the best-known alternative diet. The original version of this primarily vegetarian diet progressed in 10 increasingly restrictive stages, with the "highest level" consisting of little more than brown rice and water. The diet has since evolved to a simpler one-level regimen that emphasizes the consumption of fresh, nonprocessed food, as well as foods that are low in fat, whole grains and vegetables, and restricts the intake of fluids.[65] The composition of a macrobiotic diet may be changed depending on a person's health status and is associated with a persons' lifestyle and spiritual philosophy.[66]

Proponents tout the macrobiotic diet as a cure for a variety of illnesses, most notably cancer and cardiovascular disease. To use it as a cancer treatment, the practitioner individualizes the diet according to Eastern philosophy (yin and yang, whose symbol is shown in **Figure 3.15**) and location of the cancer. Critics say macrobiotic restrictions interfere with legitimate cancer treatment by causing weight loss and malnutrition in people who are already too thin from their illness and may potentially delay conventional treatment. Advocates of macrobiotics argue that undernutrition may help fight the cancer by starving it. It looks as if neither opinion is correct: Macrobiotic diets have not been found to prevent or cure cancer.[67]

Compared with the general public, those who follow a macrobiotic diet tend to have healthier blood lipid levels and lower blood pressure.[68] However, a diet that is low in calcium and vitamin D may contribute to the risk for osteoporosis. Pediatricians should be cautious to monitor growth and feeding patterns for children following this diet or other restrictive diets that could cause nutritional deficiencies.[69]

### Food Restrictions and Food Prescriptions

Societies throughout the world commonly use dietary changes to treat or prevent illness. The specifics vary from place to place, however, which suggests that they are based on cultural factors rather than science.

In recent years, we have seen yeast-free diets, dairy-free diets, sugar-free diets, white-flour-free diets, both low-carbohydrate and high-carbohydrate diets, both low-red-meat and high-red-meat diets, caffeine-free diets, salicylate-free diets, and more. We have been advised to load up on molasses, yogurt, honey, vinegar, oysters, mushrooms, and soy nuts. People with subjective symptoms such as headaches, fatigue, or back pain have been instructed to avoid irrational lists of "allergenic foods" based on "blood screening." We've also seen illogical instructions on how to combine foods, such as "don't eat applesauce and asparagus at the same meal." For weight loss, we've had grapefruit diets, hard-boiled-egg diets, cottage-cheese diets, water diets, high-fat diets, low-fat diets, and blue-foods-only diets; the list goes on and on.

Such fad diets come and go. Most often they are not based on science and eventually fail to interest people when they don't work. Those few that prove effective and have a scientific basis become integrated into conventional nutrition and diet therapy. (See **Figure 3.16**.)

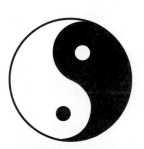

**Figure 3.15** **The symbol of yin and yang.** In traditional Chinese medicine, practitioners strive to balance the opposing life forces of yin and yang through the use of food and herbs.

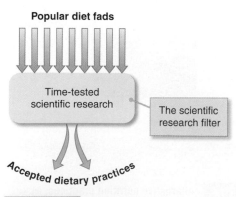

**Figure 3.16** **Many apply but few are chosen.** Dietary practices with a scientific basis and proven efficacy are incorporated into conventional nutrition and diet therapy.

**Key Concepts** *Many types of diets can be described as alternative. Their origins and claims vary, and their proponents often cannot show that they improve health. Some alternative diets can actually be harmful by restricting foods and thereby lowering the body's intake of necessary nutrients.*

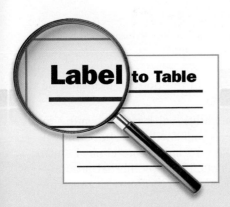

**Label to Table**

If you picked up a multivitamin/mineral container from your drugstore shelf, would you know how to read the label? Look at this Supplement Facts panel from a basic multivitamin/mineral supplement. Here are some questions that you might have.

1. If you were a 20-year-old woman who knew she wasn't consuming enough calcium, would this supplement allow you to get your recommended intake?
2. If 25 percent of the vitamin A in this supplement comes from beta-carotene, where does the rest come from?
3. What trend do you see in the amounts of B vitamins?
4. What trend do you see in the amounts of bone minerals?
5. What trend do you see in the amounts of antioxidant vitamins?

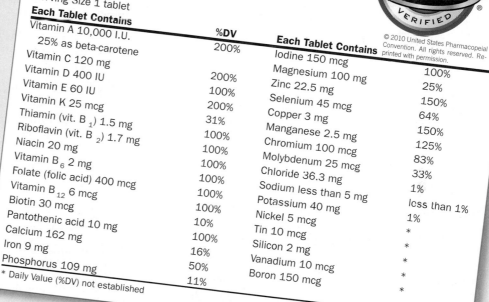

**Supplement Facts**
**Daily Multivitamin/Mineral Dietary Supplement**

USP  USP has tested and verified ingredients, potency, and manufacturing process. USP sets official standards for Dietary Supplements. For more information, go to www.uspverified.org.

Serving Size 1 tablet
**Each Tablet Contains**

| | %DV |
|---|---|
| Vitamin A 10,000 I.U. | 200% |
| 25% as beta-carotene | |
| Vitamin C 120 mg | 200% |
| Vitamin D 400 IU | 100% |
| Vitamin E 60 IU | 200% |
| Vitamin K 25 mcg | 31% |
| Thiamin (vit. B₁) 1.5 mg | 100% |
| Riboflavin (vit. B₂) 1.7 mg | 100% |
| Niacin 20 mg | 100% |
| Vitamin B₆ 2 mg | 100% |
| Folate (folic acid) 400 mcg | 100% |
| Vitamin B₁₂ 6 mcg | 100% |
| Biotin 30 mcg | 10% |
| Pantothenic acid 10 mg | 100% |
| Calcium 162 mg | 16% |
| Iron 9 mg | 50% |
| Phosphorus 109 mg | 11% |

* Daily Value (%DV) not established

© 2010 United States Pharmacopeial Convention. All rights reserved. Reprinted with permission.

**Each Tablet Contains**

| | |
|---|---|
| Iodine 150 mcg | 100% |
| Magnesium 100 mg | 25% |
| Zinc 22.5 mg | 150% |
| Selenium 45 mcg | 64% |
| Copper 3 mg | 150% |
| Manganese 2.5 mg | 125% |
| Chromium 100 mcg | 83% |
| Molybdenum 25 mcg | 33% |
| Chloride 36.3 mg | 1% |
| Sodium less than 5 mg | less than 1% |
| Potassium 40 mg | 1% |
| Nickel 5 mcg | * |
| Tin 10 mcg | * |
| Silicon 2 mg | * |
| Vanadium 10 mcg | * |
| Boron 150 mcg | * |

**Answers to Questions**

1. No. This supplement provides only 162 milligrams, and the Adequate Intake (AI) for a 20-year-old woman is 1,000 milligrams. You may need a calcium supplement if you can't eat enough calcium-rich foods.
2. The other 7,500 IU of vitamin A is most likely retinol in the form of retinyl acetate or retinyl palmitate; check the list of ingredients.

3. With the exception of biotin, this supplement provides 100 percent of the Daily Value (100%DV) for the B vitamins. And, the 30 micrograms of biotin provides 100 percent of the current AI.
4. This supplement contains very low percentages of the Daily Values for calcium, magnesium, and phosphorus (16 percent, 11 percent, and 25 percent, respectively). Adding more of these minerals would make

the pill huge and impossible to swallow! A nutritious diet should provide the rest of these minerals.
5. This supplement contains 200 percent of the Daily Value for each of the antioxidant vitamins C and E, and one-fourth (50%DV) of its vitamin A content comes from the antioxidant beta-carotene.

# Learning Portfolio

## Key Terms

## Study Points

- A functional food is considered to be a food that may provide a health benefit beyond basic nutrition.

- Phytochemicals are plant chemicals responsible for the health-promoting properties of many functional foods.

- Consumption of plant foods containing multiple antioxidants is strongly associated with health benefits. Scientific evidence strongly supports eating at least five servings of fruits and vegetables daily and emphasizing whole grains.

- The federal government reviews the safety of new additives before they can be used in foods sold on the market.

- The Delaney Clause is a controversial food law that prohibits the approval of an additive if it has been found to cause cancer in humans or laboratory animals, even if massive doses are required to produce the disease.

- Dietary supplements encompass vitamins, minerals, herbal products, amino acids, glandular extracts, enzymes, and many other products.

- Vitamin and mineral supplements may be warranted in certain circumstances, although the preferred mode of obtaining adequate nutrition is through foods.

- Megadose vitamin or mineral therapy has not been proved effective in the treatment of cancer, colds, or heart disease. Moreover, such megadoses act more like drugs than nutrients in the body and should be approached with caution.

- Herbal medicine is a traditional form of healing in many cultures. Some herbal medicines have shown enough promise to warrant large-scale clinical studies involving supplements. However, herbal products can have side effects and can interfere with prescription medications.

- Dietary supplements are regulated according to the provisions of the Dietary Supplement Health and Education Act of 1994. Unlike drugs and additives, dietary supplements do not need premarket approval.

- Claims for dietary supplements can include health claims, structure/function claims, and nutrient content claims.

- Dietary supplements must have a Supplement Facts panel on the label.

- Consumers should carefully evaluate claims and evidence for dietary supplements and consult their physician before taking a supplement.

- Complementary and alternative medicine (CAM) comprises practices outside the medical mainstream that are becoming increasingly popular. CAM includes a broad range of therapies, many of which include nutrition. People seek them for a variety of reasons, including environmental concerns and a fear of aging.

## Study Questions

1. What are phytochemicals, and how do they benefit plants and humans?

2. Name three chronic diseases that consuming functional foods may help prevent.

3. What purpose(s) do additives serve?

4. What is the purpose of the Delaney Clause? What are the complications surrounding this food law?

5. How do you know a product is a dietary supplement?

6. If a dietary supplement product label contains the words "High in vitamin E," what type of claim is it making? What other claims can a supplement make?

7. What things should someone do before purchasing supplements?

8. What are some of the possible complications involved in using herbal medicines?

9. What is a macrobiotic diet?

# Try This

## Finding Functional Beverages

This exercise will familiarize you with the many beverages that contain functional ingredients now available to consumers. Take a trip to your grocery store and spend some time in the beverage aisles. You may want to check out the chilled juice section in addition to the bottled teas and juice beverages. Pick out about 10 different products that have either a nutrient or herbal compound added and try to identify how many have nutrient content claims, health claims, and structure/function claims. Note the prices of these products. How does their nutritional content compare to a 100 percent fruit juice like orange juice? How does it compare to soda?

## Take a Walk on the "Web Side"

This exercise will familiarize you with various websites that promote and sell supplements. Log on to the Internet and start doing searches with key words affiliated with supplements. Try *vitamins*, *minerals*, *supplements*, *herbs*, and even some specific terms like *chromium picolinate* and *ginseng*. On the websites you visit, how is the nutrition information presented? Do the supplement's benefits sound too good to be true? See if you can spot a fraud. Use the information in the "Fraudulent Products" section of this chapter to identify the accuracy of the product information you find.

# References

1 PriceWaterhouseCoopers. Leveraging growth in the emerging functional foods industry: trends and market opportunities. 2009. http://download.pwc.com/ie/pubs/pwc_leveraging_growth_in_the_emerging.pdf. Accessed 6/11/11.

2 US Department of Agriculture, US Department of Health and Human Services. *Dietary Guidelines for Americans, 2010.* 7th ed. Washington, DC: US Government Printing Office; December 2010.

3 US Department of Agriculture. MyPlate. http://www.choosemyplate.gov. Accessed 10/1/11.

4 Mordente A, Guantario B, Meucci E, et al. Lycopene and cardiovascular diseases: an update. *Curr Med Chem.* 2011;18(8):1146–1163.

5 Andres S, Abraham K, Appel KE, Lampen A. Risks and benefits of dietary isoflavones for cancer. *Crit Rev Toxicol.* 2011;41(6):463–506.

6 Ibid.

7 Hilakivi-Clarke L, Andrade JE, Helferich W. Is soy consumption good or bad for the breast? *J Nutr.* 2010;140(12):2326S–2334S.

8 Wong IY, Koo SC, Chan CW. Prevention of age-related macular degeneration. *Int Ophthalmol.* 2011;31(1):73–82; and Olson JH, Erie JC, Bakri SJ. Nutritional supplementation and age-related macular degeneration. *Semin Ophthalmol.* 2011;26(3):131–136.

9 US Food and Drug Administration. Labeling and nutrition: food labeling and nutrition overview. Updated 3/23/11. http://www.fda.gov/Food/Labeling-Nutrition/default.htm. Accessed 6/17/11.

10 Percival SS, Turner RE. Applications of herbs to functional foods. In: Wildman REC, ed. *Handbook of Nutraceuticals and Functional Foods.* 2nd ed. Boca Raton, FL: CRC Press; 2006.

11 US Food and Drug Administration. Letter to manufacturers regarding botanicals and other novel ingredients in conventional foods. January 30, 2001. Updated 6/18/09. http://www.fda.gov/Food/DietarySupplements/GuidanceComplianceRegulatoryInformation/ucm103443.htm. Accessed

6/17/11; and US Food and Drug Administration. Inspections, compliance, enforcement, and criminal investigations. Warning letters. Updated 6/17/11. http://www.fda.gov/ICECI/EnforcementActions/WarningLetters/default.htm. Accessed 6/17/11.

12 US Food and Drug Administration. Appendix C: health claims. Updated 5/23/11. http://www.fda.gov/Food/GuidanceComplianceRegulatoryInformation/GuidanceDocuments/FoodLabelingNutrition/FoodLabelingGuide/ucm064919.htm. Accessed 6/19/11.

13 Silverglade B, Ringel Heller I. Food labeling chaos. The case for reform. 2010. Center for Science in the Public Interest, Washington, DC. http://cspinet.org/new/pdf/food_labeling_chaos_report.pdf. Accessed 6/19/11.

14 National Institutes of Health, Office on Dietary Supplements. How to evaluate health information on the Internet: questions and answers. http://ods.od.nih.gov/Health_Information/How_To_Evaluate_Health_Information_on_the_Internet_Questions_and_Answers.aspx. Accessed 6/20/11.

15 Position of the Academy of Nutrition and Dietetics: nutrient supplementation. *J Am Diet Assoc.* 2009;109:2073–2085.

16 Ibid.

17 *Physicians' Desk Reference 2011.* 65th ed. Montvale, NJ: Thomson Healthcare; 2010.

18 Carmel R. Cobalamin (vitamin $B_{12}$). In: Shils ME, Shike M, Ross AC, Caballero B, Cousins RJ, eds. *Modern Nutrition in Health and Disease.* 10th ed. Philadelphia: Lippincott Williams & Wilkins; 2006.

19 *Physicians' Desk Reference 2011.* Op. cit.

20 Jacqui W. Trial of niacin alongside statin is stopped early. *BMJ.* 2011;342:d3400. http://www.bmj.com/content/342/bmj.d3400.extract. Accessed 6/21/11.

21 Krishnadev N, Meleth AD, Chew EY. Nutritional supplements for age-related macular degeneration. *Curr Opin Ophthalmol.* 2010;21(3):184–189.

22 American Heart Association. Vitamin and mineral supplements. AHA scientific position. Updated 11/23/10. http://www.heart.org/HEARTORG/GettingHealthy/NutritionCenter/Vitamin-and-Mineral-Supplements_UCM_306033_Article.jsp. Accessed 6/21/11.

23 *Alternative Medicine, Expanding Medical Horizons.* A report to the National Institutes of Health on alternative medical systems and practices in the United States. NIH publication 94-066; December 1994:230–232, 237.

24 Institute of Medicine, Food and Nutrition Board. *Dietary Reference Intakes for Vitamin C, Vitamin E, Selenium, and Carotenoids.* Washington, DC: National Academies Press; 2000.

25 Institute of Medicine, Food and Nutrition Board. *Dietary Reference Intakes for Vitamin A, Vitamin K, Arsenic, Boron, Chromium, Copper, Iron, Manganese, Molybdenum, Nickel, Silicon, Vanadium, and Zinc.* Washington, DC: National Academies Press; 2001.

26 Dietary supplements: safe, beneficial, and regulated. Council for Responsible Nutrition. Updated 3/14/11. http://www.crnusa.org/CRNRegQandA.html. Accessed 6/22/11.

27 Baseline natural health products survey among consumers, March 2005. Health Canada. Updated 2/14/11. http://www.hc-sc.gc.ca/dhp-mps/prodnatur/about-apropos/cons-eng.php. Accessed 6/22/11.

28 Silverglade B, Ringel Heller I. Op cit.

29 National Center for Complementary and Alternative Medicine. What is CAM? http://nccam.nih.gov/health/whatiscam. Accessed 10/4/11.

30 National Center for Complementary and Alternative Medicine. Herbs at a glance: St John's Wort. Updated 7/10. http://nccam.nih.gov/health/stjohnswort/ataglance.htm. Accessed 6/22/11.

31 National Center for Complementary and Alternative Medicine. Herbs at a glance: milk thistle. Updated 7/10. http://nccam.nih.gov/health/milkthistle/ataglance.htm. Accessed 6/22/11.

32 National Center for Complementary and Alternative Medicine. Herbs at a glance: ginkgo biloba. Updated 7/10. http://nccam.nih.gov/health/ginkgo. Accessed 6/22/11.

33 National Center for Complementary and Alternative Medicine. Herbs at a glance: saw palmetto. Updated 7/10. http://nccam.nih.gov/health/palmetto. Accessed 6/22/11; and Tacklind J, MacDonald R, Rutks I, et al. *Serenoa repens* for benign prostatic hyperplasia. *Cochrane Database of Systematic Reviews.* 2009; CD001423.

34 National Center for Complementary and Alternative Medicine. Herbs at a glance: cranberry. Updated 7/10. http://nccam.nih.gov/health/cranberry/ataglance.htm. Accessed 6/22/11.

35    Barbosa-Cesnik C, Brown MB, Buxton M, et al. Cranberry juice fails to prevent recurrent urinary tract infection: results from a randomized placebo-controlled trial. *Clinical Infectious Diseases*. 2011;52(1):23–30.

36    National Center for Complementary and Alternative Medicine. Herbs at a glance. Gingko biloba. Updated 7/10. http://nccam.nih.gov/health/ginkgo/ataglance.htm. Accessed 6/22/11; and Rosenblatt M, Mindel J. Spontaneous hyphema associated with ingestion of ginkgo biloba extract. *N Engl J Med*. 1997;336(15):1108.

37    Kennedy DA, Seely D. Clinically based evidence of drug–herb interactions: a systematic review. *Expert Opin Drug Saf*. 2010;9(1):79–124.

38    National Center for Complementary and Alternative Medicine. Herbs at a glance: licorice root. Updated 7/10. http://nccam.nih.gov/health/licoriceroot. Accessed 6/22/11; and Edwards C. Lessons from licorice. *N Engl J Med*. 1991;325:1242–1243.

39    Izzo AA, Ernst E. Interactions between herbal medicines and prescribed drugs: an updated systematic review. *Drugs*. 2009;69(13):1777–1798.

40    Tachjian A, Maria V, Jahangir A. Use of herbal products and potential interactions in patients with cardiovascular diseases. *J Am Coll Cardiol*. 2010; 55(6):515–525.

41    DiPaola RS, Zhang H, Lambert GH, et al. Clinical and biologic activity of an estrogenic herbal combination (PC-SPES) in prostate cancer. *N Engl J Med*. 1998;339:785–791.

42    Zhang Y, Fein EB, Fein SB. Feeding of dietary botanical supplements and teas to infants in the United States. *Pediatrics*. 2011;127(6):1060–1066; and Voelker R. Study: up to 1 in 10 infants given herbal supplements, teas by their mother. *JAMA*. 2011;305(21):2161.

43    Phillips M, Sullivan B, Snyder B, et al. Effect of enzyte on QT and QTc intervals. *Arch Intern Med*. 2010;170(15):1402–1404.

44    Marrow JD. Why the United States still needs improved dietary supplement regulation and oversight. *Clin Pharmacol Ther*. 2008;83(3):391–393.

45    US Government Accountability Office. Herbal dietary supplements. Examples of deceptive or questionable marketing practices and potentially advice: testimony before the Special Committee on Aging. Washington, DC: US Government Accountability Office; May 26, 2010.

46    Betz JM, Brown PN, Roman MC. Accuracy, precision, and reliability of chemical measurements in natural products research. *Fitoterapia*. 2011;82(1):44–52.

47    Gordon RY, Cooperman T, Obermeyer W, Becker DJ. Marked variability of monacolin levels in commercial red yeast rice products: buyer beware! *Arch Intern Med*. 2010;170(19):1722–1727.

48    Food and Drug Administration. FDA issues dietary supplements final rule. FDA press release. Released 6/22/07. http://www.fda.gov/bbs/topics/NEWS/2007/NEW01657.html. Accessed 6/22/11.

49    Liu EH, Qi LW, Li K, et al. Recent advances in quality control of traditional Chinese medicines. *Comb Chem High Throughput Screen*. 2010;13(10):869–884.

50    Federal Trade Commission. "Operation Cure All" wages new battle in ongoing war against Internet health fraud. Updated 11/08. http://www.ftc.gov/opa/2001/06/cureall.shtm. Accessed 6/22/11.

51    Food and Drug Administration. Regulatory information. Dietary Supplement Health and Education Act of 1994. Updated 5/20/09. http://www.fda. gov/RegulatoryInformation/Legislation/FederalFoodDrugandCosmeticAct FDCAct/SignificantAmendmentstotheFDCAct/ucm148003.htm. Accessed 6/22/11.

52    Food and Drug Administration. FDA 101: dietary supplements. http://www.fda.gov/ForConsumers/ConsumerUpdates/ucm050803.htm. Accessed 6/22/11.

53    Food and Drug Administration. Guidance for industry: a dietary supplement labeling guide. General dietary supplement labeling. Updated 4/05. http://www.fda.gov/Food/GuidanceComplianceRegulatoryInformation/GuidanceDocuments/DietarySupplements/DietarySupplementlabelingguide/ucm070519.htm. Accessed 6/22/11.

54    US Department of Health and Human Services. FDA structure/function claims. Updated 7/28/2010. http://www.fda.gov/Food/LabelingNutrition/LabelClaims/StructureFunctionClaims/default.htm. Accessed 6/19/11.

55    US Food and Drug Administration. Overview of dietary supplements. Updated 10/14/09. http://www.fda.gov/Food/DietarySupplements/ConsumerInformation/ucm110417.htm. Accessed 6/22/11.

56    US Food and Drug Administration. Claims that can be made for conventional foods and dietary supplements. Updated 5/14/09. http://www.fda.gov/Food/LabelingNutrition/LabelClaims/ucm111447.htm. Accessed 6/22/11.

57    Health Canada. Drugs and health products. About natural health product regulation in Canada. Updated 2/14/11. http://www.hc-sc.gc.ca/dhp-mps/prodnatur/about-apropos/index-eng.php. Accessed 6/22/11.

58    Academy of Nutrition and Dietetics. Guidelines regarding the recommendation and sale of dietary supplements. http://www.eatright.org/About/Content.aspx?id=8145. Accessed 6/23/11.

59    USP Dietary Supplementation Verification program. http://www.usp.org. Accessed 6/23/11.

60    The Alpha-Tocopherol, Beta-Carotene and Cancer Prevention Study Group. The effect of vitamin E and beta-carotene on the incidence of lung cancer and other cancers in male smokers. *N Engl J Med*. 1994;330:1029–1035.

61    Food and Drug Administration. Beware of fraudulent "dietary supplements." Updated 3/11. http://www.fda.gov/forconsumers/consumerupdates/ucm246744.htm. Accessed 6/23/11.

62    Ibid.

63    National Center for Complementary and Alternative Medicine. What is complementary and alternative medicine? Defining CAM. Updated 4/1/11. http://nccam.nih.gov/health/whatiscam/#definingcam. Accessed 6/23/11.

64    Barnes PM, Bloom B, Nahin R. Complementary and alternative medicine use among adults and children: United States, 2007. *CDC National Health Statistics Report* no. 12. Updated 12/08. http://nccam.nih.gov/news/2008/nhsr12.pdf. Accessed 6/23/11.

65    Ibid.

66    Lerman RH. The macrobiotic diet in chronic disease. *Nutr Clin Pract*. 2010; 25(6):621–626.

67    American Cancer Society. Macrobiotic diet. Updated 11/08. http://www.cancer.org/Treatment/TreatmentsandSideEffects/Complementaryand AlternativeMedicine/DietandNutrition/macrobiotic-diet. Accessed 6/24/11.

68    Lerman RH. Op. cit.

69    Kirby M, Danner E. Nutritional deficiencies in children on restricted diets. *Pediatr Clin North Am*. 2009;56(5):1085–1103.

# CHAPTER 4

# The Human Body: From Food to Fuel

**THINK About It**

1  Your friend warns you that eating some foods together is not healthful. Is this likely to change your eating behavior?

2  How good are you at identifying tastes?

3  Have you ever noticed that food sometimes tastes sweeter after you've chewed it for a while?

4  You feel particularly happy, and you find that a meal prepared by your friend tastes especially good. Any connection?

**Visit go.jblearning.com/ inseldisco4e**

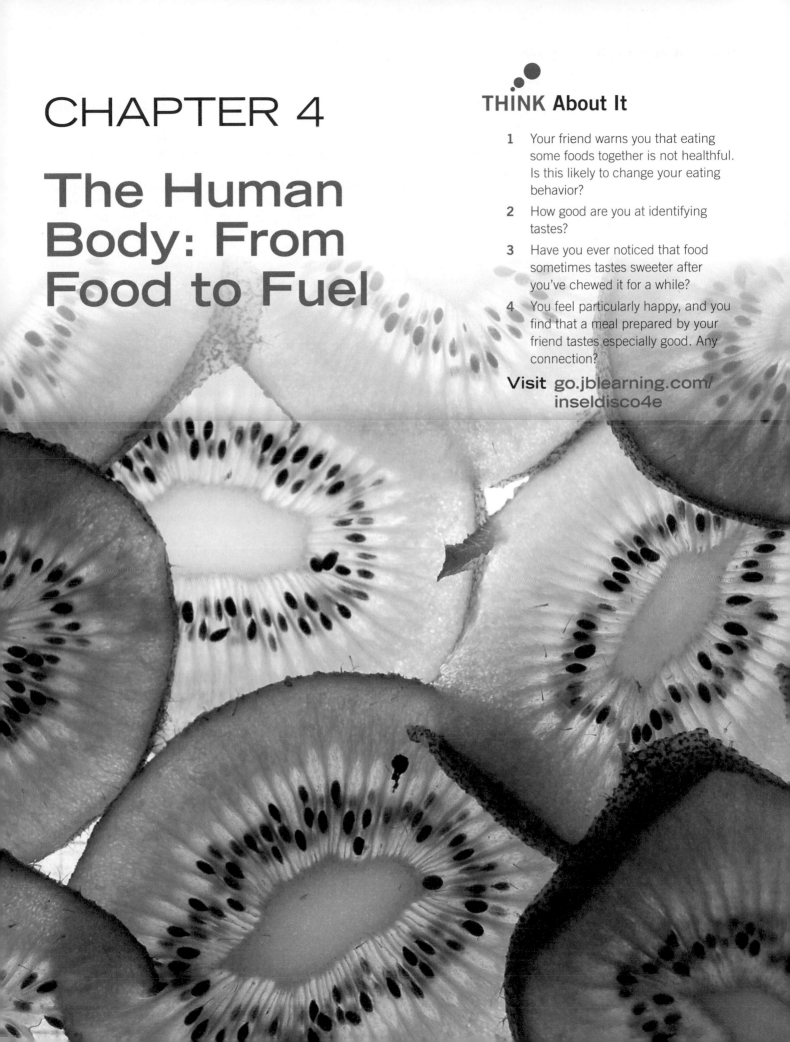

**digestion** The process of transforming the foods we eat into units for absorption.

**absorption** The movement of substances into or across tissues; in particular, the passage of nutrients and other substances into the walls of the gastrointestinal tract and then into the bloodstream.

The aroma of roasting turkey floats past your nose. You haven't eaten for six or seven hours. Anticipating a delicious experience, your mouth waters, and your digestive juices are turned on! Is this virtual reality? Not at all! Before you eat a morsel of food, fleeting thoughts from your brain signal your body to prepare for the feast to come.

Your body's mechanisms for processing food and turning it into nutrients are both efficient and elegant. The action unfolds in the digestive tract in two stages: **digestion**—the breaking apart of foods into smaller and smaller units—and **absorption**—the movement of those small units from the gut into the bloodstream or lymphatic system for circulation. Your digestive system is designed to digest carbohydrates, proteins, and fats simultaneously, while at the same time preparing other substances—vitamins, minerals, and cholesterol, for example—for absorption. Remarkably, your digestive system doesn't need any help! Despite promotions for enzyme supplements and diet books that recommend consuming food or nutrient groups separately, scientific research does not support these claims. Unless you have a specific medical condition, your digestive system is ready, willing, and able to digest and absorb the foods you eat, in whatever combination you eat them.

 THINK About It 1

But, go back to the aroma of that roast turkey for a moment. Before we begin digesting and absorbing, our senses of taste and smell first attract us to foods we are likely to consume.

## Taste and Smell: The Beginnings of Our Food Experience

You probably wouldn't eat a food if it didn't appeal in some way to your senses. Odors around us, such as the fragrance of a gardenia or the smell of bread baking, stimulate nerve cells inside the nose. In the mouth, tastes, as well as texture and temperature, combine with odors to produce a perception of flavor. It is flavor that lets us know whether we are eating a pear or an apple. You recognize flavors mainly through the sense of smell. If you hold your nose while eating chocolate, for example, you will have trouble identifying it—even though you can distinguish the food's sweetness or bitterness. That's because the familiar flavor of chocolate is sensed largely by odor, as is the well-known flavor of coffee.

 THINK About It 2

The sight, smell, thought, taste, and, in some cases, even the sound of food can trigger a set of responses that prepare the digestive tract to receive food.[1] Your mouth begins to water and stomach secretions flow. (See **Figure 4.1**.) If no food is consumed, the response diminishes, but eating prolongs the stimulation of the salivary and gastric cells.

## The Gastrointestinal Tract

If, instead of teasing the body with mere sights and smells, we actually sit down to a meal and experience the full flavor and texture of foods, the real work of the digestive tract begins. For the food we eat to nourish our bodies, we need to digest it (break it down into smaller units); absorb it (move it from the gut into circulation); and finally transport it to the tissues and cells of the body. The digestive process starts in the mouth and continues as food journeys down the gastrointestinal (GI) tract. At various points along the GI tract, nutrients are absorbed, meaning they move from the GI tract into circulatory systems so they can be transported throughout the body. If there are problems along the way, with either incomplete digestion or inadequate absorption, the cells will not receive the nutrients they need to grow, perform daily activities, fight infection, and maintain health. A closer look at the gastrointestinal tract will help you see just how amazing this organ system is.

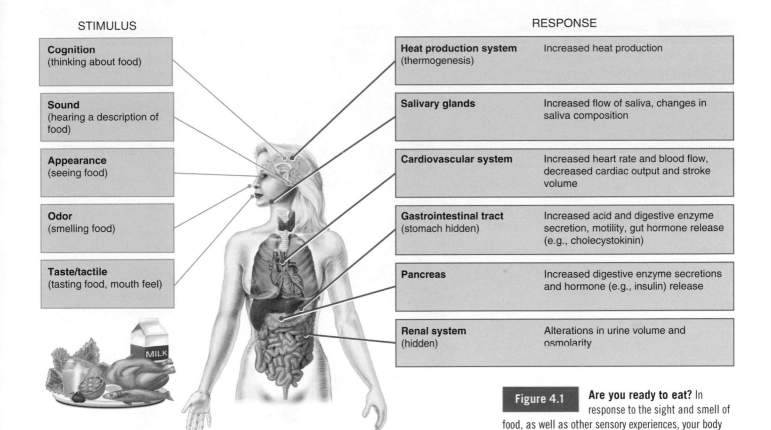

STIMULUS

**Cognition**
(thinking about food)

**Sound**
(hearing a description of food)

**Appearance**
(seeing food)

**Odor**
(smelling food)

**Taste/tactile**
(tasting food, mouth feel)

RESPONSE

| **Heat production system** (thermogenesis) | Increased heat production |
|---|---|
| **Salivary glands** | Increased flow of saliva, changes in saliva composition |
| **Cardiovascular system** | Increased heart rate and blood flow, decreased cardiac output and stroke volume |
| **Gastrointestinal tract** (stomach hidden) | Increased acid and digestive enzyme secretion, motility, gut hormone release (e.g., cholecystokinin) |
| **Pancreas** | Increased digestive enzyme secretions and hormone (e.g., insulin) release |
| **Renal system** (hidden) | Alterations in urine volume and osmolarity |

**Figure 4.1** **Are you ready to eat?** In response to the sight and smell of food, as well as other sensory experiences, your body primes its resources to better digest, absorb, and use anticipated nutrients.

## Organization of the GI Tract

The **gastrointestinal (GI) tract**, also known as the alimentary canal, is a long, hollow tube that begins at the mouth and ends at the anus. The specific parts include the mouth, esophagus, stomach, small intestine, large intestine, and rectum. (See **Figure 4.2.**) The GI tract works with assisting organs—the salivary glands, liver, gallbladder, and pancreas—to turn food into small molecules that the body can absorb and use. The GI tract has an amazing variety of functions, including:

1. Ingestion (the receipt and softening of food)
2. Transport of ingested food
3. Secretion of digestive enzymes, acid, mucus, and bile
4. Absorption of end products of digestion
5. Movement of undigested material
6. **Elimination** of digestive waste products

Because of its basic shape, the GI tract is often described as a hollow tube; however, its structure is really much more complex. As you can see in **Figure 4.3**, there are several layers to this tube. The innermost layer, called the **mucosa**, is lined with glands and absorptive cells (epithelial cells). Layers of **circular muscle** and **longitudinal muscle** help mix and move the food we eat.

At points along the tract, where one organ connects with another (e.g., where the esophagus meets the stomach) the muscles are thicker and form **sphincters**. (See **Figure 4.4.**) A sphincter acts as a valve that controls the movement of food material so that it travels through the GI tract in only one direction. By alternately contracting and relaxing, these muscular rings act

**gastrointestinal (GI) tract [GAS-troh-in-TES-tin-al]** The connected series of organs and structures used for digestion of food and absorption of nutrients; also called the *alimentary canal* or the *digestive tract.*

**elimination** The removal of undigested food from the body.

**mucosa [myu-KO-sa]** The innermost layer of a cavity. The inner layer of the gastrointestinal tract (the intestinal wall). It is composed of epithelial cells and glands.

**circular muscle** Layers of smooth muscle that surround organs, including the stomach and the small intestine.

**longitudinal muscle** Muscle fibers aligned lengthwise.

**sphincters [SFINGK-ters]** Circular bands of muscle fibers that surround the entrance or exit of a hollow body structure (e.g., the stomach) and act as valves to control the flow of material.

**Figure 4.2** **Anatomical and functional organization of the GI tract.** Although digestion begins in the mouth, most digestion occurs in the stomach and small intestine. Absorption takes place primarily in the small and large intestines.

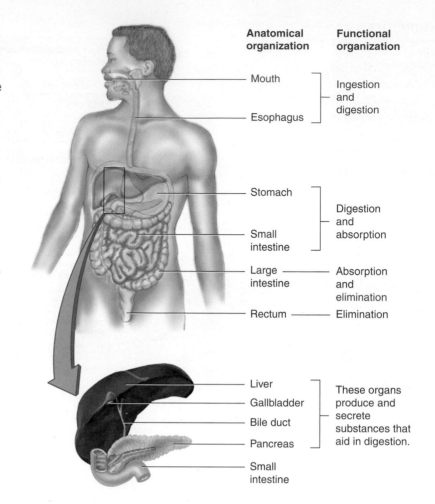

| Anatomical organization | Functional organization |
| --- | --- |
| Mouth | Ingestion and digestion |
| Esophagus | |
| Stomach | Digestion and absorption |
| Small intestine | |
| Large intestine | Absorption and elimination |
| Rectum | Elimination |
| Liver | These organs produce and secrete substances that aid in digestion. |
| Gallbladder | |
| Bile duct | |
| Pancreas | |
| Small intestine | |

**Figure 4.3** **Structural organization of the GI tract wall.** Your intestinal tract is a long hollow tube lined with mucosal cells and surrounded by layers of muscle cells.

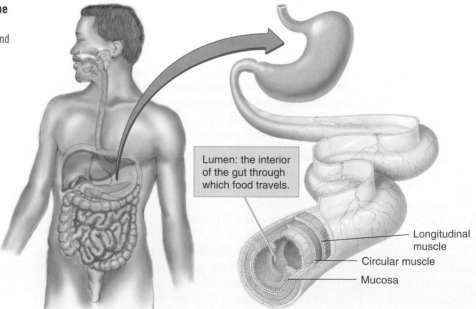

Lumen: the interior of the gut through which food travels.

Longitudinal muscle

Circular muscle

Mucosa

like one-way doors, allowing the mixture of food and digestive juices to flow into an organ but not back out.

**Key Concepts** *The gastrointestinal tract consists of the mouth, esophagus, stomach, small intestine, large intestine, and rectum. The functions of the GI tract are to ingest, digest, and absorb nutrients and to eliminate waste. The general structure of the GI tract consists of many layers, including the mucosa, the inner lining of glands and absorptive cells. Sphincters are muscular valves along the GI tract that control movement from one part to the next.*

## Overview of Digestion: Physical and Chemical Processes

The breakdown of food into smaller, absorbable nutrients involves both chemical and physical processes. The physical process comes first, as food is broken up into smaller pieces. Chewing starts the breakup, and muscular contractions of the GI tract continue it. As the GI tract breaks up food, it mixes the food with various secretions and moves the mixture (called **chyme**) along the tract. Enzymes, along with other chemicals, help complete the breakdown process and promote absorption.

### The Physical Movement and Breaking Up of Food

Distinct muscular actions of the GI tract take the food on its long journey. From mouth to anus, waves of muscular contractions, called **peristalsis**, transport food and nutrients along the length of the GI tract. Peristaltic waves from the stomach muscles occur about three times per minute. In the small intestine, circular and longitudinal bands of muscle contract approximately every four to five seconds. Peristaltic contractions of the small intestine often are continuations of contractions that began in the stomach. The large intestine uses slow peristalsis to move the waste products of digestion (feces).

**Segmentation**, a series of muscular contractions that occur in the small intestine, divides and mixes the chyme. Every few centimeters along the gut wall, alternating constrictions "chop" the contents into smaller portions. Segmentation also increases absorption by bringing chyme into contact with the intestinal wall. **Figure 4.5** shows peristalsis and segmentation.

### The Chemical Breakdown of Food

In the chemical process of digestion, enzymes divide nutrients into compounds small enough for absorption.

**Enzymes** are proteins that **catalyze**, or speed up, chemical reactions but are not themselves altered in the process. In digestion, these chemical reactions divide substances into smaller compounds by a process called **hydrolysis** (breaking apart by water), as **Figure 4.6** shows. The function of most digestive enzymes can be identified by their names, which commonly end in *–ase* (amylase, lipase, and so on). For example, the enzyme needed to digest sucro*se* is sucr*ase*.

In addition to enzymes, other chemicals are part of the digestive process. These include acid in the stomach, a neutralizing base in the small intestine, bile that prepares fat for digestion, and **mucus** secreted along the GI tract. This mucus does not break down food but lubricates it and protects the cells that line the GI tract from the strong digestive chemicals. Along the GI tract, fluids containing various enzymes and other substances are added to the consumed food. In fact, the volume of fluid secreted into the GI tract is about 7,000 milliliters (about 7½ quarts) per day.[2] Table 4.1 shows the average input and output of fluids in the GI tract each day.

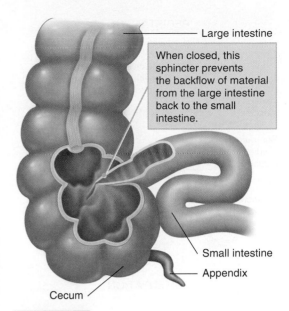

Large intestine

When closed, this sphincter prevents the backflow of material from the large intestine back to the small intestine.

Small intestine

Appendix

Cecum

**Figure 4.4** | **Sphincters in action.** Movement from one section of the GI tract to the next is controlled by muscular valves called sphincters.

**chyme [KIME]** A mass of partially digested food and digestive juices moving from the stomach into the small intestine.

**peristalsis [per-ih-STAHL-sis]** The wavelike, rhythmic muscular contractions of the GI tract that propel its contents down the tract.

**segmentation** Periodic muscle contractions at intervals along the GI tract that alternate forward and backward movement of the contents, thereby breaking apart chunks of the food mass and mixing in digestive juices.

**enzymes [EN-zimes]** Proteins in the body that speed up the rate of chemical reactions but are not altered in the process.

**catalyze** To speed up a chemical reaction.

**hydrolysis** A reaction that breaks apart a compound through the addition of water.

**mucus** A slippery substance secreted in the GI tract (and other body linings) that protects cells from irritants.

PERISTALSIS

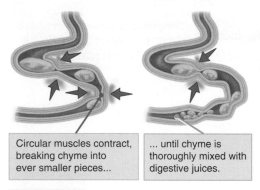

Longitudinal (lengthwise) muscles relax while circular muscles contract, pushing the bolus ahead.

Relaxed longitudinal muscles

Contracted circular muscles

Bolus

Sphincter closed

Sphincter open

SEGMENTATION

Circular muscles contract, breaking chyme into ever smaller pieces...

... until chyme is thoroughly mixed with digestive juices.

**Figure 4.5** **Peristalsis and segmentation.** Peristalsis and segmentation help break up, mix, and move food through the GI tract.

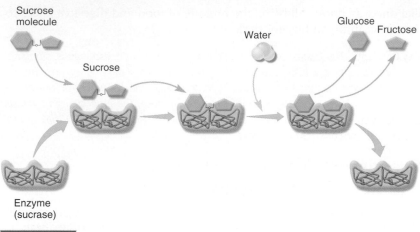

Sucrose molecule

Sucrose

Water

Glucose

Fructose

Enzyme (sucrase)

**Figure 4.6** **Water and enzymes in chemical reactions.** Enzymes speed up (catalyze) chemical reactions. When water breaks a chemical bond, the action is called hydrolysis.

**Key Concepts** *Digestion involves both physical and chemical activity. Physical activity includes chewing and the movement of muscles along the GI tract that break food into smaller pieces and mix it with digestive secretions. Chemical digestion includes the breaking of bonds in nutrients, such as carbohydrates or proteins, to produce smaller units. Enzymes—proteins that encourage chemical processes—catalyze these reactions.*

## Overview of Absorption

Food is broken apart during digestion and moved from the GI tract into circulation and on to the cells. Many of the nutrients—vitamins, minerals, and water—do not need to be digested before they are absorbed. But the energy-yielding nutrients—carbohydrate, fat, and protein—are too large to be absorbed intact and must be digested first. When ready for absorption, how are nutrients moved from the interior, or **lumen**, of the gut through the lining cells (mucosa) and into circulation?

**lumen** Cavity or hollow channel in any organ or structure of the body.

**Table 4.1** **Average Daily Fluid Input and Output**

| Source | Amount (milliliters) |
| --- | --- |
| *Fluid Input* | |
| Food and beverages | 2,000 |
| Saliva | 1,500 |
| Gastric secretions | 2,500 |
| Pancreatic secretions | 1,500 |
| Bile | 500 |
| Small intestine secretions | 1,000 |
| *Total Input* | *9,000* |
| *Fluid Output* | |
| Small intestine absorption | 7,500 |
| Large intestine absorption | 1,400 |
| Feces | 100 |
| *Total Output* | *9,000* |

**Source:** Data from Klein S, Cohn SM, Alpers DH. Alimentary tract in nutrition. In: Shils ME, Skike M, Ross AC, Cabellero B, Cousins RJ, eds. *Modern Nutrition in Health and Disease.* 10th ed. Philadelphia: Lippincott Williams & Wilkins, 2006:1115–1142.

PASSIVE DIFFUSION

FACILITATED DIFFUSION

ACTIVE TRANSPORT

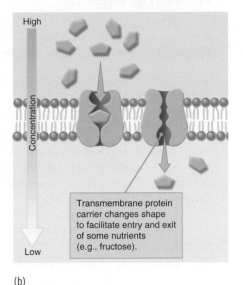

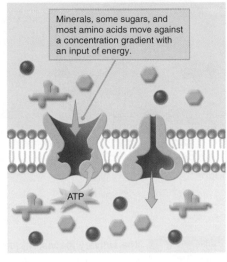

(a)                                    (b)                                    (c)

**Figure 4.7**    **(a) Passive diffusion.** Using passive diffusion, some substances easily move in and out of cells, either through protein channels or directly through the cell membrane. **(b) Facilitated diffusion.** Some substances need a little assistance to enter and exit cells. A transmembrane protein helps out by changing shape. **(c) Active transport.** Some substances need a lot of assistance to enter cells. Just as in swimming upstream, energy is needed for the substance to get through an unfavorable concentration gradient.

## The Roads to Nutrient Absorption

Three main processes allow nutrients to be absorbed from the GI tract into circulation: passive diffusion, facilitated diffusion, and active transport. (See **Figure 4.7.**) Let's take a look at each one, in turn.

**Passive diffusion** is the movement of molecules through the cell membrane without the expenditure of energy, by way of special protein channels or intermolecular gaps in the cell membrane. **Concentration gradients** (e.g., a high outside concentration and a low inside concentration of molecules) drive passive diffusion.

Because the cell membrane consists mainly of fat-soluble substances, it welcomes fats and other fat-soluble molecules. Oxygen, nitrogen, carbon dioxide, and alcohols are highly soluble in fat and readily dissolve in the cell membrane and diffuse across it. Although water crosses cell membranes easily, most water-soluble nutrients need additional help.

In **facilitated diffusion**, special protein channels help substances cross the cell membrane. The diffusing molecule becomes lightly bound to a protein channel that changes shape to open a pathway and allow diffusing molecules to enter or exit the cell.

Some substances need energy to move across a cell membrane, a process called **active transport**. Substances that usually require active transport across some cell membranes include many minerals, several sugars, and most amino acids (simple components of protein).

**Key Concepts**  *Absorption through the GI cell membranes occurs by one of three basic processes. In passive diffusion, nutrients such as water permeate the intestinal wall without a carrier or energy expenditure. In facilitated diffusion, a protein carrier helps bring substances into the absorptive intestinal cell without expending energy. Active transport requires energy to transport a substance across a cell membrane.*

**passive diffusion**  The movement of substances into or out of cells without the expenditure of energy or the involvement of transport proteins in the cell membrane. Also called *simple diffusion.*

**concentration gradients**  Differences between the solute concentrations of two solutions.

**facilitated diffusion**  A process by which carrier (transport) proteins in the cell membrane transport substances into or out of cells down a concentration gradient.

**active transport**  The movement of substances into or out of cells against a concentration gradient. Active transport requires energy (ATP) and involves carrier (transport) proteins in the cell membrane.

## Assisting Organs

The salivary glands, liver, gallbladder, and pancreas all have critical roles in the digestive process. The GI tract works in concert with these organs, which assist digestion by providing fluid, acid neutralizers, enzymes, and **emulsifiers**.

## Salivary Glands

We have three pairs of **salivary glands**, located in or near the mouth, which secrete saliva into the oral cavity. (See **Figure 4.8**.) Saliva moistens food, lubricating it for easy swallowing. Saliva also contains enzymes that begin the process of chemical digestion. We secrete approximately 1,500 milliliters (about 1½ quarts) of saliva each day. The mere sight, smell, or thought of food can start the flow of saliva.

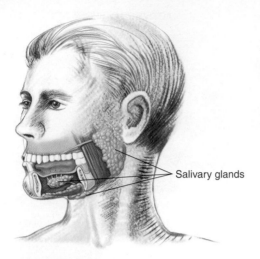

Salivary glands

**Figure 4.8**    **The salivary glands.** The three pairs of salivary glands supply saliva, which moistens and lubricates food. Saliva also contains salivary enzymes that begin the digestion of starch.

## Liver

The **liver** produces and secretes 600 to 1,000 milliliters of bile daily. **Bile** is a yellow-green, pasty material that helps digest fat. It contains water, bile salts and acids, pigments, cholesterol, phospholipids (a type of fat molecule), and electrolytes (electrically charged minerals). Bile tastes bitter, which is why the word *bile* has come to denote bitterness. Bile acts as an emulsifier by reducing large globs of fat to smaller globs, similar to how dish soap separates a layer of fat into smaller particles. This process of emulsification breaks no bonds in fat molecules, but rather increases the surface area of fat, allowing more contact between fat molecules and enzymes in the small intestine. Emulsification makes fat digestion more efficient.

Bile is stored and concentrated in your gallbladder, which releases it to the small intestine on demand. After bile has done its work, most is reabsorbed and returned to the liver for recycling. This recirculation is known as the **enterohepatic circulation** (*entero* meaning "intestines," *hepatic* referring to the liver) of bile. (See **Figure 4.9**.)

The liver also is a detoxification center that filters toxic substances from the blood and alters their chemical form. These altered substances may be sent to the kidney for **excretion** or carried by bile to the small intestine and removed from the body in feces. The liver is a "chemical factory"—performing over 500 chemical functions that include the production of blood proteins, cholesterol, and sugars. The liver is a "dynamic warehouse" that stores vitamins, hormones, cholesterol, minerals, and sugars, releasing them into the bloodstream as needed.

## Gallbladder

The primary function of the **gallbladder** is to store and concentrate bile from the liver. The gallbladder is a small, muscular, pear-shaped sac nestled in a depression on the right underside of the liver. This organ holds about a quarter of a cup of bile and is the storage stop for bile between the liver and the small intestine. The gallbladder fills with bile and thickens it, until a hormone released after eating signals the gallbladder to squirt out its colorful contents.

The gallbladder is normally relaxed and full between meals. When dietary fats enter the small intestine, they trigger the contraction of the gallbladder. Like a squeeze bulb, the gallbladder squirts bile through the common bile duct into the upper part of the small intestine. The common bile duct also carries digestive enzymes from the pancreas.

**emulsifiers**  Agents that blend fatty and watery liquids by promoting the breakup of fat into small particles and stabilizing their suspension in a watery solution.

**salivary glands**  Glands in the mouth that release saliva.

**liver**  The largest glandular organ in the body, it produces and secretes bile, detoxifies harmful substances, and helps metabolize carbohydrates, lipids, proteins, and micronutrients.

**bile**  An alkaline, yellow-green fluid that is produced in the liver and stored in the gallbladder. Bile emulsifies dietary fats, aiding fat digestion and absorption.

**enterohepatic circulation [EN-ter-oh-heh-PAT-ik]**  Recycling of certain compounds between the small intestine and the liver.

**excretion**  The process of separating and removing waste products of metabolism.

**gallbladder**  A pear-shaped sac that stores and concentrates bile from the liver.

## Pancreas

The **pancreas** secretes enzymes that affect the digestion and absorption of nutrients in the small intestine. During the course of a day, the pancreas secretes about 1,500 milliliters of fluid, which contains mostly water, bicarbonate, and digestive enzymes. The pancreas also releases hormones that are involved in other aspects of nutrient use by the body. For example, the pancreatic hormones insulin and glucagon regulate blood glucose levels. The combination of these two functions makes the pancreas one of the most important organs in the digestion and use of food.

**Key Concepts** *The salivary glands, liver, gallbladder, and pancreas all make important contributions to the digestive process. The salivary glands release saliva, which contains mucus and enzymes, into the mouth. The liver produces bile, which is stored in the gallbladder and released into the small intestine, where bile helps to prepare fats for digestion. The pancreas secretes liquid that contains bicarbonate and several types of enzymes into the small intestine.*

## Putting It All Together: Digestion and Absorption

Up to this point, we have focused on structures, mechanisms, and processes to give you a general idea of the workings of the GI tract. Now you're ready for a complete tour, a journey along the GI tract to see what happens and how digestion and absorption are accomplished.

## Mouth

THINK About It 3

As soon as you put food in your mouth the digestive process begins. As you chew, you break down the food into smaller pieces, increasing the surface area available to enzymes. Saliva contains the enzyme **salivary amylase**, which breaks down starch into small sugar molecules. Food remains in the mouth for just a short time, so only about 5 percent of the starch is completely broken down. The next time you eat a cracker or a piece of bread, chew slowly and notice the change in the way it tastes. It gets sweeter. That's the salivary amylase breaking down the starch into sugar. Salivary amylase continues to work until the strong acid content of the stomach deactivates it. To start the process of fat digestion, the cells at the base of the tongue secrete another enzyme, **lingual lipase**. The overall impact of lingual lipase on fat digestion, though, is small.

Saliva and other fluids, including mucus, blend with the food to form a **bolus**, a chewed, moistened lump of food that is soft and easy to swallow. When you swallow, the bolus slides past the epiglottis, a valvelike flap of tissue that closes off your air passages so you don't choke. The bolus then moves rapidly through the **esophagus** to the stomach, where it will be digested further. **Figure 4.10** shows the process of swallowing.

## Stomach

The bolus enters the **stomach** through the **esophageal sphincter**, also called the cardiac sphincter, which immediately closes to keep the bolus from sliding back into the esophagus. This sphincter needs to close quickly and completely to prevent the acidic stomach contents from backing up into the esophagus, causing the pain and tissue damage called **heartburn**.

### Nutrient Digestion in the Stomach

The stomach cells produce secretions that are collectively called gastric juice. Included in this mixture are water, hydrochloric acid, mucus, pepsinogen (the

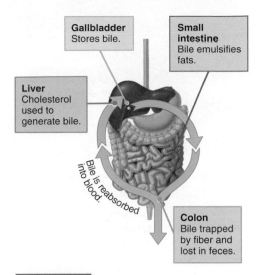

**Figure 4.9**  **Enterohepatic circulation.** During this recycling process, bile travels from the liver to the gallbladder and then to the small intestine, where it assists digestion. In the small intestine, most bile is reabsorbed and sent back to the liver for reuse.

**pancreas**  An organ that secretes enzymes that affect the digestion and absorption of nutrients and that releases hormones, such as insulin, which regulate metabolism as well as the way nutrients are used in the body.

**salivary amylase [AM-ih-lace]**  An enzyme that catalyzes the hydrolysis of amylose, a starch. Also called *ptyalin*.

**lingual lipase**  A fat-splitting enzyme secreted by cells at the base of the tongue.

**bolus [BOH-lus]**  A chewed, moistened lump of food that is ready to be swallowed.

**esophagus [ee-SOFF-uh-gus]**  The food pipe that extends from the pharynx to the stomach.

**stomach**  The enlarged, muscular, saclike portion of the digestive tract between the esophagus and the small intestine, with a capacity of about 1 quart.

**esophageal sphincter**  The opening between the esophagus and the stomach that relaxes and opens to allow the bolus to travel into the stomach, and then closes behind it. Acts as a barrier to prevent the reflux of gastric contents. Also called the *cardiac sphincter*.

**heartburn**  Burning pain behind the breastbone area caused by acidic stomach contents backing up into the esophagus.

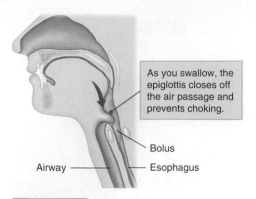

**Figure 4.10** **Swallowing.** Your epiglottis didn't completely do its job if you have ever choked on a drink that went "down the wrong pipe."

As you swallow, the epiglottis closes off the air passage and prevents choking.

Bolus

Airway

Esophagus

inactive form of the enzyme pepsin), the enzyme gastric lipase, the hormone gastrin, and intrinsic factor.

- **Hydrochloric acid (gastric acid)** makes the stomach contents extremely acidic—dropping the **pH** to 2, compared to a neutral pH of 7. (See the pH scale in **Figure 4.11**.) This acidic environment kills many pathogenic (disease-causing) bacteria that may have been ingested and also aids in the digestion of protein. Mucus secreted by the stomach cells coats the stomach lining, protecting these cells from damage by the strong gastric juice.
- Hydrochloric acid works in protein digestion in two ways. First, it demolishes the functional, three-dimensional shape of proteins, unfolding them into linear chains; this increases their vulnerability to attacking enzymes. Second, it promotes the breakdown of proteins by converting **pepsinogen**, an enzyme **precursor**, to **pepsin**, its active form.
- Pepsin then begins breaking the links in protein chains, cutting dietary proteins into smaller and smaller pieces.
- Stomach cells also produce an enzyme called **gastric lipase**. It has a minor role in the digestion of lipids, specifically butterfat.
- **Gastrin**, another component of gastric juice, is a hormone that stimulates gastric secretion and movement.

**hydrochloric acid (gastric acid)** A very strong acid of chloride and hydrogen atoms made by stomach glands and secreted intro the stomach. Also called *gastric acid*.

**pH** A measurement of the hydrogen ion concentration, or acidity, of a solution.

**pepsinogen** The inactive form of the enzyme pepsin.

**precursor** A substance that is converted into another active substance. Enzyme precursors also are called *proenzymes*.

**pepsin** A protein-digesting enzyme produced by the stomach.

**gastric lipase** An enzyme in the stomach that primarily breaks down butterfat.

**gastrin [GAS-trin]** A hormone released from the walls of the stomach and duodenum that stimulates gastric secretions and motility.

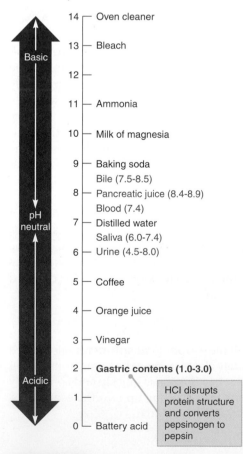

TYPICAL pHs OF COMMON SUBSTANCES

Basic

pH neutral

Acidic

| | |
|---|---|
| 14 | Oven cleaner |
| 13 | Bleach |
| 12 | |
| 11 | Ammonia |
| 10 | Milk of magnesia |
| 9 | Baking soda |
| | Bile (7.5-8.5) |
| 8 | Pancreatic juice (8.4-8.9) |
| | Blood (7.4) |
| 7 | Distilled water |
| | Saliva (6.0-7.4) |
| 6 | Urine (4.5-8.0) |
| 5 | Coffee |
| 4 | Orange juice |
| 3 | Vinegar |
| 2 | **Gastric contents (1.0-3.0)** |
| 1 | |
| 0 | Battery acid |

HCl disrupts protein structure and converts pepsinogen to pepsin

**Figure 4.11** **The pH scale.** Because pancreatic juice has a pH around 8, it can neutralize the acidic chyme, which leaves the stomach with a pH around 2.

- **Intrinsic factor** is a substance necessary for the absorption of vitamin $B_{12}$ that occurs farther down the GI tract, near the end of the small intestine. In the absence of intrinsic factor, only about one-fiftieth of ingested vitamin $B_{12}$ is absorbed.

After you swallow, salivary amylase continues to digest carbohydrates. About an hour later, acidic stomach secretions become well mixed with the food. This increases the acidity of the food and effectively blocks further salivary amylase activity.

Do you sometimes feel your stomach churning? The stomach works to continue mixing food with GI secretions and produces the semiliquid chyme. To accomplish this, the stomach has an extra layer of muscles. These diagonal muscles, along with the circular and longitudinal muscles, contract and relax to mix food completely. When the chyme is ready to leave the stomach, about 30 to 40 percent of carbohydrate, 10 to 20 percent of protein, and less than 10 percent of fat have been digested.[3] The stomach slowly releases the chyme through the **pyloric sphincter** and into the small intestine. When closed, the pyloric sphincter prevents the chyme from returning to the stomach. (See **Figure 4.12**.)

The stomach normally empties in one to four hours, depending on the types and amounts of food eaten. Carbohydrates speed through the stomach in the shortest time, followed by protein and fat. Thus, the higher the fat content of a meal, the longer it will take to leave the stomach.

**intrinsic factor**  A protein released from cells in the stomach wall that binds to and aids in the absorption of vitamin $B_{12}$.

**pyloric sphincter**  A circular muscle that forms the opening between the duodenum and the stomach. It regulates the passage of food into the small intestine.

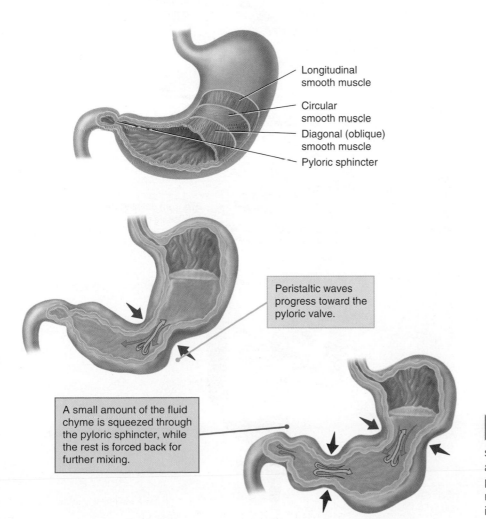

Longitudinal smooth muscle

Circular smooth muscle

Diagonal (oblique) smooth muscle

Pyloric sphincter

Peristaltic waves progress toward the pyloric valve.

A small amount of the fluid chyme is squeezed through the pyloric sphincter, while the rest is forced back for further mixing.

**Figure 4.12**  **The stomach.** The stomach churns and mixes food with stomach secretions. Hydrochloric acid unfolds proteins and stops salivary amylase action while pepsin begins protein digestion. The pyloric sphincter controls movement of chyme from the stomach to the small intestine.

> **small intestine** The tube (approximately 3 meters [10 ft] long) where the digestion of protein, fat, and carbohydrate is completed and where the majority of nutrients are absorbed. The small intestine is divided into three parts: the duodenum, the jejunum, and the ileum.

## *Nutrient Absorption in the Stomach*

Although much digestion has been accomplished by the time chyme leaves the stomach, very little absorption has occurred. The stomach absorbs weak acids, such as alcohol and aspirin, and only a few fat-soluble compounds. Chyme moves on to the small intestine, the digestive and absorptive workhorse of the gut.

## Small Intestine

The **small intestine** completes the digestion of protein, fat, and nearly all carbohydrate, and absorbs most nutrients. As you can see in **Figure 4.13**,

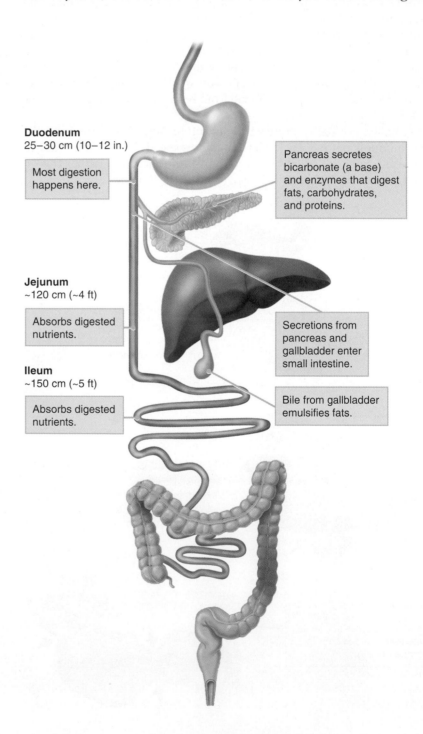

**Duodenum**
25–30 cm (10–12 in.)

Most digestion happens here.

Pancreas secretes bicarbonate (a base) and enzymes that digest fats, carbohydrates, and proteins.

**Jejunum**
~120 cm (~4 ft)

Absorbs digested nutrients.

Secretions from pancreas and gallbladder enter small intestine.

**Ileum**
~150 cm (~5 ft)

Absorbs digested nutrients.

Bile from gallbladder emulsifies fats.

**Figure 4.13**    **The small intestine.** The duodenum is mainly responsible for digesting food; the jejunum and ileum primarily deal with the absorption of nutrients. In addition to receiving the digestive juices from assisting organs, the duodenum secretes mucus, enzymes, and hormones to aid digestion. All along the intestinal walls, nutrients are absorbed into blood and lymph. Undigested materials are passed on to the large intestine.

the small intestine is a tube approximately 3 meters long (about 10 feet), divided into three parts:

- **Duodenum** (the first 25 to 30 centimeters—10 to 12 inches)
- **Jejunum** (about 120 centimeters—about 4 feet)
- **Ileum** (about 150 centimeters—about 5 feet)

Most digestion occurs in the duodenum, where the small intestine receives **digestive secretions** from the pancreas, gallbladder, and its own glands. The remainder of the small intestine primarily absorbs previously digested nutrients.

### Nutrient Digestion in the Small Intestine

In the duodenum, bicarbonate from the pancreas neutralizes the acidic chyme from the stomach. This is important because the enzymes of the small intestine need a more neutral environment to work effectively. Pancreatic juice contains a variety of digestive enzymes that help to digest fats, carbohydrates, and proteins. Secretions from the intestinal wall cells add enzymes to complete carbohydrate digestion.

The presence of fat in the duodenum stimulates the release of stored bile by the gallbladder. Lipids ordinarily do not mix with water, but bile acts as an emulsifier, keeping lipid molecules mixed with the watery chyme and digestive secretions. Without the action of bile, lipids might not come into contact with pancreatic lipase, and digestion would be incomplete.

With the pancreatic and intestinal enzymes working together, digestion progresses nicely, leaving smaller protein, carbohydrate, and lipid compounds ready for absorption. Other nutrients, such as vitamins, minerals, and cholesterol, are not digested and generally are absorbed unchanged.

Just as the small intestine accomplishes much of the nutrient digestion, it is also responsible for most nutrient absorption. Its structure makes the process of absorption efficient and complete. In most cases, more than 90 percent of ingested carbohydrate, fat, and protein is absorbed. To see how this is possible, we need to examine the structure of the small intestine.

### Absorptive Structures of the Small Intestine

The small intestine packs a gigantic surface area into a small space. As you can see in **Figure 4.14**, the interior surface of the small intestine is wrinkled into folds, tripling the absorptive surface area. These folds are carpeted with fingerlike projections called **villi** that expand the absorptive area another 10-fold. Each cell lining the surface of each villus is covered with a "brush border" containing as many as 1,000 hairlike projections called **microvilli**. The microvilli increase the surface area another 20 times. Taken together, the folds plus the villi and microvilli yield a 600-fold increase in surface area. In fact, your 10-foot- (3-meter-) long intestine has an absorptive surface area of more than 300 square yards (250 or more square meters)—equivalent to the surface of a tennis court!

### Nutrient Absorption in the Small Intestine

As nutrients journey through the small intestine, they are trapped in the folds and projections of the intestinal wall and absorbed through the microvilli into the lining cells. Depending on your diet, each day your small intestine absorbs several hundred grams of carbohydrates, 60 or more grams of fat, 50 to 100 grams of amino acids, and 7 to 8 liters of water. But the total absorptive capacity of the healthy small intestine is far greater. It actually has the capacity to absorb as much as several kilograms of carbohydrates, 500 grams of fat, 500 to 700 grams of amino acids, 3 to 5 grams of vitamins and

**duodenum [doo-oh-DEE-num]** The portion of the small intestine closest to the stomach. The duodenum is 25 to 30 cm (10 to 12 in.) long and wider than the remainder of the small intestine.

**jejunum [je-JOON-um]** The middle section of the small intestine (about 120 cm [4 ft] long), lying between the duodenum and ileum.

**ileum [ILL-ee-um]** The terminal segment of the small intestine (about 150 cm [5 ft] long), which opens into the large intestine.

**digestive secretions** Substances released at different places in the GI tract to speed the breakdown of ingested carbohydrates, fats, and proteins.

**villi** Small fingerlike projections that blanket the folds in the lining of the small intestine. Singular is *villus*.

**microvilli** Minute, hairlike projections that extend from the surface of absorptive cells facing the intestinal lumen.

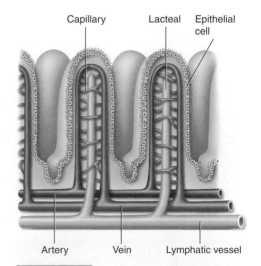

**Figure 4.14** **The absorptive surface of the small intestine.** To maximize the absorptive surface area, the small intestine is folded and lined with villi. You have a surface area the size of a tennis court packed into your gut.

**lymph**  Fluid that travels through the lymphatic system, made up of large fat particles and fluid drained from the areas between the cells.

**lacteal**  A small lymphatic vessel in the interior of each intestinal villus that picks up fat-soluble compounds from intestinal cells.

**large intestine**  The tube (about 150 cm [5 ft] long) extending from the ileum of the small intestine to the anus. The large intestine includes the appendix, cecum, colon, rectum, and anal canal.

**cecum**  The blind pouch at the beginning of the large intestine into which the ileum opens from one side and which is continuous with the colon.

**colon**  The portion of the large intestine extending from the cecum to the rectum. It is made up of four parts: the ascending, transverse, descending, and sigmoid colons.

**rectum**  The muscular final segment of the intestine, extending from the sigmoid colon to the anus.

**flatulence**  The presence of excessive amounts of air or other gases in the stomach or intestines.

minerals, and 20 or more liters of water per day.[4] Approximately 85 percent of the water absorption by the gut occurs in the jejunum.[5]

Nutrients absorbed through the intestinal lining pass into the interior of the villi. Each villus contains blood vessels (veins, arteries, and capillaries) and a **lymph** vessel (known as a **lacteal**) that transport nutrients to other parts of your body. Water-soluble nutrients are absorbed directly into the bloodstream. Fat-soluble lipid compounds are absorbed into the lymph rather than directly into the blood.

The small intestine suffers constant wear and tear as it propels and digests the chyme. The intestinal lining is renewed continually as the mucosal cells are replaced every two to five days. When the chyme has completed its 3- to 10-hour journey through the small intestine, it passes through the ileocecal valve, the connection to the large intestine.

## Large Intestine

The chyme's next stop is the **large intestine**. As **Figure 4.15** shows, this 5-foot-long tube includes the **cecum**, **colon**, **rectum**, and anal canal. As chyme fills the cecum, a local reflex signals the ileocecal valve to close, preventing material from reentering the ileum of the small intestine.

### Digestion in the Large Intestine

The peristaltic movements of the large intestine are sluggish compared with those of the small intestine. Normally 18 to 24 hours are required for material to travel its length. During that time, the colon's large population of bacteria digests small amounts of fiber,[6] providing a negligible number of calories daily. Of more significance are the other substances formed by this bacterial activity, including several vitamins, short-chain fatty acids, and various gases that contribute to **flatulence**.[7] Other than bacterial action, no further digestion occurs in the large intestine.

### Nutrient Absorption in the Large Intestine

Nutrient absorption in the large intestine is minimal, limited to water, sodium, chloride, potassium, and some of the vitamin K produced by bacteria. Although the colon's bacteria also produce vitamin $B_{12}$, it is not absorbed. The colon dehydrates the watery chyme, removing and absorbing most of the fluid. Of the approximately 1,000 milliliters of material that enters the large intestine, only about 150 milliliters remain for elimination as feces. The semisolid feces, consisting of roughly 60 percent solid matter (e.g., dietary fiber, bacteria, digestive secretions) and 40 percent water, then pass into the rectum. In the rectum, strong muscles hold back the waste until it is time to defecate. The rectal muscles then relax, and the anal sphincter opens to allow passage of the stool out the anal canal.[8]

See **Figure 4.16** for a summary of nutrient absorption along the gastrointestinal tract.

**Key Concepts**  *Digestion begins in the mouth with the action of salivary amylase. Food material next moves down the esophagus to the stomach, where it mixes with gastric secretions. Protein digestion begins with the action of pepsin, while salivary amylase action ceases due to the low pH level of the stomach. The liquid material (chyme) next moves to the small intestine. Here, secretions from the gallbladder, pancreas, and intestinal lining cells complete the digestion of carbohydrates, proteins, and fats. The end products of digestion, along with vitamins, minerals, water, and other compounds, are absorbed through the intestinal wall and into circulation. Undigested material and some liquid move on to the large intestine, where water and electrolytes are absorbed, leaving waste material to be excreted as feces.*

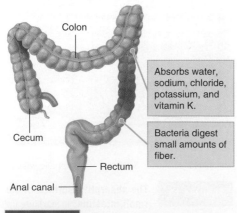

Colon

Absorbs water, sodium, chloride, potassium, and vitamin K.

Cecum

Bacteria digest small amounts of fiber.

Rectum

Anal canal

**Figure 4.15**    **The large intestine.** As the large intestine absorbs water, it forms undigested materials into feces for elimination.

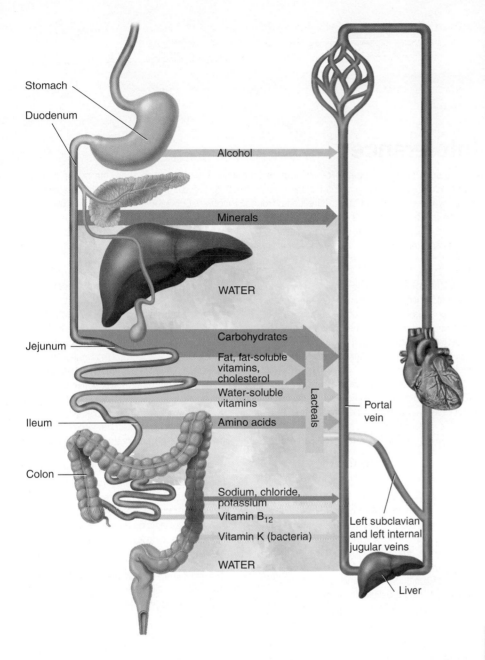

**Figure 4.16** **Nutrient absorption along the digestive tract.** Alcohol is absorbed quickly in the stomach. The small intestine is the absorptive site for carbohydrate, amino acids, fats, and most vitamins. Absorption of some vitamins and minerals takes place in the large intestine. Both the small and large intestines absorb water.

## Circulation of Nutrients

After foods are digested and nutrients are absorbed, they are transported via the vascular and lymphatic systems to specific destinations throughout the body. Let's take a closer look at how each of these circulatory systems delivers nutrients to the places they are needed.

### Vascular System

The **vascular system**, or blood circulatory system, is a network of veins and arteries through which the blood carries nutrients. (See **Figure 4.17**.) The heart is the pump that keeps the blood circulating through the body. Water-soluble nutrients are absorbed directly from intestinal cells into tiny capillary tributaries of the bloodstream, which carries them to the liver before they are dispersed throughout the body. Blood carries oxygen from the lungs and

## *Quick* Bite

**The Clever Colon**
Though it has been presumed that the colon has no digestive function, recent research shows that the human colon can be an important digestive site in patients who are missing significant sections of their small intestines. These patients can actually absorb energy from starch and nonstarch polysaccharides in the colon.

**vascular system** A network of veins and arteries through which the blood carries nutrients. Also called the *blood circulatory system*.

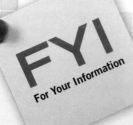

# Lactose Intolerance

If you drink a milkshake and soon afterward experience bloating, gas, abdominal pain, and diarrhea, the problem could be lactose intolerance—the incomplete digestion of the lactose in milk due to low levels of the intestinal enzyme lactase. Lactose is the primary carbohydrate in milk and other dairy foods. Nondairy foods—such as instant breakfast mixes, cake mixes, mayonnaise, luncheon meats, medications, and vitamin supplements—also may contain small amounts of lactose. Lactase enzyme is necessary to digest lactose in the small intestine. If lactase is deficient, undigested lactose enters the large intestine, where it is broken down by colonic bacteria, producing short-chain organic acids and gases (e.g., hydrogen, methane, carbon dioxide).

With the exception of infants with a rare inherited disorder in which they are born without lactase, infants have sufficient lactase. In many racial/ethnic groups, however, lactase activity declines with weaning. This normal, genetically controlled decrease in lactase activity, called lactose maldigestion, is prevalent among Asians, Native Americans, and African Americans. Among U.S. Caucasians and people from northern and central Europe, lactose maldigestion is far less common, and lactase activity tends to persist into adulthood. Lactose intolerance affects approximately 50 million American adults.[1]

In addition to primary lactose intolerance, lactose intolerance can be secondary to diseases or conditions (e.g., inflammatory bowel disease such as Crohn's disease or celiac disease; gastrointestinal surgery; certain medications) that injure the intestinal mucosa where lactase is secreted. Secondary lactose maldigestion is temporary, and lactose digestion improves once the underlying causative factor is corrected.

Many factors unrelated to lactose, including strong beliefs, can contribute to this condition. Studies have demonstrated that among self-described lactose-intolerant individuals, one-third to one-half develop few or no gastrointestinal symptoms following intake of lactose under well-controlled, double-blind conditions.

Self-diagnosis of lactose intolerance is a bad idea because it could lead to unnecessary dietary restrictions, expense, nutritional shortcomings, and failure to detect or treat a more serious gastrointestinal disorder. If lactose maldigestion is suspected, tests are available to diagnose this condition.

People with real or perceived lactose intolerance may limit their consumption of dairy foods unnecessarily and jeopardize their intake of calcium and other essential nutrients. A low intake of calcium is associated with increased risk of osteoporosis (porous bones), hypertension, and colon cancer.

With the exception of the few individuals who are sensitive to even very small amounts of lactose, avoiding all lactose is neither necessary nor recommended, because some lactase is still being produced. Lactose maldigesters need to determine the amount of lactose they can comfortably consume at any one time. Here are some strategies for including milk and other dairy foods in your diet without developing symptoms:

1. Initially, consume small servings of lactose-containing foods such as milk (e.g., ½ cup). Gradually increase the serving size until symptoms begin to appear, and then back off.
2. Consume lactose with a meal or foods (e.g., milk with cereal) to improve tolerance.
3. Adjust the type of dairy food. Whole milk may be tolerated better than low-fat milk, and chocolate milk may be tolerated better than unflavored milk. Many cheeses (e.g., cheddar, Swiss, Parmesan) contain considerably less lactose than milk. Aged cheeses generally have negligible amounts of lactose. Yogurts with live, active cultures are another option; these bacteria will digest lactose. Sweet acidophilus milk, yogurt milk, and other nonfermented dairy foods may be tolerated better than regular milk by lactose maldigesters.
4. Lactose-hydrolyzed dairy foods and/or commercial enzyme preparations (e.g., lactase capsules, chewable tablets, solutions) are another option. Lactose-reduced (70 percent less lactose) and lactose-free (99.9 percent less lactose) milks are available, although at a higher cost than regular milk.

Lactose maldigestion need not be an impediment to including milk and other dairy foods in the diet to help meet the needs for calcium and other essential nutrients.

1   National Institute of Diabetes and Digestive and Kidney Diseases. Lactose intolerance. http://digestive.niddk.nih.gov/ddiseases/pubs/lactoseintolerance. Accessed 4/28/11.

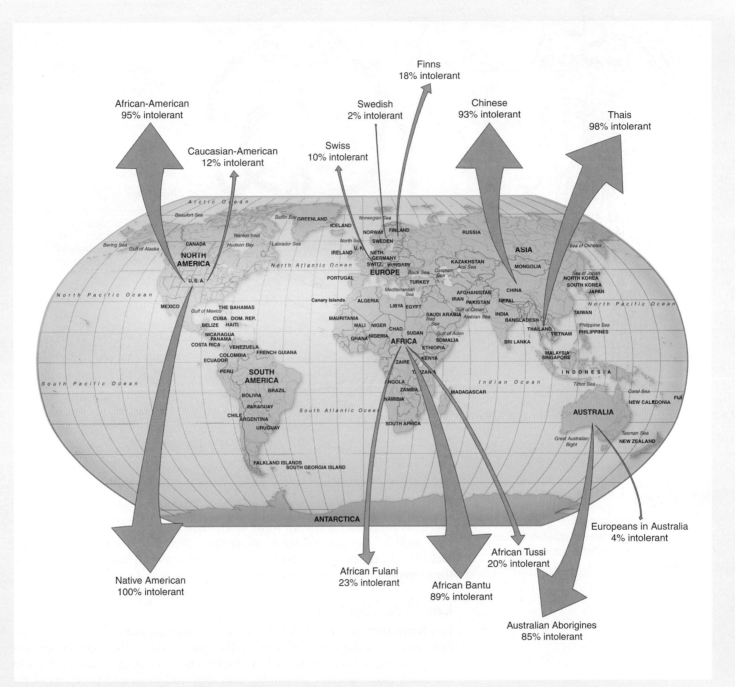

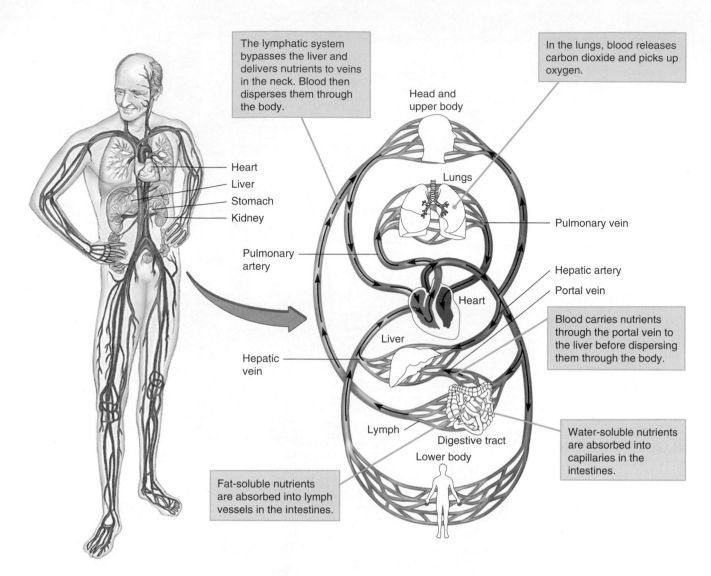

The lymphatic system bypasses the liver and delivers nutrients to veins in the neck. Blood then disperses them through the body.

In the lungs, blood releases carbon dioxide and picks up oxygen.

Head and upper body

Lungs

Heart
Liver
Stomach
Kidney

Pulmonary vein

Pulmonary artery

Hepatic artery
Portal vein

Heart

Blood carries nutrients through the portal vein to the liver before dispersing them through the body.

Liver

Hepatic vein

Lymph

Digestive tract

Lower body

Water-soluble nutrients are absorbed into capillaries in the intestines.

Fat-soluble nutrients are absorbed into lymph vessels in the intestines.

**Figure 4.17**  **Circulation.** Blood carries oxygen from the lungs and nutrients from the GI system to all body tissues. The lymphatic system, a circulatory system that bypasses the liver before connecting to the bloodstream, carries fat-soluble nutrients.

nutrients from the GI system to all body tissues. Once the destination cells have used the oxygen and nutrients, carbon dioxide and waste products are picked up by the blood and transported to the lungs and kidneys, respectively, for excretion.

## Lymphatic System

The **lymphatic system** is a network of vessels that drain lymph, the clear fluid formed in the spaces between cells. Lymph moves through this system and eventually empties into the bloodstream near the neck. Lymph vessels in the small intestine carry fat-soluble nutrients and most end products of fat digestion. After a fatty meal, lymph can become as much as 1 to 2 percent fat. Nutrients absorbed into the lymphatic system, unlike those absorbed directly into the vascular system, bypass the liver before entering the bloodstream.

Unlike the vascular system, the lymphatic system has no pumping organ. The major lymph vessels contain one-way valves; and when vessels are filled with lymph, smooth muscles in the vessel walls contract and pump the lymph forward. The succession of valves allows each segment of the vessel to act as

**lymphatic system** A system of small vessels, ducts, valves, and organized tissue (e.g., lymph nodes) through which lymph moves from its origin in the tissues toward the heart.

an independent pump. Lymph also is moved along by skeletal muscle contractions that squeeze the vessels.

The lymphatic system also performs an important cleanup function. Proteins and large particulate matter in tissue spaces cannot be absorbed directly into the blood capillaries, but they easily enter the lymphatic system, which carries them away for removal. This removal process is essential—without it a person would die within 24 hours from buildup of fluid and materials around the cells.[9]

## Excretion and Elimination

Excretion regulates the concentrations of minerals and other substances in the body and removes the waste products of metabolism. Do not confuse the metabolic waste removed by excretion with digestive waste removed by elimination. Metabolic waste arises from all the chemical reactions that take place in cells throughout the body. Digestive waste never passes into cells—it is the unabsorbed "leftovers" that pass along and out of the GI tract.

The primary organs of excretion are the lungs and kidneys. The lungs excrete water and carbon dioxide. The kidneys filter the blood and excrete substances to remove waste and maintain the body's water and ion balance. The kidneys excrete salts; nitrogen-containing wastes, such as urea; small amounts of other substances; and water. This watery mix is called urine. The kidneys vary the amount and concentration of urine to help maintain constant physiological conditions within the body.

**Key Concepts**  *Absorbed nutrients are carried by either the vascular or lymphatic system. Water-soluble nutrients are absorbed directly into the bloodstream, carried to the liver, and then distributed around the body. Fat-soluble vitamins and large lipid molecules are absorbed into the lymphatic vessels and carried by this system before entering the vascular system. The main excretory organs are the lungs and kidneys. The lungs excrete carbon dioxide and water. The kidneys excrete salts, metabolic wastes, and water.*

# Signaling Systems: Command, Control, and Defense

How does your body keep the complex processes of digestion, absorption, and nutrient transport running smoothly? The nervous system, your body's communication network, carries commands and feedback to and from tissues throughout the body. Signals delivered by the nervous system can trigger the release of hormones—chemical messengers that control and coordinate biological activities. The gastrointestinal tract also is a major player in your immune system, a coordinated system of cells and tissues that defends against invading microorganisms.

## Nervous System

Nerves carry information back and forth between tissues and the brain. Chemicals called neurotransmitters send signals to either excite or suppress nerves, thereby stimulating or inhibiting activity in various parts of the body.

The **central nervous system (CNS)** regulates GI activity in two ways. The **enteric nervous system** is a local system of nerves in the gut wall that is stimulated both by the chemical composition of chyme and by the stretching of the GI lumen that results from food in the GI tract. This stimulation leads to nerve impulses that enhance secretions and muscle movement along the tract. The enteric nervous system plays an essential role in controlling movement, blood flow, water and electrolyte transport, and acid secretion in

**central nervous system (CNS)**  The brain and the spinal cord. The central nervous system transmits signals that control muscular actions and glandular secretions along the entire GI tract.

**enteric nervous system**  A network of nerves located in the gastrointestinal wall.

the GI tract. A branch of the **autonomic nervous system (ANS)** (the portion of the CNS that controls organ function) responds to the sight, smell, and thought of food. Via the vagus nerve, this branch of the CNS carries signals to and from the GI tract and also enhances GI movement and secretion. In the past, treatments for some ulcers and other GI ailments included severing the vagus nerve, a measure that brought temporary, but not long-term, relief from pain.

## Hormonal System

Hormones also are involved in GI regulation. Hormones are chemical messengers that generally are produced at one location and travel in the bloodstream to affect another location in the body.

Gastrointestinal hormonal signals increase or decrease GI motility and secretions and influence your appetite by sending signals to the central nervous system. Some GI hormones function as growth factors for the gastrointestinal mucosa and pancreas.

Taken together, nerve cells and hormones coordinate the movement and secretions of the GI tract so that enzymes are released when and where they are needed. Chyme moves at a rate that will make digestion and absorption most efficient.

## Immune System

The immune system protects us from foreign invaders. A healthy immune system can detect and fight off potential sources of infection, recognize the difference between foreign cells and the body's own cells, recognize and react when it encounters a microbe it has seen before, and then scale back its response when the foreign agent has been dealt with.[10]

Our first line of defense is preventing infectious agents from entering the body. That's the job of the skin and the mucous membranes that line the gastrointestinal, respiratory, and reproductive systems. Of these, the gastrointestinal system is the largest barrier; about 400 square meters as compared with only about 2 square meters of skin.[11] The normal structure and activities of the gastrointestinal system are a major part of the body's defense—tight junctions between the cells that line the intestines, normal peristalsis, and intestinal secretions all work to keep foreign bodies out. Patches of smooth cells just under the lining of the intestines, called Peyer's patches, are really specialized immune cells known as gut-associated lymphoid tissue (GALT). Similar types of cell clusters are found along the lining of the tonsils and appendix. Other tissues involved in the immune system are the lymph nodes, located along the lymphatic system, and the spleen.

Different types of white blood cells carry out the immune response. Some travel the bloodstream to areas of invasion, attacking and ingesting pathogens. **Natural killer cells** attack virus-infected cells and cells that have turned cancerous. **Macrophages**, or "big eaters," take up stations in tissues and act as scavengers, devouring pathogens and worn-out cells. Macrophages congregate in the lymph nodes, where they filter bacteria and other substances from lymph. **Lymphocytes**—white blood cells of the immune system—travel in both the bloodstream and lymphatic system. Some types of lymphocytes produce **antibodies**. Others remember a prior invader, enabling the body to mount a rapid response should the same invader appear again. Upon recognizing an invasion, helper cells trigger the mass production of killer cells. When the danger is over, suppressor cells halt the immune response.

## Quick Bite

**Halt! Who Goes There?**
Be they friend or foe, antibiotics kill microorganisms in your GI tract, frequently causing diarrhea. About half of pharmaceutical drugs have gastrointestinal side effects.

**Key Concepts** *Both hormonal and nervous system signals regulate gastrointestinal activity. Nerve cells in both the enteric and autonomic nervous systems control muscle movement and secretions. Key hormones coordinate GI movement and secretion for optimal digestion and absorption of nutrients. The GI tract also is a major player in the immune system.*

## Influences on Digestion and Absorption
### Psychological Influences

The taste, smell, and presentation of foods can have a positive effect on digestion. Just the thought of food can trigger saliva production and peristalsis. Stressful emotions such as depression and fear can have the reverse effect (see **Figure 4.18**); they stimulate the brain to activate the autonomic nervous system. This results in decreased gastric acid secretion, reduced blood flow to the stomach, inhibition of peristalsis, and reduced propulsion of food.[12] The next time you sit down to a holiday meal, notice how you feel at the sight of your family's traditional foods as well as smells from your childhood. Happiness and positive memories add to the enjoyment of food, whereas unhappiness can bring on a poor appetite or stomach upset.

THINK
About It
4

### Chemical Influences

The type of protein you eat and the way it is prepared affect digestion. Plant proteins tend to be less digestible than animal proteins. Cooking food usually denatures protein (uncoils its three-dimensional structure), which increases digestibility. Cooking meat softens its connective tissue, making chewing easier and increasing the ability of digestive enzymes to break the meat down into absorbable nutrients. Food processing produces chemicals that may influence digestive secretions. For example, whereas meat extracts may stimulate digestion, frying foods in fat at very high temperatures produces small amounts of **acrolein**,[13] a chemical that decreases the flow of digestive secretions. The physical condition of a food sometimes causes problems with digestion. Cold foods may cause intestinal spasms in people who suffer from irritable bowel syndrome or Crohn's disease. Stomach contents can affect absorption. When food is consumed on an empty stomach, it has more contact with gastric secretions and will be absorbed faster than if it was consumed on a full stomach. Certain medicines may inhibit nutrient absorption, and, in turn, certain foods may interact with medicines, making the drugs less effective or even toxic.

### Bacterial Influences

In the healthy stomach, hydrochloric acid kills most bacteria. In conditions where there is a lower concentration of hydrochloric acid, more bacteria can survive and multiply. Harmful bacteria can cause gastritis (an inflammation of the stomach lining) and peptic ulcer (a wound in the mucous membranes lining the stomach or duodenum). Bacteria that cause foodborne illness can resist the germicidal effects of hydrochloric acid, so they survive to wreak havoc on the digestive process.

The large intestine maintains a large population of bacteria. These bacteria can form several vitamins and digest small amounts of fiber, producing a small amount of energy. These bacteria also synthesize gases, such as hydrogen, ammonia, and methane, as well as acids and various substances that contribute to the odor of feces. If the digestion and absorption of food in the small intestine are incomplete, the undigested material enters the large

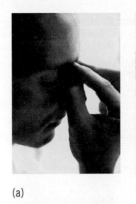
(a)

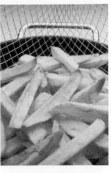
(b)

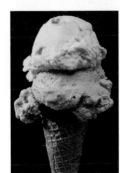
(c)

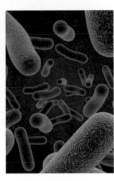
(d)

**Figure 4.18**  **Negative factors for digestion.** Several factors can reduce digestive secretions that interfere with digestion and absorption. Such factors include (a) stress, (b) high-temperature fat frying, (c) cold foods, and (d) bacteria.

**acrolein**  A pungent decomposition product of fats, generated from dehydrating the glycerol component of fats; responsible for the coughing attacks caused by the fumes released by burning fat. This toxic water-soluble liquid vaporizes easily and is highly flammable.

## Quick Bite

### Gastrointestinal Flora Abound
Your entire body has about 100 trillion cells, but this is only one-tenth the number of protective microorganisms normally living in your body. More than 500 bacterial species live in your GI tract.

**Figure 4.19** **Common GI ailments.** Beans are familiar culprits in what is perhaps the most common GI ailment—gas. Rice is the only starch that does not cause gas.

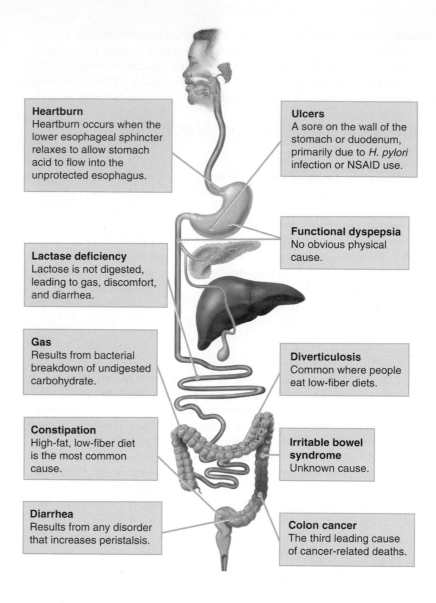

**Heartburn**
Heartburn occurs when the lower esophageal sphincter relaxes to allow stomach acid to flow into the unprotected esophagus.

**Ulcers**
A sore on the wall of the stomach or duodenum, primarily due to *H. pylori* infection or NSAID use.

**Functional dyspepsia**
No obvious physical cause.

**Lactase deficiency**
Lactose is not digested, leading to gas, discomfort, and diarrhea.

**Gas**
Results from bacterial breakdown of undigested carbohydrate.

**Diverticulosis**
Common where people eat low-fiber diets.

**Constipation**
High-fat, low-fiber diet is the most common cause.

**Irritable bowel syndrome**
Unknown cause.

**Diarrhea**
Results from any disorder that increases peristalsis.

**Colon cancer**
The third leading cause of cancer-related deaths.

intestine, where bacterial action produces excessive gas and possibly bloating and pain.

**Key Concepts** *Psychological, chemical, and bacterial factors can influence the processes of digestion and absorption. Emotions can influence GI motility and secretion. The temperature and form of food also can affect digestive secretions. Although stomach acid kills many types of bacteria, some are resistant to acid and cause foodborne illness. Helpful bacteria in the large intestine can cause bloating and gas if they receive and begin to digest food components that are normally digested in the small intestine.*

## Nutrition and GI Disorders

"I have butterflies in my stomach." "It was a gut-wrenching experience." Our language contains many references to the connection between emotional distress and the GI tract. Most of us have experienced intestinal cramping right before a big date or job interview or a queasy stomach in response to something very disgusting. Through its many neurochemical connections with the gut, the brain exerts a profound influence on GI function. Nearly all GI disorders are influenced to some degree by emotional state. However, a number of illnesses that were once attributed largely to emotional stress, such as peptic ulcer disease, have been shown to be caused primarily by infection and other physical causes. **Figure 4.19** shows some common ailments that affect the GI tract.

Although stress management might help and medical intervention might be required, we can prevent and manage most GI disorders with diet. For instance, adding fiber-rich foods (see Table 4.2) and water to the diet reduces intestinal pressure, decreases the time food by-products remain in the colon, and promotes bowel regularity. You can avoid most problems and keep your GI tract operating at peak efficiency if you regularly eat a healthful diet, exercise, and maintain a healthy weight.

## Constipation

**Constipation** is defined as having a bowel movement fewer than three times per week.[14] With constipation, stools are usually hard, dry, small in size, and difficult to eliminate. People who are constipated may find it painful to have a bowel movement and often experience straining, bloating, and the sensation of a full bowel.

Constipation is a symptom, not a disease. Almost everyone experiences constipation at some point. Although stress, inactivity, cessation of smoking, or various illnesses can lead to constipation, a poor diet (low in fiber and water and high in fats) typically is the cause. Some fibers, such as the pectins in fruits and gums in beans, dissolve easily in water and take on a soft, gel-like texture in the intestines. Other fibers, such as cellulose in wheat bran, pass almost unchanged through the intestines. The bulk and soft texture of fiber help prevent hard, dry stools that are difficult to pass. People who eat plenty of high-fiber foods are not likely to become constipated. High-fiber diets also need to include plenty of liquids to prevent dehydration. Also, regular exercise

**constipation** Infrequent and difficult bowel movements, followed by a sensation of incomplete evacuation.

## Table 4.2 Fiber Content of Foods

| Food Group | Serving Size | Fiber (g) |
|---|---|---|
| *Legumes* | | |
| Kidney beans | 1 cup, cooked | 11.3 |
| Lentils | 1 cup, cooked | 15.6 |
| Split peas | 1 cup, cooked | 16.3 |
| *Fruits* | | |
| Dried plums | ½ cup | 9.4 |
| Apple with skin | 1 small | 3.6 |
| Peach with skin | 1 large | 2.6 |
| *Vegetables* | | |
| Broccoli | 1 cup, raw | 2.4 |
| Carrot | 2 medium, raw | 3.4 |
| Tomato | 1 large | 2.2 |
| *Grains* | | |
| Wheat-bran flake cereal | 1 ounce | 5.0 |
| Bulgur wheat | ½ cup, cooked | 4.1 |
| Whole-wheat bread | 1 slice | 0.9 |
| Brown rice | ½ cup, cooked | 1.8 |
| Spaghetti, enriched white | ½ cup, cooked | 1.3 |
| White bread | 1 slice | 0.6 |
| White rice | ½ cup, cooked | 0.3 |

**Source:** Data from US Department of Agriculture, Agricultural Research Service. 2011. USDA National Nutrient Database for Standard Reference, Release 24. Nutrient Data Laboratory Home Page, http://www.ars.usda.gov/ba/bhnrc/ndl

**diarrhea** Watery stools due to reduced absorption of water.

helps keep all the body's muscles healthy, including the GI tract muscles, and will help promote regularity.

Although treatment depends on the cause, severity, and duration, in most cases dietary changes help relieve symptoms and prevent constipation.

## Diarrhea

**Diarrhea**—loose, watery stools that occur more than three times in one day—is caused by digestive products moving through the large intestine too rapidly for sufficient water to be reabsorbed.

Diarrhea is a symptom of many disorders that cause increased peristalsis. Culprits include stress, intestinal irritation or damage, side effects of medications, and intolerance to gluten (a protein in wheat), fat, or lactose (the natural sugar in milk). Eating food contaminated with bacteria or viruses often causes diarrhea when the digestive tract speeds the offending food along the alimentary canal and out of the body. (See the FYI feature "Bugs in Your Gut? Health Effects of Intestinal Bacteria.")

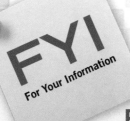

FYI
For Your Information

# Bugs in Your Gut? Health Effects of Intestinal Bacteria

Unseen and unnoticed, millions and millions of bacteria call your GI tract home. Although we often associate bacteria with illness, the right kinds of bacteria in the gut actually protect us from disease. The normal bacterial population of the gut, specifically strains of lactobacilli and bifidobacteria, have been linked to improved digestion, enhanced GI immune function, improved lactose tolerance, and even reduced risk of colorectal cancer. So how can we be good hosts to our intestinal guests, keeping them well fed and happy? The answer may be in food products and dietary supplements known as probiotics and prebiotics.

Probiotics are foods (or supplements) that contain live microorganisms such as *Lactobacillus acidophilus*. Such lactic-acid-producing bacteria have been used for centuries to break milk down into yogurt, cheeses, and other products. The bacteria convert lactose into lactic acid, which causes the milk to gel and imparts a tart flavor to the product. The resulting product has a much longer shelf life than fresh milk and is as-

sociated with good health and longevity in many societies.

The term *prebiotic* describes a nondigestible food product that stimulates the growth and/or activity of "good" gut bacteria. For example, it is thought that the composition of breast milk strongly favors the growth of lactobacilli and bifidobacteria in the newborn gut. Some scientists have found bifidobacteria to be the dominant species in breast-fed infants, while the bacterial population of bottle-fed infants is more diverse. The reduced incidence of GI infections in breast-fed infants has been attributed to the dominance of bifidobacteria. Substances that may be effective prebiotics include fructooligosaccharides, galactooligosaccharides, and inulin.

So, how does feeding your gut improve your health? Intestinal bacteria metabolize both indigestible and incompletely digested food material. Some types of bacteria produce compounds that may reduce risk of colon cancer. For example, acids produced by colon bacteria change the pH of the colon, which may interfere with carcinogen-

esis (development of cancer). "Good" bacteria can digest the lactose that enters the colon of a person with lactose intolerance, reducing symptoms and discomfort. Successful colonization of helpful bacteria allows them to outnumber (and out-eat) disease-causing bacteria, thus reducing the likelihood of foodborne illness.

Fermented milk products such as yogurt or kefir are one way to keep your gut happy. Look for a seal adopted by the National Yogurt Association to identify products that contain a minimum of 100 million live lactic acid bacteria per gram of yogurt. Not all brands of yogurt contain live, active cultures. Probiotics in supplement form must have sufficient numbers of live bacteria to be useful; currently, identification and standardization procedures are lacking. Prebiotics such as fructooligosaccharides are the subject of intense and promising research. Although results are preliminary, food and supplement sources of prebiotics may be another useful way to improve gut microflora and overall health.

Diarrhea can cause dehydration, which means the body lacks enough fluid to function properly. Dehydration is particularly dangerous in children and the elderly, and it must be treated promptly to avoid serious health problems.

A diet of broth, tea, toast, and other low-fiber foods, along with avoidance of lactose, fructose, caffeine, and sugar alcohols, such as sorbitol, can help reduce diarrhea until it subsides. As stools form, you can gradually introduce more foods. Pectin, a form of dietary fiber found in apples and citrus peel, may be helpful, along with foods high in potassium—if they are tolerated—to replace lost electrolytes. Fluid replacement also is important to avoid dehydration.

## Diverticulosis

Like an inner tube that pokes through weak places in an old tire, the colon develops small pouches that bulge outward through weak spots as people age. (See **Figure 4.20**.) Known as **diverticulosis**, this condition afflicts about half of all Americans aged 60 to 80 and almost everyone over age 80. Although it usually causes few problems, in 10 to 25 percent of these people, the pouches become infected or inflamed—a painful condition called **diverticulitis**.

Diverticulosis and diverticulitis are common in developed or industrialized countries—particularly the United States, England, and Australia—where low-fiber diets are common. Diverticular disease is rare in countries of Asia and Africa, where people eat high-fiber, vegetable-based diets.

A low-fiber diet can make stools hard and difficult to pass. If the stool is too hard, muscles must strain to move it. This is the main cause of increased pressure in the colon, which causes weak spots to bulge outward.

Increasing the amount of fiber in the diet may reduce symptoms of diverticulosis and prevent complications such as diverticulitis. Fiber keeps stools soft and lowers pressure inside the colon so bowel contents can move through easily. Additional benefits of fiber are listed in Table 4.3.

Until recently, many doctors suggested avoiding foods with small seeds, such as tomatoes or strawberries, because they believed that particles could lodge in the pouches and cause inflammation. However, this is now a controversial point, and no evidence supports this recommendation.

If cramps, bloating, and constipation are problems, the doctor may prescribe a short course of pain medication. However, many medications cause either diarrhea or constipation, undesirable side effects for people with diverticulosis.

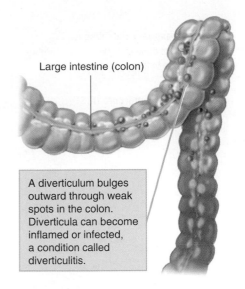

Large intestine (colon)

A diverticulum bulges outward through weak spots in the colon. Diverticula can become inflamed or infected, a condition called diverticulitis.

**Figure 4.20** **Diverticulosis.** In industrialized nations, diverticulosis is common in older people. It is unusual in developing countries where people eat high-fiber diets.

**diverticulosis [dy-vur-tik-yoo-LOH-sis]** A condition that occurs when small pouches (diverticula) push outward through weak spots in the colon.

**diverticulitis [dy-vur-tik-yoo-LY-tis]** A condition that occurs when small pouches in the colon (diverticula) become infected or irritated. Also called *left-sided appendicitis*.

**Table 4.3** **Benefits of Fiber**

- Helps control weight by delaying gastric emptying and providing a feeling of fullness.
- Improves glucose tolerance by delaying the movement of carbohydrate into the small intestine.
- Reduces risk of heart disease by binding with bile (which contains cholesterol) in the intestine and causing it to be excreted, which in turn helps to lower blood cholesterol levels.
- Promotes regularity and reduces constipation by increasing stool weight and decreasing transit time.
- Reduces the risk of diverticulosis by decreasing pressure within the colon, decreasing transit time, and increasing stool weight.

**Source:** Data from Institute of Medicine, Food and Nutrition Board. *Dietary Reference Intakes for Energy, Carbohydrate, Fiber, Fat, Fatty Acids, Cholesterol, Protein, and Amino Acids (Macronutrients)*. Washington, DC: National Academies Press; 2002.

## *Quick* Bite

**Short Bowel Syndrome**
Patients who suffer from short bowel syndrome commonly have difficulty absorbing fat-soluble vitamins. To enhance absorption, treatment includes taking a fat-soluble vitamin supplement that easily mingles with water. These patients also may need to take intramuscular shots of $B_{12}$ because they are unable to absorb this water-soluble vitamin.

**gastroesophageal reflux disease (GERD)** Tissue damage to the esophagus due to the reflux of gastric contents.

**irritable bowel syndrome (IBS)** A disruptive state of intestinal motility with no known cause.

## Heartburn and Gastroesophageal Reflux Disease

Heartburn occurs when the sphincter between the esophagus and stomach relaxes inappropriately, allowing the stomach's contents to flow back into the esophagus. Unlike the stomach, the esophagus has no protective mucous lining, so acid can damage it quickly and cause pain. Many people experience occasional heartburn, but for some, heartburn is a chronic, often daily, event and a symptom of a more serious disorder called **gastroesophageal reflux disease (GERD)**. GERD, along with obesity, is a key risk factor for esophageal cancer, a type of cancer that is on the rise in North America.[15] GERD has a variety of causes, and many treatment strategies involve lifestyle and nutrition.

Doctors recommend avoiding foods and beverages that can weaken the esophageal sphincter, including chocolate, peppermint, fatty foods, coffee, and alcoholic beverages. Foods and beverages that can irritate a damaged esophageal lining, such as citrus fruits and juices, tomato products, and pepper, also should be avoided.

Decreasing both the portion size and the fat content of meals may help. High-fat meals remain in the stomach longer than low-fat meals. This creates back pressure on the esophageal sphincter. Eating meals at least two to three hours before bedtime may reduce reflux problems by allowing partial emptying and a decrease in stomach acidity. Elevating the head of the bed or sleeping on a specially designed wedge reduces heartburn by allowing gravity to minimize reflux of stomach contents into the esophagus.

In addition, cigarette smoking weakens the esophageal sphincter, and being overweight often worsens symptoms. Smokers have various reasons to stop, including GERD, and many overweight people find relief when they lose weight.

## Irritable Bowel Syndrome

About 20 percent of people in Western countries suffer from **irritable bowel syndrome (IBS)**,[16] a poorly understood condition that causes abdominal pain, altered bowel habits (such as diarrhea or constipation), and cramps. Often IBS is just a mild annoyance, but for some people it can be disabling.

The cause of IBS remains a mystery, but emotional stress and specific foods clearly aggravate the symptoms in most sufferers.[17] Beans, chocolate, milk products, and large amounts of alcohol are frequent offenders. Fat in any form (animal or vegetable) is a strong stimulus of colonic contractions after a meal. Caffeine causes loose stools in many people, but it is more likely to affect those with IBS. Women with IBS may have more symptoms during their menstrual periods, suggesting that reproductive hormones can increase IBS symptoms.

The good news about IBS is that although its symptoms can be uncomfortable, it does not shorten life span or progress to more serious illness. IBS can usually be controlled with diet and lifestyle modifications, as well as judicious use of medication. Stress management is an important part of treatment for IBS and includes stress reduction (relaxation) training and relaxation therapies, such as meditation; counseling and support; regular exercise; changes to stressful situations in your life; and adequate sleep.[18]

## Colorectal Cancer

Colorectal cancer—cancer of the colon or rectum—is the third leading cause of cancer-related deaths in the United States.[19] According to the World Health Organization, risk for colorectal cancer is increased by high intakes of meat and fat, and decreased by high intakes of fruit, vegetables, folate, and calcium.[20] Overweight and obesity increase risk while regular physical activity reduces risk. Many studies have looked at the dietary content of red meat, processed meat and the risk of colon cancer. One large population study looked at intake of red meat and the incidence of cancer and found an increased risk of colon cancer in the population group that consumed more than 180 grams per day of red meat compared to those who consumed less than 20 grams per day.[21] In another study, red meat intake was associated with an increase of nearly 85 percent of colorectal cancer in individuals who ate red meat seven times a week compared to three times per week.[22] Although several other studies correlate the consumption of red meat with an increased risk of developing colorectal cancer,[23] it is important to realize that other dietary factors (i.e., Western lifestyle; high intake of refined sugars and alcohol; and low intake of fruits, vegetables, and fiber) and behavioral factors (i.e., low physical activity, high smoking prevalence, high body mass index) limit the ability to isolate the independent effects of red meat consumption.[24]

Observational and case control studies support the idea that fiber-rich diets reduce colorectal cancer risk, and scientists have hypothesized a number of possible ways that fiber might be protective.[25] These include dilution of carcinogens in a bulkier stool, more rapid transit of carcinogens through the GI tract, and lower colon pH due to bacterial fermentation of fiber.

Although there are logical reasons why a high fiber intake may be beneficial, studies in humans and animals fail to support these theories. Fiber has not been shown to reduce risk of colorectal cancer or to prevent recurrence of the colorectal polyps that are precursors to many cancers.[26]

## Gas

Everyone has gas and eliminates it by burping or passing it through the rectum. Gas is made primarily of odorless vapors. Flatulence has an unpleasant odor because bacteria in the large intestine release small amounts of gases that contain sulfur. Although having gas is common, it can be uncomfortable and embarrassing.

Gas in the stomach is commonly caused by swallowing air. We all swallow small amounts of air when we eat and drink. However, eating or drinking rapidly, chewing gum, smoking, or wearing loose dentures can cause us to take in more air. Burping, or belching, is the way most swallowed air leaves the stomach. The remaining gas moves into the small intestine, where it is partially absorbed. A small amount travels into the large intestine for release through the rectum. (The stomach also releases carbon dioxide when stomach acid and bicarbonate mix, but most of this gas is absorbed into the bloodstream and does not enter the large intestine.)

Frequent passage of rectal gas may be annoying, but it is seldom a symptom of serious disease. **Flatus** (lower intestinal gas) composition depends to a great extent on your carbohydrate intake and the activity of the colon's bacterial population.

Most foods that contain carbohydrates can cause gas. By contrast, fats and proteins cause little gas. In the large intestine, bacteria partially break down undigested carbohydrate, producing hydrogen, carbon dioxide, and, in about one-third of people, methane. Eventually these gases exit through the rectum.

Foods that produce gas in one person may not cause gas in another. Some common bacteria in the large intestine can destroy the hydrogen that other bacteria produce. The balance of the two types of bacteria may explain why some people have more gas than others.

**flatus**  Lower intestinal gas that is expelled through the rectum.

**ulcer** A craterlike lesion that occurs in the lining of the stomach or duodenum; also called a *peptic ulcer* to distinguish it from a skin ulcer.

Carbohydrates that commonly cause gas are (1) raffinose and stachyose, found in large quantities in beans; (2) fructose, a common sweetener in soft drinks and fruit drinks; (3) lactose; and (4) sorbitol. Most starches, including potatoes, corn, noodles, and wheat, produce gas as they are broken down in the large intestine. Rice is the only starch that does not cause gas.

The fiber in oat bran, beans, peas, and most fruits is broken down in the large intestine, where digestion causes gas. In contrast, the fiber in wheat bran and some vegetables passes essentially unchanged through the intestines and produces little gas.

## Ulcers

A gnawing, burning pain in the upper abdomen is the classic sign of a peptic **ulcer**, which also can cause nausea, vomiting, loss of appetite, and weight loss. A peptic ulcer is a sore that forms in the duodenum (duodenal ulcer) or the lining of the stomach (gastric ulcer).

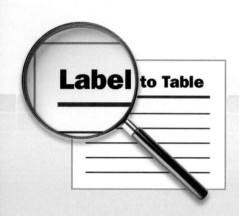

## Label to Table

As you've learned in this chapter, fiber is one of the few things you do not digest fully. Instead, fiber moves through the GI tract, and most of it leaves the body in feces. If it's not digested, then why all the fuss about eating more fiber? A healthy intake of fiber may lower your risk of cancer and heart disease and help with bowel regularity. So how do you know which foods have fiber? You have to check the food label!

This Nutrition Facts panel is from the label on a loaf of whole-wheat bread. The highlighted sections show you that every slice of bread contains 3 grams of fiber. The "12%" listed to the right of that refers to the Daily Values below. Look at the Daily Values at the bottom of the label, and note that there are two numbers listed for fiber. One (25 g) is for a person who consumes about 2,000 kilocalories per day, and the other (30 g) is for a 2,500-kilocalorie level. It should be no surprise that if you are consuming more calories, you should also be consuming more fiber. The 12 percent Daily Value (12%DV) is calculated using the 2,000-kilocalorie fiber guideline as follows:

$$\frac{3 \text{ grams fiber per slice}}{25 \text{ grams Daily Value}} = .12, \text{ or } 12 \text{ percent}$$

This means if you make a sandwich with two slices of whole-wheat bread, you're getting 6 grams of fiber and almost one-fourth (24%DV) of your fiber needs per day. Not bad! Be careful, though—many people inadvertently buy wheat bread thinking that it's as high in fiber as whole-wheat bread, but it's not. Whole-wheat bread contains the whole (complete) grain, but wheat bread is usually made of refined wheat flour that has been stripped of its fiber. Check the label before you buy your next loaf of bread!

## Nutrition Facts

Serving Size: 1 slice (43g)
Servings Per Container: 16

**Calories** 100
Calories from Fat 15

| Amount Per Serving | % Daily Value* |
| --- | --- |
| **Total Fat** 2g | 3% |
| Saturated Fat 0g | 0% |
| Trans Fat 0g | |
| **Cholesterol** 0mg | 0% |

Vitamin A 0%  •  Vitamin C 0%  •  Calcium 6%  •  Iron 6%
Thiamin 10%  •  Riboflavin 4%  •  Niacin 10%  •  Folate 10%

| Amount Per Serving | % Daily Value* |
| --- | --- |
| **Sodium** 230mg | 9% |
| **Total Carbohydrate** 18g | 6% |
| Dietary Fibers 3g | 12% |
| Sugars 2g | |
| **Protein** 5g | |

* Percent Daily Values are based on a 2,000 calorie diet. Your daily values may be higher or lower depending on your calorie needs:

| | | Calories: | 2,000 | 2,500 |
| --- | --- | --- | --- | --- |
| Total Fat | Less Than | | 65g | 80g |
| Sat Fat | Less Than | | 20g | 25g |
| Cholesterol | Less Than | | 300mg | 300mg |
| Sodium | Less Than | | 2,400mg | 2,400mg |
| Total Carbohydrate | | | 300g | 375g |
| Dietary Fiber | | | 25g | 30g |

INGREDIENTS: STONE GROUND WHOLE WHEAT FLOUR, WATER, HIGH FRUCTOSE CORN SYRUP, WHEAT GLUTEN, WHEAT BRAN. CONTAINS 2% OR LESS OF EACH OF THE FOLLOWING: YEAST, SALT, PARTIALLY HYDROGENATED SOYBEAN OIL, HONEY, MOLASSES, RAISIN JUICE CONCENTRATE, DOUGH CONDITIONERS (MAY CONTAIN ONE OR MORE OF EACH OF THE FOLLOWING: MONO- AND DIGLYCERIDES, CALCIUM AND SODIUM STEAROYL LACTYLATES, CALCIUM PEROXIDE), WHEAT GERM, WHEY, CORNSTARCH, YEAST NUTRIENTS (MONOCALCIUM PHOSPHATE, CALCIUM SULFATE, AMMONIUM SULFATE).

Ulcers used to be blamed on stress, particularly in people with "intense" personalities. Diet was also thought to be important, with spicy foods often cast as a major villain. But much to the amazement of most of the medical community, research in the 1980s and 1990s confirmed that infection with the bacterium *Helicobacter pylori* actually causes most ulcers. Excessive use of nonsteroidal anti-inflammatory drugs (NSAIDs), such as aspirin, ibuprofen, and naproxen sodium, is also a common cause of ulcers.

*H. pylori* causes 80 percent of gastric ulcers and more than 90 percent of duodenal ulcers. These bacteria weaken the protective mucous coating, allowing acid to penetrate to the sensitive lining beneath. Both the acid and the bacteria irritate the lining and cause a sore, or ulcer. *H. pylori* is able to survive in stomach acid because it secretes enzymes that neutralize the acid. This mechanism allows *H. pylori* to make its way to the "safe" area—the protective mucous lining. Once there, the bacterium's spiral shape helps it burrow through the mucous lining.[27]

NSAIDs cause ulcers by interfering with the GI tract's ability to protect itself from acidic stomach juices. Normally the stomach and duodenum employ three defenses against digestive juices: mucus that coats the lining and shields it from stomach acid, the chemical bicarbonate that neutralizes acid, and blood circulation that aids in cell renewal and repair. NSAIDs hinder all these protective mechanisms. With the defenses down, digestive juices can cause ulcers by damaging the sensitive lining of the stomach and duodenum. Fortunately, NSAID-induced ulcers usually heal once the person stops taking the medication.

If you had ulcers in the 1950s, you would have been told to quit your high-stress job and switch to a bland diet. Today, ulcer sufferers usually are treated with a program of antibiotics that can eradicate most cases of *H. pylori*.[28] Although personality and life stress are no longer considered significant factors in the development of most ulcers, relapse after treatment is more common in people who are emotionally stressed or suffering from depression.

## Functional Dyspepsia

Chronic pain in the upper abdomen that has no obvious physical cause (such as inflammation of the esophagus, peptic ulcer, or gallstones) is referred to as **functional dyspepsia**. As with IBS, the cause of functional dyspepsia is unknown. Hypersensitivity to GI stimuli, abnormal GI motility, and psychosocial problems have all been suggested as causes of dyspepsia.[29] *H. pylori* may also be a factor in some cases of functional dyspepsia.

The treatment of functional dyspepsia includes drugs that speed up the movement of food through the upper part of the intestinal tract, products that decrease stomach acid production, and antibiotics. Just as with IBS, stress-reduction techniques, such as meditation and biofeedback, can often relieve the symptoms of functional dyspepsia.

**Key Concepts** *GI disorders generally produce uncomfortable symptoms such as abdominal pain, gas, bloating, and change in elimination patterns. Some GI disorders, such as diarrhea, are generally symptoms of some other illness. Although medications are useful in reducing symptoms, many GI disorders are treatable with changes in diet, especially the addition of adequate fiber and fluids.*

As you have seen, the gastrointestinal tract is the key to turning food and its nutrients into nourishment for our bodies. **Figure 4.21** shows the sites for digestion and absorption of the macronutrients, using a piece of pizza as an example of a food that would contain substantial amounts of carbohydrate, fat, and protein. A healthy GI tract is an important factor in our overall health and well-being.

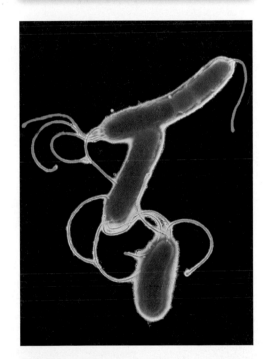

*Helicobacter pylori.*

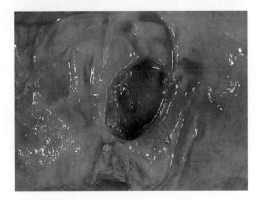

Stomach ulcer.

**functional dyspepsia** Chronic pain in the upper abdomen not due to any obvious physical cause.

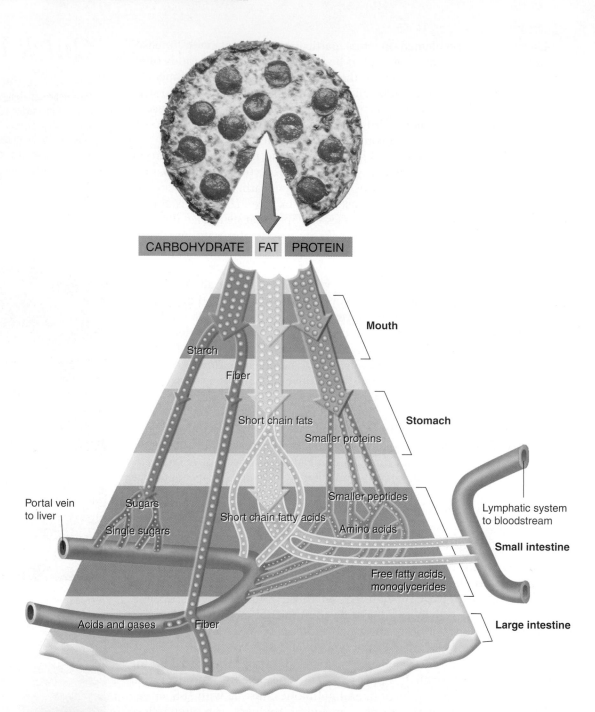

**Figure 4.21** **Fate of a piece of pizza.** When you eat a piece of pizza, what happens to the carbohydrate, fat, and protein?

- *Carbohydrate.* Enzymes in the mouth begin the breakdown of starch. Stomach acid halts carbohydrate digestion. In the small intestine, enzymes break down carbohydrate, and the products are absorbed into the blood. In the large intestine, bacteria digest small amounts of fiber. The remainder is eliminated in feces.
- *Fat.* The stomach absorbs a few short-chain fatty acids into the blood. But most fat is broken down and absorbed in the small intestine, where its products enter the lymphatic system.
- *Protein.* Stomach acid unfolds proteins, and enzymes begin protein breakdown. The small intestine completes the breakdown to amino acids, which enter the blood.

# *Learning* Portfolio

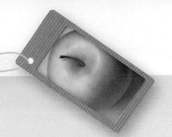

## Key Terms

## Study Points

- The GI tract is a tube that can be divided into regions: the mouth, esophagus, stomach, small intestine, large intestine, and rectum.

- Digestion and absorption of the nutrients in foods occur at various sites along the GI tract.

- Digestion involves both physical processes (e.g., chewing, peristalsis, and segmentation) and chemical processes (e.g., the hydrolytic action of enzymes).

- Absorption is the movement of molecules across the lining of the GI tract and into circulation.

- The major mechanisms involved in nutrient absorption are passive diffusion, facilitated diffusion, and active transport.

- In the mouth, food is mixed with saliva for lubrication. Salivary amylase begins the digestion of starch.

- Acid and enzyme secretions from the stomach lower the pH of stomach contents and begin the digestion of proteins.

- The pancreas and gallbladder secrete material into the small intestine to help with digestion.

- Most chemical digestion and nutrient absorption occur in the small intestine.

- Electrolytes and water are absorbed from the large intestine. Remaining material—waste—is excreted as feces.

- Both the nervous system and the hormonal system regulate GI tract processes.

- Numerous factors affect GI tract functioning, including psychological, chemical, and bacterial factors.

- Problems that occur along the GI tract can affect digestion and absorption of nutrients. Dietary changes are important in the treatment of GI disorders.

## Study Questions

1. List the organs (in order) that make up the GI tract.

2. Name the four "assisting" organs that are not part of the GI tract but are needed for proper digestion. What are their roles in digestion?

3. What substance makes the stomach contents acidic? What substance protects stomach cells from the low pH of stomach contents?

4. Where in the GI tract does the majority of nutrient digestion and absorption take place?

5. What two circulatory systems transport absorbed nutrients around the body?

6. What is gastroesophageal reflux disease?

# Try This

## The Saltine Cracker Experiment

This experiment will help you understand the effect of salivary amylase. Remember, salivary amylase is the starch-digesting enzyme produced by the salivary glands. Chew two saltine crackers until a watery texture forms in your mouth. You have to fight the urge to swallow so you can pay attention to the taste of the crackers. Do you notice a change in the taste?

The crackers first taste salty and "starchy," but as amylase is secreted it begins to break the chains of starch into sugar. As it does this, the saltines begin to taste sweet like animal crackers!

# What About Bobbie?

Because both fluid and fiber are important for a healthy gastrointestinal tract, let's check out Bobbie's intake of these. Refresh yourself with her day of eating (see the "Food Choices: Nutrients and Nourishment" chapter). How do you think Bobbie did in terms of fiber? She did pretty well! At 25 grams of fiber, she's right at the Adequate Intake (AI) for fiber for women her age—25 grams per day. Here are her best fiber sources:

| Food | Fiber Grams |
| --- | --- |
| Spaghetti (pasta) | 3.5 |
| Tortilla chips | 3 |
| Banana | 3 |
| Salsa | 2 |
| Sourdough bread | 2 |

Are you surprised by the tortilla chips and the amount of fiber they add? Don't misinterpret this to mean that tortilla chips are a great source of fiber. There are two reasons why the chips rank so high. First, the other grain choices were not whole wheat and therefore didn't contribute a lot of fiber. Second, her afternoon snack consisted of just over 200 kilocalories of tortilla chips.

What could Bobbie have done differently if she wanted to keep her fiber intake high, but reduce calories and fat by avoiding the tortilla chips? Here are a few small changes that she could make.

- By choosing a whole-wheat bagel, she'd add 4 grams of fiber.
- By having her sandwich on whole-wheat bread, she'd add at least 3 grams of fiber.
- By substituting the 2 tablespoons of croutons with 2 more tablespoons of kidney beans, she'd add 1.5 grams of fiber.

- If she ate another piece of fruit as a snack sometime during the day, it would add 1 to 3 grams of fiber.

Now let's look at Bobbie's fluid intake. Remember, when you increase your fiber intake, you need to increase your fluid intake so you don't become constipated. Here's a list of Bobbie's drinks:

| | |
| --- | --- |
| Breakfast | 10 ounces coffee |
| Snack | None |
| Lunch | 12 ounces diet soda |
| Snack | 16 ounces water |
| Dinner | 12 ounces diet soda |
| Snack | None |

How do you think she did? Her total fluid intake is 50 ounces (about 1,500 mL). Her food also contains fluids and contributes another 1,000 milliliters. The AI for total fluid intake for adult women is 2,700 milliliters per day. If Bobbie's intake is assumed to be about 2,500 milliliters, this is close to the AI. She could add another beverage with one or both of her snacks and be right on target. She could also improve her fluid choices since most contain caffeine, which is a diuretic.

What suggestions do you have that will improve Bobbie's fluid intake? Any of the following would work:

- Carry a water bottle to sip throughout the day.
- Wash down the morning banana snack with a cup or two of water.
- Consider decaffeinated coffee or decaffeinated soda.
- Drink more water with the tortilla chips in the afternoon.
- Add another beverage at dinner.
- Drink water with the piece of pizza at night.

# References

1   Smeets PA, Erkner A, deGraaf C. Cephalic phase responses and appetite. *Nutr Rev.* 2010;68(1):643–655.

2   Klein S, Cohn SM, Alpers DH. Alimentary tract in nutrition. In: Shils ME, Shike M, Ross AC, Cabellero B, Cousins RJ, eds. *Modern Nutrition in Health and Disease.* 10th ed. Philadelphia: Lippincott Williams & Wilkins; 2006:1115–1142.

3   Guyton AC, Hall JE. *Textbook of Medical Physiology.* 11th ed. Philadelphia: W.B. Saunders; 2006.

4   Ibid.

5   Klein S, Cohn SM, Alpers DH. Op. cit.

6   Scheppach W, Luehrs H, Menzel T. Beneficial health effects of low-digestible carbohydrate consumption. *Br J Nutr.* 2001;85(suppl 1):S23–S30.

7   Guyton AC, Hall JE. Op. cit.

8   Ibid.

9   Ibid.

10   Marraffini LA, Sontheimer EJ. Self versus non-self discrimination during CRISPR RNA-directed immunity. *Nature.* 2010;463(7280):568–571.

11   Jabbar A, Chang W-K, Dryden GW, McClave SA. Gut immunology and the differential response to feeding and starvation. *Nutr Clin Pract.* 2003;18:461–482.

12    Beyer PL. Digestion, absorption, transport, and excretion of nutrients. In: Mahan LK, Escott-Stump S. *Krause's Food, Nutrition and Diet Therapy*. 12th ed. Philadelphia: W.B. Saunders; 2008.

13    *Toxicological Profile for Acrolein (Update)*. Atlanta, GA: US Public Health Service, US Department of Health and Human Services, Agency for Toxic Substances and Disease Registry (ATSDR); 2007. http://www.atsdr.cdc.gov/toxprofiles/tp.asp?id=557&tid=102. Accessed 4/28/11.

14    National Digestive Diseases Information Clearinghouse. Constipation. NIH Publication No. 06-2754. February 2006. http://digestive.niddk.nih.gov/ddiseases/pubs/constipation/index.htm. Accessed 4/28/11.

15    Rubenstein JH, Scheiman JM, Sadeghi S, et al. Esophageal adenocarcinoma incidence in individuals with gastroesophageal reflux: synthesis and estimates from population studies. *Am J Gastroenterol*. 2011;106(2):254–260.

16    Doheny K. Gut feeling. *Natural Health*. 2010;40(5):46–53.

17    National Institute of Diabetes and Digestive and Kidney Diseases, National Institutes of Health. *Irritable Bowel Syndrome*. Bethesda, MD: National Digestive Diseases Information Clearinghouse; April 2003. NIH publication 03-693. http://digestive.niddk.nih.gov/ddiseases/pubs/ibs. Accessed 4/28/11.

18    Ibid.

19    Centers for Disease Control and Prevention. Colorectal (colon) cancer: basic information. http://www.cdc.gov/cancer/colorectal/basic_info. Accessed 10/27/08.

20    World Health Organization. *Diet, Nutrition and the Prevention of Chronic Diseases: A Report of a Joint WHO/FAO Expert Consultation*. Geneva, Switzerland: World Health Organization; 2003. WHO Technical Report Series 916. http://www.who.int/dietphysicalactivity/publications/trs916/intro/en. Accessed 4/28/11.

21    Brown CH, Baidas SM, Hajdenberg JJ, et al. Lifestyle interventions in the prevention and treatment of cancer. *Am J Lifestyle Med*. 2009;3(5):337–348.

22    Tavani A, La Vecchia C, Gallus S, et al. Red meat intake and cancer risk: a study in Italy. *Int J Cancer*. 2000;86:425–428.

23    Chao A, Thun MJ, Connell CJ, et al. Meat consumption and risk of colorectal cancer. *JAMA*. 2005;293:172–182; Hu J, La Vecchia C, DesMeules M, Negri E, Mery L. Canadian Cancer Registries Epidemiology Research Group. Meat and fish consumption and cancer in Canada. *Nutr Cancer*. 2008;60:313–324; and Larsson SC, Wolk A. Meat consumption and risk of colorectal cancer: a meta-analysis of prospective studies. *Int J Cancer*. 2006;119:2657–2664.

24    Alexander DD, Cushing CA. Red meat and colorectal cancer: a critical summary of prospective epidemiologic studies. *Obesity Reviews*. 2011;12(suppl):e472–e493.

25    Institute of Medicine, Food and Nutrition Board. *Dietary Reference Intakes for Energy, Carbohydrate, Fiber, Fat, Fatty Acids, Cholesterol, Protein, and Amino Acids*. Washington, DC: National Academies Press; 2002; and Cao Y, Gao X, Zhang W, et al. Dietary fiber enhances TGF-$\beta$ signaling and growth inhibition in the gut. *Am J Physiol Gastrointest Liver Physiol*. 2011;301(1):G156–164.

26    Brown CH, Baidas SM, Hajdenberg JJ, et al. Op. cit.

27    National Institute of Diabetes and Digestive and Kidney Diseases, National Institutes of Health. H. pylori *and Peptic Ulcer*. Bethesda, MD: National Digestive Diseases Information Clearinghouse; October 2004. NIH publication 05-4225. http://digestive.niddk.nih.gov/ddiseases/pubs/hpylori/index.htm. Accessed 5/1/11.

28    Ibid.

29    Barry S, Dinan TG. Functional dyspepsia: are psychosocial factors of relevance? *World J Gastro*. 2006;12(17):2701–2707.

# CHAPTER 5

# Carbohydrates: Simple Sugars and Complex Chains

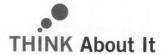

**THINK** About It

1 When you think of the word *carbohydrate*, what foods come to mind?

2 How does your dietary fiber intake stack up?

3 Is honey more nutritious than white sugar? What do you think?

4 Do you prefer artificial sweeteners to sugar? Explain your preference.

Visit **go.jblearning.com/ inseldisco4e**

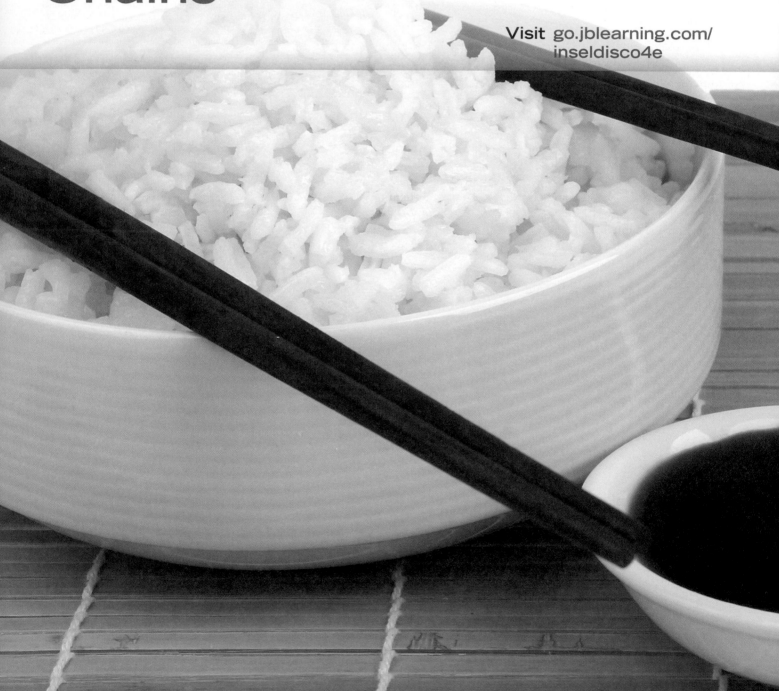

Does sugar cause diabetes? Will too much sugar make a child hyperactive? Does excess sugar contribute to criminal behavior? What about starch? Does it really make you fat? These and other questions have been raised about sugar and starch—dietary carbohydrates—over the years. But, where do these ideas come from? What is myth, and what is fact? Are carbohydrates important in the diet? Or, as some popular diets suggest, should we eat only small amounts of carbohydrates? What links, if any, are there between carbohydrates in your diet and health?

Most of the world's people depend on carbohydrate-rich plant foods for daily sustenance. Carbohydrates contain 4 kilocalories per gram, and in some countries they supply 80 percent or more of daily calorie intake. Rice provides the bulk of the diet in Southeast Asia, as does corn in South America, cassava in certain parts of Africa, and wheat in Europe and North America. (See **Figure 5.1**.) Besides providing energy, foods rich in carbohydrates, such as whole grains, legumes, fruits, and vegetables, also are good sources of vitamins, minerals, dietary fiber, and phytochemicals that can help lower the risk of chronic diseases.

THINK
About It
1

## Carbohydrates Capture Energy from the Sun

Plants produce carbohydrates (and oxygen) through photosynthesis—using carbon dioxide from the air, water from the soil, and energy from the sun. The two main types of carbohydrates in food are simple carbohydrates (sugars) and complex carbohydrates (starches and fiber).

## Simple Sugars: Monosaccharides and Disaccharides

**Simple carbohydrates** are naturally present as simple sugars in fruits, milk, and other foods. Plant carbohydrates also can be refined to produce sugar products such as table sugar or corn syrup. The two main types of sugars are monosaccharides and disaccharides. **Monosaccharides** consist of a single

**simple carbohydrates**
Monosaccharides and disaccharides; simple carbohydrates. Sugars composed of a single sugar molecule (a monosaccharide) or two joined sugar molecules (a disaccharide).

**monosaccharides** Single sugar units. The common monosaccharides are glucose, fructose, and galactose.

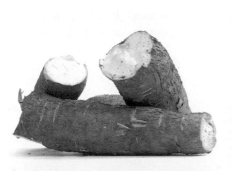
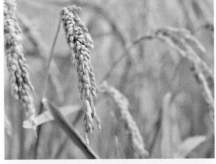
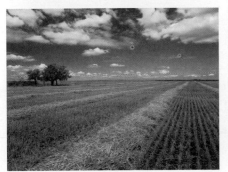
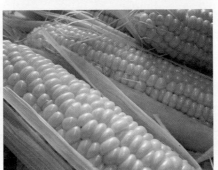

**Figure 5.1** **Cassava, rice, wheat, and corn.** These carbohydrate-rich foods are dietary staples in many parts of the world.

sugar molecule (*mono* meaning "one" and *saccharide* meaning "sugar"). **Disaccharides** consist of two sugar molecules chemically joined together (*di* meaning "two"). Monosaccharides and disaccharides give various degrees of sweetness to foods.

## Monosaccharides: The Single Sugars

The most common monosaccharides in the human diet are:

- Glucose
- Fructose
- Galactose

**Glucose**     **Fructose**     **Galactose**

### Glucose

The monosaccharide **glucose** is the most abundant simple carbohydrate unit in nature. Also referred to as dextrose, glucose plays a key role in both foods and the body. Glucose gives food a mildly sweet flavor. It doesn't usually exist as a monosaccharide in food but is instead joined to other sugars to form disaccharides, starch, or dietary fiber. Glucose makes up at least one of the two sugar molecules in every disaccharide.

In the body, glucose supplies energy to cells. The body closely regulates blood glucose (blood sugar) levels to ensure a constant fuel source for vital body functions. Glucose is virtually the only fuel used by the brain, except during prolonged starvation, when the glucose supply is low.

### Fructose

Also called levulose or fruit sugar, **fructose** tastes the sweetest of all the sugars and occurs naturally in fruits and vegetables. Although the sugar in honey is about half fructose and half glucose, fructose is the primary source of its sweet taste. Food manufacturers use high-fructose corn syrup as an additive to sweeten many foods, including soft drinks, fruit beverages, desserts, candies, jellies, and jams. The term *high fructose* is a little misleading—the fructose content of this sweetener is around 50 percent.

### Galactose

**Galactose** rarely occurs as a monosaccharide in food. It usually is chemically bonded to glucose to form lactose, the primary sugar in milk and dairy products.

## Disaccharides: The Double Sugars

Disaccharides consist of two monosaccharides linked together. The following disaccharides (see **Figure 5.2**) are important in human nutrition:

- Sucrose
- Lactose
- Maltose

### Sucrose

**Sucrose**, most familiar to us as table sugar, is made up of one molecule of glucose and one molecule of fructose. Sucrose provides some of the natural sweetness of honey, maple syrup, fruits, and vegetables. Manufacturers use a refining process to extract sucrose from the juices of sugar cane or sugar beets. Full refining removes impurities; white sugar and powdered sugar are so highly refined that they are virtually 100 percent sucrose. When a food label lists sugar as an ingredient, the term refers to sucrose.

---

**disaccharides [dye-SACK-uh-rides]** Carbohydrates composed of two monosaccharide units chemically linked. They include sucrose (common table sugar), lactose (milk sugar), and maltose.

**glucose [GLOO-kose]** A common monosaccharide that is a component of disaccharides (sucrose, lactose, and maltose) and various complex carbohydrates; present in the blood. Also known as *dextrose*.

**fructose [FROOK-tose]** A common monosaccharide naturally present in honey and many fruits. Also called *levulose* or *fruit sugar*.

**galactose [gah-LAK-tose]** A monosaccharide that has a structure similar to glucose; usually joined with other monosaccharides.

**sucrose [SOO-crose]** A disaccharide composed of one molecule of glucose and one molecule of fructose joined together. Also known as *table sugar*.

---

### DISACCHARIDES

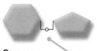

**Sucrose**

- Common table sugar
- Purified from beets or sugar cane
- A glucose-fructose disaccharide

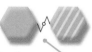

**Lactose**

- Milk sugar
- Found in the milk of most mammals
- A glucose-galactose disaccharide

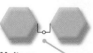

**Maltose**

- Malt sugar
- A breakdown product of starches
- A glucose-glucose disaccharide

**Figure 5.2**   **The disaccharides: sucrose, lactose, and maltose.** The three monosaccharides pair up in different combinations to form the three disaccharides.

### Lactose

**Lactose**, or milk sugar, is composed of one molecule of glucose and one molecule of galactose. Lactose gives milk and other dairy products a slightly sweet taste. Human milk has a higher concentration (approximately 7 grams per 100 milliliters) of lactose than cow's milk (approximately 4.5 grams per 100 milliliters), so human milk tastes sweeter than cow's milk.

### Maltose

**Maltose** is composed of two glucose molecules. Maltose seldom occurs naturally in foods, but is formed whenever long molecules of starch break down. Human digestive enzymes in the mouth and small intestine break starch down into maltose. When you chew a slice of fresh bread, you may detect a slightly sweet taste as starch breaks down into maltose. Starch also breaks down into maltose in germinating seeds. Maltose is fermented in the production of beer.

**Key Concepts** *Carbohydrates can be categorized as simple or complex. Simple carbohydrates include monosaccharides and disaccharides. The monosaccharides glucose, fructose, and galactose are single sugar molecules. The disaccharides sucrose, lactose, and maltose are double sugar molecules.*

> **lactose [LAK-tose]** A disaccharide composed of glucose and galactose; also called *milk sugar* because it is the major sugar in milk and dairy products.
>
> **maltose [MALL-tose]** A disaccharide composed of two glucose molecules; sometimes called *malt sugar*. Maltose seldom occurs naturally in foods but is formed whenever long molecules of starch break down.
>
> **complex carbohydrates** Chains of more than two monosaccharides. May be oligosaccharides or polysaccharides.
>
> **oligosaccharides** Short carbohydrate chains composed of 3 to 10 sugar molecules.
>
> **polysaccharides** Long carbohydrate chains composed of more than 10 sugar molecules. Polysaccharides can be straight or branched.

## Complex Carbohydrates

**Complex carbohydrates** are chains of more than two sugar molecules. Short carbohydrate chains are called oligosaccharides and contain 3 to 10 sugar molecules. Long carbohydrate chains can contain hundreds or even thousands of monosaccharide units.

### Oligosaccharides

**Oligosaccharides** (*oligo* meaning "scant") are short carbohydrate chains of 3 to 10 sugar molecules. Dried beans, peas, and lentils contain the two most common oligosaccharides—raffinose and stachyose.[1] Raffinose is formed from three monosaccharide molecules—one galactose, one glucose, and one fructose. Stachyose is formed from four monosaccharide molecules—two galactose, one glucose, and one fructose. The body cannot break down raffinose or stachyose, but they are readily broken down by intestinal bacteria and are responsible for the familiar gaseous effects of foods such as beans.

Human milk contains more than one hundred different oligosaccharides, which vary according to the length of a woman's pregnancy, how long she has been nursing, and her genetic makeup.[2] For breastfed infants, oligosaccharides serve a function similar to dietary fiber in adults—making stools easier to pass. Some of these oligosaccharides also protect infants from disease-causing agents by binding to them in the intestine. Oligosaccharides in human milk also provide sialic acid, a compound essential for normal brain development.[3]

### Polysaccharides

**Polysaccharides** (*poly* meaning "many") are long carbohydrate chains of monosaccharides. Some polysaccharides form straight chains whereas others branch off in all directions. Such structural differences affect how the polysaccharide behaves in water and with heating. The way monosaccharides are linked make them digestible (e.g., starch) or nondigestible (e.g., fiber).

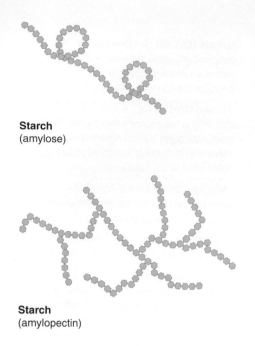

**Starch**
(amylose)

**Starch**
(amylopectin)

**Glycogen**

| Figure 5.3 | **Starch and glycogen.** Plants have two main types of starch—amylose, which has long unbranched chains of glucose, and amylopectin, which has branched chains. Animals store glucose in highly branched chains called glycogen. |

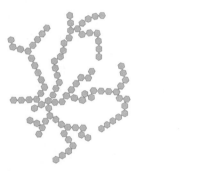

starch  The major storage form of carbohydrate in plants; starch is composed of long chains of glucose molecules in a straight (amylose) or branching (amylopectin) arrangement.

amylose [AM-ih-los]  A straight-chain polysaccharide composed of glucose units.

amylopectin [am-ih-low-PEK-tin]  A branched-chain polysaccharide composed of glucose units.

resistant starch  A starch that is not digested.

### Starch

Plants store energy as **starch** for use during growth and reproduction. Rich sources of starch include (1) grains, such as wheat, rice, corn, oats, millet, and barley; (2) legumes, such as peas, beans, and lentils; and (3) tubers, such as potatoes, yams, and cassava. Starch imparts a moist, gelatinous texture to food. For example, it makes the inside of a baked potato moist, thick, and almost sticky. The starch in flour absorbs moisture and thickens gravy.

Starch takes two main forms in plants: amylose and amylopectin. **Amylose** is made up of long, unbranched chains of glucose molecules, whereas **amylopectin** is made up of branched chains of glucose molecules. (See **Figure 5.3.**) There is usually four times as much amylopectin in plants as amylose, although this proportion can vary.[4] Wheat flour contains a higher proportion of amylose, whereas cornstarch contains a higher proportion of amylopectin.

In the body, amylopectin is digested more rapidly than amylose.[5] Although the body easily digests most starches, a small portion of the starch in plants may remain enclosed in cell structures and escape digestion in the small intestine. Starch that is not digested is called **resistant starch**.[6] Some legumes, such as white beans, contain large amounts of resistant starch. Resistant starch also is formed during the processing of starchy foods.

### Glycogen

Living animals, including humans, store carbohydrate in the form of **glycogen**, also called animal starch. When we slaughter animals for meat, their tissue enzymes break down most glycogen within 24 hours. Although some organ meats, such as kidney, heart, and liver, contain small amounts of carbohydrate, meat from muscle contains none.[7] Because plant foods also do not contain glycogen, it is a negligible carbohydrate source in our diets. Glycogen does, however, play an important role in our bodies, providing glucose when blood glucose levels get low.

Glycogen is composed of long, highly branched chains of glucose molecules. Its structure is similar to amylopectin, but glycogen is much more highly branched. When we need extra glucose, glycogen in our cells can be broken down rapidly into single glucose molecules. Because enzymes can attack only the ends of glycogen chains, the highly branched structure of glycogen multiplies the number of sites available for enzyme activity.

Most glycogen is stored in skeletal muscle and the liver. In muscle cells, glycogen provides a supply of glucose for strenuous muscular activity. Liver cells also use glycogen to regulate blood glucose levels. If necessary, liver glycogen can provide as much as 100 to 150 milligrams of glucose per minute to the blood at a sustained rate for up to 12 hours.[8] Normally, the body can store only about 200 to 500 grams of glycogen at a time.[9] Some athletes "load" carbohydrates by gradually tapering off rigorous training and emphasizing high-carbohydrate meals a few days to one week before they compete. This can increase the amount of stored glycogen by 20 to 40 percent above normal, providing a competitive edge for marathon running and other endurance events.[10]

### Fiber

The Food and Nutrition Board defined *fiber* as part of the DRI report on macronutrients. **Dietary fiber** consists of nondigestible carbohydrates and lignins that are intact and intrinsic in plants. **Functional fiber** refers to isolated, nondigestible carbohydrates that have beneficial physiological effects in humans. **Total fiber** is the sum of dietary fiber and functional fiber.

All types of plant foods—including fruits, vegetables, legumes, and whole grains—contain dietary fiber. Many types of dietary fiber resemble starches—they are polysaccharides, but are not digested in the human GI tract. Examples of these nonstarch polysaccharides include cellulose, hemicellulose, pectins, gums, and beta-glucans (ß-glucans). Oligosaccharides also are considered to be dietary fiber. Examples of functional fiber include extracted plant pectins, gums and resistant starches, chitin and chitosan, and commercially produced nondigestible polysaccharides. Fiber is not found in animal foods.

Whole-grain foods such as brown rice, rolled oats, and whole-wheat breads and cereals; legumes such as kidney beans, garbanzo beans (chickpeas), peas, and lentils; fruits; and vegetables are all rich sources of dietary fiber (see Table 5.1).

### Cellulose

In plants, **cellulose** makes the walls of cells strong and rigid. It forms the woody fibers that support tall trees. It also forms the brittle shafts of hay and straw and the stringy threads in celery. Cellulose is made up of long, straight chains of glucose molecules. (See **Figure 5.4**.) Grains, fruits, vegetables, and nuts all contain cellulose.

### Hemicelluloses

The **hemicelluloses** are a diverse group of polysaccharides that vary from plant to plant. They are mixed with cellulose in plant cell walls.[11] Hemicelluloses are composed of a variety of monosaccharides with many branching side chains. The outer bran layer on many cereal grains is rich in hemicelluloses, as are legumes, vegetables, and nuts.

### Pectins

Found in all plants, but especially fruits, **pectins** are gel-forming polysaccharides. The pectin in fruits acts like a cement that gives body to fruits and helps them keep their shape. When fruit becomes overripe, pectin breaks down into monosaccharides and the fruit becomes mushy. When mixed with sugar and acid, pectin forms a gel that the food industry uses to add firmness to jellies, jams, sauces, and salad dressings.

**glycogen [GLY-ko-jen]** A very large, highly branched polysaccharide composed of multiple glucose units. Sometimes called *animal starch*, glycogen is the primary storage form of glucose in animals.

**dietary fiber** Carbohydrates and lignins that are naturally in plants and are nondigestible; that is, they are not digested and absorbed in the human small intestine.

**functional fiber** Isolated nondigestible carbohydrates, including some manufactured carbohydrates, that have beneficial effects in humans.

**total fiber** The sum of dietary fiber and functional fiber.

**cellulose [SELL-you-los]** A straight-chain polysaccharide composed of hundreds of glucose units linked by beta bonds. It is nondigestible by humans and a component of dietary fiber.

**hemicelluloses [hem-ih-SELL-you-los-es]** A group of large polysaccharides in dietary fiber that are fermented more easily than cellulose.

**pectins** A type of dietary fiber found in fruits.

### Table 5.1   Foods Rich in Dietary Fiber

| Fruits | | Nuts and Seeds | |
|---|---|---|---|
| Apples | Grapefruit | Almonds | Sesame seeds |
| Bananas | Mango | Peanuts | Sunflower seeds |
| Berries | Oranges | Pecans | Walnuts |
| Cherries | Pears | *Legumes* | |
| Cranberries | | Most legumes | |
| *Vegetables* | | *Grains* | |
| Asparagus | Green peppers | Brown rice | Wheat-bran cereals |
| Broccoli | Red cabbage | Oat bran | Wheat-bran breads |
| Brussels sprouts | Spinach | Oatmeal | |
| Carrots | Sprouts | | |

**Source:** Adapted from Shils ME, Shike M, Ross AC, Cabellero B, Cousins RJ, eds. *Modern Nutrition in Health and Disease.* 10th ed. Philadelphia: Lippincott Williams & Wilkins; 2006.

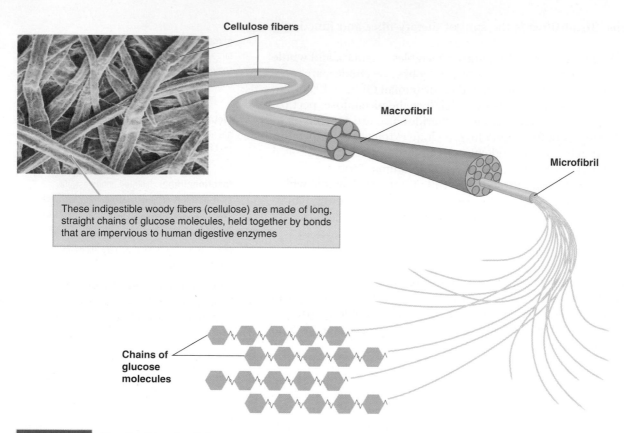

Cellulose fibers

Macrofibril

Microfibril

These indigestible woody fibers (cellulose) are made of long, straight chains of glucose molecules, held together by bonds that are impervious to human digestive enzymes

Chains of glucose molecules

**Figure 5.4** **The structure of cellulose.** Cellulose forms the nondigestible, fibrous component of plants and is part of grasses, trees, fruits, and vegetables.

**gums** Dietary fibers, which contain galactose and other monosaccharides, found between plant cell walls.

**mucilages** Gelatinous soluble fibers containing galactose, mannose, and other monosaccharides; found in seaweed.

**psyllium** The dried husk of the psyllium seed.

**lignins [LIG-nins]** Insoluble fibers composed of multiring alcohol units that constitute the only noncarbohydrate component of dietary fiber.

**beta-glucans** Functional fiber, consisting of branched polysaccharide chains of glucose, that helps lower blood cholesterol levels. Found in barley and oats.

**chitin** A long-chain structural polysaccharide of slightly modified glucose. Found in the hard exterior skeletons of insects, crustaceans, and other invertebrates; also occurs in the cell walls of fungi.

**chitosan** Polysaccharide derived from chitin.

## Gums and Mucilages

Like pectin, **gums** and **mucilages** are thick, gel-forming fibers that help hold plant cells together. The food industry uses plant gums (gum Arabic, guar gum, locust bean gum, and xanthan gum, for example) and mucilages (such as carrageenan) to thicken, stabilize, or add texture to foods such as salad dressings, puddings, pie fillings, candies, sauces, and even drinks. **Psyllium** (the husk of psyllium seeds) is a mucilage that becomes very viscous when mixed with water. It is the main component in the laxative Metamucil and is being added to some breakfast cereals.

## Lignins

Not actually carbohydrates, **lignins** are nondigestible substances that make up the woody parts of vegetables such as carrots and broccoli and the seeds of fruits such as strawberries.

## Beta-glucans

**Beta-glucans** are polysaccharides of branched glucose units. These fibers are found in large amounts in barley and oats. Beta-glucan fiber is especially effective in lowering blood cholesterol levels (see the "Carbohydrates and Health" section later in this chapter).

## Chitin and Chitosan

**Chitin** and **chitosan** are polysaccharides found in the exoskeletons of crabs and lobsters, and in the cell walls of most fungi. Chitin and chitosan are primarily consumed in supplement form. Although they are marketed as being useful for weight control, published research does not support this claim.[12] Chitosan supplements may impair the absorption of fat-soluble vitamins and some minerals.

**Key Concepts** *Complex carbohydrates include starch, glycogen, and fiber. Starch is composed of straight or branched chains of glucose molecules and is the storage form of energy in plants. Glycogen is composed of highly branched chains of glucose molecules and is the storage form of energy in animals. Fibers include many different substances that cannot be digested by enzymes in the human intestinal tract and are found in plant foods, such as whole grains, legumes, vegetables, and fruits.*

## Carbohydrate Digestion and Absorption

Although glucose is a key building block of carbohydrates, you can't exactly find it on the menu at your favorite restaurant or campus hangout. You must first drink that chocolate milkshake or eat that hamburger bun so that your body can convert the food carbohydrate into glucose in the body. Let's see what happens to the carbohydrate foods you eat!

### Digestion: Breaking Down Carbohydrates to Single Sugars

**Figure 5.5** provides an overview of the digestive process. Carbohydrate digestion begins in the mouth, where the starch-digesting enzyme salivary amylase breaks down starch into shorter polysaccharides and maltose. Chewing stimulates saliva production and mixes salivary amylase with food. Disaccharides,

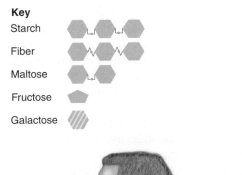

**Key**

Starch

Fiber

Maltose

Fructose

Galactose

**Figure 5.5** **Carbon digestion.** Most carbohydrate digestion takes place in the small intestine.

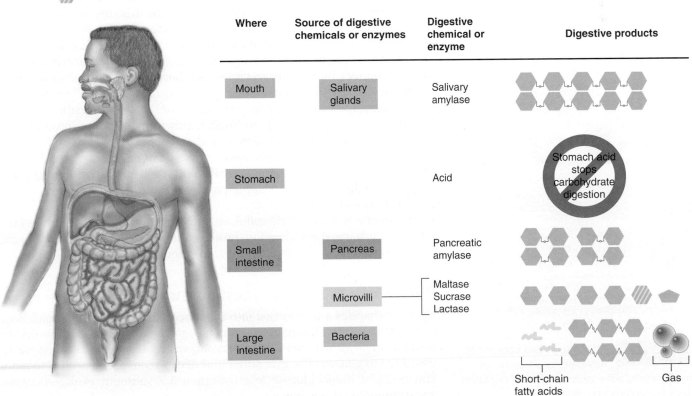

| Where | Source of digestive chemicals or enzymes | Digestive chemical or enzyme | Digestive products |
|---|---|---|---|
| Mouth | Salivary glands | Salivary amylase | |
| Stomach | | Acid | Stomach acid stops carbohydrate digestion |
| Small intestine | Pancreas | Pancreatic amylase | |
| | Microvilli | Maltase Sucrase Lactase | |
| Large intestine | Bacteria | | Short-chain fatty acids · · · Gas |

# *Quick* Bite

**Banana Facts**
You may know that bananas are high in potassium, but did you also know that they have an unusually high carbohydrate content? Before ripening, a banana is almost entirely starch. After ripening, certain bananas are almost entirely sugar—as much as 20 percent by weight.

**pancreatic amylase** Starch-digesting enzyme secreted by the pancreas.

**alpha (α) bonds** Chemical bonds linking monosaccharides, which can be broken by human intestinal enzymes, releasing the individual monosaccharides. Starch, maltose, and sucrose contain alpha bonds.

**beta (β) bonds** Chemical bonds linking monosaccharides, which sometimes can be broken by human intestinal enzymes. Lactose contains digestable beta bonds, and cellulose contains nondigestible beta bonds.

unlike starch, are not digested in the mouth. In fact, only about 5 percent of the starches in food are broken down by the time the food is swallowed.

When carbohydrate enters the stomach, the acidity of stomach juices eventually halts the action of salivary amylase by causing the enzyme (a protein) to lose its shape and function. This stops carbohydrate digestion, which will restart in the small intestine. Certain fibers, such as pectins and gums, provide a feeling of fullness and tend to delay digestive activity by slowing stomach emptying.

Most carbohydrate digestion takes place in the small intestine. As the stomach contents enter the small intestine, the pancreas secretes pancreatic amylase into the small intestine. **Pancreatic amylase** continues the digestion of starch, breaking it into many units of the disaccharide maltose.

Meanwhile, enzymes attached to the brush border (microvilli) of the mucosal cells lining the intestinal tract go to work. These digestive enzymes break disaccharides into monosaccharides for absorption. The enzyme maltase splits maltose into two glucose molecules. The enzyme sucrase splits sucrose into glucose and fructose. The enzyme lactase splits lactose into glucose and galactose.

The bonds that link glucose molecules in complex carbohydrates are called glycosidic bonds. The two forms of these bonds, **alpha (α) bonds** and **beta (β) bonds**, have important differences. (See **Figure 5.6**.) Human enzymes easily break alpha bonds, making glucose available from the polysaccharides starch and glycogen. Our bodies don't have enzymes to break most beta bonds, such as those that link the glucose molecules in cellulose, a nondigestible polysaccharide. Beta bonds also link the galactose and glucose molecules in the disaccharide lactose, but the enzyme lactase is specifically tailored to attack this small molecule. People with a sufficient supply of the enzyme lactase can break these bonds. When lactase is lacking, however, the beta bonds remain unbroken and lactose remains undigested until bacteria in the colon can attack it.

Enzymes are highly specific; they speed up only certain reactions and work on only certain molecules. Humans lack the digestive enzymes needed to break down the oligosaccharides raffinose and stachyose, for example. The commercial product Beano is an enzyme preparation. When taken immediately before eating beans or other gas-forming vegetables, Beano helps break oligosaccharides into monosaccharides so that the body can absorb them.

Some carbohydrate remains intact as it enters the large intestine. This carbohydrate may be fiber or resistant starch or the small intestine may have lacked the necessary enzymes to break it down. In the large intestine, bacteria partially ferment (break down) undigested carbohydrate and produce gas plus a few short-chain fatty acids.[13] These fatty acids are absorbed into the colon and are used for energy by the colon cells. In addition, these fatty acids may reduce the risk of developing gastrointestinal disorders, cancers, and cardiovascular disease.[14]

Some fibers, particularly cellulose and psyllium, pass through the large intestine unchanged and therefore produce little gas. Instead, these fibers add to the stool weight and water content, making it easier to pass.

## Absorption: The Small Intestine Swings into Action

Monosaccharides are absorbed into the mucosal cells lining the small intestine by two different mechanisms. Glucose, galactose, and fructose molecules travel to the liver through the portal vein, where galactose and fructose are converted to glucose. The liver stores and releases glucose as needed to maintain constant blood glucose levels. **Figure 5.7** summarizes digestion and absorption of carbohydrates.

**Starch**

Alpha bonds between glucose molecules in starch are easily broken by human digestive enzymes.

**Cellulose**

Beta bonds in dietary fibers are indigestible by human enzymes.

**Figure 5.6**    **Alpha bonds and beta bonds.** Human digestive enzymes can easily break the alpha bonds in starch, but they cannot break the beta bonds in cellulose.

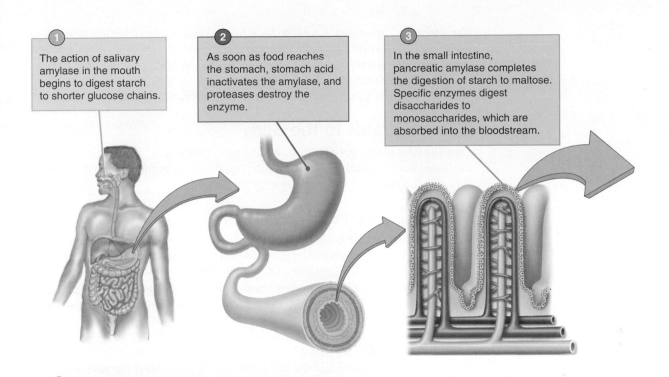

① The action of salivary amylase in the mouth begins to digest starch to shorter glucose chains.

② As soon as food reaches the stomach, stomach acid inactivates the amylase, and proteases destroy the enzyme.

③ In the small intestine, pancreatic amylase completes the digestion of starch to maltose. Specific enzymes digest disaccharides to monosaccharides, which are absorbed into the bloodstream.

④ Once in the bloodstream, the monosaccharides travel to the liver via the portal vein. The liver can convert fructose and galactose to glucose. The liver may form glucose into glycogen, burn it for energy, or release it to the bloodstream for use in other parts of the body.

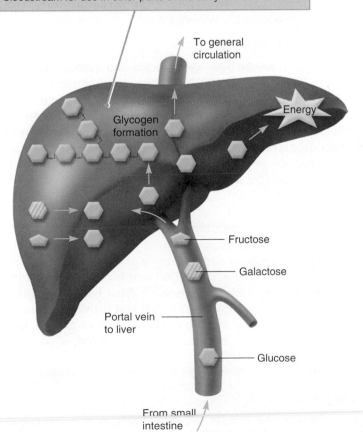

To general circulation

Glycogen formation

Energy

Fructose

Galactose

Portal vein to liver

Glucose

From small intestine

**Figure 5.7** **Travels with carbohydrate.** (1) Carbohydrate digestion begins in the mouth. (2) Stomach acid halts carbohydrate digestion. (3) Carbohydrate digestion resumes in the small intestine, where monosaccharides are absorbed. (4) The liver converts fructose and galactose to glucose, which it can assemble into chains of glycogen, release to the blood, or use for energy.

**Key Concepts** *Carbohydrate digestion takes place primarily in the small intestine, where digestible carbohydrates are broken down and absorbed as monosaccharides. Bacteria in the large intestine partially ferment resistant starch and certain types of fiber, producing gas and a few short-chain fatty acids that can be absorbed by the large intestine and used for energy. The liver converts absorbed monosaccharides into glucose.*

# Carbohydrates in the Body

Through the processes of digestion and absorption, our varied diet of carbohydrates from vegetables, fruits, grains, and milk becomes glucose. Glucose has one major role—to supply energy for the body.

## Glucose Is Your Primary Fuel

Cells throughout the body depend on glucose for energy to drive chemical processes. Although most—but not all—cells also can burn fat for energy, the body needs some glucose to burn fat efficiently.

When we eat food, our bodies immediately use some glucose to maintain normal blood glucose levels. We store excess glucose as glycogen in liver and muscle tissue.

### Using Glucose for Energy

Glucose is the primary fuel for most cells in the body and the preferred fuel for the brain, red blood cells, and nervous system, as well as for the fetus and placenta in a pregnant woman. Even when fat is burned for energy a small amount of glucose is needed to break down fat completely. To obtain energy from glucose, cells must take up glucose from the blood. Once glucose enters cells, a series of reactions breaks it down into carbon dioxide and water, releasing energy in a form the cells can use.[15]

### Storing Glucose as Glycogen

To store excess glucose, the body assembles it into the long, branched chains of glycogen. Glycogen can be broken down quickly, releasing glucose for energy as needed. Liver glycogen stores are used to maintain normal blood glucose levels and account for about one-third of the body's total glycogen stores. Muscle glycogen stores are used to fuel muscle activity and account for about two-thirds of the body's total glycogen stores.[16] The body can store only limited amounts of glycogen—usually enough to last from a few hours to one day, depending on activity level.[17]

### Sparing Body Protein

If carbohydrate is not available, both protein and fat can be used for energy. Although most cells can break down fat for energy, brain cells and developing red blood cells require a constant supply of glucose.[18] (After an extended period of starvation, the brain adapts and is able to use some by-products of fat breakdown for part of its energy needs.) What happens if glucose stores (glycogen in liver and muscles) are depleted and the diet supplies no carbohydrate? To maintain blood glucose levels and supply glucose to the brain, the body can make glucose from body proteins. Adequate consumption of dietary carbohydrate spares body proteins from being broken down and used to make glucose.

### Preventing Ketosis

Even when fat provides fuel for the body, cells require a small amount of carbohydrate to completely break down fat to release energy. When no carbohydrate is available, the liver cannot break down fat completely. Instead,

**Glucose**

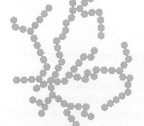

**Glycogen**

it produces small compounds called **ketone bodies**.[19] Most cells can use ketone bodies for energy.

When ketone bodies are produced more quickly than the body can use them, ketone levels build up in the blood and can cause a condition known as **ketosis**. People vulnerable to ketosis include those who consume only small amounts of carbohydrate or who cannot metabolize blood glucose normally. Ketosis is most commonly caused by very low carbohydrate diets, starvation, uncontrolled diabetes mellitus, and chronic alcoholism. Ketosis also can develop when fluid intake is too low to allow the kidneys to excrete excess ketone bodies. As the concentration of ketone bodies increases, the blood becomes too acidic. The body loses water as it excretes excess ketones in urine, and dehydration is a common consequence of ketosis. To prevent ketosis, the body needs a minimum of 50 to 100 grams of carbohydrate daily.[20]

**Key Concepts** *Glucose circulates in the blood to provide immediate energy to cells. The body stores excess glucose in the liver and muscle as glycogen. The body needs adequate carbohydrate intake so that body proteins are not broken down to fulfill energy needs. The body requires some carbohydrate to completely break down fat and prevent the buildup of ketone bodies in the blood.*

**ketone bodies** Molecules formed when insufficient carbohydrate is available to completely metabolize fat. Formation of ketone bodies is promoted by a low glucose level and high acetyl CoA level within cells. Acetone, acetoacetate, and beta-hydroxybutyrate are ketone bodies. Beta-hydroxybutyrate is sometimes improperly called a ketone.

**ketosis [kee-TOE-sis]** Abnormally high concentration of ketone bodies in body tissues and fluids.

**insulin [IN-suh-lin]** Produced by the pancreas, this hormone stimulates the uptake of blood glucose into cells, the formation of glycogen in the liver, and various other processes.

## Regulating Blood Glucose Levels

The body closely regulates blood glucose levels (also known as blood sugar levels) to maintain an adequate supply of glucose for cells. If blood glucose levels drop too low, a person becomes shaky and weak. If blood glucose levels rise too high, a person becomes sluggish and confused and may have difficulty breathing.

Two hormones produced by the pancreas tightly control blood glucose levels.[21] When blood glucose levels rise after a meal, special pancreatic cells called beta cells release the hormone insulin into the blood. **Insulin** acts like a key, "unlocking" the cells of the body and allowing glucose to enter and fuel them. It also stimulates liver and muscle cells to store glucose as glycogen. As glucose enters cells to deliver energy or be stored as glycogen, blood glucose levels return to normal. (See **Figure 5.8**.)

**Figure 5.8** **Regulating blood glucose levels.** Insulin and glucagon have opposing actions. (a) Insulin acts to lower blood glucose levels, and (b) glucagon acts to raise them.

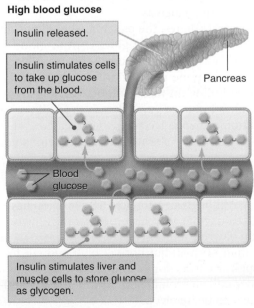

**High blood glucose**

Insulin released.

Insulin stimulates cells to take up glucose from the blood.

Pancreas

Blood glucose

Insulin stimulates liver and muscle cells to store glucose as glycogen.

(a)

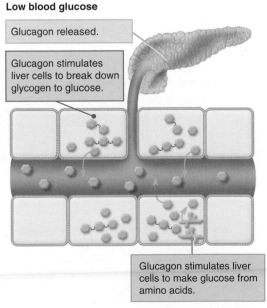

**Low blood glucose**

Glucagon released.

Glucagon stimulates liver cells to break down glycogen to glucose.

Glucagon stimulates liver cells to make glucose from amino acids.

(b)

**glucagon [GLOO-kuh-gon]** Produced by the pancreas, this hormone promotes the breakdown of liver glycogen to glucose and, thus, increases blood glucose levels.

**epinephrine** A hormone released in response to stress or sudden danger, epinephrine raises blood glucose levels to ready the body for "fight or flight." Also called *adrenaline*.

**hyperglycemia [HIGH-per-gly-SEE-me-uh]** Abnormal high concentration of glucose in the blood.

When an individual has not eaten in a while and blood glucose levels begin to fall, the pancreas releases another hormone, **glucagon**. Glucagon stimulates the body to break down stored glycogen, releasing glucose into the bloodstream (see Figure 5.8b). It also stimulates the synthesis of glucose from protein. Another hormone, **epinephrine** (also called adrenaline), exerts effects similar to glucagon to ensure that all body cells have adequate energy for emergencies. Released by the adrenal glands in response to sudden stress or danger, epinephrine is called the "fight or flight" hormone.

Different foods vary in their effect on blood glucose levels. Foods rich in simple carbohydrates or starch but low in fat or fiber tend to be digested and absorbed rapidly. This rapid absorption causes a corresponding large and rapid rise in blood glucose levels.[22] The body reacts to this rise by pumping out extra insulin, which rapidly lowers blood glucose levels. Other foods—especially those rich in dietary fiber, resistant starch, or fat—cause a less dramatic blood glucose response accompanied by smaller swings in blood glucose levels.

The glycemic index measures the effect of a food on blood glucose levels. Foods with a high glycemic index cause a faster and higher rise in blood glucose than foods with a low glycemic index. Although some experts disagree on the usefulness of the glycemic index for humans, diets that emphasize foods with a low glycemic index may offer important health benefits.[23] (For more about this debate, see the FYI feature "The Glycemic Index of Foods: Useful or Useless?")

# High Blood Glucose: Diabetes Mellitus
## What Is Diabetes?

Diabetes is a disorder of carbohydrate metabolism—the way our bodies use digested carbohydrates for growth and energy. Recall that through the processes of digestion and absorption, our varied diet of carbohydrates from vegetables, fruits, grains, and milk end up as glucose in the blood. Glucose is a major source of fuel for the body. After digestion, glucose passes into the bloodstream and into cells, where it is used for growth and energy. For glucose to enter into most types of cells, insulin must be present. Insulin is a hormone produced by the pancreas.

When we eat carbohydrates, the pancreas should automatically produce the right amount of insulin to move glucose from blood into our cells. In people with diabetes, however, the pancreas either produces little or no insulin, or the cells do not respond appropriately to the insulin that is produced. As a result, glucose builds up in the blood, causing **hyperglycemia**—an abnormally high blood glucose level that is the hallmark of diabetes mellitus. If this condition of hyperglycemia is not treated and controlled, blood glucose levels are chronically elevated, causing serious complications and possibly death.[24]

Almost everyone knows someone who has diabetes. An estimated 25.8 million people—8.3 percent of the population—in the United States have diabetes mellitus.[25] Although an estimated 18.8 million have been diagnosed, 7 million do not realize that they have this serious, lifelong condition, and another 79 million have a condition called *pre-diabetes*, where blood glucose levels are higher than normal, but not yet high enough to be diagnosed as diabetes.[26] Although scientists don't completely understand the causes of diabetes, both genetics and environmental factors (obesity and lack of exercise, for example) appear to be involved.

## Consequences of Diabetes

Hyperglycemia, or an abnormally high blood glucose level, is the hallmark of diabetes mellitus. (See **Figure 5.9**.)

Even though glucose in the blood is overabundant, it is unable to enter starving cells to fuel their needs. For this reason diabetes often is called a disease of "starvation in the midst of plenty." In an ironic twist of fate, these starving cells signal the liver to make more glucose, worsening the hyperglycemia. The kidneys are taxed beyond their capacities to reabsorb glucose, and the excess spills into the urine, where it can be detected by urine glucose tests. Thus, even though the blood contains large amounts of glucose, the body loses access to its main source of fuel.

Unable to use glucose, cells turn to other energy sources—fat and protein. But these options can lead to other problems. Excessive use of fat as an energy source, without available glucose in the cell, causes ketosis and acidosis, dangerously high acidity levels in the blood. Breaking down muscle proteins to fuel the cells causes muscle wasting and weakness. Alterations in fat and protein metabolism often accompany hyperglycemia.[27]

Over time, abnormally high blood glucose levels increase risk of high blood pressure, heart disease, and kidney disease. Excess glucose in the blood reacts with and damages body proteins and tissues, especially in the eyes, kidneys, nerves, and blood vessels. Complications of diabetes can contribute to degenerative conditions such as peripheral vascular disease (disease of blood vessels that supply the feet and legs), deterioration of the eye and eventual blindness, kidney disease, and progressive nerve damage. Diabetes is responsible for more than 60 percent of all nontraumatic amputations of the lower extremities and 44 percent of all new cases of kidney failure in adults.[28] Diabetes is also the leading cause of blindness in adults.[29] Diabetics are 40 times more likely to develop glaucoma.[30] Sixty-seven percent of people with diabetes have high blood pressure, and nearly all have one or more lipid abnormality.[31] People with diabetes are two to four times more likely to develop heart disease than people without diabetes. In the United States and Canada, diabetes is one of the leading contributors to death and disability.

## Forms of Diabetes Mellitus

Three main forms of diabetes occur:

1. *Type 1 diabetes.* **Type 1 diabetes** usually is diagnosed in children and young adults and was previously known as insulin-dependent diabetes (IDDM) or juvenile diabetes. In type 1 diabetes, the body fails to produce insulin, the hormone that "unlocks" cells, allowing glucose to enter and fuel them. Roughly 5 to 10 percent of Americans who are diagnosed with diabetes have type 1 diabetes.[32]
2. *Type 2 diabetes.* In **type 2 diabetes**, either the body does not produce enough insulin or cells ignore the insulin. Type 2 diabetes was previously known as non-insulin-dependent diabetes (NIDDM) or adult-onset diabetes. Approximately 90 to 95 percent of all Americans with diabetes mellitus have type 2 diabetes.[33]
   - *Pre-diabetes (impaired glucose tolerance or impaired fasting glucose).* **Pre-diabetes** is a condition in which a person's blood glucose levels are higher than normal but not high enough to warrant a diagnosis of type 2 diabetes. Between the years 2005–2008, 35 percent of American adults ages 20 years

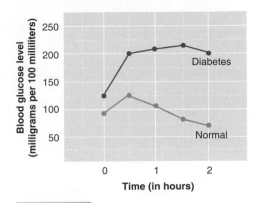

**Figure 5.9** **Glucose tolerance test.** A glucose tolerance test measures the level of glucose in the blood following consumption of a standard dose of glucose. Glucose tolerance tests are used to diagnose diabetes.

**type 1 diabetes** Diabetes that occurs when the body's immune system attacks beta cells in the pancreas, causing them to lose their ability to make insulin.

**type 2 diabetes** Diabetes that occurs when target cells (e.g., fat and muscle cells) lose the ability to respond normally to insulin.

**pre-diabetes** Blood glucose levels higher than normal but not high enough to warrant a diagnosis of diabetes.

or older had pre-diabetes, and of those age 65 and older, 50 percent had pre-diabetes.[34] Using these percentages to predict the incidence of pre-diabetes for the entire American population in the year 2010 yields an estimate that 79 million Americans ages 20 years and older will have pre-diabetes.

3. *Gestational diabetes.* **Gestational diabetes** occurs in a pregnant woman who has never had diabetes but who develops hyperglycemia during pregnancy. It affects approximately 4 percent of all pregnant women—about 135,000 cases in the United States each year.[35]

### Type 1 Diabetes Mellitus

Type 1 diabetes usually occurs in people younger than 30 and often develops suddenly. People with type 1 diabetes lack insulin, usually because an autoimmune response has destroyed insulin-producing cells of the pancreas. Symptoms include excessive thirst, frequent urination, rapid weight loss, and blurred vision.[36] When blood glucose levels rise, glucose spills into the urine, taking water with it and causing frequent urination and increased thirst. Although blood glucose levels are high, the lack of insulin prevents glucose from entering cells to be burned for energy. The result is weight loss and feelings of hunger.

People with type 1 diabetes require lifelong, daily insulin injections balanced with a healthful diet and regular exercise to maintain blood glucose levels in the normal range. Because exercise lowers blood glucose levels, individuals must consider the timing of exercise in addition to food intake and insulin injections to avoid lowering blood glucose levels excessively.

### Type 2 Diabetes Mellitus

In type 2 diabetes, glucose has trouble entering body cells because either the pancreas cannot produce enough insulin or cells in the body become resistant to the action of insulin. Although obesity contributes to **insulin resistance** in many people with type 2 diabetes, genetic factors may play a role. Type 2 diabetes usually develops in overweight individuals aged 45 and older. However, with the rising prevalence of obesity, type 2 diabetes is occurring more frequently in adolescents.

The result is the same as for type 1 diabetes—glucose builds up in the blood, and the body cannot use its main source of fuel efficiently. Type 2 diabetes often is part of a metabolic syndrome that includes obesity, elevated blood pressure, and high levels of blood triglycerides.

In contrast to the sudden onset of type 1 diabetes, the symptoms of type 2 diabetes develop gradually, and some people may not show symptoms for many years. Symptoms of type 2 diabetes may eventually include fatigue or nausea, frequent urination, unusual thirst, weight loss, blurred vision, frequent infections, and slow healing of wounds or sores.

### Pre-diabetes

Before people develop type 2 diabetes, they usually have pre-diabetes—impaired glucose tolerance that results in a blood glucose level that is higher than normal yet not high enough to be diagnosed as diabetes. Some long-term damage to the body, especially to the heart and circulatory system, may already be occurring during the pre-diabetes stage.

People who have pre-diabetes are at increased risk for developing both type 2 diabetes and heart disease. Unless they take steps toward prevention,

**gestational diabetes** A condition that results in high blood glucose levels during pregnancy.

**insulin resistance** State in which enough insulin is produced but cells do not respond to the action of insulin. Also called *insulin insensitivity.*

such as dietary changes, moderate weight loss, and regular exercise, many will develop type 2 diabetes within 10 years.

### Gestational Diabetes Mellitus

Pregnant women who have never had diabetes before but who develop impaired glucose tolerance during pregnancy are said to have gestational diabetes. Although the cause of gestational diabetes remains unknown, researchers have uncovered certain clues. The placenta produces hormones that help the baby develop. Unfortunately, these hormones also block the action of the mother's insulin in her body. This insulin resistance makes it difficult for the mother's body to use insulin and can triple the amount of insulin needed to get sufficient glucose into her cells. Gestational diabetes occurs more often in African Americans, Native Americans, and Hispanic Americans and is more common among obese women and women with a family history of diabetes.

In women with gestational diabetes, blood glucose levels usually decrease after pregnancy. Once a woman has had gestational diabetes, however, her chances are two in three that it will return in future pregnancies. In a few women, pregnancy reveals preexisting type 1 or type 2 diabetes that requires ongoing treatment after pregnancy. Forty to 60 percent of women who had gestational diabetes will develop type 2 diabetes later in life.[37] Both forms of diabetes involve insulin resistance.

## Risk Factors for Diabetes

Some people are at higher risk than others for developing diabetes. Table 5.2 lists the risk factors for type 1 and type 2 diabetes. Anyone with a family history of diabetes has an increased risk. In most cases of type 1 diabetes, people must inherit risk factors from both parents, and whites have the highest rate of this disease.[38]

A family history of type 2 diabetes is one of the strongest risk factors for getting the disease.[39] The ethnic groups at highest risk of type 2 diabetes are Native Americans, Hispanic Americans, and African Americans. An increased risk of type 2 diabetes seems to occur more frequently in people who follow a "Western" lifestyle characterized by too much fat; too few fruits, vegetables, and fiber; and not enough exercise.[40] The risk of developing type 2 diabetes increases progressively as body fat increases, especially around the midsection. The dramatic surge in obesity rates in the United States is a major reason that the incidence of type 2 diabetes has tripled since 1970.[41] Compared with a normal-weight person, an obese person has a significantly increased risk of developing type 2 diabetes.[42] More than 80 percent of adults diagnosed with type 2 diabetes are overweight or obese at the time of their diagnosis.[43]

Unfortunately, as more children and adolescents become overweight, type 2 diabetes is becoming more common in young people. Contrary to popular opinion, high sugar or high carbohydrate intake does not by itself cause diabetes as long as it does not contribute to excess energy intake and obesity. The best measures for preventing pre-diabetes and obesity-related type 2 diabetes are a healthful diet and regular exercise. (See **Figure 5.10**.) Reducing excess body fat will improve glucose tolerance and reduce related risk factors for heart disease. Regular exercise will improve carbohydrate and lipid metabolism and increase insulin sensitivity. In addition, exercise improves blood flow to the extremities, bringing blood pressure down to normal levels and reducing risk of heart disease.

Although people with diabetes have the same nutritional needs as anyone else, good diabetes control requires that they monitor their food intake care-

| Table 5.2 | Risk Factors for Type 1 and Type 2 Diabetes Mellitus |
| --- | --- |

*Risk Factors for Type 1 Diabetes*
First-degree relative (parent, sibling) with type 1 diabetes

*Risk Factors for Type 2 Diabetes*
Age ≥ 45 years
Overweight (BMI ≥ 25 kg/m²)
First-degree relative with diabetes
Sedentary lifestyle
Ethnicity: African American, Latino, Native American, Asian American, Pacific Islander
Previously identified pre-diabetes
History of gestational diabetes or delivery of a baby weighing more than 9 pounds
Hypertension (≥ 140/90 mm Hg)
HDL cholesterol level < 35 mg/dL and/or triglyceride level > 250 mg/dL
Polycystic ovary syndrome
History of vascular disease

**Sources:** American Diabetes Association. Position statement: prevention of type 1 diabetes. *Diabetes Care.* 2004;27(suppl 1):S133; and American Diabetes Association. Position statement: prevention or delay of type 2 diabetes. *Diabetes Care.* 2004;27(suppl 1):S47–S54. Copyright © 2004 American Diabetes Association. Reprinted with permission from American Diabetes Association.

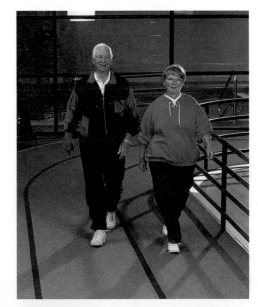

| Figure 5.10 | **Diabetes management.** |
| --- | --- |

Exercises, diet, and weight loss can have a significant impact on blood glucose levels for people with type 2 diabetes.

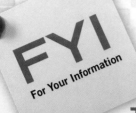

# The Glycemic Index of Foods: Useful or Useless?

Although controversial, the glycemic index is a valuable and easy-to-use concept.[1] Others suggest that although promising, more definitive data are needed before this concept should be promoted for widespread public use.[2] Several popular weight-loss diets use the glycemic index to guide food choices.

## How Is the Glycemic Index Measured?

The glycemic index is a measure of the change in blood glucose following consumption of carbohydrate-containing foods. It compares the change in blood glucose after eating a sample food to the change expected from eating an equal amount of available carbohydrate from a standard food such as white bread.[3]

Foods with a high glycemic index trigger a marked rise followed by a more or less rapid fall in blood glucose. Foods with a low glycemic index produce a smaller peak along with a more gradual decline in blood glucose.

## What Factors Affect the Glycemic Index of a Food or Meal?

The glycemic index of a food is not always easy to predict. Would you expect a sweet food such as ice cream to have a high glycemic index? Ice cream actually has a low glycemic value because its fat slows sugar absorption. On the other hand, wouldn't you expect complex carbohydrates such as bread or potatoes to have a low glycemic index? In fact, the starch in white bread and cooked potatoes is readily absorbed, so each has a high value.[4] The glycemic indices of some common foods are listed in Table A, and lower-glycemic-index substitutions are provided in Table B.

The type of carbohydrate, degree of processing, method of cooking, and the presence of fat, dietary fiber, and other food components in a meal or snack all affect the glycemic response.[5] The glycemic index of mixed meals, referred to as the glycemic load, is more important than the effect of individual foods on blood glucose.[6]

## Why Do Some Researchers Believe the Glycemic Index Is Useful?

Health benefits can be significant. Diets that emphasize low-glycemic-index foods decrease the risk of developing type 2 diabetes and improve blood glucose control in people who are already afflicted.[7] Epidemiological studies suggest that such diets also reduce the risk of colon and other

### Table A — Glycemic Index of Some Foods Compared to Pure Glucose[a]

| Food | Glycemic Index | Food | Glycemic Index |
|---|---|---|---|
| *Bakery Products* | | Skim milk | 36 |
| Angel food cake | 67 | *Fruits* | |
| Waffles | 76 | Apples | 38 |
| *Bread* | | Bananas | 52 |
| White bread | 73 | Pineapple | 59 |
| Whole-wheat bread, whole meal flour | 71 | *Legumes* | |
| | | Black-eyed peas | 42 |
| *Breakfast Cereals* | | Lentils | 29 |
| All bran | 42 | *Pasta* | |
| Corn flakes | 81 | Spaghetti | 42 |
| Oatmeal | 58 | Macaroni | 47 |
| *Cereal Grains* | | *Vegetables* | |
| Barley | 25 | Carrots | 47 |
| Sweet corn | 53 | Baked potatoes | 85 |
| White rice, long grain | 56 | Green peas | 48 |
| Bulgur | 45 | *Candy* | |
| *Dairy Foods* | | Jelly beans | 78 |
| Ice cream | 61 | Life Savers | 70 |

[a] Glycemic response to pure glucose is 100.

**Source:** Data from Foster-Powell K, Holt SHA, Brand-Miller JC. International table of glycemic index and glycemic load values: 2002. *Am J Clin Nutr.* 2002;76:5–56.

cancers[8] and may help reduce the risk of heart disease as well. Diets with a low glycemic load are associated with higher HDL cholesterol levels and reduced incidence of heart attack.[9] Also, studies indicate that the effectiveness of low-fat, high-carbohydrate diets for weight loss can be improved by reducing the glycemic load.[10]

## Why Do Some Researchers Believe the Glycemic Index Is Useless?

Some researchers question the usefulness of conclusions drawn primarily from epidemiologi-

cal studies.[11] Epidemiologic studies can show association, but they cannot prove causation. Also, researchers worry about the wide variations in measured glycemic responses to individual foods.

Some believe the glycemic index is too complex for most people to use effectively. The position of the American Diabetes Association is that the glycemic index and load may provide additional benefit in the management of diabetes over that observed when total carbohydrate is considered alone.[12]

| Table B | **Sample Substitutions for High-Glycemic-Index Foods**[a] |
|---------|------------------------------------------------------------|

| High-Glycemic-Index | Low-Glycemic-Index Alternative |
|---------------------|--------------------------------|
| Bread, wheat or Bread, white | Oat bran, rye, or pumpernickel bread |
| Processed breakfast cereal | Unrefined cereal such as oats (either museli or oatmeal) or bran cereal |
| Plain cookies and crackers | Cookies made with nuts and whole grains such as oats |
| Cakes and muffins | Cakes and muffins made with fruit, oats, or whole grains |
| Bananas | Apples |
| White potatoes | Sweet potatoes, pastas, or legumes |

[a] Low glycemic index = 55 or less; medium = 56–69; high = 70 or more.

## What Is the Bottom Line?

Like many other nutrition issues, the glycemic index needs further study. We need to continue to identify the influence of processing techniques on the glycemic index. Most researchers also call for prospective, long-term clinical trials to evaluate the effects of low-glycemic-index and low-glycemic-load diets in chronic disease risk reduction and treatment.[13] Until then, encouraging the consumption of fruits, vegetables, whole-grain, minimally refined cereal products, and other low-glycemic-index foods won't hurt, and it may help to improve health!

1   Mondazzi L, Arcelli, E. Glycemic index in sport nutrition. *J Am Coll Nutr.* 2009;28(suppl):455S–463S.

2   Thomas D, Elliott EJ. Low glycaemic index, or low glycaemic load, diets for diabetes mellitus. *Cochrane Database Syst Rev.* 2009;(1):CD006296.

3   Udani J, Singh B, Barrett M, Preuss H. Lowering the glycemic index of white bread using a white bean extract. *Nutr J.* 2009;8:52.

4   Foster-Powell K, Holt SH, Brand-Miller JC. International table of glycemic index and glycemic load values: 2002. *Am J Clin Nutr.* 2002;76:5–56.

5   Pi-Sunyer FX. Glycemic index and disease. *Am J Clin Nutr.* 2002;76(suppl):290S–298S; and Fernandes G, Velangi A, Wolever T. Glycemic index of potatoes commonly consumed in North America. *J Am Diet Assoc.* 2005;105(4):557–562.

6   Franz M, Powers M, Leontos C, et al. The evidence for medical nutrition therapy for type 1 and type 2 diabetes in adults. *J Am Diet Assoc.* 2010;110(12):1852–1889.

7   Finley C, Barlow C, Halton T, Haskell W. Glycemic index, glycemic load, and prevalence of the metabolic syndrome in the Copper Center Longitudinal Study. *J Am Diet Assoc.* 2010;110(12):1820–1829.

8   Cari K. Low-glycemic load diets: how does the evidence for prevention of disease measure up? *J Am Diet Assoc.* 2010;110(12):1818–1819.

9   Ibid.

10  Ibid.

11  Raben A. Should obese patients be counseled to follow a low-glycaemic index diet? *No Obes Rev.* 2002;3(4):245–256; and Pi-Sunyer FX. Op. cit.

12  American Diabetes Association. Nutrition recommendations and interventions for diabetes: a position statement of the American Diabetes Association. *Diabetes Care.* 2007;30(suppl 1):S48–S65.

13  Ludwig DS, Eckel RH. The glycemic index at 20 y. *Am J Clin Nutr.* 2002;76(suppl):264S–265S.

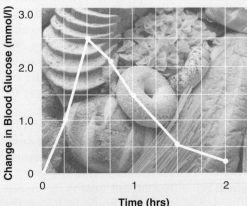

**Time (hrs)**
HIGH GLYCEMIC INDEX

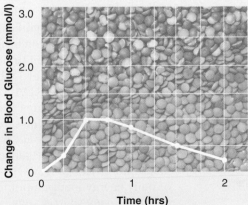

**Time (hrs)**
LOW GLYCEMIC INDEX

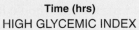

fully. By eating well-balanced meals in the correct amounts, people can keep their blood glucose levels as close to normal (nondiabetes level) as possible. People with diabetes can use Exchange Lists to plan their diets.

## Low Blood Glucose Levels: Hypoglycemia

Excess insulin results in low blood sugar, or **hypoglycemia**. Too much glucose enters cells, lowering blood glucose levels too far. When blood glucose levels drop too low, nervousness, irritability, hunger, headache, shakiness, rapid heartbeat, and weakness can develop. A further drop in blood glucose levels can cause coma and death.

A person with diabetes can develop hypoglycemia in response to an overdose of insulin or vigorous exercise. In nondiabetic individuals, two types of hypoglycemia occur. **Reactive hypoglycemia** occurs about one hour after eating carbohydrate-rich food. The body overreacts and produces too much insulin in response to the food. Individuals can prevent reactive hypoglycemia by eating frequent, smaller meals to smooth out blood glucose responses to food. **Fasting hypoglycemia** occurs because the body produces too much insulin even when no food is eaten. Pancreatic tumors can cause fasting hypoglycemia.

**Key Concepts**  *In healthy individuals, two hormones produced by the pancreas closely regulate blood glucose levels. Insulin allows glucose to enter cells and stimulates storage of glucose as glycogen, lowering blood glucose levels. Glucagon stimulates the release of glucose from glycogen and the formation of glucose from protein. Some individuals lack the ability to regulate blood glucose levels properly, resulting in diabetes, which is characterized by hyperglycemia (high blood glucose) or hypoglycemia (low blood glucose). Individuals with type 1 diabetes cannot make insulin; individuals with type 2 diabetes are resistant to the action of insulin or make inadequate amounts.*

# Carbohydrates in Your Diet

What foods supply our dietary carbohydrates? **Figure 5.11** shows many foods rich in carbohydrates. Plant foods are our main dietary sources of carbohydrates: Grains, legumes, and vegetables provide starches and fibers; fruits provide sugars and fibers. Additional sugar (mainly lactose) is found in dairy foods, and various sugars are found in sweeteners, beverages, jams, jellies, and candy.

## Recommendations for Carbohydrate Intake

The minimum amount of carbohydrate required by the body is based on the brain's requirement for glucose. This glucose can come either from dietary carbohydrate or from synthesis of glucose from protein in the body. Because adaptation to using protein for glucose and ketone bodies for energy may be incomplete relying on protein alone is not recommended.[44] Therefore, an RDA for carbohydrate of 130 grams per day has been set for individuals age 1 year and older. The RDA for carbohydrate rises to 175 grams per day for pregnancy and 210 grams per day during lactation.

The *Dietary Guidelines for Americans* suggest that we "reduce the intake of added sugars."[45] One key recommendation is to choose and prepare foods and beverages with little added sugar. Although the Acceptable Macronutrient Distribution Range (AMDR) for added sugars is no more than 25 percent of daily energy intake, a point at which the micronutrient quality of the diet declines, many sources suggest that added sugar intake should be lower. The *Dietary Guidelines for Americans* also recommends that we choose foods such

**hypoglycemia [HIGH-po-gly-SEE-mee-uh]** Abnormally low concentration of glucose in the blood; any blood glucose value below 40 to 50 mg/dL of blood.

**reactive hypoglycemia** A type of hypoglycemia that occurs about one hour after eating carbohydrate-rich food. The body overreacts and produces too much insulin in response to food, rapidly decreasing blood glucose.

**fasting hypoglycemia** A type of hypoglycemia that occurs because the body produces too much insulin even when no food is eaten.

**germ** The innermost part of a grain that can grow into a new plant. Germ is rich in protein, oils, vitamins, and minerals.

**endosperm** The middle portion of a grain kernel; high in starch to provide food for the growing plant embryo.

**bran** The layers of protective coating around the grain kernel that are rich in dietary fiber and nutrients.

**husk** The inedible covering of grain; also known as the *chaff*.

as whole grains, vegetables, fruits, and cooked dry beans and peas as staples in our diet and to consume at least half of all grains as whole grains.[46] Fruits, vegetables, and whole grains, along with legumes, are good sources of fiber. The Adequate Intake (AI) value for total fiber is 38 grams per day for men aged 19 to 50 years and 25 grams per day for women in the same age group. This AI value is based on a level of intake (14 grams per 1,000 kilocalories) that provides the greatest risk reduction for heart disease.[47] The Daily Value for fiber used on food labels is 25 grams.

## Current Consumption: How Much Carbohydrate Do You Eat?

THINK
About It
2

The AMDR for carbohydrate is 45 to 65 percent of kilocalories. For an adult who eats about 2,000 kilocalories daily, this represents 225 to 325 grams of carbohydrate. The Daily Value for carbohydrates is 300 grams per day, representing 60 percent of the calories in a 2,000-kilocalorie diet.

Adult Americans currently consume about 49 to 50 percent of their energy intake as carbohydrate; however, this does not account for the quality of the carbohydrates consumed. According to National Health and Nutrition Examination Survey (NHANES) data, 13 percent of the population has an added sugar intake of more than 25 percent of calories, with a mean equivalent of added sugar intake of about 83 grams per day.[48] About one-third of Americans added sugar intake comes from nondiet soft drinks. This is of concern because as soft drink consumption rises, energy intake increases, but milk consumption and the vitamin and mineral quality of the diet decline.[49] Many studies suggest that rising soft drink consumption is a factor in overweight and obesity, even among very young children.[50] Regular soft drinks, sugary sweets, sweetened grains, and regular fruitades/drinks comprise 72 percent of the intake of added sugar.[51]

Most Americans do not consume enough dietary fiber, with usual intakes averaging only 15 grams per day.[52] With the exception of older women (51 years and older), only 0 to 5 percent of individuals in all other life stage groups have fiber intakes meeting or exceeding the AI.[53] The major sources of dietary fiber in the American diets are white flour and potatoes, not because they are concentrated fiber sources but because they are widely consumed.[54]

## Choosing Carbohydrates Wisely

The *Dietary Guidelines for Americans* encourages us to increase our intake of fruits, vegetables, whole grains, and fat-free or low-fat milk while keeping calorie intake under control. These foods are all good sources of carbohydrates and many other nutrients. Choosing a variety of fruits and vegetables, and particularly including choices from all five vegetable subgroups (dark green vegetables, orange vegetables, legumes, starchy vegetables, and other vegetables) provides vitamin A, vitamin C, folate, potassium, and fiber.

## Strategies for Increasing Fiber Intake

Along with fruits and vegetables, whole grains are important sources of fiber. Whole kernels of grain consist of four parts: germ, endosperm, bran, and husk. (See **Figure 5.12**.) The **germ**, the innermost part at the base of the kernel, is the portion that grows into a new plant. It is rich in protein, oils, vitamins, and minerals. The **endosperm** is the middle portion (and largest part) of the grain kernel. It is high in starch and provides food for the growing plant embryo. The **bran** is composed of layers of protective coating around the grain kernel and is rich in dietary fiber. The **husk** is an inedible covering.

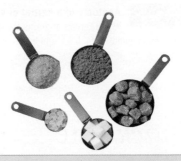

Table sugar, corn syrup, and brown sugar are rich in sucrose, a simple carbohydrate.

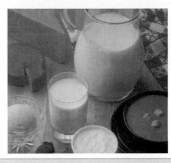

Milk and milk products are rich in lactose, a simple carbohydrate.

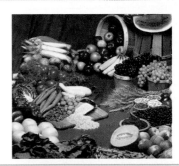

Fruits and vegetables provide simple sugars, starch, and fiber.

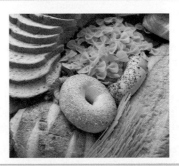

Bread, flour, cornmeal, rice, and pasta are rich in starch and, sometimes, dietary fiber.

**Figure 5.11** **Sources of carbohydrates.**

**Figure 5.12**   **Anatomy of a kernel of grain.** Whole kernels of grains consist of four parts: germ, endosperm, bran, and husk.

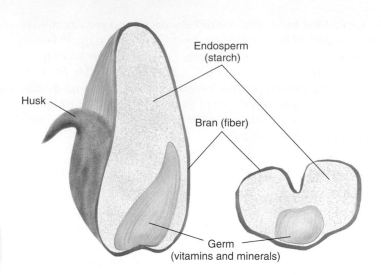

## Quick Bite

### Carbohydrate Companions
The word *companion* comes from the Latin word *companio*, meaning "one who shares bread."

**Table 5.3**   **High-Carbohydrate Foods**

| High in Complex Carbohydrates | High in Simple Carbohydrates |
| --- | --- |
| Bagels | **Naturally Present** |
| Tortillas | Fruits |
| Cereals | Fruit juices |
| Crackers | Skim milk |
| Rice cakes | Plain nonfat yogurt |
| Legumes | **Added** |
| Corn | Angel food cake |
| Potatoes | Soft drinks |
| Peas | Sherbet |
| Squash | Syrups |
| Popcorn | Sweetened nonfat yogurt |
| | Candy |
| | Jellies |
| | Jams |
| | Gelatin |
| | High-sugar breakfast cereals |
| | Cookies |
| | Frosting |

## Quick Bite

### Liquid Candy
In the United States, corn sweeteners are primarily consumed in carbonated soft drinks (25.4 pounds per year), fruitades and drinks (8.2 pounds), and syrup and sweet toppings (4.1 pounds). In all, 36.3 percent of sugar and corn sweeteners are consumed in carbonated soft drinks, fruitades, and other nonalcoholic drinks.

When grains are refined—making white flour from wheat, for example, or making white rice from brown rice—the process removes the outer husk and bran layers and sometimes the inner germ of the grain kernel. Because the bran and germ portions of the grain contain much of the dietary fiber, vitamins, and minerals, the nutrient content of whole grains is far superior to that of refined grains. Although food manufacturers add iron, thiamin, riboflavin, and niacin back to white flour through enrichment, they usually do not add back lost dietary fiber and nutrients such as vitamin $B_6$, calcium, phosphorus, potassium, magnesium, and zinc, which are lost in processing.

Read labels carefully to choose foods that contain whole grains. Terms such as *whole-wheat, whole-grain, rolled oats,* and *brown rice* indicate that the entire grain kernel is included in the food. Even better, look for the words *100 percent whole grain* or *100 percent whole wheat.*

To increase your fiber intake:

- Eat more whole-grain breads, cereals, pasta, and rice as well as more fruits, vegetables, and legumes.
- Eat fruits and vegetables with the peel, if possible. The peel is high in fiber.
- Add fruits to muffins and pancakes.
- Add legumes—such as lentils and pinto, navy, kidney, and black beans—to casseroles and mixed dishes as a meat substitute.
- Substitute whole-grain flour for all-purpose flour in recipes whenever possible.
- Use brown rice instead of white rice.
- Substitute oats for flour in crumb toppings.
- Choose high-fiber cereals.
- Choose whole fruits rather than fruit juices.

When increasing your fiber intake, do so gradually and drink plenty of fluids to allow your body to adjust. Add just a few grams a day; otherwise, abdominal cramps, gas, bloating, and diarrhea or constipation may result. Parents and caregivers should also emphasize foods rich in fiber for children older than 2 years but must take care that these foods do not fill a child up before energy and nutrient needs are met. Table 5.3 lists various foods that are high in simple and complex carbohydrates.

Although health food stores, pharmacies, and even grocery stores sell many types of fiber supplements, most experts agree that you should get fiber from food rather than from a supplement. Foods rich in dietary fiber contain a variety of fibers as well as vitamins, minerals, and other phytochemicals that offer important health effects.

## Moderating Your Sugar Intake

Most of us enjoy the taste of sweet foods, and there's no reason why we should not. But for some individuals, habitually high sugar intake crowds out foods that are higher in fiber, vitamins, and minerals.

To reduce added sugars in your diet:

- Use less of all added sugars, including white sugar, brown sugar, honey, and syrups.
- Limit use of soft drinks, high-sugar breakfast cereals, candy, ice cream, and sweet desserts.
- Use fresh or frozen fruits and fruits canned in natural juices or light syrup for dessert and to sweeten waffles, pancakes, muffins, and breads.

Read ingredient lists carefully. Food labels list the total grams of sugar in a food, which includes both sugars naturally present in foods and sugars added to foods. Many terms for added sweeteners appear on food labels. Foods likely to be high in sugar list some form of sweetener as the first, second, or third ingredient on labels. Table 5.4 lists various forms of sugar used in foods.

Sugar substitutes can help you lower sugar intake, but foods with these substitutes may not provide less energy than similar products containing nutritive sweeteners. Rather than sugar, other energy-yielding nutrients, such as fat, are the primary source of the calories in these foods. Also, as sugar substitute use in the United States has increased, so has sugar consumption—an interesting paradox!

**Key Concepts** *Current recommendations suggest that Americans consume at least 130 grams of carbohydrate per day. An intake of total carbohydrates representing between 45 and 65 percent of total energy intake and a fiber intake of 14 grams per 1,000 kilocalories are associated with reduced heart disease risk. Added sugar should account for no more than 25 percent of daily energy and ideally should be much less. Americans generally eat too little fiber. An emphasis on consuming whole grains, legumes, fruits, and vegetables would help to increase fiber intake.*

### Nutritive Sweeteners

**Nutritive sweeteners** are digestible carbohydrates and therefore provide energy. They include monosaccharides, disaccharides, and **sugar alcohols** from either natural or refined sources. White sugar, brown sugar, honey, maple syrup, glucose, fructose, xylitol, sorbitol, and mannitol are just some of the many nutritive sweeteners used in foods. One slice of angel food cake, for example, contains about 5 teaspoons of sugar. Fruit-flavored yogurt contains about 7 teaspoons of sugar. Even two sticks of chewing gum contain about 1 teaspoon of sugar. Whether sweeteners are added to foods or are present naturally, all are broken down in the small intestine and absorbed as monosaccharides and provide energy. Because all these absorbed monosaccharides end up as glucose, the body cannot tell whether these monosaccharides came from honey or table sugar.

THINK
About It
3

The sugar alcohols in sugarless chewing gums and candies are also nutritive sweeteners, but the body does not digest and absorb them fully, so they provide only about 2 kilocalories per gram, compared with the 4 kilocalories per gram that other sugars provide.

**Natural Sweeteners** Natural sweeteners such as honey and maple syrup contain monosaccharides and disaccharides that make them taste sweet. Honey

| Table 5.4 | **Forms of Sugar Used in Foods** |
|---|---|

Brown rice syrup
Brown sugar
Concentrated fruit juice sweetener
Confectioners' sugar
Corn syrup
Dextrose
Galactose
Glucose
Granulated sugar
High-fructose corn syrup
Invert sugar
Lactose
Levulose
Maltose
Mannitol
Maple sugar
Molasses
Natural sweeteners
Raw sugar
Sorbitol
Turbinado sugar
White sugar
Xylitol

## *Quick* Bite

### Why Is Honey Dangerous for Babies?
Because honey and Karo syrup (corn syrup) can contain spores of the bacterium *Clostridium botulinum*, they should never be fed to infants younger than 1 year of age. Infants do not produce as much stomach acid as older children and adults, so *C. botulinum* spores can germinate in an infant's GI tract and cause botulism, a deadly foodborne illness.

**nutritive sweeteners** Substances that make foods sweet and can be absorbed and yield energy in the body.

**sugar alcohols** Compounds formed from monosaccharides; commonly used as nutritive sweeteners. Also called *polyols*.

**refined sweeteners** Substances composed of monosaccharides and disaccharides that have been extracted and processed from other foods.

**polyols** See *sugar alcohols*.

**non-nutritive sweeteners** Substances that impart sweetness to foods but supply little or no energy to the body; also called artificial or alternative sweeteners. They include acesulfame, aspartame, saccharin, and sucralose.

## *Quick* Bite

### The Discovery of Saccharin

A German student named Constantine Fahlberge discovered saccharin in 1879 while working with organic chemicals in the lab of Ira Remsen at Johns Hopkins University. One day, while eating some bread, he noticed a strong sweet flavor. He deduced that the flavor came from the compound on his hands, $C_6H_4CONHSO_2$. Fahlberg then patented saccharin himself, without Remsen.

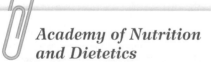

### *Academy of Nutrition and Dietetics*

#### Use of Nutritive and Non-nutritive Sweeteners

It is the position of the Academy of Nutrition and Dietetics that consumers can safely enjoy a range of nutritive and non-nutritive sweeteners when consumed in a diet that is guided by current federal nutrition recommendations, such as the *Dietary Guidelines for Americans* and the Dietary Reference Intakes, as well as individual health groups.

**Source:** Reproduced from Position of the American Dietetic Association: use of nutritive and non-nutritive sweeteners. *J Am Diet Assoc.* 2004;104(2):255–275.

contains a mix of fructose and glucose—the same two monosaccharides that make up sucrose. Bees make honey from the sucrose-containing nectar of flowering plants. Real maple syrup contains primarily sucrose and is made by boiling and concentrating the sap from sugar maple trees. Most maple-flavored syrups sold in grocery stores, however, are made from corn syrup with maple flavoring added.

Many fruits also contain sugars that impart a sweet taste. Usually the riper the fruit, the higher its sugar content—a ripe pear tastes sweeter than an unripe one.

**Refined Sweeteners  Refined sweeteners** are monosaccharides and disaccharides that have been extracted from plant foods. White table sugar is sucrose extracted from either sugar beets or sugar cane. Molasses is a by-product of the sugar-refining process. Most brown sugar is really white table sugar with molasses added for coloring and flavor.

Manufacturers make high-fructose corn syrup by treating cornstarch with acid and enzymes to break down the starch into glucose. Then different enzymes convert about half the glucose to fructose. High-fructose corn syrup has about the same sweetness as table sugar but costs less to produce. An increase in high-fructose corn syrup (HFCS) in soft drinks and other processed foods accounts for much of the increased use of sweeteners in the United States since the 1970s.[55] High HFCS consumption may contribute to obesity and high triglyceride levels.[56] On average, Americans consume 132 calories of HFCS each day, which is nearly 200 more calories a day than in the 1970s. HFCS can be found in approximately 40 percent of items purchased at local grocery stores.[57]

**Sugar Alcohols**  The sugar alcohols sorbitol, xylitol, and mannitol occur naturally in a wide variety of fruits and vegetables and are commercially produced from other carbohydrates such as sucrose, glucose, and starch. Also known as **polyols**, these sweeteners are not as sweet as sucrose, but they do have the advantage of being less likely to cause tooth decay. The body does not digest and absorb sugar alcohols fully, so they provide only 2 kilocalories per gram compared with the 4 kilocalories per gram that other sugars provide. When sugar alcohols are used as the sweetener, the product may be sugar- (sucrose-) free, but it is not calorie-free. Check the label to be sure. Manufacturers use sugar alcohols to sweeten sugar-free products, such as gum and mints, and to add bulk and texture, provide a cooling sensation in the mouth, and retain moisture in foods. An excess intake of sugar alcohols may cause diarrhea.[58]

### Non-nutritive Sweeteners

Gram for gram, most **non-nutritive sweeteners** (also called *artificial sweeteners*) are many times sweeter than nutritive sweeteners. As a consequence, food manufacturers can use much less artificial sweetener to sweeten foods. **Figure 5.13** compares the sweetness of sweeteners. Although some non-nutritive sweeteners do provide energy, their energy contribution is minimal given the small amount used.

The most common non-nutritive sweeteners in the United States are saccharin, aspartame, acesulfame K, and sucralose. Cyclamates, which were banned in the United States in 1969 because of cancer concerns, are still used in Canada and many other countries. For people who want to decrease their intake of sugar and energy while still enjoying sweet foods, non-nutritive sweeteners offer an alternative. Also, non-nutritive sweeteners do not contribute to tooth decay.

THINK
About It
4

**Saccharin** Discovered in 1879 and used in foods ever since then, **saccharin** tastes about 300 times sweeter than sucrose. In the 1970s, research indicated that very large doses of saccharin were associated with bladder cancer in laboratory animals. As a result, in 1977 the U.S. Food and Drug Administration (FDA) proposed banning saccharin from use in food. Widespread protests by consumer and industry groups, however, led Congress to impose a moratorium on the saccharin ban. Every few years, the moratorium was extended, and products containing saccharin had to display a warning label about saccharin and cancer risk in animals. In 2000, convincing evidence of safety led to saccharin's removal from the National Toxicology Program's list of potential cancer-causing agents,[59] and the U.S. Congress repealed the warning label requirement. In Canada, although saccharin is banned from food products, it can be purchased in pharmacies and carries a warning label.

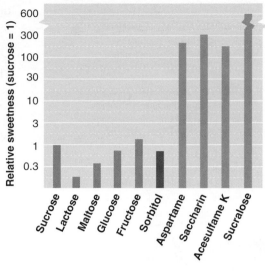

**Figure 5.13** **Comparing the sweetness of sweeteners.** Non-nutritive sweeteners are much sweeter than table sugar.

**Aspartame** The artificial sweetener **aspartame** is a combination of two amino acids, phenylalanine and aspartic acid. When digested and absorbed, it provides 4 kilocalories per gram. However, aspartame is so many times sweeter than sucrose that the amount used to sweeten foods contributes virtually zero calories to the diet, and it does not promote tooth decay. The FDA approved aspartame for use in some foods in 1981 and for use in soft drinks in 1983. More than 90 countries allow aspartame in products such as beverages, gelatin desserts, gums, and fruit spreads. Because heating destroys the sweetening power of aspartame, this sweetener cannot be used in products that require cooking.

Several safety concerns have been raised regarding aspartame. Some groups claim that aspartame could cause high blood levels of phenylalanine. In reality, high-protein foods, such as meats, contain much more phenylalanine than foods sweetened with aspartame. The amount of phenylalanine in aspartame-sweetened foods is not high enough to cause concern for most people. However, people with a genetic disease called **phenylketonuria (PKU)** cannot properly metabolize the amino acid phenylalanine, so they must carefully monitor their phenylalanine intake from all sources, including aspartame.

Although some people report headaches, dizziness, seizures, nausea, or allergic reactions with aspartame use, scientific studies have failed to confirm these effects, and most experts believe aspartame is safe for healthy people.[60] The FDA sets a maximum allowable daily intake of aspartame of 50 milligrams per kilogram of body weight.[61] This amount of aspartame equals the amount in sixteen 12-ounce diet soft drinks for adults and eight diet soft drinks for children.

**Acesulfame K** Marketed under the brand name Sunette, **acesulfame K** is about 200 times sweeter than table sugar. The FDA approved its use in the United States in 1988. Acesulfame K provides no energy, because the body cannot digest it. Food manufacturers use acesulfame K in chewing gum, powdered beverage mixes, nondairy creamers, gelatins, and puddings. Heat does not affect acesulfame K, so it can be used in cooking.

**Sucralose** Sold under the trade name Splenda, **sucralose** was approved for use in the United States in 1998 and has been used in Canada since 1992. Sucralose is made from sucrose, but the resulting compound is non-nutritive and about 600 times sweeter than sugar. Sucralose has been approved for use in a wide variety of products, including baked goods, beverages, gelatin

**saccharin [SAK-ah-ren]** An artificial sweetener that tastes about 300 to 700 times sweeter than sucrose. Neither digested nor absorbed, saccharin contributes no calories to the diet.

**aspartame [AH-spar-tame]** An artificial sweetener composed of two amino acids. It is 200 times sweeter than sucrose and sold by the trade name NutraSweet.

**phenylketonuria (PKU)** An inherited disorder that causes a lack of the enzyme that metabolizes phenylalanine.

**acesulfame K [ay-see-SUL-fame]** An artificial sweetener that is 200 times sweeter than common table sugar (sucrose). Because it is not digested and absorbed by the body, acesulfame contributes no calories to the diet and yields no energy when consumed.

**sucralose** An artificial sweetener made from sucrose. Sucralose is non-nutritive and about 600 times sweeter than sugar.

**D-tagatose** An artificial sweetener derived from lactose that has the same sweetness as sucrose with only half of the calories.

**trehalose** A disaccharide of two glucose molecules but with a linkage different from maltose. Used as a food additive and sweetener.

desserts, and frozen dairy desserts. It also can be used as a tabletop sweetener, with consumers adding it directly to food.

### Other Sweeteners

The FDA has accepted manufacturers' determinations that the sweet substances known as **D-tagatose** and **trehalose** are GRAS and can be added to foods. Small amounts of tagatose are found naturally in some dairy foods, and tagatose is derived from lactose. Although it has only 75 to 92 percent of the sweetness of sugar, tagatose is incompletely absorbed and provides only 1.5 kilocalories per gram. Trehalose, which is only half as sweet as sucrose, is found naturally in mushrooms, lobster, shrimp, and foods produced

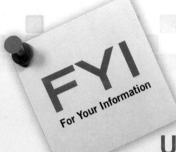

FYI
For Your Information

# Unfounded Claims Against Sugars

Sugar has become the vehicle used by some diet zealots to create a new soapbox. Cut sugar to trim fat! Bust sugar! Break the sugar habit! These battle cries demonize sugar as a dietary villain. But what are the facts?

### Sugar and Obesity

Many people believe that sugar is fattening and causes obesity. Sugar is a carbohydrate, and carbohydrates provide 4 kilocalories per gram. High intake of added sugar is associated with increased total energy intake and decreased nutrient intake.[1] Sugar-sweetened beverages, particularly soda, are associated with weight gain and obesity.[2] These beverages have low satiety, provide little nutritional benefit, and should be limited. Water, low-fat milk, and small quantities of fruit juice have greater nutritional value than sugary beverages.

High fat intakes are also associated with obesity.[3] Fat is a more concentrated source of energy and provides 9 kilocalories per gram. However, many foods high in sugar, such as doughnuts and cookies, are also high in fat. Excess energy intake from any source will cause obesity. The increased availability of low-fat and fat-free foods has not reduced obesity rates in the United States; in fact, the incidence of obesity is still climbing. Some speculate that consumers equate fat-free with calorie-free and eat more of these foods, not realizing that fat-free foods often have a higher sugar content, which makes any calorie savings negligible. Also, foods high in added sugars often have low nutrient value and become "extras" in the diet.

### Sugar and Heart Disease

Risk factors for heart disease include a genetic predisposition, smoking, high blood pressure, high blood cholesterol levels, diabetes, and obesity. Sugar by itself does not cause heart disease.[4] However, if intake of high-sugar foods contributes to obesity, then risk for heart disease increases. In addition, excessive intake of refined sugar can alter blood lipids in carbohydrate-sensitive people, increasing their risk for heart disease. However, a high fat intake is more likely to promote obesity than a high sugar intake. Thus, total fats, saturated fat, cholesterol, and obesity have a significantly more important relationship to heart disease than sugar.

### Sugar and Behavior

Parents continue to talk about kids "bouncing off the walls" at birthday parties because of "all that sugar." So, what's going on? Most likely, the event (e.g., a party, trick-or-treating for Halloween, a carnival) is enhancing kids' normal levels of excitement and enthusiasm. From a brain chemistry perspective, carbohydrates actually have a calming effect by increasing production of the sleep-inducing chemical serotonin! Well-controlled research studies have found no link between sugar and hyperactivity, so blame the excitement of the party, but not the sugar, for kids' "wild" behavior.[5]

In 1978, Dan White gunned down the mayor of San Francisco and blamed the act on his emotional state—created, he said, by eating too many Hostess Twinkies. This legal strategy

became known as the "Twinkie defense." Claims that sugar causes criminal behavior in adults are unfounded. Studies show no association between high sugar intake and aggressive behavior.[6]

1    Austin GL, Ogden LG, Hill JO. Trends in carbohydrate, fat, and protein intakes and association with energy intake in normal-weight, overweight, and obese individuals: 1971–2006. *Am J Clin Nutr.* 2011;93(4):836–843.

2    Mucci L, Santilli F, Cuccurullo C, Davi, G. Cardiovascular risk and dietary sugar intake: is the link so sweet? *Intern Emerg Med.* 2011 May 5.

3    Smilowitz JT, German JB, Zivkovic AM. *Food Intake and Obesity: The Case of Fat. Frontiers in Neuroscience.* Boca Raton, FL: CRC Press; 2010, Chapter 22.

4    World Health Organization. Carbohydrates in Human Nutrition: Report of a Joint FAO/WHO Expert Consultation, Rome, 1997. FAO Food and Nutrition Paper 66; 1997.

5    Benton D. Sucrose and behavioral problems. *Crit Rev Food Sci Nutr.* 2008;48(5):385–401.

6    White JW, Wolraich M. Effect of sugar on behavior and mental performance. *Am J Clin Nutr.* 1995;62:S242–S249; and Wolraich ML, Lindgren SD, Stumbo PJ, et al. Effects of diets high in sucrose or aspartame on the behavior and cognitive performance of children. *N Engl J Med.* 1994;330:301–307.

using baker's or brewer's yeast. It is made commercially from starch. In foods, trehalose is probably used more often for its textural properties than for its sweetness. Trehalose is absorbed completely and provides 4 kilocalories per gram but produces a lower glycemic response than glucose.[62]

**Neotame** was approved as a food additive in 2002. It can be used as a tabletop sweetener or added to foods. Neotame is a derivative of a dipeptide containing aspartic acid and phenylalanine—the same two amino acids that make up aspartame. However, chemical modifications to the structure make it 30 to 40 times sweeter than aspartame, or about 7,000 to 13,000 times sweeter than sucrose.

**Stevioside** (also known as **stevia**) is derived from the stevia plant found in South America. This plant's leaves have been used for centuries to sweeten beverages and make tea. In Japan, stevioside has been used as a sweetener since the 1970s. This substance is 300 times sweeter than sucrose, but its metabolism in the body has been incompletely investigated. Because the FDA has not approved stevioside as an additive nor accepted it as a GRAS substance, it cannot be used in food in the United States. Although stevia may be sold as a dietary supplement, its labels may not promote its use as a sweetener.

**Key Concepts** *Sweeteners add flavor to foods. Nutritive sweeteners provide energy, whereas non-nutritive sweeteners provide little or no energy. The body cannot tell the difference between sugars derived from natural and refined sources.*

## Carbohydrates and Health

Carbohydrates contribute both positively and negatively to health. On the upside, foods rich in fiber help keep the gastrointestinal tract healthy and may reduce the risk of heart disease and cancer. On the downside, excess sugar can contribute to weight gain, poor nutrient intake, and tooth decay. (See the FYI feature "Excessive Sugar in the American Diet.")

### Sugar and Dental Caries

High sugar intake contributes to **dental caries**, or cavities. (See **Figure 5.14.**) When bacteria in your mouth feed on sugars, they produce acids that eat away tooth enamel and dental structure, causing dental caries. Although these bacteria quickly metabolize sugars, they feed on any carbohydrate, including starch.

The longer a carbohydrate remains in the mouth, or the more frequently it is consumed, the more likely it is to promote dental caries. Foods that stick to your teeth, such as caramel, licorice, crackers, sugary cereals, and cookies, are more likely to cause dental caries than foods that are quickly washed out of your mouth. If you sip high-sugar beverages such as soft drinks over an extended period of time, you will be more likely to have problems with dental caries. A baby should never be put to bed with a bottle, because the warm milk or juice may remain in the mouth all night, providing a ready source of carbohydrate for bacteria to break down.

Snacking on high-sugar foods throughout the day provides a continuous supply of carbohydrates that nourish the bacteria in your mouth, promoting the formation of dental caries. Good dental hygiene, adequate fluoride, and a well-balanced diet for strong tooth formation can help prevent such cavities.[63]

### Fiber and Obesity

Foods rich in fiber usually are low in fat and energy. They offer a greater volume of food for fewer calories, take longer to eat, and are filling. Once eaten, foods high in dietary fiber take longer to leave the stomach and they attract water, adding to the feeling of fullness. Consider, for example, three apple

**neotame** An artificial sweetener similar to aspartame, but one that is sweeter and does not require a warning label for people with phenylketonuria.

**stevioside** A dietary supplement, not approved for use as a sweetener, that is extracted and refined from *Stevia rebaudiana* leaves.

**stevia** See *stevioside.*

**dental caries [KARE-ees]** Destruction of the enamel surface of teeth caused by acids resulting from bacterial breakdown of sugars in the mouth.

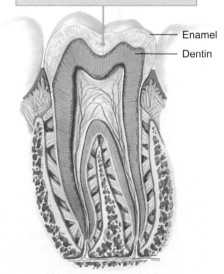

Bacteria feeding on sugar and other carbohydrates produce acids that eat away tooth enamel.

— Enamel
— Dentin

**Figure 5.14** **Dental health.** Good dental hygiene, adequate fluoride, and proper nutrition help maintain healthy teeth. A well-balanced diet contains vitamins and minerals crucial for healthy bones and teeth. To help prevent dental caries, avoid continuous snacking on high-sugar foods, especially those that stick to the teeth.

## Quick Bite

### Sugar Overload

Americans consume very large quantities of carbonated soft drinks each year. Soft drink manufacturers produce enough of the sweet beverage to provide 557 12-ounce cans to every man, woman, and child in the United States each year. That equals over 52 gallons of soft drink each year! Today, adults consume nearly twice as many ounces of sugar-sweetened sodas as milk. Children's milk consumption was more than three times that of their soda consumption in the late 1970s, but today children consume roughly equal amounts of each.

products with the same energy but different fiber content: a large apple (5 grams fiber), ½ cup of applesauce (2 grams fiber), and ¾ cup of apple juice (0.2 grams fiber). Most of us would find the whole apple more filling and satisfying than the applesauce or apple juice.

Studies show that people who consume more fiber weigh less than those who consume less fiber, suggesting that fiber intake has a role in weight control. Although research supports a role for dietary fiber in reducing hunger and promoting satiety, studies on specific types of fiber have produced inconsistent results.[64]

### Fiber and Type 2 Diabetes

People who consume plenty of dietary fiber, especially the fiber in whole grains and cereal, have a low incidence of type 2 diabetes.[65] Evidence suggests that intake of certain fibers may delay glucose uptake and smooth out the blood glucose response, thus providing a protective effect against diabetes.[66] Current dietary recommendations for people with type 2 diabetes advise a high intake of foods rich in dietary fiber.[67]

### Fiber and Cardiovascular Disease

High blood cholesterol levels increase the risk for heart disease. Dietary trials using high doses of oat bran, which is high in dietary fiber, show blood cholesterol reductions of 2 percent per gram of intake.[68] Because every 1 percent decrease in blood cholesterol levels decreases the risk of heart disease by 2 percent, high fiber intake can decrease the risk of heart disease substantially. Studies show a 20 to 40 percent difference in heart disease risk between the highest and lowest fiber-intake groups.[69]

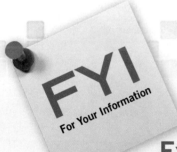

FYI
For Your Information

# Excessive Sugar in the American Diet

Foods high in sugar are popular in American diets. These empty-calorie foods (e.g., candy, caloric soft drinks, sweetened gelatin, some desserts) provide energy but contain little or no dietary fiber, vitamins, or minerals. Data from the 1999–2004 NHANES study indicate that the average American consumes 22.5 teaspoons of added sugars per day. American adults consume 21.6 teaspoons of added sugars per day, and children (ages 2–19) consume 24.9 teaspoons. Caloric sweetened sodas and fruit drinks (containing less than 100% juice by volume) are major sources of added sugars in American diets, contributing an average of 10.58 teaspoons of added sugars each day. Children consume 11.96 teaspoons of added sugars from sodas and fruit drinks per day (47% of their total intake of added sugars).[1]

Studies have linked the increasing prevalence of obesity in children to consumption of sugar-sweetened drinks.[2] Consider that one 12-ounce soft drink contains 10 to 12 teaspoons of sugar. Would you add that much sugar to a glass of iced tea?

People with high energy needs, such as active teenagers and young adults, can afford to get a bit more of their calories from high-sugar foods. People with low energy needs, such as some elderly or sedentary people or people trying to lose weight, cannot afford as many calories from high-sugar foods. Most people can include moderate amounts of sugar in their diet and still meet other nutrient needs. But, as the amount of added sugar in the diet increases, intake of vitamins and minerals tends to decrease.[3]

1    Smith T, Lin B-H, Lee J-Y. Taxing caloric sweetened beverages: potential effects on beverage consumption, calorie intake, and obesity. 2010. USDA Economic Research Report no. 100. http://www.ers.usda.gov/Publications/err100/err100.pdf. Accessed 5/13/11.

2    Evans AE, Springer AE, Evans MH, et al. A descriptive study of beverage consumption among an ethnically diverse sample of public school students in Texas. *J Am Coll Nutr.* 2010;29(4):387–396.

3    Smith T, Lin B-H, Lee J-Y. Op. cit.

Fiber from oat bran, legumes, and psyllium can lower blood cholesterol levels. Your body uses cholesterol to make bile, which is secreted into the intestinal tract to aid fat digestion. Most bile is reabsorbed and recycled. In the gastrointestinal tract, fiber can bind bile and reduce the amount available for reabsorption. With less reabsorbed bile, the body makes up the difference by removing cholesterol from the blood and making new bile. The short-chain fatty acids produced from bacterial breakdown of fiber in the large intestine also may prevent cholesterol formation.[70] Studies also show a relationship between high intake of whole grains and low risk of heart disease.[71] Whole grains contain fiber as well as antioxidants and other compounds that may protect against cellular damage that promotes heart disease. It is likely that the combination of compounds found in grains, rather than any one component, explains the protective effects against heart disease.[72] Consuming at least three 1-ounce servings of whole grains each day can reduce heart disease risk.[73]

## Fiber and Gastrointestinal Disorders

Eating plenty of dietary fiber, especially the types found in cereal grains, helps promote healthy gastrointestinal functioning. Diets rich in fiber add bulk and increase water in the stool, softening the stool and making it easier to pass. Fiber also accelerates passage of food through the intestinal tract, promoting regularity. If fluid intake is also ample, high fiber intake helps prevent and treat constipation, hemorrhoids (swelling of rectal veins), and diverticular disease (development of pouches on the intestinal wall).

## Negative Health Effects of Excess Fiber

Despite its health advantages, high fiber intake can cause problems, especially for people who drastically increase their fiber intake in a short period of time. If you increase your fiber intake, you also need to increase your water intake to prevent the stool from becoming hard and impacted. A sudden increase in fiber intake also can cause increased intestinal gas and bloating. You can prevent these problems both by increasing fiber intake gradually over several weeks and by drinking plenty of fluids.

Just as fiber binds cholesterol, it also can bind small amounts of minerals in the GI tract and prevent them from being absorbed. Fiber binds the minerals zinc, calcium, and iron. For people who get enough of these minerals, however, the recommended amounts of dietary fiber do not affect mineral status significantly.[74]

Some people, such as young children and the elderly who eat high-fiber diets, may feel full before meeting energy and nutrient needs. Because of a limited stomach capacity, they must be careful that fiber intake does not interfere with their ability to consume adequate energy and nutrients.

Due to the bulky nature of fibers, excess consumption is likely to be self-limiting. Although a high fiber intake may cause occasional adverse gastro-intestinal symptoms, serious chronic adverse effects have not been observed. As part of an overall healthy diet, a high intake of fiber will not produce significant deleterious effects in healthy people. Therefore, a Tolerable Upper Intake Level (UL) is not set for fiber.

**Key Concepts** *High sugar intake promotes dental caries and can contribute to nutrient deficiencies by replacing other more nutritious foods in the diet. High intake of foods rich in dietary fiber offers many health benefits, including reduced risk of obesity, type 2 diabetes, cardiovascular disease, and gastrointestinal disorders. Increase fiber intake gradually while drinking plenty of fluids; children and the elderly with small appetites should take care that energy needs are still met. The DRIs do not set a UL for fiber.*

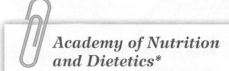

*Academy of Nutrition and Dietetics\**

**Health Implications of Dietary Fiber**
It is the position of the American Dietetic Association that the public should consume adequate amounts of dietary fiber from a variety of plant foods.

**Source:** Reproduced from Slavin JL. Position of the Academy of Nutrition and Dietetics: health implications of dietary fiber. *J Am Diet Assoc.* 2008;108(10):1716–1731.

\* Formerly the American Dietetic Association

*Quick* Bite

**Fierce Fiber and Flatulence**
The Jerusalem artichoke surpasses even dry beans in its capacity for facilitating flatulence. This artichoke contains large amounts of nondigestible carbohydrate. After passing through the small intestine undigested, the fiber is attacked by gas-generating bacteria in the colon.

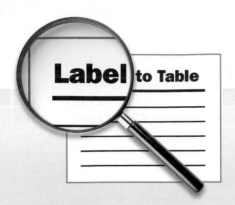

This label highlights all the carbohydrate-related information you can find on a food label. Look at the center of the Nutrition Facts label and you'll see the Total Carbohydrates along with two of the carbohydrate "subgroups"—Dietary Fiber and Sugars. Recall that carbohydrates are classified into simple carbohydrates and the two complex carbohydrates starch and fiber.

Using this food label, you can determine all three of these components. There are 19 total grams of carbohydrate, with 14 grams coming from sugars and 0 grams from fiber. This means the remaining 5 grams must be from starch, which is not required to be listed separately on the label. Without even knowing what food this label represents, you can decipher that it contains a high proportion of sugar (14 of the 19 grams) and is probably sweet. If this is a fruit juice, that level of sugar would be expected; but, if this is cereal, you'd be getting a lot more sugar than complex carbohydrates and probably wouldn't be making the best choice!

Do you see the "6%" listed to the right of "Total Carbohydrate"? This doesn't mean that the food item contains 6 percent of its calories from carbohydrate. Instead, it refers to the Daily Value for carbohydrates listed at the bottom of the la-bel. There you can see that a person consuming 2,000 kilocalories per day should consume 300 grams of carbohydrates each day. This product contributes 19 grams per serving, which is just 6 percent of the Daily Value of 300 grams per day. Note that the Percent Daily Value for fiber is "0%" because this food item lacks fiber.

The last highlighted section on this label, at the bottom of some Nutrition Facts labels, is the number of calories in a gram of carbohydrate. Recall that carbohydrates contain 4 kilocalories per gram. Armed with this information and the product's calorie information, can you calculate the percentage of calories that come from carbohydrate?

Here's how:

**19 g carbohydrate × 4 kcal per g**

**= 76 carbohydrate kcal**

**76 carbohydrate kcal ÷ 154 total kcal**

**= 0.49, or 49 percent carbohydrate kcal**

## Nutrition Facts

Serving Size: 1 cup (248g)
Servings Per Container: 4

**Amount Per Serving**

**Calories** 154 Calories from fat 35

| | % Daily Value* |
|---|---|
| **Total Fat** 4g | |
| Saturated Fat 2.5g | 6% |
| Trans Fat 0.5g | 12% |
| **Cholesterol** 20mg | |
| **Sodium** 170mg | 7% |
| **Total Carbohydrate** 19g | 7% |
| Dietary Fiber 0g | 6% |
| Sugars 14g | 0% |
| **Protein** 11g | |

| | | |
|---|---|---|
| Vitamin A 4% | • | Vitamin C 6% |
| Calcium 40% | • | Iron 0% |

* Percent Daily Values are based on a 2,000 calorie diet. Your daily values may be higher or lower depending on your calorie needs:

| | | Calories: | 2,000 | 2,500 |
|---|---|---|---|---|
| Total Fat | Less Than | | 65g | 80g |
| Sat Fat | Less Than | | 20g | 25g |
| Cholesterol | Less Than | | 300mg | 300mg |
| Sodium | Less Than | | 2,400mg | 2,400mg |
| Total Carbohydrate | | | 300g | 375g |
| Dietary Fiber | | | 25g | 30g |

Calories per gram:
Fat 9 • Carbohydrate 4 • Protein 4

# Learning Portfolio

## Key Terms

## Study Points

- Carbohydrates include the simple sugars and complex carbohydrates.
- Monosaccharides are the building blocks of carbohydrates.
- Three monosaccharides are important in human nutrition: glucose, fructose, and galactose.
- The monosaccharides combine to make disaccharides: sucrose, lactose, and maltose.
- Starch, glycogen, and fiber are long chains (polysaccharides) of monosaccharide units; starch and glycogen contain only glucose.

- Carbohydrates are digested by enzymes from the mouth, pancreas, and small intestine and absorbed as monosaccharides.
- The liver converts the monosaccharides fructose and galactose to glucose.
- Blood glucose levels rise after eating and fall between meals. Two pancreatic hormones, insulin and glucagon, regulate blood glucose levels, preventing extremely high or low levels.
- In diabetes, insulin either is not produced or is ineffective, resulting in hyperglycemia. Diabetes is treated with diet, exercise, and medication, including insulin injections in some cases.
- Hypoglycemia results when blood glucose levels fall too low.
- The main function of carbohydrates in the body is to supply energy. In this role, carbohydrates spare protein for use in making body proteins and allow for the complete breakdown of fat as an additional energy source.
- Carbohydrates are found mainly in plant foods as starch, fiber, and sugar.
- In general, Americans consume more sugar and less starch and fiber than is recommended.
- Carbohydrate intake can affect health. Excess sugar can contribute to low nutrient intake, excess energy intake, and dental caries.
- Diets high in complex carbohydrates, including fiber, have been linked to reduced risk for GI disorders, heart disease, and cancer.

## Study Questions

1. What are the differences between a monosaccharide, disaccharide, and polysaccharide?
2. What advantage does the branched-chain structure of glycogen provide compared to a straight chain of glucose?
3. Describe the difference between starch and fiber.
4. Which blood glucose regulation hormone is secreted in the fed state? The fasting state?
5. Which foods contain carbohydrates?
6. What are the most common non-nutritive sweeteners used in the United States?
7. How will eating excessive amounts of added sugars affect health?
8. List the benefits of eating more fiber. What are the consequences of eating too much? Too little?

## Try This

### Banana Basics

Purchase one banana that is covered with brown spots (if necessary, let it sit on the counter for several days). Purchase another banana with a yellow skin, possibly with a greenish tinge, and no brown spots. Note that this may require two trips to the market.

Now it's time for the taste test. Mash each banana separately so both have the same consistency and texture. Taste each one. Which is sweeter?

As ripening begins, starch is converted to sugar. As fruit continues to ripen, sugar content increases. The sugar content of ripe, spotted bananas is higher than that of a green banana—by 20 percent or more!

### The Sweetness of Soda

This experiment is to help you understand the amount of sugar found in a can of soda. Take a glass and fill it with 12 ounces (1½ cups) of water. Using a measuring spoon, add 10 to 12 teaspoons of sugar to the water. Stir the sugar water until all the sucrose has dissolved. Now sip the water. Does it taste sweet? It shouldn't taste any sweeter than a can of regular soda. This is the amount of sugar found in one 12-ounce can!

## What About Bobbie?

Let's examine Bobbie's day of eating (see the "Food Choices: Nutrients and Nourishment" chapter) using the guidelines you've learned in this chapter. How well did Bobbie do? Did she consume 45 to 65 percent of her calories from carbohydrates? Was her diet made up mostly of complex carbohydrates or simple sugars? Let's take a look.

Her overall carbohydrate intake was 292 grams, or 1,168 kilocalories. Her total energy intake was 2,300 kilocalories, which means 51 percent of her calories were from carbohydrates. This is within the Acceptable Macronutrient Distribution Range (AMDR) for carbohydrate. Here are the biggest contributors, which supply more than 80 percent of Bobbie's carbohydrate intake:

| Food | Carbohydrate (g) | Percentage of Calorie Intake |
|---|---|---|
| Spaghetti | 60 | 10 |
| Bread (lunch and dinner) | 53 | 9 |
| Bagel | 39 | 7 |
| Banana | 27 | 5 |
| Tortilla chips | 27 | 5 |
| Pizza | 24 | 4 |
| Spaghetti sauce | 10 | 1.7 |
| Cookie | 9 | 1.5 |

Review the list of Bobbie's foods again. Do you think her carbohydrate intake comes mostly from complex sources or simple sugars? Very few of her carbohydrate sources are high in sugars—just the banana, the sugar for the coffee, and the chocolate chip cookie.

Let's take a closer look at Bobbie's food sources of carbohydrates. Which food groups contribute the most to her carbohydrate intake? To answer this, let's divide her carbohydrate-dense foods into the three carbohydrate-rich food groups.

| Food Group | Amount | |
|---|---|---|
| | Bobbie's | Recommended[a] |
| **Grains Group** | | |
| Bagel | 2 | |
| Bread (lunch) | 2 | |
| Bread (dinner) | 1 | |
| Tortilla chips | 2 | |
| Pasta | 3 | |
| Pizza | 1 | |
| Total | 11 oz-eq | 7 oz-eq (3.5 whole grain) |
| **Fruit Group** | | |
| Banana | 1 cup | |
| Total | 1 cup | 2 cups |
| **Vegetable Group** | | |
| Lettuce | 1 cup | |
| Sandwich and salad toppings | ½ cup | |
| Salsa | ½ cup | |
| Green beans | ½ cup | |
| Total | 2½ cups | 3 cups |

[a] Based on MyPlate recommendations.

So, now that you've reviewed Bobbie's food group totals, what can you conclude about her carbohydrate intake? Her total carbohydrate calories are within the recommended range, but her diet could use some improvement. Bobbie has plenty of servings for grains, but no whole grains. She is low in fruits, and her vegetable choices could be a little more varied. Adding a half a cup of orange juice for breakfast and another piece of fresh fruit during the day would help. Choosing spinach or romaine lettuce for her salad would broaden her vegetable choices, and a whole-wheat bagel instead of cinnamon raisin would be a good start for adding more whole grains.

## References

1   Biesiekierski JR, Rosella O, Rose R, et al. Quantification of fructans, galacto-oligosacharides and other short-chain carbohydrates in processed grains and cereals. *J Hum Nutr Diet*. 2011;24(2):154–176.

2   Ninonuevo MR, Perkins PD, Francis J, et al. Daily variations in oligosaccharides of human milk determined by microfluidic chips and mass spectrometry. *J Agric Food Chem*. 2008;56(2):618–626.

3   Lacomba R, Salcedo J, Alegría A, et al. Effect of simulated gastrointestinal digestion on sialic acid and gangliosides present in human milk and infant formulas. *J Agric Food Chem*. 2011;59(10):5755–5762.

4   Eliasson AC. *Carbohydrates in Food*. New York: Marcel Dekker; 1996; and GMO Compass. Amylose, amylopectin (starch). http://www.gmo-compass.org/eng/glossary/104.amylose-amylopectin-starch.html. Accessed 5/15/11.

5   Institute of Medicine, Food and Nutrition Board. *Dietary Reference Intakes for Energy, Carbohydrate, Fiber, Fat, Fatty Acids, Cholesterol, Protein, and Amino Acids.* Washington, DC: National Academies Press; 2002.

6   Murphy M, Spungen Douglass J, Birkett A. Resistant starch intakes in the United States. *J Am Diet Assoc.* 2008;108(1):67–78.

7   Meat processing. *Encyclopedia Britannica* [online]. http://www.britannica.com/eb/article?eu5120856. Accessed 5/13/11.

8   Décombaz J, Jentjens R, Ith M, et al. Fructose and galactose enhance post-exercise human liver glycogen synthesis. *Med Sci Sports Exerc.* 2011;43(10):1964–1971; and Rapoport B. Metabolic factors limiting performance in marathon runners. *PLoS Comput Biol.* 2010;6(10). doi: 10.1371/journal.pcbi.1000960. Accessed 5/12/11.

9   Rapoport B. Ibid.

10  Kerksick C, Harvey T, Stout J, et al. International Society of Sports Nutrition position stand: nutrient timing. *J Int Soc Sports Nutr.* 2008;5:17; and Sedlock DA, the latest on carbohydrate loading: a practical approach. *Current Sports Medicine Reports.* 2008;7(4):209–213.

11  Schisti C, Richter A, Blandr A, Richt A. Hemicellulose concentration and composition in plant cell walls under extreme carbon source-sink imbalances. *Physiologia Plantarum.* 2010;139(3):241–255.

12  Sarubin Fragakis A. *The Health Professional's Guide to Popular Dietary Supplements.* 3rd ed. Chicago: Academy of Nutrition and Dietetics; 2007.

13  Grabitske H, Slavin J. Low-digestible carbohydrates in practice. *J Am Diet Assoc.* 2008;108(10):1677–1681.

14  Ibid.

15  Martini FH. *Fundamentals of Anatomy and Physiology.* 8th ed. San Francisco. Benjamin Cummings; 2008.

16  Ibid.

17  Ibid.

18  Ibid.

19  Position of the Academy of Nutrition and Dietetics: weight management. *J Am Diet Assoc.* 2009;109(2):330–346.

20  Ibid.

21  Franz MJ, Powers MA, Leontos C, et al. The evidence for medical nutrition therapy for type 1 and type 2 diabetes in adults. *J Am Diet Assoc.* 2010;110(12):1852–1889.

22  Institute of Medicine, Food and Nutrition Board. Op cit.

23  Jenkins DJA, Kendall CWC, Augustin LSA, et al. Glycemic index: overview of implications in health and disease. *Am J Clin Nutr.* 2002;76(suppl):266S–273S.

24  National Diabetes Information Clearinghouse. National Diabetes Statistics, 2007. NIH Publication No. 08-3892. June, 2008. http://diabetes.niddk.nih.gov/dm/pubs/statistics/index.htm. Accessed 5/14/11.

25  Academy of Nutrition and Dietetics. Diabetes statistics. http://www.diabetes.org/diabetes-basics/diabetes-statistics. Accessed 5/17/11.

26  Ibid.

27  Gropper SS, Smith JL, Groff JL. *Advanced Nutrition and Human Metabolism.* 5th ed. Belmont, CA: Wadsworth; 2009.

28  National Institute of Diabetes and Digestive and Kidney Diseases. National diabetes statistics, 2011. http://diabetes.niddk.nih.gov/DM/PUBS/statistics/index.htm. Accessed 5/17/11.

29  Ibid.

30  National Institute of Diabetes and Digestive and Kidney Diseases, 2011. Op. cit.

31  Ibid.

32  Ibid.

33  Ibid.

34  Ibid.

35  Ibid.

36  American Diabetes Association. Diagnosis and classification of diabetes mellitus. *Diabetes Care.* 2007;30(suppl 1):S42–S47.

37  National Institute of Diabetes and Digestive and Kidney Diseases, 2011. Op. cit.

38  American Diabetes Association. Genetics of diabetes. http://www.diabetes.org/diabetes-basics/genetics-of-diabetes.html. Accessed 5/17/11.

39  Ibid.

40  Ibid.

41  Diabetes Prevention Program Research Group. Reduction in the incidence of type 2 diabetes with lifestyle intervention or metformin. *N Engl J Med.* 2002;346:393–403.

42  Church T. Exercise in obesity, metabolic syndrome, and diabetes. *Prog Cardiovasc Dis.* 2011;53(6):412–418.

43  National Diabetes Information Clearinghouse. Diabetes overview. http://diabetes.niddk.nih.gov/dm/pubs/overview. Accessed 5/17/11.

44  Institute of Medicine, Food and Nutrition Board. Op. cit.

45  US Department of Agriculture, US Department of Health and Human Services. *Dietary Guidelines for Americans, 2010.* 7th ed. Washington, DC: US Government Printing Office; December 2010.

46  Ibid.

47  Institute of Medicine, Food and Nutrition Board. Op. cit.

48  Report of the Dietary Guidelines Advisory Committee on the *Dietary Guidelines for Americans, 2010.* Part D, Section 5: Carbohydrates. http://www.cnpp.usda.gov/Publications/DietaryGuidelines/2010/DGAC/Report/D-5-Carbohydrates.pdf. Accessed 5/12/11.

49  Report of the Dietary Guidelines Advisory Committee on the *Dietary Guidelines for Americans, 2010.* http://www.cnpp.usda.gov/dgas2010-dgacreport.htm. Accessed 5/12/11.

50  Nayga RM. Childhood obesity and unhappiness: the influence of soft drinks and fast food consumption. *Journal of Happiness Studies.* 2010;11(3):261–275.

51  Marriott BP, Olsho L, Hadden L, Connor P. Intake of added sugars and selected nutrients in the United States, National Health and Nutrition Examination Survey (NHANES) 2003–2006. *Cr Rev Food Sci Nutr.* 2010;50:228–258.

52  Report of the Dietary Guidelines Advisory Committee on the *Dietary Guidelines for Americans, 2010.* Part D, Section 5: Carbohydrates. Op. cit.

53  Marriott BP, et al. Op. cit.

54  Report of the Dietary Guidelines Advisory Committee on the *Dietary Guidelines for Americans, 2010.* Part D, Section 5: Carbohydrates. Op. cit.

55  Coulston AM, Johnson RK. Sugar and sugars: myths and realities. *J Am Diet Assoc.* 2002;102:351–353.

56  White J, Foreyt J, Elanson K, Angelopoulos T. High-fructose corn syrup: controversies and common sense. *Am J Lifestyle Med.* 2010;4(6):515–520.

57  Bray GA. Fructose: pure, white, and deadly? Fructose, by any other name, is a health hazard. *J Diabetes Sci Technol.* 2010;4(4):1003–1007.

58  Position of the Academy of Nutrition and Dietetics: use of nutritive and non-nutritive sweeteners. *J Am Diet Assoc.* 2004;104(2):255–275.

59  US Department of Health and Human Services. National Toxicology Program. *Report on Carcinogens, Appendx B: Agents, Substances, Mixtures or Exposure Circumstances Delisted from Report on Carcinogens.* 11th ed. January 31, 2005. http://ntp.niehs.nih.gov/roc/eleventh/append/appb.pdf. Accessed 5/12/11.

60  Whitehouse C, Boullata J, McCauley LA. The potential toxicity of artificial sweeteners. *AAOHN J.* 2008;56(6):251–259.

61  Academy of Nutrition and Dietetics, 2004. Op. cit.

62  Ibid.

63  US Department of Agriculture, US Department of Health and Human Services. Op. cit.

64  Slavin JL. Position of the Academy of Nutrition and Dietetics: health implications of dietary fiber. *J Am Diet Assoc.* 2008;108(10):1716–1731.

65  Ibid.

66  Ibid.

67  American Diabetes Association, 2007. Op. cit.

68  Institute of Medicine, Food and Nutrition Board. Op. cit.

69  Ibid.

70  Wong JM, de Souza R, Kendall CW, et al. Colonic health: fermentation and short chain fatty acids. *J Clin Gastroenterol.* 2006;40(3)235–243.

71  Maki KC, Beiseigel JM, Jonnalagadda SS, et al. Whole-grain ready-to-eat oat cereal, as part of a dietary program for weight loss, reduces low-density lipoprotein cholesterol in adults with overweight and obesity more than a dietary program including low-fiber control foods. *J Am Diet Assoc.* 2010;110(2):205–214.

72  Slavin JL. Op. cit.

73  Ibid.

74  Institute of Medicine, Food and Nutrition Board. Op. cit.

# Spotlight on Alcohol

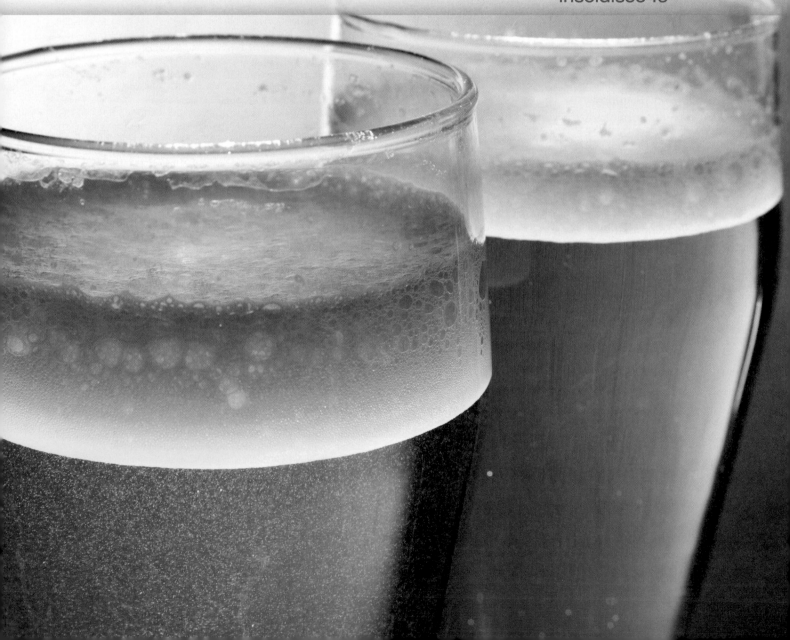

**THiNK About It**

1   In a word or two, how would you describe alcohol? Is it a nutrient?

2   What's your impression of the alcohol content of wine compared with that of beer? How about compared with vodka?

3   Have you ever thought of alcohol as a poison?

4   After a night of drinking and carousing, your friend awakens with a splitting headache and asks you for a pain reliever. What would you recommend?

**Visit go.jblearning.com/inseldisco4e**

Think about alcohol. What image comes to mind: Champagne toasts? Elegant gourmet dining? Hearty family meals in the European countryside? Or, do you think of wild parties? Sick, out-of-control drunks? Violence? Car accidents? Broken homes? No other food or beverage has the power to elicit such strong, disparate images—images that reflect both the healthfulness of alcohol in moderation, the devastation of excess, and the political, social, and moral issues surrounding alcohol.

Alcohol has a long and checkered history. More drug than food, alcoholic beverages produce druglike effects in the body while providing little, if any, nutrient value other than energy. Yet it is still important to consider alcohol in the study of nutrition. Alcohol is common to the diets of many people. In moderation, it may impart significant health benefits, yet even small quantities can raise risks for birth defects and breast cancer. In large amounts, it interferes with our intake of nutrients as well as the body's ability to use them, and it causes significant damage to every organ system in the body. The *Dietary Guidelines for Americans* advises, "If alcohol is consumed, it should be consumed in moderation—up to one drink per day for women and two drinks per day for men—and only by adults of legal drinking age."[1]

For most people, alcohol consumption is a pleasant social activity. Moderate alcohol use does not harm most adults. Nonetheless, many people have serious trouble with drinking. Episodes of heavy drinking are common among adult populations and are on the rise.[2] Adult excessive drinkers and underage drinkers account for half of all alcohol consumption and half of consumer spending on alcohol.[3] Heavy drinking can increase the risk for certain cancers. It can also cause liver cirrhosis, brain damage, and harm to the fetus during pregnancy. In addition, drinking increases the number of deaths from automobile crashes, recreational accidents, on-the-job accidents, homicide, and suicide. A recent analysis found that alcohol use is the third leading actual cause of death in the United States after (1) tobacco use and (2) poor diet and/or inactivity.[4]

Many young people are experiencing the consequences of drinking too much, at too early an age. Underage alcohol use is more likely to kill young people than all illegal drugs combined,[5] and it is a serious public health problem. A recent analysis found that the leading causes of death for those ages 12 to 19 years are accidents (unintentional injuries), homicide, and suicide.[6] In adolescents, alcohol is the leading contributor to accidents and injury deaths.[7]

## History of Alcohol Use

Alcohol has had a prominent role throughout history. Old religious and medical writings frequently recommend its use, although with warnings for moderation. Thanks to alcohol's antiseptic properties, fermented drinks were safer than water during the centuries before modern sanitation, especially as people moved to towns and villages where water supplies were contaminated. Even mixing alcohol with dirty water afforded some protection from bacteria.[8]

At a time when life was filled with physical and emotional hardships, people valued alcohol for its analgesic and euphoric qualities. People relied on it to lift spirits, ease boredom, numb hunger, and dull the discomfort, even pain, of daily routine. Before the twentieth century, it was one of the few painkillers available in the Western world.

In sharp contrast to what is allowed today, drinking was often encouraged at the work site. Workers might be given alcohol as an inducement to do boring, painful, or dangerous jobs. Distilled spirits, beer, and wine accompanied

*Quick* **Bite**

**Preferred Beverages**
Beer is the national beverage of Germany and Britain. Wine is the national beverage of Greece and Italy.

*Quick* **Bite**

**Nutrients in Beer?**
Most of the carbohydrate used in the production of alcohol is converted to ethanol. In beer, however, some carbohydrate remains, along with a little protein and some vitamins. So although it is technically correct to say there are nutrients in beer, the amounts are small when beer is consumed at recommended low levels.

**alcohol** Common name for ethanol or ethyl alcohol. As a general term, it refers to any organic compound with one or more hydroxyl (–OH) groups.

**ethanol** Chemical name for drinking alcohol. Also known as ethyl alcohol.

**ethyl alcohol** See *ethanol*.

**methanol** The simplest alcohol. Also known as methyl alcohol and wood alcohol.

**methyl alcohol** See *methanol*.

**wood alcohol** Common name for methanol.

**fermentation** The anaerobic conversion of various carbohydrates to carbon dioxide and an alcohol or organic acid.

**Methanol**
(wood alcohol)

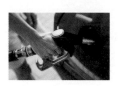

Methanol is an alcohol used as an alternative car fuel and in paint strippers, duplicator fluid, and model airplane fuels.

**Ethanol**
(EtOH)

Ethanol is the alcohol in beer, wine, and liquor.

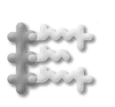

**Glycerol**

Glycerol is the alcohol that forms the backbone of triglyceride molecules.

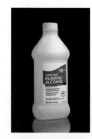

**Isopropanol**
(rubbing alcohol)

Isopropanol is an alcohol that is used as a disinfectant or solvent, and in making many commercial products.

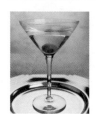

**Figure SA.1** **Alcohols.** Ethanol is not the only alcohol people consume. When people eat fat, they consume the alcohol glycerol. Consuming the alcohol methanol or isopropanol can be deadly.

sailors and passengers on all long voyages, supplying relatively pathogen-free fluid and calories. Legend has it that even the Puritans, a group known for rigid morality, disembarked at Plymouth Rock because their beer supply was depleted.[9]

## The Character of Alcohol

Although there are many types of alcohol, the term **alcohol** commonly refers to the specific alcohol compound in beer, wine, and spirits. (See **Figure SA.1**.) Its technical name is **ethanol**, or **ethyl alcohol**. Ethanol is commonly abbreviated to "EtOH," shorthand often preferred by health professionals. In this chapter, when we use the term *alcohol*, we are referring to ethanol.

Other types of alcohol are unsafe to drink. The simplest alcohol is **methanol**, also called **methyl alcohol** or **wood alcohol**, a solvent used in paints and for woodworking. Some years ago, down-on-their-luck alcoholics thought they had discovered a way to save money—wood alcohol, used at that time to heat chafing dishes, was intoxicating but considerably cheaper than beer or wine. Unfortunately, methanol caused blindness and death. Methanol is no longer used in these products, but methanol poisoning from other sources still occurs.[10] Today, methanol is used in a number of consumer products, including paint strippers, duplicator fluid, model airplane fuel, and dry gas. Most windshield washer fluids are 50 percent methanol.

## Alcohol: Is It a Nutrient?

Alcohol eludes easy classification. Like fat, protein, and carbohydrate, it provides energy when metabolized. Laboratory experiments in the nineteenth century demonstrated that upon oxidation pure alcohol releases 7 kilocalories per gram, but many people doubted it actually produced energy in the body. These doubts were the basis of the controversial conclusion that alcohol was not food—a conclusion used by early Prohibitionists in their fight against alcohol. (See **Figure SA.2**.) However, a classic series of experiments by energy researchers Francis Atwater and Wilbur Benedict showed that alcohol did indeed produce 7 kilocalories per gram in the body—findings that were a great disappointment to the Temperance Movement, because they showed that alcohol was a food.[11]

But alcohol's status as a nutrient is more questionable. It is certainly different from any other substance in the diet. It provides energy but is not essential, performing no necessary function in the body. Unlike the nutrients, alcohol is not stored in the body. And for no nutrient are the dangers of overconsumption so dramatic and the window of safety so narrow. In the small amounts most people usually consume, alcohol acts as a drug, producing a pleasant euphoria. For some people, it is addictive, with the characteristics of tolerance, dependence, and withdrawal symptoms. Certainly, alcohol is a substance available in the diet, but it does not meet the technical definition of a nutrient.

THINK
About It
1

**Key Concepts** *Alcohol, or more specifically, the compound ethyl alcohol, has been part of people's diets for thousands of years. Although it provides calories, alcohol performs no essential function in the body and, therefore, is not a nutrient.*

## Alcohol and Its Sources

When yeast cells metabolize sugar, they produce alcohol and carbon dioxide by a process called **fermentation**. If little oxygen is present, these cells produce more alcohol and less carbon dioxide. **Figure SA.3** shows living yeast cells.

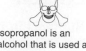
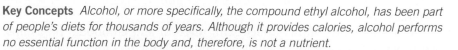

Fermentation can occur spontaneously in nature—all that's needed is sugar, water, a warm environment, and yeast (whose spores are present in air and soil). Human experience with alcohol probably began at least 10,000 years ago with spontaneously fermented fruits or honey. Because all humans possess the enzymes to metabolize at least minimal amounts of alcohol,[12] it's reasonable to assume that humans have always had small quantities of alcohol in their diets. Very small amounts of alcohol are even produced by the microorganisms in our intestines.

Humans probably learned to make wine from fruits, mead from honey, and beer from grain about 5,000 years ago. In some areas, people made alcohol-containing dairy products. Using simple yeast fermentation, they could not produce beverages with alcohol levels exceeding 16 percent—the point at which alcohol kills off the yeast, halting alcohol production. Later, seventh-century Egyptian chemists discovered how to use distillation to capture concentrated alcohol, which could be added to drinks to boost alcohol content. Distilled alcoholic beverages (such as rum, gin, and whiskey) are called spirits, liquor, or hard liquor.

## Quick Bite

**First Wine?**
Wine residue has been found on pottery shards that date back to about 3,000 B.C.E. They came from the ancient village of Godin Tepe in the Zagros Mountains of western Iran.

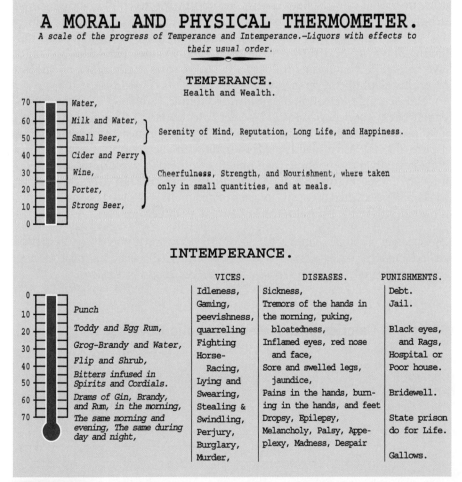

**Figure SA.2** **A moral and physical thermometer of temperance and intemperance.** As part of a late eighteenth century temperance movement, Philadelphian Dr. Benjamin Rush (1745–1813) created the *Moral and Physical Thermometer* and distributed it to the clergy in a campaign against heavy drinking.

**Source:** Reprinted with permission from *Quarterly Journal of Studies on Alcohol*, vol 4, pp. 321–341, 1943 (presently *Journal of Studies on Alcohol*). Copyright Alcohol Research Documentation, Inc., Rutgers Center of Alcohol Studies, Piscataway, NJ 08854.

## Quick Bite

**Energy Drinks + Alcohol = A Recipe for Trouble**
Think twice before mixing energy drinks with alcohol. These drinks not only increase the risk of alcohol toxicity, but they also increase the risk of serious injury, sexual assault, drunk driving, heart rhythm problems, nervous system problems, impaired judgment, shortness of breath, dizziness, disorientation, and rapid heartbeat.

**congeners** Biologically active compounds in alcoholic beverages that include nonalcoholic ingredients as well as other alcohols such as methanol. Congeners contribute to the distinctive taste and smell of the beverage and may increase intoxicating effects and subsequent hangover.

**standard drink** One serving of alcohol (about 15 grams) is equal to 12 ounces of beer, 4 to 5 ounces of wine, or 1.5 ounces of liquor.

**binge drinking** Consuming excessive amounts of alcohol in short periods of time.

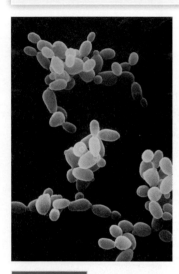

| Figure SA.3 | **A micrograph of yeast.** |

Distillation can yield more than just ethanol. Traces of other compounds, such as methanol, evaporate and then condense in the distilled product. Called **congeners**, these biologically active compounds help to create the distinctive taste, smell, and appearance of alcoholic beverages such as whiskey, brandy, and red wine. But congeners are also suspected of causing or contributing to hangovers[13] and may play a role in alcohol's relationship to cancer.

THINK
About It

2

Beer, wine, and liquor have different alcohol levels: Most beer is up to 5 percent alcohol, although some beers exceed 6 percent; wine is 8 to 14 percent alcohol; and hard liquor is typically 35 to 45 percent alcohol. Beer and wine are labeled with the percentage of alcohol, but hard liquor is labeled by "proof," which is twice the alcohol percentage (an 80 proof whiskey is 40 percent alcohol).

Pure alcohol—a clear, colorless liquid used in chemistry labs—is 95 percent alcohol. (Even "pure" alcohol contains some water.) The beverage closest to pure alcohol is vodka, which is alcohol, water, and almost nothing else; gin is similar but flavored with juniper berries. Scotch, rum, rye, whiskey, and other liquors have residual flavor traces of the grain from which they were fermented or flavors introduced during storage. All liquors, however, offer little nutritional value besides energy. Beer and wine do contain unfermented carbohydrates and a trace of protein but, like liquor, have negligible minerals. With the exception of niacin in beer (a 12-ounce beer contains 1.8 milligrams of niacin, nearly 10 percent of the Daily Value), alcoholic beverages have negligible vitamins as well. Table SA.1 shows the number of calories in various alcoholic beverages.

One serving of alcohol, or a **standard drink**, is defined as 12 ounces of regular beer, 5 ounces of wine (12 percent alcohol), or 1.5 ounces (a "jigger") of 80 proof liquor.[14] All contain roughly 15 grams (1 measuring tablespoon) of pure alcohol. Most health professionals who speak of "moderate alcohol intake" usually mean no more than one (for women) or two (for men) servings in a day.[15] (See **Figure SA.4**.) Moderate intake is not an average of seven drinks per week when there are six days of abstinence followed by seven drinks in one night! That's **binge drinking**, and it's dangerous.

**Key Concepts** *Alcohol is formed when yeast ferments sugars to yield energy. Distillation methods produce concentrated solutions, containing up to 95 percent alcohol. A typical serving of beer, wine, or distilled spirits contains about 15 grams of alcohol.*

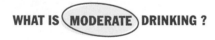

WHAT IS MODERATE DRINKING?

*Women:*
No more than **1** drink a day

*Men:*
No more than **2** drinks a day

COUNT AS A DRINK...

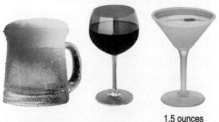

12 ounces of regular beer

5 ounces of wine

1.5 ounces of 80-proof distilled spirits

| Figure SA.4 | **Moderate drinking.** |

**Source:** USDA Center for Nutrition Policy and Promotion.

## Table SA.1    Calories in Selected Alcoholic Beverages

| Beverage | Serving Size | Approximate Kcalories |
|---|---|---|
| Beer (regular) | 12 fl oz | 153 |
| Beer (light) | 12 fl oz | 103 |
| White wine | 5 fl oz | 121 |
| Red wine | 5 fl oz | 125 |
| Sweet dessert wine | 3.5 fl oz | 165 |
| 80 proof distilled spirits (gin, rum, vodka, whiskey) | 1.5 fl oz | 97 |

**Note:** This table is a guide to estimate the caloric intake from various alcoholic beverages. Higher alcohol content and mixing alcohol with other beverages, such as calorically sweetened soft drinks, tonic water, fruit juice, or cream, increases the amount of calories in the beverage. Alcoholic beverages supply calories but provide few essential nutrients.

**Source:** US Department of Agriculture, Agricultural Research Service. USDA National Nutrient Database for Standard Reference, Release 20. 2007. http://www.ars.usda.gov/main/site_main.htm?modecode=12-35-45-00. Accessed 5/23/11.

## Alcohol Absorption

When small quantities enter the bloodstream alcohol absorption begins immediately in the mouth and esophagus. Although alcohol absorption continues in the stomach, the small intestine efficiently absorbs most of the alcohol a person consumes.[16] (See **Figure SA.5**.)

You've heard it before: "Don't drink on an empty stomach." Eating before or with a drink slows down the advance of alcohol into the bloodstream in several ways. Food, especially if it contains fat, delays emptying of the stomach into the small intestine. The delay also provides a longer opportunity for oxidizing stomach enzymes to work. And food dilutes the stomach contents, lowering the concentration of alcohol and its rate of absorption.

About 80 to 95 percent of alcohol is absorbed unchanged. However, some oxidation does take place in the digestive tract, mainly in the stomach, and products of this metabolism join alcohol as it diffuses into the gut cells.[17] These products travel via the portal vein directly to the liver, where most alcohol metabolism takes place. When all goes well, metabolism achieves two goals: energy production and protection from the damaging effects of alcohol and its even more toxic metabolite **acetaldehyde**.

## Alcohol Metabolism

The body cannot store potentially harmful alcohol, and so it works extra hard to get rid of it. To prevent alcohol from accumulating and destroying cells and organs, the body quickly metabolizes it and removes it from the blood. The liver selectively metabolizes alcohol before other compounds and has alternative pathways to handle excess consumption.

### Metabolizing Small Amounts of Alcohol

**Alcohol dehydrogenase (ADH)** is a zinc-containing enzyme that catalyzes the conversion of small to moderate amounts of alcohol to acetaldehyde, a toxic substance. To avoid toxic buildup, another enzyme, **aldehyde dehydrogenase (ALDH)**, quickly and effectively converts acetaldehyde to acetate. (See **Figure SA.6**.) People differ in their ability to eliminate toxic acetaldehyde, and small amounts of it are found in the blood of intoxicated people.[18]

Dehydrogenases in the gastrointestinal tract and the liver are responsible for almost all alcohol metabolism. Probably about 4 to 9 percent, but possibly as much as 20 percent, of alcohol is changed to acetaldehyde in the digestive tract.[19] Gastrointestinal aldehyde dehydrogenase does not completely convert acetaldehyde to acetate, however. The remaining acetaldehyde is more destructive than alcohol itself and can damage the mucous membranes lining the gut.[20]

Alcohol breakdown always takes priority over the breakdown of carbohydrates, proteins, and fats. Liver cells detoxify alcohol and use the products to synthesize fatty acids, which are assembled into fats. Fat accumulation in the liver can be seen after a single bout of heavy drinking, and fatty acid synthesis accelerates with chronic alcohol consumption. **Fatty liver** is the first stage of liver destruction in alcoholics.

### Metabolizing Large Amounts of Alcohol

Large amounts of alcohol can overwhelm the alcohol dehydrogenase system, the usual metabolic path. As alcohol builds up, the body identifies it as a foreign substance and routes it into the primary overflow pathway, the

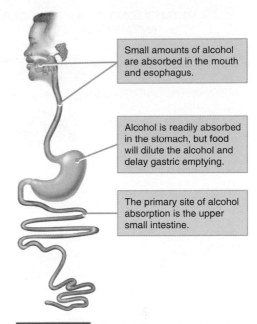

**Figure SA.5** **Alcohol absorption.** Alcohol easily diffuses in and out of cells, so most alcohol is absorbed unchanged.

Small amounts of alcohol are absorbed in the mouth and esophagus.

Alcohol is readily absorbed in the stomach, but food will dilute the alcohol and delay gastric emptying.

The primary site of alcohol absorption is the upper small intestine.

## Quick Bite

**Alcohol Aversion Therapy**
In alcohol aversion therapy, the medication disulfiram (Antabuse) deliberately blocks the conversion of toxic acetaldehyde to acetate (acetic acid). Even small amounts of alcohol trigger the highly unpleasant Antabuse–alcohol reaction, which includes a throbbing headache, breathing difficulties, nausea, copious vomiting, flushing, vertigo, confusion, and a drop in blood pressure.

**acetaldehyde** A toxic intermediate compound formed by the action of the alcohol dehydrogenase enzyme during the metabolism of alcohol.

**alcohol dehydrogenase (ADH)** The enzyme that catalyzes the oxidation of ethanol and other alcohols.

**aldehyde dehydrogenase (ALDH)** The enzyme that catalyzes the conversion of acetaldehyde to acetate, which forms acetyl CoA.

**fatty liver** Accumulation of fat in the liver, a sign of increased fatty acid synthesis.

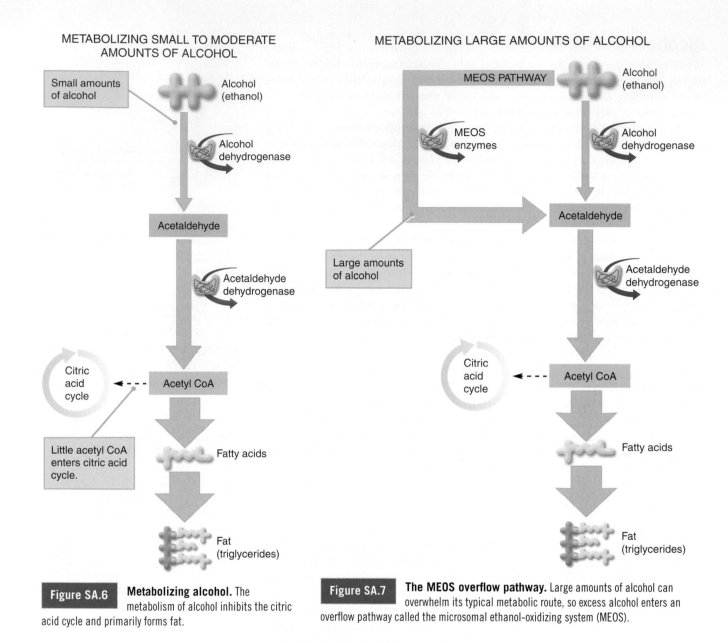

METABOLIZING SMALL TO MODERATE AMOUNTS OF ALCOHOL

Small amounts of alcohol

Alcohol (ethanol)

Alcohol dehydrogenase

Acetaldehyde

Acetaldehyde dehydrogenase

Citric acid cycle

Acetyl CoA

Little acetyl CoA enters citric acid cycle.

Fatty acids

Fat (triglycerides)

METABOLIZING LARGE AMOUNTS OF ALCOHOL

MEOS PATHWAY

Alcohol (ethanol)

MEOS enzymes

Alcohol dehydrogenase

Large amounts of alcohol

Acetaldehyde

Acetaldehyde dehydrogenase

Citric acid cycle

Acetyl CoA

Fatty acids

Fat (triglycerides)

**Figure SA.6**   **Metabolizing alcohol.** The metabolism of alcohol inhibits the citric acid cycle and primarily forms fat.

**Figure SA.7**   **The MEOS overflow pathway.** Large amounts of alcohol can overwhelm its typical metabolic route, so excess alcohol enters an overflow pathway called the microsomal ethanol-oxidizing system (MEOS).

microsomal ethanol-oxidizing system (MEOS). (See **Figure SA.7**.) The liver ordinarily uses the MEOS bypass pathway to metabolize drugs and detoxify "foreign" substances. Chronic heavy drinking appears to activate MEOS enzymes, which may be responsible for transforming the pain reliever acetaminophen into chemicals that can damage the liver.

To transform alcohol into acetaldehyde, the MEOS pathway uses different enzymes than the alcohol dehydrogenase system. When repeatedly exposed to large doses of alcohol, the MEOS pathway increases its capacity and processing speed. Whether alcoholics metabolize alcohol differently from nonalcoholics is unknown. Clearly, chronic ingestion of alcohol leads to changes in the liver, and the alcohol abuser acquires an increased tolerance to alcohol and to drugs such as sedatives, tranquilizers, and antibiotics.

## Removing Alcohol from Circulation

Despite its multiple alcohol-processing pathways, the liver can metabolize only a certain amount of alcohol per hour, regardless of the amount in the

**microsomal ethanol-oxidizing system (MEOS)** An energy-requiring enzyme system in the liver that normally metabolizes drugs and other foreign substances. When the blood alcohol level is high, alcohol dehydrogenase cannot metabolize it fast enough, and the excess alcohol is metabolized by the MEOS.

bloodstream. The rate of alcohol metabolism depends on several factors, including the amount of metabolizing enzymes in the liver, and varies greatly between individuals. In general, after one standard drink, the amount of alcohol in the drinker's blood (blood alcohol concentration, or BAC) peaks in 30 to 45 minutes. (See **Figure SA.8**.) When absorption exceeds the liver's capacity, a bottleneck develops, and alcohol enters the general circulation. Alcohol diffuses rapidly, dispersing equally into all body fluids, including cerebrospinal fluid and the brain and, during pregnancy, into the placenta and fetus. About 10 percent of circulating alcohol is lost in urine, through the lungs, and through skin. Consequently, urine tests and breathalyzer tests both reflect concentrations of blood alcohol as well as alcohol levels in the brain and can indicate how much a person's mental and motor functions may be impaired.

Even after a person stops drinking, alcohol in the stomach and small intestine continues to enter the bloodstream and circulate throughout the body. Blood alcohol concentration continues to rise, and it is dangerous to assume the person will be fine by sleeping it off. Rapid binge drinking (which often happens as a result of a bet or a dare) is especially dangerous, because the victim can ingest a fatal dose of alcohol before becoming unconscious. Even if the victim lives, an alcohol overdose can lead to irreversible brain damage.

Excessive alcohol consumption deprives the brain of oxygen. The struggle to deal with an overdose of alcohol and lack of oxygen eventually causes the brain to shut down functions that regulate breathing and heart rate. This shutdown leads to a loss of consciousness and, in some cases, coma and death. When a drinker passes out, the body is actually protecting itself: When you lose consciousness, you can't add more alcohol to your system. When you hear of an **alcohol poisoning** death, it usually is the result of consuming such a large quantity of alcohol in such a short period of time that the brain of the victim is overwhelmed. Heart and lung functions shut down, and the person dies.

THINK
About It
3

**alcohol poisoning** An overdose of alcohol. The body is overwhelmed by the amount of alcohol in the system and cannot metabolize it fast enough.

## *Quick* Bite

### How to Shock Your Surgeon

If a former alcoholic neglects to disclose past alcohol use before undergoing surgery, the surgeon could be in for a big surprise. Even if the patient is now a teetotaler, his MEOS could still act like that of an alcoholic—operating at the faster speed it once needed to process alcohol quickly. The overactive MEOS would deplete anesthesia much quicker than expected. Theoretically, the patient could wake up in the middle of surgery, much to the shock of the surgeon. That's why anesthesiologists and surgeons ask their patients about alcohol use, past and present.

Blood alcohol concentration peaks at about 40 minutes after drinking; all drinks absorbed within 1 hour.

It takes another 6 hours to metabolize absorbed alcohol.

Blood Alcohol Concentration (%)

0.40 min.

Time (hours)

— One drink    0.10% - - -
— Two drinks    0.05% - - -
— Three drinks
— Four drinks

**Figure SA.8** **Blood alcohol concentration over time.** Because the body metabolizes alcohol at a relatively constant rate, it clears small amounts faster than large amounts.

**Source:** Reproduced from Wilkinson PK, et al. Pharmacokinetics of ethanol after oral administration in the fasting state. J *Pharmacokinet Biopharm.* 1977;5(3):207–224.

**hangover** The collection of symptoms experienced by someone who has consumed a large quantity of alcohol. Symptoms can include pounding headache, fatigue, muscle aches, nausea, stomach pain, heightened sensitivity to light and sound, dizziness, and possibly depression, anxiety, and irritability.

## Hangover Symptoms

*Constitutional*—fatigue, weakness, and thirst
*Pain*—headache and muscle aches
*Gastrointestinal*—nausea, vomiting, and stomach pains
*Sleep and biological rhythms*—decreased sleep, decreased dreaming when asleep
*Sensory*—vertigo and sensitivity to light and sound
*Cognitive*—decreased attention and concentration
*Mood*—depression, anxiety, and irritability
*Sympathetic hyperactivity*—tremor, sweating, increased pulse, and blood pressure

## Possible Contributing Factors

Direct effects of alcohol
- Dehydration
- Electrolyte imbalance
- Gastrointestinal disturbances
- Low blood sugar
- Sleep and biological rhythm disturbances

Alcohol withdrawal
Alcohol metabolism (i.e., acetaldehyde toxicity)
Nonalcohol factors
- Compounds other than alcohol in beverages, especially the congener methanol
- Use of other drugs, especially nicotine
- Personality traits such as neuroticism, anger, and defensiveness
- Negative life events and feelings of guilt about drinking
- Family history for alcoholism

**Figure SA.9** **Hangovers.** Factors other than just alcohol contribute to the misery of a hangover.

## The Morning After

After a night of heavy alcohol consumption, the drinker may suffer from a pounding headache, fatigue, muscle aches, nausea, and stomach pain as well as a heightened sensitivity to light and noise—a **hangover** in full force. The sufferer may be dizzy, have a sense that the room is spinning, and be depressed, anxious, and irritable. Usually a hangover begins within several hours after the last drink, when the blood alcohol level is dropping. Symptoms normally peak about the time the alcohol level reaches zero, and they may continue for an entire day.[21]

What causes a hangover? Scientists have identified several causes of the painful symptoms of a hangover. (See **Figure SA.9**.) Alcohol causes dehydration, which leads to headache and dry mouth. Alcohol directly irritates the stomach and intestines, contributing to stomach pain and vomiting. The sweating, vomiting, and diarrhea that can accompany a hangover cause additional fluid loss and electrolyte imbalance. Alcohol's hijack of the metabolic process diverts liver activity away from glucose production and can lead to low blood glucose (hypoglycemia), causing light-headedness and lack of energy. Alcohol also disrupts sleep patterns, interfering with the dream state and contributing to fatigue. The symptoms of a hangover are largely due to inflammation. During a hangover, blood levels of C-reactive protein are elevated and strongly associated with hangover severity.[22] In general, the greater the amount of alcohol consumed, the more likely a hangover will strike. However, some people experience a hangover after only one drink, whereas some heavy drinkers do not have hangovers.[23]

In addition, factors other than alcohol may contribute to the hangover. A person with a family history of alcoholism has increased vulnerability to hangovers. Mixing alcohol and drugs also is suspected of increasing the likelihood of a hangover. The congeners in most alcoholic beverages can contribute to more vicious hangovers. Research shows that gin and vodka—beverages that contain less of these biologically active compounds—cause fewer headaches.[24]

## Treating a Hangover

So what can you do about a hangover? Few treatments have undergone rigorous, scientific investigation. Time is the most effective treatment—symptoms usually disappear in 8 to 24 hours. Eating bland foods that contain complex carbohydrates, such as toast or crackers, can combat low blood glucose and possibly nausea. Sleep can ease fatigue, and drinking nonalcoholic beverages can alleviate dehydration. Limited research suggests that taking vitamin $B_6$ or an extract from *Optunia ficus indica* (a type of prickly pear cactus) before drinking may reduce the severity of hangover symptoms.[25] The prickly pear cactus extract may reduce three symptoms of hangover—nausea, dry mouth, and loss of appetite.[26] The best way to prevent a hangover, of course, is to abstain from alcohol.

Certain medications also can relieve some symptoms. Antacids, for example, may relieve nausea and stomach pains. Aspirin may reduce headache and muscle aches, but could increase stomach irritation. Avoid acetaminophen, because alcohol metabolism enhances its toxicity to the liver.[27] In fact, people who drink three or more alcoholic beverages per day should avoid all over-the-counter pain relievers and fever reducers. These heavy drinkers may have an increased risk of liver damage and stomach bleeding from medicines that contain aspirin, acetaminophen (Tylenol), ibuprofen (Advil), naproxen sodium (Aleve), or ketoprofen (Orudis KT and Actron).[28]

People with hangovers should avoid "the hair of the dog that bit you," a remedy that calls for drinking more alcohol. Additional drinking only enhances

THINK
About It

4

the toxicity of the alcohol previously consumed and extends the recovery time.

## Individual Differences in Alcohol Metabolism

Individuals vary in their ability to metabolize alcohol and acetaldehyde. As a consequence, they differ in their susceptibility to intoxication, hangover, and, in the long term, addiction and organ damage.

The result of individual differences is easiest to see in acute responses to alcohol. For example, when people of Asian descent drink alcohol, about half experience flushing around the face and neck, probably as a result of high blood acetaldehyde levels.[29] These individuals lack gastric alcohol dehydrogenase, and their livers have an inefficient form of aldehyde dehydrogenase. This may explain why their ancestors depended on boiled water (for teas) as a source of safe fluid. In contrast, Europeans are able to metabolize larger quantities of alcohol and historically have relied on fermentation to produce fluids that were safer to drink.[30]

Elderly people often find their tolerance for alcohol is less than it used to be. Due to decreased tolerance, the effects of alcohol, such as impaired coordination, occur at lower intakes in the elderly than in younger people, whose tolerance increases with increased consumption. This reduced tolerance is compounded by an age-related decrease in body water, so that blood alcohol concentrations in older people are likely to rise higher after drinking.[31]

### Women and Alcohol

Men and women respond differently to alcohol. (See **Figure SA.10**.) Blood alcohol rises faster in women, so they become more intoxicated than men with an equivalent dose of alcohol.[32] Accordingly, moderate drinking is usually defined as "two standard drinks for men and one for women."[33] Women also metabolize alcohol more slowly than men. Several factors are responsible for alcohol's greater effect on women.

### Body Size and Composition

Women, on average, are smaller than men and have smaller livers; thus they have less capacity for metabolizing alcohol. Women also have lower total body water and higher body fat than men of comparable size. After alcohol is consumed, it diffuses uniformly into all body water, both inside and outside cells. Because of their smaller quantity of body water, women have higher concentrations of alcohol in their blood than men do after drinking equivalent amounts of alcohol.[34]

### Less Enzyme Activity

Women also have less alcohol dehydrogenase (the primary enzyme involved in the metabolism of alcohol) activity than men—about 40 percent less.[35] This contributes to higher blood alcohol concentrations and lengthens the time needed to metabolize and eliminate alcohol. The gender difference in blood alcohol levels is due mainly to the significantly lower activity of gastric enzymes in women.[36]

### Chronic Alcohol Abuse

Alcoholism and other abuses exact a greater physical toll on women than men. Female alcoholics have death rates 50 to 100 percent higher than those of male alcoholics. Furthermore, a higher percentage of female alcoholics die from suicides, alcohol-related accidents, circulatory disorders, and cirrhosis of the liver.

*Quick* Bite

**Is the Alcohol Beverage Industry Addicted to Alcohol Abuse?**
The combined value of illegal and underage drinking and adult alcohol abuse to the alcoholic beverage industry is estimated to be at least $48.3 billion, or 37.5 percent of consumer expenditures for alcohol in 2001. Other estimates suggest the value may be closer to $62.9 billion (48.8 percent of expenditures).

**Body composition**
Women have a higher percentage of fat than men and thus have less water to dilute alcohol.

**Less enzyme activity**
Alcohol dehydrogenase, the primary enzyme involved in the metabolism of alcohol, is up to 40% less active in women than in men.

**Body size**
Women are smaller on average than men (smaller livers and less total water).

**Hormonal fluctuations**
Women typically have a heightened response to alcohol which is increased when they are about to have their periods, or when taking birth control pills.

**Figure SA.10**    **Women and men respond differently to alcohol.** Women tend to have a lower capacity for alcohol than men.

*Quick* Bite

**Ancient Hangover Helpers**
According to the ancient Persians, eating five almonds could prevent a hangover. The Romans and Greeks had a different solution: celery.

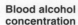

**Blood alcohol concentration**

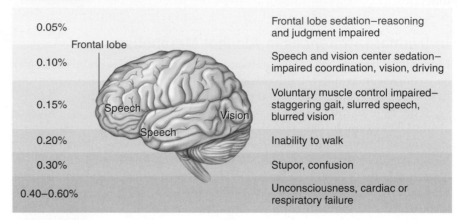

| | |
|---|---|
| 0.05% | Frontal lobe sedation–reasoning and judgment impaired |
| 0.10% | Speech and vision center sedation–impaired coordination, vision, driving |
| 0.15% | Voluntary muscle control impaired–staggering gait, slurred speech, blurred vision |
| 0.20% | Inability to walk |
| 0.30% | Stupor, confusion |
| 0.40–0.60% | Unconsciousness, cardiac or respiratory failure |

**Figure SA.11** **Effects of alcohol on the brain.** As blood alcohol concentration rises, different parts of the brain are affected.

**Key Concepts** *Alcohol does not need to be digested prior to absorption and moves easily across the GI tract lining into the bloodstream. Once alcohol is absorbed, the liver metabolizes it. The primary metabolic enzymes are alcohol dehydrogenase and aldehyde dehydrogenase. When large amounts of alcohol are consumed, some is metabolized by the MEOS pathway. Genetic and gender differences in the amount and activity levels of alcohol-metabolizing enzymes influence a person's response to consuming alcohol.*

# When Alcohol Becomes a Problem

Alcohol affects every organ system in the body. In the short term, small amounts of alcohol change the levels of neurotransmitters in the brain, reducing inhibitions and physical coordination. In the long term, chronic intake of large amounts of alcohol damages the heart, liver, GI tract, and brain. When a pregnant woman drinks, alcohol can have a devastating effect on the development of her baby.

## Alcohol in the Brain and the Nervous System

Alcohol diffuses readily into the brain, and because a small amount is absorbed from the mouth directly into circulating blood, its effects can be almost immediate, reaching the brain in as little as one minute after consumption. Alcohol can produce detectable impairments in memory after only a few drinks and, as the amount of alcohol increases, so does the degree of impairment. Large quantities of alcohol, especially when consumed quickly and on an empty stomach, can produce a blackout, that is, an interval of time for which the intoxicated person cannot recall key details of events, or even entire events. **Figure SA.11** shows the effects alcohol has on the brain.

Because alcohol is soluble in fat, it can easily cross the protective fatty membrane of nerve cells. There, it disrupts the brain's complex system for communicating between nerve cells. Neurotransmitters that excite nerve cells and those that inhibit nerve cells are thrown out of balance. Excess of some neurotransmitters produces sleepiness; high levels of others cause a loss of coordination; an imbalance of others impairs judgment and mental ability; and still other neurotransmitters perpetuate the desire to keep drinking, even when it's clearly time to stop. Changes in these messengers are suspected of leading to addiction and symptoms of alcohol withdrawal.[37] In the short run, they probably contribute to a hangover.

Alcohol's short-term effects are related to how much a person drinks. One or two drinks typically bring alcohol blood levels to 0.04 percent and usually cause only mild, pleasant changes in mood and release of inhibitions. With more drinks and rising blood alcohol levels, coordination, judgment, reaction time, and vision are increasingly impaired. In the United States and Canada, it is illegal for a person whose blood level of alcohol has reached or exceeds 0.08 percent to drive a motor vehicle. A review of 112 studies concludes that certain skills required to drive a motor vehicle can become significantly impaired at a blood alcohol concentration as low as 0.05 percent.[38] For commercial drivers, a BAC of 0.04 percent is illegal nationwide. Table SA.2 shows the effects various amounts of alcohol have on mood and behavior.

The acute effect of a large alcohol intake—swallowed accidentally by children, for example—is hypoglycemia (low blood glucose) severe enough to kill.[39] Binge drinking, especially following several days of little food, also can be deadly. The lack of food depletes glycogen stores, and heavy drinking suppresses gluconeogenesis. The resulting severe hypoglycemia is a medical emergency with the potential for coma and death.

**Table SA.2**  **Alcohol Impairment Chart**

### Men

| Drinks | 100 | 120 | 140 | 160 | 180 | 200 | 220 | 240 | |
|--------|-----|-----|-----|-----|-----|-----|-----|-----|---|
| 0 | .00 | .00 | .00 | .00 | .00 | .00 | .00 | .00 | Only Safe Driving Limit |
| 1 | .04 | .03 | .03 | .02 | .02 | .02 | .02 | .02 | Impairment Begins |
| 2 | .08 | .06 | .05 | .05 | .04 | .04 | .03 | .03 | Driving Skills Affected |
| 3 | .11 | .09 | .08 | .07 | .06 | .06 | .05 | .05 | |
| 4 | .15 | .12 | .11 | .09 | .08 | .08 | .07 | .06 | Possible Criminal Penalties |
| 5 | .19 | .16 | .13 | .12 | .11 | .09 | .09 | .08 | |
| 6 | .23 | .19 | .16 | .14 | .13 | .11 | .10 | .09 | |
| 7 | .26 | .22 | .19 | .16 | .15 | .13 | .12 | .11 | Legally Intoxicated |
| 8 | .30 | .25 | .21 | .19 | .17 | .15 | .14 | .13 | |
| 9 | .34 | .28 | .24 | .21 | .19 | .17 | .15 | .14 | Criminal Penalties |
| 10 | .38 | .31 | .27 | .23 | .21 | .19 | .17 | .16 | |

Body Weight in Pounds. Approximate Blood Alcohol Percentage.

### Women

| Drinks | 90 | 100 | 120 | 140 | 160 | 180 | 200 | 220 | 240 | |
|--------|----|-----|-----|-----|-----|-----|-----|-----|-----|---|
| 0 | .00 | .00 | .00 | .00 | .00 | .00 | .00 | .00 | .00 | Only Safe Driving Limit |
| 1 | .05 | .05 | .04 | .03 | .03 | .03 | .02 | .02 | .02 | Impairment Begins |
| 2 | .10 | .09 | .08 | .07 | .06 | .05 | .05 | .04 | .04 | Driving Skills Affected |
| 3 | .15 | .14 | .11 | .10 | .09 | .08 | .07 | .06 | .06 | Possible Criminal Penalties |
| 4 | .20 | .18 | .15 | .13 | .11 | .10 | .09 | .08 | .08 | |
| 5 | .25 | .23 | .19 | .16 | .14 | .13 | .11 | .10 | .09 | |
| 6 | .30 | .27 | .23 | .19 | .17 | .15 | .14 | .12 | .11 | |
| 7 | .35 | .32 | .27 | .23 | .20 | .18 | .16 | .14 | .13 | Legally Intoxicated |
| 8 | .40 | .36 | .30 | .26 | .23 | .20 | .18 | .17 | .15 | |
| 9 | .45 | .41 | .34 | .29 | .26 | .23 | .20 | .19 | .17 | Criminal Penalties |
| 10 | .51 | .45 | .38 | .32 | .28 | .25 | .23 | .21 | .19 | |

Body Weight in Pounds. Approximate Blood Alcohol Percentage.

**Note:** Your body can get rid of one drink per hour. One drink is 1.25 oz of 80 proof liquor, 12 oz of beer, or 5 oz of table wine.

**Source:** Reproduced with permission of the Pennsylvania Liquor Control Board's Bureau of Alcohol Education using data from The National Clearinghouse for Alcohol and Drug Information, Substance Abuse and Mental Health Services Administration.

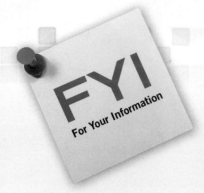

# Changing the Culture of Campus Drinking

From car crashes to alcohol poisoning, the culture of drinking on many college campuses puts students at grave risk. Alcohol use is pervasive among college students, many of whom are younger than the legal drinking age.

Annually, at least 1,700 student deaths and nearly 600,000 unintentional injuries involve alcohol.[1] From 2001 to 2005, excessive alcohol use was the third leading preventable cause of death in the United States.[2] College students who drink are more likely to drink and drive, have failing grades, and have medical and legal problems. Increased rates of crime, traffic crashes, rapes and assaults, property damage, and other alcohol-related consequences affect both drinking and nondrinking students, as well as members of the surrounding community. Each year, for example, students who have been drinking assault more than 696,000 of their classmates.[3]

## The Culture of College Drinking

On many campuses, alcohol consumption is a rite of passage, and the influence of peers is an especially powerful force driving college problem drinking.[4] Traditions and beliefs handed down through generations of college drinkers reinforce the perception that alcohol is a necessary component of social success.[5] Many students arrive at college with a history of alcohol consumption and positive expectations about alcohol's effects. Thirty percent of twelfth-graders, for example, report heavy episodic drinking in high school, slightly more report having "been drunk," and almost three-fourths report drinking in the past year.[6]

Rates of excessive alcohol use are highest at colleges and universities where fraternities and sororities are popular, where sports teams have a prominent role, and at schools located in the Northeast.[7] In the local community, tolerance of student drinking may permit alcoholic beverage outlets and advertising to be located near campus. Due to lax enforcement, selling alcohol to students below the legal drinking age often has few consequences. Also, underage students who are caught using fake IDs to obtain alcohol are seldom penalized.[8] Just look at the advertising and sale of alcoholic beverages on or near campuses, and the role of alcohol in college life is evident.

## Alcohol Use and Abuse by College Students

Approximately 70 percent of college students consumed some alcohol within 30 days of being surveyed.[9] Although some of these students are problem drinkers (e.g., frequent heavy episodic drinkers or those who display symptoms of dependence), others may drink moderately or may misuse alcohol only occasionally (e.g., drink and drive infrequently). Surveys of drinking patterns show that college students are more likely than nonstudents of similar age to consume any alcohol, to drink heavily, and to engage in heavy episodic drinking. Young people who are not in college, however, are more likely to consume alcohol every day.[10] Even though college students

tend to drink more, they are not at greater risk of alcohol-related problems.[11]

Results from the Fall 2010 American College Health Association National College Health Assessment revealed that 60 percent of college students reported using alcohol within the past 30 days.[12] Another recent survey questioned students about patterns and consequences of their alcohol use.[13] Thirty-two percent reported symptoms associated with alcohol abuse (e.g., drinking in hazardous situations, alcohol-related school problems), and 6 percent reported three or more symptoms of alcohol dependence (e.g., drinking more or longer than initially planned, experiencing increased tolerance to alcohol's effects). Binge drinkers consumed 91 percent of all the alcohol that students reported drinking, and 68 percent of alcohol was consumed by frequent binge drinkers. What happens when these student imbibers leave college? Surprisingly, most high-risk student drinkers reduce their consumption of alcohol. Nevertheless, some continue frequent, excessive drinking, leading to alcoholism or medical problems associated with chronic alcohol abuse.[14]

## Binge Drinking

Binge drinking is especially worrisome, and it is widespread on college campuses. What is binge drinking? Binge drinking is defined as the consumption of at least five drinks in a row for men or four drinks in a row for women. Just over two in five students (44 percent) report binge drinking behaviors, and about one in four (23 percent) report bingeing frequently, defined as three or more times in a two-week period. Frequent binge drinkers average more than 14 drinks per week and account for more than 90 percent of the alcohol consumed by college students.[15] Most college binge drinkers drink not for sociability, but solely and purposefully to get drunk.

Binge drinkers often do something they later regret—argue with friends, make fools of themselves, get sick, engage in unplanned (and often unprotected) sexual activity, or drive drunk. Afterward they may forget where they were or what they did, but the consequences of the binge

remain. These consequences may include alienated friends, a hangover, and embarrassment. Or the consequences could be much more serious—sexually transmitted disease, hospitalization, permanent injury, rape, pregnancy, or death.

## Abstaining

There is a polarizing trend in college drinking, with binge drinkers at one extreme and abstainers at the other. The number of college students who drink no alcohol is rising and now nearly equals the number who binge frequently. About one in five students (19 percent) report consuming no alcohol within the past year.[16] In a survey, one in three college campuses reported banning the use of alcohol on campus by all students regardless of age.[17]

## Prevention Strategies and Changing the Culture of Drinking

Changing the culture of college drinking represents the first step toward an effective prevention strategy, according to a task force of college presidents, alcohol researchers, and students established by the National Institute on Alcohol Abuse and Alcoholism. The report emphasizes the need for collaboration between academic institutions, researchers, and the community to effect lasting change.[18]

The task force strongly supports the use of a "3-in-1 Framework" to target three primary audiences simultaneously: (1) individual students, including high-risk drinkers; (2) the student body as a whole; and (3) the surrounding community.[19] The task force reviewed potentially useful preventive interventions, grouping them into "tiers" according to evidence for their effectiveness.

### Tier 1: Strategies Effective Among College Students

Strong evidence supports the following strategies:

1. Simultaneously address alcohol-related attitudes and behaviors (e.g., refuting false beliefs about alcohol's effects while teaching students how to cope with stress without resorting to alcohol).

2. Use survey data to counter students' misperceptions about their fellow students' drinking practices and attitudes toward excessive drinking.
3. Increase student motivation to change drinking habits by providing nonjudgmental advice and progress evaluations.
4. Programs that combine these three strategies have proved effective in reducing alcohol consumption.[20]

## Tier 2: Strategies Effective Among the General Population That Could Be Applied to College Environments

These strategies have proved successful in populations similar to those found on college campuses. Measures include the following:

1. Increase enforcement of minimum legal drinking age laws.[21]
2. Implement, enforce, and publicize other laws to reduce alcohol-impaired driving, such as zero-tolerance laws that reduce the legal blood alcohol concentration for underage drivers to near zero.[22]
3. Increase the prices or taxes on alcoholic beverages.[23]
4. Institute policies and training for servers of alcoholic beverages to prevent sales to underage or intoxicated patrons.[24]
5. Use the secondhand smoke campaign as a model to change the culture of alcohol abuse on campus.[25]

## Tier 3: Promising Strategies That Require Research

These strategies make sense intuitively or show theoretical promise, but their usefulness requires further testing. They include more consistent enforcement of campus alcohol regulations and increasing the severity of penalties for violating them, regulating happy hours, enhancing awareness of personal liability for alcohol-related harm to others, establishing alcohol-free dormitories, restricting or eliminating alcohol-industry sponsorship of student events while promoting alcohol-free student activities, and conducting social norms campaigns to correct exaggerated estimates of the overall level of drinking among the student body.

## How Can I Say No to Drinking Alcohol and Still Fit in with My Friends?

Drinking alcohol is a personal decision. It is best to make your decision of whether or not to drink based on your own feelings, knowledge, and experiences. You may want to consider the following before you are put in a position where drinking alcohol is encouraged:[26]

- If you choose to abstain, make up your mind to say no before you are ever in the situation.
- Tell people that you feel better when you drink less.
- Stay away from people who give you a hard time about not drinking.
- Learn to hold a glass or beer bottle for a long time, and refill it with whatever you want (such as water or club soda).

1 Hingson RW, Heeren T, Winter M, et al. Magnitude of alcohol-related mortality and morbidity among US college students ages 18–24: changes from 1998 to 2001. *Ann Rev Pub Health.* 2005;26:259–279.
2 Centers for Disease Control and Prevention (CDC). Vital signs: binge drinking among high school students and adults—United States, 2009. *MMWR.* 2010;59(39):1274–1279.
3 Hingson RW, Heeren T, Winter M, et al. Op. cit.
4 Ham LS, Hope DA. Incorporating social anxiety into a model of college student problematic drinking. *Addict Behav.* 2005;30(1):127–150.
5 National Institute on Alcohol Abuse and Alcoholism (NIAAA). *A Call to Action: Changing the Culture of Drinking at U.S. Colleges.* Bethesda, MD: NIAAA; 2002. NIH publication 02-5010; and NIAAA. *Young Adult Drinking.* Bethesda, MD: NIAAA; 2006. Alcohol Alert No. 68.
6 CDC. Op. cit.
7 Carter AC, Brandon KO, Goldman MS. The college and noncollege experience: a review of the factors that influence drinking behavior in young adulthood. *J Stud Alcohol Drugs.* 2010;71(5):742–750.
8 Toomey TL, Lenk KM, Wagenaar AC. Environmental policies to reduce college drinking: an update of research findings. *J Stud Alcohol Drugs.* 2007;68(2):208–219.
9 Wagoner K, Rhodes S, Lentz A, Wolfson M. Community organizing goes to college: a practice-based model to implement environmental strategies to reduce high-risk drinking on college campuses. *Health Promot Pract.* 2010;11(6):817–827.
10 Slutske WS. Alcohol use disorders among US college students and their non-college-attending peers. *Arch Gen Psychiatry.* 2005;62:321–327.
11 Ibid.
12 American College Health Association. *National College Health Assessment II. Reference Group Executive Summary. Fall 2010.* http://www.achancha.org/docs/ACHA-NCHA-II_ReferenceGroup_ExecutiveSummary_Fall2010.pdf. Accessed 5/23/11.
13 Wechsler H, Nelson TF. What we have learned from the Harvard School of Public Health College Alcohol Study: focusing attention on college student alcohol consumption and the environmental conditions that promote it. *J Stud Alcohol Drugs.* 2008;69(4):481–490.
14 McMambridge J, McAlaney J, Rowe R. Adult consequences of late adolescent alcohol consumption: a systematic review of cohort studies. *PLoS Med.* 2011;8(2).
15 Wechsler H, Nelson TF. Op. cit.
16 Wechsler H, Lee JE, Kuo M, et al. Trends in college binge drinking during a period of increased prevention efforts: findings from 4 Harvard School of Public Health College Alcohol Study Surveys: 1993–2001. *J Am Coll Health.* 2002;50(5):203–217.
17 Wechsler H, Seibring M, Liu IC, Ahl M. Colleges respond to student binge drinking: reducing student demand or limiting access. *J Am Coll Health.* 2004;52(4):159–168.
18 NIAAA. Op. cit.
19 Hingson RW, Howland J. Comprehensive community interventions to promote health: implications for college-age drinking problems. *J Studies Alcohol.* 2002;(suppl 14):226–240; and Holder HD, Gruenewald PJ, Ponicki WR, et al. Effect of community-based interventions on high-risk drinking and alcohol-related injuries. *JAMA.* 2000;284: 2341–2347.
20 Larimer ME, Cronce JM. Identification, prevention, and treatment: a review of individual-focused strategies to reduce problematic alcohol consumption by college students. *J Studies Alcohol.* 2002;(suppl 14):148–163.
21 Wagenaar AC, Toomey TL. Effects of minimum drinking age laws: review and analyses of the literature from 1960 to 2000. *J Studies Alcohol.* 2002;(suppl 14):206–225.
22 Wagenaar A, O'Malley P, LaFond L. Lowered legal blood alcohol limits for young drivers: effects on drinking, driving, and driving-after-drinking behaviors in 30 states. *Am J Pub Health.* 2001;91(5): 801–804.
23 Cook PJ, Moore MJ. The economics of alcohol abuse and alcohol-control policies. *Health Affairs.* 2002;21(2):120–133.
24 Toomey TL, Wagenaar AC. Op. cit.
25 Misch DA. Changing the culture of alcohol abuse on campus: lessons learned from secondhand smoke. *J Am Coll Health.* 2010;59(3):232–234.
26 Anderson J, Vitale T. *Eat Right! Healthy Eating in College and Beyond.* San Francisco: Pearson Benjamin Cummings; 2007.

A person who drinks heavily over a long period of time may have brain deficits that persist well after he or she achieves sobriety. Exactly how alcohol affects the brain and the likelihood of reversing the impact of heavy drinking on the brain remain hot topics in alcohol research today.[40] Chronic alcoholism produces many different mental disorders. Malnutrition is a probable factor in most of these, even when diet appears adequate. After years of drinking, brain cells become permanently damaged and unable to metabolize nutrients properly.

## Alcohol's Effect on the Gastrointestinal System

Years of heavy drinking and ongoing contact with alcohol and acetaldehyde eventually damage the gastrointestinal system, which, in turn, discourages eating, affects absorption of protective nutrients, and leaves the digestive lining even more vulnerable to damage as the vicious cycle continues.

Chronic irritation from alcohol and acetaldehyde erodes protective mucosal linings, causing inflammation and release of destructive free radicals. **Esophagitis** (inflammation of the esophagus), esophageal stricture (closing), and swallowing difficulties are common among alcoholics. When the stomach is exposed repeatedly to alcohol at high concentrations, **gastritis** (inflammation of the stomach) often develops. Alcoholics frequently have diarrhea and malabsorption, evidence of intestinal damage. The mouth, throat, esophagus, stomach, and small and large intestines are all at greatly increased risk of cancer.[41] Smoking dramatically multiplies this risk.

## Alcohol and the Liver

Metabolizing and detoxifying alcohol is almost entirely the responsibility of the liver. So it's not surprising that too much drinking hurts the liver more than any other site in the body. In the United States, heavy alcohol use is considered the most important risk factor for chronic liver disease. During 2007, the number of deaths from chronic liver disease or cirrhosis in the United States was over 29,000 (nearly 10 deaths per 100,000 persons), according to the Centers for Disease Control and Prevention.[42]

The earliest evidence of liver damage is fat accumulation, which can appear after only a few days of heavy drinking. Fatty liver (see **Figure SA.12**) recedes with abstinence but persists with continued drinking. Is fatty liver in and of itself harmful? The answer is controversial among liver researchers, with some experts suggesting it's a benign condition. However, studies show that 5 to 15 percent of people with alcoholic fatty liver who continue to drink develop liver fibrosis (excessive fibrous tissue) or cirrhosis (scarring) in only 5 to 10 years.[43]

Fat accumulation is one of several factors resulting in alcoholic liver disease. With regular, high intakes of alcohol, alcohol and acetaldehyde continually irritate and inflame the liver, producing alcoholic hepatitis (persistent inflammation of the liver) in 10 to 35 percent of heavy drinkers. The inflammatory process also generates free radicals that batter away at liver cells.[44] The destruction of liver cells becomes self-perpetuating, especially if antioxidant nutrients are unavailable to help break the cycle. If the intestines also have been damaged, toxins, including those produced by the gut's microorganisms, may be able to cross the intestinal barrier into circulation, worsening inflammation.[45]

Alcoholic hepatitis may be treatable, but it's often fatal. Alcoholic hepatitis also predisposes a person to liver cancer and cirrhosis, conditions that are usually fatal. With continued inflammation, the liver makes excessive collagen and becomes fibrous (fibrotic liver disease) and scarred (cirrhosis). This

**esophagitis** Inflammation of the esophagus.

**gastritis** Inflammation of the stomach.

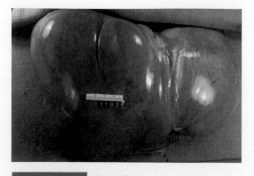

Figure SA.12    **Fatty liver.**

ultimately kills liver cells by choking off tiny blood vessels that nourish them. About 10 to 20 percent of heavy drinkers develop cirrhosis.[46]

Dietary changes may be helpful in treating liver disease, but abstinence from alcohol is essential. Reducing dietary fats somewhat reduces fat accumulation in the liver. Consuming adequate micronutrients and a healthful balance of macronutrients probably speeds recuperation from liver diseases in their earlier stages.[47] In late-stage liver disease, dietary restrictions, often of proteins, may slow disease progression or improve symptoms.

## Fetal Alcohol Syndrome

**Fetal alcohol syndrome** is perhaps the saddest result of alcohol consumption. Victims of this syndrome suffer a variety of congenital defects: mental retardation, coordination problems, and heart, eye, and genitourinary malformations, as well as low birth weight and slowed growth rate. Most apparent are characteristic facial abnormalities. Severe cases of fetal alcohol syndrome are rare, but subtle damage with one or two abnormalities, sometimes called "fetal alcohol effects," is probably much more widespread. Symptoms of the syndrome may not emerge until months after birth and are apt to go undiagnosed.[48] This disorder, a major cause of mental retardation in the United States, is preventable.

Alcohol is especially damaging in the early weeks of pregnancy, before a woman may know she's pregnant. It crosses the placenta into the tiny body of the fetus, where its effects are grossly magnified. Both the congeners in alcoholic beverages and the associated disturbed metabolism of vitamin A and folic acid—nutrients clearly required for fetal growth and development—can interfere with embryonic development.[49]

Relatively small amounts of alcohol may cause fetal alcohol syndrome. A safe level during pregnancy is not known; therefore, pregnant women should abstain from alcohol consumption. Unlike most other alcohol-related diseases, fetal alcohol damage does not require chronic intake. A binge—even having several drinks at a party—at the wrong moment of pregnancy can cause serious problems. However, population studies show that babies with neurodevelopmental problems are more common among women who drink more frequently during pregnancy.[50]

Official health advisories warn women against drinking alcohol if they are pregnant or considering becoming pregnant. Labels on alcoholic beverages must carry a warning for pregnant women. The Centers for Disease Control and Prevention reports that from 1991 to 2005 more than 12 percent of pregnant women consumed alcohol in the past 30 days. Those women most likely to report any alcohol use were 35 to 44 years of age (17.7 percent) and college graduates (14.4 percent).[51] **Figure SA.13** shows the prevalence of alcohol consumption by women of childbearing age.

**Key Concepts** *Alcohol affects every organ system of the body. In the brain and nervous system, alcohol impairs coordination, judgment, reaction time, and vision. In the GI tract, alcohol damages cells of the esophagus and stomach and increases the risk for GI cancers. The liver is most affected by alcohol consumption, culminating in alcoholic hepatitis and cirrhosis after years of alcohol abuse. Alcohol intake during pregnancy can have devastating effects on fetal development.*

## Alcoholics and Malnutrition

In the United States and Canada, where food is plentiful and fortification of foods with vitamins and minerals is common, overt nutrient deficiencies are rare—except among alcoholics. The results of their poor diet interact with

**fetal alcohol syndrome** A set of physical and mental abnormalities observed in infants born to women who abuse alcohol during pregnancy. Affected infants exhibit poor growth, characteristic abnormal facial features, limited hand–eye coordination, and mental retardation.

*Quick* Bite

**Are Alcoholics More Likely to Get Food Poisoning?**
When alcohol inhibits the breakdown of another toxin, the effect can be dramatic. Consider seafood toxins, for example. The alcoholic who sits down for a good fish dinner should be extra careful about seafood because alcoholic liver disease makes him or her 200 times more likely to die from *Vibrio vulnificus*, a bacterium found in raw oysters. Alcohol also accentuates the symptoms of ciguatera, or "fish poisoning," a relatively common food poisoning in tropical areas where people eat large fish from infected waters.

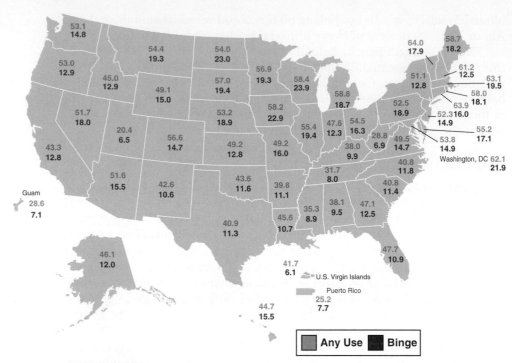

| 53.1 14.8 |
| 53.0 12.9 |
| 45.0 12.9 |
| 54.4 19.3 |
| 54.0 23.0 |
| 56.9 19.3 |
| 58.4 23.9 |
| 64.0 17.9 | 58.7 18.2 |
| 61.2 12.5 | 63.1 19.5 |

Guam 28.6 7.1

Puerto Rico 25.2 7.7

U.S. Virgin Islands 41.7 6.1

46.1 12.0

44.7 15.5

Any Use ■ Binge

**Figure SA.13** **Prevalence of frequent alcohol consumption among women of childbearing age (18–44 years).** Alcohol is especially damaging to the fetus during the early weeks of pregnancy—before a woman may know she is pregnant.

**Source:** Courtesy of the Centers for Disease Control and Prevention.

the results of alcohol's toxicity—which include diarrhea, malabsorption, liver malfunction, bleeding, bone marrow changes, and hormonal changes—to worsen malnutrition. (See **Figure SA.14**.) In general, the more a person drinks, the worse the malnutrition.

## *Poor Diet*

A nationally representative study found that as alcohol quantity increased, diet quality worsened, but as alcohol frequency increased, diet quality improved. Diet quality was poorest among the highest-quantity, lowest-frequency drinkers and best among the lowest-quantity, highest-frequency drinkers.[52]

Disordered eating is common among heavy drinkers, especially among alcoholic women.[53] Factors responsible for the poor diet of alcoholics are much easier to identify than to correct. Economic factors include poverty, lack of cooking facilities, and homelessness. Anxiety, depression, loneliness, and isolation are all characteristic of alcoholism, and all contribute to loss of appetite. So can physical pain. Lack of interest in food is common. There may be an aversion to many specific foods or to eating in general, especially after the experience of diarrhea, painful indigestion, or difficulty swallowing.

Heavy drinkers who get about half their calories from alcohol cannot eat enough to obtain adequate vitamins and minerals. Severely malnourished alcoholics often have multiple deficiencies.

## Vitamin Deficiencies

Inadequate intake, poor absorption, increased vitamin destruction in the body, and urinary losses all contribute to vitamin deficiencies in the alcoholic. Alcohol also interferes with the conversion of vitamin precursors to active forms.

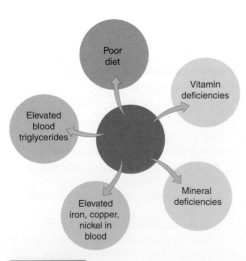

**Figure SA.14** **Alcoholism and malnutrition.** Alcoholics' poor diets interact with alcohol's toxicity to worsen their malnutrition.

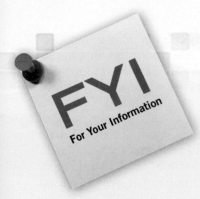

# Myths About Alcohol

Myths and misunderstandings just keep circulating about alcohol. Some of these statements are partly true, but most are completely false. You may have heard some of the following:

- *Drinking isn't all that dangerous.* Wrong! One in three 18- to 24-year-olds admitted to emergency rooms for serious injuries is intoxicated. Alcohol use is also associated with homicides, suicides, and drownings.
- *I can manage to drive well enough after a few drinks.* No. About one-half of all fatal traffic crashes among 18- to 24-year-olds involve alcohol.

- *I can sober up quickly if needed.* No. It takes about three hours to eliminate the alcohol content of two drinks, depending on your weight and other factors. Nothing can speed up this process—not even coffee or cold showers.
- *Alcohol is a stimulant.* No. It's actually a depressant, but its initial depressing effect on inhibitions and judgment may make it seem stimulating.
- *Alcohol keeps you warm.* Partly true. It dilates blood vessels near the body's surface, giving a feeling of warmth. But as body heat escapes, alcohol cools the inner body.

- *Alcohol is an aphrodisiac.* Partly true. By suppressing inhibitions, it may loosen behavior. However, sexual function is often compromised by alcohol.
- *Most alcoholics live on skid row.* No. The highly visible skid-row alcoholic represents only a minority of alcoholics.
- *Beer is a source of vitamins.* Partly true. Beer does contain a fair amount of niacin. But you'd need about 1 liter to fulfill daily niacin requirements. Levels of other vitamins are much lower.
- *Alcohol helps you sleep.* No. Alcohol disrupts sleep patterns, leading to a restless, unsatisfying sleep.

- *Laboratory animals love to drink.* No. Alcohol is usually given by tube feeding because most animals refuse to drink it willingly.
- *It's good to have a beer before breastfeeding.* No. Alcohol may be relaxing and allow milk to flow more readily, but alcohol concentrations in breast milk are similar to those in the mother's blood. Alcohol in breast milk reduces milk production by reducing the intensity of the infant's suckling.

Folate, thiamin, and vitamin A are most often affected by alcoholism. Folate deficiency contributes to malabsorption, anemia, and nerve damage— all of which worsen malnutrition. Vitamin A deficiency also creates a vicious cycle by damaging gastrointestinal lining and by impairing immunity, leaving the victim susceptible to infections. Thiamin deficiency contributes to classic diseases of alcoholism: the brain damage of Wernicke-Korsakoff syndrome, polyneuropathy (nerve inflammation), and cardiomyopathy (heart inflammation). Alcoholics can have overt scurvy from vitamin C deficiency. Vitamin $B_6$ and vitamin $B_{12}$ deficiencies are less common.

Alcohol metabolism interferes with the normal metabolism of vitamins and other nutrients. For example, metabolism of ethanol uses up the dehydrogenase enzyme that is also used for metabolism of retinol.[54] Retinol (vitamin A) uses that enzyme for its conversion to other active forms of vitamin A, and the disruption of its metabolism is probably one way that alcohol increases cancer risk. The same disruption may produce fetal birth defects when pregnant women drink.

Alcohol-induced fat malabsorption and metabolic abnormalities contribute to the depletion of fat-soluble vitamins A, D, E, and K. Blood-clotting factors drop with depleted vitamin K, increasing risk of bleeding and anemia. Vitamin E deficiency is not generally recognized as a complication of alcoholism, but its depletion due to fat malabsorption is possible. Optimal vitamin E status is necessary to quench free radicals generated during alcohol metabolism.[55]

## Mineral Deficiencies

Alcoholics are commonly deficient in minerals such as calcium, magnesium, iron, and zinc. Alcohol itself does not seem to affect their absorption. Rather,

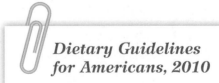

*Dietary Guidelines for Americans, 2010*

**Key Recommendation**
- If alcohol is consumed, it should be consumed in moderation—up to one drink per day for women and two drinks per day for men—and only by adults of legal drinking age.

fluid losses and an inadequate diet are the primary culprits. Magnesium deficiency causes "shakes" similar to that seen in alcohol withdrawal. Chronic diarrhea and loss of epithelial tissue (caused by skin rashes or sloughing off of the digestive lining) may seriously deplete zinc, a mineral needed for immune function. In cases of bleeding, especially gastrointestinal blood loss, iron levels fall.

Not all minerals are lower in heavy drinkers than in nondrinkers. If there is no bleeding, a heavy drinker's iron levels tend to be higher than normal in the blood and liver, potentially contributing to harmful oxidation. Copper and nickel levels also may be elevated in advancing disease, but the reason and the effects are unclear.[56]

## Macronutrients

Animal experiments can demonstrate a number of ways that alcohol alters digestion and metabolism of carbohydrate, fat, and protein, but the relevance to humans at usual levels of intake is not certain. Alcohol interferes with amino acid absorption, but its overall effect on protein balance appears minimal. It inhibits gluconeogenesis and lowers blood glucose levels, probably contributing to hangovers and, at the most extreme, causing acute, potentially lethal hypoglycemia if a person who drinks heavily neglects to eat.[57]

Alcohol's most dramatic effect is on fats. You have seen that alcohol causes fatty liver. On the one hand, excess alcohol has the undesirable effect of raising blood triglyceride levels, often significantly. Hyperlipidemia (high blood fats) is common among heavy drinkers. Abstinence and a balanced diet can usually return blood lipids to normal.[58] On the other hand, moderate alcohol use increases protective high-density lipoproteins (HDL, or "good cholesterol"), an important factor in alcohol's relationship to the reduced risk for coronary artery disease.

## Body Weight

Although alcoholic beverages provide minimal nutrient value, they do provide calories; alcohol contains 7 kilocalories per gram. Does alcohol consumption contribute to obesity? It appears likely. In an analysis of data collected from more than 37,000 people, researchers found that overweight drinkers consumed more drinks than leaner drinkers on the days that they drank.[59] Men and women who infrequently consume the greatest quantity of alcohol weigh more than those who frequently drink small amounts. Because smoking and drinking interact to influence body weight, the researchers looked only at current drinkers who had never smoked.

Drinking patterns are important. Alcohol consumption consists of two components: (1) the amount consumed on drinking days (quantity) and (2) how often drinking days occur (frequency). Although previous studies of the relation between drinking alcohol and body weight have been inconsistent, these studies looked at average consumption. A given average volume, however, can result from widely varying drinking patterns. An average volume of 2 drinks per day, for example, may result from consuming 2 drinks every day, 4 drinks every other day, 14 drinks on one day per week, or 30 drinks on two days per month. Body weight is more sensitive to drinking patterns than average volume.

**Key Concepts**  *Alcohol interferes with normal nutrition by reducing the intake of nutrient-dense foods and by affecting the absorption, metabolism, and excretion of many vitamins and minerals. Alcohol contains a significant number of calories (7 kilocalories per gram), and heavy episodic drinkers tend to weigh more than light drinkers.*

# Does Alcohol Have Benefits?

Can a potentially harmful drink like alcohol play a role in a healthful diet? The consensus of health experts is that it can—but not for everyone. The question continues to arouse much debate, however, and even those supporting alcohol's usefulness often have reservations. Public health statements on alcohol are typically accompanied by plenty of "ifs" and "buts."

Consistent epidemiological evidence suggests that low to moderate drinking reduces mortality among some groups.[60] (Table SA.3 gives definitions of different levels of drinking.) Compared with nondrinkers or heavy drinkers, middle-aged and older adults who drink moderate amounts of alcohol have a lower risk of mortality from all causes.[61] This includes people with heart disease,[62] diabetes,[63] high blood pressure,[64] or a prior heart attack.[65]

**Table SA.3** **How Much Is Too Much?**

| Term | Criterion |
|---|---|
| Moderate drinking (NIAAA) | Men: ≤ 2 drinks per day<br>Women: ≤ 1 drink per day<br>Over 65: ≤ 1 drink per day |
| At-risk drinking (NIAAA) | Men: > 14 drinks per week or > 4 drinks per occasion<br>Women: > 7 drinks per week or > 3 drinks per occasion |
| Alcohol abuse (APA) | Maladaptive pattern of alcohol use leading to clinically significant impairment or distress, manifested within a 12-month period by one or more of the following:<br>• Failure to fulfill role obligations at work, school, or home<br>• Recurrent use in hazardous situations<br>• Legal problems related to alcohol<br>• Continued use despite alcohol-related social or interpersonal problems<br>• Symptoms have never met criteria for alcohol dependence |
| Alcohol dependence (APA) | Maladaptive pattern of alcohol use leading to clinically significant impairment or distress, manifested within a 12-month period by three or more of the following:<br>• Tolerance (either increasing amounts used or diminished effects with the same amount)<br>• Withdrawal (withdrawal symptoms or use to relieve or avoid symptoms)<br>• Use of larger amounts over a longer period than intended<br>• Persistent desire or unsuccessful attempts to cut down or control use<br>• Great deal of time spent obtaining or using or recovering from use<br>• Important social, occupational, or recreational activities given up or reduced<br>• Use despite knowledge of alcohol-related physical or psychological problems |
| Hazardous use (WHO) | Person at risk for adverse consequences |
| Harmful use (WHO) | Use resulting in physical or psychological harm |

**Note:** NIAAA, National Institute on Alcohol Abuse and Alcoholism; APA, American Psychiatric Association; WHO, World Health Organization.

Research also suggests that moderate intake of alcohol can protect against other diseases, such as cancer, diabetes, inflammatory liver disease, and lower extremity arterial disease, as well as have positive effects on bone density in elderly women.[66] Consistent and growing evidence shows that alcohol reduces insulin resistance and may protect against heart disease by improving "good" cholesterol levels and reducing blood clotting.[67]

No evidence has suggested that moderate drinking harmed the people in the studies. In fact, analysis of data from the Nurses' Health Study, which involves more than 12,000 participants, suggests that in women, up to one drink per day does not impair mental functioning and may actually decrease the risk of mental decline with age.[68]

Tracked against alcohol intake, death rates typically follow what statisticians describe as a "U-shaped" curve. Compared with people who rarely or never drink, people who drink slightly or moderately have lower total mortality rates. The lowest rate is seen in people who consume one drink per week. Increasing the number of drinks confers no additional benefit. In fact, as the number of drinks increases, the mortality rate rises. People who consume two drinks per day have about the same mortality rate as nondrinkers.[69] Beyond three drinks per day, the death rate rises dramatically.[70] Heavy alcohol consumption increases the risk of stroke, for example, whereas light or moderate drinking appears to reduce that risk.[71] Alcohol's primary benefit is to raise protective HDL cholesterol levels. It may also inhibit formation of blood clots, but this connection is less clear.[72] In addition, alcohol may have subjective benefits such as stress relief and relaxation.

In most studies, wine, beer, and spirits appear equal in offering protection against heart disease. Findings of reduced rates of nonfatal heart attacks among moderate drinkers support the view that protective benefits are due to alcohol itself rather than other substances in alcoholic beverages.[73] However, international comparisons that highlight unexpectedly low rates of heart disease in France, despite a high-fat diet (the **French paradox**), suggest that red wine may have a unique protective effect. The apparent benefits of red wine may result from overall healthier behavior of people who drink red wine. As yet, a direct connection between red wine and health benefits remains unproven.[74] Nevertheless, recognizing that alcohol generally confers moderate protection and noting the possibility that wine has a particular benefit, the Bureau of Alcohol, Tobacco, and Firearms granted permission for wine labels to include one of the following statements:[75]

- "The proud people who made this wine encourage you to consult your family doctor about the health effects of wine consumption."
- "To learn the health effects of wine consumption, send for the Federal Government's *Dietary Guidelines for Americans. . . .*"

Because of the many harmful effects of alcohol (see **Figure SA.15**), public health agencies and organizations caution against inappropriate drinking. Although low to moderate alcohol use may offer some benefit, these groups advise people to discuss their alcohol intake with their doctors, and they urge moderation. The U.S. Preventive Services Task Force recommends that primary care doctors routinely screen patients for unhealthy alcohol use and, when appropriate, intervene with a brief counseling session to reduce alcohol misuse.[76] Public health officials also point out that numerous groups should not drink any alcohol:[77]

- People who cannot restrict their alcohol intake to moderate levels
- Anyone younger than the legal drinking age
- People taking prescription or over-the-counter medications that can interact with alcohol

**French paradox** The phenomenon observed in the French, who have a lower incidence of heart disease than people whose diets contain comparable amounts of fat. Part of the difference has been attributed to the regular and moderate drinking of red wine.

- People who have an alcohol-related illness or another illness that will be worsened by alcohol, such as liver disease, hypertriglyceridemia, or pancreatitis
- People who plan to drive, operate machinery, or take part in other activities that require attention, skill, or coordination or participate in situations where impaired judgment could cause injury or death (e.g., swimming)
- Women who are pregnant or may become pregnant
- Women who are breastfeeding
- People with a personal or strong family history of alcoholism

**American Heart Association**

**Alcohol**

If you drink alcohol, do so in moderation. This means an average of one to two drinks per day for men and one drink per day for women. Drinking more alcohol increases such dangers as alcoholism, high blood pressure, obesity, stroke, breast cancer, suicide, and accidents. Also, it's not possible to predict in which people alcoholism will become a problem. Given these and other risks, the American Heart Association cautions people NOT to start drinking . . . if they do not already drink alcohol. Consult your doctor on the benefits and risks of consuming alcohol in moderation.

**Source:** Reproduced with permission, www.heart.org, © 2011 American Heart Association, Inc.

**Addiction**
Alcohol addiction destroys lives, families, and communities. Researchers are trying to learn why some people, and not others, become addicted.

**Accidents and violence**
These result from impairment of mental function and coordination.

**Birth defects**
Fetal alcohol syndrome can occur when pregnant women drink.

**Emotional and social**
Emotional, social, and economic problems are associated with heavy drinking.

**Cardiomyopathy**
Inflammation of the heart muscle is much more common in heavy drinkers.

**Brain**
Acute effect is drunkenness. Long-term effects of chronic alcohol excess are dementia, memory loss, and generalized impairment of mental function.

**Liver disease**
Heavy drinking can lead to alcoholic fatty liver, alcoholic hepatitis, cirrhosis, and liver cancer.

**Gastritis**
Continued contact with excess alcohol irritates and inflames the stomach lining.

**Pancreatitis**
Both chronic and acute pancreatitis are increased by alcoholism.

**Cancer**
Excess alcohol increases the risk of gastrointestinal, liver, and breast cancers. Smoking further increases these risks.

**Anemia**
Heavy drinkers often have poor diets and may bleed from the digestive tract.

**Osteoporosis**
Heavy drinking contributes to bone loss, especially in older women.

**Peripheral neuropathy**
Painful nerve inflammation in hands, arms, feet, and legs is common in long-time heavy alcohol users.

**Figure SA.15**  **Harmful effects of alcohol.** Because excess alcohol reaches all parts of the body, it causes a wide array of physical problems. Here are some of the ways alcohol can harm.

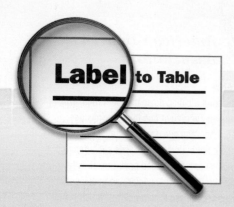

Have you ever wondered how much protein, carbohydrate, and fat are in a can of beer? If you've ever looked at a beer label, you know it's quite different from a food label. Look at the following information from a can of light beer and see if you can calculate the calories from carbohydrate, fat, and protein.

Serving size = 12 fl oz
Calories = 103 (kcal)
Carbohydrate = 5 g
Protein = 1 g
Fat = 0 g

First, to figure out how many calories come from the three macronutrients, multiply the number of grams by their respective calorie contribution per gram:

5 g carbohydrate × 4 kcal/g = 20 kcal from carbohydrate
1 g protein × 4 kcal/g = 4 kcal from protein
0 g fat × 9 kcal/g = 0 kcal from fat

Uh oh. Is this adding up correctly? So far we have accounted for only 24 of the 103 kilocalories in this beer. Where are the other 79 kilocalories? Don't forget that many of the calories in beer come from alcohol, and it's easy to calculate just how many grams are in this can of light beer. Remember, alcohol has 7 kilocalories per gram, so the remaining 79 kilocalories come from 11 grams of alcohol (79 ÷ 7 = 11.3).

So, for the 103 kilocalories this beer provides, you get very little (if any) protein, carbohydrate, or fat. Instead, a majority of the calories come from alcohol. This holds true for the micronutrients as well—beer contains negligible amounts of vitamins or minerals.

This is why people say alcoholic beverages have only "empty calories." They provide calories but almost no nutrient value!

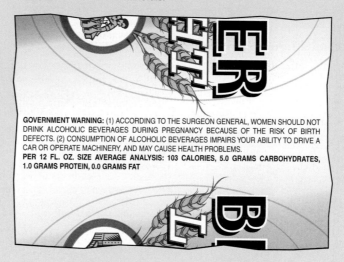

GOVERNMENT WARNING: (1) ACCORDING TO THE SURGEON GENERAL, WOMEN SHOULD NOT DRINK ALCOHOLIC BEVERAGES DURING PREGNANCY BECAUSE OF THE RISK OF BIRTH DEFECTS. (2) CONSUMPTION OF ALCOHOLIC BEVERAGES IMPAIRS YOUR ABILITY TO DRIVE A CAR OR OPERATE MACHINERY, AND MAY CAUSE HEALTH PROBLEMS. PER 12 FL. OZ. SIZE AVERAGE ANALYSIS: 103 CALORIES, 5.0 GRAMS CARBOHYDRATES, 1.0 GRAMS PROTEIN, 0.0 GRAMS FAT

## *Quick* Bite

### A What?
An oenologist is an expert in the science of wine and wine making.

**Key Concepts** *Although alcohol has the potential to reduce risk for heart disease, most health organizations recommend moderate to no drinking. It is too early in the scientific investigation of alcohol's benefits to recommend alcohol intake for all adults. Some people, such as pregnant women, should not drink any alcohol.*

# *Learning* Portfolio

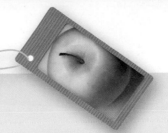

## Key Terms

## Study Points

- Alcohol provides 7 kilocalories per gram but no essential function for the body; therefore, alcohol is not a nutrient.

- Alcohol requires no digestion and is absorbed easily all along the gastrointestinal tract.

- Fatty liver is apparent even after one night of binge drinking.

- Different rates of alcohol metabolism can be attributed to different levels of the alcohol-metabolizing enzymes; these differences are due to genetic and gender variations.

- Alcohol affects all organs in the body, but the most obvious effects are in the brain and the nervous system, the GI system, and the liver.

- Malnutrition among alcoholics is common due to poor food choices and alcohol's interference with the absorption, metabolism, and excretion of nutrients.

- Fetal alcohol syndrome is one of the most devastating consequences of alcohol consumption, and it is preventable.

- Moderate alcohol consumption has been linked to reduced risk of heart disease.

- The potential benefits of moderate alcohol consumption may be related to effects on lipoprotein levels and the antioxidant components of beverages such as wine.

- Health organizations recommend moderate to no alcohol consumption.

## Study Questions

1. How much alcohol is in beer, wine, and liquor?
2. List the ways food helps to delay or avoid inebriation.
3. Where does alcohol metabolism take place?
4. What causes a hangover? Is there any way to relieve one?
5. List some factors that affect our ability to metabolize alcohol.
6. Why do healthcare professionals advise pregnant women not to drink alcohol?
7. List the positive and the negative effects of alcohol.

## Try This

### Cruising Through the Medicine Cabinet

This exercise will increase your awareness of the amounts of alcohol in over-the-counter medications. Look through your medicine cabinet and check the ingredient lists of all the products there. In particular, take a close look at any mouthwash or cough syrup. Which products contain alcohol? How much? What do you think its purpose is in these medicines?

## References

1. US Department of Agriculture and US Department of Health and Human Services. *Dietary Guidelines for Americans, 2010.* 7th ed. Washington, DC: US Government Printing Office; 2010.

2. Courtney KE, Polich J. Binge drinking in young adults: Data, definitions, and determinants. *Psychol Bull.* 2009;135(1):142–156.

3. Ham LS, Hope DA. Incorporating social anxiety into a model of college student problematic drinking. *Addict Behav.* 2005;30(1):127–150.

4. Johnston LD, O'Malley PM, Bachman JG. *Monitoring the Future: National Survey Results on Drug Use, 1975–2000.* Volume 1: Secondary School Students. Bethesda, MD: National Institute on Drug Abuse; 2001. NIH publication 01-4924.

5. National Institute on Alcohol Abuse and Alcoholism. *A Call to Action: Changing the Culture of Drinking at U.S. Colleges.* Bethesda, MD: NIAAA; 2002. NIH publication 02-5010; National Institute on Alcohol Abuse and Alcoholism (NIAAA). *Young Adult Drinking.* Bethesda, MD: NIAAA; 2006 Alcohol Alert No. 68; and NIAAA. *Underage Drinking. Why Do Adolescents Drink, What Are the Risks, and How Can Underage Drinking Be Prevented?* Bethesda, MD: NIAAA; 2006. Alcohol Alert No. 67.

6. Minino AM. *Mortality Among Teenagers Aged 12–19 Years: United States, 1999–2006.* Hyattsville, MD: National Center for Health Statistics, Data Brief No. 37; 2010.

7. National Institute on Alcohol Abuse and Alcoholism. *Underage Drinking.* Op. cit.

8. Presley CA, Meilman PW, Leichliter JS. College factors that influence drinking. *J Studies Alcohol.* 2002;(suppl 14):82–90.

9. Toomey TL, Wagenaar AC. Environmental policies to reduce college drinking: options and research findings. *J Studies Alcohol.* 2002;(suppl 14):193–205.

10. Paasma R, Hovda KE, Jacobsen D. Methanol poisoning and long-term sequelae—a six-year follow-up after a large methanol outbreak. *BMC Clin Pharmacol.* 2009;9:5.

11  Slutske WS. Alcohol use disorders among US college students and their non-college-attending peers. *Arch Gen Psychiatry*. 2005;62:321–327.

12  Haseba T, Ohno Y. A new view of alcohol metabolism and alcoholism—role of the high-$K_m$ class III alcohol dehydrogenase (ADH3). *Int J Environ Res Pub Health*. 2010;7(3):1076–1092.

13  Mitchinson A. Hangovers: uncongenial congeners. *Nature*. 2009;462(7276):992.

14  US Department of Agriculture and US Department of Health and Human Services. Op. cit.

15  Ibid.

16  Seitz HK, Oneta CM. Gastrointestinal alcohol dehydrogenase. *Nutr Rev*. 1998;56:52–60.

17  Zakhari S. Overview: How is alcohol metabolized by the body? *Alcohol Res Health*. 2006;29(4):245–254.

18  Pontes Ferreira M, Weems MKS. Alcohol consumption by aging adults in the United States: health benefits and detriments. *J Am Diet Assoc*. 2008;108(10):1668–1676.

19  Seitz HK, Oneta CM. Op. cit.

20  Ibid.

21  Verster JC, Penning R. Treatment and prevention of alcohol hangover. *Curr Drug Abuse Rev*. 2010;3(2):103–109.

22  Wiese J, McPherson S, Odden MC, et al. Effect of *Opuntia ficus indica* on symptoms of the alcohol hangover. *Arch Intern Med*. 2004;164:1334–1340.

23  Piasecki TM, Robertson BM, Epler AJ. Hangover and risk for alcohol use disorders: existing evidence and potential mechanisms. *Curr Drug Abuse Rev*. 2010;3(2):92–102.

24  Swift R, Davidson D. Alcohol hangover: mechanisms and mediators. *Alcohol Health Res World*. 1998;22:54–60.

25  Wiese JG, McPherson S, Odden MC, et al. Op. cit.; Verster JC, Penning R, Op. cit.

26  Ibid.

27  Fruchter LL, Alexopoulou I, Lau KK. Acute interstitial nephritis with acetaminophen and alcohol intoxication. *Ital J Pediatr*. 2011;15(37):17.

28  Ibid.

29  Nishimura FT, Kimura Y, Abe S, Fukunaga T, Minami J, Tanii H, Saijoh K. Effects of functional polymorphisms related to catecholaminergic systems on changes in blood catecholamine and cardiovascular measures after alcohol ingestion in the Japanese population. *Alcohol Clin Exp Res*. 2008;32(11):1937–1946.

30  Vallee BL. Alcohol in the Western world. *Scientific American*. June 1998;80–85.

31  National Institute on Alcohol Abuse and Alcoholism. *Alcohol and Aging*. Bethesda, MD: NIAAA; 1998. Alcohol Alert No. 40.

32  Dufour MC. What is moderate drinking? *Alcohol Res Health*. 1999;23(1):1–14.

33  US Department of Health and Human Services and US Department of Agriculture. Op. cit.

34  National Institute on Alcohol Abuse and Alcoholism. *Alcohol—An Important Women's Health Issue*. Bethesda, MD: NIAAA; 2004. Alcohol Alert No. 62.

35  Swift R, Davidson D. Op. cit.

36  Baraona E, Abbittan CS, Dohmen K, et al. Gender differences in pharmacokinetics of alcohol. *Alcohol Clin Exp Res*. 2001;25:502–507.

37  Pinel JP. *Biopsychology*. Boston: Allyn & Bacon; 2006.

38  Friedman TW, Robinson SR, Yelland GW. Impaired perceptual judgment at low blood alcohol concentrations. *Alcohol*. 2011;45(7):711–718.

39  National Institutes of Health. *Hypoglycemia*. Bethesda, MD: NIH; 2006. NIH Publication No. 03-3926.

40  Parada M, Corral M, Caamano-Isorna F, et al. Binge drinking and declarative memory in university students. *Alcohol Clin Exp Res*. 2011;35(8):1475–1484.

41  Boffetta P, Hashibe M. Alcohol and cancer. *Lancet Oncol*. 2006;7(2):149–156.

42  Centers for Disease Control and Prevention. FastStats. Chronic Liver Disease or Cirrhosis. http://www.cdc.gov/nchs/fastats/liverdis.htm. Accessed 5/22/11.

43  Lieber CS. Alcoholic fatty liver: its pathogenesis and mechanism of progression to inflammation and fibrosis. *Alcohol*. 2004;34(1):9–19.

44  Dey A, Cederbaum AI. Alcohol and oxidative liver damage. *Hepatology*. 2006;43(2 suppl.):S63–S74.

45  University of Maryland Medical Center. Liver disease: alcohol-induced liver disease. http://www.umm.edu/liver/alcohol.htm. Accessed 5/22/11.

46  Ibid.

47  Teli MR, Day CP, Burt AD, et al. Determinants of progression to cirrhosis or fibrosis in pure alcoholic fatty liver. *Lancet*. 1995;346:987–990.

48  Identification of children with fetal alcohol syndrome and opportunity for referral of their mother for primary prevention, Washington, 1993–1997. *MMWR*. 1998;47:861–864.

49  Thompson BL, Levitt P, Stanwood GD. Prenatal exposure to drugs: effects on brain development and implications for policy and education. *Neuroscience*. 2009;10(4):303–312.

50  Alcohol consumption among pregnant and childbearing-aged women—United States, 2002. *MMWR*. 2004;53:1178–1181.

51  Centers for Disease Control and Prevention. Fetal Alcohol Spectrum Disorders (FASDs). http://www.cdc.gov/ncbddd/fasd/data.html. Accessed 5/21/11.

52  Breslow RA, Guenther PM, Juan W, Graubard B. Alcoholic beverage consumption, nutrient intakes, and diet quality in the US adult population, 1999–2006. *J Am Diet Assoc*. 2010;110(4):551–562.

53  Harrop EN, Marlatt GA. The comorbidity of substance use disorders and eating disorders in women: Prevalence, etiology, and treatment. *Addict Behav*. 2010;35(5):392–398.

54  Seitz HK, Oneta CM. Op. cit.; and Wang XD. Chronic alcohol intake interferes with retinoid metabolism and signaling. *Nutr Rev*. 1999;57:51–59.

55  Lieber CS. Nutrition and diet in alcoholism. In: Shils ME, Olson JA, Shike M, eds. *Modern Nutrition in Health and Disease*. 10th ed. Philadelphia: Lippincott Williams & Wilkins; 2005.

56  Ibid.

57  Ibid.

58  Ibid.

59  Pontes Ferreira M, Weems MKS. Op. cit.

60  Klatsky AL. Should patients with heart disease drink alcohol? *JAMA*. 2001;285:2004–2006; and Doll R, Peto R, Boreham J, Sutherland I. Mortality in relation to alcohol consumption: a prospective study among male British doctors. *Int J Epidemiol*. 2005;34:199–204.

61  Pontes Ferreira M, Weems MKS. Op. cit.

62  Klatsky AL. Op. cit.

63  Ajani UA, Gaziano JM, Lotufo PA, et al. Alcohol consumption and risk of coronary heart disease by diabetes status. *Circulation*. 2000;102:500–505; and Solomon CG, Hu FB, Stampfer MJ, et al. Moderate alcohol consumption and risk of coronary heart disease among women with type 2 diabetes mellitus. *Circulation*. 2000;102:494–499.

64  Malinski MK, Sesso HD, Lopez-Jimenez F, et al. Alcohol consumption and cardiovascular mortality in hypertensive patients. Paper presented at 41st Annual Conference on Cardiovascular Disease Epidemiology and Prevention; March 2, 2001; San Antonio, TX.

65  Muntwyler J, Hennekens CH, Buring JE, et al. Mortality and light to moderate alcohol consumption after myocardial infarction. *Lancet*. 1998;352:1882–1885.

66  Pontes Ferreira M, Weems MKS. Op. cit.

67  Fagrell B, De Faire U, Bondy S, et al. The effects of light to moderate drinking on cardiovascular diseases. *J Intern Med*. 1999;246:331–340; and Paoletti R, Klatsky AL, Poli A, Zahari S, eds. *Moderate Alcohol Consumption and Cardiovascular Disease*. Dordrecht: Kluwer; 2000.

68  Stampfer MJ, Kand JH, Chen J, et al. Effects of moderate alcohol consumption on cognitive function in women. *N Engl J Med*. 2005;352:245–253.

69  Gaziano JM, Gaziano TA, Glynn RJ, et al. Light-to-moderate alcohol consumption and mortality in the Physicians' Health Study enrollment cohort. *J Am Coll Cardiol*. 2000;35:96–105.

70  Pearson TA. Alcohol and heart disease. *Circulation*. 1996;94:3023–3025.

71  Reynolds K, Lewis BL, Nolen JD, et al. Alcohol consumption and risk of stroke. *JAMA*. 2003;289:579–588.

72  Van Horn L, McMoin M, Kris-Etherton PM, et al. The evidence for dietary prevention and treatment of cardiovascular disease. *J Am Diet Assoc*. 2008;108(2):287–331.

73  Ibid.

74  Peregrin T. Wine—a drink to your health? *J Am Diet Assoc*. 2005;105(7):1053–1054.

75  Treasury announces actions concerning labeling of alcoholic beverages. US Treasury Department, Bureau of Alcohol, Tobacco and Firearms press release; February 5, 1999.

76  Saitz R. Unhealthy alcohol use. *N Engl J Med*. 2005;352:596–607.

77  US Department of Health and Human Services and US Department of Agriculture. Op. cit.

# CHAPTER 6

# Lipids:
# Not Just Fat

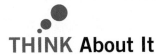

## THINK About It

1    How important is fat to the foods you find tasty?

2    What's your view about the value of body fat?

3    What's your take on the differences between fat and cholesterol?

4    What's your understanding of "good" versus "bad" cholesterol?

**Visit** go.jblearning.com/
inseldisco4e

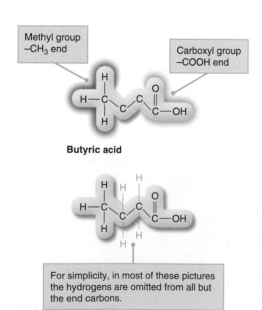

**Fat**

Triglycerides (fat)

Sterols

Phospholipids

Glycerols

**Water**

Maria and Rachel are trying to lose weight. Maria swears by a new diet program that allows you to eat all the fat you want but no high-carbohydrate, "starchy" foods. Her new diet is working—she's already lost 10 pounds! Then there's Rachel, whose goal in life is to eat zero grams of fat. She's fat-obsessed—insisting on "fat-free" everything and driving her friends nuts with information about the number of fat grams in whatever they eat. As you listen to the two of them compare dieting stories, you wonder which one has the right approach to fat consumption—or even if there is a right approach. On one hand, it seems you hear about American high-fat diets and high rates of obesity and heart disease. On the other hand, can a "no-fat" diet be healthy? Are all low-fat and no-fat products really more nutritious?

Fat is an essential nutrient that provides energy and helps transport fat-soluble nutrients to destinations throughout the body. Triglycerides—the fats we associate with fried foods, cream cheese, vegetable oil, or salad dressing—are one type of a larger group of compounds called lipids. Cholesterol, another lipid, is familiar to most Americans, but you may not realize that your body makes cholesterol and that the cholesterol you eat contributes only a small portion of the total amount in your body. All lipids have important roles, but at the same time, too much triglyceride or too much cholesterol can increase the risk for chronic disease.

Fats contribute greatly to the flavor and texture of foods. When food manufacturers remove fat to produce a low-fat product, they often have to boost the flavor with sugar, sodium, or other additives to create a tasty product. This means that fat-free foods sometimes aren't any lower in calories than regular food—so Rachel can't eat the whole box of fat-free cookies and still expect to lose weight!

THINK
About It

1

## What Are Lipids?

The term *lipids* applies to a variety of substances, including triglycerides, phospholipids, and sterols. Triglycerides are the most abundant lipid. In the body, fat cells store triglycerides in adipose tissue. In foods, we call triglycerides "fats and oils," with fats usually being solid and oils being liquid at room temperature. Overall, however, the choice of terms—fat, triglyceride, oil—is somewhat arbitrary, and these words often are used interchangeably. In this chapter, when we use the word *fat* or *oil*, we are referring to triglycerides.

About 2 percent of dietary lipids are phospholipids. They are found in foods of both plant and animal origin, and the body can make them. Unlike other lipids, phospholipids are soluble in both fat and water. These versatile molecules play crucial roles as major components of cell membranes and in blood and body fluids, where they help keep fats suspended.

Only a small percentage of our dietary lipids are sterols, yet one infamous member, cholesterol, causes much public concern. The body makes cholesterol, which is an important component of cell membranes and a precursor of sex hormones, adrenal hormones (e.g., cortisol), vitamin D, and bile salts.

## Fatty Acids Are Key Building Blocks

Fatty acids determine the characteristics of a fat, such as whether it is solid or liquid at room temperature. The basic structure of a fatty acid is a chain of carbon atoms with a carboxyl (acid) group (–COOH) at one end and a methyl group (–CH$_3$) at the other end. (See **Figure 6.1**.) Fatty acids that are not attached to other compounds are sometimes called "free" fatty acids. Some free fatty acids have their own distinct flavor. Butyric acid, for example, gives butter its flavor. Caproic, caprylic, and capric acids, all named after the Greek word for "goat," have the undesirable "goaty" flavors and odors that their names suggest. These "goaty" fatty acids contribute to the strong unpleasant odor of spoiled foods.

Methyl group
–CH$_3$ end

Carboxyl group
–COOH end

**Butyric acid**

For simplicity, in most of these pictures the hydrogens are omitted from all but the end carbons.

**Figure 6.1**   **Fatty acid structure.** The basic structure of a fatty acid is a carbon chain with a methyl end (–CH$_3$) and an acid (carboxyl) end (–COOH). Butyric acid (shown here) is a fatty acid found in butter fat.

## Chain Length

Fatty acids differ in **chain length** (the number of carbons in the chain). Foods contain fatty acids with chain lengths of 4 to 24 carbons, and most have an even number of carbons. Fatty acids are grouped as short-chain (fewer than 6 carbons), medium-chain (6 to 10 carbons), and long-chain (12 or more carbons). (See **Figure 6.2**.) The shorter the carbon chain, the more liquid the fatty acid becomes (the lower its melting point). (See **Figure 6.3**.) Shorter

**chain length** The number of carbons that a fatty acid contains. Foods contain fatty acids with chain lengths of 4 to 24 carbons, and most have an even number of carbons.

**Short-chain fatty acid**
(2–4 carbons)

Butyric acid C4:0

**Medium-chain fatty acid**
(6–10 carbons)

Caprylic acid C8:0

**Long-chain fatty acid**
(12 or more carbons)

Palmitic acid C16:0

**Very-long-chain fatty acid**
(20 or more carbons)

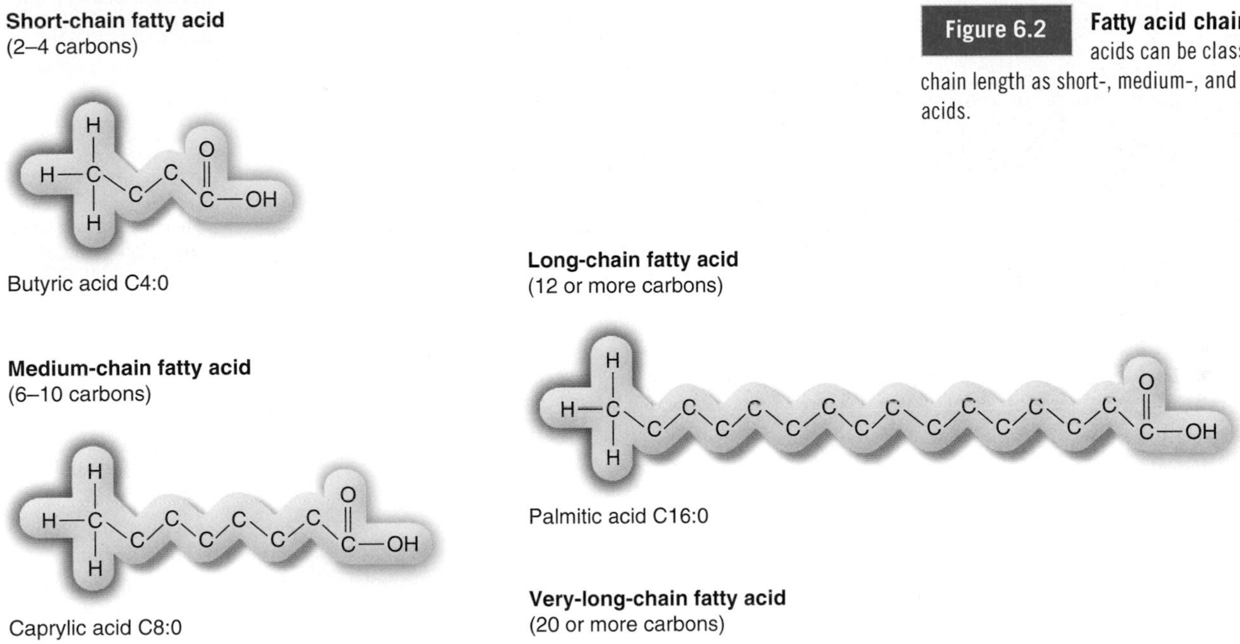

**Figure 6.2** **Fatty acid chain lengths.** Fatty acids can be classified by their chain length as short-, medium-, and long-chain fatty acids.

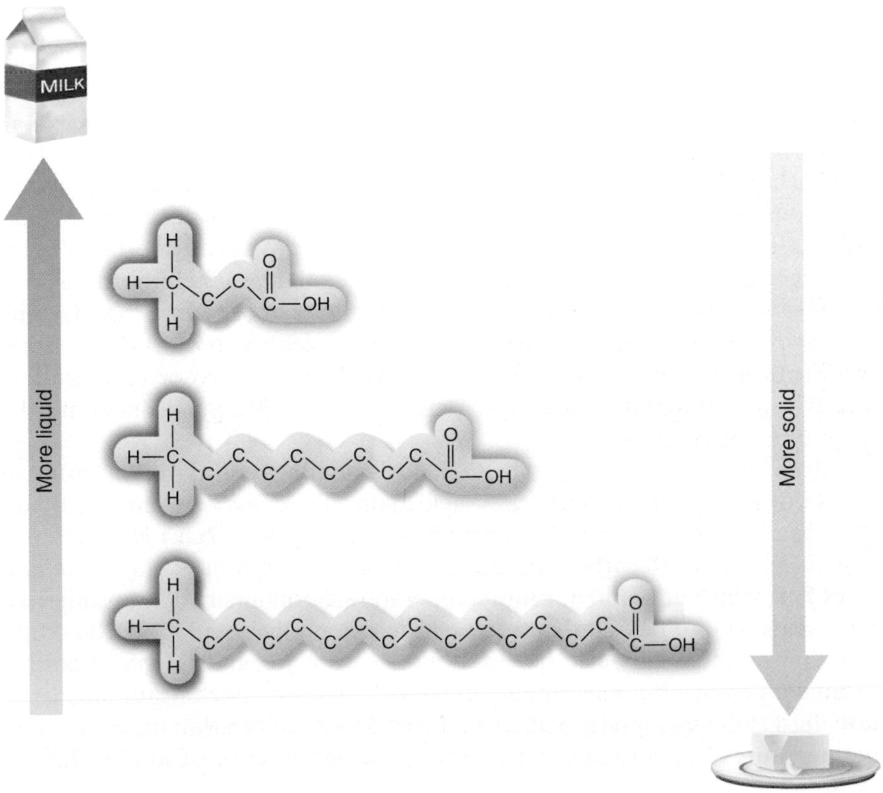

**Figure 6.3** **Fatty acid chain lengths and liquidity.** As the chain length of saturated fatty acids increase, fats tend to become more solid at room temperature.

More liquid

More solid

MILK

**Type of fatty acid**                    **Name and chemical structure**

Saturated

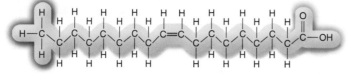

Stearic acid

Monounsaturated

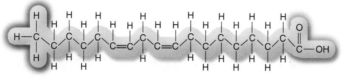

Oleic acid

Polyunsaturated

Linoleic acid

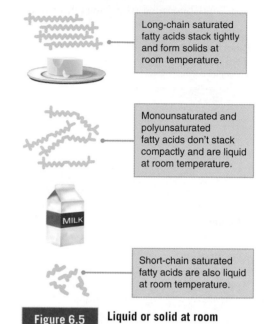

Long-chain saturated fatty acids stack tightly and form solids at room temperature.

Monounsaturated and polyunsaturated fatty acids don't stack compactly and are liquid at room temperature.

Short-chain saturated fatty acids are also liquid at room temperature.

**Figure 6.4**    **Saturated, monounsaturated, and polyunsaturated fatty acids.** Hydrogens saturate the carbon chain of a saturated fatty acid. Unsaturated fatty acids have fewer hydrogens and have one (mono) or more (poly) carbon–carbon double bonds.

**Figure 6.5**    **Liquid or solid at room temperature?** Short-chain and unsaturated fatty acids cannot pack tightly together and tend to be more liquid than long-chain saturated fatty acids.

**saturated fatty acid** A fatty acid completely filled by hydrogen, with all carbons in the chain linked by single bonds.

**unsaturated fatty acid** A fatty acid in which the carbon chain contains one or more double bonds.

**monounsaturated fatty acid** A fatty acid in which the carbon chain contains one double bond.

**polyunsaturated fatty acid** A fatty acid in which the carbon chain contains two or more double bonds.

**linoleic acid [lin-oh-LAY-ik]** An essential *omega*-6 fatty acid that contains 18 carbon atoms and 2 carbon–carbon double bonds (18:2); a thin liquid at room temperature.

**conjugated linoleic acid (CLA)** A polyunsaturated fatty acid in which the position of the double bonds has moved so that a single bond alternates with two double bonds.

fatty acids also are more water-soluble, a property that affects their absorption in the digestive tract.

## Saturation

The carbons in a fatty acid chain are attached to each other and to hydrogen atoms. If all the bonds between the carbon atoms in a fatty acid chain are single bonds (C–C), then the fatty acid is called a **saturated fatty acid**. Hydrogen atoms completely fill (saturate) all the other available bonding sites. If one or more bonds between carbon atoms is a double bond (C=C), the fatty acid is an **unsaturated fatty acid**. A fatty acid with one double bond is a **monounsaturated fatty acid** (MUFA); one with two or more double bonds is a **polyunsaturated fatty acid** (PUFA). **Figure 6.4** illustrates the three types of fatty acids.

Even though we refer to olive oil, for example, as a monounsaturated fat, food fats are a mixture of fatty acid types. Foods rich in saturated fatty acids tend to be solid at room temperature. (See **Figure 6.5**.) For example, stearic acid is an 18-carbon saturated fatty acid abundant in chocolate and meat fats, which are solid at room temperature. Food fats rich in unsaturated fatty acids tend to be liquid at room temperature. Oleic acid is an 18-carbon monounsaturated fatty acid plentiful in olive oil. Olive oil is a thick liquid at room temperature but may solidify under refrigeration. Polyunsaturated **linoleic acid** is the major fatty acid of soybean oil, which is a thin liquid at room temperature. One form of linoleic acid, **conjugated linoleic acid (CLA)**, is

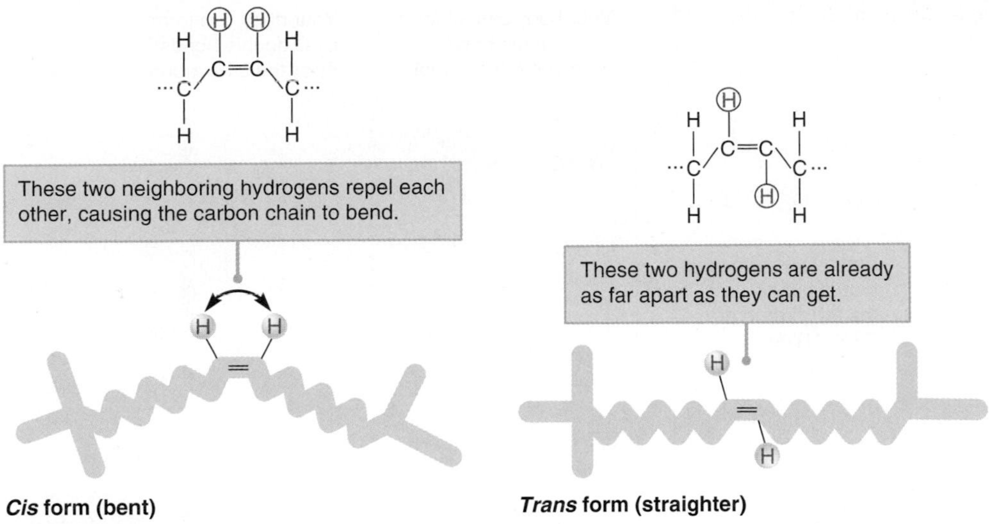

**Cis form (bent)**

**Trans form (straighter)**

These two neighboring hydrogens repel each other, causing the carbon chain to bend.

These two hydrogens are already as far apart as they can get.

| Figure 6.6 | *Cis* and *trans* **fatty acids.** Fatty acids with the bent *cis* form are more common in food than the *trans* form. *Trans* fatty acids most commonly are found in hydrogenated fats, such as those in stick margarine, shortening, and deep-fat-fried foods. |

under study for potential anticancer benefits.[1] Another polyunsaturated fatty acid, **alpha-linolenic acid** (don't confuse linole_n_ic with linoleic), is abundant in flaxseed oil, a very thin liquid at room temperature.

**Key Concepts** *The term* lipids *refers to a group of substances that includes triglycerides, phospholipids, and sterols. Fatty acids are key building blocks of both triglycerides and phospholipids. Fatty acids are carbon chains of varying lengths. Fatty acids filled with hydrogen are called saturated, while those with missing hydrogen are unsaturated fatty acids.*

## *Cis* Versus *Trans*

Otherwise identical unsaturated **fatty acids** can have different shapes. The carbon chain of a ***cis* fatty acid** is bent, and the chain of a ***trans* fatty acid** is straighter. (See **Figure 6.6.**) Most naturally occurring unsaturated fatty acids are *cis* fatty acids. While there are small amounts of *trans* fatty acids in meats and dairy products from cows and sheep, a commercial process called **hydrogenation** creates most *trans* fatty acids in our diets. Hydrogenation adds hydrogen to an unsaturated fatty acid, making it more saturated. This process also straightens the fatty acid to a *trans* configuration. *Trans* fatty acids have been shown to raise LDL ("bad") cholesterol and lower HDL ("good") cholesterol levels. Because they can increase one's risk for heart disease, *trans* fatty acids have become a health concern.

## Nonessential and Essential Fatty Acids

The body is a good chemist, synthesizing many fatty acids as needed. Because it is not essential to have these fatty acids in your diet, they are called **nonessential fatty acids**. Don't confuse "nonessential" with "unimportant"—you must have an adequate supply of nonessential fatty acids, either by making or eating them.

Because the body cannot make all types of fatty acids it needs, some must come from food. These fatty acids are called **essential fatty acids (EFAs)**. (See **Figure 6.7.**) There are two families of essential fatty acids: *omega*-**3**

**alpha-linolenic acid [al-fah-lin-oh-LEN-ik]** An essential *omega*-3 fatty acid that contains 18 carbon atoms and 3 carbon–carbon double bonds (18:3).

**fatty acids** Compounds containing a long hydrocarbon chain with a carboxyl group (–COOH) at one end and a methyl group (–$CH_3$) at the other end.

***cis* fatty acid** An unsaturated fatty acid with a bent carbon chain. Most naturally occurring unsaturated fatty acids are *cis* fatty acids.

***trans* fatty acid** An unsaturated fatty acid with a straighter chain than a *cis* fatty acid, usually as a result of hydrogenation; *trans* fatty acids are more solid than *cis* fatty acids.

**hydrogenation [high-dro-jen-AY-shun]** A chemical reaction in which hydrogen atoms are added to a fat; hydrogenation produces more saturated fatty acids and converts some unsaturated fatty acids from a *cis* form to a *trans* form.

**nonessential fatty acids** Fatty acids that your body can make when they are needed. It is not necessary to consume them in the diet.

**essential fatty acids (EFAs)** Fatty acids that the body needs but cannot synthesize and must obtain from the diet.

***omega*-3 fatty acid** An essential fatty acid; alpha-linolenic acid is the major type.

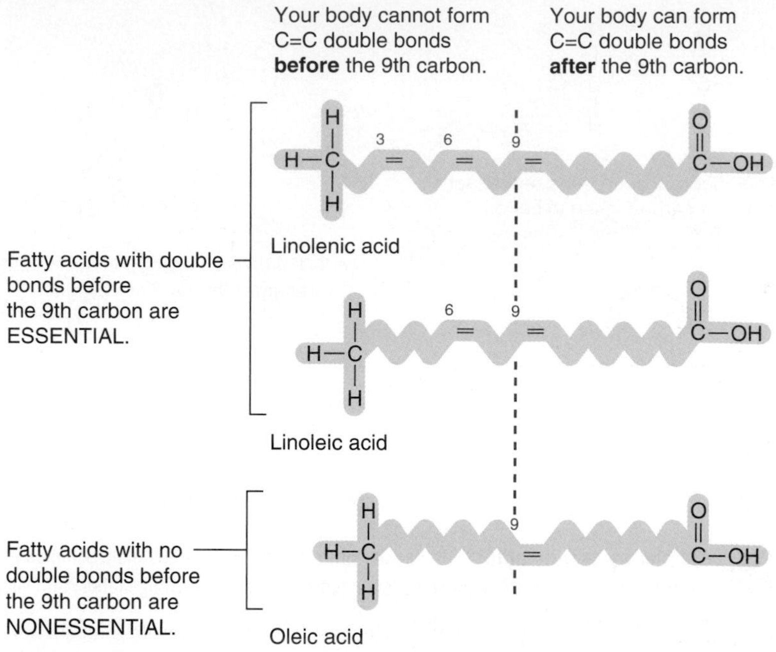

Your body cannot form C=C double bonds **before** the 9th carbon.

Your body can form C=C double bonds **after** the 9th carbon.

Fatty acids with double bonds before the 9th carbon are ESSENTIAL.

Linolenic acid

Linoleic acid

Fatty acids with no double bonds before the 9th carbon are NONESSENTIAL.

Oleic acid

**Figure 6.7** **Essential and nonessential fatty acids.** Your body makes some types of fatty acids, but others are essential in your diet.

*omega*-**6 fatty acid** An essential fatty acid; linoleic acid is the primary type.

**eicosanoids** A class of hormonelike substances formed in the body from long-chain essential fatty acids.

and ***omega*-6**. These numbers refer to the location of the first double bond in these unsaturated fatty acids, counting from the carbon in the methyl (*omega*) end. Alpha-linolenic is the major *omega*-3 fatty acid, and linoleic is the major *omega*-6 fatty acid. Arachidonic acid, a longer *omega*-6 fatty acid, was once thought to be essential, but our bodies can make it from linoleic acid.

Essential fatty acids deficiency is extremely rare. It typically occurs only with severe fat malabsorption or prolonged intravenous feeding without supplemental fat. A lack of linoleic acid leads to a scaly skin rash and dermatitis, poor growth in children, and a lowered immune response. In the few human cases where alpha-linolenic acid was lacking, neuropathy, visual problems, and poor growth were the results.[2]

Essential fatty acids are precursors to hormonelike compounds called **eicosanoids**. Eicosanoids formed from the *omega*-6 fatty acid arachidonic acid can increase blood pressure, heart rate, blood clotting, immune response, and inflammation. Eicosanoids formed from the *omega*-3 fatty acid alpha-linolenic acid have opposing "heart healthy" effects.

**Key Concepts** *Unsaturated fatty acids can have* cis *or* trans *double bonds. The body can make many, but not all, types of the fatty acids it needs. A fatty acid the body can make is a nonessential fatty acid, and one that must come from the diet is an essential fatty acid.*

## Triglycerides

Triglycerides are the major lipids in the diet and in the body. Triglycerides add flavor and texture (and calories!) to foods and are an important source of energy.

### Triglyceride Structure

Most fatty acids in food and in the body exist as part of a triglyceride molecule. A triglyceride consists of three fatty acids attached to a glycerol backbone.

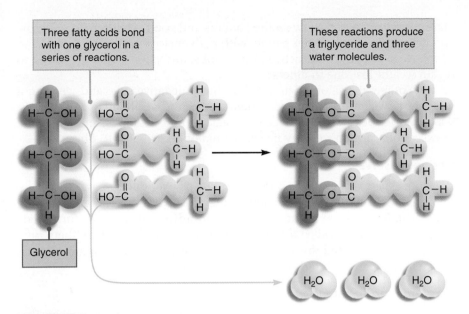

Three fatty acids bond with one glycerol in a series of reactions.

These reactions produce a triglyceride and three water molecules.

Glycerol

$H_2O$  $H_2O$  $H_2O$

**Figure 6.8**  **Forming a triglyceride.** Reactions attach three fatty acids to a glycerol backbone to form a triglyceride. These reactions release water.

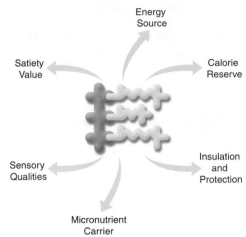

Energy Source

Satiety Value

Calorie Reserve

Sensory Qualities

Insulation and Protection

Micronutrient Carrier

**Figure 6.9**  **Functions of triglycerides.** Fat performs a number of essential functions in the body.

Alone, **glycerol** is a thick, smooth liquid often used by the food industry. **Figure 6.8** illustrates the formation of a triglyceride.

Two fatty acids attached to a glycerol form a **diglyceride**. A **monoglyceride** has one fatty acid attached to glycerol. Our foods contain relatively small amounts of mono- and diglycerides, mostly as food additives used for their emulsifying or blending qualities.

**glycerol [GLISS-er-ol]** The backbone of mono-, di-, and triglycerides; alone, it is a thick, smooth liquid.

**diglyceride** A molecule of glycerol combined with two fatty acids.

**monoglyceride** A molecule of glycerol combined with one fatty acid.

## Triglyceride Functions

Although some of us, like Rachel at the beginning of this chapter, think of fat as something to avoid, fat is a key nutrient with important body functions. **Figure 6.9** shows the functions of triglycerides.

### Energy Source

Fat is a rich and efficient source of calories. Under normal circumstances, dietary and stored fats supply about 60 percent of the body's resting energy needs. Like carbohydrate, fat is protein-sparing; that is, fat is burned for energy, saving valuable proteins for their important roles as muscle tissue, enzymes, antibodies, and the like. Different body tissues prefer different sources of calories. While muscle tissue at rest prefers to burn fat (see **Figure 6.10**), brain cells rely almost exclusively on glucose except during prolonged starvation. During physical activity, glucose and glycogen join fat in supplying energy to muscles.

High-fat foods are higher in calories than either high-protein or high-carbohydrate foods. One gram of fat contains 9 kilocalories, compared with only 4 kilocalories in a gram of carbohydrate or protein, or 7 kilocalories per gram of alcohol. For example, a tablespoon of corn oil (pure fat) has 120 kilocalories, whereas a tablespoon of sugar (pure carbohydrate) has only 50 kilocalories.

We welcome the high caloric density of fat when our energy needs are high. An infant, for example, who needs ample energy for fast growth but whose stomach can hold only a limited amount of food, needs the high-fat content of breast milk or infant formula to get enough calories. When

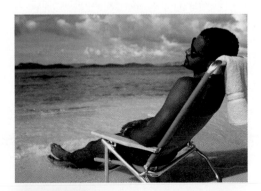

**Figure 6.10**  **Fat is an important energy source.** When at rest, muscles prefer to use fat for fuel.

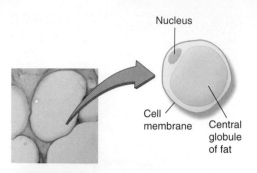

**Figure 6.11**    **Adipose cells store fat.** Adipocytes (fat cells) in adipose (fat) tissue store fat as an energy reserve. These are simple cells with just a nucleus, cell membrane, and fat droplet.

---

**adipocytes**  Fat cells.

**adipose tissue**  Body fat tissue.

**visceral fat**  Fat stores that cushion body organs.

**subcutaneous fat**  Fat stores under the skin.

**lanugo [lah-NEW-go]**  Soft, downy hair that covers a normal fetus from the fifth month but is shed almost entirely by the time of birth. It also appears on semistarved individuals who have lost much of their body fat, serving as insulation normally provided by body fat.

---

## *Quick* Bite

**The Marvelous Storage Efficiency of Fat**
Why do you think we don't store all our extra energy as readily available glycogen? It would take more than 6 pounds of glycogen to store the same energy as 1 pound of fat. Just imagine how much bulkier we would be! How cumbersome it would be to move about! That's why only a very small portion of the body's energy reserve is glycogen.

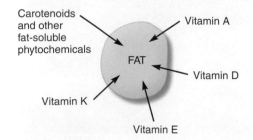

**Figure 6.12**    **Fat is a micronutrient carrier.** Fat holds more than just energy. It also carries important nutrients, such as fat-soluble vitamins and carotenoids.

---

inappropriately put on a low-fat diet, infants and young children do not grow and develop properly. Other people with high-energy needs include athletes, people who are physically active in their jobs, and people who are trying to regain weight lost due to illness.

Of course, the caloric density of fat has a negative side, and we do not welcome it when we are trying to maintain a healthy weight. In practical terms, 9 kilocalories per gram makes it easy to eat too many calories, and dietary fat in excess of a person's energy needs is a major contributor to obesity.

### Energy Reserve

We store excess dietary fat as body fat to tide us over during periods of calorie deficit. Because fat is calorie-dense, it can store a lot of energy in a small space. The fat is stored inside fat cells called **adipocytes**, which form body fat tissue, technically called **adipose tissue**. (See **Figure 6.11**.) Hibernating animals have perfected this process; the fat stores they build in autumn can see them through a winter's fast.

### Insulation and Protection

Fat tissue usually accounts for about 15 to 30 percent of body weight. Part of this is **visceral fat**, adipose tissue around organs. Visceral fat cushions and shields delicate organs, especially the kidneys. Women have extra fat, most noticeably in the breasts and hips, to help shield their reproductive organs and to guarantee adequate calories during pregnancy. Other fat tissue is **subcutaneous**, lying under the skin, where it protects and insulates the body. Perhaps nowhere is fat's structural role more dramatic than in the brain, which is 60 percent fat.[3]

Can a person have too little body fat? Just ask someone whose body fat has been depleted by illness. It hurts to sit and it hurts to lie down. For people without enough body fat, cool temperatures are intolerable, and even room temperature may be uncomfortably cool. Women stop menstruating and become infertile. Children stop growing. Skin deteriorates from pressure sores or from fatty acid deficiency and may become covered with fine hair called **lanugo**. Illness, involuntary starvation, and famine can deplete fat to this extent, as can excessive dieting and exercise.

THINK About It 2

### Carrier of Fat-Soluble Compounds

Dietary fats dissolve and transport micronutrients, such as fat-soluble vitamins (A, D, E, and K) and fat-soluble phytochemicals (carotenoids, for example). (See **Figure 6.12**.) Dietary fats carry fat-soluble substances through the digestive process, improving intestinal absorption.[4] For example, the body absorbs more lycopene, the healthful red-colored phytochemical in tomatoes, if the tomatoes are served with oil or salad dressing.

Removing a food's lipid portion—for example, removing butterfat from milk—also removes fat-soluble vitamins. In most dairy products, manufacturers replace vitamin A. Refining wheat grain to white flour extends shelf life but removes the lipid-rich germ portion. Vitamin E is lost with the germ and is not replaced. Processing fats may destroy fat-soluble vitamins; for example, some vitamin E is lost in processing vegetable oils.

### Sensory Qualities

Fat contributes greatly to the flavor, odor, and texture of food. Simply put, it makes food taste good. (See **Figure 6.13**.) Flavorful chemicals dissolve in the fat of a food; heat sends them into the air, producing mouth-watering odors that perk up appetites. Fats have a rich, satisfying feeling in the mouth. Fats make baked goods tender and moist. And fats can be heated to high temperatures for frying, which seals in flavors and cooks food quickly. These are all good qualities—but too good for many people who find high-fat foods irresistible and eat too much of them. Alas, fat's most appealing attributes also are serious drawbacks to maintaining a healthful diet.

**Key Concepts** *Triglycerides are formed when a glycerol molecule combines with three fatty acids. Dietary triglycerides add texture and flavor to food and are a concentrated source of calories. The body stores excess calories as adipose tissue. While storing energy, adipose tissue also insulates the body and cushions its organs. The fats in food carry valuable fat-soluble nutrients into the body and help with their absorption.*

## Triglycerides in Food

Dietary triglycerides are found in a variety of fats and oils as well as in foods that contain them, such as salad dressing and baked goods. Some food fats are obvious, such as butter, margarine, cooking oil, and the fat along a cut of meat or under the skin of chicken. Baked goods, snack foods, nuts, and seeds also provide fat, but it is less noticeable.

Fats and oils are mixtures of many triglycerides, but we often classify them by their most prevalent type of fatty acid—saturated, monounsaturated, or polyunsaturated. (See **Figure 6.14**.) Canola oil, for example, often is classified as a monounsaturated fat. Most fatty acids in canola oil are monounsaturated oleic acid, although about 10 percent is polyunsaturated alpha-linolenic acid.

### Sources of Omega-3 Fatty Acids

Plant foods are generally rich in polyunsaturated fatty acids. Soybean oil, canola oil, and walnuts contain alpha-linolenic acid, an essential *omega*-3 fatty acid. However, the most generous source is flaxseed oil, which is more than 50 percent alpha-linolenic acid. Longer-chain *omega*-3s are found in fatty fish (e.g., salmon, tuna, mackerel) and in fish oil supplements. Because fish oil supplements can have potent effects, children, pregnant women, and nursing mothers should not take them without medical supervision.[5] (See the FYI feature "Fats on the Health Food Store Shelf.")

### Sources of Omega-6 Fatty Acids

Good sources of the *omega*-6 fatty acid linoleic acid include seeds, nuts, and the richest source, common vegetable oils such as corn oil. Small amounts of arachidonic acid, a longer *omega*-6 fatty acid, are found in meats, poultry, and eggs but not in plant foods.

### Commercial Processing of Fats

In earlier times, people could obtain concentrated fats and oils only through simple processing: removing fats from meats and poultry, skimming or churning the butterfat from milk, skimming the oil from ground nuts, or pressing a few oil-rich plant parts such as coconuts or olives.

In the 1920s, new technology began producing pure vegetable oils.[6] Processing vegetable oils reduces waste, prevents spoilage during normal use, and increases the worldwide availability of calorie-rich oils. Processing removes damaging free fatty acids and certain destructive enzymes. Processing also adds antioxidants such as vitamin E to delay rancidity and extend shelf life. Without protection, unsaturated fats exposed to air undergo **oxidation** and rapidly turn rancid. People fortunately avoid bad-tasting rancid fats. Oxidized fats damage body tissues, particularly blood vessels.[7] Exposure to light increases the rate of oxidation and shortens shelf life.

Unfortunately, processing has a negative side. To achieve stability and uniform taste, processing removes potentially healthful phospholipids, plant

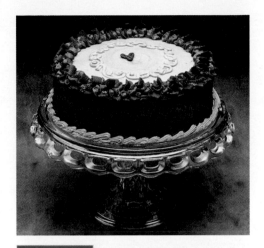

**Figure 6.13** **Sensory decadence.** Fat imparts a rich texture and smooth mouth feel to food.

**oxidation** Oxygen attaches to the double bonds of unsaturated fatty acids. Oxidation causes fats to become rancid.

SATURATED FATS AND OILS

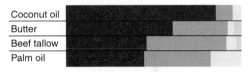

Coconut oil
Butter
Beef tallow
Palm oil

MONOUNSATURATED OILS

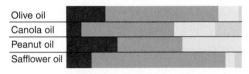

Olive oil
Canola oil
Peanut oil
Safflower oil

POLYUNSATURATED OILS

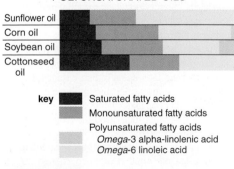

Sunflower oil
Corn oil
Soybean oil
Cottonseed oil

**key**
Saturated fatty acids
Monounsaturated fatty acids
Polyunsaturated fatty acids
*Omega*-3 alpha-linolenic acid
*Omega*-6 linoleic acid

**Figure 6.14** **The diversity of fats.** Fats contain a mix of saturated and unsaturated fatty acids. Depending on which type of fatty acid is most prevalent, the fat is classified as saturated, monounsaturated, or polyunsaturated.

**Source:** Adapted from *Nutrition Today*, May/June 1996;31(3).

sterols, and other phytochemicals; a significant portion of the natural vitamin E also is lost. Oils have become so familiar that we often forget they are highly processed, highly refined foods. Further processing of oils into solid fats, such as margarine or shortening, also produces some undesirable changes, such as increasing the proportion of *trans* fatty acids.

To get a liquid vegetable oil to act like a solid fat, hydrogenation adds hydrogen to unsaturated fatty acids. This process produces a harder, more saturated fat—one that is more effective for making baked goods and snack foods and one that spreads like butter. (Most of us recoil at the thought of putting pure corn oil on toast!) Although hydrogenation protects the fat from oxidation and rancidity, it also straightens the fatty acids to become *trans* fatty acids. Combined with the increase in saturated fatty acids, this might lead you to wonder whether margarine is a better alternative to butter. (See the FYI feature "Which Spread for Your Bread?")

**Key Concepts** *Triglycerides are found mainly in foods we think of as fats and oils but also in nuts, seeds, meats, and dairy products. Saturated fatty acids are found mainly in animal foods and tropical oils, whereas polyunsaturated fatty acids are found in vegetable oils and other plant foods. Unsaturated fatty acids are susceptible to spoilage by oxidation. Hydrogenation of oils protects fats from oxidation but creates* trans *fatty acids, which increase the risk for heart disease.*

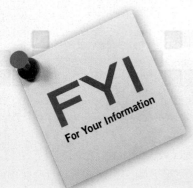

# Fats on the Health Food Store Shelf

Many claims made for lipid products sold as supplements may not hold up under scientific scrutiny. You may not even recognize these products as lipids, especially because their long, complicated names are often abbreviated. The amount of lipid and calories in most of these products is quite small.

### EPA and DHA in Fish Oil Capsules

These *omega*-3 fatty acids are thought to help lower blood pressure, reduce inflammation, reduce blood clotting, and lower high serum triglyceride levels.[1] Some studies indicate that nutrition intake that includes *omega*-3 fatty acids is a viable treatment alternative in patients with psoriasis.[2] EPA (eicosapentaenoic acid) and DHA (docosahexaenoic acid) usually make up only about one-third of the fatty acids in fish oil capsules, and research studies often use multiple doses. These should not be taken without close medical supervision, because their blood-thinning properties can cause bleeding. Because fish oil is highly unsaturated, antioxidant vitamins are included to prevent oxidation. Another problem, though not health related, is that fish oil capsules often leave a fishy aftertaste. The aftertaste can be avoided by taking the fish oil capsules with meals or at bedtime. A concentrated, purified FDA-approved prescription form of *omega*-3 fatty acids has been developed that has a minimal aftertaste.[3]

### Flaxseed Oil Capsules

Flaxseed oil is an unusually good source of *omega*-3 alpha-linolenic acid, which accounts for about 55 percent of its fatty acids. Like fish oil, flaxseed oil is highly unsaturated and thus very susceptible to rancidity. Capsules protect the oil from oxygen, but limit the dose. A half-tablespoon of canola oil has about as much *omega*-3 as a capsule of flaxseed oil but adds more calories. DHA and EPA are considered more potent *omega*-3 fatty acids than alpha-linolenic.

### GLA in Borage, Evening Primrose, or Black Currant Seed Oil Capsules

These oils contain 9 to 24 percent gamma-linolenic acid (GLA), an *omega*-6 derivative of linoleic acid. Studies of GLA's effects on skin diseases and heart conditions have been disappointing, and research on potential benefits

of GLA supplements in rheumatoid arthritis has been conflicting.[4]

### Medium-Chain Triglycerides Oil

Medium-chain triglycerides (MCT) can be purchased as such or found as ingredients in "sports" drinks and foods. Because MCT are absorbed easily, they are marketed to athletes as a

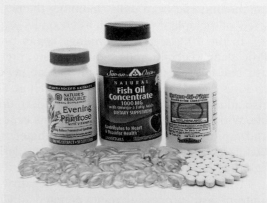

# Phospholipids

Like triglycerides, **phospholipids** contain glycerol and fatty acids. However, phospholipids also contain other substances that give them entirely different properties and functions. Our bodies can make phospholipids, so we do not need them in our diets.

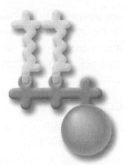

A generic phospholipid

## Phospholipid Structure

A phospholipid looks like a triglyceride, except that one fatty acid is replaced by another compound. Phospholipids are diglycerides—two fatty acids attached to a glycerol backbone. A **phosphate group** with a nitrogen-containing component occupies the third attachment site. **Figure 6.15** shows the structure of a phospholipid.

The phosphate–nitrogen component of phospholipids is soluble in water, so a phospholipid is compatible with both fat and water. The fatty acids in the diglyceride area attract fats, and the phosphate–nitrogen component attracts water-soluble substances.

> **phospholipids** Compounds that consist of a glycerol molecule bonded to two fatty acid molecules and a phosphate group with a nitrogen-containing component. Phospholipids have both water-soluble and fat-soluble regions, which makes them good emulsifiers.
>
> **phosphate group** A chemical group that contains phosphate ($-PO_4$) attached to a larger molecule. Attaching a phosphate group, along with two fatty acids, to a glycerol backbone forms a phospholipid.

## Phospholipid Functions

Because phospholipids have both water-soluble and fat-soluble parts, they are ideal emulsifiers (compounds that help keep fats suspended in a watery

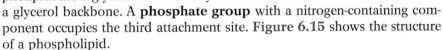

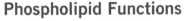

noncarbohydrate source of quick, concentrated energy. However, they have no specific performance benefits. A tablespoon of MCT contains about 100 kilocalories.

### Lecithin Oil or Granules

Lecithin supplements are a mixture of phospholipids derived from soybeans. They often are promoted as emulsifiers that lower cholesterol, but, because dietary phospholipids are broken down by the enzyme lecithinase in the intestine, they cannot have this effect. They may be useful as a source of choline. Because choline is the precursor of acetylcholine (a neurotransmitter), lecithin is promoted for treating Parkinson's and Alzheimer's diseases, which are associated with low levels of acetylcholine in the brain. Unfortunately, these claims have little scientific support.[5]

### Monolaurin Capsules

Monolaurin is a type of lauric acid, a 12-carbon fatty acid found in coconut oil. Lauric acid is said to protect against infection, but the amount in these capsules is probably too small to be significant.

### CLA

Conjugated linoleic acid (CLA) is linoleic acid with a different pattern of chemical bonds. It is pro-

moted as an aid for reducing body fat and has been suggested to have anticancer properties. Studies show promising results, but more work is needed to identify specific functions of CLA and evaluate its long-term safety.[6]

### DHEA

Dehydroepiandrosterone (DHEA) is a testosterone precursor formed from cholesterol. It is present in the body in large quantities during adolescence, peaks in the 20s, and gradually declines with age. Many elderly people have low levels, and levels also dip during serious illnesses. With only a few exceptions, attempts to use DHEA for illnesses or to slow aging have been disappointing. Researchers generally use doses many times greater than those in over-the-counter supplements, levels that may cause hairiness in women and, more seriously, a risk of liver problems.[7]

### Squalene Capsules and Shark Liver Oil

Squalene, an intermediary compound in the synthesis of cholesterol in the body, and shark liver oil, which contains squalene, are said to help liver, skin, and immune function. The basis for these claims is unclear.

1   Meyer BJ. Are we consuming enough long chain *omega*-3 polyunsaturated fatty acids for optimal health? *Prostaglandins Leukot Essent Fatty Acids.* 2011;85(5):275–280.

2   Ricketts JR, Rothe MJ, Grant-Kels JM. Nutrition and psoriasis. *Clin Dermatol.* 2010;28(6):615–626.

3   Abete P, Testa G, Galizia G, et al. PUFA for human health: diet or supplementation? *Curr Pharm Des.* 2009;15(36):4186–4190.

4   Cameron M, Gagnier JJ, Crubasik S. Herbal therapy for treating rheumatoid arthritis. *Cochrane Database Syst Rev.* 2011 Feb 16;(2):CD002948.

5   Sarubin Fragakis A, Tomson CA. *The Health Professional's Guide to Popular Dietary Supplements.* 3rd ed. Chicago: Academy of Nutrition and Dietetics; 2006.

6   Racine NM, Watras AC, Carrel AL, et al. Effect of conjugated linoleic acid on body fat accretion in overweight or obese children. *Am J Clin Nutr.* 2010;91(5):1157–1164.

7   Christensen JJ, Bruun JM, Christiansen JS, et al. Long-term dehydroepiandrosterone substitution in female adrenocortical failure, body composition, muscle function, and bone metabolism—a randomized trial. *Eur J Endocrinol.* 2011;165(2):293–300.

**choline** A nitrogen-containing compound that is part of phosphatidylcholine, a phospholipid. Choline also is part of the neurotransmitter acetylcholine. The body can synthesize choline from the amino acid methionine.

**lecithin** In the body, a phospholipid with the nitrogen-containing component choline. In foods, lecithin is a blend of phospholipids with different nitrogen-containing components.

environment). In foods, phospholipids can keep oil and water mixed. This same property makes phospholipids a perfect structural element for cell membranes—able to communicate with the watery environments of blood and cell fluids, yet with a lipid portion that allows other lipids to enter and exit cells.

### Cell Membranes

Phospholipids are major components of cell membranes. Cell membranes are a double layer of phospholipids that selectively allow both fatty and water-soluble substances into the cell. (See **Figure 6.16**.) They also store fatty acids temporarily, donating them when the body has short-term energy needs or must make regulatory chemicals (e.g., eicosanoids). One phospholipid, phosphatidylcholine, whose **choline** component eventually becomes part of the major neurotransmitter acetylcholine, plays an especially important role in nerve cells. By keeping fatty acids, choline, and other biologically active substances bound in phospholipids and freeing them only as needed, the body can regulate them closely.

### Lipid Transport

The ability of phospholipids to combine both fatty and watery substances comes in handy throughout the body. In the stomach, dietary phospholipids help break fats into tiny particles for easier digestion. In the intestine, phospholipids from bile continue emulsifying. And in the watery environment of blood, phospholipids coat the surface of the lipoproteins that carry lipid particles to their destinations in the body.

### Emulsifiers (Lecithin)

In the body and in foods of animal origin, phosphatidylcholine also is called **lecithin**. However, for food additives or supplements, the term *lecithin* is used for a mix of phospholipids derived from plants (usually soybeans). Understandably, this inconsistent terminology has caused confusion.

The food industry uses lecithin as an emulsifier to combine two ingredients that don't ordinarily mix, such as oil and water. (See **Figure 6.17**.) In high-fat powdered products (e.g., dry milk, milk replacers, coffee creamers), lecithin helps mix fatty compounds with water. Lecithin in salad dressing, chili,

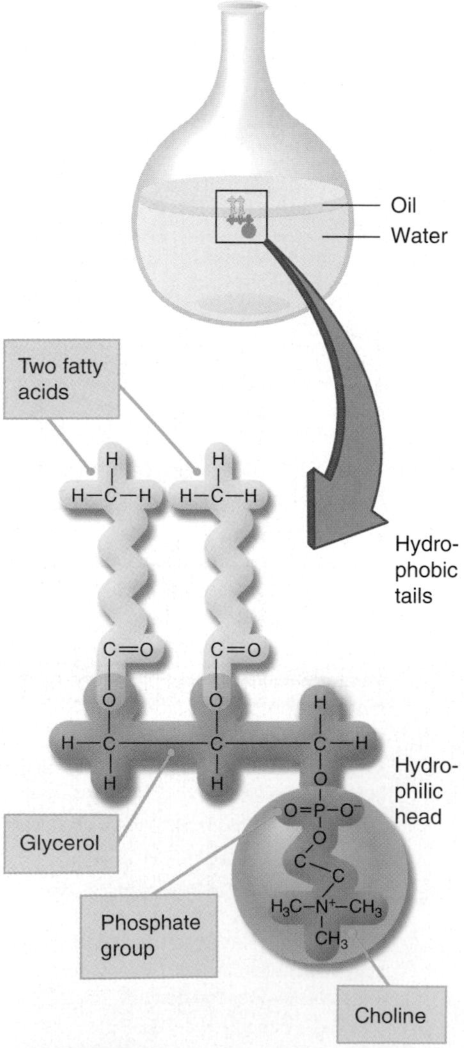

Oil
Water

Two fatty acids

Hydro-phobic tails

Glycerol

Hydro-philic head

Phosphate group

Choline

**Figure 6.15** **Phospholipid.** A phospholipid is compatible with both oil and water. This is a useful property for transporting fatty substances in the body's watery fluids.

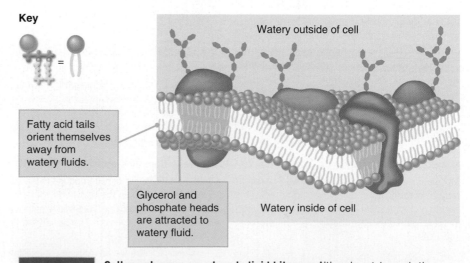

**Key**

Fatty acid tails orient themselves away from watery fluids.

Glycerol and phosphate heads are attracted to watery fluid.

Watery outside of cell

Watery inside of cell

**Figure 6.16** **Cell membranes are phospholipid bilayers.** Although proteins and other substances are embedded in cell membranes, these membranes primarily consist of phospholipids.

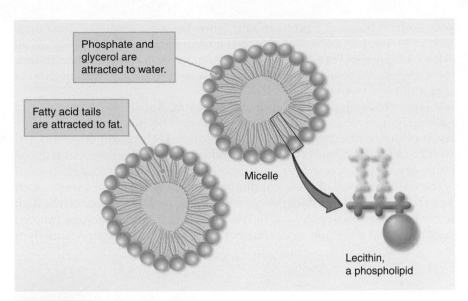

**Figure 6.17** **Lecithin and emulsification.** Lecithin, a phospholipid, forms water-soluble packages called micelles that suspend fat-soluble compounds in watery mediums. In a micelle, the lecithin molecules form into a water-soluble ball with a fatty core. The water-soluble head of each lecithin molecule points outward in contact with the watery medium, whereas the fat-soluble tails point inward in contact with the fatty core.

and sloppy-joe mixes allows the ingredients to mix well and remain mixed, avoiding separation. Lecithin is even added to chewing gum to increase shelf life, prolong flavor release, and prevent the gum from sticking to teeth and dental work.

## Phospholipids in Food

Phospholipids occur naturally throughout the plant and animal world, but in much smaller amounts than triglycerides. They are most abundant in egg yolks, liver, soybeans, and peanuts. Although food processing often removes some phospholipids, other phospholipids are common food additives. Overall, a typical diet contains only about 2 grams per day. Because your body can make phospholipids, they are not a dietary essential.

**Key Concepts** *Phospholipids are diglycerides (glycerol plus two fatty acids) with a phosphate–nitrogen compound attached at the third attachment point of glycerol. This structure makes phospholipids compatible with both fat and water. Phospholipids are major components of cell membranes and act as emulsifiers. They also store fatty acids for release into the cell and serve as a source of choline. Because the body can make phospholipids, they are not needed in the diet.*

## Sterols

THINK
About It
**3**
Although sterols are lipids, they are quite different from triglycerides and phospholipids. Whereas triglycerides and phospholipids have a glycerol backbone and fingerlike fatty acid structures, **sterols** have a multiple-ring structure. (See **Figure 6.18**.) Unlike triglycerides and phospholipids, most sterols contain no fatty acids.

**Cholesterol**

**Figure 6.18** **Sterols.** Sterols are multiple-ring structures. Because of cholesterol's role in heart disease, it has become the best-known sterol.

## Cholesterol Functions

Because of the publicity generated by its role in heart disease, **cholesterol** is the best-known sterol. But cholesterol is a necessary, important substance in your body; it becomes a problem only when excessive amounts accumulate in your blood. Like phospholipids, it is a major structural component of all cell membranes and is especially abundant in nerve and brain tissue. In fact, most cholesterol resides in body tissue, not in the blood serum or plasma that is routinely tested for cholesterol levels.

High blood cholesterol levels are common, but it also is possible to have undesirably low cholesterol levels. Although it's not common, very low levels of cholesterol (usually defined as less than 160 mg/dL) are associated with some kinds of stroke; lung, liver, and behavioral illnesses; and reduced immunity.[8] As yet, researchers have not determined whether low cholesterol is the cause or result of these conditions. Declining cholesterol levels often signal deteriorating health in people with cancer or AIDS.[9] Conversely, high levels of dietary cholesterol are linked to increased risk of various cancers, suggesting that a diet low in cholesterol may play a role in the prevention of

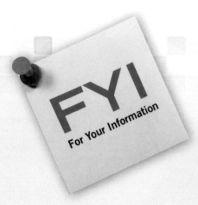

# Which Spread for Your Bread?

Okay, it's time to see if you can put some of your new knowledge about lipids to work. You're standing in front of the dairy case ready to pick out the best spread. But, wow! So many choices. Of course, there's butter, the traditional spread—wholesome, natural, and creamy; sometimes there's just no substitute for the real thing. Margarine is the choice of many and has come to be more familiar than butter to some consumers. Then what's this "vegetable oil spread"? Here's one that says it "helps promote healthy cholesterol levels."

## Butter

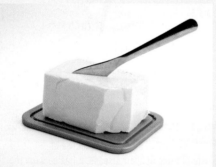

When it comes to heart health, butter has some serious disadvantages: (1) Butter is high in cholesterol-raising saturated fat, (2) it contains cholesterol, and (3) like other fats, it's high in calories.

Here are the facts: one tablespoon of butter provides the following:

- 100 kcals
- 11 g fat
- 7 g saturated fat
- 0 g *trans* fat
- 30 mg cholesterol
- 85 mg sodium
- 8 percent of the Daily Value for vitamin A

The ingredients are simple: "cream, salt, annatto (added seasonally)." Annatto is a natural coloring (a carotenoid) that is used to keep the color of butter consistent, despite what dairy cows might have been grazing on.

If you like the taste of butter, but want a bit less saturated fat and cholesterol, you can buy "whipped butter." The ingredients are the same, but the incorporation of air reduces calories, fat, saturated fat, cholesterol, and sodium by 30 to 40 percent.

## Margarine

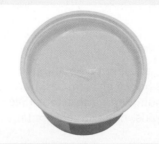

Margarine was developed to be a substitute for butter. Made from vegetable oils, it appears to be more healthful; as a plant-derived food, it's certainly cholesterol-free, and vegetable oils contain

more unsaturated fatty acids than butter. Inconveniently, though, unsaturated oils are liquid, and without extra processing, margarine would run right off any slice of bread. Hydrogenated oils are needed to produce a spreadable consistency. But, as you know, hydrogenation increases the number of saturated and *trans* fatty acids in a fat, and both of these are associated with higher blood cholesterol levels.

Looking at the label of a standard stick of margarine, you'll find the following per tablespoon:

- 100 kcals
- 11 g fat
- 2 g saturated fat
- 2 g *trans* fat
- 3.5 g polyunsaturated fat
- 3.5 g monounsaturated fat
- 0 mg cholesterol
- 115 mg sodium
- 10 percent of the Daily Value for vitamin A

Compared with butter, margarine has the same amount of calories and fat (a fact unknown to many consumers!), less saturated fat and cholesterol, and a bit more sodium and vitamin A. The PUFA and MUFA content of butter is not listed because these are not required elements of the Nutrition Facts label.

cancers such as stomach, colon, rectum, pancreas, lung, breast, kidney, and bladder.[10]

Cholesterol is a precursor of important substances. For example, your body can use cholesterol to make vitamin D. Cholesterol also is the precursor of five major classes of sterol hormones: progesterone, glucocorticoids, mineralocorticoids, androgens, and estrogens. (See **Figure 6.19**.) When making testosterone (an androgen) from cholesterol, our bodies form an intermediate compound called dehydroepiandrosterone (DHEA). DHEA has become a popular nutritional supplement, marketed with the largely unfulfilled promise that it will boost potency and restore youth.

The liver uses cholesterol to manufacture bile salts, which are secreted in bile. The gallbladder stores and concentrates the bile. On demand, the gallbladder releases the bile into the small intestine, where bile salts emulsify dietary fats.

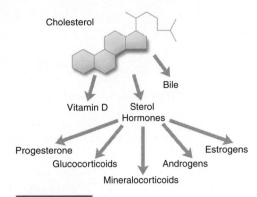

**Figure 6.19** **Cholesterol has important roles.** Cholesterol is a precursor of vitamin D and sterol hormones. The liver uses cholesterol to make bile.

Turning to the list of ingredients, we find "liquid soybean oil, partially hydrogenated soybean oil, water, whey, salt, soy lecithin, and vegetable mono- and diglycerides (emulsifiers), sodium benzoate (a preservative), vitamin A palmitate, beta carotene (color)." Nothing terribly unusual, especially now that you know what lecithin and mono- and diglycerides are.

### Spreads and Other Butter Imitators

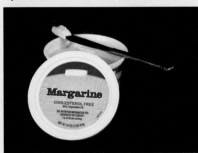

Beyond the traditional stick margarine, there are a growing number of "light," "soft," "whipped," "squeeze," "spray," and "spread" products. These items do not fit the legal definition of "margarine," and so the term *vegetable oil spread* is generally used. In terms of ingredients, these products have more liquid oil and water and less partially hydrogenated oil. More emulsifiers may be needed, along with flavors (including salt) and colors. The result typically is fewer calories, less saturated fat, and still no cholesterol.

Some products tout the inclusion of canola or olive oil for more healthful MUFA. Others in-

dicate "no *trans* fatty acids" and have no hydrogenated oils on the list. Several spreads contain plant sterols or stanols that reduce intestinal absorption of cholesterol.[1]

### Cholesterol-Lowering Margarines

Stanols are plant sterols similar in structure to cholesterol. Ingested plant sterols compete with and inhibit cholesterol absorption. Studies have shown that consumption of stanols reduces total blood cholesterol levels and LDL cholesterol levels[2] whereas HDL cholesterol levels increase or remain unchanged.[3] Stanols are available in a variety of foods, drinks, and soft gel capsules. The "cholesterol-lowering" margarines Benecol and Take Control contain plant stanol esters and plant sterols. Research on the extent of the ability for products such Benecol and Take Control to improve cholesterol levels is split. Although some studies show a benefit secondary to their use, others have found that the agents have a modest ability to lower LDL cholesterol and are not effective in all conditions, nor do they have an effect on HDL cholesterol or triglyceride levels.[4] Caution and communication with a physician should be used in persons who choose to use stanol- or sterol-ester-containing margarines in an effort to improve cholesterol levels.

### Making Choices

The spread you choose may depend on your purpose. There are times, and foods, where nothing but real butter will do. If you've ever tried baking cookies with a soft, reduced-fat spread, you know

the outcome . . . and probably will use butter, margarine, or vegetable shortening next time.

Remember, your goal is to limit total fats as well as saturated and *trans* fatty acids. Using less butter or margarine overall will do that. Choosing a margarine or spread with liquid vegetable oil as the first ingredient (meaning that the amount of hydrogenated oil is less) will reduce not only saturated fat, but *trans* fat as well. Moderation is the key—making choices that consider your whole diet will help you stay in line with heart-healthy recommendations.

1   Clifton P. Lowering cholesterol—a review on the role of plant sterols. *Aust Fam Physician*. 2009;38(4):218–221.

2   Calpe-Berdiel L, Escola-Gil JC, Blanco-Vaca F. New insights into the molecular actions of plant sterols and stanols in cholesterol metabolism. *Atherosclerosis*. 2009;203(1):18–31.

3   Ketomäki A, Gylling H, Miettinen TA. Noncholesterol sterols in serum, lipoproteins, and red cells in statin-treated FH subjects off and on plant stanol and sterol ester spreads. *Clin Chim Acta*. 2005;353:75–86; and Patch CS, Tapsell LC, Williams PG. Plant sterol/stanol prescription is an effective treatment strategy for managing hypercholesterolemia in outpatient clinical practice. *J Am Diet Assoc*. 2005;105:46–53.

4   Doggrell SA. Lowering LDL cholesterol with margarine containing plant stanol/sterol esters: is it still relevant in 2011? *Complement Ther Med*. 2011;19(1):37–46.

## Cholesterol Synthesis

Because your body can make cholesterol, you do not need cholesterol in your diet. Although researchers believe that all cells synthesize at least some cholesterol, the liver is the primary cholesterol-manufacturing site, and the intestines contribute appreciable amounts. In fact, your body produces approximately 1,000 milligrams of cholesterol per day, far more than is found in the average diet. This production level attests to cholesterol's biological importance. In the lens of the eye, which has a high concentration of cholesterol, on-site cholesterol synthesis may be essential for preventing cataracts.[11] Animal studies suggest that the brain makes almost all the cholesterol incorporated into it during development.[12]

Increasing dietary cholesterol reduces synthesis somewhat, but not by an equivalent amount.[13] When we eat frequent small meals our bodies produce less cholesterol than when we eat a few large meals. Fasting markedly reduces cholesterol production.[14]

## Sterols in Food

Only foods of animal origin contain cholesterol. The brain has the highest cholesterol content, liver and other organ meats are high, and muscle tissue contains moderate amounts. Egg yolks are high in cholesterol, with about 212 milligrams per large egg (the egg white contains no cholesterol), and breast milk is moderately high, suggesting the importance of cholesterol during early growth and development.[15] Dairy products also contain cholesterol, which

| Table 6.1 | **Cholesterol in Selected Foods** |
| --- | --- |

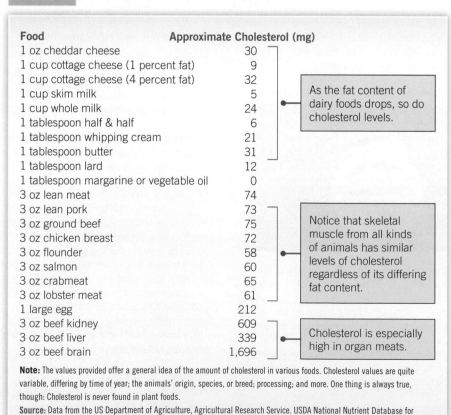

| Food | Approximate Cholesterol (mg) |
| --- | --- |
| 1 oz cheddar cheese | 30 |
| 1 cup cottage cheese (1 percent fat) | 9 |
| 1 cup cottage cheese (4 percent fat) | 32 |
| 1 cup skim milk | 5 |
| 1 cup whole milk | 24 |
| 1 tablespoon half & half | 6 |
| 1 tablespoon whipping cream | 21 |
| 1 tablespoon butter | 31 |
| 1 tablespoon lard | 12 |
| 1 tablespoon margarine or vegetable oil | 0 |
| 3 oz lean meat | 74 |
| 3 oz lean pork | 73 |
| 3 oz ground beef | 75 |
| 3 oz chicken breast | 72 |
| 3 oz flounder | 58 |
| 3 oz salmon | 60 |
| 3 oz crabmeat | 65 |
| 3 oz lobster meat | 61 |
| 1 large egg | 212 |
| 3 oz beef kidney | 609 |
| 3 oz beef liver | 339 |
| 3 oz beef brain | 1,696 |

As the fat content of dairy foods drops, so do cholesterol levels.

Notice that skeletal muscle from all kinds of animals has similar levels of cholesterol regardless of its differing fat content.

Cholesterol is especially high in organ meats.

**Note:** The values provided offer a general idea of the amount of cholesterol in various foods. Cholesterol values are quite variable, differing by time of year; the animals' origin, species, or breed; processing; and more. One thing is always true, though: Cholesterol is never found in plant foods.

**Source:** Data from the US Department of Agriculture, Agricultural Research Service. USDA National Nutrient Database for Standard Reference, Release 20. 2007. http://www.ars.usda.gov/nutrientdata. Accessed 11/2/07.

is found in the butterfat portion. Table 6.1 lists the amounts of cholesterol in some common foods.

Aside from cholesterol and vitamin D, few dietary sterols have been found to have nutritional significance. Whale liver and plants contain the cholesterol precursor **squalene**. Although whale liver is not a common item in grocery stores, squalene capsules are sold as dietary supplements with the unproved claim that squalene speeds healing. Plants contain a number of other sterols (**phytosterols**) that are poorly absorbed. Because phytosterols reduce intestinal absorption of cholesterol, they have attracted much interest and are used as a cholesterol-lowering food ingredient in certain vegetable oil spreads.

**Key Concepts** *Sterols have ring structures and contain no fatty acids. Cholesterol is the best-known sterol; other sterols are hormones or hormone precursors. Cholesterol is an important precursor compound and is a key component of cell membranes. High levels of blood cholesterol increase the risk of heart disease. Cholesterol is found only in foods of animal origin; because the body can make all it needs, cholesterol is not a dietary essential.*

## Lipid Digestion and Absorption

Like the other macronutrients (carbohydrates and proteins), most lipids are broken into smaller compounds for absorption. (See **Figure 6.20**.) However, because lipids generally are not water-soluble and digestive secretions are all water-based, the body must treat lipids a bit differently.

### Digestion of Triglycerides and Phospholipids

Triglycerides are not soluble in water, but the enzymes that digest them are found only in a watery environment. Don't worry! Your digestive system is equal to the task. Physical actions (e.g., chewing, peristalsis, segmentation),

**squalene** A cholesterol precursor found in whale liver and plants.

**phytosterols** Sterols found in plants. Phytosterols are poorly absorbed by humans and reduce intestinal absorption of cholesterol. They recently have been introduced as a cholesterol-lowering food ingredient.

## *Quick* Bite

**Would You Pay More for Cholesterol-Free Mushrooms?**
Several years ago, some plant foods were promoted with labels claiming they were "cholesterol free." As you might expect, the FDA found this misleading, because plant foods never contain cholesterol unless an animal product such as butter or egg has been added. Regulations no longer allow the implication that cholesterol has been removed from a naturally cholesterol-free food. Rather than saying "cholesterol-free mushrooms," labels must now say "mushrooms, a cholesterol-free food."

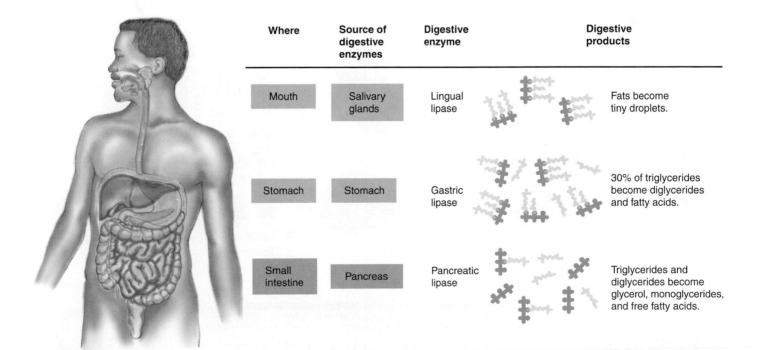

| Where | Source of digestive enzymes | Digestive enzyme | | Digestive products |
|---|---|---|---|---|
| Mouth | Salivary glands | Lingual lipase | | Fats become tiny droplets. |
| Stomach | Stomach | Gastric lipase | | 30% of triglycerides become diglycerides and fatty acids. |
| Small intestine | Pancreas | Pancreatic lipase | | Triglycerides and diglycerides become glycerol, monoglycerides, and free fatty acids. |

**Figure 6.20** **Triglyceride digestion.** Most triglyceride digestion takes place in the small intestine.

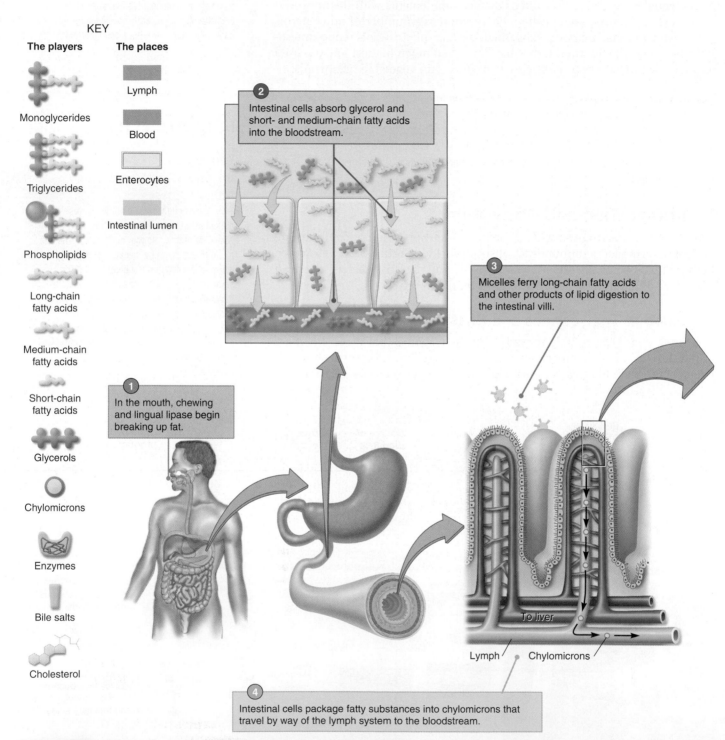

**KEY**

**The players**

Monoglycerides

Triglycerides

Phospholipids

Long-chain fatty acids

Medium-chain fatty acids

Short-chain fatty acids

Glycerols

Chylomicrons

Enzymes

Bile salts

Cholesterol

**The places**

Lymph

Blood

Enterocytes

Intestinal lumen

**2** Intestinal cells absorb glycerol and short- and medium-chain fatty acids into the bloodstream.

**1** In the mouth, chewing and lingual lipase begin breaking up fat.

**3** Micelles ferry long-chain fatty acids and other products of lipid digestion to the intestinal villi.

**4** Intestinal cells package fatty substances into chylomicrons that travel by way of the lymph system to the bloodstream.

To liver

Lymph    Chylomicrons

**Figure 6.21**    **Digestion and absorption of lipids.** Minimal fat digestion takes place in the mouth and stomach. In the small intestine, bile salts and lecithin break up and disperse fatty lipids in tiny globules. Enzymes attack these globules, breaking down triglycerides and phospholipids to fatty acids and other component parts. Glycerol, short- and medium-chain fatty acids are absorbed directly into the bloodstream. Bile salts surround the remaining products of fat digestion, forming water-soluble micelles that carry fat to intestinal cells, where it is absorbed and repackaged for transport by the lymphatic system.

combined with various emulsifiers, allow digestive enzymes to do their work. The digestion of triglycerides and phospholipids is similar and breaks these molecules down to their component parts—fatty acids, glycerol, and, in the case of phospholipids, a component containing phosphate and nitrogen.

In the mouth, a combination of chewing and the work of lingual lipase starts the digestive process rolling, with the small amount of dietary phospholipid providing emulsification. In the stomach, gastric lipase joins in, and the stomach's churning and contractions keep the fat dispersed. Diglycerides that form in the breakdown process become emulsifiers, too. After two to four hours in the stomach, digestion has broken down about 30 percent of dietary triglycerides to diglycerides and free fatty acids.[16]

Fat in the small intestine stimulates the gallbladder to contract, sending bile down the bile duct to the small intestine. The pancreas releases pancreatic juice rich in pancreatic lipase, which joins bile in the bile duct just before it reaches the small intestine.

Bile contains a large quantity of bile salts and the phospholipid lecithin. These key elements emulsify fat, breaking globules into smaller pieces so water-soluble pancreatic lipase can attack the surface. Emulsification increases the total surface area of fats by as much as 1,000-fold.[17] (Many common household detergents use emulsification to remove grease from dishes or clothing.) Pancreatic juice contains enormous amounts of pancreatic lipase. Within minutes, it breaks down nearly all accessible triglycerides to monoglycerides and free fatty acids. (See **Figure 6.21.**)

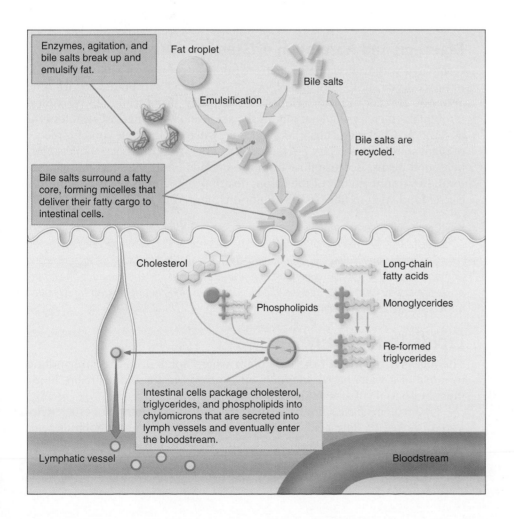

Enzymes, agitation, and bile salts break up and emulsify fat.

Fat droplet

Bile salts

Emulsification

Bile salts are recycled.

Bile salts surround a fatty core, forming micelles that deliver their fatty cargo to intestinal cells.

Cholesterol

Long-chain fatty acids

Phospholipids

Monoglycerides

Re-formed triglycerides

Intestinal cells package cholesterol, triglycerides, and phospholipids into chylomicrons that are secreted into lymph vessels and eventually enter the bloodstream.

Lymphatic vessel

Bloodstream

**micelles** Tiny emulsified fat packets. They are composed of emulsifier molecules (phospholipids) oriented with their fat-soluble part facing inward and their water-soluble part facing outward toward the surrounding aqueous environment.

**lipoprotein** A complex that transports lipids in the lymph and blood. Lipoproteins consist of a central core of triglycerides and cholesterol surrounded by a shell composed of proteins, cholesterol, and phospholipids. The various types of lipoproteins differ in size, composition, and density.

**chylomicron [kye-lo-MY-kron]** A large lipoprotein formed in intestinal cells following the absorption of dietary fats. A chylomicron has a central core of triglycerides and cholesterol surrounded by phospholipids and proteins.

## Lipid Absorption

In the small intestine, bile salts surround monoglycerides and free fatty acids, forming **micelles**—water-soluble globules with a fatty core. Micelles carry monoglycerides and long-chain fatty acids through the watery intestinal environment to the surfaces of the microvilli, even penetrating the recesses between individual microvilli. Here, the monoglycerides and long-chain fatty acids immediately diffuse into the intestinal cells, and the bile salts return to the interior of the small intestine to form another micelle. The last section of the small intestine absorbs bile salts for recycling. The bile salts return via the portal vein to the liver, where they are once again secreted as part of bile. This bile recycling pathway—the liver to the intestine and the intestine to the liver—is called enterohepatic circulation.

Inside intestinal cells, monoglycerides and fatty acids re-form triglycerides. These triglycerides, as well as cholesterol and phospholipids, join protein carriers to form a **lipoprotein**. When this assemblage leaves the intestinal cell, it is called a **chylomicron**. Chylomicrons make their way to the interior of the villi, where they enter the lymph system, which eventually empties into veins in the neck.

Short- and medium-chain fatty acids are more water-soluble than long-chain fatty acids. Intestinal cells absorb them, along with glycerol, directly into the bloodstream, bypassing the lymph system. One or two hours after you eat, dietary fat begins to appear in the bloodstream. Fat levels peak after three to five hours, and fats are generally cleared by 10 hours. That's why health professionals instruct people to fast for 12 hours before having blood drawn for lipid testing.

## Digestion and Absorption of Sterols

Compared with triglycerides, which are poorly absorbed, digestion does little to break down cholesterol and other sterols. Overall, our bodies absorb only about 50 percent of dietary cholesterol, and that proportion falls as cholesterol intake increases. Dietary fat in the small intestine increases cholesterol absorption. Cholesterol absorption declines when the intestine contains plenty of plant sterols and dietary fiber, especially fiber from fruits, vegetables, oats, peas, and beans. Because fiber from these foods binds bile salts and cholesterol, carrying them out of the colon, health professionals often recommend eating foods rich in fiber to lower blood cholesterol.

**Key Concepts** *Digestion breaks most lipids down into glycerol, free fatty acids, monoglycerides, and, in the case of phospholipids, a compound containing phosphate and nitrogen. In the small intestine, long-chain fatty acids and monoglycerides are absorbed primarily into the lymphatic system while glycerol, short-chain, and medium-chain fatty acids are absorbed directly into the blood. Sterols are mostly unchanged by digestion and their absorption is relatively poor.*

## Lipids in the Body

The digestive tract is not the only place where lipids need special handling to move in a water-based environment. To travel in the bloodstream, lipids must be specially packaged into lipoprotein carriers.

Lipoproteins have a lipid core of triglycerides and cholesterol esters (cholesterol linked to fatty acids) surrounded by a shell of phospholipids with embedded proteins and cholesterol. They can carry water-insoluble lipids through the watery environment of the bloodstream. Lipoproteins differ mainly by size, density, and the composition of their lipid cores. In general, as

## *Quick* Bite

### How Do Cholesterol-Lowering Medications Work?

One class of cholesterol-lowering medications, the "bile-acid sequestrants," works by combining bile acid and cholesterol in the intestine to form compounds that the body cannot absorb. Because this cholesterol is then lost in the feces, cholesterol must be taken from the blood to make more bile, thus lowering the blood cholesterol level.

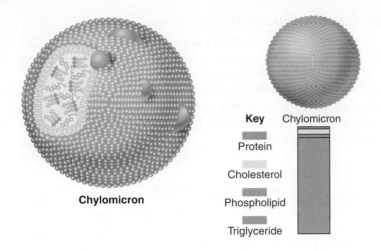

**Key** Chylomicron

Protein

Cholesterol

Phospholipid

Triglyceride

**Chylomicron**

Phospholipid — Protein

Cholesterol
Triglyceride

**Chylomicron**

**Key** Chylomicron VLDL IDL LDL HDL

Protein

Cholesterol

Phospholipid

Triglyceride

**Figure 6.22** **Lipoprotein sizes and composition.** Lipoproteins become less dense as they increase in size. LDL is about double the size of HDL. VLDL is about 60 times larger than HDL. Chylomicrons range from 500 to 1,000 times larger than HDL.

the percentage of triglyceride drops, the density increases. A lipoprotein with a small core that contains little triglyceride is much denser than a lipoprotein with a large core composed mostly of triglycerides. To get a feel for relative sizes, you can think of the different lipoproteins as a huge beach ball, softball, baseball, golf ball, and ¾-inch steel ball bearing. (See **Figure 6.22**.)

## Chylomicron

Chylomicrons formed in the intestinal tract enter the lymphatic system, which empties into the bloodstream at the jugular veins of the neck. When chylomicrons enter the bloodstream, they are large, fatty lipoproteins—think of a beach ball 3 to 6 feet in diameter. Chylomicrons are about 90 percent fat, but, as they circulate through the capillaries, they gradually give up their triglycerides.

An enzyme located on the capillary walls, called **lipoprotein lipase**, attacks the chylomicrons and removes triglyceride, breaking it into free fatty acids and glycerol. These components enter adipose cells as needed, where they are reassembled into triglycerides. Alternatively, fatty acids may be taken up by muscle and oxidized for energy or may remain in circulation and return to the liver.[18] After about 10 hours, little is left of a circulating chylomicron except cholesterol-rich remnants. It is as if the air was let out of our beach ball, shrinking it to about the size of a softball 4½ inches in diameter. The liver picks up these chylomicron remnants and uses them as raw material to build very-low-density lipoproteins.

## Very-Low-Density Lipoprotein

The liver and intestines assemble **very-low-density lipoproteins (VLDL)** with a triglyceride-rich core—for relative size, think of a softball. VLDL has a very low density because it is nearly two-thirds triglyceride. As with chylomicrons, lipoprotein lipase splits off and breaks down triglycerides as VLDL circulates through the capillaries. As VLDL loses triglycerides, it becomes denser, gradually becoming an intermediate-density lipoprotein. Our softball has shrunk to about the size of a baseball, 2¾ inches in diameter. When the diet is high in saturated and *trans* fat, more VLDL and triglycerides are released from the liver.[19]

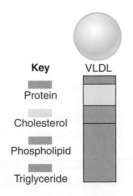

**Key** VLDL

Protein

Cholesterol

Phospholipid

Triglyceride

**lipoprotein lipase** The major enzyme responsible for the breakdown of lipoproteins and triglycerides in the blood.

**very-low-density lipoproteins (VLDL)** The triglyceride-rich lipoproteins formed in the liver. VLDL enters the bloodstream and is gradually acted upon by lipoprotein lipase, releasing triglyceride to body cells.

**intermediate-density lipoproteins (IDL)** The lipoproteins formed when lipoprotein lipase strips some of the triglycerides from VLDL.

**low-density lipoproteins (LDL)** The cholesterol-rich lipoproteins that result from the breakdown and removal of triglycerides from intermediate-density lipoprotein. LDL cholesterol sometimes is called "bad cholesterol."

**atherosclerosis** A type of "hardening of the arteries" in which cholesterol and other substances in the blood build up in the walls of arteries. As the process continues, the arteries to the heart may narrow, cutting down the flow of oxygen-rich blood and nutrients to the heart.

**high-density lipoproteins (HDL)** The blood lipoproteins that contain high levels of protein and low levels of triglycerides. Synthesized primarily in the liver and small intestine, HDL picks up cholesterol released from dying cells and other sources and transfers it to other lipoproteins. HDL cholesterol sometimes is called "good cholesterol."

## Intermediate-Density Lipoprotein

**Intermediate-density lipoproteins (IDL)** are about 40 percent triglyceride. As IDL travels through the bloodstream, it acquires cholesterol from another lipoprotein (HDL; see the "High-Density Lipoprotein" section), and circulating enzymes remove some phospholipids. IDL returns to the liver, where liver cells convert it to low-density lipoproteins.

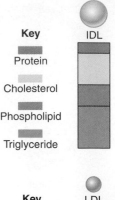

## Low-Density Lipoprotein

Elevated levels of **low-density lipoproteins (LDL)** in the blood increase the risk of artery and heart disease, earning LDL cholesterol the nickname "bad cholesterol." LDL delivers cholesterol to body cells, which use it to synthesize membranes, hormones, and other vital compounds. LDL is more than half cholesterol and cholesterol esters; triglycerides make up only 6 percent. For a relative size, think of a golf ball about 1⅝ inches in diameter.

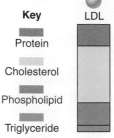

Special receptors on the cell walls bind low-density lipoproteins, which the cell engulfs and ingests. Once inside, the cell breaks down LDL, releasing LDL's load of cholesterol.

When the LDL receptors on liver cells bind LDL, they help control blood cholesterol levels.[20] A lack of LDL receptors reduces the uptake of cholesterol, forcing it to remain in circulation at dangerously high levels. Some research suggests that saturated fats block LDL receptors, limiting their clearance from the blood.[21] However, the main effect of saturated (and also *trans*) fats appears to be on VLDL production, which then leads to elevated LDL levels in the blood.[22]

The process by which LDL affects the blood vessels takes place over a number of years. When smoking, diabetes, high blood pressure, or infections injure blood vessel walls, the body's emergency repair team swings into action. It mobilizes white blood cells, which travel to the site of the injury, where they bury themselves in the blood vessel wall. Certain white blood cells bind and ingest LDL, especially altered (oxidized) LDL, which degrades and releases cholesterol. Over several decades, cholesterol accumulates as plaque thickens and narrows the artery, a condition known as **atherosclerosis**.

## High-Density Lipoprotein

**High-density lipoproteins (HDL)** appear to protect against atherosclerosis, earning HDL cholesterol the nickname "good cholesterol." The liver and intestines make HDL, which is about 5 percent triglyceride, a fat content similar to LDL. Much less than LDL, which is more than 50 percent cholesterol HDL is only about 20 percent cholesterol and has a higher protein content than any other lipoprotein. For a relative size, think of a steel ball bearing about ¾ inch in diameter.

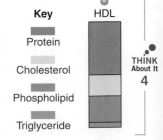

THINK
About It

4

In the bloodstream, HDL picks up cholesterol from arterial plaques, reducing their accumulation. HDL also picks up cholesterol released by dying cells and from cell membranes as they are renewed. HDL hands off cholesterol to other lipoproteins, especially IDL, which return cholesterol to the liver for recycling. Low HDL levels are thought to increase risk for atherosclerotic heart disease, whereas high HDL levels have a protective effect.[23]

**Key Concepts**  *Lipoprotein carriers transport lipids in the blood. Chylomicrons, formed in the intestinal mucosal cells, transport lipids from the digestive tract into circulation. VLDL carries lipids from the liver to the other body tissues, delivering triglycerides and gradually becoming IDL. The liver takes up IDL and assembles LDL, the main carrier of cholesterol. High blood levels of LDL, the "bad cholesterol," have been shown to be a risk factor for heart disease. Circulating HDL picks up cholesterol and sends it back to the liver for recycling or excretion. A relatively high level of HDL, the "good cholesterol," reduces risk for heart disease.*

## Lipids in the Diet

Now that you know something about lipids and their importance in the body, you can see that Rachel's no-fat approach to life has serious flaws. However, consumption of too much dietary fat can contribute unwanted calories, and high intake of saturated and *trans* fat has been linked to heart disease. Read on for a discussion of the recommended amounts and balance of lipids in a healthful diet.

### Recommended Intakes

As interest in the relationship between fat intake and health grew in the 1970s and 1980s, the American Heart Association (AHA), the National Cholesterol Education Program (NCEP) of the National Institutes of Health, and the Dietary Guidelines for Americans set intake guidelines for lipids. These guidelines set limits on total fat and saturated fat intake as a percentage of calories and on the total amount of cholesterol in the diet.

AHA guidelines (see Table 6.2) focus on overall eating patterns rather than specific percentages of dietary fat. The four main goals of the guidelines

**Table 6.2    AHA Dietary Guidelines**

The 2006 American Heart Association Diet and Lifestyle Goals are designed to assist individuals in reducing cardiovascular disease risk.

*Consume an Overall Healthy Diet*
- Consume a diet rich in vegetables and fruits.
- Choose whole-grain, high-fiber foods.

*Aim for a Healthy Body Weight*
- Balance calorie intake and physical activity to achieve or maintain a healthy body weight.

*Aim for Recommended Levels of LDL Cholesterol, HDL Cholesterol, and Triglycerides*
- Limit the intake of saturated fat to < 7 percent of energy, *trans* fat to < 1 percent of energy, and cholesterol to <300 mg per day by:
  - Choosing lean meats and vegetable alternatives
  - Selecting fat-free (skim), 1 percent fat, and low-fat dairy products
  - Minimizing intake of partially hydrogenated fats
- Consume fish, especially oily fish, at least twice a week.

*Aim for Normal Blood Pressure*
- Choose and prepare foods with little or no salt.
- If you consume alcohol, do so in moderation.

*Aim for a Normal Blood Glucose Level*
- Minimize intake of beverages and foods with added sugars.

*Be Physically Active*

*Avoid Use of and Exposure to Tobacco Products*

**Source:** Adapted from *Circulation.* 2006;114:82–96.

## Dietary Guidelines for Americans, 2010

### Key Recommendations

- Consume less than 10 percent of calories from saturated fatty acids by replacing them with monounsaturated and polyunsaturated fatty acids.
- Consume less than 300 milligrams per day of dietary cholesterol
- Keep *trans* fatty acid consumption as low as possible by limiting foods that contain synthetic sources of *trans* fats, such as partially hydrogenated oils, and by limiting other solid fats.

### Recommendations for Specific Population Groups

- Children and adolescents. Keep total fat intake between 30 to 35 percent of calories for children 2 to 3 years of age and between 25 to 35 percent of calories for children and adolescents 4 to 18 years of age, with most fats coming from sources of polyunsaturated and monounsaturated fatty acids, such as fish, nuts, and vegetable oils.

Cholesterol: no more than 300 mg/day

Saturated fat intake

10%

Maximum 20–35% total fat intake

Total kcal intake

**Figure 6.23** **Recommended fat intake.** The *Dietary Guidelines for Americans, 2010* recommends a fat intake of 20 to 35 percent of total calories. Saturated fat should supply no more than 10 percent of our total calories, or about one-third of our fat calories. Dietary cholesterol intake should be less than 300 milligrams per day.

are to help Americans (1) achieve an overall healthy eating pattern, (2) achieve and maintain an appropriate body weight, (3) achieve and maintain a desirable blood cholesterol profile, and (4) achieve and maintain a desirable blood pressure. One of the most significant changes from prior guidelines was a recommendation to consume two weekly servings (a total of 8 to 12 ounces) of fatty fish, such as tuna or salmon.

Researchers also have focused on the balance of calories from fat and carbohydrate rather than just targeting a reduction in fat. A high-fat, low-carbohydrate diet tends to contribute extra calories that lead to weight gain. When high-fat diets are high in saturated and *trans* fat, increased LDL cholesterol levels and higher heart disease risk result.[24] In contrast, low-fat, high-carbohydrate diets are associated with lower HDL cholesterol and higher blood triglyceride levels—also increasing heart disease risk. Very low fat intake can make it difficult to get adequate amounts of vitamin E and essential fatty acids.[25]

In 2002, the National Academy of Sciences published its report on Dietary Reference Intakes (DRI) for the macronutrients.[26] This report recommends an Acceptable Macronutrient Distribution Range (AMDR) for fat of 20 to 35 percent of calories for adults. This is balanced with 45 to 65 percent of calories from carbohydrates and 10 to 35 percent of calories from protein. Because children have higher energy needs, the AMDR for younger ages is more liberal: 30 to 40 percent of calories from fat for children aged 1 to 3 years and 25 to 35 percent of calories from fat for those aged 4 to 18 years. For infants, the Adequate Intake (AI) for fat is 31 grams per day for birth to 6 months of age and 30 grams per day for ages 7 to 12 months. AIs or RDAs were not set for older children and adults because there is no defined fat intake level that promotes optimal growth, maintains fat balance, or reduces chronic disease risk. In short, humans can adapt to a wide range of fat intakes.

Many nutritionists were surprised to find that the DRI committee did not set Tolerable Upper Intake Levels (ULs) for fat or cholesterol. The committee concluded that there were no defined levels of intake that separated "healthful" from "harmful" and that any increase in saturated fat, *trans* fat, or cholesterol in the diet increased LDL cholesterol levels and heart disease risk. Because it would be virtually impossible to completely exclude these lipids from the diet, the committee recommended that saturated fat, *trans* fat, and cholesterol intake be minimized. Substituting monounsaturated and polyunsaturated sources improves blood lipid values, with the most favorable results produced by replacing saturated fat with monounsaturated fat.[27]

The *Dietary Guidelines for Americans, 2010* merged recommendations from the DRI committee with those of the American Heart Association. (See **Figure 6.23.**) The recommendation for total fat intake is the AMDR: 20 to 35 percent of calories for adults. Saturated fat should be limited to no more than 10 percent of calories, and cholesterol intake limited to less than 300 milligrams per day. The *Dietary Guidelines* also suggest that we keep *trans* fat intake as low as possible. The Daily Values on food labels are 65 grams of total fat (29 percent of the calories in a 2,000-kilocalorie diet), 20 grams of saturated fat (9 percent of calories), and 300 milligrams of cholesterol. Although *trans* fat information is now required on all food labels, no Daily Value has been set; consumers should choose foods to minimize *trans* fat intake along with saturated fat and cholesterol.[28]

## Essential Fatty Acid Requirements

Although too much fat in the diet is not healthful, we still need to get enough fat to meet our need for essential fatty acids. Because essential fatty acid deficiency is virtually nonexistent in the United States and Canada, the DRI committee relied on median intake levels of essential fatty acids to set AI levels. For adults aged 19 to 50, the AI for linoleic acid is 17 grams per day for men and 12 grams per day for women. The AI for alpha-linolenic acid is 1.6 grams per day for men and 1.1 grams per day for women. To fulfill our need for *omega*-6 fatty acids, linoleic acid should provide about 2 percent of our calories. Average U.S. consumption is much more than that. Two teaspoons of corn oil, which is a little more than half linoleic acid, would supply more than 2 percent of the calories in a 2,000-kilocalorie diet.

Because science has recognized the importance of *omega*-3 fatty acids only recently, we know less about our requirements.

## *Omega*-6 and *Omega*-3 Balance

The AIs for essential fatty acids reflect the balance of *omega*-6 linoleic acid and *omega*-3 alpha-linolenic acid in our modern food supply. Before commercial processing made large quantities of vegetable oils widely available, *omega*-6 linoleic acid was hard to come by. In contrast, availability of *omega*-3s in the food supply is relatively unchanged. As a result, the ratio of *omega*-3 to *omega*-6 in the American diet has fallen. The low intake of *omega*-3 fatty acids in relation to the high intake of *omega*-6 fatty acids has caused concerns about an unhealthy imbalance in the eicosanoids these fatty acids produce.

Some researchers suggest that to gain the benefits of EPA and DHA in reducing cardiovascular disease risk we should get about 0.75 percent of our calories as alpha-linolenic acid (about 1.7 grams per day for a 2,000-kilocalorie diet) and increase EPA and DHA intake to 0.25 to 0.5 percent of calories, or about 500 to 1,000 milligrams per day for a 2,000-kilocalorie diet.[29] A ratio of 6:1 for *omega*-6 fatty acids to *omega*-3 fatty acids is also recommended.[30] Along the same lines are the *Dietary Guidelines for Americans, 2010* recommendations that encourage a diet rich in *omega*-3 fatty acids as provided by seafood, which is a good source of *omega*-3 fatty acids, eicosapentaenoic acid (EPA), and docasahexaenoic acid (DHA). Moderate evidence shows that consumption of about 8 ounces per week of a variety of seafood, which provide an average consumption of 250 milligrams per day of EPA and DHA, is associated with reduced cardiac deaths among individuals with and without pre-existing cardiovascular disease.[31] To meet these recommendations for *omega*-3 fatty acids, we would need about 1½ to 2 tablespoons of canola or soybean oil per day along with four fatty fish–containing meals each week—a threefold increase in current U.S. fish consumption! **Figure 6.24** gives an overview of the dietary sources of fatty acids. Because shark, swordfish, king mackerel, and tilefish contain high levels of mercury, the FDA and EPA recommend that women who may become pregnant, pregnant women, nursing mothers, and young children avoid eating these fish.[32]

It is important to remember that consuming too much of the *omega*-3 fatty acids can suppress immune function and prolong bleeding time, so we should be cautious about the high levels of these fatty acids found in some supplements. The DRI committee set an AMDR for *omega*-6 fatty acids of 5 to 10 percent of energy and an AMDR for alpha-linolenic acid of 0.6 to 1.2 percent of energy.

**BASIC FATTY ACIDS**

**Saturated**
Animal products (including dairy products), palm and coconut oils, and cocoa butter.

**Polyunsaturated**
Sunflower, corn, soybean, and cottonseed oils.

**Monounsaturated**
Most nuts and olive, canola, peanut, and safflower oils.

**TRANS FATTY ACIDS**
Stick margarine (not soft or liquid margarine) and many fast foods and baked goods.

**ESSENTIAL FATTY ACIDS**

**Omega-3 fatty acids**
*Alpha-linolenic acid*
Canola oil, soybeans, olive oil, many nuts (e.g., walnuts, peanuts, filberts, pistachios, pecans, almonds), seeds, and purslane (a green, leafy vegetable).

*DHA and EPA*
Fish such as mackerel, tuna, salmon, herring, trout, and cod liver oil. The fish with the lowest amount of total fat include Atlantic cod, haddock, and pink salmon. Other fish high in omega-3 but also high in total fat are sardines and bluefish. Human milk.

**Omega-6 fatty acids**
*Linoleic acid*
Plants (flax) and some vegetable oils (soybean and canola oil).

**Figure 6.24**    Overview of dietary sources of fatty acids.

**Source:** Adapted from Cancer smart. *Scientific American.* 1998;4(3):9.

**fat replacers** Compounds that imitate the functional and sensory properties of fats but contain less available energy than fats.

**olestra** A fat replacer made from a sucrose backbone with six to eight fatty acids attached. The fatty acid arrangement prevents breakdown by the digestive enzyme lipase, so the fatty acids are not absorbed. Olestra can withstand heat and is stable at frying temperatures. Its trade name is Olean.

## Current Dietary Intakes

Currently, Americans are eating about 33 percent of their total calories each day from fat.[33] Recall that the acceptable range for total fat intake for adults is between 20 and 35 percent. Fat intake as a percentage of calories is down from 36 percent in the early 1970s, and down markedly from 45 percent in 1965. See "What About Bobbie?" at the end of this chapter to see how to calculate the percentage of calorie intake from fat.

Although the percentage of calories from fat dropped, average calorie intake increased, which means Americans are actually consuming more total grams of fat. Current intake of saturated fat is about 11 percent of calories, a little higher than recommended. Major sources of saturated fatty acids in the American diet include regular cheese; pizza; grain-based desserts; chicken and chicken mixed dishes; and sausage, franks, bacon, and ribs.[34] Cholesterol intake averages 341 milligrams per day for adult men and 242 milligrams per day for adult women.[35] Intake of linoleic acid is estimated to be 6 percent of calories, with alpha-linolenic acid providing 0.75 percent of calories and EPA plus DHA another 0.1 percent of calories. By keeping total fat intake within the AMDR and getting most of our fat from vegetable oils, fish, and nuts, we can move closer to meeting recommendations.

## Role of Fat Replacers

The food industry responded to the public health challenge of the 1990s to lower fat intake by making low-fat, low-calorie goodies that still taste good. More than 15 different types of **fat replacers** have been developed, and over the years thousands of fat-free, low-fat, and reduced-fat foods have hit grocery shelves.[36]

### Fat Replacers: What Are They Made Of?

Some fat replacers are carbohydrates: generally starches and fibers such as vegetable gums, cellulose, maltodextrins, and Oatrim (a fat replacer made from oats). Some are more digestible than others, but all provide far fewer than 9 kilocalories per gram. They also bind water and incorporate it into foods, further diluting calories. With their moist, thick textures, they mimic fat's richness and smooth "mouth feel."

Proteins are the raw ingredients of other fat replacers. Food manufacturers can modify egg whites and whey from milk so they become thick and smooth and hold water. Because this protein and water combination has fewer calories per gram than fat, it cuts calories. However, high heat changes protein structures, which changes the properties of these replacers and limits their usefulness. Manufacturers used the protein-based product Simplesse in frozen desserts, but it was not well accepted by consumers.

The most high-tech fat replacers—and the most controversial—are the "fat-based" replacers. This group includes Olean, Caprenin, and Salatrim (or Benefat). Caprenin is a blend of medium-chain fatty acids and a 22-carbon fatty acid. Salatrim is primarily a blend of 18-carbon stearic acid and short-chain fatty acids. For both Caprenin and Salatrim, the fatty acids are arranged on glycerol in a way that inhibits digestion. They provide about half the calories of fat, although this is only an estimate because people differ in their ability to digest them. Manufacturers use these fat replacers in reduced-fat candies and baked goods.

One advantage of fat-based fat replacers is their ability to withstand heat. That's fortunate for **olestra** (Olean) because few food ingredients have had to take as much heat from consumer advocacy groups. Olestra has a sucrose (instead of glycerol) backbone with six to eight fatty acids attached (instead of triglyceride's three). (See **Figure 6.25**.) Manufacturers can alter the characteristics of the fatty acids—their number, length, arrangement, and saturation, for example—to vary properties such as melting point and consistency. Digestive enzymes do not recognize the fatty acid arrangement, so olestra is not broken down and absorbed. This makes olestra calorie-free, even though its fatty acids give it the flavor and cooking performance of fat. It is stable even at frying temperatures.

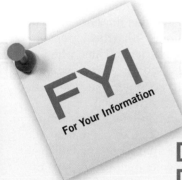

## Does "Reduced Fat" Reduce Calories? It Depends on the Food

Experts often tell us to reduce fat in our diets to help reduce risk for heart disease, cancer, and obesity. Given that fat is our most concentrated source of calories, we would expect a reduced-fat or low-fat food to have fewer calories than its unmodified counterpart. But is this always true?

Sometimes low-fat and fat-free foods make a big difference in calories.

| Food | Kilocalories |
|---|---|
| 1 oz American cheese | 105 |
| 1 oz low-fat cheese product | 50 |
| 2 oz bologna | 180 |
| 2 oz fat-free bologna | 45 |
| 1 tablespoon mayonnaise | 100 |
| 1 tablespoon fat-free mayonnaise/dressing | 12 |

But sometimes they make almost no difference at all.

| Food | Kilocalories |
|---|---|
| 1 cup canned chicken vegetable soup | 75 |
| 1 cup reduced-fat chicken vegetable soup | 95 |
| 3 chocolate chip cookies (30 g) | 145 |
| 3 reduced-fat chocolate chip cookies (30 g) | 135 |
| 2 tablespoon peanut butter | 190 |
| 2 tablespoon reduced-fat peanut butter | 170 |
| 1 oz potato chips | 150 |
| 1 oz reduced-fat potato chips | 135 |

Many reduced-fat products contain added sugar. Although sugar has fewer calories per gram than fat, the amount added may negate any difference in calories. If fat is your concern, low-fat or fat-free products make sense. But, if you're trying to reduce fat *and* calories, modified products may not be a big help. So, be a smart shopper—check the label before you check out with a cartload of reduced-fat foods.

**Source:** US Department of Agriculture, Agricultural Research Service. 2007. USDA National Nutrient Database for Standard Reference, Release 20. 2007. http://www.ars.usda.gov/nutrientdata. Accessed 11/11/07.

Light mayonnaise

**Nutrition Facts**
Serving Size: 1 Tbsp (14g)
Servings: 32

| | | %DV |
|---|---|---|
| **Calories** 50 | | |
| Fat Cal 45 | | |
| **Amount/serving** | | |
| **Total Fat** 5g | | 8% |
| Saturated Fat 1g | | 4% |
| Trans Fat 0g | | |
| **Cholesterol** 5mg | | 2% |
| **Sodium** 115mg | | 5% |
| **Total Carbohydrate** 0g | | 0% |
| **Protein** 0g | | |

* Percent Daily Values (DV) are based on a 2,000 calorie diet.

Not a significant source of dietary fiber, vitamin A, vitamin C, calcium, and iron.

INGREDIENTS: WATER, SOYBEAN OIL, VINEGAR, FOOD STARCH-MODIFIED*, EGG YOLKS, SALT, LEMON JUICE, MUSTARD FLOUR, XANTHAN GUM*, BETA-CAROTENE (COLOR)*, AND NATURAL FLAVORS, POTASSIUM SORBATE, AND CALCIUM DISODIUM SULFATE EDTA USED TO PROTECT QUALITY.

*INGREDIENTS NOT FOUND IN MAYONNAISE.

Regular mayonnaise

**Nutrition Facts**
Serving Size: 1 Tbsp (14g)
Servings: 32

| | | %DV |
|---|---|---|
| **Calories** 100 | | |
| Fat Cal 100 | | |
| **Amount/serving** | | %DV |
| **Total Fat** 11g | | 17% |
| Saturated Fat 1.5g | | 8% |
| Trans Fat 0g | | |
| **Cholesterol** 5mg | | 2% |
| **Sodium** 80mg | | 3% |
| **Total Carbohydrate** 0g | | 0% |
| **Protein** 0g | | |

* Percent Daily Values (DV) are based on a 2,000 calorie diet.

INGREDIENTS: SOYBEAN OIL, WHOLE EGGS AND EGG YOLKS, WATER, VINEGAR, SALT, SUGAR, LEMON JUICE, NATURAL FLAVORS, CALCIUM DISODIUM SULFATE EDTA USED TO PROTECT QUALITY.

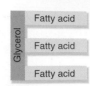

A triglyceride has three fatty acids attached to a glycerol backbone.

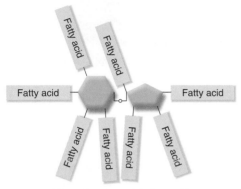

Olestra has six to eight fatty acids attached to a sucrose backbone.

**Figure 6.25** **The structure of olestra is unlike the structure of a triglyceride.** Olestra adds the savory qualities of fat, but your digestive enzymes cannot break it down.

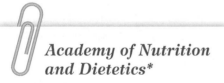

### *Academy of Nutrition and Dietetics**

**Fat Replacers**

It is the position of the American Dietetic Association that the majority of fat replacers, when used in moderation by adults, can be safe and useful adjuncts to lowering the fat content of foods and may play a role in decreasing total dietary energy and fat intake. Moderate use of low-calorie, reduced-fat foods, combined with low total energy intake, could potentially promote dietary intake consistent with the objectives of *Healthy People 2010* and the *Dietary Guidelines for Americans, 2005.*

**Source:** Reproduced from Position of the Academy of Nutrition and Dietetics: fat replacers. *J Am Diet Assoc.* 2005;105(20):266–275.

* Formerly the American Dietetic Association

### The Olestra Controversy: Are Fat Replacers Safe?

Consumers have expressed few safety concerns about carbohydrate- and protein-based fat replacers. Most concerns center on olestra, which aroused controversy long before it received FDA approval as a food additive in January 1996. The approval process itself was lengthy and controversial,[37] and, even after FDA approval, olestra continues to evoke strong, conflicting opinions.[38]

Olestra is a mixture of sucrose and long-chain fatty acids. Unlike the glycerol backbone of fatty acids, olestra contains six to eight fatty acids connected to sucrose. The enzymes that normally break apart fatty acids during digestion cannot separate the sucrose from its fatty acids, and, therefore, olestra moves through the GI tract unabsorbed. Because the GI tract does not absorb olestra, some people suffer fat malabsorption symptoms—diarrhea, gas, and cramps. Olestra also acts as a solvent for fat-soluble nutrients. Thus, when it leaves the body unabsorbed, it carries these nutrients with it. Manufacturers are required to replace fat-soluble vitamins, but critics counter that healthful phytochemicals such as the carotenoids are lost and not replaced.

The FDA, concerned about malabsorption and nutrient loss, limits olestra's use to a few snack foods. Critics would like to see olestra eliminated, while the food industry wants to expand its usage. Postmarketing surveillance (mandated by the FDA) shows that only a small percentage (5 percent) of those surveyed were "heavy consumers," with an average intake of more than 2.0 grams per day.[39] On average, intake for those who use olestra as part of a weight management diet is about 0.75 grams per day.[40] The calorie savings from even a small amount (1 to 2 grams per day) of fat replacement with olestra may be enough to prevent gradual weight gain in adulthood.[41] Surveillance also has not found significant evidence of reduced blood levels of carotenoids and fat-soluble vitamins.[42]

The "power of suggestion" brought on by adverse publicity may be responsible for some consumers' digestive discomfort after eating olestra-containing chips. In fact, in a large double-blind study of volunteers eating olestra-containing chips or regular chips, more people had indigestion after eating the regular chips. Will using olestra subtly encourage people to eat more? In another study, when subjects ate unlabeled olestra-containing potato chips, they ate fewer total calories and less fat than when they ate unlabeled regular potato chips. But when they knew the chips they were eating were fat-free, the subjects ate more.[43] If consumers overeat olestra-containing snacks, they may be more likely to suffer side effects.

When used in moderation, we think that fat replacers pose no specific risks to adult consumers. There is still a need for research to determine whether long-term consumption increases health risks or if there are specific risks to children.[44]

### Do Fat Replacers Save Calories? Do They Reduce Total Fat Intake?

Considering the American population as a whole, the answer to these questions seems to be "no." American fat and calorie intakes have not declined with the growth in the fat-replacer market. It is clear that fat replacers won't help if people treat them simply as an excuse to eat more. Nor should "low-fat foods" be confused with "low-calorie foods"; the calories saved by eating low-fat foods are often negligible.[45]

## Lipids and Health

Moderation and balance are the keys to a healthful diet. If your diet is consistently high in fat, you may have several problems. High-fat diets are typically high in calories and contribute to weight gain and obesity. High intakes of saturated fat and *trans* fat increase risk for heart disease, and high-fat diets have been linked to several types of cancer, although the evidence is not as strong.[46] If you follow the dietary recommendations discussed earlier, you should reduce your risk for these conditions.

## Obesity

**Obesity** is defined as the excessive accumulation of body fat leading to a body weight in relation to height that is substantially greater than some accepted standard. Approximately 34 percent of American adults are obese; 17 percent of children and teens are obese.[47]

Eating large amounts of dietary fat contributes to this obesity epidemic. Fat is a dense source of calories, it makes food taste good, and it's often unnoticed or "hidden" in restaurant and convenience foods. Table 6.3 shows how fat increases the calorie content of foods. Standard advice to Americans trying to attain or maintain normal weight usually includes cutting back on fats and fatty foods, along with increasing physical activity and eating fewer calories.

## Heart Disease

Heart disease and stroke are the principal types of **cardiovascular disease (CVD)**, which is the leading cause of death in the United States and Canada, claiming one life every minute. Given the current state of diet behavior, nearly half of all Americans alive today will die from CVD. Although we typically think of CVD as primarily affecting men and older adults, heart attack is the number one killer of American women.[48] Every year approximately 785,000 Americans have a first heart attack. Another 470,000 who have already had one or more heart attacks have another attack.[49] But not all the news is bad. In the past 50 years, lifestyle changes and medical advances have led to significant progress in the fight against CVD. According to a recent report by the U.S. National Heart, Lung, and Blood Institute, deaths from coronary heart disease have declined in women from one in three to one in four.[50]

### Atherosclerosis

High blood cholesterol, or **hypercholesterolemia**, along with smoking and high blood pressure are principal risk factors for CVD. High blood cholesterol

**obesity** Excessive accumulation of body fat leading to a body weight in relation to height that is substantially greater than some accepted standard.

**cardiovascular disease (CVD)** General term for all disorders affecting the heart and blood vessels.

**hypercholesterolemia** High blood cholesterol (total cholesterol).

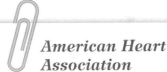

### *American Heart Association*

**Cardiovascular Disease Risk Reduction**

- Balance calorie intake and physical activity to achieve or maintain a healthy body weight.
- Consume a diet rich in vegetables and fruits.
- Choose whole-grain, high-fiber foods.
- Consume fish, especially oily fish, at least twice a week.
- Limit your intake of saturated fat to < 7 percent of energy, *trans* fat to < 1 percent of energy, and cholesterol to < 300 mg per day by:
  - Choosing lean meats and vegetable alternatives
  - Selecting fat-free (skim), 1 percent fat, and low-fat dairy products
  - Minimizing intake of particularly hydrogenated fats
- Minimize your intake of beverages and foods with added sugars.
- Choose and prepare foods with little or no salt.
- If you consume alcohol, do so in moderation.
- When you eat food that is prepared outside the home, follow the AHA Diet and Lifestyle Recommendations.

**Source:** Reproduced from Diet and lifestyle recommendations revision 2006: a scientific statement from the American Heart Association Nutrition Committee. Circulation. 2006;114(1):82-96.

| Table 6.3 | **Fat Can Markedly Increase Calories in Food** |
|---|---|

| | Approximate Kcalories | Approximate Fat (g) |
|---|---|---|
| 4 oz fried potatoes | 153 | 5.9 |
| 4 oz boiled potatoes | 99 | 0.1 |
| ½ cup creamed cottage cheese | 108 | 4.7 |
| ½ cup 1 percent low-fat cottage cheese | 81 | 1.2 |
| ½ cup green beans with 1 teaspoon butter | 56 | 5.0 |
| ½ cup green beans without butter | 22 | 0.2 |
| 3 oz T-bone steak, untrimmed | 260 | 19.4 |
| 3 oz T-bone steak, trimmed | 161 | 7.4 |
| ½ cup vanilla ice cream | 133 | 7.3 |
| ½ cup light vanilla ice cream | 125 | 3.7 |

**Source:** Data from US Department of Agriculture, Agricultural Research Service. USDA National Nutrient Database for Standard Reference, Release 20. 2007. http://www.ars.usda.gov/main/site_main.htm?modecode=12-35-45-00. Accessed 5/23/11.

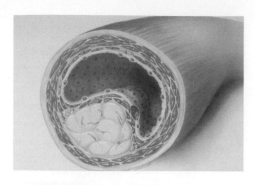

**Figure 6.26** **Development of atherosclerosis.** Atherosclerotic plaque is formed by a buildup of fatty material in the wall of an artery. An artery narrowed by plaque is vulnerable to blockage by a blood clot, causing a heart attack or stroke.

levels promote atherosclerosis, the slow, progressive hardening and narrowing of the arteries that often causes heart attacks or strokes. (See **Figure 6.26**.)

Total cholesterol levels do not tell the entire story. The levels of LDL and HDL cholesterol provide a more accurate prediction of a person's risk for developing atherosclerosis. High LDL cholesterol increases risk more than high total cholesterol, with some kinds of LDL being more dangerous than others. Low HDL cholesterol levels increase the risk of a future cardiovascular event, as do high levels of triglycerides.[51]

**Lipoprotein a [Lp(a)]** is a low-density lipoprotein that seems especially harmful to the cardiovascular system. High levels prevent the normal breakup of blood clots that cause heart attack or stroke. Although Lp(a) is associated with heart attack, it cannot be influenced sufficiently by diet or by drug therapy to reduce its harmful effects.[52]

### Inflammation and Atherosclerosis

Laboratory evidence and study findings suggest that inflammation is important in the development of atherosclerosis. No one knows for sure what causes the low-grade inflammation that seems to put otherwise healthy people at risk. However, findings are consistent with the hypothesis that an infection—possibly one caused by a bacteria or a virus—might contribute to or even cause atherosclerosis.

During systemic (whole body) inflammation, the body releases several proteins, including **C-reactive protein (CRP)**. Testing CRP levels in the blood may be a new way to assess cardiovascular disease risk. Recent studies show that the higher the CRP levels, the higher the risk of a cardiovascular event, such as heart attack.[53]

## Dietary and Lifestyle Factors for Reducing Atherosclerosis Risk

The American Heart Association (AHA) has identified that the best weapons to fight cardiovascular disease are a healthy diet and a healthy lifestyle. AHA recommends that all persons over the age of 2 years can find benefit in following these simple steps: (1) consume an overall healthy diet; (2) aim for a healthy body weight; (3) aim for a desirable lipid profile as defined by the National Cholesterol Education Program (NCEP) of the National Heart, Lung, and Blood Institute (NHLBI) (see Table 6.4); (4) aim for a normal blood pressure; (5) aim for a normal blood glucose level; (6) be physically active; and (7) avoid use of and exposure to tobacco products. The AHA recommendations plus other risk-reducing factors are summarized below.

### Balance Calorie Intake and Physical Activity to Achieve or Maintain a Healthy Body Weight

Obesity is an independent risk factor for cardiovascular disease, and weight gain during the teen years and adulthood is associated with increased risk of heart disease.[54] To avoid weight gain, calorie intake must match calorie output. Awareness of the calorie content of foods and beverages and control of portion sizes are major steps toward calorie control.

By expending calories and increasing fitness, physical activity helps reduce cardiovascular disease risk.[55] Current recommendations advocate at least 30 minutes of moderate-intensity activity on most days of the week; more activity would reduce heart disease risk further.

### Consume a Diet Rich in Fruits and Vegetables

A diet that emphasizes fruits and vegetables lowers cardiovascular disease risk factors. Fruits and vegetables not only are rich in nutrients and fiber, but they are also low in calories. Brightly colored vegetables and fruits also are

**lipoprotein a [Lp(a)]** A substance that consists of an LDL "bad cholesterol" part plus a protein (apoprotein a) whose exact function is currently unknown.

**C-reactive protein (CRP)** A protein released by the body in response to acute injury, infection, or other inflammatory stimuli. CRP is associated with future cardiovascular events.

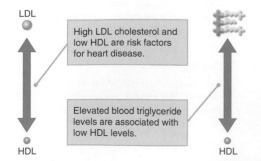

High LDL cholesterol and low HDL are risk factors for heart disease.

Elevated blood triglyceride levels are associated with low HDL levels.

**Table 6.4**   **Adult Blood Cholesterol and Triglyceride Levels**

| Total Cholesterol | | LDL Cholesterol | |
|---|---|---|---|
| Desirable | < 200 | Optimal | < 100 |
| Borderline high | 200–239 | Near optimal/ | 100–129 |
| High | ≥ 240 | above optimal | |
| | | Borderline high | 130–159 |
| | | High | 160–189 |
| | | Very high | ≥ 190 |
| **Triglyceride** | | **Triglyceride** | |
| Normal | < 150 | High | 160–189 |
| Borderline high | 150–199 | Very high | ≥ 190 |
| High | 200–499 | **HDL Cholesterol** | |
| Very high | ≥ 500 | Low | < 40 |
| | | High | ≥ 60 |

**Note:** All units are mg/dL.

**Source:** National Cholesterol Education Program. *Third Report of the Expert Panel on Detection, Evaluation, and Treatment of High Blood Cholesterol in Adults (Adult Treatment Panel III), Final Report.* Washington, DC: US Department of Health and Human Services; 2003. NIH publication 02-5215.

good sources of phytochemicals, including antioxidants. Choose a variety of vegetables and fruits, with an emphasis on whole, unprocessed sources, and use preparation methods that do not add calories, saturated or *trans* fats, sugar, and salt.

## Choose Whole-Grain, High-Fiber Foods

Diets that emphasize whole grains and other foods rich in fiber have also been linked to improved overall diet quality and reduced cardiovascular disease risk.[56] Note that certain types of fiber can bind to bile acids in the gastrointestinal tract. These bile acids are excreted via the feces rather than recycled and reused. Additional bile acids must then be made from cholesterol, lowering the total amount in the body. In the large intestine, intestinal bacteria partially digest fiber and then produce short-chain fatty acids, some of which are linked to reduced cholesterol synthesis.[57] The Adequate Intake (AI) level for fiber (14 grams per 1,000 kilocalories) is based on the amount of fiber that has been shown to reduce CVD risk.[58] People who eat more whole grains (two and a half servings each day) are 21 percent less likely to have heart disease than those who eat fewer than two servings a week.[59] The AHA and the *Dietary Guidelines for Americans, 2010* recommend that at least half of daily grain intake come from whole grains.[60]

## Consume Fish, Especially Oily Fish, at Least Twice a Week

In the 1970s, a study of the Inuit (Greenland Eskimos) focused attention on the beneficial effects of EPA and DHA, the *omega*-3 fatty acids in fish fats.[61] Researchers were puzzled: This group of people had a high intake of fat, saturated fat, and cholesterol from marine mammals and fish, yet they showed little evidence of atherosclerosis. The Inuit were compared to the Danes, among whom atherosclerosis was common and whose diet was similarly high in fat, but from meats and dairy products. It became clear that the high EPA and DHA content of fish in the Inuit diet protects against heart disease by discouraging blood cells from clotting and from sticking to artery walls and by reducing inflammation.

Other studies continue to support the idea that consuming *omega*-3s from fish and fish oils protects against heart disease and its many complications.[62] The Nurses' Health Study showed that higher consumption of fish or *omega*-3 fatty acids reduces the risk of stroke caused by blood clots.[63]

*Omega*-3 fatty acids have been shown to decrease arrhythmias, triglyceride levels, and rate of atherosclerotic plaque as well as to slightly lower blood pressure and reduce the incidence of CVD.[64]

Scientists also are investigating whether *omega*-3s may help some chronic inflammatory conditions such as rheumatoid arthritis, asthma, inflammatory bowel disease as well as renal disease, bone density, cognitive function, metabolic syndrome, and diabetes, although research in these areas is still inconclusive.[65] All in all, there are certainly enough positive results to encourage further study and recommend regular consumption of cold-water fish (e.g., salmon, cod) for EPA and DHA as well as plant foods with alpha-linolenic acid.[66]

### Limit Intake of Saturated and Trans *Fat and Cholesterol*

Saturated and *trans* fatty acids raise total and LDL cholesterol and should be minimized in a heart-healthy diet. These two types of fat have opposite effects on HDL cholesterol levels, however. The difference: Saturated fats raise HDL cholesterol whereas *trans* fats have been shown to lower HDL cholesterol,[67] making them twice as troublesome. The AHA recommends limiting saturated fat intake to less than 7 percent of total calories and *trans* fat intake to less than 1 percent. The *Dietary Guidelines* recommends keeping *trans* fatty acid consumption "as low as possible." Replacing saturated fats with monounsaturated or *omega*-3 polyunsaturated fatty acids lowers both total and LDL cholesterol. Research also shows that consuming monounsaturated fats, such as olive oil, lowers total and LDL cholesterol without lowering HDL.[68]

This positive effect of olive oil may explain why Greeks, Turks, Italians, and others around the Mediterranean who eat a diet high in fat still have low rates of heart disease. Their overall diet pattern seems to model AHA recommendations: ample fresh fruits, vegetables, pasta, and whole grains; small amounts of meat and poultry; and generous use of olive oil. Favorable results from both epidemiological and intervention studies have made the Mediterranean diet popular.[69]

Does the total amount of fat consumed make a difference? The AHA supports recommendations put forth by the Institute of Medicine (the DRI values) and the NCEP for limiting total fat intake to 25 to 35 percent of energy intake. What about cholesterol intake? Some evidence links cholesterol intake to blood cholesterol levels, and because cholesterol is not essential in the diet, it should be limited. When people reduce their saturated fat intake by limiting fat from dairy products and meats, cholesterol intake usually goes down. The AHA recommends limiting cholesterol intake to less than 300 milligrams per day.

### Minimize Intake of Beverages and Foods with Added Sugars

Consumption of foods and beverages with added sugars continues to rise. A high intake of added sugars can contribute to weight gain, which, in turn, increases CVD risk. Reducing consumption of added sugars reduces calorie intake and improves the nutrient quality of the diet. Being aware of and limiting sources of added sugars will help people achieve their weight goals.

In the United States, consumption of sugar-sweetened carbonated beverages (i.e., soft drinks) has increased dramatically over the past three decades.[70] Accumulating evidence has linked soft drink intake and poor diet quality, such as higher intake of saturated fat and lower intake of key nutrients.[71] This finding agrees with the trend that Americans are also consuming more added sugars through intake of fruit juice, food mixtures (e.g., prepared and convenience foods), grain snacks, and pastries.[72]

## Choose and Prepare Foods with Little or No Salt

Hypertension is one of the major risk factors for cardiovascular disease, and blood pressure tends to rise as salt intake increases. The AHA suggests that reducing sodium intake to 2,300 milligrams per day or less is an achievable goal. The *Dietary Guidelines, 2010* recommend that persons who are 51 years and older and those of any age who are African American or have hypertension, diabetes, or chronic disease should reduce intake to 1,500 milligrams per day.

## If You Consume Alcohol, Do So in Moderation

Numerous studies associate moderate alcohol consumption with a substantial decrease in heart disease risk.[73] Although the positive effects of alcohol are generally associated with wine, and particularly red wine, consumption, the benefits also are found with other forms of alcohol.[74] Alcohol is addictive, however, and high intake can have adverse effects on the body. The AHA recommends limiting alcohol intake to no more than one drink per day for women and two drinks per day for men, ideally with meals.

The positive effects of alcohol on reducing heart disease risk provide at least a partial explanation for the "French paradox"—the fact that the French eat rich cheeses and fatty meats yet still have low rates of heart disease. They also have relatively high intakes of fruits, vegetables, and red wine—all rich sources of antioxidant phytochemicals.[75] Antioxidants and moderate alcohol consumption may offset some of the adverse effects of poor food choices and perhaps protect against heart disease. In addition to its heart-protective effects, these antioxidant phytochemicals may also have anticancer, anti-inflammatory, and anti-aging benefits.

## When You Eat Food That Is Prepared Outside of the Home, Follow the AHA 2006 Diet and Lifestyle Recommendations

More and more of our meals are either eaten away from home or brought home as "take-out" food. All too often, our choices away from home are high in saturated and *trans* fats, cholesterol, added sugars, and sodium and low in fiber, fruits, and vegetables. Also, portion sizes at restaurants are typically more than those recommended by MyPlate. Consumers need to make wise choices both at home and when away from home. Splitting entrée portions with a companion, choosing steamed vegetables instead of a loaded baked potato, or substituting a salad with low-fat dressing for french fries will help individuals follow the AHA guidelines.

## Other Dietary Factors

Vitamins and other foods, such as soy, have been studied for their influence on heart disease risk.

**B Vitamins** Folate and vitamins $B_6$ and $B_{12}$ are involved in pathways that convert one amino acid, homocysteine, to another amino acid, methionine. As noted earlier, high levels of homocysteine may contribute to heart disease by promoting atherosclerosis, excessive blood clotting, and blood vessel rigidity. Folate and vitamins $B_6$ and $B_{12}$ can help reduce destructive levels of homocysteine. Researchers think that consumption of a diet rich in fruits, vegetables, and low-fat dairy products, which are good sources of these vitamins, helps prevent blood vessel damage from homocysteine.[76]

**Soy** Soy-based foods, such as soy milks, soy burgers, tofu, and tempeh, have become popular items in grocery stores. Replacing animal-based foods with

*Quick* Bite

**NCEP Tips for Healthful Eating Out**
- Choose restaurants that have low-fat, low-cholesterol menu items.
- Don't be afraid to ask for foods that follow your eating pattern.
- Select poultry, fish, or meat that is broiled, grilled, baked, steamed, or poached rather than fried.
- Choose lean deli meats like fresh turkey or lean roast beef instead of higher-fat cuts like salami or bologna.
- Look for vegetables seasoned with herbs or spices rather than butter, sour cream, or cheese. Ask for sauces on the side.
- Order a low-fat dessert like sherbet, fruit ice, sorbet, or low-fat frozen yogurt.
- Control serving sizes by asking for a small serving, sharing a dish, or taking some home.
- At fast-food restaurants, go for grilled chicken and lean roast beef sandwiches or lean plain hamburgers (but remember to hold the fatty sauces), salads with low-fat salad dressing, low-fat milk, and low-fat frozen yogurt. Pizza topped with vegetables and minimum cheese is another good choice.

soy products may offer advantages, and not just in reducing saturated and total fat intake. Soy protein, a complete protein, has been shown to lower blood levels of both total and LDL cholesterol. Based on studies showing that 25 grams of soy protein per day has a cholesterol-lowering effect, the FDA approved a health claim for food labels about the role of soy protein in reducing the risk of cardiovascular disease.[77]

Soy also contains isoflavones, a group of compounds often referred to as *phytoestrogens* because of their hormonelike effects. Phytoestrogens also are found in lignins from flax seed, whole grains, and some fruits. A number of health benefits, including a lowered risk of osteoporosis, heart disease, breast cancer, and menopausal symptoms, are frequently attributed to phytoestrogens, but many also are considered endocrine disruptors, indicating that they have the potential to cause adverse health effects as well.[78]

## Metabolic Syndrome

One in four adults in the United States has **metabolic syndrome**, and the prevalence will continue to grow because of the tendency toward a sedentary lifestyle.[79] Metabolic syndrome is a cluster of at least three of the following signs:[80]

**metabolic syndrome**  A cluster of at least three of the following risk factors for heart disease: hypertriglyceridemia (high blood triglycerides), low HDL cholesterol, hyperglycemia (high blood glucose), hypertension (high blood pressure), and excess abdominal fat.

**cancer**  A term for diseases in which abnormal cells divide without control. Cancer cells can invade nearby tissues and can spread through the bloodstream and lymphatic system to other parts of the body.

- Excess abdominal fat: for most men, a 40-inch waist or greater; for women, a waist of 35 inches or greater
- High blood glucose: at least 100 mg/dL after fasting
- High serum triglycerides: at least 150 mg/dL
- Low HDL cholesterol: less than 40 mg/dL for men; less than 50 mg/dL for women
- Blood pressure of 130/85 mm Hg or higher

Taken individually, each risk factor may not look particularly serious. When you put them together, however, health risks rise dramatically—people with metabolic syndrome have the greatest risk of death from heart attack.

## Putting It All Together

*Healthy People 2010* objectives target reducing deaths from heart disease and stroke as well as reducing the number of adults with high blood cholesterol levels. To accomplish these goals, dietitians recommend lowering total fat intake, lowering saturated and *trans* fat intake, maintaining a healthy body weight, and exercising on a regular basis. Eating fruits, vegetables, legumes, and grains that contain fiber helps lower cholesterol levels, too. These foods contain antioxidants and B vitamins, such as $B_6$ and folate, that may also reduce the risk of heart disease. Substituting fish or soy foods for high-fat meats and cheeses can be beneficial as well.

**Key Concepts**  *To reduce your risk of heart disease, don't smoke, get regular exercise, and control your weight. Dietary changes you can make to reduce your heart disease risk include eating less fat, saturated and trans fat, and cholesterol while increasing intake of fruits, vegetables, and whole grains. Look for sources of omega-3 fatty acids and fiber in your food choices. Metabolic syndrome is a cluster of risk factors that dramatically elevates heart disease risk.*

## Cancer

In the United States and Canada, **cancer** is the second leading cause of death and climbs to the leading cause for American adults aged 40 to 80 years.[81] Reducing both the number of new cancer cases and the death rates from cancer are key objectives of *Healthy People 2010*. There are more than 100 types of cancer; each involves the uncontrolled division of the body's cells. Although cancer can develop in virtually any of the body's tissues, and each type of cancer has its unique features, the basic processes that produce cancer are quite similar in all forms of the disease. Cancer develops in a multistage process that occurs over many years. There are typically three phases of development:

1. *Initiation*, when something alters a cell's genetic structure and prepares it to act abnormally during later stages
2. *Promotion*, a reversible stage when a chemical or other factor encourages initiated cells to become active
3. *Progression*, when promoted cells multiply and may invade surrounding healthy tissue

Cancer usually develops over time. It results from a complex mix of factors related to lifestyle, heredity, and environment. Researchers have identified a number of factors that increase a person's chance of developing cancer. Many types of cancer are related to the use of tobacco, items that people eat and drink, exposure to ultraviolet (UV) radiation from the sun, and exposure to cancer-causing agents (**carcinogens**) in the environment and the workplace. Some people are more sensitive than others to factors that cause cancer. Nevertheless, some people who develop cancer have none of the known risk factors. And some people who do have risk factors do not develop the disease. Researchers have learned that cancer is caused by changes (called *mutations* or *alterations*) in genes that control normal cell growth and cell death. Most cancer-causing gene changes are generated by factors in a person's lifestyle or the environment. However, some alterations that may lead to cancer are inherited; that is, they are passed from parent to child. Having such an inherited gene alteration increases the risk of cancer, but it does not mean that the person is certain to develop cancer.

Although evidence suggests that between 30 and 40 percent of cancers are due to poor food choices and physical inactivity, the role of nutrition and diet in cancer development is complex. Some dietary factors may act as promoters; many others may have protective roles, blocking the cellular changes in one of the developmental stages.

High-fat diets have been associated with an increase in the risk of cancers of the colon and rectum, prostate, and endometrium. The association between high-fat diets and breast cancer appears to be much weaker. The Nurses' Health Study followed more than 121,000 women for 14 years and found no evidence that higher total fat intake was associated with an increased risk of breast cancer.[82] High intake of red meat (beef, pork, lamb) and processed meat (bacon, sausage, hotdogs, lunchmeat) is associated with some types of colorectal cancer; long-term consumption of poultry and fish is associated with reduced risk.[83]

### Dietary and Lifestyle Factors for Reducing Cancer Risk

To reduce your cancer risk, eat a moderately low-fat diet and increase your consumption of fruits, vegetables, and whole grains. Maintain a healthy weight, exercise regularly, don't smoke, and don't use alcohol excessively. If these recommendations are beginning to sound familiar, you're right—the same lifestyle changes that reduce the risk of atherosclerosis and hypertension can reduce the risk of cancer.

The American Cancer Society guidelines—*Nutrition and Physical Activity Guidelines for Cancer Prevention*—emphasize physical activity and weight control and suggest how communities can provide opportunities for Americans to be physically active.[84] The guidelines offer four major recommendations for individual choices. Notice how similar these guidelines are to those for reducing the risk of heart disease:

**carcinogens [kar-SIN-o-jins]** Any substances that cause cancer.

## *Quick* Bite

**What Does the Color of Beef Fat Reveal?**
Yellow-tinged fat indicates that a steer was grass fed. White fat suggests that the animal was fed corn or cereal grain, at least during its final months. Thus, steak surrounded by pearly white fat should be more tender and, consequently, more expensive.

1. Maintain a healthful weight throughout life and balance caloric intake with physical activity.
2. Adopt a physically active lifestyle.
   - For adults: at least 30 minutes of moderate to vigorous activity per day for at least five days of the week; 45 to 60 minutes of intentional physical activity are preferable.
   - For children and adolescents: at least 60 minutes per day of moderate to vigorous activity at least five days of the week.
3. Consume a healthy diet, with an emphasis on plant sources.
   - Choose foods and beverages in amounts that help achieve and maintain a healthy weight.
   - Eat at least five servings of a variety of vegetables and fruits each day.
   - Choose whole grains in preference to processed (refined) grains.
   - Limit consumption of processed and red meats.
4. If you drink alcoholic beverages, limit consumption.
   - Limit intake to no more than two drinks per day for men and one drink per day for women.

**Key Concepts** *Although the evidence linking dietary fats with cancer is contradictory, many other dietary factors play key roles in reducing risk. Strategies for reducing cancer risk include eating more fruits, vegetables, and whole grains; increasing physical activity; maintaining a healthy weight; and limiting alcohol consumption.*

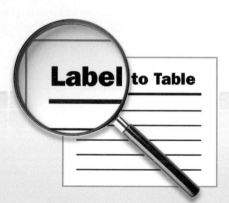

**Label** to Table

The Nutrition Facts panel shown here highlights all of the lipid-related information you can find on a food label. Look at the top of the label, where it states that this product contains 35 calories from fat. Do you know how you can estimate this number from another part of the label? Recall that each gram of fat contains 9 kilocalories (or look at the bottom of the label). If this food item has 4 grams of fat, then it should make sense that there are approximately 36 kilocalories provided by fat.

Total fat is the second thing you'll see, along with saturated and *trans* fat. Manufacturers are required to list only saturated and *trans* fat content on the label, but they can voluntarily list monounsaturated and polyunsaturated fat. Using this food label, you can estimate the amount of unsaturated fat by simply looking at the highlighted sections. There are 4 total grams of fat—2.5 are saturated and 0.5 are *trans*. That means the remaining 1.0 grams are either polyunsaturated, monounsaturated, or a mix of both. Without even knowing what food item this label represents, you can see that it contains more saturated and *trans* fat than unsaturated fat (3.0 grams versus 1.0 gram).

Do you see the "6%" to the right of "Total Fat"? This does not mean that the food item contains 6 percent of its calories from fat. In fact, this food item contains 23 percent of its calories from fat (35 fat kilocalories ÷ 154 total kilocalories = 0.23, or 23 percent fat kilocalories). The 6 percent refers to the Daily Values. You can see that a person who consumes 2,000 kilocalories per day could consume up to 65 grams of fat per day. This product contributes just 4 grams per serving, which is 6 percent of that amount (4 ÷ 65 = 0.06, or 6 percent). Note that the Percent Daily Value (%DV) for saturated fat is 12 percent, so just a few servings of this food can contribute quite a bit of saturated fat to your diet. There is no %DV for *trans* fat, but intake should be kept as low as possible. Cholesterol also is highlighted on this label (20 milligrams), along with its Daily Value contribution (7 percent).

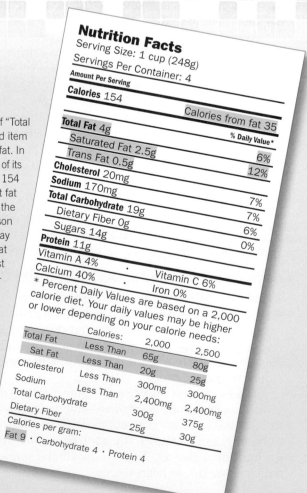

**Nutrition Facts**
Serving Size: 1 cup (248g)
Servings Per Container: 4

**Amount Per Serving**

**Calories** 154 | Calories from fat 35

| | % Daily Value * |
|---|---|
| **Total Fat** 4g | 6% |
| Saturated Fat 2.5g | 12% |
| Trans Fat 0.5g | |
| **Cholesterol** 20mg | 7% |
| **Sodium** 170mg | 7% |
| **Total Carbohydrate** 19g | 6% |
| Dietary Fiber 0g | 0% |
| Sugars 14g | |
| **Protein** 11g | |

Vitamin A 4% • Vitamin C 6%
Calcium 40% • Iron 0%

* Percent Daily Values are based on a 2,000 calorie diet. Your daily values may be higher or lower depending on your calorie needs:

| | | Calories: | 2,000 | 2,500 |
|---|---|---|---|---|
| Total Fat | Less Than | | 65g | 80g |
| Sat Fat | Less Than | | 20g | 25g |
| Cholesterol | Less Than | | 300mg | 300mg |
| Sodium | Less Than | | 2,400mg | 2,400mg |
| Total Carbohydrate | | | 300g | 375g |
| Dietary Fiber | | | 25g | 30g |

Calories per gram:
Fat 9 • Carbohydrate 4 • Protein 4

# Learning Portfolio

## Key Terms

## Study Points

- There are three main classes of lipids: triglycerides, phospholipids, and sterols.
- Fatty acids are components of both triglycerides and phospholipids.
- Saturated fatty acids have no double bonds between carbon atoms in their carbon chains, monounsaturated fatty acids have one double bond, and polyunsaturated fatty acids have more than one double bond in their carbon chains.
- Two polyunsaturated fatty acids, linoleic acid and alpha-linolenic acid, are essential and must be supplied in the diet. Phospholipids and sterols are made in the body and do not have to be supplied in the diet.
- Essential fatty acids are precursors of hormonelike compounds called eicosanoids. These compounds regulate many body functions, including blood pressure, heart rate, inflammation, and immune response.
- Triglycerides are food fats and storage fats. They are composed of glycerol and three fatty acids.
- In the body, triglycerides are an important source of energy. Stored fat provides an energy reserve.
- Phospholipids are made of glycerol, two fatty acids, and a compound containing phosphate and nitrogen.
- Phospholipids are components of cell membranes and lipoproteins. Having both fat- and water-soluble components allows them to be effective emulsifiers in foods and in the body.
- Cholesterol is found in cell membranes and is used to synthesize vitamin D, bile salts, and steroid hormones. High levels of blood cholesterol are associated with increased heart disease risk.
- For adults, the Acceptable Macronutrient Distribution Range (AMDR) for fat is 20 to 35 percent of calories.
- Diets high in fat and saturated fat tend to increase blood levels of LDL cholesterol and increase risk for heart disease.
- Excess fat in the diet is linked to obesity, heart disease, and some types of cancer.

## Study Questions

1. What do the terms *saturated*, *monounsaturated*, and *polyunsaturated* mean with regard to fatty acids?
2. What does the hardness or softness of a fat typically signify?
3. Name the two essential fatty acids.
4. What is the most common form of lipid found in food?
5. List the many functions of triglycerides.
6. What are the positive and negative consequences of hydrogenating a fat?

7. Which foods contain cholesterol?

8. Describe the difference between LDL and HDL in terms of cholesterol and protein composition.

9. List the recommendations for intake of total fat, saturated fat, and cholesterol.

## Try This

### The Fat = Fullness Challenge

The goal of this experiment is to see whether fat affects your desire to eat between meals. Do this experiment for two consecutive breakfasts. Each meal is to include only the foods listed below. Try to eat normally for the other meals of the day and eat around the same time of day. Each of these breakfasts has approximately the same calories, but one has a high percentage of them from fat, the other from carbohydrate. After each breakfast, take note of how many hours pass before you feel hungry again.

| Day 1 (~420 kcal; 1.5 grams of fat) | Day 2 (~430 kcal; 28 grams of fat) |
|---|---|
| 1 3-oz bagel with 3 tablespoon of jelly | 2 eggs, fried |
| | 1 biscuit (2½ inch diameter) with 1 teaspoon butter or margarine |

### The Salad Dressing Experiment

You can learn a lot from oil-and-vinegar dressing! The purpose of this experiment is twofold. First, you will understand better what it means to say that lipids are insoluble (or not water-soluble). Second, you will be able to experience how fat acts based on its density. Go to your local grocery store and purchase a seasoning packet for Italian (oil and vinegar) dressing. Make sure you also purchase the amount of oil (any type is fine) and vinegar (any type is fine) you need based on the directions. Once home, prepare the dressing. Shake the dressing as if you were to pour it on a salad and then let it stand. What happens to the dressing? What explains this action? Once the dressing settles, which ingredient is found on top—the oil or the vinegar? What property of fat explains this?

## What About Bobbie?

Let's take a look at Bobbie's fat intake. Review her day of eating (see the "Food Choices: Nutrients and Nourishment" chapter) and pay special attention to the foods you know contain fat. What percentage of her calories do you think came from fat? Did she eat more saturated or unsaturated fat? How about her cholesterol intake? Do you think she came in below the guideline?

Bobbie's total fat intake was 86 grams. Here are the foods that contributed the most fat:

| Food | Fat (g) |
|---|---|
| Salad dressing | 13 |
| Meatballs | 11 |
| Tortilla chips | 11 |
| Garlic bread | 10 |
| Cream cheese | 8 |
| Mayonnaise | 7 |
| Pizza | 6 |

Bobbie's diet has 34 percent of its calories from fat, which is within the AMDR for fat.

**86 g fat × 9 kcal/g = 774 kcal fat**
**774 kcal fat ÷ 2,300 total kcal = 0.34, or 34% kcal from fat**

Are you surprised her fat intake is on the high end of the recommended range? Her intake doesn't look too unusual, but you can see how the "extras" along the way add up. Look at the list of fat-containing foods again. Do you think her diet is higher in saturated or unsaturated fat? Well, three of the foods listed are animal products (meatballs, pizza, and cream cheese), so you know they contribute to the amount of saturated fat. Both the tortilla chips and garlic bread contain a mixture of saturated and unsaturated fats, and the Italian dressing contains mostly unsaturated fat. Her overall saturated fat intake is 27 grams. That's about 11 percent of her caloric intake, which is more than recommended by the *Dietary Guidelines for Americans* (no more than 10 percent of energy as saturated fat).

If Bobbie wanted to lower her saturated fat and total fat intake, what changes could she make? Here are some suggestions.

Bobbie can lower her saturated fat intake by:

- Topping her bagel with peanut butter instead of cream cheese
- Decreasing the number of meatballs on her pasta
- Snacking on pizza less often

Bobbie can lower her overall fat intake by:

- Using cream cheese on only half her bagel and using jelly on the other half
- Using only mustard on her sandwich, not mustard and mayonnaise
- Reducing the amount of tortilla chips she eats by half and having a piece of fruit in their place
- Reducing the amount of Italian dressing she puts on her salad (2 tablespoons contain 11 grams of fat and more than 100 kilocalories!)

- Having a plain piece of bread with dinner, not the garlic bread made with butter or margarine
- When dining out, selecting a baked potato topped with salsa rather than butter and sour cream

In terms of cholesterol, how do you think Bobbie did? She consumed 261 milligrams in this day. If she follows the above tips to lower her saturated fat intake, she'll find her overall cholesterol intake will be cut in half!

# References

1 Goncalves DC, Lira FS, Carnevali LC Jr, et al. Conjugated linoleic acid: good or bad nutrient. *Diabetol Metab Syndr*. 2010;2:62.

2 Anderson BM, Ma DW. Are all *n*-3 polyunsaturated fatty acids created equal? *Lipids Health Dis*. 2009;8:33.

3 Der G, Batty GD, Deary IJ. Effect of breastfeeding on intelligence in children: prospective study, sibling pairs analysis, and meta-analysis. *BMJ*. 2006;333:945–949.

4 Sathe MN, Patel AS. Update in pediatrics: focus on fat-soluble vitamins. *Nutr Clin Prac*. 2010;25(4):340–346.

5 American Heart Association. Fish and omega-3 fatty acids. http://www.heart.org/HEARTORG/GettingHealthy/NutritionCenter/HealthyDietGoals/Fish-and-Omega-3-Fatty-Acids_UCM_303248_Article.jsp. Accessed 5/24/11.

6 Sharma A, Khare SK, Gupta MN. Three phase partitioning for extraction of oil from soybean. *Bioresour Technol*. 2002;85:327–329.

7 Heinecke JW. Oxidative stress: new approaches to diagnosis and prognosis in atherosclerosis. *Am J Cardiol*. 2003;91(suppl):12A–16A.

8 Wiviott SD, Cannon CP, Morrow DA, et al. Can low-density lipoprotein be too low? The safety and efficacy of achieving very low low-density lipoprotein with intensive statin therapy. *J Am Coll Cardiol*. 2005;46:1411–1416.

9 El-Sadr WM, Mullin CM, Carr A, et al. Effects of HIV disease on lipid, glucose and insulin levels: results from a large antiretroviral-naïve cohort. *HIV Medicine*. 2005;6:114–121.

10 Hu J, La Vecchia C, de Groh M, et al. Dietary cholesterol intake and cancer. *Ann Oncol*. 2001;May 4.

11 Vejux A, Samadi M, Lizard G. Contribution of cholesterol and oxysterols in the physiopathology of cataract: implication for the development of pharmacological treatment. *J Ophthalmol*. 2011;2011:471947.

12 Dooley R, Harvey BJ, Thomas W. The regulation of cell growth and survival by aldosterone. *Front Biosci*. 2011;16:440–457; and Saher G, Brugger B, Lappe-Siefke C, et al. High cholesterol level is essential for myelin membrane growth. *Nat Neurosci*. 2005;8:468–475.

13 Castro Cabezas M, de Vries JHM, Antonie JH, et al. Effects of stanol-enriched diet on plasma cholesterol and triglycerides in patients treated with statins. *J Am Diet Assoc*. 2006;106(10):1564–1569.

14 Ibid.

15 Ohlsson L. Dairy products and plasma cholesterol levels. *Food Nutr Res*. 2010;19:54.

16 Jones PJH, Kubow S. Lipids, sterols and their metabolites. In: Shills ME, Shike M, Ross CA, Caballero B, Cousins, RJ, eds. *Modern Nutrition in Health and Disease*. 10th ed. Philadelphia: Lippincott Williams & Wilkins; 2006:92–135.

17 Guyton AC, Hall JE. *Textbook of Medical Physiology*. 11th ed. Philadelphia: W.B. Saunders; 2006.

18 Dean JT, Rizk ML, Tan Y, et al. Ensemble modeling of hepatic fatty acid metabolism with a synthetic glyoxylate shunt. *Biophys J*. 2010; 98(8):1385–1395.

19 Lin J, Yang R, Tarr PT. Hyperlipidemic effects of dietary saturated fats mediated through PGC-1b coactivation of SREBP. *Cell*. 2005;120:261–273.

20 Zhao Z, Michaely P. Role of an intramolecular contact on lipoprotein uptake by the LDL receptor. *Biochem Biophys Acta*. 2011;1811(6):397–408.

21 Kolovou GD, Anagnostopoulou KK, Cokkinos DV. Pathophysiology of dyslipidaemia in the metabolic syndrome. *Postgrad Med J*. 2005;81:358–366.

22 Wijendran V, Hayes KC. Dietary *n*-6 and *n*-3 fatty acid balance and cardiovascular health. *Ann Rev Nutr*. 2004;24:597–615.

23 Kleber ME, Grammer TB, Marz W. High-density lipoprotein (HDL) and cholesteryl ester transfer protein (CETP): role in lipid metabolism and clinical meaning. *MMW Fortschr Med*. 2010;152(suppl 2):47–55.

24 US Department of Agriculture, US Department of Health and Human Services. *Dietary Guidelines for Americans, 2010*. 7th ed. Washington, DC: US Government Printing Office; 2010.

25 Ibid.

26 Institute of Medicine, Food and Nutrition Board. *Dietary Reference Intakes for Energy, Carbohydrate, Fiber, Fat, Fatty Acids, Cholesterol, Protein, and Amino Acids*. Washington, DC: National Academies Press; 2005.

27 Ibid.

28 Ibid.

29 Egert S, Kannenberg F, Somoza V, et al. Dietary alpha-linolenic acid, EPA, and DHA have differential effects on LDL fatty acid composition but similar effects on serum lipid profiles in normolipidemic humans. *J Nutr*. 2009;139(5):861–868.

30 Wijendran V, Hayes KC. Op. cit.; and Egert S, Kannenberg F, Somoza V. Op. cit.

31 US Department of Agriculture, US Department of Health and Human Services. Op. cit.

32 US Department of Health and Human Services, Environmental Protection Agency. What You Need to Know About Mercury in Fish and Shellfish. March 2004. http://www.fda.gov/Food/FoodSafety/Product-SpecificInformation/Seafood/FoodbornePathogensContaminants/Methylmercury/ucm115662.htm. Accessed 5/24/11.

33 Wright JD, Wang C-H. Trends in Intake of Energy and Macronutrients in Adults from 1999–2000 Through 2007–2008. US Department of Health and Human Services, Centers for Disease Control and Prevention. http://www.cdc.gov/nchs/data/databriefs/db49.pdf. Accessed 5/23/11.

34 US Department of Agriculture, US Department of Health and Human Services. Op. cit.

35 Briefel RR, Johnson CL. Secular trends in dietary intake in the United States. *Ann Rev Nutr*. 2004;24:401–431.

36 Position of the Academy of Nutrition and Dietetics: fat replacers. *J Am Diet Assoc*. 2005;105:266–275; and Phelan S, Lang W, Jordan D, Wing RR. Use of artificial sweeteners and fat-modified foods in weight loss maintainers and always-normal weight individuals. *Int J Obes*. 2009;33(10):1183–1190.

37 Neuhouser ML, Rock CL, Kristal AR, et al. Olestra is associated with slight reductions in serum carotenoids but does not markedly influence serum fat-soluble vitamin concentrations. *Am J Clin Nutr*. 2006;83:624–631.

38 Position of the Academy of Nutrition and Dietetics: fat replacers. *J Am Diet Assoc*. 2005;105(2):266–275.

39 Satia-Abouta J, Kristal AR, Patterson RE, et al. Is olestra consumption associated with changes in dietary intake, serum lipids, and body weight? *Nutrition*. 2003;19:754–759.

40 Neuhouser ML, Rock CL, Kristal AR, et al. Olestra is associated with slight reductions in serum carotenoids but does not markedly influence serum fat-soluble vitamin concentrations. *Am J Clin Nutr*. 2006;83(3):624–631.

41 Ibid.

42 Ibid.

43 Miller DL, Casteollanos VH, Shide DJ, et al. Effect of fat-free potato chips with and without nutrition labels on fat and energy intakes. *Am J Clin Nutr*. 1998;68:282–290.

44 Position of the Academy of Nutrition and Dietetics: fat replacers. Op. cit.

45 Ibid.

46 Prentice RL, Caan B, Chlebowski RT, et al. Low-fat dietary pattern and risk of invasive breast cancer: the Women's Health Initiative Randomized Controlled Dietary Modification Trial. *JAMA*. 2006;295:629–642.

47 Centers for Disease Control and Prevention. Overweight and Obesity. http://www.cdc.gov/nccdphp/dnpa/obesity/index.htm. Accessed 5/23/11.

48 Goldie MP. Heart disease: the number one killer of women. *Int J Dent Hyg*. 2007;5(2):122–123.

49 Lloyd-Jones D, Adams RJ, Brown TM, et al. *Heart Disease and Stroke Statistics—2010 Update. A Report from the American Heart Association Statistics Committee and Stroke Statistics Subcommittee*. 2010; page 121.

50    Mehta PK, Wenger NK. Coronary heart disease in women: battle is won, but the war remains. *Minerva Med*. 2007;98(5):459–478.

51    Goldenberg I, Benderly M, Sidi R, et al. Relation of clinical benefit of raising high-density lipoprotein cholesterol to serum levels of low-density lipoprotein cholesterol in patients with coronary heart disease (from the Bezafibrate Infarction Prevention Trial). *Am J Cardiol*. 2009;103(1):41–45.

52    Kassner U, Vogt A, Rosada A, et al. Designing a study to evaluate the effect of apheresis in patients with elevated lipoprotein(a). *Atheroscler*. 2009;10(5):85–88.

53    Calabro P, Galia E, Yeh ET. Role of C-reactive protein in acute myocardial infarction and stroke: possible therapeutic approaches. *Curr Pharm Biotechnol*. 2011;Apr 6.

54    Walvoord EC. The timing of puberty: is it changing? Does it matter? *J Adolesc Health*. 2010;47(5):433–439.

55    World Health Organization. *Diet, Nutrition and the Prevention of Chronic Disease*. WHO Technical Report Series, no. 913. Geneva: World Health Organization; 2002.

56    Craig WJ. Nutrition concerns and health effects of vegetarian diets. *Nutr Clin Pract*. 2010;25(6):613–620.

57    Wong J, de Souza R, Kendall C, et al. Colonic health: fermentation and short chain fatty acids. *J Clin Gastroenterol*. 2006;40(3):235–243.

58    Institute of Medicine, Food and Nutrition Board. Op. cit.

59    Mellen PB, Walsh TF, Herrington DM. Whole grain intake and cardiovascular disease: a meta-analysis. *Nutr Metab Cardiovasc Dis*. 2008;18(4):283–290.

60    Institute of Medicine, Food and Nutrition Board. Op. cit.

61    Bang HO, Dyerberg J. The composition of food consumed by Greenlandic Eskimos. *Acta Med Scand*. 1973;200:69–73.

62    Harris WS. *Omega*-3 fatty acids and cardiovascular disease: A case for *omega*-3 index as a new risk factor. *Pharm Research*. 2007;55:217–223.

63    He K, Song Y, Daviglus ML, et al. Fish consumption and incidence of stroke: a meta-analysis of cohort studies. *Stroke*. 2004;35:1538–1542.

64    Egert S, Kannenberg F, Somoza V, et al. Dietary alpha-linolenic acid, EPA, and DHA have differential effects on LDL fatty acid composition but similar effects on serum lipid profiles in normolipidemic humans. *J Nutr*. 2009;139(5):861–868.

65    National Institutes of Health, Office of Dietary Supplements. *Omega*-3 fatty acids and health. http://ods.od.nih.gov/factsheets/Omega3FattyAcidsandHealth. Accessed 5/31/11.

66    American Heart Association. Fish and *omega*-3 fatty acids. Updated 11/7/2010. http://www.heart.org/HEARTORG/General/Fish-and-Omega-3-Fatty-Acids_UCM_303248_Article.jsp. Accessed 10/20/2011.

67    Brouwer IA, Wanders AJ, Katan MB. Effect of animal and industrial *trans* fatty acids on HDL and LDL cholesterol levels in humans—a quantitative review. *PLoS One*. 2010;5(3).

68    Siri-Tarino PW, Sun Q, Hu FB, Krauss RM. Saturated fat, carbohydrate, and cardiovascular disease. *Am J Clin Nutr*. 2010;91(3):502–509.

69    Bhupathiraju SN, Tucker KL. Coronary heart disease prevention: Nutrients, foods, and dietary patterns. *Clin Chim Acta*. 2011;412(17–18):1493–1514.

70    Yamada M, Murakami K, Sasaki S, et al. Soft drink intake is associated with diet quality even among young Japanese women with low soft drink intake. *J Am Diet Assoc*. 2008;108(12):1997–2004.

71    Ibid.

72    Wright JD, Wang C-H. Op. cit.; and Briefel RR, Johnson CL. Op. cit.

73    Lippi G, Franchini M, Favaloro EJ, Targher G. Moderate red wine consumption and cardiovascular disease risk: beyond the "French paradox." *Semin Thromb Hemost*. 2010;36(1):59–70.

74    Lucas DL, Brown RA, Wassef M, Giles TD. Alcohol and the cardiovascular system: research challenges and opportunities. *J Am Coll Cardiol*. 2005;45;1916–1924.

75    Khoo HE, Prasad KN, Kong KW, et al. Carotenoids and their isomers: color pigments in fruits and vegetables. *Molecules*. 2011;16(2):1710–1738.

76    McCully KS. Homocysteine, vitamins, and vascular disease prevention. *Am J Clin Nutr*. 2007;86:1563S–1568S.

77    FDA Talk Paper. New Health Claim Proposed for Relationship of Soy Protein and Coronary Heart Disease. November 10, 1998, Food and Drug Administration, US Department of Health and Human Services, Rockville, MD.

78    Patisaul HB, Jefferson W. The pros and cons of phytoestrogens. *Front Neuroendocrinol*. 2010;31(4):400–419.

79    Finley CE, Barlow CE, Halton TL, Haskell WL. Glycemic index, glycemic load, and prevalence of the metabolic syndrome in the Copper Center Longitudinal Study. *J Am Diet Assoc*. 2010;110(12):1820–1829.

80    Ibid.

81    Center for Disease Control and Prevention. Deaths and mortality. Final 2007 data. http://www.cdc.gov/nchs/fastats/deaths.htm. Accessed 5/23/11.

82    Holmes MD, Hunter DJ, Colditz GA, et al. Association of dietary intake of fat and fatty acids with risk of breast cancer. *JAMA*. 1999;281:914–920.

83    Randi G, Edefonti V, Ferraroni M, et al. Dietary patterns and the risk of colorectal cancer and adenomas. *Nutr Rev*. 2010;68(7):389–408.

84    Kushi L, Byers T, Doyle C, et al., and the American Cancer Society 2006 Nutrition and Physical Activity Guidelines Advisory Committee. American Cancer Society Guidelines on Nutrition and Physical Activity for Cancer Prevention. Reducing the risk of cancer with healthy food choices and physical activity. *CA Cancer J Clin*. 2006;55:254–281.

# CHAPTER 7

# Proteins and Amino Acids: Function Follows Form

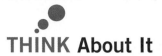

**THINK About It**

1 What's your understanding of the term *protein-sparing*?

2 What percentage of your energy intake do you think comes from protein?

3 Do you take amino acid supplements? If so, do you know how well they are absorbed?

4 Do you follow a vegetarian type diet, or have you ever considered it?

**Visit go.jblearning.com/inseldisco4e**

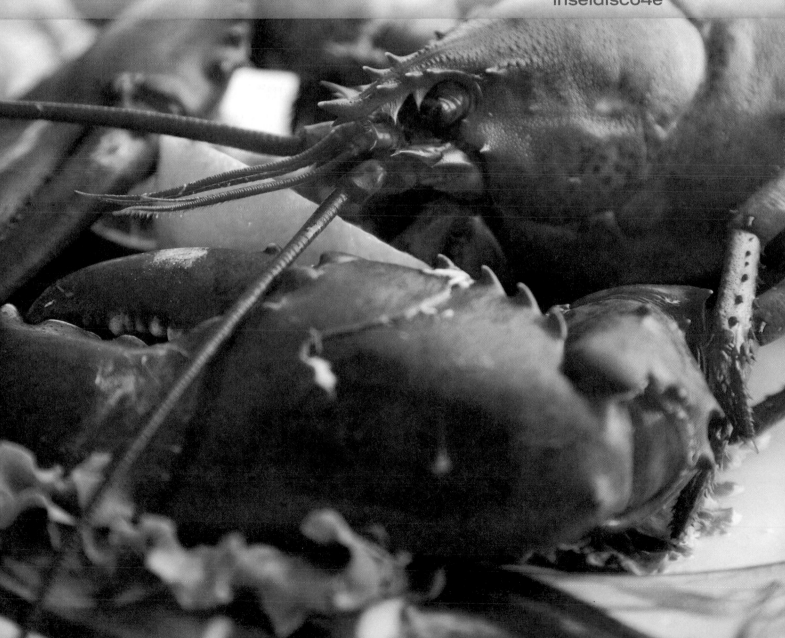

## *Quick* Bite

**A Bugburger Anyone?**
Did you know that bugs provide 10 percent of the protein consumed worldwide? What creepy crawler would you choose for your dinner plate? A grasshopper is 15 to 60 percent protein. Pound for pound, spiders have more protein than any other bug.

Think of your favorite meal—perhaps a holiday feast, the foods you always ask for on your birthday, or something from a special restaurant. If you're like most Americans, you've probably conjured up something along the lines of steak and baked potato; lobster and corn on the cob; turkey with dressing, mashed potatoes, and all the trimmings; or maybe something simpler—a juicy hamburger and fries. What do all these meals have in common? In each case, you imagine a meat or fish item as the focus of the meals, surrounded by various grain or vegetable accompaniments.

From a young age, we're taught that meat is an important source of protein and that protein helps us grow big and strong. Many traditional diets emphasize meat as the most important ingredient of the meal and protein as the most important nutrient. But do such meals meet your body's needs? Could a different style of eating be more healthful? For example, what about adding just a small amount of meat to a stir-fry of vegetables over rice? Or what about eliminating meat entirely from the diet? What makes the most sense nutritionally?

From the body's perspective, protein is critically important. Protein is part of every cell, is needed in thousands of chemical reactions, and keeps us "together" structurally. But, as you are about to learn, the human body is so good at using the protein we feed it that our actual needs for dietary protein are relatively small—meat doesn't need to be at the center of the plate to keep you healthy!

## Why Is Protein Important?

The word *protein* was coined by the Dutch chemist Gerardus Mulder in 1838 and comes from the Greek word *protos*, meaning "of prime importance." Second only to water, Mulder discovered that proteins are a major component of all plant and animal tissues. Today we know that these intricately constructed molecules are vital to many aspects of health and play an essential role in every living cell. Our bodies use protein for functions such as replacing skin cells that slough off over time, producing antibodies to fight infections, and assisting in the essential body processes of water balance, nutrition transport, and muscle contractions.[1] Proteins are a source of energy and help keep skin, hair, and nails healthy.[2] Protein is absolutely critical for overall good health. Our bodies constantly assemble, break down, and use proteins, so we count on our diet to provide enough protein each day to replace what is being used. When we eat more protein than we need, the excess is either used to make energy or stored as fat.

Most people associate protein with animal foods such as beef, chicken, fish, or milk. However, plant foods such as dried beans and peas, grains, nuts, seeds, and vegetables also provide protein. Many protein-rich plant foods are also rich in vitamins and minerals. These plant foods usually are low in fat and calories.

People living in poverty may suffer from a shortage of both protein and energy in the diet. When the diet lacks protein, the body breaks down tissue such as muscle and uses it as a protein source. This causes loss, or **wasting**, of muscles, organs, and other tissues. Protein deficiency also affects the immune system, making people more vulnerable to infection, and impairs digestion and absorption of nutrients. In the United States and other industrialized countries, most people are able to get more than enough protein to meet the body's needs. In fact, a more common problem in these areas is excess intake of protein.

**wasting** The breakdown of body tissue, such as muscle and organ, for use as a protein source when the diet lacks protein.

# Amino Acids Are the Building Blocks of Proteins

Just as glucose is the basic building block of carbohydrates, **amino acids** are the basic building blocks of proteins. Proteins are sequences of amino acids. When building these sequences, your body has 20 different amino acids from which to choose. Nine of these amino acids are called **indispensable**, or **essential**, **amino acids** because your body cannot make them and must get them through the diet. Your body can manufacture the remaining 11 amino acids, called **dispensable**, or **nonessential**, **amino acids**, when enough nitrogen, carbon, hydrogen, and oxygen are supplied in the diet. Dispensable amino acids do not need to be supplied in your diet.

Some dispensable amino acids may become conditionally indispensable amino acids if the body cannot make them because of illness or in certain circumstances where the body lacks the necessary precursors or enzymes to make them. Tyrosine and cysteine are both considered **conditionally indispensable amino acids**. Under normal circumstances, your body makes tyrosine from the indispensable amino acid phenylalanine and cysteine from either methionine or serine. If a disease or condition interferes with the body's ability to synthesize tyrosine or cysteine from their amino acid precursors, then it will need tyrosine or cysteine from the diet. Table 7.1 lists the indispensable, dispensable, and conditionally indispensable amino acids.

Tyrosine becomes an indispensable amino acid for individuals with the rare genetic disorder phenylketonuria (PKU). Because people with PKU lack sufficient amounts of an enzyme needed to convert phenylalanine to tyrosine, tyrosine must be supplied in their diets. Phenylalanine intake must be carefully controlled because excess phenylalanine can build up and contribute to irreversible brain damage.[3] When babies with PKU receive treatment starting at birth, their IQ development is unaffected. Without treatment, however, they suffer severe mental retardation.

Other amino acids can become indispensable under certain circumstances. The amino acid glutamine is the main fuel for rapidly dividing cells and plays a key role in transporting nitrogen between organs.[4] Although normally considered dispensable, glutamine can become indispensable if the body's need for it increases substantially, such as when a person suffers trauma or becomes critically ill.[5] The amino acid arginine can become indispensable when a person is ill or experiencing severe physiological stress.[6]

**amino acids** The building blocks of protein.

**indispensable (essential) amino acids** Amino acids the body cannot make at all or cannot make in sufficient quantities to meet the body's needs. Indispensable amino acids must be supplied in the diet.

**dispensable (nonessential) amino acids** Amino acids the body can make if supplied with adequate nitrogen. Dispensable amino acids do not need to be supplied in the diet.

**conditionally indispensable amino acids** Amino acids that are normally made in the body (dispensable) but become indispensable under certain circumstances, such as during critical illness. Also called *conditionally essential amino acids*.

**Table 7.1** **Indispensable, Dispensable, and Conditionally Indispensable Amino Acids**

| Indispensable | Dispensable | Conditionally Indispensable |
|---|---|---|
| Histidine | Alanine | |
| Isoleucine | Arginine | Arginine |
| Leucine | Asparagine | |
| Lysine | Aspartic acid | |
| Methionine | Cysteine | Cysteine |
| Phenylalanine | Glutamic acid | |
| Theronine | Glutamine | Glutamine |
| Tryptophan | Glycine | Glycine |
| | Proline | Proline |
| | Serine | |
| | Tyrosine | Tyrosine |

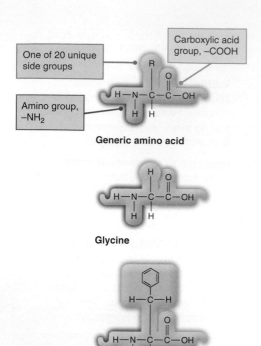

**Figure 7.1**  **Structure of an amino acid.**
All amino acids have a similar structure. Attached to a carbon atom is a hydrogen (H), an amino group (–NH$_2$), an acid group (–COOH), and a side group (R). The side group gives each amino acid its unique identity.

**peptide bond**  The bond between two amino acids formed when a carboxyl (–COOH) group of one amino acid joins an amino (–NH$_2$) group of another amino acid, releasing water in the process.

**dipeptide**  Two amino acids joined by a peptide bond.

**tripeptide**  Three amino acids joined by peptide bonds.

**oligopeptide**  Four to 10 amino acids joined by peptide bonds.

**polypeptide**  More than 10 amino acids joined by peptide bonds.

**hemoglobin [HEEM-oh-glow-bin]**  The oxygen-carrying protein in red blood cells that consists of four heme groups and four globin polypeptide chains. The presence of hemoglobin gives blood its red color.

## Amino Acids Are Identified by Their Side Groups

Amino acids (with the exception of proline) have a central carbon atom attached to one hydrogen atom (H), one carboxylic acid group (–COOH), one amino (nitrogen-containing) group (–NH$_2$), and one side group unique to each amino acid (R). The side group gives each amino acid its identity. It can vary from a simple hydrogen atom, as in glycine, to a complex ring of carbon and hydrogen atoms, as in phenylalanine. The variations in side groups mean that individual amino acids differ in shape, size, composition, electrical charge, and pH. When amino acids link together to form a protein, these characteristics work together to determine that protein's specific function. **Figure 7.1** shows the structure of an amino acid.

**Key Concepts**  *Amino acids, which consist of a central carbon atom bonded to a hydrogen, a carboxyl group, an amino group, and a side group, are the building blocks of proteins. Indispensable amino acids cannot be made by the body and must be supplied in the diet. Dispensable amino acids can be made by the body, given an adequate supply of nitrogen, carbon, hydrogen, and oxygen. Conditionally indispensable amino acids are normally dispensable but become indispensable under certain physiological conditions.*

## Protein Structure: Unique Three-Dimensional Shapes and Functions

Proteins are very large molecules. Just as we combine letters of the alphabet in different sequences to form a nearly infinite variety of words, the body combines amino acids in different sequences to form a nearly infinite variety of proteins. For this reason, protein molecules are more varied than those of either carbohydrates or lipids. (See the FYI feature "Scrabble Anyone?")

### Amino Acid Sequence

Amino acids link in specific sequences to form strands of protein (often called *peptides*) up to hundreds of amino acids long. Each amino acid is joined to the next by a **peptide bond**. (See **Figure 7.2**.) A **dipeptide** is two amino acids joined by a peptide bond, and a **tripeptide** is three amino acids joined by peptide bonds. The term **oligopeptide** refers to a chain of 4 to 10 amino acids, and a **polypeptide** contains more than 10 amino acids.[7] A chain with more than 50 amino acids is called a protein. Proteins in the body and in the diet are long polypeptides, most with hundreds, or even thousands of linked amino acids.

### Protein Shape

As a cell assembles amino acids into a protein, the protein assumes a unique three-dimensional shape that stems from the sequence and properties of its amino acids. This three-dimensional shape determines the protein's function and the way it interacts with other molecules. As an example, **Figure 7.3** illustrates the unique folded and twisted shape of **hemoglobin**, the iron-carrying protein in red blood cells. In the lungs, hemoglobin binds oxygen and releases carbon dioxide. It then travels throughout the body, delivering oxygen to other tissues and picking up carbon dioxide for the return trip to the lungs.

## Protein Denaturation: Destabilizing a Protein's Shape

The chemical links that hold a protein's three-dimensional shape can be disrupted. Changes in the acidity or alkalinity of the protein's environment, high temperatures, alcohol, oxidation, and agitation can all cause a protein to unfold and lose its shape (denature), as shown in **Figure 7.4**. Because a protein's shape determines its function, denatured proteins lose their ability to function properly.

If you've ever cooked an egg, you've witnessed protein **denaturation**. As the egg cooks, some of its protein bonds break. As these proteins unfold, they bump into and bind to each other. Eventually, as these interconnections increase, the liquid egg coagulates to form a solid. Raw egg white proteins denature and stiffen as they are whipped, and milk proteins denature and curdle when acid is added.

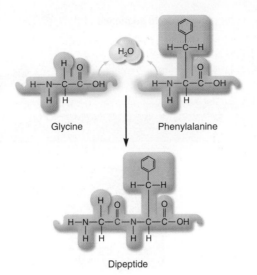

Glycine    Phenylalanine

Dipeptide

**Figure 7.2**  **Forming a peptide bond.** When two amino acids join together, the acid group of one amino acid is matched with the amino group of another. When amino acids are joined, the reaction forms a peptide bond and releases water.

**denaturation** A change in the three-dimensional structure of a protein resulting in an unfolded polypeptide chain that cannot fulfill the protein's function. Treatment with heat, acid, alkali, or extreme agitation can denature most proteins.

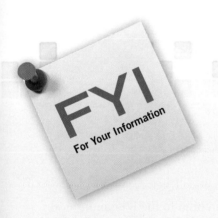

# Scrabble Anyone?

Making a meaningful word from available Scrabble tiles is a good analogy for the making of a functional protein chain from available amino acids. Just as we can make many different words from the same tiles, cells can make many different proteins from the same amino acids.

If your cells have all 20 amino acids at their disposal, these can be arranged in a bewildering number of combinations to create tens of thousands of different protein chains, just as all the letters of the alphabet can be used to make an almost unlimited number of words.

**Scrabble tile = amino acid**

**word = protein chain**

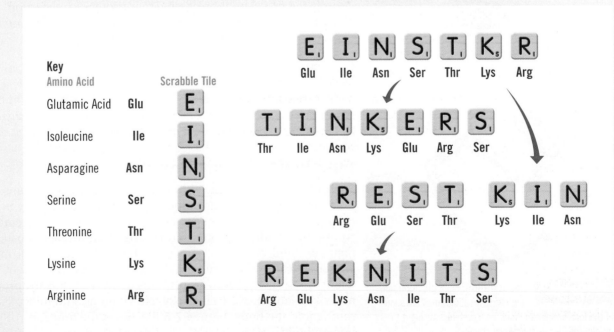

| Key | | Scrabble Tile |
|---|---|---|
| Amino Acid | | |
| Glutamic Acid | Glu | E₁ |
| Isoleucine | Ile | I₁ |
| Asparagine | Asn | N₁ |
| Serine | Ser | S₁ |
| Threonine | Thr | T₁ |
| Lysine | Lys | K₅ |
| Arginine | Arg | R₁ |

E₁ I₁ N₁ S₁ T₁ K₅ R₁
Glu  Ile  Asn  Ser  Thr  Lys  Arg

T₁ I₁ N₁ K₅ E₁ R₁ S₁
Thr  Ile  Asn  Lys  Glu  Arg  Ser

R₁ E₁ S₁ T₁ K₅ I₁ N₁
Arg  Glu  Ser  Thr  Lys  Ile  Asn

R₁ E₁ K₅ N₁ I₁ T₁ S₁
Arg  Glu  Lys  Asn  Ile  Thr  Ser

**Amino acid sequence**

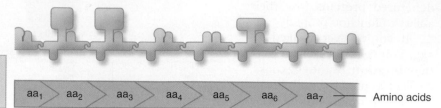

A simple illustration of a protein just shows the sequence of amino acids that form one or more polypeptide chains.

aa₁ > aa₂ > aa₃ > aa₄ > aa₅ > aa₆ > aa₇ > — Amino acids

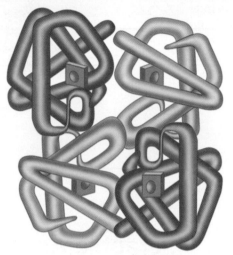

A more complex illustration of a protein shows its three-dimensional structure. This molecule of hemoglobin is composed of four polypeptide chains. The square plates represent nonprotein portions of the molecule (heme) that carry oxygen.

**Three-dimensional structure**

**Figure 7.3** **Protein structure.** The simplest depiction of a protein reveals its unique sequence of amino acids. Each protein becomes folded, twisted, and coiled into a shape all its own. This shape defines how a protein functions in your body.

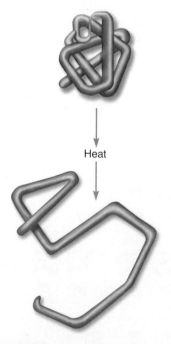

Heat

**Figure 7.4** **Denaturation.** Heat, pH, oxidation, and mechanical agitation are some of the forces that can denature a protein, causing it to unfold and lose its functional shape.

If an egg is eaten raw, its avidin protein can bind to the B vitamin biotin in the digestive tract, making the vitamin unavailable for absorption. Cooking the egg denatures the avidin and destroys its ability to bind biotin. Denaturation is the first step in breaking down protein for digestion. Stomach acids denature protein, uncoiling the structure into a simple amino acid chain that digestive enzymes can start breaking apart.

**Key Concepts** *Proteins are large molecules made up of amino acids joined in various sequences. Amino acids are joined by peptide bonds. Each protein assumes a unique three-dimensional shape depending on the sequence of its amino acids and properties of their side groups. Acid, alkali, heat, alcohol, and agitation can disrupt chemical forces that stabilize proteins, causing the proteins to denature, or lose their shape.*

## Functions of Body Proteins

Each of the human body's thousands of different proteins has a specific function determined by its unique shape. Some act as enzymes, speeding up chemical reactions. Others act as hormones, a kind of chemical messenger. Antibodies made of protein protect us from foreign substances. Proteins maintain fluid balance by pumping molecules across cell membranes and attracting water. They maintain the acid and base balance of body fluids by taking up or giving off hydrogen ions as needed. Finally, proteins transport many key substances, such as oxygen, vitamins, and minerals, to target cells throughout the body. **Figure 7.5** illustrates the functions of proteins in the human body.

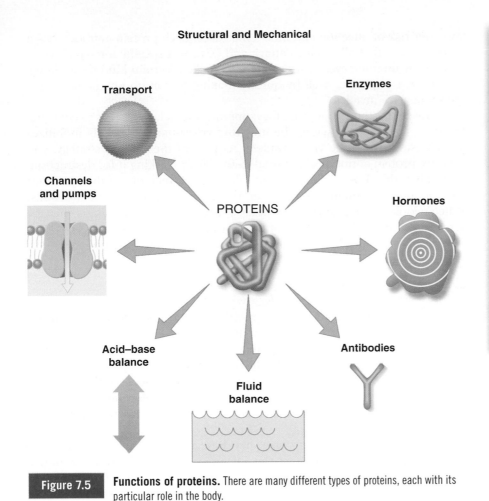

**Structural and Mechanical**

**Transport**

**Enzymes**

**Channels and pumps**

PROTEINS

**Hormones**

**Acid–base balance**

**Antibodies**

**Fluid balance**

**Figure 7.5** **Functions of proteins.** There are many different types of proteins, each with its particular role in the body.

> **collagen** The most abundant fibrous protein in the body. Collagen is the major constituent of connective tissue, forms the foundation for bones and teeth, and helps maintain the structure of blood vessels and other tissues.
>
> **keratin** A water-insoluble fibrous protein that is the primary constituent of hair, nails, and the outer layer of the skin.
>
> **motor proteins** Proteins that use energy and convert it into some form of mechanical work. Motor proteins are active in processes such as cell division, muscle contraction, and sperm movement.
>
> **antibodies [AN-tih-bod-eez]** Infection-fighting protein molecules in blood or secretory fluids that tag, neutralize, and help destroy pathogenic microorganisms (e.g., bacteria, viruses) or toxins.

## Structural and Mechanical Functions

Structures such as bone, skin, and hair owe their physical properties to unique proteins. **Collagen**, which under the microscope looks like a densely packed long rod, is the most abundant protein in mammals and gives skin and bone their elastic strength. Hair and nails are made of **keratin**, which is another dense protein made of coiled shapes. Because protein is essential for building these structures, protein deficiencies during a child's development can be disastrous.

**Motor proteins** turn energy into mechanical work. In fact, these proteins are the final step in converting our food into physical work. When you bike down a road or up a mountain, you are using your stored food energy to power your muscles. Acting like tiny "motors," protein filaments slide past each other as they shorten (contract) your muscle. As you pump the pedals, proteins turn that energy bar you ate into work! Similarly, specialized motor proteins also are involved in cell division, sperm movement, and other processes.

## Immune Function

Proteins play an important role in the immune system, which is responsible for fighting invasion and infection by foreign substances. **Antibodies** are blood proteins that attack and inactivate bacteria and viruses that cause infection. When your diet does not contain enough protein, your body cannot make as many antibodies as it needs. Your immune response is weakened,

*Quick* Bite

**How to Beat the Stiffest Egg Whites**
Whenever you want the greatest possible lightness or fluffiness, beat egg whites alone. A single drop of yolk or fat may reduce the foam's maximum volume by as much as two-thirds. Also avoid plastic bowls because plastics tend to retain fatty material on their surfaces.

**immune response** A coordinated set of steps, including production of antibodies, that the immune system takes in response to an antigen.

and your risk of infection and illness increases. Each protein antibody has a specific shape that allows it to attack and destroy a specific foreign invader. Once your immune system learns how to make a certain kind of antibody, your body can protect itself by quickly making that antibody the next time the same germ invades.

Viruses, like those that cause the common cold, take over cells to replicate. In a series of steps known as the **immune response**, your body mobilizes its defenses against the viral invaders. As part of the defense strategy, you produce protein antibodies that bind to the virus, marking it for destruction. Even when the virus is gone, special cells retain a memory of the particular virus so a faster immune response can be mounted against future invasions. When people are immunized for a disease such as measles or mumps, they are actually getting a small amount of dead or inactivated virus in the injection. The dead virus cannot cause infection, but it does allow the body to make antibodies to the disease.

## Enzymes

Enzymes are proteins that catalyze, or speed up, chemical reactions without being destroyed in the process. (See **Figures 7.6a** and **7.6b**.) Every cell contains thousands of types of enzymes, each with its own purpose. During digestion, for example, enzymes help break down carbohydrates, proteins, and fats into monosaccharides, amino acids, and fatty acids so the body can absorb them. Cellular enzymes release energy from these nutrients to fuel thousands of body processes. Enzymes also trigger the reactions that build muscle and tissue.

Our foods also contain enzymes, but these are inactivated (denatured) by cooking. Stomach acid denatures the enzymes in raw foods. You may notice special purified enzymes being sold as supplements to enhance digestion. Most of the time, stomach acid denatures these enzymes, so they are unable to

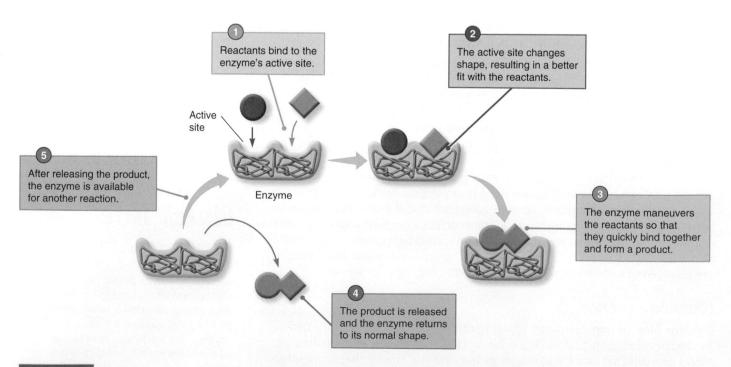

**1** Reactants bind to the enzyme's active site.

**2** The active site changes shape, resulting in a better fit with the reactants.

Active site

Enzyme

**5** After releasing the product, the enzyme is available for another reaction.

**3** The enzyme maneuvers the reactants so that they quickly bind together and form a product.

**4** The product is released and the enzyme returns to its normal shape.

**Figure 7.6a**   Enzymes catalyze (speed up) reactions that make or change substances (reactants).

function in the intestinal tract. However, some enzyme supplements are coated with a special substance to protect them from stomach acid. For example, a specially coated tablet form of the enzyme lactase can help people with lactose intolerance. Such coated enzymes temporarily help break down foods in the small intestine but eventually are digested themselves.

## Hormones

Hormones are chemical messengers that are made in one part of the body but act on cells in other parts of the body. Protein hormones perform many important regulatory functions. Insulin, for example, is a protein hormone that plays a key role in regulating the amount of glucose in the blood. It is released from the pancreas in response to a rise in blood glucose levels and works to lower those levels.

People with type 1 diabetes must take insulin injections to control blood glucose levels. If people with diabetes tried to take insulin as a pill, it would be denatured and digested just like any other protein.

## Acid–Base Balance

Measured on a scale of 0 to 14, pH indicates the concentration of hydrogen ions in a substance. The higher the concentration of hydrogen ions, the lower the pH. Acids, which have a high concentration of hydrogen ions, have a pH lower than 7; bases, which have a low concentration of hydrogen ions, have a pH higher than 7. The lower the pH, the stronger the acid. The higher the pH, the stronger the base. The body works hard to keep the pH of the blood near 7.4, or nearly neutral. We can tolerate only small blood pH fluctuations without disastrous consequences. Only a few hours with a blood pH above 8.0 or below 6.8 will cause death.

Proteins help maintain stable pH levels in body fluids by serving as **buffers**; they pick up extra hydrogen ions when conditions are acidic, and they donate hydrogen ions when conditions are alkaline. If proteins are not available to buffer acidic or alkaline substances, the blood can become too acidic or too alkaline, resulting in either **acidosis** or **alkalosis**. Both condi-

**buffers** Compounds that can take up and release hydrogen ions to keep the pH of a solution constant. The buffering action of proteins and bicarbonate in the bloodstream plays a major role in maintaining the blood pH at 7.35 to 7.45.

**acidosis** An abnormally low blood pH (below about 7.35) due to increased acidity.

**alkalosis** An abnormally high blood pH (above about 7.45) due to increased alkalinity.

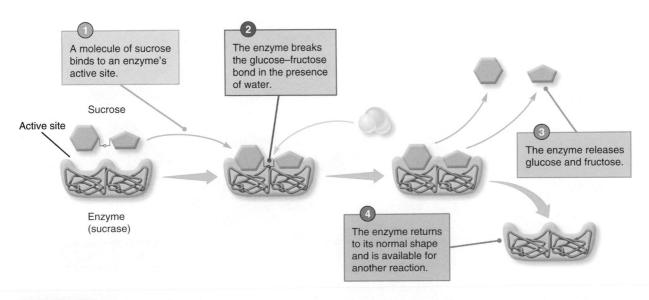

1. A molecule of sucrose binds to an enzyme's active site.

2. The enzyme breaks the glucose–fructose bond in the presence of water.

3. The enzyme releases glucose and fructose.

4. The enzyme returns to its normal shape and is available for another reaction.

Sucrose

Active site

Enzyme (sucrase)

**Figure 7.6b**    Enzymes catalyze reactions that break down molecules.

**intracellular fluid** The fluid in the body's cells. It usually is high in potassium and phosphate and low in sodium and chloride. It constitutes about two-thirds of total body water.

**extracellular fluid** The fluid located outside of cells. It is composed largely of the liquid portion (plasma) of the blood and the fluid between cells in tissues (interstitial fluid), with fluid in the GI tract, eyes, joints, and spinal cord contributing a small amount. It constitutes about one-third of body water.

**interstitial fluid [in-ter-STISH-ul]** The fluid between cells in tissues, usually high in sodium and chloride. Also called *intercellular fluid*.

**intravascular fluid** The fluid portion (plasma) of the blood contained in arteries, veins, and capillaries. It accounts for about 15 percent of the extracellular fluid.

tions can be serious—either can cause proteins to denature, which can lead to coma or death.

## Transport Functions

Many substances pass in and out of cells through proteins that cross cell membranes and act as channels and pumps. Some protein channels allow substances to flow rapidly through the membranes without an input of energy. Other channels are protein pumps that use energy to drive substances across membranes.

Proteins also act as carriers, transporting many important substances in the bloodstream for delivery throughout the body. Lipoproteins, for example, package proteins with lipids so lipid particles can be carried in the blood. Other proteins carry fat-soluble vitamins, such as vitamin A and certain other vitamins and minerals. Because protein carries vitamin A in the blood, protein deficiency contributes to vitamin A deficiency. The protein transferrin carries iron in the blood.

## Fluid Balance

Fluids in the body are found inside cells (**intracellular fluid**) or outside cells (**extracellular fluid**). There are two types of extracellular fluid—fluid between cells (called *intercellular fluid*, or **interstitial fluid**) and fluid in the blood (**intravascular fluid**). Whereas fluid within cells is usually high in potassium and phosphate, fluid between cells is usually high in sodium and chloride. These interior and exterior fluid levels must stay in balance for body processes to work properly.

Proteins in the blood help to maintain appropriate fluid levels in the vascular system. (See **Figure 7.7**.) When your heart beats, the force pushes

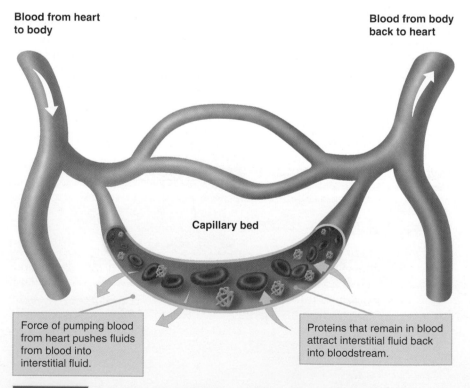

**Blood from heart to body**

**Blood from body back to heart**

Capillary bed

Force of pumping blood from heart pushes fluids from blood into interstitial fluid.

Proteins that remain in blood attract interstitial fluid back into bloodstream.

**Figure 7.7** **Proteins in the blood.** Blood proteins attract fluid into capillaries. This counteracts the force of the heart beating, which pushes fluid out of capillaries.

fluid and nutrients from the capillaries out into the fluid surrounding the cells. But blood proteins such as albumin and globulin are too large to leave the capillary beds. These proteins remain in the capillaries, where they attract fluid to replace what has been pushed out. This system maintains a balance of fluids in the vascular system.

If the diet lacks enough protein to maintain normal levels of blood proteins, fluid will leak into the surrounding tissue and cause swelling, also called **edema**. Children with protein malnutrition often suffer from severe edema. Reestablishing a diet adequate in protein and energy will allow the edema to subside.

> **edema**  Swelling caused by the buildup of fluid between cells.
>
> **deamination**  The removal of the amino group ($-NH_2$) from an amino acid.
>
> **proteases [PRO-tea-aces]**  Enzymes that break down protein into peptides and amino acids.
>
> **proenzymes**  Inactive precursors of enzymes.

## Source of Energy and Glucose

THINK About It 1

Although your body prefers to burn carbohydrate and fat for energy, if necessary it can use protein for energy or to make glucose. Thus, carbohydrate and fat are protein-sparing: They spare amino acids from being burned for energy and allow them to be used for protein synthesis.

If the diet does not provide enough energy for vital functions, the body will sacrifice its own protein from enzymes, muscle, and other tissues to make energy and glucose for use by the brain, lungs, and heart. This is what happens in cases of starvation.

When the body uses protein for energy, it first breaks the protein into individual amino acids. A process called **deamination** removes the nitrogen group, which is released in urine, and reduces the amino acid to its carbon skeleton. This carbon skeleton can be used for energy, and most amino acids yield carbon skeletons that can be used to make glucose.

If your diet contains more protein than you need for protein synthesis, your body converts most of the excess to glucose or stores it as fat. So taking protein supplements or eating high-protein diets as a means of increasing muscle mass may instead add to body fat.

**Key Concepts**  *In the body, proteins perform numerous vital functions that are determined by each protein's shape. Protein antibodies protect the body from infection and illness. As enzymes, proteins speed up chemical reactions; as hormones, they are chemical messengers. Proteins also maintain fluid balance and acid–base balance and transport substances throughout the body. If needed, protein can also be used as a source of energy or glucose.*

# Protein Digestion and Absorption

Before your body can make a body protein from food protein, it must digest and absorb the protein you eat. **Figure 7.8** shows the process of protein digestion and absorption.

## Protein Digestion

The first step in using dietary protein is breaking down its long polypeptide chains into amino acids. As with the other energy-yielding nutrients, digestion of protein requires enzymes from a number of sources. Cells produce and secrete most **proteases** (protein-digesting enzymes) as **proenzymes**, inactive forms of enzymes, for later activation in the intestine. If a cell produced active forms of a protease, it could digest itself and break down its own cellular protein. Delaying the activation of proteases protects the integrity of cells.

### In the Stomach

Digestion of protein begins in the stomach. Here, hydrochloric acid (HCl) denatures a protein, unfolding it and making the amino acid chain more

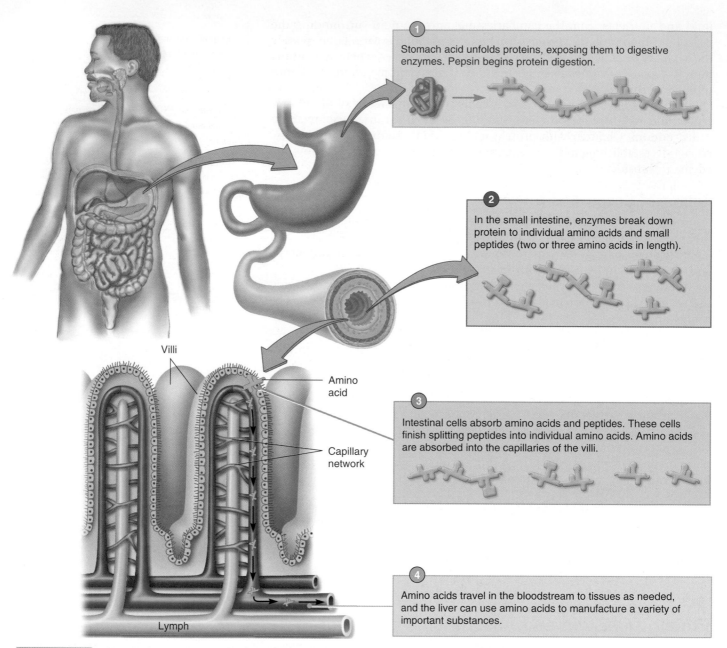

**1** Stomach acid unfolds proteins, exposing them to digestive enzymes. Pepsin begins protein digestion.

**2** In the small intestine, enzymes break down protein to individual amino acids and small peptides (two or three amino acids in length).

**3** Intestinal cells absorb amino acids and peptides. These cells finish splitting peptides into individual amino acids. Amino acids are absorbed into the capillaries of the villi.

**4** Amino acids travel in the bloodstream to tissues as needed, and the liver can use amino acids to manufacture a variety of important substances.

Villi

Amino acid

Capillary network

Lymph

**Figure 7.8** **Digestion and absorption of protein.** Digestion breaks down protein to amino acids and small peptides for absorption. Amino acids are absorbed into the capillaries of the villi and transported in the bloodstream.

accessible to the action of enzymes. Glands in the stomach lining produce the proenzyme pepsinogen, the inactive precursor of the enzyme pepsin. When pepsinogen comes in contact with hydrochloric acid, it is converted to the active enzyme pepsin. Gastric juices must be acidic for this enzyme to be active. By the time dietary protein leaves the stomach, pepsin has broken it down into individual amino acids and shorter polypeptides of various lengths that then travel to the small intestine for further digestion. Pepsin is responsible for about 10 to 20 percent of protein digestion.[8]

### In the Small Intestine

From the stomach, amino acids and polypeptides pass into the small intestine, where most protein digestion takes place. In the small intestine, activated

*Quick* Bite

**Softening Tough Meat**
Cooking tough meat in liquid for hours helps dissolve the source of its toughness, fibrous protein called *connective tissue.*

proteases from the pancreas and intestinal lining cells break down large peptides into smaller peptides. Pancreatic enzymes completely digest only a small percentage of proteins into individual amino acids; enzymes on the surface of the small intestine split the remaining larger polypeptides into tripeptides and dipeptides, and some are even split all the way into amino acids. The intestinal cells absorb these smaller units and break down virtually all the remaining dipeptides and tripeptides into individual amino acids for absorption into the bloodstream.

## Amino Acid and Peptide Absorption

More than 99 percent of protein enters the bloodstream as individual amino acids. Peptides are rarely absorbed, and whole proteins that escape digestion are almost never absorbed. Once absorbed, most amino acids and the few absorbed peptides travel via the portal vein to the liver, which releases them into general circulation. Intestinal cells retain some amino acids to synthesize enzymes and make new cells.

## Undigested Protein

Any parts of proteins not digested and absorbed in the small intestine continue through the large intestine and pass out of the body in the feces. Normally, the body efficiently digests and absorbs protein. Diseases of the intestinal tract, however, decrease the efficiency of absorption and increase protein losses in the feces.[9] People with **celiac disease**, for example, cannot properly digest gluten—a protein found in wheat, rye, and barley. Unless treated with a gluten-free diet, people with celiac disease show poor growth, weight loss, and other symptoms resulting from poor absorption of protein and other nutrients.[10] When people have **cystic fibrosis**, thick, sticky mucus prevents digestive enzymes, including proteases, from reaching the small intestine, resulting in poor digestion and absorption of protein and other nutrients.[11] Special enzyme preparations that contain protease, lipase, and amylase are needed to prevent malnutrition.

**Key Concepts** *Protein digestion begins in the stomach, where hydrochloric acid (HCl) denatures protein, and then the enzyme pepsin breaks proteins into smaller peptides. Digestion continues in the small intestine, where proteases break polypeptides into smaller peptide units, which are then absorbed into cells where additional enzymes complete digestion to amino acids. So cells do not digest themselves, proteases (protein-digesting enzymes) are synthesized and secreted as inactive proenzymes.*

# Proteins in the Body

Once in the bloodstream, amino acids are transported throughout the body and are available for synthesizing cellular proteins. To build proteins, cells use peptide bonds to link amino acids.

## Protein Synthesis

Genetic material in the nucleus of every cell provides the blueprint for the thousands of proteins needed to perform life functions. To synthesize a protein, cells assemble amino acids in a specific sequence.

Just as one missing part of a car can stop an entire auto assembly line, one missing amino acid can stop synthesis of an entire protein in the cell. If a dispensable amino acid is missing during protein synthesis, the cell will either make that amino acid or obtain it from the liver via the bloodstream, and protein synthesis will continue. If an indispensable amino acid is missing,

**celiac disease [SEA-lee-ak]** A disease that involves an inability to digest gluten, a protein found in wheat, rye, and barley. If untreated, it causes flattening of the villi in the intestine, leading to severe malabsorption of nutrients. Symptoms include diarrhea, fatty stools, swollen belly, and extreme fatigue.

**cystic fibrosis** An inherited disorder that causes widespread dysfunction of the exocrine glands, resulting in chronic lung disease, abnormally high levels of electrolytes (e.g., sodium, potassium, chloride) in sweat, and deficiency of pancreatic enzymes needed for digestion.

**amino acid pool** The amino acids in body tissues and fluids that are available for new protein synthesis.

the body may break its own protein down to supply the missing amino acid. If a missing indispensable amino acid is unavailable, protein synthesis halts, and the partially completed protein is broken down into individual amino acids for use elsewhere in the body.

Genetic defects can cause problems in protein synthesis. People who have sickle cell anemia cannot construct the correct sequence to form the protein hemoglobin. A genetic error causes the amino acid valine to be substituted for glutamic acid in two locations in the protein chain. This simple error causes the shape of hemoglobin to change so much that the red blood cell becomes stiff and sickle-shaped instead of soft and disk-shaped. Because this faulty protein cannot carry oxygen efficiently, it causes serious medical problems.

## The Amino Acid Pool and Protein Turnover

Cells throughout the body constantly and simultaneously synthesize and break down protein. When cells break down protein, the protein's amino acids return to circulation. (See **Figure 7.9**.) These available amino acids, found throughout body tissues and fluids, are collectively referred to as the **amino acid pool**.[12] Some of these amino acids may be used for protein synthesis,

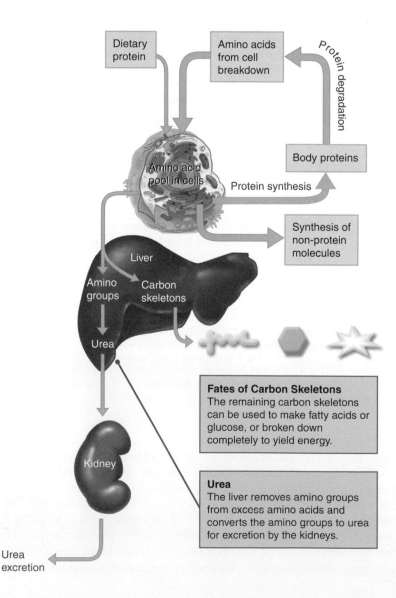

**Figure 7.9** **Protein turnover.** Cells draw upon their amino acid pools to synthesize new proteins. These small pools turn over quickly and must be replenished by amino acids from dietary protein and the degradation (breakdown) of body protein. Dietary protein supplies about one-third and the breakdown of body protein supplies about two-thirds of the amino acids needed to synthesize roughly 300 grams of body protein daily. When dietary protein is inadequate, increased degradation of body protein replenishes the amino acid pool. This can lead to the breakdown of essential body tissue.

such as the rebuilding of skin cells every 25 to 45 days;[13] others may have their amino group removed and be used to produce energy or nonprotein substances such as glucose.

The constant recycling of proteins in the body is known as **protein turnover**.[14] Each day, more amino acids in your body are recycled than are supplied in your diet. Of the approximately 300 grams of protein synthesized by the body each day, 200 grams are made from recycled amino acids. The protein in the intestine and the liver, which are two tissue types with rapid rates of degradation and resynthesis, account for as much as 50 percent of this protein turnover.[15] This remarkable recycling capacity is the reason we need so little protein in our diet. Although our requirements are small, dietary protein is extremely important. When dietary protein is inadequate, body protein is broken down faster to replenish the amino acid pool. This can lead to the loss of essential body tissue.

## Synthesis of Nonprotein Molecules

Amino acids do more than help build peptides and proteins; they are precursors of many molecules with important biological roles. Your body makes nonprotein molecules from amino acids and the nitrogen they contain. The vitamin niacin, for example, is made from the amino acid tryptophan. Precursors of DNA, RNA, and many coenzymes are formed in part from amino acids. Your body also uses amino acids to make **neurotransmitters**, chemicals that send signals from nerve cells to other parts of the body. The neurotransmitter serotonin, which helps regulate mood, is made from tryptophan. Norepinephrine and epinephrine (also called *noradrenaline* and *adrenaline*, respectively), which get the body ready for action, are neurotransmitters made from tyrosine. Your body also uses tyrosine to make the skin pigment melanin and the hormone thyroxin. The simple amino acid glycine combines with many toxic substances to make less harmful substances that the body can eliminate. Your body uses the amino acid histidine to make histamine, which dilates blood vessels and is a culprit in allergic reactions.

## Protein and Nitrogen Excretion

Cells break down and recycle amino acids. Amino acid breakdown yields amino groups ($-NH_2$). This $NH_2$ molecule is unstable, and the body quickly converts it to ammonia ($NH_3$). However, ammonia is toxic to cells, so it is expelled into the bloodstream as a waste product and is carried to the liver. In the liver, an amino group and an ammonia group react with carbon dioxide (through a series of reactions known collectively as the urea cycle) to produce **urea** and water. The nitrogen-rich urea is transported from the liver by way of the bloodstream to the kidneys, where it is filtered from the blood and sent to the bladder for excretion in the urine. Small amounts of other nitrogen-containing compounds, such as ammonia, uric acid, and creatinine, are excreted in the urine as well. Some nitrogen is also lost through skin, sloughed-off GI cells, mucus, hair and nail cuttings, and body fluids.

## Nitrogen Balance

Because nitrogen is excreted as proteins are recycled or used, we can use the balance of nitrogen in the body to evaluate whether the body is getting enough protein. (See **Figure 7.10**.) We can estimate the balance of nitrogen, and therefore protein, in the body by comparing nitrogen intake to the sum of all sources of nitrogen output (urine, feces, skin, hair, and body fluids).[16]

**nitrogen balance = grams of nitrogen intake − grams of nitrogen output**

**protein turnover** The constant breakdown and synthesis of proteins in the body.

**neurotransmitters** Substances released at the end of a stimulated nerve cell that diffuse across a small gap and bind to another nerve cell or muscle cell, stimulating or inhibiting it.

**urea** The main nitrogen-containing waste product in mammals. Formed in liver cells from ammonia and carbon dioxide, urea is carried via the bloodstream to the kidneys, where it is excreted in the urine.

**nitrogen balance** Nitrogen intake minus the sum of all sources of nitrogen excretion.

**nitrogen equilibrium** Nitrogen intake equals the sum of all sources of nitrogen excretion; nitrogen balance equals zero.

**positive nitrogen balance** Nitrogen intake exceeds the sum of all sources of nitrogen excretion.

**negative nitrogen balance** Nitrogen intake is less than the sum of all sources of nitrogen excretion.

If nitrogen intake equals nitrogen output, **nitrogen balance** is zero and the body is in **nitrogen equilibrium**. If nitrogen intake exceeds nitrogen output, the body is said to be in **positive nitrogen balance**. Positive nitrogen balance means that the body is adding protein; growing children, pregnant women, or people recovering from protein deficiency or illnesses should be in positive nitrogen balance. If nitrogen output exceeds nitrogen intake, the body is in **negative nitrogen balance**. This means that the body is losing protein. People who are starving or on extreme weight-loss diets or who suffer from fever, severe illnesses, or infections are in a state of negative nitrogen balance. Healthy adults are in nitrogen equilibrium, which means that they take in enough protein to maintain and repair tissue. They have no net gain or loss of body protein, and they simply excrete excess dietary nitrogen.

**Key Concepts** *Cells throughout the body constantly synthesize and break down protein simultaneously, a process known as protein turnover. Nitrogen-containing end products of protein metabolism are excreted in urine via the kidneys. Comparison of nitrogen intake (from dietary protein) to nitrogen excretion gives a measure of nitrogen balance and indicates protein status in the body.*

## Proteins in the Diet

Many government and health organizations have made recommendations about the amount of protein in a healthful diet, just as they have for other nutrients. Meat, eggs, milk, legumes, grains, and vegetables are all sources of protein. Fruits contain minimal amounts and, along with fats, are not considered protein sources. **Figure 7.11** shows some good sources of protein.

### Recommended Intakes of Protein

In the United States and Canada, the Recommended Dietary Allowance (RDA) is the accepted dietary standard for protein. RDAs are set to meet the

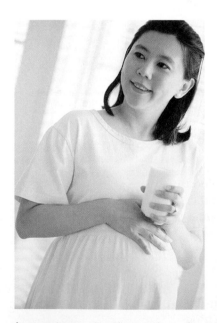

A pregnant woman is adding protein, so she has a positive nitrogen balance.

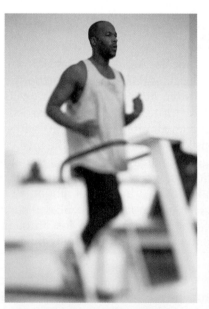

A healthy person who is neither gaining nor losing protein is in nitrogen equilibrium (zero balance).

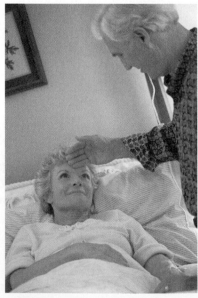

A person who is severely ill and losing protein has a negative nitrogen balance.

**Figure 7.10** **Nitrogen balance.** Nitrogen balance reflects whether a person is gaining or losing protein.

nutritional needs of most healthy people, so most of us actually require somewhat less protein than the RDA. RDA values also assume we are consuming adequate energy and other nutrients to allow our bodies to use dietary protein for protein synthesis, rather than for energy.

Based on evidence of increased heart disease risk when diets are low in fat and high in carbohydrate, and increased risk of obesity and heart disease when diets are high in fat, the Food and Nutrition Board developed Acceptable Macronutrient Distribution Ranges (AMDRs) for the energy-yielding nutrients.[17] For adults, the AMDR for fat is 20 to 35 percent of energy intake, and the AMDR for carbohydrate is 45 to 65 percent of energy intake. This leaves about 10 to 35 percent of energy intake from protein, a level that is typically higher than the RDA.

### Adults

For adults, the RDA for protein intake is 0.8 gram per kilogram of body weight.[18] Using a reference body weight of 57 kilograms for adult women and 70 kilograms for adult men, this translates into a daily protein recommendation of 46 grams for women and 56 grams for men. The RDA for adults works out to be about 8 to 11 percent of average energy intake.

### Other Life Stages

Infants have the highest protein needs relative to body weight of any time of life. (See Table 7.2.) Protein is needed to support rapid growth during infancy. The Adequate Intake (AI) value for infants 0 to 6 months of age is based on the protein content of human milk and the average milk consumption of breastfed babies. Protein requirements per kilogram body weight gradually fall throughout childhood and adolescence until a person reaches adulthood. (See **Figure 7.12**.)

Both pregnancy and breastfeeding increase a woman's need for protein. The RDA for pregnant and lactating women is 1.1 grams per kilogram. This is an increase of about 25 grams per day over the female RDA for protein. Most American women already consume more than enough protein to support pregnancy and breastfeeding.

Some nutritionists suggest that people older than 50 should consume up to 1.2 grams of protein per kilogram body weight. Although elderly people on average have less lean body mass to maintain than younger people, the body becomes less efficient at digesting, absorbing, and using protein as it ages.[19] However, because a statistical analysis of nitrogen balance studies found no significant effect of age on protein requirements,[20] the RDA for this age group is the same as for younger adults—0.8 grams per kilogram.

| Convert weight to kg |
| --- |
| (pounds ÷ 2.2) |
| Multiply kg by 0.8 = Protein RDA in g |

Male, 19–24 years old, 70 kg (154 lb)

70 kg × 0.8 g/kg = 56 g protein

Female, 19–24 years old, 57 kg (125 lb)

57 kg × 0.8 g/kg = 46 g protein

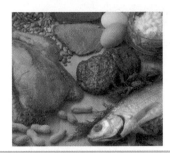

Rich sources of protein include meats, fish, poultry, eggs, dairy products, legumes, and nuts.

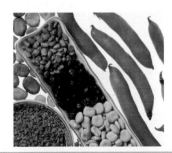

Legumes and nuts are important sources of protein for vegetarians.

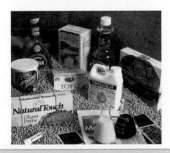

Soybeans and soy products are the only plant sources of complete protein.

**Figure 7.11**   **Protein sources.** Meat, fish, eggs, dairy products, and soy are excellent protein sources. Legumes, grain products, starchy vegetables, nuts, and seeds also are good sources.

### Table 7.2    Protein AI or RDA for Infants, Children, and Teens

| Age | Protein AI or RDA (g/kg body weight) |
| --- | --- |
| 0 to 6 months | 1.52 |
| 7 to 12 months | 1.5 |
| 1 to 3 years | 1.1 |
| 4 to 8 years | 0.95 |
| 9 to 13 years | 0.95 |
| 14 to 18 years | 0.85 |

**Source:** Data from Institute of Medicine, Food and Nutrition Board. *Dietary Reference Intakes for Energy, Carbohydrate, Fiber, Fat, Fatty Acids, Cholesterol, Protein, and Amino Acids (Macronutrients)*. Washington, DC: National Academies Press; 2005.

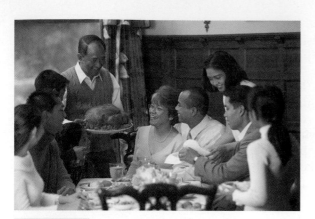

**Figure 7.12** **Protein needs change as we age.** Growing children have higher protein needs (as grams per kilogram body weight) than older adults.

But, because energy needs decline with age, protein should provide a larger percentage of energy intake.

### Physical Stress

Severe physical stress can increase your body's need for protein. Infections, burns, fevers, and surgery all increase protein losses, and the diet must replace that lost protein. A severe infection can increase protein requirements by one-third. Severe burns can increase requirements two to four times. Less severe physical stressors, such as a viral illness with a mild fever lasting only a few days, rarely increase protein requirements. Muscle-building activities, such as intense weight training, increase protein needs much less than most people think. In fact, the typical American diet supplies an ample amount of protein for most people, even for bodybuilders. (See the FYI feature "Do Athletes Need More Protein?")

## Protein Consumption in the United States

According to national survey data, the median daily intake of protein for adults ages 19 to 30 years ranges from about 70 to 110 grams, decreasing to about 50 to 85 grams in the elderly. This is approximately 0.71 to 1.56 grams per kilogram using a reference body weight of 70 kilograms.[21] The intake of protein as a percentage of calories ranges from about 13 percent in children to 16 percent in adults.[22] Individual intake of protein has a large range, but, based on average intake data, Americans are generally eating within the recommended range of 10 to 35 percent of calories from protein.

**Key Concepts** *Infants, who are growing rapidly, have the highest protein needs in proportion to body weight. The recommended intakes, AIs or RDAs, decline from 1.52 grams per kilogram for infants under 6 months old to 0.8 grams per kilogram for adults. Pregnancy, lactation, and severe physical stress all can alter protein requirements. Adults currently consume about 16 percent of their energy as protein, a level that provides ample protein for most people.*

## Protein Quality

Although both animal and plant foods contain protein, the quality of protein in these foods differs. Foods that supply all the indispensable amino acids in the proportions needed by the body are called *high-quality proteins*, or **complete proteins**. Foods that lack adequate amounts of one or more indispensable amino acids are called *low-quality proteins*, or **incomplete proteins**.

Because we typically eat a variety of foods that provides ample dietary protein, we don't ordinarily worry about protein quality. But for people with marginal protein or energy intake and for people who use only one or a few plant foods as their main dietary protein source, protein quality is a critical issue.

### Complete Proteins

Animal foods generally provide complete protein; that is, they provide all the indispensable amino acids in approximately the right proportions. One exception is gelatin, a protein derived from animal collagen that lacks the indispensable amino acid tryptophan.

Red meats, poultry, fish, eggs, milk, and milk products (all animal foods) contain complete protein. Protein supplies more than 20 percent of the energy content of these foods. In water-packed tuna, protein provides about 80 percent of the energy. The protein isolated from soybeans, unlike protein from

**complete proteins** Proteins that supply all of the indispensable amino acids in the proportions the body needs. Also known as *high-quality proteins*.

**incomplete proteins** Proteins that lack one or more indispensable amino acids. Also called *low-quality proteins*.

other plant foods, is a complete, high-quality protein comparable to that of animal protein.[23] Although, compared with animal protein, soy protein contains lower proportions of the amino acids cysteine and methionine, the amount of soy typically consumed provides sufficient quantities. Moreover, soybeans contain no cholesterol or saturated fat.

Americans, on the average, get about 63 percent of their protein intake from animal foods.[24] (See Table 7.3.) In other parts of the world, animal proteins play a smaller role. In Africa and East Asia, for example, animal foods provide only 20 percent of protein intake.[25] Now more than ever, America is a nation of meat eaters. Beef, chicken, and pork top the list of animal protein sources, with total consumption of beef averaging 67 pounds of beef

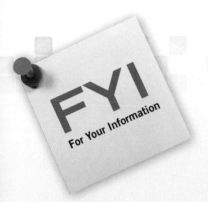

## Do Athletes Need More Protein?

Athletes not only pump iron these days, they also pump protein supplements in hopes of building muscle and improving performance. Look inside many sports magazines, and you'll see ads for protein or amino acid supplements aimed at athletes. You cannot force your body to build muscle by pumping in more protein than you need, any more than you can make your car run faster by adding more gas to a full tank. Extra protein does not build muscles; only regular workouts fueled by a mix of nutrients can do that.

### Protein Requirements for Athletes

Many people assume that because muscle fibers are protein, building muscle must require protein. This is only partially true. The heavy resistance-type exercise that is needed to stimulate muscle growth must first be fueled by glucose and fatty acids (glucose will be the predominant fuel). Little protein is used as a fuel source in resistance-type exercise. Some studies have shown that men who consume the RDA for protein (0.8 grams per kilogram body weight) and engage in heavy resistance exercise go into negative nitrogen balance. However, other studies have show positive nitrogen balance and muscle hypertrophy during resistance training with intake at the RDA.[1] The DRI committee reviewing evidence on macronutrients concluded that a higher RDA was not warranted for healthy adults doing resistance or endurance exercise.[2]

Because Americans, on average, consume much more protein than they actually need, any increased need for athletes most likely is being met already. An athlete in training (let's make him 70 kilograms) might consume as many as 5,000 kilocalories per day. Even if his diet contained only 10 percent of calories as protein (the low side of the AMDR for protein, and lower than average), he would be getting about 126 grams of protein daily—about 1.8 grams per kilogram. It is unlikely that an athlete would not be able to meet his or her protein needs from a normal, mixed diet. Adequate intake and appropriate timing of

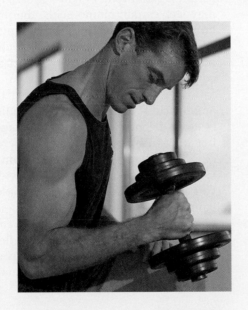

protein ingestion has been shown to be beneficial in multiple exercise modes, including endurance, anaerobic, and strength exercise.[3]

### Risks of Supplements

Maybe there's no benefit to taking protein or amino acid supplements, but there's no harm either, right? Not necessarily. If excess protein means excess calories, it adds weight as fat, not muscle, which can slow down your performance. Purified protein supplements can contribute to

calcium losses, thereby harming bone health. Excess protein means excess nitrogen that must be excreted. This can place an extra burden on kidneys and pose a risk for dehydration if fluid intake is inadequate. Supplements of single amino acids can interfere with absorption of other amino acids and can affect neurotransmitter activity.

If you are a weekend athlete, there's no need to increase the protein in your diet, and no reason to expect that doing so will help your performance. If you are a competitive athlete, choosing adequate calories from a wide variety of foods will ensure an adequate protein intake. Supplements are unnecessary, and expensive, and they may disrupt normal protein balance in the body. Play it safe—choose a healthful diet to fuel your exercise.

1   Vieillevoye S, Poortmans JR, Duchateau J, Carpentier A. Effects of a combined essential amino acid/carbohydrate supplementation on muscle mass, architecture and maximal strength following heavy-load training. *Eur J Appl Physiol.* 2010;110(3):479–488.

2   Institute of Medicine, Food and Nutrition Board. *Dietary Reference Intakes for Energy, Carbohydrate, Fiber, Fat, Fatty Acids, Cholesterol, Protein, and Amino Acids.* Washington, DC: National Academies Press; 2005.

3   Kreider RB, Campbell B. Protein for exercise and recovery. *Phys Sports Med.* 2009;37(2):12–21.

| Table 7.3 | Top 10 Sources of Protein in the United States |
|---|---|

| Rank | Food | Percentage of Protein Contributed |
|---|---|---|
| 1 | Beef | 18 |
| 2 | Poultry | 14 |
| 3 | Milk | 9 |
| 4 | Yeast bread | 7 |
| 5 | Cheese | 6 |
| 6 | Fish/shellfish[a] | 4 |
| 7 | Eggs | 3 |
| 8 | Pork, fresh | 3 |
| 9 | Ham | 3 |
| 10 | Pasta | 2 |

[a] Does not include tuna.

**Source:** US Department of Agriculture, Agricultural Research Service. *1989–1991 Continuing Survey of Food Intake by Individuals.*

**complementary protein** Two or more incomplete food proteins whose assortment of amino acids make up for, or complement, each other so the combination provides sufficient amounts of all the indispensable amino acids.

per person per year.[26] Annual beef consumption per person is highest in the Midwest (73 pounds) and lowest in the Northeast (63 pounds).[27]

### Incomplete and Complementary Proteins

With the exception of soy protein, the protein in plant foods is incomplete; that is, it lacks one or more indispensable amino acids and does not match the body's amino acid needs as closely as animal foods do. (See the FYI feature "High-Protein Plant Foods.") Although the protein in one plant food may lack certain amino acids, the protein in another plant food may be a **complementary protein** that completes the amino acid pattern. The protein of one plant food can provide the indispensable amino acid(s) that the other plant food is missing. Table 7.4 lists some examples of complementary food combinations.

For example, grain products such as pasta are low in the indispensable amino acid lysine but high in the indispensable amino acids methionine and cysteine. Legumes such as kidney beans are low in methionine and cysteine but high in lysine. In a dish that combines these foods, such as a pasta–kidney bean salad, the protein from pasta complements the protein from kidney beans, so together they provide a complete protein. Generally, when you combine grains with legumes or legumes with nuts or seeds, you will get complete, high-quality protein.

Small amounts of animal foods can also complement the protein in plant foods. For example, Asians often flavor rice with small amounts of beef, chicken, or fish, complementing the protein in the rice. Americans eat breakfast cereal with milk, which complements the protein in the cereal.

| Table 7.4 | Examples of Complementary Food Combinations |
|---|---|

Beans and rice
Beans and corn or wheat tortilla
Rice and lentils
Rice and black-eyed peas
Pea soup with bread or crackers
Hummus (garbanzo beans [chickpeas] with sesame paste)
Pasta with beans
Peanut butter on bread

If you consume little or no animal protein, you should pay attention to complementary proteins. Consuming a wide variety of plant protein sources is the key to obtaining adequate amounts of all the indispensable amino acids. When protein and energy intakes are adequate, there is no need to plan complementary proteins at each meal.[28] In the past, it was mistakenly believed that complementary proteins needed to be eaten at the same meal for your body to use them together. Now studies show that your body can combine complementary proteins that are eaten within the same day.[29]

Boosting your intake of plant protein foods is less costly and can provide excellent health benefits. High-protein plant foods are usually rich in vitamins, minerals, and dietary fiber. Plant foods contain no cholesterol and little fat, and they usually cost less than animal foods high in protein. Lentil loaf, for example, is substantially cheaper to make than meat loaf.

### Evaluating Protein Quality

A high-quality protein (1) provides all the indispensable amino acids in the amounts the body needs, (2) provides enough other amino acids to serve as nitrogen sources for making dispensable amino acids, and (3) is easy to digest. If a food protein contains the right proportion of amino acids but cannot be digested and absorbed, it is useless to the body. Protein quality might be assessed to plan a special diet or develop a new product, such as infant formula.

A simple way to determine a food's protein quality is to compare its amino acid composition to that of a reference pattern of amino acids. The reference pattern closely reflects the amounts and proportions of amino acids humans need. The **protein digestibility-corrected amino acid score (PDCAAS)** accounts for both the amino acid composition of a food and the digestibility of the protein.

The U.S. Food and Drug Administration (FDA) recognizes the PDCAAS as the official method for determining the protein quality of most food.[30] If the percent Daily Value (%DV) for protein is listed on a food label, it must be based on the food's PDCAAS. It would be misleading to say that, for example, 8 grams of protein from tuna and 8 grams of protein from kidney beans would contribute equally to amino acid needs. Consequently, even though the number of grams of protein per serving might be the same, the %DV would be different for these two foods.

## Proteins and Amino Acids as Additives and Supplements

Proteins contribute to the structure, texture, and taste of food. They often are added to foods to enhance these properties. The milk protein casein is added to frozen dessert toppings. Gelatin is added to yogurt and fillings. **Protein hydrolysates**—proteins that have been broken down into amino acids and shorter peptides—are added to many foods as thickeners, stabilizers, or flavor enhancers.

Amino acids also are used as additives. Monosodium glutamate (sodium bound to the amino acid glutamic acid) is a flavor enhancer added to many foods. The artificial sweetener aspartame is a dipeptide composed of aspartic acid and phenylalanine.

Protein and amino acid supplements are sold to dieters, athletes, and people who suffer from certain diseases. Despite a lack of scientific evidence, some people buy the amino acid lysine for cold sores and the amino acid tryptophan in hopes that it will relieve pain, depression, and sleep disorders. Some protein powders and amino acid cocktails are marketed with the claims that they enhance muscle building and exercise performance. Although the anecdotal evidence (stories from friends and health food store clerks) for these products may be convincing, few scientific studies back up these claims.

**protein digestibility-corrected amino acid score (PDCAAS)** A measure of protein quality that takes into account the amino acid composition of the food and the digestibility of the protein.

**protein hydrolysates** Proteins that have been treated with enzymes to break them down into amino acids and shorter peptides.

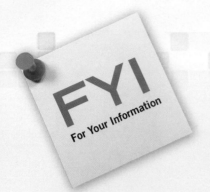

# High-Protein Plant Foods

Of the top 10 sources of protein in the American diet, only 2—yeast breads and pasta—are plant-based. (See Table 7.3.) Lentils, a dense source of plant protein, don't even make the list. Yet look at the comparison between the nutritional profile of lentils and the profile of beef in Table A.

When we consider these two foods in light of the *Dietary Guidelines for Americans*, it's no contest. To reduce fat, saturated fat, and cholesterol while increasing fiber, the lentils win hands down! With all that lentils have going for them, you'd think more Americans would be eating them. Yet dried beans, peas, and lentils combined contribute less than 1 percent of the daily protein intake of Americans, while beef contributes 17.7 percent.

High-protein plant foods also contribute complex carbohydrates, dietary fiber, vitamins, and minerals. Because these plant foods contain little fat, they are nutrient dense; that is, they provide a high amount of protein and nutrients in proportion to their energy contribution.

## Sources of Plant Protein

Grains and grain products, legumes (lentils and dried beans and peas such as kidney beans or chickpeas), starchy vegetables, and nuts and seeds all provide protein (see Table B). A serving of a grain product or starchy vegetable provides about 5 grams of protein, a serving of legumes provides 10 to 20 grams of protein, and a serving of vegetables provides about 3 grams of protein. Although a serving of these foods contains less protein than a serving of meat, you can eat more plant protein foods for fewer calories.

## Complementing Plant Proteins

It's important to remember that plant proteins lack one or more of the indispensable amino acids needed to build body proteins, so individual plant proteins need to complement each other. A simple rule to remember in complementing plant proteins is that combining grains and legumes or combining legumes and nuts or seeds provides complete, high-quality protein.

## Soy Protein

The protein in soybeans is a notable exception to the rule that most plant proteins are incomplete. Soy provides complete, high-quality protein comparable to that in animal foods. In addition, soybeans provide no saturated fat or cholesterol, and are rich in isoflavonoids—phytochemicals that help reduce risk of heart disease and cancer and improve bone health.

Isoflavonoids act as antioxidants, protecting cells and tissues from damage. One specific isoflavonoid, genistein, inhibits growth of both breast and prostate cancer cells in the laboratory. Isoflavonoids protect LDL cholesterol (the kind of cholesterol associated with greater risk of heart disease) from oxidation. Oxidized LDL cholesterol contributes to the plaque buildup in arteries. The isoflavonoids in soybeans also act as phytoestrogens, helping to protect older women from cardiovascular disease and osteoporosis. Soy foods that contain most or all of the bean, such as soymilk, sprouts, flour, and tofu, are the best sources of these phytochemicals.

It is easy to incorporate a variety of soy foods into your diet. Tofu, tempeh, ground soy, soymilk, soy flour, and textured soy protein are soy-based products that can be included in many meals and snacks (see Table C).

The nutritional benefits of plant protein sources such as soy foods and other legumes, grains, and vegetables deserve a closer look. Most Americans would benefit from emphasizing plant protein foods in their diet. Next time you plan to make a meat loaf, make a lentil loaf instead.

### Table A — How Do Lentils Stack Up Against Beef?

|  | Cooked Lentils | Lean Broiled Sirloin |
|---|---|---|
| Amount | 1 cup | 5 ounces |
| Energy | 226 kcalories | 259 kcalories |
| Protein | 18 grams | 43 grams |
| Fat | 1 gram | 8 grams |
| Saturated fat | 0 | 3 grams |
| Cholesterol | 0 | 82 milligrams |
| Carbohydrate | 39 grams | 0 |
| Dietary fiber | 16 grams | 0 |
| Percent of calories from fat | 3 percent | 28 percent |

**Source:** US Department of Agriculture, Agricultural Research Service. USDA Nutrient Database for Standard Reference, Release 20. 2007. http://www.ars.usda.gov/ba/bhnrc/ndl. Accessed 11/9/08.

Remember, muscle work builds muscle strength and size, and muscles prefer carbohydrate to fuel this type of work.

There is no evidence that consuming large amounts of individual amino acids is beneficial, and the risks are unknown. An excess of a single amino acid in the digestive tract can impair absorption of certain other amino acids. This could cause a deficiency of one or more amino acids and an unhealthy excess of the supplemented amino acid.

THINK
About It

3

| Table B | **Plant Sources of Protein** |

| Plant Protein Source | Grams of Protein | Kilocalories |
| --- | --- | --- |
| *Grain Products* | | |
| 1 oat bran bagel (3-inch diameter) | 6 | 145 |
| 1 whole English muffin, mixed grain | 6 | 155 |
| 1 large flour tortilla (10-inch diameter) | 6 | 218 |
| 1 cup cooked spaghetti | 8 | 221 |
| 1 cup cooked brown rice | 5 | 216 |
| 1 cup cooked oatmeal | 6 | 166 |
| 2 slices whole-wheat bread | 7 | 138 |
| ½ cup low-fat granola | 4 | 186 |
| *Starchy Vegetables* | | |
| 1 cup cooked corn | 5 | 177 |
| 1 cup baked hubbard squash | 5 | 102 |
| 1 medium baked potato with skin | 4 | 161 |
| *Legumes* | | |
| ½ cup tofu | 10 | 94 |
| 1 cup cooked lentils | 18 | 230 |
| 1 cup cooked kidney beans | 16 | 129 |
| *Vegetables* | | |
| 1 cup cooked broccoli | 4 | 55 |
| 1 cup cooked cauliflower | 2 | 29 |
| 1 cup cooked Brussels sprouts | 4 | 56 |
| *Nuts and Seeds* | | |
| 2 tablespoons peanut butter | 8 | 188 |
| ¼ cup peanuts | 10 | 216 |
| ¼ cup sunflower seeds | 7 | 200 |

**Source:** US Department of Agriculture, Agricultural Research Service. USDA Nutrient Database for Standard Reference, Release 20. 2007. http://www.ars.usda.gov/ba/bhnrc/ndl. Accessed 11/9/08.

| Table C | **Soy Food Products and Uses** |

| | |
| --- | --- |
| Tofu | A solid cake of curdled soymilk similar to soft cheese. Tofu comes in hard and soft varieties. It absorbs flavors of the foods it is mixed with. Soft tofu can be substituted for cheese in pasta dishes, stuffed in large shell pasta, blended with fruit, or used to make pie filling. Hard tofu can be used in salads and shish kebabs and can replace meat in stir-fry or mixed dishes. |
| Tempeh | Tempeh is a flat cake made from fermented soybeans. It has a mild flavor and chewy texture. Tempeh can be grilled, included in sandwiches, or combined in casseroles. |
| Meat analogs | Meat analogs are meat alternatives made primarily of soy protein. Flavored and textured to resemble chicken, beef, and pork, they can be substituted for meat in mixed dishes, pizza, tacos, or sloppy joes. |
| Soymilk | Soymilk is the liquid of the soybean. It comes in regular and low-fat versions and in different flavors. Soymilk can be used plain or substituted for regular milk on cereals, in hot cocoa, puddings, or desserts. |
| Soy flour | Soy flour is made from roasted soybeans ground into flour. Soy flour can replace up to one-quarter of the regular flour in a recipe. |
| Textured soy protein | Textured soy protein resembles ground beef. It can be rehydrated and substituted for ground beef in any recipe. |

**Key Concepts**  *In general, animal foods provide complete protein that contains the right mix of all the indispensable amino acids. With the exception of soybean protein, plant foods contain incomplete protein; that is, protein lacking one or more indispensable amino acids. Plant foods can be combined to complement each other's amino acid patterns. The FDA uses the protein digestibility-corrected amino acid score (PDCAAS) as the official method for determining protein quality. Supplements of protein or amino acids are rarely necessary and might even be harmful.*

| Table 7.5 | Religious Groups with Vegetarian Dietary Practices | |
|---|---|---|

| Religious Group | Dietary Practices |
|---|---|
| Buddhism | Some sects lacto-vegetarian, other sects vegan. |
| Hinduism | Generally lacto-vegetarian but mutton or pork eaten occasionally. |
| Seventh-Day Adventists | Lacto-ovo-vegetarian, emphasizing whole-grain foods. Also avoid alcohol, tobacco, and caffeine. |

## The Pros and Cons of Vegetarian Eating

What did Socrates, Plato, Albert Einstein, Leonardo da Vinci, William Shakespeare, Charles Darwin, and Mahatma Gandhi have in common? They all advocated a vegetarian lifestyle.[31] George Bernard Shaw, vegetarian, famous writer, and political analyst of the early 1900s, wrote, "A man fed on whiskey and dead bodies cannot do the finest work of which he is capable."[32]

Meat-eaters often argue that vegetarian diets don't provide enough protein and other essential nutrients, but this isn't necessarily so. With careful planning, a diet that contains no animal products can be nutritionally complete and offer many health benefits. Poorly planned vegetarian diets, however, can pose health risks.

### Why People Become Vegetarians

In parts of the world where food is scarce, vegetarianism is not a choice but a necessity. Where food is abundant, people choose vegetarianism for many reasons such as religious beliefs, concern for the environment, a desire to reduce world hunger and to make better use of scarce resources, an aversion to eating another living creature, or concerns about cruelty to animals. Still others become vegetarians because they believe it is healthier. The number of vegetarians in the United States has doubled in the last 10 years. Table 7.5 shows three religious groups and their vegetarian practices. Today, about 3 percent of Americans consistently follow a vegetarian diet, and close to 1 percent are vegans.[33]

THINK
About It

4

### Types of Vegetarians

Although all vegetarians share the common practice of not eating meat and meat products, they differ greatly in specific dietary practices. Lacto-ovo-vegetarians use animal products such as milk, cheese, and eggs but don't eat the flesh of animals. Vegans eat no animal-based foods and usually avoid products, such as cosmetics, made with animal-based ingredients. Fruitarians eat only raw fruit, nuts, and green foliage.

Some people eat a semi-vegetarian diet, avoiding red meats but eating small amounts of chicken or fish. The Mediterranean diet, known for reducing the risk of heart disease, is a semi-vegetarian diet rich in grains, pasta, vegetables, cheeses, and olive oil supplemented with small amounts of chicken and fish. Table 7.6 lists different types of vegetarian diets and the foods typically included and excluded.

Zen macrobiotic diets are mostly vegan and stress whole grains, locally grown vegetables, beans, sea vegetables, and soups. Extreme Zen macrobiotic diets can be very limited, consisting, for example, primarily of brown rice.

**Table 7.6   Types of Vegetarian Diets**

| Type | Animal Foods Included | Foods Excluded |
| --- | --- | --- |
| Semi-vegetarian | Dairy products, eggs, chicken, and fish | Red meats (beef and pork) |
| Pesco-vegetarian | Dairy products, eggs, and fish | Beef, pork, and poultry |
| Lacto-ovo-vegetarian | Dairy products and eggs | All animal flesh |
| Lacto-vegetarian | Dairy products | Eggs and all animal flesh |
| Ovo-vegetarian | Eggs | Dairy products and all animal flesh |
| Vegan | None | All animal products |
| Fruitarian | None | All foods except raw fruits, nuts, and green foliage |

## Health Benefits of Vegetarian Diets

Vegetarian diets usually contain less fat, saturated fat, *trans* fat, and cholesterol and more magnesium and folate than nonvegetarian diets.[34] Vegetarian diets that emphasize fresh fruits and vegetables contain high amounts of antioxidants such as beta-carotene and vitamins C and E, which protect the body's cells and tissues from damage. Fruits and vegetables also contain dietary fiber and phytochemicals; although these substances are not essential in the diet, they can have important health effects.

On average, vegetarians have lower blood cholesterol levels and are less likely to develop heart disease than nonvegetarians. Vegetarian diets low in fat and saturated fat combined with other healthful lifestyle habits can reverse the clogging of arteries that eventually can lead to heart attack or stroke.[35]

Vegetarians usually weigh less for their height than nonvegetarians, partly because their diets provide less energy and partly because of other healthful lifestyle factors such as regular exercise. High blood pressure occurs less frequently among vegetarians than among nonvegetarians, regardless of body weight or sodium intake. Vegetarians, especially vegans, have lower rates of cancer than nonvegetarians, particularly for prostate and colorectal cancer.[36] Vegetarian diets generally include more fruits, vegetables, phytochemicals, and fiber, and less fat. Also, intake of red meat has been linked to higher risk of colorectal cancer.

## Health Risks of Vegetarian Diets

Although vegetarian diets offer many health benefits, certain types of vegetarian diets pose some unique nutritional risks. The more limited the vegetarian diet, the more likely it is to cause nutritional problems. Lacto-ovo-vegetarian diets that contain a variety of foods generally are nutritionally adequate but can be high in fat and cholesterol. Iron content may be low if the diet contains large amounts of milk products.

Poorly planned vegan diets tend to be low in zinc, calcium, vitamin D, riboflavin, and vitamin $B_{12}$.[37] The best sources of these nutrients are animal foods—red meat for zinc; milk for calcium; vitamin D, riboflavin, and chicken for vitamin $B_6$; and any animal foods for $B_{12}$. Because plant foods contain a form of iron that is not as well absorbed as the iron in animal foods, vegetarians need to include more iron in their diets. Vitamin C and other compounds in fruits and vegetables aid iron absorption into the body.

## *Quick* Bite

### Paleolithic Protein

Didn't our ancestors eat a lot of meat, too? Researchers estimate that hunter-gatherers had diets that were about one-third meat and two-thirds vegetable. The meat from wild game, however, averages only one-seventh the fat of domesticated beef (about 4 grams of fat per 100 grams of wild meat, compared with 29 grams of fat per 100 grams of domestic meat). In addition, compared with the meat at your local supermarket, the fat contained in game animals that graze on the free range has five times as much polyunsaturated fat.

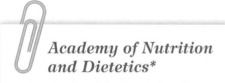

### *Academy of Nutrition and Dietetics**

**Vegetarian Diets**

It is the position of the American Dietetic Association that appropriately planned vegetarian diets are healthful, nutritionally adequate, and provide health benefits in the prevention and treatment of certain diseases.

**Source:** Reproduced from Position of the Academy of Nutrition and Dietetics and Dietitians of Canada: vegetarian diets. *J Am Diet Assoc.* 2003;103(6):748–765.

* Formerly the American Dietetic Association

---

Vegans tend to have higher intakes of phytates (found in whole grains, bran, and soy products), oxalates (found in spinach, rhubarb, and chocolate), and tannins (found in tea). These compounds can bind minerals, making them less available to the body for absorption.

Very limited vegan diets, such as fruitarian diets or extreme Zen macrobiotic diets, pose the greatest nutritional risks. These diets are likely to be lacking in many essential nutrients.

For most people, vegetarian diets readily provide sufficient nutrients. But for some, especially infants, young children, and pregnant or breastfeeding women, vegetarian diets must be carefully planned to meet the needs of rapid growth. The nutritional areas of concern for vegetarian children include:

- Providing sufficient energy and nutrients for normal growth
- Providing an adequate iron intake to prevent iron-deficiency anemia
- Identifying adequate sources of vitamin $B_{12}$ to prevent deficiency
- Obtaining sufficient vitamin D and calcium to prevent rickets
- Ensuring a plentiful supply of long-chain ($n$–3) fatty acids from nonmeat sources, such as seeds and nuts
- Having food in an appropriate form and combination to ensure that nutrients can be digested and absorbed by the child

### Dietary Recommendations for Vegetarians

Dietitians from the United States and Canada have developed a food guide for use in planning vegetarian diets.[38] This food guide includes the following food groups: grains, vegetables, fruits, legumes, nuts and other protein-rich foods, fats, and calcium-rich foods. Vegetarians who include milk, milk products, and eggs in their diet can easily meet their nutritional needs for protein and other essential nutrients but must take care to choose low-fat milk products and limit eggs to avoid excess saturated fat and cholesterol.

Because grains, vegetables, and legumes (dried beans and peas) all provide protein, vegans who eat a variety of foods also can meet their protein needs easily. Although most plant foods do not contain complete protein, eating complementary plant protein sources during the same day adequately meets the body's needs for protein production.

Vegans who avoid all animal products must supplement their diets with a reliable source of vitamin $B_{12}$, such as fortified soymilk. Although bacteria in some fermented foods and in the knobby growths of some seaweeds produce vitamin $B_{12}$, most vegans do not eat enough seaweeds and fermented foods to meet their vitamin $B_{12}$ needs. Vegans also need a dietary source of vitamin D when sun exposure is limited.

The Academy of Nutrition and Dietetics gives the following nutritional guidelines for vegetarians:

1. Choose a variety of foods, including whole grains, vegetables, fruits, legumes, nuts, seeds, and, if desired, dairy products and eggs.
2. Choose whole, unrefined foods often and minimize the intake of highly sweetened, fatty, and heavily refined foods.
3. Choose a variety of fruits and vegetables.
4. If animal foods such as dairy products and eggs are used, choose lower-fat dairy products and use both eggs and dairy products in moderation.
5. Include a regular source of vitamin $B_{12}$ and, if sun exposure is limited, of vitamin D.[39]

**Key Concepts** *Vegetarian diets eliminate animal products to various degrees. Lacto-ovo-vegetarians include milk and eggs in their diets, whereas vegans eat no animal foods. Vegetarian diets tend to be low in fat and high in fiber and phytochemicals, which may help reduce chronic disease risks. Careful diet planning is necessary for vegans and growing children to ensure that all nutrient needs are met.*

## The Health Effects of Too Little or Too Much Protein

Because protein plays such a vital role in so many body processes, protein deficiency can wreak havoc in numerous body systems. If your body doesn't have enough available protein, it will not have the indispensable amino acids needed to synthesize body proteins.

Protein deficiency occurs when energy and/or protein intake is inadequate. Adequate energy intake spares dietary and body proteins so they can be used for protein synthesis. Without adequate energy intake, the body burns dietary protein for energy rather than using it to make body proteins. Protein deficiency can occur even in people who eat seemingly adequate amounts of protein if the protein they eat is of poor quality or cannot be absorbed.

Although protein deficiency is widespread in poverty-stricken communities and in some nonindustrialized countries, most people in industrialized countries face the opposite problem—protein excess. The RDA for a 70-kilogram (154-pound) person is 56 grams, but the average American man consumes approximately 110 grams of protein daily, and the average woman about 70 grams.[40] Many meat-loving Americans eat far more protein.

Some research suggests that high protein intake contributes to risk for heart disease, cancer, and osteoporosis. However, because high protein intake often goes hand in hand with high intakes of saturated fat and cholesterol, the independent effects of high protein intake are difficult to determine.

### Protein-Energy Malnutrition

Childhood malnutrition is prevalent around the world and contributes to one-third of all deaths worldwide.[41] Death for these children results from a condition called **protein-energy malnutrition (PEM)**, a deficiency of protein, energy, or both.

Protein and energy intakes are difficult to separate because diets adequate in energy usually are adequate in protein, and diets inadequate in energy inhibit the body's use of dietary protein for protein synthesis. When both calories and protein are inadequate, dietary protein is used for energy rather than for other necessary functions, forcing the body to break down its own protein to be used as needed. Because protein is a key component for so many different functions in the body, chronic protein deficiency can lead to a number of health problems.

Many situations contribute to PEM, including poverty, insufficient food intake, poor food quality, unsanitary living condition, and improper feeding of infants and young children.[42] Although it can occur at all stages of life, PEM is most common during childhood, when protein is needed to support rapid growth. Symptoms of PEM can be mild or severe and exist in either acute or chronic forms.

Protein-energy malnutrition occurs in all parts of the world but is most common in Africa, South and Central America, East and Southeast Asia, and the Middle East. In industrialized countries, PEM occurs most often among people living in poverty, in the elderly, and in hospitalized patients with other conditions such as anorexia nervosa, AIDS, cancer, or malabsorption syndromes.

In some instances, either calorie or protein deficiency exists without the other. Severe protein deficiency is called **kwashiorkor**, whereas severe calo-

**protein-energy malnutrition (PEM)** A condition resulting from long-term inadequate intakes of protein and energy that can lead to wasting of body tissues and increased susceptibility to infection.

**kwashiorkor** A type of malnutrition that occurs primarily in young children who have an infectious disease and whose diets supply marginal amounts of energy and very little protein. Common symptoms include poor growth, edema, apathy, weakness, and susceptibility to infections.

**marasmus** A type of malnutrition resulting from chronic inadequate consumption of protein and energy that is characterized by wasting of muscle, fat, and other body tissue.

rie deficiency is called **marasmus**.[43] In general, marasmus is an insufficient energy intake that does not meet the body's requirements. As a result, the body draws on its own stores, resulting in emaciation. In kwashiorkor, adequate carbohydrate consumption and decreased protein intake lead to decreased synthesis of visceral proteins. The resulting hypoalbuminemia contributes to extravascular fluid accumulation and the appearance of a bloated or enlarged abdomen.[44] See **Figure 7.13** for signs and symptoms of kwashiorkor and marasmus.

### Kwashiorkor

The term *kwashiorkor* is a Ghanian word that describes the "evil spirit that infects the first child when the second child is born." In many cultures, babies are breastfed until the next baby comes along. When the new baby arrives, the first baby is weaned from nutritious breast milk and placed on a watered-down version of the family's diet. In areas of poverty, this diet is often low in protein, or the consumed protein is not digested and absorbed easily.

One symptom of kwashiorkor that sets it apart from marasmus is edema, or swelling of body tissue, usually in the feet and legs. Lack of blood proteins reduces the force that keeps fluid in the bloodstream, allowing fluid to leak out into the tissues. Because proteins are unavailable to transport fat, it accumulates in the liver. Combined with edema, this accumulation produces a bloated belly. Other features of kwashiorkor include stunted weight and height, increased susceptibility to infection, dry and flaky skin, and sometimes skin sores; dry, brittle, and unnaturally blond hair; and changes in skin color. Because the energy deficit is usually not as severe (or as long-standing) in kwashiorkor as in marasmus, people with kwashiorkor may still have some body fat stores left.

Kwashiorkor usually develops in children between 18 and 24 months of age, about the time weaning occurs. Its onset can be rapid and is often triggered by an infection or illness that increases the child's protein needs. In hospital settings, kwashiorkor can develop in situations where protein needs are extremely high (e.g., trauma, infection, burns) but dietary intake is poor.

Kwashiorkor is associated with extreme poverty in developing countries and except for people with chronic illness is rarely seen in affluent countries. Some cases, however, can be explained by nutritional ignorance and food faddism.[45] A number of cases of kwashiorkor induced in infants by dietary restriction of "well-meaning" parents have been reported in the U.S. literature.[46] In one case, for example, the mother of an 8-month old infant had placed the child on a severely restrictive diet, consisting only of RICE DREAM milk (which is low in protein), sweet potatoes, and bananas, with the assumption that it would help his rash.[47] The results were severe protein-calorie malnutrition, a condition that is often under diagnosed or misdiagnosed even in the United States.[48]

### Marasmus

Marasmus is derived from the Greek word *marasmos*, which means "withering" or "to waste away." It develops more slowly than kwashiorkor and results from chronic PEM. Protein, energy, and nutrient intakes are all grossly inadequate, depleting body fat reserves and severely wasting muscle tissue, including vital organs like the heart. Growth slows or stops, and children are both short and very thin for their age. Metabolism slows and body temperature drops as the body tries to conserve energy. Children with marasmus are apathetic, often not even crying in an effort to conserve energy. Their hair is sparse and falls out easily. Because muscle and fat are used up, a child with marasmus often looks like a frail, wrinkled, elderly person.

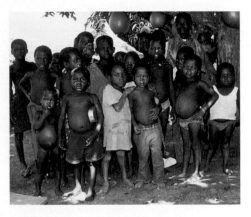
(a)

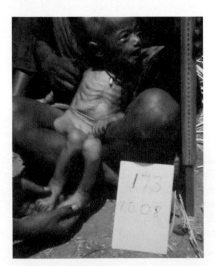
(b)

**Figure 7.13** **Kwashiorkor and marasmus.** (a) Edema in the feet and legs and a bloated belly are symptoms of kwashiorkor. (b) Children with marasmus are short and thin for their age and can appear frail and wrinkled.

Marasmus occurs most often in infants and children 6 to 18 months of age who are fed diluted or improperly mixed formulas. Because this is a time of rapid brain growth, marasmus can permanently stunt brain development and lead to learning disabilities. Marasmus also occurs in adults who have cancer or are experiencing starvation, including the self-imposed starvation of the eating disorder known as anorexia nervosa.

### Nutritional Rehabilitation

To recover, people with PEM need gradual and careful refeeding to correct protein, energy, fluid, and vitamin and mineral imbalances.[49] As a result of diarrhea, people with PEM are often dehydrated and have low body potassium stores. These imbalances in fluids and electrolytes are corrected first to raise blood pressure and strengthen the heart. Once that is achieved, the patient receives protein and other nutrients in small amounts that are gradually increased as tolerated.

## Excess Dietary Protein

In industrialized countries, an excess of protein and energy is more common than a deficiency. Generally, self-selected diets do not contain more than 40 percent of calories from protein.[50] Although high protein intake has been suggested to contribute to kidney problems, osteoporosis, heart disease, and cancer (see **Figure 7.14**), the Food and Nutrition Board decided that evidence to support these links was not strong enough to set a UL for protein.[51]

### Kidney Function

Because the kidneys must excrete the products of protein breakdown, high protein intake can strain kidney function and is especially harmful for people with kidney disease or diabetes.

To prevent dehydration, it is important to drink plenty of fluids to dilute the byproducts of protein breakdown for excretion. Human infants should

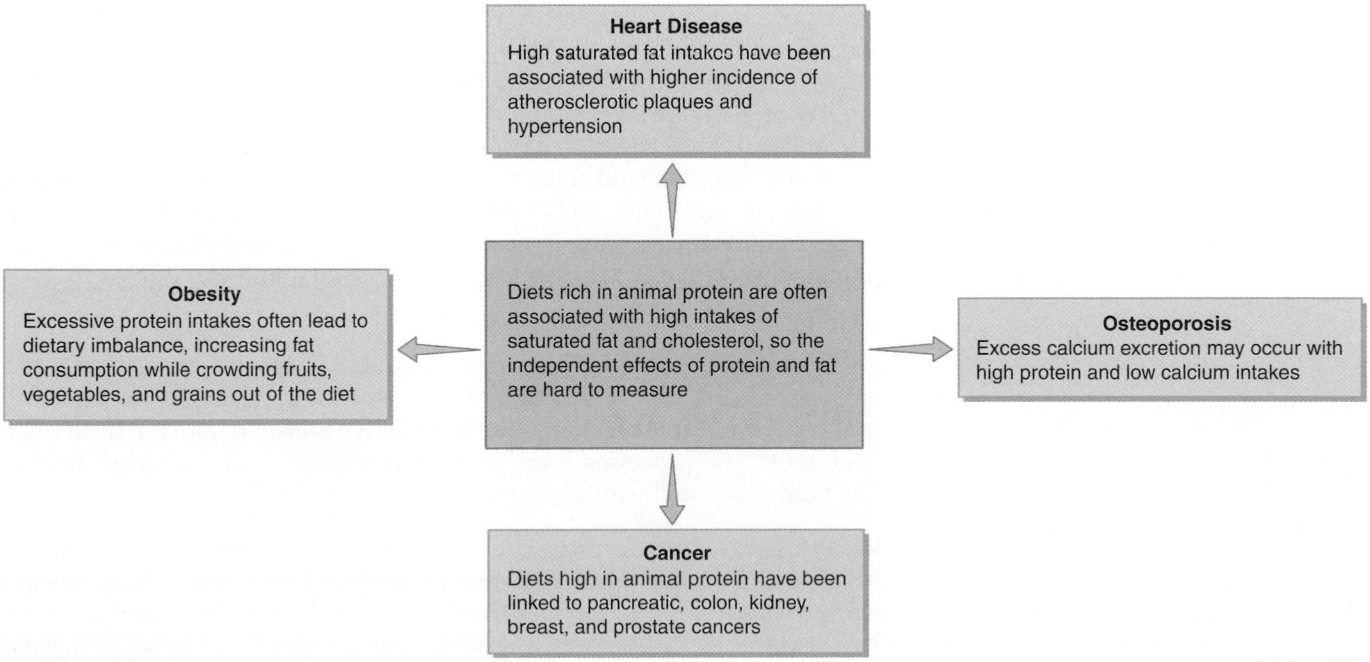

*Quick* Bite

**The Source of Salisbury Steak**

Dr. James Salisbury, a London physician who lived in the late 1800s, believed man to be two-thirds carnivorous and one-third herbivorous. He recommended a diet low in starch and high in lean meat, with lots of hot water to rinse out the products of fermentation. His diet regimen included broiled, lean, minced beef three times a day. Although we call it Salisbury steak as a courtesy to Dr. Salisbury's heritage, minced beef patties are really more like hamburgers.

**Heart Disease**
High saturated fat intakes have been associated with higher incidence of atherosclerotic plaques and hypertension

**Obesity**
Excessive protein intakes often lead to dietary imbalance, increasing fat consumption while crowding fruits, vegetables, and grains out of the diet

Diets rich in animal protein are often associated with high intakes of saturated fat and cholesterol, so the independent effects of protein and fat are hard to measure

**Osteoporosis**
Excess calcium excretion may occur with high protein and low calcium intakes

**Cancer**
Diets high in animal protein have been linked to pancreatic, colon, kidney, breast, and prostate cancers

**Figure 7.14** **Excess protein.** In developed countries, excess protein and energy are a greater problem than protein deficiency.

not be fed unmodified cow's milk until they are at least 1 year of age because the high protein concentration in cow's milk combined with an immature kidney system can cause excessive fluid losses and dehydration.

### Mineral Losses

The link between high-protein diets and osteoporosis is based on studies showing that a high protein intake increases calcium excretion, which could then contribute to bone mineral losses. However, these studies generally used purified proteins rather than food proteins. Studies of healthy postmenopausal women with an increase in dietary protein from 10 to 20 percent of energy slightly improved calcium absorption compared to a low-calcium diet, nearly compensating for the slight increase in urinary calcium excretion.[52] Other studies have found favorable effects on bone mineral density from increasing intake of protein in the presence of adequate dietary calcium and acid-neutralizing fruits and vegetables.[53]

### Obesity

Some epidemiological studies have shown a correlation between high protein intake and body fatness.[54] High-protein foods often are high in fat. A diet high in fat and protein may provide too much energy, contributing to obesity. Large amounts of high-protein foods will displace fruits, vegetables, and grains—foods that contain fewer calories. Researchers have suggested that high dietary protein intake alters hormones and the body's response to hormones, including leptin, which regulates feeding centers in the brain to reduce food intake.[55] Some studies suggest that because of this effect on hormones, a high protein intake early in life increases the risk of obesity later in life.[56]

### Heart Disease

Research has linked high intake of foods rich in animal protein to high blood cholesterol levels and increased risk of heart disease. Foods high in animal protein are also high in saturated fat and cholesterol. Whether protein alone—independent of fat—plays a role in the development of heart disease is less clear. Soy protein foods contain no saturated fat or cholesterol, and the FDA approved a health claim saying that soy protein is beneficial in reducing the risk of heart disease. Some epidemiologic studies, however, found that consuming soy protein has little or no effect on the risk factors for heart disease.[57] The researchers suggested that consuming soy protein products, such as tofu, soy butter, soy nuts, and some soy burgers, should be beneficial because of their low saturated fat content and high content of polyunsaturated fats, fiber, vitamins, and minerals. Using these and other soy foods to replace foods high in animal protein can reduce intake of saturated fat and cholesterol.[58]

### Cancer

Some studies suggest a link between a diet high in animal protein foods and an increased risk for certain types of cancers, with a strong link between animal protein and colon cancer.[59] Prolonged high intake of both red meat (e.g., beef, pork) and processed meat (e.g., ham, smoked meats, sausage, bacon) has been associated with increased colon cancer risk.[60]

**Key Concepts** *Protein-energy malnutrition (PEM) is a common form of malnutrition in the developing world, with potentially devastating effects for children. PEM can take two forms: kwashiorkor and marasmus. Among other symptoms, kwashiorkor is characterized by edema, or swelling of the tissues. Marasmus results from chronic PEM and is characterized by severe wasting of body fat and muscles. Intake of too much protein may contribute to obesity, heart disease, and certain forms of cancer. These links, however, may be attributed to the high fat intake that often accompanies high protein intake.*

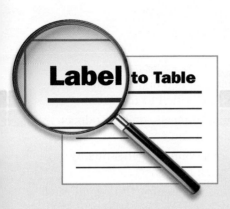

**Label to Table**

Have you ever visited a health food store and noticed all the protein powders, amino acid supplements, and high-protein bars? Do you believe claims like "protein boosts your energy level" or "amino acid *x* helps you build muscle" or "protein shakes are the best pre-workout fuel"? You know from this chapter that protein is an important nutrient and it's used to build and repair tissue. But do you need one of these supplements? Before reaching into your wallet, check out the Nutrition Facts of this protein powder and determine whether it's a good buy.

Look at this label and note how far down protein is on the list of nutrients. This placement is intentional and attempts to encourage consumers to de-emphasize protein in their diets. You may recall that most Americans eat more protein than they need, and because much of that protein comes from animal foods, they are also getting excess saturated fat. Although there is a Daily Value (DV) for protein (50 grams), to determine %DV for protein, manufacturers first would have to use the PDCAAS method to determine the food protein's quality. Manufacturers are not required to give the %DV for protein on food labels.

Do protein and amino acid supplements do what they claim to do? In terms of building muscle, exercise physiologists agree that it takes consistent muscle work (i.e., weight lifting) and a healthful diet that meets the body's calorie needs. Building muscle does not depend on extra protein. In fact, muscles mainly use carbohydrate and fat for fuel, not protein, so these other nutrients are more important for effective workouts.

In terms of protein's ability to boost your energy level, recall that anything with calories (carbohydrates, proteins, and fats) provides the body with "energy." In fact, unlike carbohydrates and fats, only a small amount of protein is used for energy expenditure. Research shows that the best thing to eat before a workout is carbohydrate, not protein, because carbohydrate provides glucose to the muscle cells. Review this label again. What percentage of this protein powder's calories comes from protein?

**154 kcalories**

**11 grams protein × 4 kcalories per gram**

**= 44 protein kcalories**

**44 ÷ 154 = 0.28, or 28% protein kcalories**

Surprise! Surprise! Only about one-quarter of the powder's calories are protein anyway, so it's okay as a pre-workout fuel, not because of its protein content but because of its ample carbohydrate!

**Nutrition Facts**

Serving Size: 2 scoops
Servings Per Container: 18

**Amount Per Serving**

**Calories** 154   Calories from fat 35

| | % Daily Value* |
|---|---|
| **Total Fat** 4g | 6% |
| Saturated Fat 2.5g | 12% |
| Trans Fat 0g | |
| **Cholesterol** 20mg | 7% |
| **Sodium** 170mg | 7% |
| **Total Carbohydrate** 17g | 6% |
| Dietary Fiber 0g | 0% |
| Sugars 14g | |
| **Protein** 11g | |

Vitamin A 4%    •    Vitamin C 6%

Calcium 40%    •    Iron 0%

* Percent Daily Values are based on a 2,000 calorie diet. Your daily values may be higher or lower depending on your calorie needs:

| | | Calories: | 2,000 | 2,500 |
|---|---|---|---|---|
| Total Fat | Less Than | | 65g | 80g |
| Sat Fat | Less Than | | 20g | 25g |
| Cholesterol | Less Than | | 300mg | 300mg |
| Sodium | Less Than | | 2,400mg | 2,400mg |
| Total Carbohydrate | | | 300g | 375g |
| Dietary Fiber | | | 25g | 30g |

Calories per gram:
Fat 9    •    Carbohydrate 4    •    Protein 4

# Learning Portfolio

## Key Terms

## Study Points

- Many vital compounds are proteins, including enzymes, hormones, transport proteins, and regulators of both acid–base and fluid balance.
- Proteins are long chains of amino acids.
- Amino acids are composed of a central carbon atom bonded to hydrogen, carboxyl, amino, and side groups.
- Twenty amino acids are important in human nutrition; nine of these amino acids are considered indispensable (must come from the diet), whereas the body can make the other 11 (dispensable) amino acids.
- The amino acid sequence of a protein determines its shape and function.
- Denaturing proteins changes their shape and therefore their functional properties.
- Hydrochloric acid in the stomach denatures proteins so the enzyme pepsin can begin their digestion.
- Proteins are completely digested in the small intestine and, after absorption, are carried to the liver.
- Dietary protein is found in meats, dairy products, legumes, nuts, seeds, grains, and vegetables.
- In general, animal foods contain higher-quality protein than is found in plant foods.
- Protein needs are highest when growth is rapid, such as during infancy, childhood, and adolescence.
- The protein intake of most Americans exceeds their RDA.
- Protein deficiency is most common in developing countries and often results in marasmus and kwashiorkor.
- Protein excess is also harmful and may affect risk for osteoporosis, heart disease, and cancer.

## Study Questions

1. Describe the differences among indispensable, dispensable, and conditionally indispensable amino acids.
2. List the functions of body proteins.
3. How is protein related to immune function?
4. What is meant by nitrogen balance? Give examples of conditions associated with positive and negative nitrogen balance.
5. What are complementary proteins? List three examples of food combinations that contain complementary proteins.
6. Describe a vegan diet.
7. List the potential health benefits of a vegetarian diet.
8. What health effects occur if you are protein deficient?
9. What health effects can occur over time from consuming too much protein?

## Try This

### The Sweetness of NutraSweet

The purpose of this experiment is to see the effect of high temperatures on the dipeptide known as NutraSweet (aspartame). Make a cup of hot tea (or coffee) and add one packet of Equal (one brand of aspartame). Stir and taste the tea; note its sweetness. Reheat the tea (via a microwave or stovetop) so it boils for 30 to 60 seconds.

After the tea cools, taste it. Does it still taste sweet? Why or why not?

## The Vegetarian Challenge

The purpose of this activity is to eat a completely vegan diet for one day. Begin by making a list of your typical meals and snacks. Once the list is complete, review each food item and determine whether it contains animal products. Cross off items that contain animal products and circle the remaining vegan-friendly options. Double-check the circled list with a friend or roommate. You may have missed something! Create a full day's worth of meals and snacks using your circled foods as well as additional vegan options. Make sure your menu looks complete and nutritionally balanced. Try to stick to this menu for at least one day. Pay attention to deviations you make and determine whether these are vegan food choices.

# What About Bobbie?

Take a minute to review Bobbie's food intake (see the "Food Choices: Nutrients and Nourishment" chapter) with a special eye on protein. How do you think she did? Do you think she's lower or higher than her RDA? Let's first calculate her protein RDA. Because Bobbie weighs 155 pounds, her protein RDA is as follows:

**155 pounds ÷ 2.2 pounds = 70.5 kilograms**

**70.5 kilograms × 0.8 grams protein = 56.4 grams**

Her protein intake is 96 grams. This is quite high compared to her RDA! Are you surprised to learn she eats nearly twice as much protein as she needs? Her diet doesn't look that high in protein, does it? Here are the foods that contribute the most protein to her diet:

| Food | Protein Grams |
|---|---|
| Meatballs | 24 |
| Turkey breast | 17 |
| Spaghetti | 10 |
| Pizza | 9 |
| Bagel | 7 |

Another way to evaluate Bobbie's protein intake is in terms of calories. If her total protein intake is 96 grams, then 384 kilocalories come from protein. Remember, her total kilocalorie intake is 2,300, which means protein makes up 17 percent of her energy intake. General guidelines recommend that 10 to 35 percent of energy come from protein.

So what's the deal? Is Bobbie eating way too much protein or just the right amount? She's certainly high compared to her RDA of 56 grams, but, using the AMDR, she could consume as much as 200 grams at her current energy intake level! Bobbie's diet could certainly use more servings of fruits and vegetables.

# References

1 Lesk AM. *Introduction to Protein Science: Architecture, Function, and Genomics*. 2nd ed. New York: Oxford University Press; 2010.
2 Ibid.
3 Ribas GS, Sitta A, Wajner M, Vargas CR. Oxidative stress in phenylketonuria: what is the evidence? *Cell Mol Neurobiol*. 2011;31(5):653–662.
4 Oliveira GP, Dias CM, Pelosi P, Rocco PR. Understanding the mechanisms of glutamine action in critically ill patients. *Ann Acad Bras Cienc*. 2010;82(2):417–430.
5 Ibid.
6 Mizock BA. Immunonutrition and critical illness: an update. *Nutrition*. 2010;26(7–8):701–707.
7 Gropper SS, Smith JL, Groff JL. *Advanced Nutrition and Human Metabolism*. 5th ed. Belmont, CA: Wadsworth; 2009.
8 Hall J. *Guyton and Hall Textbook of Medical Physiology*. 12th ed. Philadelphia: Saunders/Elsevier; 2011.
9 Gropper SS, Smith JL, Groff JL. Op. cit.
10 Ibid.
11 Olveira G, Olverira C, Casado-Miranda E, et al. Markers for the validation of reported dietary intake in adults with cystic fibrosis. *J Am Diet Assoc*. 2009;109(10):1704–1711.
12 Stipanuk M. *Biochemical, Physiological, and Molecular Aspects of Human Nutrition*. 2nd ed. Philadelphia: Elsevier; 2006.
13 Marieb E, Hoehn K. *Human Anatomy and Physiology*. 8th ed. Upper Saddle River, NJ: Pearson Benjamin Cummings; 2008.
14 Medeiros D, Wildman R. *Advanced Human Nutrition*. 2nd ed. Burlington, MA: Jones & Bartlett Learning; 2012.
15 Institute of Medicine, Food and Nutrition Board. *Dietary Reference Intakes for Energy, Carbohydrate, Fiber, Fat, Fatty Acids, Cholesterol, Protein, and Amino Acids*. Washington, DC: National Academies Press; 2005.
16 Jordan LY, Hickey MS, Miller BR, et al. Nitrogen balance in older individuals in energy balance depends on timing of protein intake. *J Gerontol*. 2010;65A(10):1068–1076.
17 Institute of Medicine, Food and Nutrition Board. http://www.iom.edu/About-IOM/Leadership-Staff/Boards/Food-and-Nutrition-Board.aspx. Accessed 6/15/11.
18 Institute of Medicine, Food and Nutrition Board. http://iom.edu/Activities/Nutrition/SummaryDRIs/~/media/Files/Activity%20Files/Nutrition/DRIs/DRI_Macronutrients.ashx. Accessed 6/15/11.
19 Koopman R, van Loon LJ. Aging, exercise, and muscle protein metabolism. *J Appl Physiol*. 2009;106(6):2040–2048.
20 Campbell WW, Johnson CA, McCabe GP, Carnell NS. Dietary protein requirements of younger and older adults. *Am J Clin Nutr*. 2008;88(5):1322–1329.
21 Fulgoni V. Current protein intake in America: analysis of the National Health and Nutrition Examination Survey, 2003–2004. *Am J Clin Nutr*. 2008;87(5):1554S–1557S.
22 Ibid.
23 Van Horn L, McCoin M, Kris-Etherton PM, et al. The evidence for dietary prevention and treatment of cardiovascular disease. *J Am Diet Assoc*. 2008;108(2):287–331.
24 US Department of Agriculture. Nutrient content of the US food supply. http://www.cnpp.usda.gov/Publications/FoodSupply/FoodSupply2005Report.pdf. Accessed 6/15/11.
25 Ibid.
26 USDA Economic Research Service. Dietary quality and food consumption: who eats what, where, and how much. http://www.ers.usda.gov/Briefing/DietQuality/whoeats.htm#other. Accessed 6/15/11.
27 Ibid.
28 Position of the Academy of Nutrition and Dietetics: vegetarian diets. *J Am Diet Assoc*. 2009;109(7):1266–1282
29 Centers for Disease Control and Prevention. Protein. http://www.cdc.gov/nutrition/everyone/basics/protein.html. Accessed 7/15/11.
30 US Food and Drug Administration. Nutrition labeling; questions G1 through P8. *Guidance for Industry: A Food Labeling Guide*; October 2009.

31    Ballenntine R. *Transition to Vegetarianism: An Evolutionary Step*. Honesdale, PA: Himalayan International Institute of Yoga Science and Philosophy; 1987; and Null G. *The Vegetarian Handbook: Eating Right for Total Health*. New York: St. Martin's Press; 1987.

32    Null G. Op. cit.

33    Position of the Academy of Nutrition and Dietetics: vegetarian diets. *J Am Diet Assoc*. 2009;109(7):1266–1282.

34    Ibid.

35    Ibid.

36    Ibid.

37    Ibid.

38    US Department of Agriculture. Tips and resources. Vegetarian diets. http://www.choosemyplate.gov/tipsresources/vegetarian_diets.html. Accessed 6/15/11.

39    Position of the Academy of Nutrition and Dietetics: vegetarian diets. Op. cit.

40    Fulgoni V. Op. cit.

41    Imdad A, Sadig K, Bhutta ZA. Evidence-based prevention of childhood malnutrition. *Curr Opin Clin Nutr Metab Care*. 2011;14(3):276–285.

42    World Health Organization. WHO Global Database on Child Growth and Malnutrition Introduction. 2008. http://www.who.int/nutgrowthdb/en. Accessed 6/15/11.

43    Bandsma RH, Spoelstra MN, Mari A, et al. Impaired glucose absorption in children with severe malnutrition. *J Pediatr*. 2011;158(2):282–287.

44    Scheinfeld N. Protein-energy malnutrition. *Medscape Reference Drugs, Diseases & Procedures*. http://emedicine.medscape.com/article/1104623-overview#a0104. Accessed 6/15/11.

45    Grover Z, Ee LC. Protein energy malnutrition. *Pediatr Clin North Am*. 2009;56(5):1055–1068.

46    Tierney EP, Sage R, Shwayder T. Kwashiorkor from a severe dietary restriction in an 8-month infant in Detroit, Michigan: case report and review of the literature. *Int J Dermatol*. 2010;49(7):54.

47    Grover Z, Ee LC. Op. cit.

48    Ibid.

49    Kohn MR, Madden S, Clarke SD. Refeeding in anorexia nervosa: increased safety and efficiency through understanding the pathophysiology of protein calorie malnutrition. *Curr Opin Pediatr*. 2011;23(4):390–394.

50    Institute of Medicine, Food and Nutrition Board. *Dietary Reference Intakes for Energy, Carbohydrate, Fiber, Fat, Fatty Acids, Cholesterol, Protein, and Amino Acids*. Op. cit.

51    Ibid.

52    Hunt JR, Johnson LK, Fariba Roughead ZK. Dietary protein and calcium interact to influence calcium retention: a controlled feeding study. *Am J Clin Nutr*. 2009;89(5):1357–1365.

53    Thrope MP, Evans EM. Dietary protein and bone health: harmonizing conflicting theories. *Nutr Rev*. 2011;69(4):215–230.

54    KD Hall. Predicting metabolic adaptation, body weight change, and energy intake in humans. *Am J Physiol Endocrin Metab*. 2010;298(3):E449–E466.

55    Gautron L, Elmquist JK. Sixteen years and counting: an update on leptin in energy balance. *J Clin Invest*. 2011;121(6):2087–2093.

56    Gunther AL, Remer T, Kroke A, Buyken AE. Early protein intake and later obesity risk: which protein sources at which time points throughout infancy and childhood are important for body mass index and body fat percentage at 7 y of age? *Am J Clin Nutr*. 2007;86(6):1765–1772.

57    Messina M. Insights gained from 20 years of soy research. *J Nutr*. 2010;140(12):2289S–2295S.

58    Patisaul HB, Jefferson W. The pros and cons of phytoestrogens. *Front Neuroendocrinol*. 2010;31(4):400–419.

59    Satia JA, Tseng M, Galanko JA, Sandler RS. Dietary patterns and colon cancer risk in Whites and African Americans in the North Carolina Colon Cancer Study. *Nutr Cancer*. 2009;61(2):179–193.

60    Corpet DE. Red meat and colon cancer: Should we become vegetarians, or can we make meat safer? *Meat Sci*. 2011;89(3):310–316; and Hu J, La Vecchia C, Morrison H, et al. Salt, processed meat and the risk of cancer. *Eur J Cancer Prev*. 2011;20(2):132–139.

# Spotlight on Metabolism

## THiNK About It

1  You are driving on "the energy highway." You stop at the tollbooth. What kind of currency do you need to pay the toll?

2  When you think of "cell power," what comes to mind?

3  What do you think is meant by the saying "Fat burns in a flame of carbohydrate"?

4  When it comes to fasting, what's your body's first priority?

**Visit** go.jblearning.com/
inseldisco4e

Your body is a wonderfully efficient factory. It accepts raw materials (food), burns some to generate power, uses some to produce finished goods, routes the rest to storage, and discards waste and byproducts. Constant turnover of your stored inventory keeps it fresh. Your body draws on these stored raw materials to produce compounds, and nutrient intake replenishes the supply.

Do you ever wonder how your biological factory responds to changing supply and demand? Under normal circumstances, the body hums along nicely with all processes in balance. When supply exceeds demand, your body stores the excess raw materials. When supply fails to meet demand, your body draws on these stored materials to meet its needs. Your biological factory never stops; even though a storage or energy-production process may dominate, all your factory operations are active at all times.

Collectively, we call these processes **metabolism**. (See **Figure SM.1**.) While some metabolic reactions break down molecules to extract energy, others synthesize building blocks to produce new molecules. To carry out metabolic processes, thousands of chemical reactions occur every moment in cells throughout your body. The most active metabolic sites include your liver, muscle, and brain cells.

## Energy: Fuel for Work

To operate, machines need energy. Cars use gasoline for fuel, factory machinery uses electricity, and windmills rely on wind power. So what about you? All cells require energy to sustain life. Even during sleep your body uses energy for breathing, pumping blood, maintaining body temperature, delivering oxygen to tissues, removing waste products, synthesizing new tissue for growth, and repairing damaged or worn-out tissues. When awake, you need additional energy for physical movement (such as standing, walking, and talking) and for the digestion and absorption of foods.

Where does the energy come from to power your body's "machinery"? Our cells get their energy from **chemical energy** held in the molecular bonds of carbohydrates, fats, and proteins—the energy macronutrients—as well as alcohol.[1] The chemical energy in food and beverages originates as light energy from the sun. Green plants use light energy to make carbohydrate in a process called **photosynthesis**. In photosynthesis, carbon dioxide ($CO_2$) from the air combines with water ($H_2O$) from the earth to form a carbohydrate, usually glucose ($C_6H_{12}O_6$), and oxygen ($O_2$). Plants store glucose as starch and release oxygen into the atmosphere. Plants such as corn, peas, squash, turnips, potatoes, and rice store especially high amounts of starch in their edible parts. When our bodies extract energy from food and convert it to a form that our cells can use, we lose more than half of the total food energy as heat.[2]

## Transferring Food Energy to Cellular Energy

Our bodies extract energy from food in three stages (see **Figure SM.2**):[3]

- *Stage 1: Digestion, absorption, and transport.* Digestion breaks food down into small subunits—simple sugars, fatty acids, monoglycerides, glycerol, and amino acids—that the small intestine can absorb. The circulatory system then transports these nutrients to tissues throughout the body.
- *Stage 2: Breakdown of many small molecules to a few key metabolites.* Inside individual cells, chemical reactions convert simple sugars, fatty acids, glycerol, and amino acids into a few

**metabolism** All chemical reactions within organisms that enable them to maintain life. The two main categories of metabolism are catabolism and anabolism.

**chemical energy** Energy contained in the bonds between atoms of a molecule.

**photosynthesis** The process by which green plants use light energy from the sun to produce carbohydrates from carbon dioxide and water.

key **metabolites** (products of metabolic reactions). This process liberates a small amount of usable energy.

- *Stage 3: Transfer of energy to a form that cells can use.* The complete breakdown of metabolites to carbon dioxide and water liberates large amounts of energy. The reactions during this stage are responsible for converting more than 90 percent of the available food energy to a form of energy our bodies can use.

**metabolites** Substances produced during metabolism.

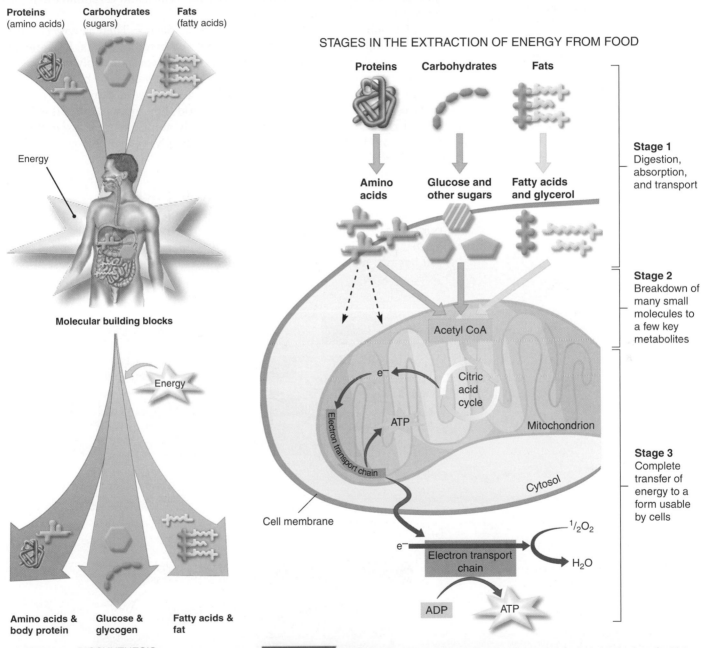

EXTRACTION OF ENERGY

**Proteins** (amino acids)   **Carbohydrates** (sugars)   **Fats** (fatty acids)

Energy

**Molecular building blocks**

Energy

**Amino acids &** **body protein**   **Glucose &** **glycogen**   **Fatty acids &** **fat**

BIOSYNTHESIS

STAGES IN THE EXTRACTION OF ENERGY FROM FOOD

**Proteins**   **Carbohydrates**   **Fats**

**Amino** **acids**   **Glucose and** **other sugars**   **Fatty acids** **and glycerol**

**Stage 1** Digestion, absorption, and transport

Acetyl CoA

**Stage 2** Breakdown of many small molecules to a few key metabolites

e⁻

Citric acid cycle

ATP

Mitochondrion

Electron transport chain

Cytosol

Cell membrane

**Stage 3** Complete transfer of energy to a form usable by cells

e⁻

$^1/_2O_2$

Electron transport chain

$H_2O$

ADP   ATP

**Figure SM.1** **Metabolism.** Cells use metabolic reactions to extract energy from food and to form building blocks for biosynthesis.

**Figure SM.2** **Energy extraction from food.** In the first stage, the body breaks down food into amino acids, monosaccharides, and fatty acids. In the second stage, cells degrade these molecules to a few simple units, such as acetyl CoA, that are widespread in metabolism. In the third stage, the oxygen-dependent reactions of the citric acid cycle and electron transport chain liberate large amounts of energy in the form of ATP.

**metabolic pathway** A series of chemical reactions that either break down a large compound into smaller units (catabolism) or synthesize more complex molecules from smaller ones (anabolism).

**catabolism [ca-TA-bol-iz-um]** Any metabolic process whereby cells break down complex substances into simpler, smaller ones.

**anabolism [an-A-bol-iz-um]** Any metabolic process whereby cells build complex substances from simple, smaller units.

**cells** The basic structural units of all living tissues. Cells have two major parts—the nucleus and the cytoplasm.

**nucleus** The primary site of genetic information in the cell, enclosed in a double-layered membrane.

# What Is Metabolism?

*Metabolism* is a general term that encompasses all chemical changes occurring in living organisms. The term **metabolic pathway** describes a series of chemical reactions that either break down a large compound into smaller units (**catabolism**) or build more complex molecules from smaller ones (**anabolism**).[4] For example, when you eat bread or rice, the GI tract breaks down the starch into glucose units. Cells can further catabolize these glucose units to release energy for activities such as muscle contractions. Conversely, anabolic reactions take available glucose molecules and assemble them into glycogen for storage. (See **Figure SM.3**.)

Metabolic pathways are never completely inactive. Their activity continually ebbs and flows in response to internal and external events. Imagine, for example, that your instructor keeps you late and you have only five minutes to get to your next class. As you hustle across campus, your body ramps up energy production to fuel the demand created by your rapidly contracting muscles. As you sit in your next class, your body continues to break down and extract glucose from the banana you recently ate. Your body assembles the glucose into branched chains to replenish the glycogen stores you depleted running across campus.

## The Cell Is the Metabolic Processing Center

**Cells** are the "work centers" of metabolism. (See **Figure SM.4**.) Although our bodies are made up of different types of cells (e.g., liver cells, brain cells, kidney cells, muscle cells), most have a similar structure. The basic animal cell has two major parts—the cell **nucleus** and a membrane-enclosed space

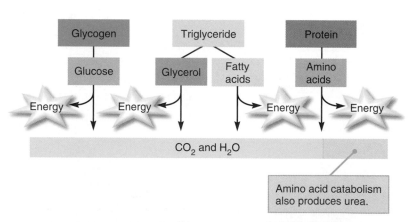

(a)

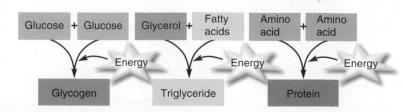

(b)

**Figure SM.3**  **Catabolism and anabolism.** (a) Catabolic reactions break down molecules and release energy. (b) Anabolic reactions consume energy as they assemble complex molecules.

called the **cytoplasm**. As we zoom in for a closer look, we see that the semi-fluid **cytosol** fills the cytoplasm. Floating in the cytosol are many organelles, small units that perform specialized metabolic functions. A large number of these **organelles**—the capsulelike **mitochondria**—are power generators that contain many important energy-producing pathways.

To remember the major parts of a cell, think about a bowl of thick vegetable soup with a single meatball floating in it. For our example, think of

**cytoplasm** The material of the cell, excluding the cell nucleus and cell membranes. The cytoplasm includes the semifluid cytosol, the organelles, and other particles.

**cytosol** The semifluid inside the cell membrane, excluding organelles. The cytosol is the site of glycolysis and fatty acid synthesis.

**organelles** Various membrane-bound structures that form part of the cytoplasm. Organelles perform specialized metabolic functions.

**mitochondria (mitochondrion)** The sites of aerobic production of ATP, where most of the energy from carbohydrate, protein, and fat is captured. Called the "power plants" of the cell, the mitochondria are where the citric acid cycle and electron transport chain are located. A human cell contains about 2,000 mitochondria.

## Organelles
**Endoplasmic reticulum (ER)**
- An extensive membrane system extending from the nuclear membrane.
- Rough ER: The outer membrane surface contains ribosomes.
- Smooth ER: Devoid of ribosomes, the site of lipid synthesis.

**Golgi apparatus**
- A system of stacked membrane-encased discs.
- The site of extensive modification, sorting, and packaging of compounds for transport.

**Lysosome**
- Vesicle containing enzymes that digest intracellular materials and recycle the components.

**Mitochondrion**
- Contains two highly specialized membranes, an outer membrane and a highly folded inner membrane. Membranes are separated by narrow intermembrane space. Inner membrane encloses space called mitochondrial matrix.
- Often called the power plant of the cell. Site where most of the energy from carbohydrate, protein, and fat is captured in ATP (adenosine triphosphate).
- About 2,000 mitochondria in a cell.

**Ribosome**
- Site of protein synthesis.

## Nucleus
- Contains genetic information in the DNA of chromosomes.
- Site of RNA synthesis—RNA needed for protein synthesis.
- Enclosed in a double-layered membrane.

## Cytoplasm
- Enclosed in the cell membrane and separated from the nucleus by the nuclear membrane.
- Filled with particles and organelles that are dispersed in a clear semiliquid fluid called cytosol.

**Cytosol**
- The semifluid inside the cell membrane.
- Site of glycolysis and fatty acid synthesis.

## Cell Membrane
- A double-layered sheet, made up of lipid and protein, that encases the cell.
- Controls the passage of substances in and out of the cell.
- Contains receptors for hormones and other regulatory compounds.

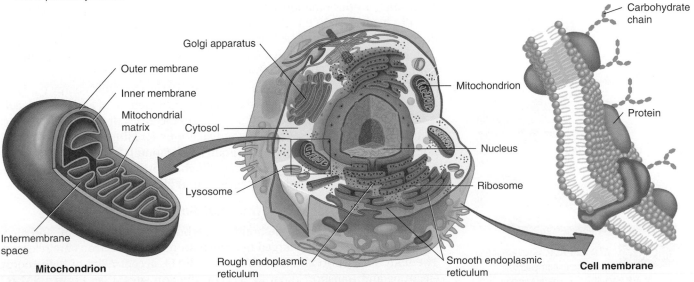

**Figure SM.4** **Cell structure.** Liver cells, brain cells, kidney cells, muscle cells, and so forth, all have a similar structure.

**cofactors** Compounds required for an enzyme to be active. Cofactors include coenzymes and metal ions such as iron, copper, and magnesium.

**coenzymes** Organic compounds, often derived from B vitamins, that combine with inactive enzymes to form active enzymes.

**adenosine triphosphate (ATP) [ah-DEN-oh-seen try-FOS-fate]** A high-energy compound composed of adenosine and three phosphate groups. ATP is the main direct fuel that cells use to synthesize molecules, contract muscles, transport substances, and perform other tasks. Breaking down ATP to adenosine diphosphate (ADP) releases energy, and forming ATP from ADP captures energy.

**adenosine diphosphate (ADP) [ah-DEN-oh-seen di-FOS-fate]** A molecule composed of adenosine and two phosphate groups.

**NAD⁺** Nicotinamide adenine dinucleotide (NAD⁺), a coenzyme derived from the B vitamin niacin, becomes NADH as it accepts a pair of high-energy electrons for transport in cells.

**FAD** Flavin adenine dinucleotide (FAD), a coenzyme derived from the B vitamin riboflavin, becomes FADH₂ as it accepts a pair of high-energy electrons for transport in cells.

the broth as having a runny, jellylike consistency and the bowl as a thin, flexible structure with the consistency of a wet paper bag. The bowl surrounds and holds the mixture, similar to the way a cell membrane encloses a cell. The meatball represents the cell nucleus, and the remaining mixture is the cytoplasm. This cytoplasmic soup is made up of a thick, semiliquid fluid (cytosol) and vegetables (organelles). Among the vegetables, think of those kidney beans as mitochondria.

Enzymes speed up chemical reactions in metabolic pathways. Many enzymes are inactive unless they are combined with certain smaller molecules called **cofactors**, which usually are derived from a vitamin or mineral. Vitamin-derived cofactors also are called **coenzymes**. All the B vitamins form coenzymes used in metabolic reactions.

**Key Concepts** *Metabolism encompasses the many reactions that take place in cells to build tissue, produce energy, break down compounds, and do other cellular work. Anabolism refers to reactions that build compounds, such as protein or glycogen. Catabolism is the breakdown of compounds to yield energy. Mitochondria, the power plants within cells, contain many of the breakdown pathways that produce energy.*

## Who Are the Key Energy Players?

Certain compounds have recurring roles in metabolic activities. Adenosine triphosphate (ATP) is the fundamental energy molecule used to power cellular functions, so it is known as the universal energy currency. Two other molecules, NADH and FADH₂, are important couriers that carry energy for the synthesis of ATP.

### ATP: The Body's Energy Currency

To power its needs, your body must convert the energy in food to a readily usable form called **adenosine triphosphate (ATP)**. (See **Figure SM.5.**) ATP—the body's universal energy currency—kick-starts many energy-releasing processes, such as the breakdown of glucose and fatty acids, and powers energy-consuming processes, such as the building of glycogen from glucose. By breaking one of the high-energy bonds in an ATP molecule, cells can release usable energy as they convert high-energy ATP to lower-energy **adenosine diphosphate (ADP)**. That energy can then be used to make large molecules from smaller ones (anabolism).

THINK About It

1

Production of ATP is the fundamental goal of metabolism's energy-producing pathways. Just as the ancient Romans could claim that all roads lead to Rome, you can say that, with a few exceptions, your body's energy-producing pathways lead to ATP production.

The body's pool of ATP is a small, immediately accessible energy reservoir rather than a long-term energy reserve. The typical lifetime of an ATP molecule is less than one minute, and ATP production increases or decreases in direct relation to energy needs. At rest, you use about 40 kilograms of ATP in 24 hours (an average rate of about 28 grams per minute). In contrast, if you are exercising strenuously, you can use as much as 500 grams per minute! On average, you turn over your body weight in ATP every day.[5]

### NAD⁺ and FAD: The Body's Transport Shuttles

During the breakdown of the bonds in carbohydrate, fat, protein, and alcohol, protons (positively charged hydrogen atoms) and electrons are released. The body's transport shuttles, **NAD⁺** and **FAD**, accept pairs of high-energy electrons and transport them to ATP production sites. (See **Figure SM.6.**) When the empty shuttle molecules (NAD⁺ and FAD) pick up their high-energy electron cargo, they also pick up hydrogen and become NADH + H⁺ and

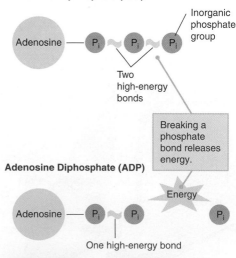

**Figure SM.5** **ATP and ADP.** When extracting energy from nutrients, the formation of ATP from ADP + P_i captures energy. Breaking a phosphate bond in ATP to form ADP + P_i releases energy for biosynthesis and work.

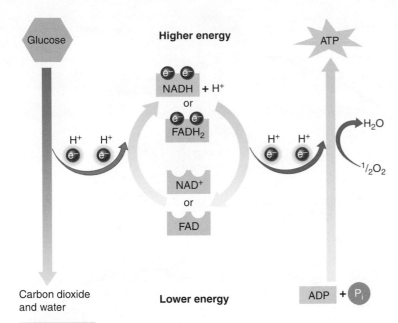

| Figure SM.6 | **Energy transfer.** As energy moves from glucose to ATP, molecules become high-energy or low-energy as they collect and transfer protons (positively charged hydrogen atoms) and high-energy electrons. |

$FADH_2$. These shuttle molecules highlight the importance of B vitamins in metabolism. $NAD^+$ is derived from the B vitamin niacin, and FAD is derived from the B vitamin riboflavin.

**Key Concepts** *ATP is the energy currency of the body. Your body extracts energy from food to produce ATP. As energy-yielding compounds break down, the shuttle molecules $NAD^+$ and FAD transport high-energy electrons to ATP production sites.*

## Breakdown and Release of Energy

Bang! The starter's gun echoes in your ears as you leap out of the blocks. With legs pumping, you race to the finish 200 meters away. As you cross the finish line, you congratulate yourself on your best race yet.

Where did the energy come from to power your muscles at peak effort? Your stores of readily available ATP are used up within the first few seconds. To power the remainder of the race, **anaerobic** reactions (reactions that do not require oxygen) partially break down glucose. Needy cells gobble up glucose and rapidly pour out ATP. Although partial breakdown produces only a small amount of ATP per glucose molecule, it is extremely fast and powers maximal effort for short events.

Bang! The starter's gun signals the beginning of the marathon and you commence running at a moderate pace. For 26 miles, your feet pound the pavement over and over again. Rather than sprinting, you settle into a rhythm. The minutes and hours pass as you maintain your steady pace until reaching the finish.

While anaerobic reactions can power a short, maximal burst of energy for a sprint, they cannot fuel a prolonged event. To sustain muscle contractions during endurance events, **aerobic** reactions (reactions that require oxygen) complete the breakdown of glucose. These aerobic pathways also extract energy from fat and a bit of protein. Compared with anaerobic energy production, aerobic metabolism produces much more energy but at a slower,

**anaerobic [AN-ah-ROW-bic]** Referring to the absence of oxygen or the ability of a process to occur in the absence of oxygen. Glycolysis is an anaerobic pathway.

**aerobic [air-ROW-bic]** Referring to the presence of or need for oxygen. The complete breakdown of glucose, fatty acids, and amino acids to carbon dioxide and water occurs only via aerobic metabolism. The citric acid cycle and electron transport chain are aerobic pathways.

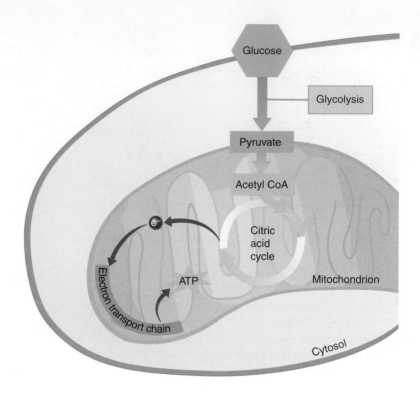

| Figure SM.7 | **Obtaining energy from carbohydrate.** The complete breakdown of glucose uses four major metabolic pathways: glycolysis, pyruvate to acetyl CoA, the citric acid |

cycle, and the electron transport chain. Glycolysis takes place in the cytosol of the cell. The remaining reactions take place in the mitochondria.

more easily maintained rate. Anaerobic metabolism may be fast, but, for a single glucose molecule, complete aerobic breakdown produces more than 15 times as much ATP.

Although different pathways initiate the breakdown of carbohydrate, fat, and protein, complete breakdown of these nutrients eventually proceeds along two shared catabolic pathways—the citric acid cycle and the electron transport chain. The next section first describes the pathways that catabolize glucose. Then it discusses the breakdown of fat and protein.

## Extracting Energy from Carbohydrate

Cells extract usable energy from carbohydrate via four main pathways: glycolysis, pyruvate to acetyl CoA, the citric acid cycle, and the electron transport chain. (See **Figure SM.7.**) Of these four pathways, the electron transport chain is the major ATP production site.

### Glycolysis

**Glycolysis** (glucose splitting), the first few steps in the "burning" of glucose, does not require oxygen. In the cytosol, this sequence of reactions splits one six-carbon glucose molecule into two three-carbon **pyruvate** molecules while producing a relatively small amount of energy. Just as a pump requires priming, glycolysis requires the input of two ATP to get started. Using several reactions, glycolysis then transfers high-energy electrons to NAD$^+$ shuttle molecules and produces four ATP. Finally, it forms two pyruvate molecules. (See **Figure SM.8.**)

**glycolysis [gligh-COLL-ih-sis]** The anaerobic pathway that breaks down a glucose molecule into two molecules of pyruvate and yields two molecules of ATP and two molecules of NADH. Glycolysis occurs in the cytosol of a cell.

**pyruvate** The three-carbon compound that results from glycolysis. Cells also can make glucose from pyruvate, but this process requires energy and several enzymes not involved in glycolysis. Pyruvate also can be derived from glycerol and some amino acids.

What about the other simple sugars, fructose and galactose? In liver cells, glycolysis also breaks them down.[6] Although fructose and galactose enter glycolysis at intermediate points, the breakdown of each sugar yields the same results as the breakdown of glucose.

Once glycolysis is complete, the two pyruvate molecules easily pass from the cytosol to the interior of the mitochondria, the cell's power generators, for further processing.

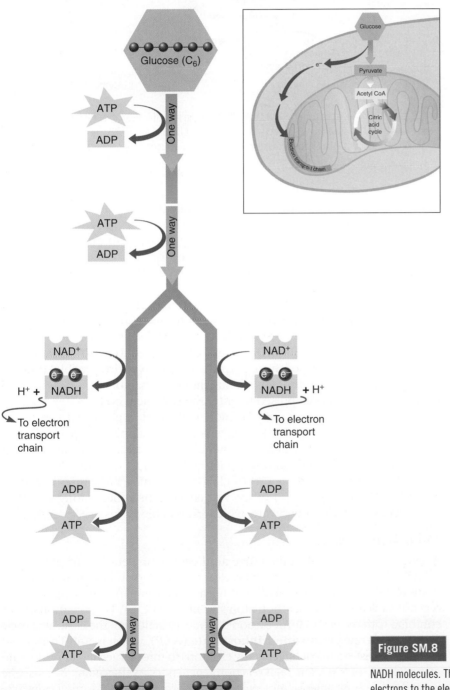

**Figure SM.8**    **Glycolysis.** The breakdown of one glucose molecule yields two pyruvate molecules, a net of two ATP and two NADH molecules. The two NADH molecules shuttle pairs of high-energy electrons to the electron transport chain for ATP production. Glycolytic reactions do not require oxygen, and some steps are irreversible.

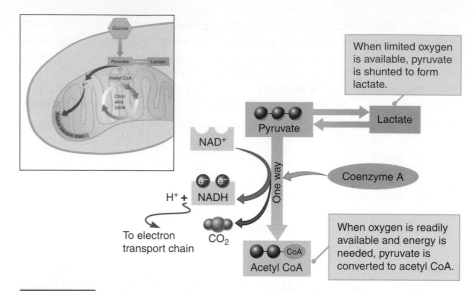

When limited oxygen is available, pyruvate is shunted to form lactate.

When oxygen is readily available and energy is needed, pyruvate is converted to acetyl CoA.

NAD⁺

Pyruvate

Lactate

Coenzyme A

One way

H⁺ + NADH

To electron transport chain

$CO_2$

Acetyl CoA

**Figure SM.9** **Pyruvate to acetyl CoA.** When oxygen is readily available, each pyruvate formed from glucose yields one acetyl CoA, one $CO_2$, and one NADH. The NADH shuttles high-energy electrons to the electron transport chain for ATP production.

## Pyruvate to Acetyl CoA

When a cell requires energy, and oxygen is readily available, an aerobic reaction in the mitochondria converts each pyruvate molecule to an **acetyl CoA** molecule and transfers a pair of high-energy electrons to an NAD⁺ shuttle. (See **Figure SM.9**.) The shuttle carries the electrons to the electron transport chain. To form acetyl CoA, reactions remove one carbon from the three-carbon pyruvate and add **coenzyme A**, a molecule derived from the B vitamin pantothenic acid. After combining with oxygen, the carbon is released as part of carbon dioxide. Because glucose splits into two pyruvate molecules, two acetyl CoA molecules are produced from each molecule of glucose.

Although many metabolic pathways can proceed forward or backward, the formation of acetyl CoA from pyruvate is a one-way (irreversible) process. Acetyl CoA cannot exit through the mitochondrial membrane, so it is trapped inside the mitochondria, poised to enter the citric acid cycle.

In rapidly contracting muscles such as those that propelled you to the finish of your 200-meter sprint, oxygen is in short supply, and pyruvate cannot form acetyl CoA. Instead, pyruvate is rerouted to form lactate, another three-carbon compound. **Lactate** is an alternative fuel that muscle cells can use or that liver cells can convert to glucose. (See the FYI feature "Lactate Is Not a Metabolic Dead End.") When oxygen again becomes readily available, lactate converts back to pyruvate, which irreversibly forms acetyl CoA.

## Citric Acid Cycle

A series of reactions called the **citric acid cycle** completes the breakdown of acetyl CoA. To begin the citric acid cycle, acetyl CoA combines with **oxaloacetate** to form citrate (citric acid) and release coenzyme A (CoA). Subsequent reactions release the two carbon atoms from acetyl CoA. These carbon atoms combine with oxygen to form carbon dioxide. Reactions of the citric acid cycle also produce one **guanosine triphosphate (GTP)**, which readily converts to ATP, and transfer pairs of high-energy electrons to three molecules of NAD⁺ and one molecule of FAD. The final reaction regenerates oxaloacetate. Because the breakdown of one glucose molecule produces two acetyl CoA molecules, the citric acid cycle will make two complete "turns"—one for each acetyl CoA.

**acetyl CoA** A key intermediate product in the metabolic breakdown of carbohydrates, fatty acids, and amino acids. It consists of a two-carbon acetate group linked to coenzyme A, which is derived from pantothenic acid.

**coenzyme A** A cofactor derived from the vitamin pantothenic acid.

**lactate** A three-carbon compound that is produced when insufficient oxygen is present in cells to break down pyruvate to acetyl CoA. Often called *lactic acid*.

**citric acid cycle** The aerobic metabolic pathway in mitochondria that breaks down acetyl CoA to yield two molecules of carbon dioxide, one molecule of GTP, and pairs of high-energy electrons. It transfers the electrons to three molecules of NAD⁺ (yielding three NADH) and one molecule of FAD (yielding one FADH₂). Also known as the *Krebs cycle* and the *tricarboxylic acid cycle*.

**oxaloacetate** A four-carbon intermediate compound in the citric acid cycle. Acetyl CoA combines with free oxaloacetate in the mitochondria, forming citric acid and beginning the cycle.

**GTP (guanosine triphosphate)** A high-energy compound, similar to ATP but with three phosphate groups linked to guanosine instead of adenosine.

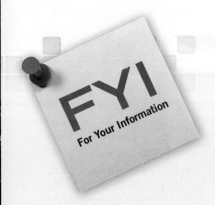

# Lactate Is Not a Metabolic Dead End

Today's race is 200 meters, and you are in the lead. The crowd roars with excitement and your coach screams hoarsely as your feet slam over and over on the hard gray cinder track. Other runners are close behind, and you can feel them breathing and pounding at your heels. Air whistles in and out of your wheezing lungs as you doggedly push to stay ahead. Your muscles are screaming, but they carry you across the finish line. A winner!

As you slump in exhaustion, you wonder how your limp muscles carried you through to the end. Each leg seemed to weigh a thousand pounds. As your muscles tire, lactate levels rise and the pH in your muscle cells drops. Scientists, coaches, and athletes have long believed that lactate was a useless, even toxic, dead-end substance. Research proves otherwise. It is the overall acidification of the muscle tissue, rather than a buildup of lactate, that primarily causes muscle fatigue. Also, lactate is now recognized as a fuel in its own right. In addition to acting as a metabolic shunt, lactate is a useful fuel produced and consumed under all conditions of oxygen availability, while exercising or at rest.

Without the energy supplied by the lactic acid energy system, you would never have crossed the finish line. While your body anaerobically burned muscle glycogen, it produced large amounts of lactate. Where does this lactate come from, and how does your body handle it?

### Cori Cycle

During vigorous exercise, your contracting muscle cells quickly extract small amounts of ATP from glucose. This simple pathway, called *glycolysis*, splits glucose into pyruvate molecules faster than the oxygen energy system can accept them for further processing. Cells divert excess pyruvate to lactate to help alleviate the backup.

Lactate accumulates rapidly in muscle cells, which receive a boost of energy by burning some lactate with oxygen—a strategy that yields far more energy than glycolysis alone.[1] Most lactate easily diffuses through muscle cell membranes into the bloodstream. The liver picks up the circulating lactate and converts it back to pyruvate. Using energy-demanding reactions, the liver transforms pyruvate to glucose. Glucose enters the bloodstream and travels back to the skeletal muscle cells, where it reenters energy-producing pathways.

This recurring circular pathway is called the *Cori cycle*. When pyruvate is backed up in muscle cells, the Cori cycle buys time with a detour through the liver. When oxygen becomes readily available, the oxygen energy system becomes the main pathway.

### Lactate Shuttle

The pathways of the Cori cycle are an important, but incomplete, part of the lactate picture. The use of the Cori cycle as a holding pattern led to the mistaken belief that lactate was simply a metabolic dead end. More recent studies described a more extensive role for this long-maligned substance.

Researchers now recognize lactate as an important means of distributing carbohydrate energy sources after a meal and during sustained physical exercise. Lactate's advantage is its ability to move rapidly between cells. It is a small molecule and, unlike glucose, does not need insulin to cross a cell membrane.

Under resting conditions of plentiful carbohydrate and oxygen, diverse tissues such as skeletal muscle, liver, and skin produce lactate.[2] In these conditions, the supply of raw materials, rather than limited oxygen, drives the formation of lactate.

According to the lactate shuttle hypothesis, lactate formed in muscle cells becomes an energy source at other sites, either adjacent or remote. Skeletal muscle, once thought simply to produce lactate, also directly uses lactate as a fuel. At times, skeletal muscle actually removes more lactate than it produces. The heart muscle is fully aerobic, but it both produces and consumes lactate. Studies suggest that during exercise lactate is the major fuel for the heart and the preferred fuel for certain muscle fibers.[3]

The next time you complain about sore, tired muscles, don't blame lactate. Instead, think about the daily usefulness of lactate and how this little-respected substance helped power you to the finish.

1    Hashimoto T, Hussien R, Brooks GA. Colocalization of MCT1, CD147, and LDH in mitochondrial inner membrane of L6 muscle cells: evidence of a mitochondrial lactate oxidation complex. *Am J Physiol Endocrinol Metab.* 2006;290(6):E1237–E1244.

2    van Hall G. Lactate kinetics in human tissues at rest and during exercise. *Acta Physiol* (Oxf). 2010;199(4):499–508.

3    Brooks GA. Cell–cell and intracellular lactate shuttles. *J Physiol.* 2009;587:5591–5600.

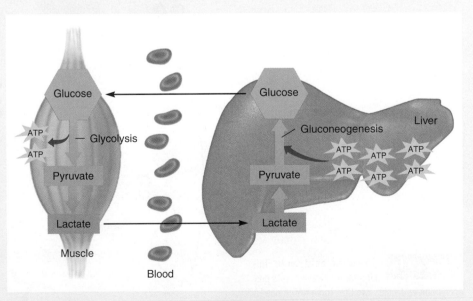

**The Cori cycle.** The Cori cycle shifts some of the metabolic burden of contracting muscle to the liver. Lactate formed in contracting muscle travels to the liver, which uses it to form glucose. This glucose returns to the muscle to fuel further contractions.

# *Quick* Bite

## When Glycolysis Goes Awry

Red blood cells do not have mitochondria, so they rely on glycolysis as their only source of ATP. They use ATP to maintain the integrity and shape of their cell membranes. A defect in red blood cell glycolysis can cause a shortage of ATP, which leads to deformed red blood cells. Destruction of these cells by the spleen leads to a type of anemia called *hemolytic anemia.*

To help visualize the citric acid cycle, think of a merry-go-round at an amusement park. This is a special ride that completes only one revolution per rider and on which the ticket agent rides along. Acetyl CoA is the rider, and oxaloacetate is the ticket agent. Oxaloacetate welcomes acetyl CoA and, hand in hand, they climb aboard. Acetyl CoA's ticket (coenzyme A) is dropped into the recycling box. As the merry-go-round whirls by, two NAD⁺ shuttles swoop in and grab pairs of high-energy electrons as two carbons combine with oxygen and fly off the ride as carbon dioxide molecules. Who is jumping off in mid-cycle? It's GTP, a molecule similar to ATP. An FAD shuttle swoops in and grabs another pair of high-energy electrons. Nearing the end of the ride, a third NAD⁺ shuttle departs with a final pair of high-energy electrons. As the merry-go-round returns to the beginning, a new oxaloacetate beckons to the next acetyl CoA waiting in line. The cycle is ready to begin again. **Figure SM.10** shows an overview of the citric acid cycle.

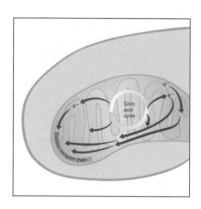

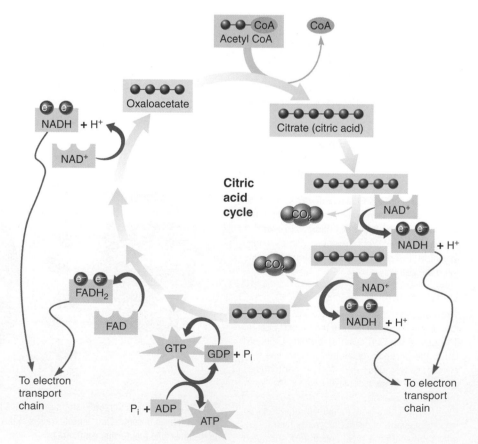

**Figure SM.10** **The citric acid cycle.** This circular pathway accepts one acetyl CoA and yields two CO₂, three NADH, one FADH₂, and one GTP (readily converted to ATP). The electron shuttles NADH and FADH₂ carry high-energy electrons to the electron transport chain for ATP production.

The citric acid cycle also is an important source of building blocks for the **biosynthesis** of amino acids and fatty acids. Many of the cycle's intermediate molecules may be used for biosynthesis rather than the completion of the cycle. Oxaloacetate, for example, may be converted to glucose or to amino acids for protein synthesis.

### Electron Transport Chain

The final step in glucose breakdown is a sequence of linked reactions that take place in the **electron transport chain**, which is located in the inner **mitochondrial membrane**. Most ATP is produced here, and the outpouring of energy can fuel exercise for hours, such as during your marathon race. Because the mitochondrion is the site of both the citric acid cycle and the electron transport chain, it truly is the energy power plant of the cell.

When NAD⁺ accepts a pair of electrons, it becomes NADH. Similarly, FAD accepts electrons to become FADH$_2$. These shuttle molecules, NADH and FADH$_2$, deliver their cargo of high-energy electrons to the electron transport chain. As the electrons travel along the electron transport chain, they give up energy to power the production of ATP. At the end of the chain, an oxygen "basket" accepts the energy-depleted electrons and combines with hydrogen to form water (H$_2$O). (See **Figure SM.11**.)

THINK
About It
2

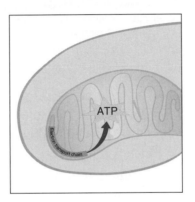

**biosynthesis** Chemical reactions in which complex biomolecules, especially carbohydrates, lipids, and proteins, are formed from simple molecules.

**electron transport chain** An organized series of protein carrier molecules located in mitochondrial membranes. As high-energy electrons delivered by NADH and FADH$_2$ traverse the electron transport chain to oxygen, it produces ATP and water.

**mitochondrial membrane** The mitochondria are enclosed by a double shell separated by an intermembrane space. The outer membrane acts as a barrier and gatekeeper, selectively allowing some molecules to pass through while blocking others. The inner membrane is where the electron transport chain is located.

**Krebs cycle** See *citric acid cycle.*

**tricarboxylic acid (TCA) cycle** See *citric acid cycle.*

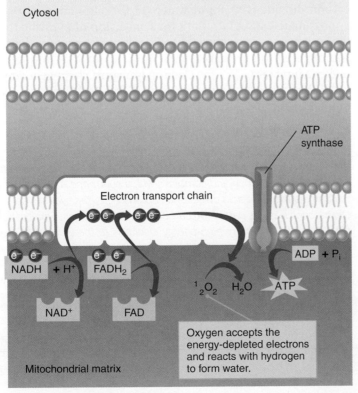

Cytosol

Outer mitochondrial membrane

Inner mitochondrial membrane

Electron transport chain

ATP synthase

NADH + H⁺    FADH$_2$

NAD⁺    FAD

$\frac{1}{2}$O$_2$    H$_2$O    ATP

ADP + P$_i$

Oxygen accepts the energy-depleted electrons and reacts with hydrogen to form water.

Mitochondrial matrix

**Figure SM.11**    **Electron transport chain.** This pathway produces most of the ATP available from glucose. NADH shuttles deliver pairs of high-energy electrons to the beginning of the chain. The pairs of high-energy electrons carried by FADH$_2$ enter this pathway farther along and produce fewer ATP than electron pairs carried by NADH. Water is the final product of the electron transport chain.

| Table SM.1 | Summary of the Major Metabolic Pathways in Glucose |

| Phase | Location | Type | Summary | Starting Materials | End Products |
|---|---|---|---|---|---|
| Glycolysis | Cytosol | Anaerobic | A series of reactions that converts one glucose to two pyruvate molecules. | Glucose, ATP | Pyruvate, ATP, NADH |
| Pyruvate to acetyl CoA | Mitochondria | Aerobic | Pyruvate from glycolysis combines with coenzyme A to form acetyl CoA while releasing carbon dioxide. | Pyruvate, coenzyme A | Acetyl CoA, carbon dioxide, NADH |
| Citric acid cycle | Mitochondria | Aerobic | This cycle of reactions degrades the acetyl portion acetyl CoA and releases the coenzyme A portion. This cycle releases carbon dioxide and produces most of the energy-rich molecules, NADH and $FADH_2$, generated by the breakdown of glucose. | Acetyl CoA | Carbon dioxide, NADH, $FADH_2$, GTP |
| Electron transport chain | Mitochondria (membrane) | Aerobic | As the electrons from NADH and $FADH_2$ pass along this chain of transport proteins, they release energy to power the generation of ATP. Oxygen is the final electron acceptor and combines with hydrogen to form water. | NADH, $FADH_2$ | ATP, water |

Without oxygen, ATP production would stop, halting the supply of power for our body's essential functions. If our oxygen supply is not restored rapidly, we die.

### End Products of Glucose Catabolism

Now you've seen all the steps in glucose breakdown. What has the cell produced from glucose? In the end, the complete breakdown of glucose to carbon dioxide ($CO_2$) and water ($H_2O$) takes about 30 steps and creates approximately 32 ATP.[7] Both the conversion of pyruvate to acetyl CoA and the citric acid cycle produce $CO_2$. The electron transport chain produces water. Although glycolysis makes small amounts of ATP and the citric acid cycle makes a little (as GTP), the electron transport chain generates the vast majority of this universal energy currency. Table SM.1 summarizes the pathways of glucose metabolism.

**Key Concepts** *Extracting energy from glucose requires several steps. Glycolysis breaks the six-carbon glucose molecule into two pyruvate molecules. After glycolysis, the remaining breakdown pathways are used twice—once for each pyruvate molecule. Each pyruvate loses a carbon and combines with a coenzyme A to form an acetyl CoA, which then enters the citric acid cycle. Two carbons enter the cycle as part of acetyl CoA, and two carbons leave as part of two carbon dioxide molecules. Finally, the shuttle molecules NADH and $FADH_2$ carry high-energy electrons to the electron transport chain, where ATP and water are produced. When completely oxidized, each glucose molecule yields carbon dioxide, water, and ATP.*

## Extracting Energy from Fat

To extract energy from fat, the body first breaks down triglycerides into their component parts, glycerol and fatty acids. Glycerol, a small three-carbon molecule, carries a relatively small amount of energy, and the liver can convert it to pyruvate or glucose. Most of the energy stored in a triglyceride is in the fatty acids.

The breakdown of fatty acids takes place inside the mitochondria. **Carnitine** has the unique task of ferrying fatty acids across the mitochondrial membrane, from the cytosol to the interior of the mitochondrion. Because of this role, some people claim carnitine supplements act as "fat burners." However, research has shown that carnitine supplementation has little or no effect on fatty acid oxidation rates or athletic performance in healthy individuals.[8]

### Beta-Oxidation

Once inside a mitochondrion, a process called **beta-oxidation** disassembles the fatty acid chain. Like scissors, enzymes snip the chain into two-carbon "links." Reactions convert each link to acetyl CoA and transfer pairs of high-energy electrons to $NAD^+$ and FAD shuttles. (See **Figure SM.12**.) These shuttle molecules (now NADH and $FADH_2$) transport their high-energy cargo to the electron transport chain.

### Completing Fatty Acid Breakdown

Beta-oxidation of a fatty acid produces a flood of acetyl CoA. The citric acid cycle and electron transport chain complete the extraction of energy from fatty acids. Just as they processed acetyl CoA, NADH, and $FADH_2$ from glucose, these same pathways use acetyl CoA, NADH, and $FADH_2$ from fatty acids to produce ATP.

The end products of fatty acid breakdown are the same as those of glucose breakdown: carbon dioxide, water, and ATP. The exact amount of ATP depends on the length of the fatty acid chain. Because longer chains have more carbons than shorter chains, beta-oxidation of longer chains produces more acetyl CoA and thus more ATP. The complete breakdown of an 18-carbon fatty acid, for example, produces 120 ATP, whereas a 10-carbon fatty acid would produce only 66 ATP. A triglyceride, with its three fatty acids and glycerol, contains many more carbon atoms than a molecule of glucose, and thus produces substantially more ATP. In a single triglyceride with three 18-carbon fatty acids, completely breaking down the fatty acids produces 360 ATP—over 10 times the 32 ATP from glucose.

### Fat Burns in a Flame of Carbohydrate

Acetyl CoA from beta-oxidation can enter the citric acid cycle only when fat and carbohydrate breakdown are synchronized. Without available oxaloacetate, acetyl CoA cannot start the citric acid cycle. Conditions such as starvation and very-low-carbohydrate diets can deplete oxaloacetate, blocking acetyl CoA from entry. This reroutes the acetyl CoA to form a family of compounds called *ketone bodies*. (See the section, "Making Ketone Bodies" later in this chapter.) Excess production of ketone bodies can occur with popular high-protein diets that are low in carbohydrate but high in fat.

**THINK About It 3**

For fatty acid oxidation to continue efficiently, reactions in the mitochondria help ensure a reliable supply of oxaloacetate. These reactions convert some pyruvate directly to oxaloacetate rather than to acetyl CoA. Because carbohydrate (glucose) is the original source of the pyruvate and, hence, this oxaloacetate, scientists coined the saying "Fat burns in a flame of carbohydrate."

**Key Concepts** *Extracting energy from fat involves several steps. First, triglycerides are separated into glycerol and three fatty acids. Glycerol forms pyruvate and can be broken down to yield a small amount of energy. Beta-oxidation breaks down fatty acid chains to two-carbon links that form acetyl CoA, which enters the citric acid cycle. Beta-oxidation and the citric acid cycle transfer electrons to $NAD^+$ and FAD. As NADH and $FADH_2$, these shuttle molecules carry high-energy electrons to the electron transport chain, where ATP and water are made. The complete breakdown of a triglyceride yields water, carbon dioxide, and substantially more ATP than one glucose molecule.*

**carnitine [CAR-nih-teen]** A compound that transports fatty acids from the cytosol into the mitochondria, where they undergo beta-oxidation.

**beta-oxidation** The breakdown of a fatty acid into numerous molecules of the two-carbon compound acetyl coenzyme A (acetyl CoA).

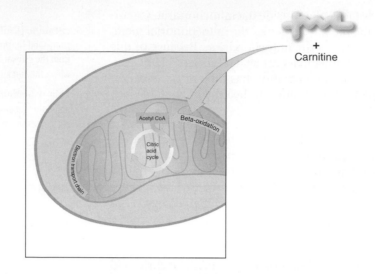

+
Carnitine

Enzymes clip a two-carbon link from the end of the chain.

**Activated Stearic Acid**
(an 18-carbon fatty acid)

CoA    FAD    NAD⁺

The two-carbon link becomes part of acetyl CoA as electrons are transferred to shuttle molecules.

CoA + CoA + FADH₂ + NADH + H⁺

The chain is clipped another seven times, making acetyl CoA while transferring electrons.

Repeated beta-oxidation cycles

7 CoA + 7 FADH₂ + 7 NADH + 7 H⁺

The final two-carbon link becomes part of acetyl CoA without a transfer of electrons.

CoA

Total            9 acetyl CoA + 8 FADH₂ + 8 NADH + 8 H⁺

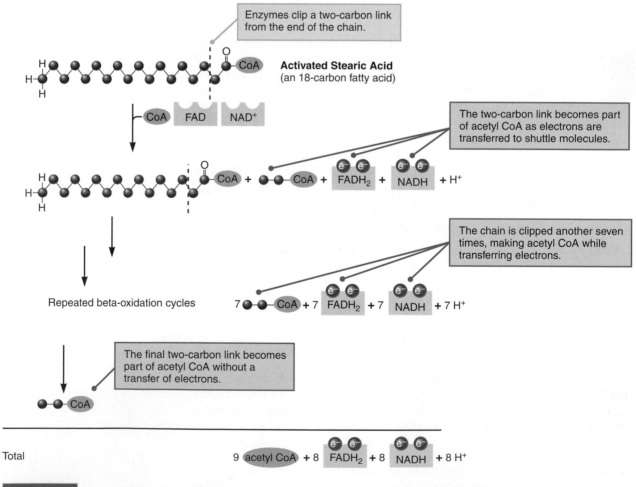

**Figure SM.12**  **Beta-oxidation.** Beta-oxidation reactions repeatedly clip two carbons from the end of a fatty acid until it is degraded entirely to molecules of acetyl CoA.

# Extracting Energy from Protein

Protein has vital structural and functional roles, so proteins and amino acids are not considered primary sources of energy. However, if energy production falters due to a lack of available carbohydrate and fat, protein comes to the rescue. During starvation, for example, energy needs take priority, so the body breaks down protein and extracts energy from the amino acid building blocks.

Our bodies can't use the nitrogen-containing portion of an amino acid in energy production, so a process called *deamination* strips down the amino acid to a "carbon skeleton" (see **Figure SM.13**) while producing a nitrogen byproduct that becomes urea. When you eat more protein than you need, your kidneys excrete urea in urine, and your liver uses carbon skeletons to produce energy, glucose, or fat. Much to the dismay of bodybuilders, when they attempt to build muscle by drinking pricey protein drinks, they can end up gaining fat instead!

## Carbon Skeletons Enter Pathways at Different Points

Carbon skeletons—unlike glucose—can enter the breakdown pathways at several different points. Imagine arriving at an amusement park with five entrance gates. The ticket agent hands you a ticket that allows you to enter at your designated gate. Similarly, the structure of an amino acid's carbon skeleton determines which "entrance gate" it uses to enter the breakdown pathways. Some carbon skeletons directly enter the citric acid cycle, others enter at pyruvate, and still others at acetyl CoA. (See **Figure SM.14**.)

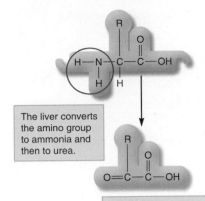

The liver converts the amino group to ammonia and then to urea.

The structure of the remaining carbon skeleton determines where it can enter the energy-producing pathways.

**Figure SM.13**   **Deamination.** A deamination reaction strips the amino group from an amino acid.

**Amino acid oxidation**
The amount of ATP that an amino acid produces depends upon where it enters the breakdown pathways.

Pyruvate

(e.g., alanine)

Acetyl CoA

Oxaloacetate

(e.g., asparagine)

(e.g., leucine)

(e.g., tyrosine)

(e.g., methionine)

(e.g., glutamic acid)

**Figure SM.14**   **Extracting energy from amino acids.** The carbon skeletons of amino acids have several different entrances to the breakdown pathways. Compared with glucose and fatty acids, amino acids yield much smaller amounts of energy (ATP).

The complete breakdown of an amino acid yields urea, carbon dioxide, water, and ATP. The carbon skeleton's point of entry to the breakdown pathways determines the amount of ATP it produces. Whereas the complete breakdown of alanine, for example, produces 12.5 ATP, methionine produces only 5 ATP. Compared with glucose and fatty acids, no amino acid produces much ATP.

**Key Concepts** *To extract energy from amino acids, cells strip them down to carbon skeletons (deamination). The remaining nitrogen becomes urea, which is removed by the kidneys. The carbon skeleton structure determines where it enters the catabolic pathways. Some carbon skeletons become pyruvate, others become acetyl CoA, and still others become intermediate compounds of the citric acid cycle. Complete breakdown of amino acids yields water, carbon dioxide, urea, and ATP.*

## Biosynthesis and Storage

Uh oh! Surveying the results of those holiday dinners and treats, you cringe with regret. Your clothes no longer fit, and you hate the idea of stepping on the scale. Your biosynthetic pathways have been hard at work, building fat stores from your excess intake of energy.

You head for the gym. After sweating through many workouts, your body begins to firm. You drop fat and add muscle. Now any problem with clothes fitting is due to muscle gain, not fat gain. To build muscle protein, different biosynthetic pathways have been busy making amino acids and assembling proteins.

Perhaps you've heard of "carbo loading." This strategy uses high-carbohydrate meals to pack carbohydrate into your muscle glycogen stores before a competition. Biosynthetic pathways assemble glucose into glycogen chains for storage. When needed, your body also can make glucose from certain amino acids and other precursors.

Both the breakdown and biosynthetic pathways are active at all times. While some cells are breaking down carbohydrate, fat, and protein to extract energy, other cells are busy building glucose, fatty acids, and amino acids. When your body needs energy, the breakdown pathways prevail. When it has an excess of nutrients, the biosynthetic pathways dominate. The activities in these pathways ebb and flow so they proceed at just the right rate, not too fast and not too slowly. **Figure SM.15** illustrates the interconnections among the metabolic pathways.

## Making Carbohydrate (Glucose)

Your body sets a high priority on maintaining an adequate amount of glucose circulating in the bloodstream. Blood glucose is the primary source of energy for your brain, central nervous system, and red blood cells. In fact, while you're at rest, your brain consumes about 60 percent of the energy consumed by your entire body.

### Gluconeogenesis: Pathways to Glucose

When you are exercising intensely or when you aren't taking in enough carbohydrate such as a typical overnight fast, your body can make glucose by using a clever strategy called **gluconeogenesis**. Gluconeogenesis is a pathway essential for the survival of humans that enables the body to maintain blood glucose levels after dietary sources of carbohydrate have been used up. Your liver is the major site of gluconeogenesis, accounting for about 90 percent of glucose production. Your kidneys make the rest.

*Quick* Bite

**Sweet Origins**
The word *gluconeogenesis* is derived from the Greek words *glyks*, meaning "sweet"; *neo*, meaning "new"; and *genesis*, meaning "origin" or "generation."

gluconeogenesis [gloo-ko-nee-oh-JEN-uh-sis] Synthesis of glucose within the body from noncarbohydrate precursors such as amino acids, lactic acid, and glycerol. Fatty acids cannot be converted to glucose.

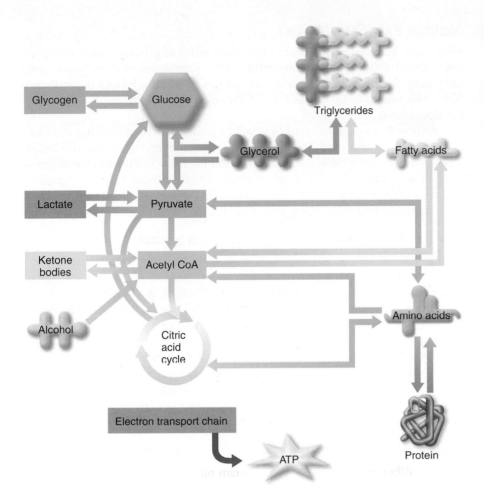

**Figure SM.15** **Overview of metabolic pathways.** As if they were traveling a maze of city streets, molecules move through a network of breakdown and biosynthetic pathways. Not all pathways are available to a molecule. Just as traffic lights and one-way streets regulate traffic flow, cellular mechanisms control the flow of molecules in metabolic pathways. These mechanisms include hormones, irreversible reactions, and locations of reactions in the cell.

Gluconeogenesis and glycolysis share many—but not all—reactions. During gluconeogenesis, reactions flow in the opposite direction as during glycolysis. Because some reactions of glycolysis flow only one way, gluconeogenesis must use energy-consuming detours to bypass them. Thus gluconeogenesis is *not* simply a reversal of glycolysis.

Your body can make glucose from pyruvate, lactate, and some noncarbohydrate sources—glycerol and most amino acids. Although gluconeogenesis can use the glycerol portion of fat, it cannot make glucose from fatty acids.

If the carbon skeleton of an amino acid can be made into glucose, the amino acid is called **glucogenic**. Glucogenic amino acids provide carbon skeletons that become pyruvate or they may directly enter the citric acid cycle at intermediate points other than forming acetyl CoA. If a carbon skeleton of an amino acid directly forms acetyl CoA (which your body can convert to ketone bodies but not glucose), the amino acid is called **ketogenic** (see the "Ketogenesis" section).

### Storage: Glucose to Glycogen

By using a pathway called **glycogenesis**, our bodies store glucose as glycogen in the liver and muscles. Liver glycogen serves as a glucose reserve for the blood, and muscle glycogen supplies glucose to exercising muscle tissue. Glycogen stores are limited; fasting or strenuous exercise can deplete them rapidly.

**glucogenic** A term describing an amino acid whose carbon skeleton can be used in gluconeogenesis to form glucose.

**ketogenic** A term describing an amino acid broken down to acetyl CoA (which can be converted into ketone bodies).

**glycogenesis** The formation of glycogen from glucose.

lipogenesis [lye-poh-JEN-eh-sis] Synthesis of fatty acids from acetyl CoA derived from the metabolism of fats, alcohol, and some amino acids.

ketone bodies Molecules formed from fat when cells do not have enough available carbohydrate to break down fat completely. Sometimes improperly called *ketones*.

ketones [KEE-tonez] Organic compounds that contain a chemical group consisting of C=O (a carbon–oxygen double bond) bound to two hydrocarbons. Pyruvate and fructose are examples of ketones. Acetone and acetoacetate are both ketones and ketone bodies. Although beta-hydroxybutyrate is not a ketone, it is a ketone body.

## *Quick* Bite

### Will the Smelly Body Please Stand Up?

Ketone bodies (sometimes incorrectly called **ketones**) include three compounds: acetoacetate, beta-hydroxybutyrate, and acetone. Acetoacetate and beta-hydroxybutyrate are acids, so they may be called *keto acids*. You may recognize the term *acetone*, which also is a common solvent. In fact, you can smell the strong odor of acetone on the breath of people with high levels of ketone bodies in their blood; their breath smells like nail polish remover!

## Making Fat (Fatty Acids)

Your body can make long-chain fatty acids using a process called **lipogenesis**. To do this, your body assembles two-carbon acetyl CoA "links" into fatty acid chains. Where do these acetyl CoA building blocks come from? Ketogenic amino acids, alcohol, and fatty acids themselves supply acetyl CoA for lipogenesis.

Although you can think of fatty acid synthesis as reassembling the links broken apart by beta-oxidation, lipogenesis is not the reversal of beta-oxidation. These pathways use different reactions and take place in different locations— fatty acid synthesis occurs in the cytosol, whereas beta-oxidation operates inside the mitochondria. Your body assembles surplus fatty acids and glycerol to form triglycerides for storage as body fat.

### *Storage: From Dietary Energy to Stored Triglyceride*

When you overeat, your body uses body fat as a long-term energy storage depot. When you eat an excess of fat, most extra dietary fatty acids head straight to your fat stores. If you eat more protein than your tissues can use, your body converts most of the excess protein to body fat. Interestingly, excess carbohydrate does not readily become fat. In research studies, massive over-feeding of carbohydrate in normal men caused only minimal amounts of fat synthesis. So are carbohydrate calories "free"? Unfortunately not. Although excess carbohydrate does not dramatically increase fat synthesis, it shifts your body's fuel preferences so it burns more carbohydrate and fewer fatty acids.[9] Thus, eating excess carbohydrate still can make you fat by allowing the fat you eat to go directly to storage rather than to make ATP. (See Table SM.2.)

**Key Concepts** *Your body can make glucose from pyruvate, lactate, glucogenic amino acids, and glycerol but not from fatty acids. The main storage form of glucose is glycogen. When your diet supplies an excess of energy, your body makes fatty acids and triglycerides. Excess dietary carbohydrate is not readily converted to fat but instead shifts the body's selection of fuel and encourages the accumulation of dietary fat in body fat stores.*

## Making Ketone Bodies

**Ketone bodies** include three compounds, acetoacetate, beta-hydroxybutyrate, and acetone. Your body makes and uses small amounts of ketone bodies at all times. Although long considered to be just an emergency energy source or the result of an abnormal condition such as starvation or uncontrolled

## Table SM.2 Summary of Energy Yield and Interconversions

| Dietary Nutrient | Yields Energy? | Convertible to Glucose? | Convertible to Amino Acids and Body Proteins? | Convertible to Fat? |
|---|---|---|---|---|
| Carbohydrate (glucose, fructose, galactose) | Yes | Yes | Yes, can yield certain amino acids when amino groups are available | Insignificant |
| Fat (triglycerides) | | | | |
| Fatty acids | Yes, large amounts | No | No | Yes |
| Glycerol | Yes, small amounts | Small amounts | Yes (see carbohydrate) | Insignificant |
| Protein (amino acids) | Yes, generally not much (see starvation in text) | Yes, if insufficient carbohydrate is available | Yes | Yes, from some amino acids |
| Alcohol (ethanol) | Yes | No | No | Yes |

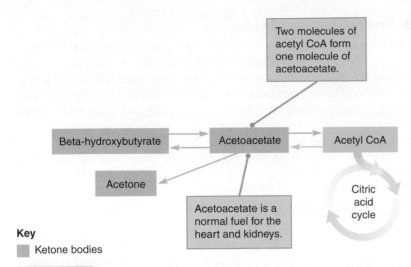

**Figure SM.16** **Ketogenesis (ketone body formation).** For acetyl CoA from fatty acid oxidation to enter the citric acid cycle, fat and carbohydrate metabolism must be synchronized. When acetyl CoA cannot enter the citric acid cycle, it is shunted to form ketone bodies, a process called ketogenesis.

*Quick* Bite

**Why Didn't My Cholesterol Levels Drop?**
Your body can make cholesterol from acetyl CoA by way of ketones. In fact, all 27 carbons in synthesized cholesterol come from acetyl CoA. The rate of cholesterol formation is highly responsive to cholesterol levels in cells. If levels are low, the liver makes more. If levels are high, synthesis decreases. This is why dietary cholesterol in the absence of dietary fat often has little impact on blood cholesterol levels.

diabetes, ketone bodies are normal, everyday fuel source for many tissues such as cardiac muscle, skeletal muscle, and the brain.[10]

### Ketogenesis: Pathways to Ketone Bodies

During the breakdown of fatty acids, not all acetyl CoA enters the citric acid cycle. Your body converts some acetyl CoA to ketone bodies, a process called **ketogenesis**. (See **Figure SM.16**.) When a person has uncontrolled diabetes or is starving, ketone bodies help provide emergency energy to all body tissues, especially the brain and the rest of the central nervous system. Other than glucose, ketone bodies are your central nervous system's only effective fuel.[11]

To dispose of excess ketone bodies, your kidneys excrete them in urine and your lungs exhale them. If this removal process cannot keep up with the production process, ketone bodies accumulate in the blood—a condition called *ketosis*. There are two types of ketosis, normal ketosis that occurs with fasting, and the medically dangerous hyperketonemia of diabetic **ketoacidosis**.[12] During even a brief overnight fast, the catabolism of fat and protein increases the production of ketone bodies. Hyperketonemia can occur in uncontrolled type 1 diabetes mellitus. In this situation, blood acidity rises quickly, leading to ketoacidosis, which can cause brain damage and eventually death if left untreated.[13] During a short fast, ketoacidosis rarely occurs.

Because "fat burns in a flame of carbohydrate," a very-high-fat, low-carbohydrate diet promotes ketosis. The lack of carbohydrate inhibits formation of oxaloacetate, slowing entry of acetyl CoA into the citric acid cycle and rerouting acetyl CoA towards the formation of ketone bodies. Given time, however, the body can adapt to a very-high-fat, low-carbohydrate diet and avoid ketosis. Eskimos, for example, sometimes live almost entirely on fat but do not develop ketosis.[14]

**Key Concepts** *Three types of ketone bodies—acetoacetate, beta-hydroxybutyrate, and acetone—can be made from the precursor acetyl CoA. Ketone bodies are an important fuel source during starvation because they are able to be used in place of glucose by the brain. In uncontrolled type 1 diabetes mellitus, an accumulation of ketone bodies can acidify the blood, resulting in ketoacidosis.*

**ketogenesis** The process in which excess acetyl CoA from fatty acid oxidation is converted into ketone bodies.

**ketoacidosis** Acidification of the blood caused by a buildup of ketone bodies. It is primarily a consequence of uncontrolled type 1 diabetes mellitus and can be life threatening.

## Making Protein (Amino Acids)

Your body rebuilds proteins from a pool of amino acids in your cells. But how is that amino acid pool replenished? Your diet supplies some amino acids, the breakdown of body proteins supplies some, and your cells make some. During protein synthesis, your cells can make dispensable amino acids and retrieve indispensable amino acids from the bloodstream. Your cells cannot make indispensable amino acids, however. If a cell lacks an indispensable amino acid and your diet doesn't supply it, protein synthesis stops. The cell breaks down this incomplete protein into its constituent amino acids, which are returned to the bloodstream.

### Biosynthesis: Making Amino Acids

To synthesize dispensable amino acids, your body uses many different pathways. Each pathway is short, involving just a few steps, and builds amino acids from carbon skeletons. Pyruvate and other compounds involved in glycolysis and the citric acid cycle supply the carbon skeletons.

**Key Concepts** *Proteins are made from combinations of indispensable and dispensable amino acids. The body synthesizes dispensable amino acids from pyruvate, other compounds involved in glycolysis, and compounds from the citric acid cycle.*

# Special States

Now you can put your new knowledge of metabolism to work by evaluating what happens when feasting or fasting. What do you think happens to your metabolism in each situation?

## Feasting

You're stuffed. You just ate a huge holiday dinner: two servings of turkey with a big ladle of gravy and ample servings of dressing, mashed potatoes, caramelized sweet potatoes, green peas, and two bread rolls. To top it off, you ate a piece of pumpkin pie with whipped cream. You meant to stop there; you loudly proclaimed, "I'm so full—I can't eat another bite!" But, eventually your grandmother convinced you to taste her special pecan pie. Gosh, that was good! But now you are lying on the couch, uncomfortable and bloated, with your belt loosened. Your feasting may be finished for now, but your body's work has just begun.

Your meal led to a huge influx of carbohydrate, fat, and protein—a plentiful supply for your tissues and far more energy than you need for life as a couch potato. The influx of food signals your cells to "store, store, store!" Consequently, much of your holiday dinner will wind up stored as fat. The surplus carbohydrate first enters glycogen stores, filling their limited capacity. In the short term, excess carbohydrate adjusts your body's fuel preferences to maximize its use of carbohydrate and minimizes its use of fat, thereby promoting fat storage. Carbohydrate in excess of energy needs will be converted to fatty acids and stored in adipose tissue to provide an available source of fuel during fasting.[15]

What happens to the surplus fat and protein? Fat tissue is the perfect energy storage package for both. Although some ATP is produced from dietary fat, nearly all excess dietary fat becomes body fat. Excess protein, beyond what's needed to replenish the overall body pool of amino acids, also heads to fat storage. (See **Figure SM.17**.)

### The Return to Normal

After this frenzied bout of storage, the amount of glucose and triglyceride circulating in the bloodstream drops to the fasting level roughly three to four hours after eating. The level of amino acids in the blood also returns to baseline.

Hours later, after a nap, and perhaps a game of touch football, a further decline in blood glucose levels triggers the signal "release the glucose!" and your body swings into action to counteract falling blood glucose levels. The body breaks down liver glycogen to glucose, which is released into the bloodstream. Synthesis and storage of glycogen and fatty acids slow. The body breaks down muscle glycogen to form glucose that muscles can use.

If low blood glucose levels persist for hours or days, most cells start shifting their fuel usage from glucose to fatty acids. Gluconeogenesis begins to ramp up and make glucose from circulating amino acids.[16] The body's metabolic pathways work in concert to maintain blood glucose levels and ensure a constant supply of glucose for the central nervous system and red blood cells[17]—until it is time to attack the leftovers!

**Key Concepts** *Feasting, or taking in too many calories, stimulates anabolic processes such as glycogen and fat synthesis. After a meal that contains dietary fat, carbohydrate and protein, dietary fat will be deposited as fatty acids in adipose tissue. Dietary amino acids in excess of what is needed for protein synthesis and carbohydrate in excess of what is needed for glycogen synthesis and energy will also be converted to fatty acids and deposited in adipose tissue leading to the accumulation of fat stores.*

## Fasting

Feasting on a holiday dinner floods your body with excess energy that is stored for future use. In contrast, fasting and starvation deprive you of energy, so your body must employ an opposing strategy—the mobilization of fuel. (See **Figure SM.18**.) Whether

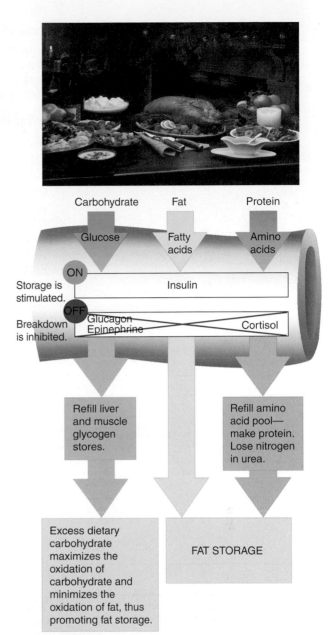

**Figure SM.17** **Feasting.** Your body deals with a large influx of nutrients by increasing cellular uptake of glucose and promoting fat storage.

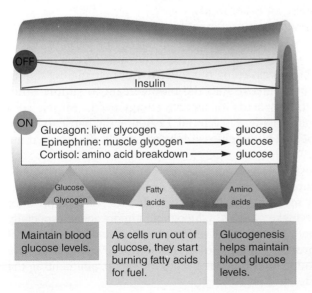

**Figure SM.18** **Short-term fasting.** During a short fast, cells first break down liver glycogen to maintain blood glucose levels. They also burn fatty acids and ramp up the production of glucose from amino acids.

starvation occurs in a child during a famine, a young woman with anorexia nervosa, a patient with AIDS wasting syndrome, or a person intentionally fasting, the body responds in the same way. Some people deprive themselves of food for a particular purpose—to lose weight, to stage a political protest, to participate in a religious fast, or to "cleanse" their bodies.

### Survival Priorities and Potential Energy Sources

Starvation confronts your body with several dilemmas. Where will it get energy to fuel survival needs? Which should it burn first—fat, protein, or carbohydrate? Can it conserve its energy reserves? Which tissues should it sacrifice to ensure survival?

Your body's first priority is to preserve glucose-dependent tissue: red blood cells, brain cells, and the rest of the central nervous system. Your brain will not tolerate even a short interruption in the supply of adequate energy. Once your body depletes its carbohydrate reserves, it begins sacrificing readily available circulating amino acids to make glucose and ATP.

THINK
About It
4

Your body's second priority is to maintain muscle mass. In the face of danger, we rely upon our ability to mount a "fight or flight" response. This survival mechanism requires a large muscle mass, allowing us to move quickly and effectively. Your body grudgingly uses muscle protein for energy and breaks it down rapidly only in the final stages of starvation.

Although your body stores most of its energy reserve in body fat, triglycerides are a poor source of glucose. Your body can make a small amount of glucose from the glycerol backbone, but it cannot make any glucose from fatty acids. As a consequence, your body's primary energy stores—fat—are incompatible with your body's paramount energy priority—glucose for your brain. To meet this metabolic challenge, your body's antistarvation strategies include a glucose-sparing mechanism. Your body shifts to fatty acids and ketone bodies for its primary fuel needs. In time, even your brain adapts as most, but not all, of its cells come to rely on ketone bodies for fuel.

### The Prolonged Fast: In the Beginning

What happens during the fasting state? Let's take a metabolic look at Fasting Frank, a political activist determined to make a dramatic statement. Frank begins fasting at sundown, planning to drink nothing but water and to consume no other foods.

The first few hours are no different from your nightly fast between dinner and breakfast. As blood glucose drops to fasting baseline levels, the liver breaks down glycogen to glucose. Gluconeogenesis becomes highly active and begins churning out glucose from circulating amino acids. The liver pours glucose into the bloodstream to supply other organs and shifts to fatty acids for its own energy needs. Muscle cells also start burning fatty acids. After about 12 hours, the battle to maintain a constant supply of blood glucose exhausts nearly all carbohydrate stores.[18]

During the next few days, fat and protein are the primary fuels. To preserve structural proteins, especially muscle mass, Frank's body first turns to easily metabolized amino acids. It uses some to produce ATP and others to make glucose. Glucogenic amino acids, especially alanine, furnish about 90 percent of the brain's glucose supply. Glycerol from triglyceride breakdown supplies the remaining 10 percent. After a couple of days, production of ketone bodies ramps up, augmenting the fuel supply. (See **Figure SM.19.**)

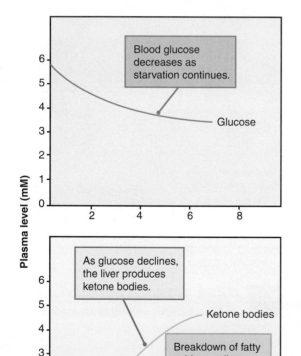

**Figure SM.19** **Shifting fuel selection during starvation.** To fuel its needs as blood glucose levels decline, the body shifts from glucose to fatty acids and ketone bodies.

### The Early Weeks

As starvation continues, Frank's body initiates several energy-conservation strategies. It ratchets down its energy use by lowering body temperature, pulse rate, blood pressure, and resting metabolism. Frank becomes lethargic, reducing the amount of energy expended in activity. He may begin to have detectable signs of mild vitamin deficiencies as his body depletes its small reserves of vitamin C and some B vitamins.

If Frank's body continued to rapidly break down protein, he would survive less than three weeks. To avoid such a quick demise, protein breakdown slows drastically and gluconeogenesis drops significantly.[19] To pick up the slack, Frank's body doubles the rate of fat breakdown to supply fatty acids for fuel and glycerol for glucose. Ketone bodies pour into the bloodstream and provide an important glucose-sparing energy source for the brain and red blood cells. After about 10 days of fasting, ketone bodies meet most of the nervous system's energy needs. Some brain cells, however, can use only glucose. To maintain a small, but essential, supply of blood glucose, protein breakdown crawls along, supplying small amounts of amino acids for gluconeogenesis.

### Several Weeks of Fasting

The main determinant of survival during prolonged fasting is the amount of body fat at the start of the fast. An average adult has about two months' worth of stored fat.[20] As the later stages of starvation exhaust the final fat stores, the body turns again to protein, its sole remaining fuel source. (See **Figure SM.20**.) You can see some of the effects of accelerated protein breakdown in

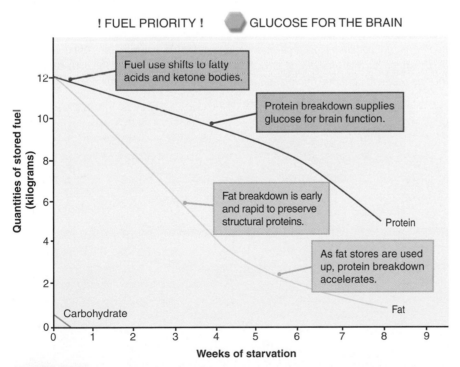

! FUEL PRIORITY !    GLUCOSE FOR THE BRAIN

- Fuel use shifts to fatty acids and ketone bodies.
- Protein breakdown supplies glucose for brain function.
- Fat breakdown is early and rapid to preserve structural proteins.
- As fat stores are used up, protein breakdown accelerates.

Protein

Fat

Carbohydrate

Quantities of stored fuel (kilograms)

Weeks of starvation

**Figure SM.20** **Starvation and fuel sources.** During starvation, stored carbohydrate (glycogen) is exhausted quickly, and fat becomes the primary fuel. Burning fat without available carbohydrate produces ketone bodies, a byproduct that the body can use as fuel. Glucose produced from amino acids and the glycerol portion of fatty acids help fuel the brain. The body conserves protein and breaks it down rapidly only after most fat stores are depleted.

starving children suffering from kwashiorkor. The loss of blood proteins leads to the swollen limbs and bulging stomachs that typify this type of protein-energy malnutrition (PEM).

### The End Is Near

In the final stage of protein depletion, the body deteriorates rapidly. You can see the severe muscle atrophy and emaciation in photos of Holocaust victims. Their bodies sacrificed muscle tissue in attempts to preserve brain tissue. Even organ tissues were not spared. The final stage of starvation attacks the liver and intestines, greatly depleting them. It moderately depletes the heart and kidneys and even mounts a small attack on the nervous system. Amazingly, starving people can cling to life until they lose about half their body proteins, after which death generally occurs.[21]

How long can a person survive total starvation? Several years ago, some Irish prisoners starved themselves to death—the average time was 60 days.[22] Most people survive total starvation for one to three months. Starvation survival factors include:

- *Starting percentage of body fat.* Ample fat tissue prolongs survival.
- *Age.* Middle-aged people survive longer than children and the elderly.
- *Gender.* Women fare better due to their higher proportion of body fat.
- *Energy expenditure levels.* Increased activity leads to an earlier death.

**Key Concepts**  *Fasting, or underconsumption of energy (calories), favors catabolic pathways. The body first obtains fuel from stored glycogen, then from stored fat and body proteins, such as muscle. Over time, the body adapts to using more and more ketone bodies as fuel because limited carbohydrate is available. Larger stores of fat in adipose tissue extend survival time during starvation. In prolonged starvation, the body catabolizes muscle tissue to continue minimal production of glucose from amino acids.*

# *Learning* Portfolio

## Key Terms

## Study Points

- Energy is necessary to do any kind of work. The body converts chemical energy from food sources—carbohydrates, proteins, and fats—into a form usable by cells.

- Anabolic reactions (anabolism) build compounds. These reactions require energy.

- Catabolic reactions (catabolism) break compounds into smaller units. These reactions produce energy.

- Adenosine triphosphate, ATP, is the energy currency of the body.

- NAD+ and FAD accept pairs of high-energy electrons, becoming NADH and $FADH_2$ and shuttling the electrons to the electron transport chain to make ATP.

- Cells extract energy from carbohydrate via four main pathways: glycolysis, pyruvate to acetyl CoA, the citric acid cycle, and the electron transport chain.

- The citric acid cycle and electron transport chain require oxygen. Glycolysis does not.

- The electron transport chain produces more ATP than other catabolic pathways.

- To extract energy from fat, first triglycerides are separated into glycerol and fatty acids. Next, beta-oxidation breaks down the fatty acids to yield acetyl CoA and high-energy electrons that are shuttled to the electron transport chain. The acetyl CoA enters the citric acid cycle, which yields one GTP and more high-energy electrons. In the electron transport chain, the high-energy electrons give up energy to produce ATP.

- To extract energy from an amino acid, first the amino group is removed. Depending on the structure of the remaining carbon skeleton, it enters the catabolic pathways at pyruvate, acetyl CoA, or a citric acid cycle intermediate. The citric acid cycle and the electron transport chain complete the extraction of energy and production of ATP.

- The liver converts the nitrogen portion of amino acids to urea, which the kidneys excrete.

- Tissues differ in their preferred source of fuel. The brain, nervous system, and red blood cells rely primarily on glucose whereas other tissues use a mix of glucose, fatty acids, and ketone bodies as fuel sources.

- When carbohydrate is available, glucose can be stored as glycogen in liver and muscle tissue.

- Glucose can be produced from the noncarbohydrate precursors glycerol and some (glucogenic) amino acids but not from fatty acids.

- Feasting, or overconsumption of energy, leads to glycogen and triglyceride storage.

- Fasting, or underconsumption of energy, leads to the mobilization of liver glycogen and stored triglycerides. Starvation, the state of prolonged fasting, leads to protein breakdown as well and can be fatal.

## Study Questions

1. What is the "universal energy currency"?

2. In the catabolic pathways, what two molecules accept electrons? Where are these electrons carried?

3. What four pathways are involved in extracting energy from carbohydrate? Which of these pathways are anaerobic, and which are aerobic?

4. What molecule does beta-oxidation form from the two-carbon links it "clips" off a fatty acid chain? What else does beta-oxidation produce that is important to producing ATP?

5. What dictates whether an amino acid is considered glucogenic or ketogenic?

6. What are ketone bodies, and when are they produced?

7. Name the three tissues where energy is stored. Which contains the largest store of energy?

8. Define *gluconeogenesis* and *lipogenesis*. Under what conditions do they predominantly occur? What are their primary inputs and outputs?

# Try This

## Comparing Fad Diets

The purpose of this exercise is to have you evaluate two fad diets in regard to their metabolic consequences. The two diets, Cabbage Soup and Super Protein, are described here. Once you've reviewed them, answer the following questions.

Will these diets result in weight loss? On the seventh day of each diet, which of the following metabolic pathways will be highly active?

- Glycogen breakdown
- Fat breakdown
- Gluconeogenesis
- Ketogenesis

### Diet 1: The Cabbage Soup Diet

A person following the Cabbage Soup diet eats only a water-based soup made out of cabbage and a few other vegetables. Three to four meals per day of this restricted diet supply approximately 500 kilocalories per day. The diet is devoid of protein and fat and gets its calories from the small amount of carbohydrate in the vegetables. Think about what happens during starvation.

### Diet 2: The Super Protein Diet

In the Super Protein diet, a person can eat an unlimited amount of protein-rich foods, such as meat, poultry, eggs, and seafood, but no added fats or carbohydrates are allowed. The average person can consume about 1,400 kilocalories if he or she eats three or four small meals each day. Think about what happens when little carbohydrate is available as a person metabolizes fat and protein.

## Fasting for Ketones

The purpose of this experiment is to see whether a day without eating will cause your body to produce measurable ketones in your urine. Before starting your fast, check with your physician to be sure this won't pose any health risks. Go to your local pharmacy and ask the pharmacist for urine ketone strips (often called *Ketostix*). Bring them home and read the directions. Before you start your one-day fast, test your urine to see whether it has a detectable amount of ketones. Start a 24-hour fast (or fast for as long as you can go without food or calorie-containing fluids but no longer than 24 hours) and test your urine at 6-hour intervals. Do you detect a color change on the strips as the day goes on? Why? What has happened metabolically as the day progresses?

*Remember to drink lots of water!*

# References

1  Gropper SS, Smith JL, Groff JL. *Advanced Nutrition and Human Metabolism*. 5th ed. Belmont, CA: Wadsworth; 2009.

2  Butte NF, Cabellero B. Energy needs: assessment and requirements. In: Shils ME, Shike M, Ross AC, Cabellero B, Cousins RJ, eds. *Modern Nutrition in Health and Disease*. 10th ed. Philadelphia: Lippincott Williams & Wilkins; 2006:136–148.

3  Stipanuk MH. *Biochemical and Physiological Aspects of Human Nutrition*. 2nd ed. Philadelphia: WB Saunders; 2006.

4  Nelson DL, Cox MM. *Principles of Biochemistry*. 5th ed. New York: WH Freeman and Co.; 2008.

5  Berg JM, Tymoczko JL, Stryer L. *Biochemistry*. 7th ed. New York: WH Freeman and Co.; 2010.

6  Gropper SS, Smith JL, Groff JL. Op. cit.

7  Devlin TM. *Textbook of Biochemistry with Clinical Correlations*. 7th ed. Hoboken, NJ: John Wiley and Sons, Inc.; 2011.

8  Sarubin Fragakis A. *The Health Professional's Guide to Popular Dietary Supplements*. 3rd ed. Chicago: Academy of Nutrition and Dietetics; 2007.

9  Gropper SS, Smith JL, Groff JL. Op. cit.

10  Devlin TM. Op. cit.

11  Ibid.

12  Ibid.

13  Anderson JW. Diabetes mellitus: medical nutrition therapy. In: Shils ME, Shike M, Ross AC, Cabellero B, Cousins RJ, eds. *Modern Nutrition in Health and Disease*. 10th ed. Philadelphia: Lippincott Williams & Wilkins; 2006:1043–1066.

14  Guyton AC, Hall JE. *Textbook of Medical Physiology*. 11th ed. Philadelphia: Elsevier Health Sciences; 2010.

15  Gropper SS, Smith JL, Groff JL. Op. cit.

16  Nelson DL, Cox MM. Op. cit.

17  Martini FH, Nath JL. *Fundamentals of Anatomy and Physiology*. 9th ed. San Francisco: Benjamin Cummings; 2011.

18  Gropper SS, Smith JL, Groff JL. Op. cit.

19  Ibid.

20  Hoffer LJ. Metabolic consequences of starvation. In: Shils ME, Shike M, Ross AC, Cabellero B, Cousins RJ, eds. *Modern Nutrition in Health and Disease*. 10th ed. Philadelphia: Lippincott Williams & Wilkins; 2006.

21  Ibid.

22  Ganong WF. *Review of Medical Physiology*. 23rd ed. New York: McGraw-Hill; 2009.

# CHAPTER 8

# Energy Balance and Weight Management: Finding Your Equilibrium

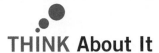

**THINK About It**

1 How often are you tempted by dessert after a big meal?

2 When it comes to body fat distribution, what is your body shape? Are you an apple or a pear?

3 What does it mean to be metabolically fit?

4 How much time do you spend talking with your friends about weight?

**Visit** go.jblearning.com/inseldisco4e

## Quick Bite

Your body is in the energy exchange business. Here's how it works. You balance the energy you expend with energy you take in from the food that you eat. If you do a fairly good job of equalizing intake and expenditure, your body does the rest—maintaining energy equilibrium, or "balance," and keeping your weight stable. But suppose you bring in more energy than your body can handle? It banks the excess energy as fat, and you gain weight. If your "account" grows too big, you become overweight and, perhaps, even obese. Losing that extra weight—withdrawing the fat from your account—is not always easy. Thus, weight management is a balancing act between energy intake and energy expenditure.

**Energy intake** is the amount of fuel you consume through the food you eat (i.e., carbohydrate, protein, fat, and alcohol). **Energy output** is the amount you expend. As will be described in detail later in this chapter, energy expenditure includes more than just physical activity. Your body cells use large amounts of energy in order to carry out basic bodily functions. In addition, the processing of food requires energy. An average adult consumes 1,800 to 3,000 kilocalories per day. In one year, that adds up to 657,000 to 1,095,000 kilocalories! Amazingly, despite such a huge intake of energy over time, most people maintain relatively stable body weights during most of their adult lives.

People who maintain a relatively constant weight are in **energy equilibrium**, such that, on average, the calories they consume are approximately equal to the calories they expend. Your body can be in energy equilibrium even if your energy intake is very high, as long as your expenditure also is high. Conversely, your body can be in energy equilibrium when you don't expend much energy, as long as your energy intake also is low.

When you consume more calories than you expend, you have a situation of **positive energy balance**. The surplus in calories will be stored as fat—the major energy reserve—and you will see the number on the bathroom scale go up. Now, positive energy balance is not always a bad thing. Pregnant women and growing children need a positive energy balance to increase energy stores. Strength and power athletes need to be in positive energy balance to increase lean body mass (e.g., muscle). But the positive energy balance that results from overeating and inactivity, a common occurrence in the United States and Canada, leads to unneeded weight gain.

When you consume fewer calories than you expend (or conversely, expend more calories than you consume), you are said to be in **negative energy balance**. To obtain the fuel it needs, your body uses its stores of glycogen and fat (and breaks down body protein, too, if the deficit is extreme), and body weight goes down. Thus, body weight change reflects overall **energy balance**. **Figure 8.1** shows three people with different ratios of energy intake to energy expenditure.

**Key Concepts** *Energy balance is the relationship between energy intake and energy output. Energy intake is the number of calories consumed. Energy output is the number of calories expended, mainly for basic body functions, the processing of food, and physical activity.*

## Energy In

We know that energy intake is the number of calories consumed. But how does the body know how much energy it needs? A complex interaction between internal and external cues is believed to help the body regulate food intake and, thus, maintain energy equilibrium. Internal cues involve interactions and feedback mechanisms among neuropeptides, hormones, and other

**energy intake** The caloric or energy content of food provided by the sources of dietary energy: carbohydrate (4 kcal/g), protein (4 kcal/g), fat (9 kcal/g), and alcohol (7 kcal/g).

**energy output** The use of calories or energy for basic body functions, physical activity, and processing of consumed foods.

**energy equilibrium** A balance of energy intake and output that results in little or no change in weight over time.

**positive energy balance** Energy intake exceeds energy expenditure, resulting in an increase in body energy stores and weight gain.

**negative energy balance** Energy intake is lower than energy expenditure, resulting in a depletion of body energy stores and weight loss.

**energy balance** The balance in the body between amounts of energy consumed and expended.

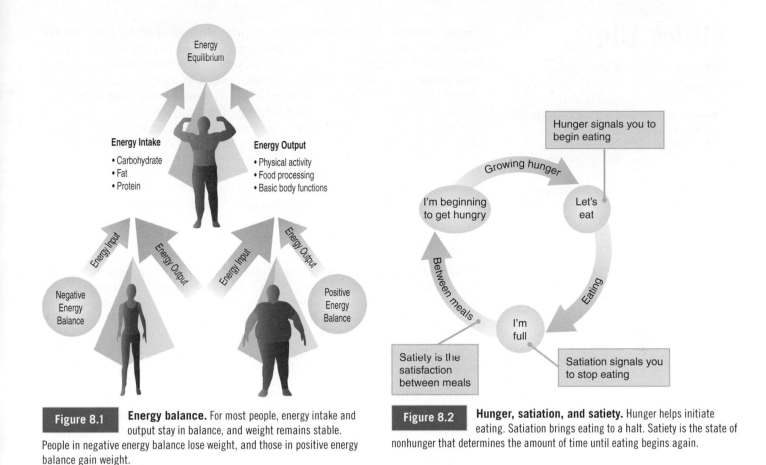

**Figure 8.1** **Energy balance.** For most people, energy intake and output stay in balance, and weight remains stable. People in negative energy balance lose weight, and those in positive energy balance gain weight.

**Figure 8.2** **Hunger, satiation, and satiety.** Hunger helps initiate eating. Satiation brings eating to a halt. Satiety is the state of nonhunger that determines the amount of time until eating begins again.

hormonelike compounds and organ systems. External cues are stimuli in the eating environment and include the sight, smell, and taste of food. Although these internal and external cues generally work together to ensure that we eat enough to survive, they can be readily overridden, such that we eat more than we need, resulting in positive energy balance and weight gain.

## Hunger, Satiation, and Satiety

The internal cues that govern our energy intake are frequently classified as three distinct sensations, although there is some fundamental overlap in how we experience them. (See **Figure 8.2**.) The first, **hunger**, prompts eating ("I'm hungry"). Most of us recognize hunger as the empty or gnawing feeling in our stomachs, lightheadedness, and even headaches that signal the physiological need to eat. **Satiation**, the second internal cue, tells you when you've had enough to eat ("I'm full"). Finally, **satiety** represents the length of time that satiation lasts and generally tells you when you are ready to eat again ("I'm not ready to eat yet" or "I just ate an hour ago and I'm hungry already").

## Appetite

External cues can stimulate **appetite**, which complicates the workings of hunger, satiation, and satiety. Appetite is the psychological desire to eat and is related to pleasant sensations associated with food. The eating environment often influences appetite. For example, exposure to a variety of tasty foods (such as at a buffet) can stimulate you to eat more than if you are served a

**hunger** The internal, physiological drive to find and consume food. Unlike appetite, hunger is often experienced as a negative sensation, often manifesting as an uneasy or painful sensation; the recurrent and involuntary lack of access to food that may produce malnutrition over time.

**satiation** Feeling of satisfaction and fullness that terminates a meal.

**satiety** The effects of a food or meal that delay subsequent intake. Feeling of satisfaction and fullness following eating that quells the desire for food.

**appetite** A psychological desire to eat that is related to the pleasant sensations often associated with food.

## Quick Bite

**Why Do We Have Hunger Pangs?**

When the stomach has been without food for at least three hours, intense stomach contractions can begin, sometimes lasting two to three minutes. Healthy young people have the strongest contractions, due to good muscle tone in the GI tract. After 12 to 24 hours, contractions of an empty stomach can cause painful hunger pangs.

limited number of foods. Hunger is the physiological need for food. In this sense, whereas appetite reflects our eating experiences, hunger is a basic drive. When you are truly hungry, any food will do, but your appetite can trigger your desire for a specific food or type of food, even though you may not be hungry. For example, after a big meal of steak, potato, salad, and bread, you probably wouldn't want a second helping of these foods. But you might be tempted by the dessert cart! That's appetite. Even when we are hungry, illness and medication can cause loss of appetite and a lack of interest in food.

THINK About It

1

**Key Concepts** *Food intake is regulated by sensations of hunger, a physiological drive to eat; satiation, feelings of satisfaction that lead to ending a meal; and satiety, continued feelings of fullness that delay the start of the next meal. Appetite is the psychological urge to eat and often has no relation to hunger.*

## Control by Committee

What, then, stimulates hunger, satiation, satiety, and appetite? Internal responses in the digestive tract, central nervous system, and general circulation influence your eating behavior. Sites throughout the body monitor energy status and send reports to the brain, which can then stimulate feelings of hunger, satiety, and satiation. Externally, the eating environment—where we are eating, what we are eating, who we are eating with—can all influence what and how much we eat.

### Gastrointestinal Sensations

As food fills your stomach and small intestine, they stretch and trigger signals to the brain. Your sense of fullness suppresses your urge to eat. Just passing a reasonable amount of food through the mouth can satisfy hunger temporarily—even if the food never reaches the stomach. When researchers fed large amounts of food to a person with a hole in the esophagus, hunger decreased, even though the food never reached the stomach. As we taste, salivate, chew, and swallow, the brain probably measures the passage of food, much as a water meter measures the flow of water. After a certain amount of food passes through the mouth, hunger diminishes for 20 to 40 minutes.[1]

### Neurological and Hormonal Factors

More than 50 different chemicals are thought to be involved in the regulation of feeding. Determining the way these chemical factors work is an active research area that may lead to improved therapies for both the overweight and underweight.

Hormones, hormonelike factors, and some drugs (including appetite suppressants) influence eating behavior through their direct or indirect effects on the brain.[2] **Neuropeptide Y (NPY)** is a hormonelike factor in the brain and a powerful appetite stimulator that has been shown to cause people to hoard food.[3] Although a number of signals can affect NPY activity, opposing signals from the hormones **ghrelin** and **leptin** link NPY secretion to daily feeding patterns.[4]

Ghrelin, sometimes called the "hunger hormone," is produced in the stomach. Ghrelin levels rise prior to a meal and fall quickly after food is consumed. The rise in ghrelin levels appears to stimulate NPY, thus encouraging feeding.

Leptin, sometimes called the "satiety hormone," is produced in fat cells in direct proportion to the amount of fat stored. Leptin signals the brain for the regulation of fat storage.[5] A rise in leptin levels appears to inhibit NPY, thus suppressing appetite. Leptin also appears to signal pathways that enhance energy production to keep body weight in a normal range. Administering

**neuropeptide Y (NPY)** A neurotransmitter widely distributed throughout the brain and peripheral nervous tissue. NPY activity has been linked to eating behavior, depression, anxiety, and cardiovascular function.

**ghrelin** A hormone produced by the stomach that stimulates feeding by increasing release of neuropeptide Y.

**leptin** A hormone produced by adipose cells that signals the amount of body fat content and influences food intake.

leptin to obese experimental animals lacking the hormone causes them to become normal weight.

Unfortunately, when body weight is high, these regulators act inconsistently. Obese people tend to have lower fasting ghrelin levels (suggesting that they would experience lower levels of hunger before a meal) and smaller reductions of ghrelin levels after a meal (suggesting that overeating may be due to lower levels of satiation).[6] This situation may be a result of a combination of factors, including body weight and diet composition. People with increased body weight tend to have diets high in sugar and low in fiber. When these individuals consume a high-sugar/low-fiber diet, leptin levels rise following a meal. However, this rise in leptin is not accompanied by an increase in satiety and limiting of food intake.[7] Because high-sugar/low-fiber meals may inhibit leptin's ability to signal satiety effectively, this eating pattern may play a role in the current obesity epidemic by increasing energy intake.[8]

**Key Concepts** *The interaction of internal factors, such as gastrointestinal sensations, hormonal responses, and neurological signals, helps regulate our feeding behavior. In obese people, these regulators can act inconsistently.*

### Diet Composition

The energy density (kilocalories per gram of food), balance of energy sources (carbohydrates, lipids, and protein), and the form (liquid vs. solid) of your foods affect your energy intake. Overall, people tend to eat a fairly constant amount of food. If your diet includes a lot of energy-dense foods (typically high-fat, high-sugar, low-fiber foods), the way you eat likely will result in excess energy consumption, and in turn, weight gain.

Dietary protein and fiber may help control energy intake. Protein appears to make a stronger contribution to satiety than fats or carbohydrates.[9] Adding fiber to low-energy-dense foods may be an effective way to suppress appetite and control food intake.[10] Some types of fiber enhance satiation by slowing the rate at which the stomach empties, whereas others seem to enhance satiation by creating bulk.[11]

Liquid sources of calories (e.g., juices, soft drinks) generally have a lower satiety value than solid food with the same amount of energy.[12] Sugared beverages can represent a significant source of calories, and because they are less satiating than solid foods, this could result in weight gain.

Epidemiological studies have linked beverage consumption (such as soda) to the growing obesity rates in the United States.[13] In young children, research indicates that regular consumption of sugar-sweetened beverages between meals increases risk for becoming overweight.[14]

### Sensory Properties

The aroma of freshly baked bread or the warmth and chewiness of chocolate chip cookies right out of the oven can encourage us to eat more than our hunger dictates. Food's sensory properties—flavor, texture, color, temperature, and presentation—influence its appeal, and such external cues affect food intake.[15] (See **Figure 8.3**.) Taste often is the reason why people choose a particular food, and we are more likely to overconsume a food that tastes good.

### Portion Size

Portion size plays a role in how much we eat, with larger portions generally leading to an increase in energy intake.[16] Over the past two decades, portion sizes have increased for virtually all foods and beverages prepared for immediate consumption, including fast food, individually packaged food, and ready-to-eat prepared food.[17] (See Table 8.1.)

## Quick Bite

**Supersize Me!**
Morgan Spurlock wrote, directed, produced, and is the lead character in *Supersize Me*, a film that documents Spurlock's consumption of a 30-day, McDonald's-only diet. Whenever offered the option to "supersize" his order, Spurlock always selected the larger portion size. Starting at 185 pounds, the 6-foot, 2-inch Spurlock packed on 25 pounds and weighed 210 by the end of his experiment. His total cholesterol shot up from 165 to 230, his libido flagged, and he suffered headaches and depression.

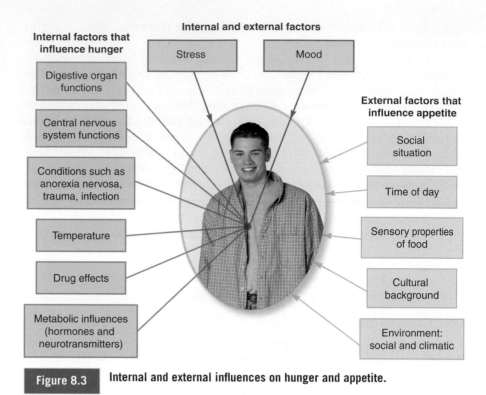

| **Figure 8.3** | **Internal and external influences on hunger and appetite.** |

Several studies have documented a "portion distortion" phenomenon. In a controlled study of adults, people served a 1,000-gram portion (approximately 33 ounces) of macaroni and cheese for lunch ate 30 percent more than when they were served 500 grams (approximately 17 ounces).[18] It didn't matter whether the portions were served on individual plates or whether people served themselves from a serving dish. In another study, young adults were given pieces of candy that had been cut into two pieces to make the food-item smaller in size. The participants ate the same number of pieces but half as much candy overall, thus decreasing the total energy intake during that snacking occasion.[19]

When people select their own portions, the size of the serving bowl may affect the amount consumed. In a study of snack food consumption, adults presented with food in a large serving bowl took more food (and consumed about 140 more kilocalories) than when an equal amount of food was pre-

| Table 8.1 | **Comparison of Common Portion Sizes 20 Years Ago Versus Today** |

| Food Item | 20 Years Ago | | Today | |
|---|---|---|---|---|
| | *Portion* | *Calories* | *Portion* | *Calories* |
| Bagel | 3-inch diameter | 140 | 6-inch diameter | 350 |
| Cheeseburger | 1 | 333 | 1 | 590 |
| Spaghetti with meatballs | 1 cup sauce and 3 small meatballs | 500 | 2 cups sauce and 3 large meatballs | 1,020 |
| Soda | 6.5 oz | 82 | 20 oz | 250 |
| Muffin | 1.5 oz | 210 | 5 oz | 500 |

**Source:** National Heart, Lung, and Blood Institute; National Institutes of Health; US Department of Health and Human Services. Portion distortion and serving size. http://www.nhlbi.nih.gov/health/public/heart/obesity/wecan/eat-right/distortion.htm. Accessed 11/28/11.

sented in a smaller bowl.[20] Children also are susceptible to the temptation of big portions, eating 25 percent more when served a double portion[21] but consuming less when they serve themselves. We tend to respond visually to the amount of food on a plate and consider that "normal" rather than paying attention to internal feelings of satiation.[22]

Americans are living in a "super-size" culture in which portion sizes keep getting larger. Buffets, fast-food restaurants, and convenience stores offer "value meals" providing more food for less money. Consumers indicate that value for money is important when purchasing food and that large portion sizes offer more value for money than small portion sizes.[23] This dramatic increase in portion sizes eaten both at home and at restaurants[24] may be a major contributing factor to excess energy intake and weight gain.

### Environmental and Social Factors

We tend to eat more in cold weather and less in hot weather. Systems in the **hypothalamus** that regulate body temperature and food intake probably interact to link temperature and eating behavior. In cold temperatures, increased food intake helps us survive—increasing the metabolic rate, which helps generate heat, and increasing fat stores, which provide insulation to reduce heat loss.[25]

Plate size and shape, package sizes, lighting, color, convenience, and socializing are other factors that influence consumption.[26] Any change in our surroundings that inhibits our self-monitoring of consumption tends to increase the volume that we eat. Larger plates and bowls encourage larger servings. We tend to eat more in dimly lit situations than when the lights are brighter, perhaps because we are less inhibited and self-conscious.[27]

The best predictor of the amount of food that will be eaten at a given time is the number of people present. Studies show that meals eaten with other people last longer and tend to increase consumption by at least one-third compared with eating alone.[28]

### Emotional Factors

Many people use food to cope with stress and negative emotions. Eating can provide a powerful distraction from loneliness, anger, boredom, anxiety, shame, sadness, and inadequacy. To combat low moods, low energy levels, and low self-esteem, people often turn to the refrigerator. When we use food and eating to cope with our emotions, binge eating or other disturbed eating patterns can develop.

**Key Concepts** *External factors such as portion size, aroma, weather, social circumstances, and emotions can enhance or suppress appetite. Our eating behaviors are determined by a complex interplay of physiological and psychological influences.*

## Energy Out: Fuel Uses

Our bodies use fuel (expend energy) for three primary purposes:

1. To maintain basic physiological functions such as breathing and blood circulation
2. To process the food we eat
3. To power physical activity

We also expend energy to support growth, stay warm in cold environments, metabolize drugs, and deal with physical trauma, fever, and psychological stress. The sum of all energy expended is the **total energy expenditure (TEE)**. **Figure 8.4** illustrates the major components of energy expenditure.

**hypothalamus [high-po-THAL-ah-mus]** A region of the brain involved in regulating hunger and satiety, respiration, body temperature, water balance, and other body functions.

**total energy expenditure (TEE)** The total of the resting energy expenditure (REE), energy used in physical activity, and energy used in processing food (TEF); usually expressed in kilocalories per day.

**resting metabolic rate (RMR)** A clinical measure of resting energy expenditure performed three to four hours after eating or performing significant physical activity.

**resting energy expenditure (REE)** The minimum energy needed to maintain basic physiological functions (e.g., heartbeat, muscle function, respiration). The resting metabolic rate (RMR) extrapolated to 24 hours.

**lean body mass** The portion of the body exclusive of stored fat, including muscle, bone, connective tissue, organs, and water.

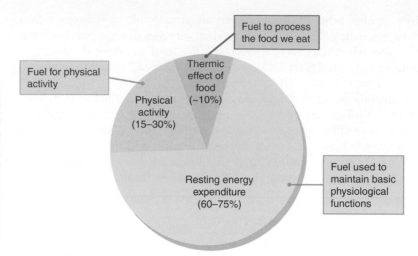

Fuel to process the food we eat

Fuel for physical activity

Thermic effect of food (~10%)

Physical activity (15–30%)

Resting energy expenditure (60–75%)

Fuel used to maintain basic physiological functions

**Figure 8.4** **Major components of energy expenditure.** You expend most of your energy to maintain basic body functions. Energy expended in physical activity can be significant and is the most variable component of total energy expenditure. The thermic effect of food is the energy needed to digest, absorb, transport, metabolize, and store ingested food.

## Major Components of Energy Expenditure

### Energy Expenditure at Rest

We generally expend most of our energy on the basic body functions needed to sustain life at rest. This resting energy expenditure is the energy needed to maintain heartbeat, respiration, nervous function, muscle tone, body temperature, and other bodily functions. Resting energy expenditure accounts for approximately 60 to 75 percent of total energy expenditure.[29]

The rate of energy expended at rest (kcal/hour) is called the **resting metabolic rate (RMR)**. Extrapolating the RMR over 24 hours (kcal/hr × 24) determines the **resting energy expenditure (REE)**.[30]

Energy expended by the vital organs (e.g., liver, brain, heart, kidneys, pancreas) and skeletal muscle makes up the greatest proportion of RMR. Other tissues, such as fat, have lower metabolic activity and consume less energy. The vital organs and skeletal muscle, along with bones and fluids, make up most of what is known as the **lean body mass**—the total mass of the body that isn't fat. An extremely muscular person will generally have more total lean body mass and, thus, a higher RMR than someone who weighs the same but has a higher proportion of body fat.

Lean body mass tends to decline as we age, and body fat tends to rise. Keeping physically active helps slow this age-related loss of lean tissue and discourages accumulation of fat so we maintain a higher RMR.

Women usually have lower RMRs than men. Women tend to be smaller, and pound for pound they generally have less lean body mass. A woman's RMR also varies during the menstrual cycle, fluctuating from a low point about one week before ovulation to a high point just before the onset of menstruation.[31] **Figure 8.5** shows the factors that affect RMR.

**Key Concepts** *We use energy to fuel basic body functions, process the food we eat, and support physical activity. The energy used in these basic functions is called resting energy expenditure, or REE. Factors that affect resting energy expenditure include body composition, age, and gender.*

### Energy Expenditure in Physical Activity

Physical activity encompasses more than just exercise and participation in sports. It includes the activity you do at work, during leisure activities, and

**Increase RMR**

- Total body weight
- Large body surface area
- Hot and cold ambient temperature
- Fever
- Hyperthyroidism
- Stress

- Caffeine
- Smoking
- Increased lean body mass
- Rapid growth
- Pregnancy and lactation

- Genetics
- Some medications

- Aging
- Female gender
- Fasting/starvation
- Hypothyroidism
- Sleep

**Decrease RMR**

**Figure 8.5** **Factors that affect RMR.** Inherited traits determine whether you have a generally high or low RMR. Many environmental and physiological factors may temporarily raise RMR, and other factors may temporarily lower it.

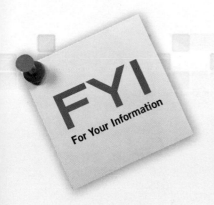

# What's Neat About NEAT?

It seems Jan only has to look at food to gain weight. Yet her friend Molly doesn't seem to gain weight no matter what she eats. Both have the same height and frame, eat about the same amount of calories, and get about the same amount of exercise. So what's missing? Recent research suggests that fidgeting and movements such as posture adjustments may be part of the answer.

Studies in the early 1900s first suggested that weight gained in response to overeating wasn't proportional to the extra calories ingested. Following experiments on himself, the German scientist R. O. Neumann coined the term *luxuskonsumption* to describe his observation that excess calories did not result in weight gain and therefore must be lost as heat.[1] Further studies supported this idea, showing wide individual variation in response to overfeeding. Some suggest that the ease of weight gain is genetically based.[2]

A study at the Mayo Clinic attributes differences in weight gain in response to overfeeding to a mechanism described as NEAT: nonexercise activity thermogenesis.[3] According to the researchers, NEAT is "the thermogenesis [heat production] that accompanies physical activities other than volitional [intentional] exercise, such as the activities of daily living, fidgeting, spontaneous muscle contraction, and maintaining posture when not recumbent."

In the NEAT study, 16 volunteers (12 men and 4 women) were given an extra 1,000 kilocalories per day—roughly equivalent to two double cheeseburgers—for a period of eight weeks. Before the study began, careful measurements were made over a two-week period to determine each participant's maintenance energy requirements. Physical activity during the study was controlled, and meals were provided only through the Mayo Clinic General Clinical Research Center. Questionnaires and interviews were done to ensure compliance.

The average weight gained by the study participants was 4.7 kilograms (10.3 pounds), but some gained as much as 7.2 kilograms (15.8 pounds), whereas others added only 1.4 kilograms (3.1 pounds). The theoretical expected weight gain from an eight-week excess of 56,000 kilocalories would be 7.3 kilograms (16.0 pounds) to 9.1 kilograms (20.0 pounds)—more than the maximum weight gain of any participant!

After accounting for RMR, TEF, and energy used in physical activity, the remaining energy expenditure was attributed to NEAT. The amount of energy expended as NEAT varied among the participants by nearly 800 kilocalories per day. Participants with higher NEAT resisted weight gain, suggesting that people who can effectively activate NEAT tend not to gain weight, even with overeating. Further, this suggests that obese people may not effectively activate NEAT.

In another study, the Mayo Clinic researchers found that obese individuals sat for two hours longer than lean individuals.[4] This pattern of activity (or lack thereof) didn't change when obese individuals lost weight or lean individuals gained weight.

So, is the take-home message "fidget more, stand up straight, and you won't gain weight"? Not exactly. The researchers did not account for factors such as the extra energy needed to move a higher body weight in activity. In addition, they relied on self-reports that may have been inaccurate. Attributing the entire difference in energy expenditure to NEAT ignores heat production by brown adipose tissue, a type of fat tissue that tends to "waste" energy.[6] Clearly, though, some individuals are able to resist weight gain, even when overeating, while others cannot. Further studies to better understand NEAT and the factors that regulate it may help to better understand

conditions of energy imbalance—not only obesity but also anorexia nervosa.[7]

1   Neumann RO. Experimentalle Beitrage zur Lehre von dem taglichen Nahrungsbedarf der Menschen unter besonder Berucksichtigung der notwendigen Eisewissmenge. *Arch Hyg*. 1902;45:1–2.

2   Dian C. New insights into the genetics of body weight. *Curr Opin Clin Nutr Metab Care*. 2008;11(4):378–384.

3   Levine JA, Eberhardt NL, Jensen MD. Role of nonexercise activity thermogenesis in resistance to fat gain in humans. *Science*. 1999;283:212–214.

4   Levine JA, Lanningham-Foster LM, McCrady SK, et al. Interindividual variation in posture allocation: possible role in human obesity. *Science*. 2005;307:584–586.

5   Ravussin E, Danforth E. Beyond sloth—physical activity and weight gain. *Science*. 1999;283:184–185.

6   Ravussin E, Galgani JE. The implication of brown adipose tissue for humans. *Annu Rev Nutr*. 2011;31:33–47.

7   Levine JA. Nonexercise activity thermogenesis (NEAT): environment and biology. *Am J Physiol Endocrinol Metab*. 2004;286:E675–E685.

other everyday activities—even fidgeting. For most individuals, the energy expended in physical activity accounts for 15 to 30 percent of total daily energy expenditure (depending on whether you are mostly sedentary or very physically active).[32] For some elite athletes, training several hours each day, the energy expended in physical activity may be as high as 50 percent of total daily energy expenditure.

The energy cost of an activity depends on its type (i.e., walking, running, or typing, for example), duration, and intensity. Table 8.2 shows the amounts of energy expended in specific activities. Body size affects energy cost, too—it takes more energy to move a bigger mass, so a large person expends more kilocalories per minute than a smaller person doing the same activity. Fitness level has an effect as well. A fit person exercises more efficiently, with lower

## *Quick* Bite

**Brrr! Shivering Away Calories**

Cold weather increases energy needs. Shivering alone can increase the RMR by 2.5 times. Although shivering bodies use both fat and carbohydrate, carbohydrates are the preferred fuel. In addition, people with less body fat shiver more in the cold.

## Table 8.2    Amount of Energy Expended in Specific Activities

| Description | kcal/hr/kg | kcal/hr/lb | 50 kg (110 lb) | 57 kg (125 lb) | 68 kg (150 lb) | 80 kg (175 lb) | 91 kg (200 lb) |
|---|---|---|---|---|---|---|---|
| **Aerobics** | | | | | | | |
| Light | 3.0 | 1.36 | 150 | 170 | 205 | 239 | 273 |
| Moderate | 8.0 | 2.27 | 250 | 284 | 341 | 398 | 455 |
| Heavy | 8.0 | 3.64 | 400 | 455 | 545 | 636 | 727 |
| **Bicycling** | | | | | | | |
| Leisurely (<10 mph) | 4.0 | 1.82 | 200 | 227 | 273 | 318 | 364 |
| Light (10–11.9 mph) | 6.0 | 2.73 | 300 | 341 | 409 | 477 | 545 |
| Moderate (12–13.9 mph) | 8.0 | 3.64 | 400 | 455 | 545 | 636 | 727 |
| Fast (14–15.9 mph) | 10.0 | 4.55 | 500 | 568 | 682 | 795 | 909 |
| Racing (16–19 mph) | 12.0 | 5.45 | 600 | 682 | 818 | 955 | 1,091 |
| BMX or mountain | 8.5 | 3.86 | 425 | 483 | 580 | 676 | 773 |
| **Daily Activities** | | | | | | | |
| Sleeping | 1.2 | 0.55 | 60 | 68 | 82 | 95 | 109 |
| Studying, reading, writing | 1.8 | 0.82 | 90 | 102 | 123 | 143 | 164 |
| Cooking, food preparation | 2.5 | 1.14 | 125 | 142 | 170 | 199 | 227 |
| Home Activities | | | | | | | |
| House painting, outside | 4.0 | 1.82 | 200 | 227 | 273 | 318 | 364 |
| General gardening | 5.0 | 2.27 | 250 | 284 | 341 | 398 | 455 |
| Shoveling snow | 6.0 | 2.73 | 300 | 341 | 409 | 477 | 545 |
| **Running** | | | | | | | |
| Jogging | 7.0 | 3.18 | 350 | 398 | 477 | 557 | 636 |
| Running 5 mph | 8.0 | 3.64 | 400 | 455 | 545 | 636 | 727 |
| Running 6 mph | 10.0 | 4.55 | 500 | 568 | 682 | 795 | 909 |
| Running 7 mph | 11.5 | 5.23 | 575 | 653 | 784 | 915 | 1,045 |
| Running 8 mph | 13.5 | 6.14 | 675 | 767 | 920 | 1,074 | 1,227 |
| Running 9 mph | 15.0 | 6.82 | 750 | 852 | 1,023 | 1,193 | 1,364 |
| Running 10 mph | 16.0 | 7.27 | 800 | 909 | 1,091 | 1,273 | 1,455 |
| **Sports** | | | | | | | |
| Frisbee, ultimate | 3.5 | 1.59 | 175 | 199 | 239 | 278 | 318 |
| Hacky sack | 4.0 | 1.82 | 200 | 227 | 273 | 318 | 364 |
| Wind surfing | 4.2 | 1.91 | 210 | 239 | 286 | 334 | 382 |
| Golf | 4.5 | 2.05 | 225 | 256 | 307 | 358 | 409 |
| Skateboarding | 5.0 | 2.27 | 250 | 284 | 341 | 398 | 455 |
| Rollerblading | 7.0 | 3.18 | 350 | 398 | 477 | 557 | 636 |
| Soccer | 7.0 | 3.18 | 350 | 398 | 477 | 557 | 636 |
| Field hockey | 8.0 | 3.64 | 400 | 455 | 545 | 636 | 727 |
| Swimming, slow to moderate laps | 8.0 | 3.64 | 400 | 455 | 545 | 636 | 727 |
| Skiing downhill, moderate effort | 6.0 | 2.73 | 300 | 341 | 409 | 477 | 545 |
| Skiing cross country, moderate effort | 8.0 | 3.64 | 400 | 455 | 545 | 636 | 727 |
| Tennis, doubles | 6.0 | 2.73 | 300 | 341 | 409 | 477 | 545 |
| Tennis, singles | 8.0 | 3.64 | 400 | 455 | 545 | 636 | 727 |
| **Walking** | | | | | | | |
| Strolling (<2 mph), level | 2.0 | 0.91 | 100 | 114 | 136 | 159 | 182 |
| Moderate pace (~3 mph), level | 3.5 | 1.59 | 175 | 199 | 239 | 278 | 318 |
| Moderate pace (~3 mph), uphill | 6.0 | 2.73 | 300 | 341 | 409 | 477 | 545 |
| Brisk pace (~3.5 mph), level | 4.0 | 1.82 | 200 | 227 | 273 | 318 | 364 |
| Very brisk pace (~4.5 mph), level | 4.5 | 2.05 | 225 | 256 | 307 | 358 | 409 |

*Table header: Kcal/hr at Different Body Weights*

**Source:** Adapted from Nieman DC. *Exercise Testing and Prescription*. 4th ed. Mountain View, CA: Mayfield Publishing; 1999.

energy costs. However, fit people also can exercise with greater intensity and duration, burning more kilocalories overall. **Figure 8.6** shows how energy expenditure is measured during exercise.

Mental activity—such as studying for an exam—uses little energy. But if you fidget when you study, you may expend a significant amount of energy. The acronym **NEAT** stands for **nonexercise activity thermogenesis**, which is the energy associated with activities other than exercise, such as fidgeting, maintenance of posture, and similar contributors to energy expenditure.[33] (See the FYI feature "What's Neat About NEAT?")

### Energy Expenditure to Process Food

Our bodies expend energy to digest, absorb, and metabolize the nutrients we take in, and these processes generate heat. This energy output is collectively called the **thermic effect of food (TEF)**. TEF peaks about one hour after eating and normally dissipates within five hours. For a typical mixed diet, TEF accounts for between 6 and 10 percent of total energy expenditure.[34] The daily TEF is determined primarily by the number of kilocalories an individual consumes—a higher intake of energy requires more energy for digestion, absorption, and metabolism. Research also suggests that TEF may be reduced in obese individuals[35] and may be reduced by irregular meal patterns.[36] It's possible to increase the TEF by altering the macronutrient composition of the diet but not by much—only about 50 kilocalories or so daily.

**Key Concepts**  *An individual's fitness level and weight and the type, duration, and intensity of activity affect the amount of energy expended in physical activity. The thermic effect of food is the energy needed to process the food we eat and is influenced by the amount and mix of nutrients in the diet.*

## Estimating Total Energy Expenditure

An adult's REE can be estimated using an abbreviated method. The 1.0 and 0.9 factors used in this method for kilocalories per kilogram reflect the differences in body composition between men and women. As previously described, men have proportionally more lean body mass and thus burn more kilocalories per kilogram of body weight. This abbreviated method dramatically underestimates children's REE, however, and somewhat overestimates the REE of elders.

The abbreviated method estimates only REE. To determine total energy expenditure (TEE), energy expended in physical activity and the thermic effect of food must be included. Energy expended in physical activity can be estimated as a percentage of REE based on a person's general activity level. (See Table 8.3.) Most adults in the United States and Canada have a light or moderate activity level. The thermic effect of food can be estimated as roughly 6 to 10 percent of the sum of REE plus energy expended in physical activity. Summing the three estimated components—REE, physical activity, and TEF—delivers the estimated total energy expenditure. See the FYI feature "How Many Calories Do I Burn?" for an example of these estimates in action.

## DRIs for Energy: Estimated Energy Requirements

Just as there are DRIs for nutrients, there are also DRIs for energy, called Estimated Energy Requirements (EERs).[37] The EER is defined as the energy intake predicted to maintain energy balance in a healthy person of normal weight. The EER equations for adults (see Table 8.4) predict TEE from age, height, weight, gender, and physical activity level. Separate equations have been developed for infants, children, and teens, and adjustments are made for pregnancy and lactation.

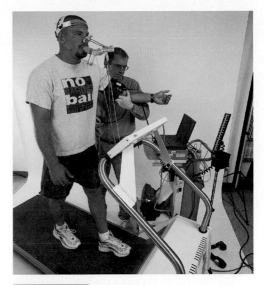

| Figure 8.6 | **Measuring energy expended in physical activity.** A |

technician can collect respiratory gases and indirectly calculate energy expenditure during exercise.

**Abbreviated Method to Estimate REE**

**For adult men**

REE = weight (kg) × 1.0 kcal/kg × 24 hr/day

REE = weight (kg) × 1.0 × 24

**For adult women**

REE = weight (kg) × 0.9 kcal/kg × 24 hr/day

REE = weight (kg) × 0.9 × 24

**nonexercise activity thermogenesis (NEAT)**  The output of energy associated with fidgeting, maintenance of posture, and other minimal physical exertions.

**thermic effect of food (TEF)**  The energy used to digest, absorb, and metabolize energy-yielding foodstuffs. It constitutes about 10 percent of total energy expenditure but is influenced by various factors.

*Quick* Bite

**The Fattest Mammals**
Among mammals, humans carry the largest percentage of weight as body fat.

| Table 8.3 | Estimating Energy Expended in Physical Activity |

| Percentage of REE | Activity Level | Description |
| --- | --- | --- |
| 20–30 | Sedentary | Mostly resting with little or no activity |
| 30–45 | Light | Occasional unplanned activity (e.g., going for a stroll) |
| 45–65 | Moderate | Daily planned activity (e.g., brisk walks) |
| 65–90 | Heavy | Daily workout routine requiring several hours of continuous exercise |
| 90–120 | Exceptional | Daly vigorous workouts for extended hours; training for competition |

**Source:** Data from Institute of Medicine, Food and Nutrition Board. *Dietary Reference Intakes for Energy, Carbohydrate, Fiber, Fat, Fatty Acids, Cholesterol, Protein, and Amino Acids (Macronutrients)*. Washington, DC: National Academies Press; 2005.

| Table 8.4 | Estimated Energy Requirements for Adults |

**Males**
$$EER = 662 - 9.53 \times age\ [yr] + PA \times (15.91 \times weight\ [kg] + 539.6 \times height\ [m])$$

| PA = | 1.0 | Sedentary |
| --- | --- | --- |
| | 1.11 | Low active |
| | 1.25 | Active |
| | 1.48 | Very active |

**Females**
$$EER = 354 - 6.91 \times age\ [yr] + PA \times (9.36 \times weight\ [kg] + 726 \times height\ [m])$$

| PA = | 1.0 | Sedentary |
| --- | --- | --- |
| | 1.12 | Low active |
| | 1.27 | Active |
| | 1.45 | Very active |

**Source:** Modified with permission from Institute of Medicine, Food and Nutrition Board. *Dietary Reference Intakes for Energy, Carbohydrate, Fiber, Fat, Fatty Acids, Cholesterol, Protein, and Amino Acids (Macronutrients)*. Copyright © 2005 by the National Academy of Sciences, courtesy of the National Academies Press, Washington, DC.

**body composition** The chemical or anatomical composition of the body. Commonly defined as the proportions of fat, muscle, bone, and other tissues in the body.

**body mass index (BMI)** Body weight (in kilograms) divided by the square of height (in meters), expressed in units of kg/m$^2$.

**To calculate BMI**

$$BMI = \frac{weight\ (kg)}{height\ (m)^2}\ , or$$

$$BMI = \frac{weight\ (lb)}{height\ (in)^2} \times 704.5.$$

# Body Composition: Understanding Fatness and Weight

Stepping onto a scale provides quick and easy feedback about your body weight. Yet many people have a distorted notion of their weight—thinking they're too fat when they aren't or thinking their weight is just fine when it isn't. In terms of your health risks, body composition is more important than body weight.

**Body composition** is the relative amount of fat and lean body mass. Excess body fatness is linked with increased risk for heart disease, hypertension, cancer, diabetes, and other chronic diseases. Two people with the same high weight and height may have very different health risks. One may be obese and have many weight-related health risks. The other could be very fit and muscular, with no increased disease risk.

## Assessing Body Weight

The **body mass index (BMI)** has become the accepted method for assessing body weight for height. This index, which is a ratio of weight to height squared, correlates reasonably well with body fatness and health risks.[38] To determine your BMI, accurately measure your height without shoes and your weight with minimal clothing. Then plug these numbers into the equation in the margin. For adults, the NHLBI (National Heart, Lung, and Blood Institute) defines **underweight**, **normal weight**, **overweight**, and **obesity** as follows:[39]

- *Underweight:* BMI < 18.5 kg/m$^2$
- *Normal weight:* 18.5 kg/m$^2$ ≤ BMI < 25 kg/m$^2$
- *Overweight:* 25 kg/m$^2$ ≤ BMI < 30 kg/m$^2$
- *Obese:* BMI ≥ 30 kg/m$^2$

Table 8.5 can help you determine whether your weight is a healthy weight according to the *Dietary Guidelines for Americans*.

As **Figure 8.7** shows, correlating BMI with mortality produces a J-shaped curve. Studies indicate that underweight (BMI less than 18.5 kg/m$^2$) is associated with increased mortality, as is obesity (BMI greater than or equal to 30 kg/m$^2$). Normal weight and overweight are not associated with excess overall mortality.[40]

Although your BMI can give you a general idea of your overall health risks, it still doesn't tell you enough about whether you are carrying muscle weight or excess fat and/or where that excess fat is (i.e., around your midsection or in your hips and thighs). A classic example is the heavy football player or bodybuilder with a large muscle mass who has a BMI greater than 30 kg/m$^2$ but is not overfat. For someone who has lost muscle mass, perhaps an older adult, BMI can underestimate health risks associated with excess body fat. BMI measurements should be interpreted cautiously when used for people who are petite, who have large body frames, or who are highly muscular.[41]

**underweight** BMI less than 18.5 kg/m$^2$.

**normal weight** BMI at or above 18.5 kg/m$^2$ and less than 25 kg/m$^2$.

**overweight** BMI at or above 25 kg/m$^2$ and less than 30 kg/m$^2$.

**obesity** BMI at or above 30 kg/m$^2$.

## *Quick* Bite

### Is Shaq Too Fat?
Although BMI has become the standard reference for determining overweight and obesity, it has limitations at the extremes of body size and composition. Consider the former NBA center, Shaquille O'Neal. At 7 feet, 1 inch, and 325 pounds, Shaq has a BMI of 32.7 kg/m$^2$—well into the range for obesity. LaDanian Tomlinson, star NFL running back, also could be considered obese based on his BMI of 31.8 kg/m$^2$ (5 feet, 10 inches, and 221 pounds)!

| Table 8.5 | **Adult BMI Chart** |
| --- | --- |

| BMI | 19 | 20 | 21 | 22 | 23 | 24 | 25 | 26 | 27 | 28 | 29 | 30 | 31 | 32 | 33 | 34 | 35 |
|---|---|---|---|---|---|---|---|---|---|---|---|---|---|---|---|---|---|
| **Height** | | | | | | | **Weight in Pounds** | | | | | | | | | | |
| 4'10" | 91 | 96 | 100 | 105 | 110 | 115 | 119 | 124 | 129 | 134 | 138 | 143 | 148 | 153 | 158 | 162 | 167 |
| 4'11" | 94 | 99 | 104 | 109 | 114 | 119 | 124 | 128 | 133 | 138 | 143 | 148 | 153 | 158 | 163 | 168 | 173 |
| 5' | 97 | 102 | 107 | 112 | 118 | 123 | 128 | 133 | 138 | 143 | 148 | 153 | 158 | 163 | 158 | 174 | 179 |
| 5'1" | 100 | 106 | 111 | 116 | 122 | 127 | 132 | 137 | 143 | 148 | 153 | 158 | 164 | 169 | 174 | 180 | 185 |
| 5'2" | 104 | 109 | 115 | 120 | 126 | 131 | 136 | 142 | 147 | 153 | 158 | 164 | 169 | 175 | 180 | 186 | 191 |
| 5'3" | 107 | 113 | 118 | 124 | 130 | 135 | 141 | 146 | 152 | 158 | 163 | 169 | 175 | 180 | 186 | 191 | 197 |
| 5'4" | 110 | 116 | 122 | 128 | 134 | 140 | 145 | 151 | 157 | 163 | 169 | 174 | 180 | 186 | 192 | 197 | 204 |
| 5'5" | 114 | 120 | 126 | 132 | 138 | 144 | 150 | 156 | 162 | 168 | 174 | 180 | 186 | 192 | 198 | 204 | 210 |
| 5'6" | 118 | 124 | 130 | 136 | 142 | 148 | 155 | 161 | 167 | 173 | 179 | 186 | 192 | 198 | 204 | 210 | 216 |
| 5'7" | 121 | 127 | 134 | 140 | 146 | 153 | 159 | 166 | 172 | 178 | 185 | 191 | 198 | 204 | 211 | 217 | 223 |
| 5'8" | 125 | 131 | 138 | 144 | 151 | 158 | 164 | 171 | 177 | 184 | 190 | 197 | 203 | 210 | 216 | 223 | 230 |
| 5'9" | 128 | 135 | 142 | 149 | 155 | 162 | 169 | 176 | 182 | 189 | 196 | 203 | 209 | 216 | 223 | 230 | 236 |
| 5'10" | 132 | 139 | 146 | 153 | 160 | 167 | 174 | 181 | 188 | 195 | 202 | 209 | 216 | 222 | 229 | 236 | 243 |
| 5'11" | 136 | 143 | 150 | 157 | 165 | 172 | 179 | 186 | 193 | 200 | 208 | 215 | 222 | 229 | 236 | 243 | 250 |
| 6' | 140 | 147 | 154 | 162 | 169 | 177 | 184 | 191 | 199 | 206 | 213 | 221 | 228 | 235 | 242 | 250 | 258 |
| 6'1" | 144 | 151 | 159 | 166 | 174 | 182 | 189 | 197 | 204 | 212 | 219 | 227 | 235 | 242 | 250 | 257 | 265 |
| 6'2" | 148 | 155 | 163 | 171 | 179 | 186 | 194 | 202 | 210 | 218 | 225 | 233 | 241 | 249 | 256 | 264 | 272 |
| 6'3" | 152 | 160 | 168 | 176 | 184 | 192 | 200 | 208 | 216 | 224 | 232 | 240 | 248 | 256 | 264 | 272 | 279 |
| | **Healthy Weight** | | | | | | **Overweight** | | | | | **Obese** | | | | | |

Locate the height of interest in the leftmost column, and read across the row for that height to the weight of interest. Follow the column of the weight up to the top row that lists the BMI. A BMI of 19 to 24 is in the healthy range, a BMI of 25 to 29 is in the overweight range, and a BMI of 30 and above is in the obese range. Due to rounding, these ranges vary slightly from the NHLBI values.

A calculator for adult BMI is available at http://www.nhlbisupport.com/bmi. A child and adolescent BMI calculator is available at http://apps.nccd.cdc.gov/dnpabmi.

**Source:** US Departments of Agriculture and Health and Human Services. *Dietary Guidelines for Americans.* 6th ed. Washington, DC: US Government Printing Office; 2005.

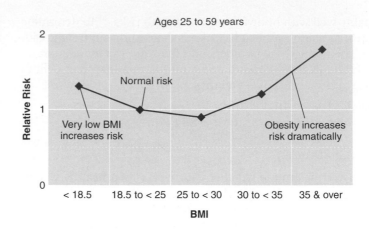

**Figure 8.7** **BMI and mortality.** People with a high or very low BMI have a higher relative risk of mortality.

**Source:** Adapted from Flegal KM, Graubard BI, Williamson DF, Gail MH. Excess deaths associated with underweight, overweight, and obesity. *JAMA*. 2005;293:1861–1867.

For children and teens, height and weight measurements can be compared to standard growth charts to see if the child is growing and gaining weight at the appropriate rate. For children and teens (2 to 20 years old), pediatric growth charts include age- and sex-specific percentile curves for BMI.[42] A BMI-for-age at or above the 95th percentile indicates overweight and the need for further evaluation and possible treatment. Further evaluation may also be indicated if the child's BMI-for-age is at or above the 85th percentile and is accompanied by other risk factors, such as high blood pressure, high blood cholesterol, diabetes, and family history of obesity-related disease.[43] A BMI-for-age below the 5th percentile suggests the child is underweight.

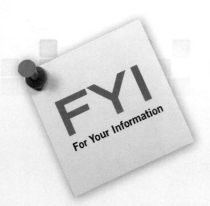

# How Many Calories Do I Burn?

You can estimate the amount of energy you use each day by using some simple equations. Remember that there will be quite a lot of individual variation in actual energy output, and so these calculated values are just estimates.

1. Convert your weight in pounds to weight in kilograms. For example, Carol is a 120-pound female. Her weight is 54.5 kilograms (54.5 = 120 ÷ 2.2).

$$\frac{\phantom{xxxxxxx}}{\text{weight (lbs)}} \div 2.2 = \frac{\phantom{xxxxxxx}}{\text{weight (kg)}}$$

2. Estimate your personal REE.

**For adult women:**

$$REE = \frac{\phantom{xxxxxx}}{\text{weight (kg)}} \times 0.9 \times 24$$

**For adult men:**

$$REE = \frac{\phantom{xxxxxx}}{\text{weight (kg)}} \times 1.0 \times 24$$

For example, Carol has an estimated REE of 1,177 kilocalories (1,177 = 54.5 × 0.9 × 24).

3. Estimate your energy expended in physical activity (see Table 8.2).

$$energy_{\text{physical activity}} = \frac{\phantom{xxxxxxx}}{\text{from Table 8.2}} \times REE$$

For example, Carol has a light to moderate physical activity level. She expends about 530 kilocalories in physical activity (530 = 0.45 × 1,177).

4. Estimate your thermic effect of food (TEF).

$$TEF = 0.1 \times \left( \frac{\phantom{xxxx}}{energy_{\text{physical activity}}} + \frac{\phantom{xx}}{REE} \right)$$

For our example, Carol's thermic effect of food is about 171 kilocalories (171 = 0.1 × [530 + 1,177]).

5. Estimate your personal total energy expenditure (TEE).

$$TEE = \frac{\phantom{xx}}{REE} + \frac{\phantom{xxxx}}{energy_{\text{physical activity}}} + \frac{\phantom{xx}}{TEF}$$

For our example, Carol's total energy expenditure is about 1,878 kilocalories (1,177 + 530 + 171).

**Key Concepts** *Body composition is a key element in determining energy expenditure and is an important factor in disease risk. Weight and height measures can be used to calculate BMI, which is correlated with body fatness and health risks. Elevated BMI in adults or children can increase health risks.*

## Assessing Body Fatness

Fat that is stored in adipose tissue that lies directly under the skin is referred to as *subcutaneous fat*, whereas fat that surrounds internal organs is called *visceral fat*. Healthy adult females typically have 20 to 35 percent of total body weight; for adult men, the typical range is 8 to 24 percent. Risk of chronic disease appears to rise when body fat exceeds these levels.

Densitometry is the measure of body density (body mass divided by body volume). Because fat and lean tissues have different densities, if we know the person's volume and weight we can calculate the ratio of fat to lean body mass. The density of fat doesn't vary, but hydration status, age, gender, and ethnicity all influence the density of lean body mass. For example, bone loss in the elderly leads to a lower density of lean body mass.

Body fatness can be assessed by a number of methods. The current "gold standard" for measuring composition and determining body fatness is dual energy x-ray absorptiometry (DXA).[44] Originally developed for the measurement of bone mineral density (to test for osteoporosis), DXA is unique in that it measures the body's mineral content (bone), fat mass, and lean body mass (protein and water). Unfortunately, the equipment is expensive and not readily available, limiting its use to research settings. Another technique frequently used in research settings is **underwater weighing**, also called **hydrostatic weighing**. Because fat is less dense than muscle, a person with more body fat will have a lower underwater weight than a person with the same body weight but less fat. The newer **BodPod** uses the same principle of density, but it measures displacement of air to determine relative amounts of fat and fat-free mass. **Figure 8.8** illustrates underwater weighing, and **Figure 8.9** shows the BodPod.

**Skinfold measurements** are a low-tech method for assessing body fatness. Special calipers are used to measure the thickness of fat deposits directly underneath the skin at several locations around the body. Done correctly, body composition estimates from skinfolds correlate well with those from underwater weighing, but an inexperienced or careless technician can easily make large errors. Skinfold measurements usually work better for assessing malnutrition than for identifying overweight and obesity.

Many health clubs and fitness centers use **bioelectrical impedance analysis (BIA)** to measure body fatness. A technician uses special equipment to pass a small electric current through the body and measure how well the body conducts electricity. Because lean tissue contains more water than fat tissue, it is a better conductor of electricity, whereas fat produces a greater "impedance." Measurements are used to determine the amounts of lean and fat mass. Unfortunately this method is readily affected by hydration status, with dehydration producing a falsely elevated impedance and overestimation of body fatness. Thus, the many factors that can impact hydration status (exercise, eating, drinking, medications, etc.) render this measure unreliable and inaccurate.

## Body Fat Distribution

Measurements of body fatness tell you more about your health risks than your weight does, but they still don't tell the whole story. Where the fat is located—**body fat distribution**—can be an independent risk factor.[45]

**underwater weighing** Determining body density by measuring the volume of water displaced when the body is fully submerged in a specialized water tank. Also called *hydrostatic weighing*.

**hydrostatic weighing** See *underwater weighing*.

**BodPod** A device used to measure the density of the body based on the volume of air displaced as a person sits in a sealed chamber of known volume.

**skinfold measurements** A method to estimate body fat by measuring the thickness of a fold of skin and subcutaneous fat.

**bioelectrical impedance analysis (BIA)** Technique to estimate amounts of total body water, lean tissue mass, and total body fat. It uses the resistance of tissue to the flow of an alternating electric current.

**body fat distribution** The pattern of fat distribution on the body.

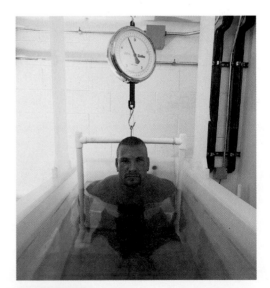

**Figure 8.8** **Underwater weighing.** During underwater weighing, the subject must exhale completely, submerge without taking a breath, and remain motionless until the water is still and the scale is steady.

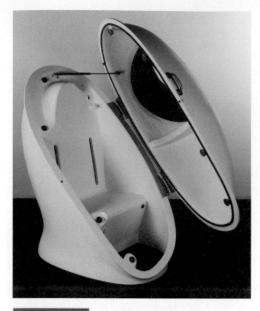

| Figure 8.9 | **BodPod.** By using air displacement, the BodPod provides |

an alternative to underwater weighing that is easier, cheaper, and of similar accuracy.

**gynoid obesity** Excess storage of fat located primarily in the buttocks and thighs. Also called *gynecoid obesity*.

**android obesity [AN-droyd]** Excess storage of fat located primarily in the abdominal area.

**waist circumference** The waist measurement, as a marker of abdominal fat content, can be used to indicate health risks.

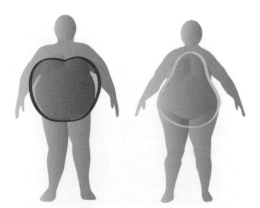

| Figure 8.10 | **Differences in body fat distribution.** Men tend to carry |

excess fat around their abdomen (android obesity). Women tend to accumulate excess fat in their hips and thighs (gynoid obesity).

The "pear shape," or **gynoid obesity**, which is more common in women, has fat distributed predominantly around the hips and thighs. The "apple shape," or **android obesity**, typical of men, has extra fat distributed higher up, around the abdomen. You are at greater health risk with the apple pattern than with the pear pattern of fat distribution. In fact, excess abdominal fat may increase breast cancer risk for women.[46] **Figure 8.10** shows the gynoid and android distributions of body fat.

If your **waist circumference** increases, you are probably gaining abdominal fat. National Institutes of Health (NIH) clinical guidelines suggest that for people with a BMI of 25 kg/m² to 34.9 kg/m², a waist circumference greater than 40 inches (102 centimeters) in men or greater than 35 inches (88 centimeters) in women is a sign of increased health risk. When BMI is 35 kg/m² or higher, waist circumference measures do not accurately predict health risks. Combining measures of BMI and waist circumference is more predictive of cardiovascular disease risk than either measure alone.[47]

**Key Concepts** *Excess body fatness is associated with increased risk for chronic diseases, including heart disease and diabetes. Researchers use a number of different methods to assess body fatness. Skinfold measurements are better suited for assessing malnutrition than for detecting excess fat. Distribution of body fat is important in evaluating the risk of disease. Excess body fat around the abdomen (even with normal to slightly elevated BMI) is associated with higher disease risk than is excess fat around the hips and thighs. Waist circumference can be used to assess body fat distribution.*

## Overweight and Obesity

Obesity has become a global problem[48] and has emerged as the most important contributor to ill health, displacing undernutrition and infectious diseases.[49] Not only is obesity prevalent in Europe and the Americas,[50] but it also is on the rise in Southeast Asia, where Japan and China have seen a marked increase. In North Africa, about 39 percent of women in Morocco and Tunisia are overweight or obese,[51] and, in the Middle East, the United Arab Emirates now recognizes obesity as a major public health problem.[52]

In the United States, the prevalence of overweight and obesity has increased dramatically over the past three decades, jumping from 47 percent of the adult population to over 65 percent![53] Moreover, much of this increase is attributed to an increase in the number of individuals who are obese (vs. just overweight). Perhaps most disconcerting is the rapidly increasing prevalence of overweight and obesity among America's youth. Nearly one of six children and teens (ages 6 to 19) are overweight (double the rate from 20 years earlier), and a similar number are at risk of becoming overweight.[54] This escalating problem is blamed on overconsumption of energy-dense foods, along with decreased physical activity. The goal of *Healthy People 2020* is to reduce the proportion of adults, adolescents, and children who are obese by 10 percent.[55]

As overweight and obesity have increased, so has society's emphasis on thinness, as well as efforts at weight management. Every year, the diet industry rakes in more than $60 billion from weight-loss programs, diet books, pills, videos, and supplements.[56] Various reports and surveys reveal that 33 to 55 percent of U.S. adults are trying to lose weight.[57] Children and adolescents also are concerned about weight. In studies of grade-school girls from various socioeconomic backgrounds, 68 percent reported that they have attempted to lose weight because they very often worried about being fat.[58] Attempts to lose weight can be very costly and offer virtually no long-term assurance of keeping the weight off. Reports suggest that approximately 80 percent of

THINK About It

2

people who intentionally lose weight regain the weight and that 50 percent of the weight is regained within the first year.[59]

**Key Concepts** *Worldwide, the number of overweight or obese people has increased markedly in recent years. The rising rates among children are especially disturbing. At the same time, more people are engaging in weight-control efforts and starting to do so at younger ages.*

## Factors in the Development of Obesity

At its simplest, obesity results from a chronic positive energy balance—energy intake regularly exceeds energy expenditure, and weight is gained. But, although the cause of weight gain may be simple, the factors that contribute to the energy imbalance are highly complex. As we learn more about the factors that regulate feeding behavior and energy metabolism, scientists are beginning to unravel the specific mechanisms at work and, from there, to determine what may go wrong in people who are obese. The reality is that obesity is a complex disorder that probably involves several regulatory mechanisms and the way they interact and respond to biological factors, such as heredity, age, and sex; social and environmental factors; and behavior and lifestyle choices.[60]

### Biological Factors

Genetics researchers have long recognized heredity patterns of obesity. For example, when both parents are morbidly obese (body weight 100 percent above normal), the probability that their children will be obese is high (80 percent); when neither parent is obese, the probability that their children will be obese is relatively low (less than 10 percent). One might question then whether this is truly evidence of a genetic predisposition or simply the influence of family lifestyle and, thus, more related to environment. The answer is probably both.[61] Studies using monozygotic (identical) and dizygotic (fraternal) twins confirm that gene–environment interactions do impact energy balance.[62] Researchers estimate that genes alone generally account for 50 to 90 percent of variations in the amount of stored body fat.[63]

**Fat Cell Development** The number and size of fat cells in the body help determine how easily a person gains or loses fat. People with **hypercellular obesity**, an above-average number of fat cells, may have been born with them or may have developed them at certain "critical times" in their lives because of overeating. In **hypertrophic obesity**, fat cells are larger than normal. Fat cells continue to expand as they fill with more fat; when their capacity is reached, the body generates more cells. (See **Figure 8.11**.) Once body fat reaches three to five times the normal amount, fat tissue is likely to have both bigger fat cells and more of them, a condition called **hyperplastic obesity** (hyperplasia).

Even with weight loss, the number of fat cells does not decline (though presumably some could be removed by liposuction). Fat cells do become smaller, but beyond a certain point they resist further shrinking and the body strives to refill them with fat, making it difficult to maintain weight loss.

**Sex and Age** The prevalence of obesity among men and women in the United States is similar: 33.8 percent of men are obese and 35.5 percent of women are obese.[64] Despite the similarities in obesity statistics, men and women seem to set different weight standards for themselves. Beginning in grade school, boys are less likely than girls to consider themselves overweight; in fact, males of all ages accept some degree of overweight. Boys typically are

*Quick* Bite

**Island Obesity**
Some of the most obese people in the world live in the islands of Micronesia. Among these populations, the Naurus are the most obese.

**hypercellular obesity** Obesity due to an above-average number of fat cells.

**hypertrophic obesity** Obesity due to an increase in the size of fat cells.

**hyperplastic obesity (hyperplasia)** Obesity due to an increase in both the size and number of fat cells.

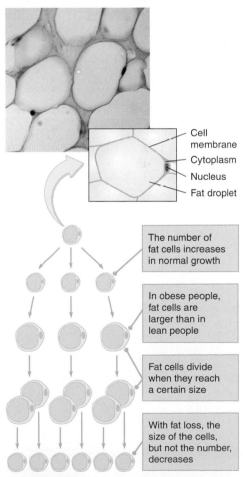

- Cell membrane
- Cytoplasm
- Nucleus
- Fat droplet

The number of fat cells increases in normal growth

In obese people, fat cells are larger than in lean people

Fat cells divide when they reach a certain size

With fat loss, the size of the cells, but not the number, decreases

**Figure 8.11** **The formation of fat cells.** As body fat accumulates, fat cells enlarge and divide. Fat loss reduces the size of fat cells but not their number.

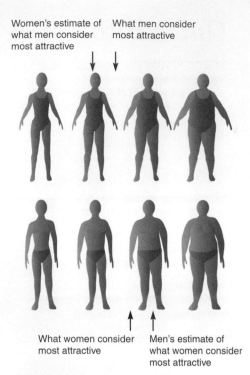

Women's estimate of
what men consider
most attractive

What men consider
most attractive

What women consider
most attractive

Men's estimate of
what women consider
most attractive

**Figure 8.12** **What men and women consider attractive.** Compared with men, women perceive slimmer shapes to be more attractive.

**Source:** Data from Bully P, Elosua P. Changes in body dissatisfaction relative to gender and age: the modulating character of BMI. *Span J Psychol.* 2011;14(1):313–322.

more concerned about becoming taller and more muscular. As adolescents and young adults, most of us worry about body weight and appearance. A survey of dietetics majors aspiring to become registered dietitians, for example, found that most dieters in this group wanted to lose weight to improve appearance and increase self-esteem.[65]

By early adulthood, about the same number of men want to lose or gain weight, whereas almost all women want to lose weight. As adults, males tend to see themselves as overweight at higher weights, whereas females describe themselves as overweight when they are closer to a healthy body weight. (See **Figure 8.12**.) Adult women feel thin only when they weigh less than 90 percent of desirable body weight, whereas men rate themselves as thin even when they are above a healthy body weight.[66]

As we age, we become more concerned with our weight as it relates to health. Both men and women gain the most weight between 25 and 34 years of age. After that, we gain weight more slowly and then start to lose it after we reach age 55.[67] However, it's often important for seniors to maintain weight.

**Race and Ethnicity** In the United States, the prevalence of obesity and attitudes about weight differ among racial and ethnic groups. Black and Hispanic women are more likely to be overweight than white women.[68] Rates of overweight are similar for black, Hispanic, and white men. Because of cultural factors, African Americans, Hispanic Americans, Native Americans, and Pacific Islanders typically value thinness less than white Americans do.[69]

### Social and Environmental Factors

**Socioeconomic Status** Americans are more likely to be obese if they have low socioeconomic status, and the stigma of obesity can impede their upward mobility. For people living with lower social economic status, food insecurity has been associated with being overweight or obese, especially among women.[70] The relationship of obesity and food insecurity may be related to the low cost of energy-dense foods and reinforced by the satisfying taste of sugar and fat; however, food-insecure women do not seem to consume more high-fat, high-sugar, empty-calorie foods than their food-secure counterparts.[71] Periods of overeating when food is available, including binge-like patterns of eating or changes in eating habits that promote a metabolic-adaptive response, also may account for overweight and obesity among adults from food-insecure households.[72] The trend in increased childhood obesity can be seen in low-income preschool-age children as well. Approximately one in seven low-income, preschool-aged children is obese.[73]

Where you live also may affect your weight. Rural women tend to be heavier than women living in metropolitan areas, and Southern women are the most likely to be overweight.[74] Among the U.S. states, the prevalence of adult obesity in 2010 ranged from 21 percent in Colorado to 34 percent in Mississippi.[75] A total of 36 states had a prevalence of obesity greater than or equal to 25 percent, and 12 of those states had a prevalence of obesity greater than 30 percent. All states continued to have high obesity rates, and no state met the *Healthy People 2010* target of 15 percent. In fact, none were below 20 percent. (See the FYI feature "U.S. Obesity Trends: 1985 to 2010" for more information.)

Some studies suggest that employed women are thinner than those not in the labor force.[76] Changing jobs, losing a job, or retiring often changes eating patterns and subsequently body weight as well.

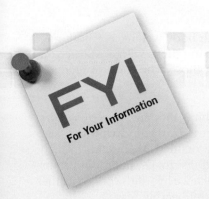

# U.S. Obesity Trends: 1985 to 2010

During the past 20 years, there has been a dramatic increase in obesity in the United States, and rates remain high. The maps in **Figures A** and **B** illustrate this trend by showing the increased prevalence of obesity across each of the states. In 2010, no state had a prevalence of obesity less than 20 percent. Thirty-six states had a prevalence of 25 percent or more; 12 of these states (Alabama, Arkansas, Kentucky, Louisiana, Michigan, Mississippi, Missouri, Oklahoma, South Carolina, Tennessee, Texas, and West Virginia) had a prevalence of 30 percent or more (see Table A). Refer to the following website for a complete slide show of each year during this time period: http://www.cdc.gov/obesity/data/trends.html.

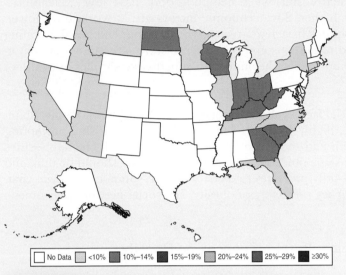

No Data | <10% | 10%–14% | 15%–19% | 20%–24% | 25%–29% | ≥30%

**Figure A**  Percentage of obesity (BMI ≥ 30) in U.S. adults, 1985.

**Source:** Centers for Disease Control and Prevention. Overweight and obesity: data and statistics. Trends by state, 1985–2010. http://www.cdc.gov/obesity/data/trends.html. Accessed 11/24/11.

**Table A**  ### 2010 State Obesity Rates

| State | Percent | State | Percent |
|---|---|---|---|
| Alabama | 32.2 | Illinois | 28.2 |
| Alaska | 24.5 | Indiana | 29.6 |
| Arizona | 24.3 | Iowa | 28.4 |
| Arkansas | 30.1 | Kansas | 29.4 |
| California | 24.0 | Kentucky | 31.3 |
| Colorado | 21.0 | Louisiana | 31.0 |
| Connecticut | 22.5 | Maine | 26.8 |
| Delaware | 28.0 | Maryland | 27.1 |
| District of Columbia | 22.2 | Massachusetts | 23.0 |
| Florida | 26.6 | Michigan | 30.9 |
| Georgia | 29.6 | Minnesota | 24.8 |
| Hawaii | 22.7 | Mississippi | 34.0 |
| Idaho | 26.5 | Missouri | 30.5 |
| Montana | 23.0 | Rhode Island | 25.5 |
| Nebraska | 26.9 | South Carolina | 31.5 |
| Nevada | 22.4 | South Dakota | 27.3 |
| New Hampshire | 25.0 | Tennessee | 30.8 |
| New Jersey | 23.8 | Texas | 31.0 |
| New Mexico | 25.1 | Utah | 22.5 |
| New York | 23.9 | Vermont | 23.2 |
| North Carolina | 27.8 | Virginia | 26.0 |
| North Dakota | 27.2 | Washington | 25.5 |
| Ohio | 29.2 | West Virginia | 32.5 |
| Oklahoma | 30.4 | Wisconsin | 26.3 |
| Oregon | 26.8 | Wyoming | 25.1 |
| Pennsylvania | 28.6 | | |

**Source:** Centers for Disease Control and Prevention. Overweight and obesity: data and statistics. Trends by state, 1985–2010. http://www.cdc.gov/obesity/data/trends.html. Accessed 11/24/11.

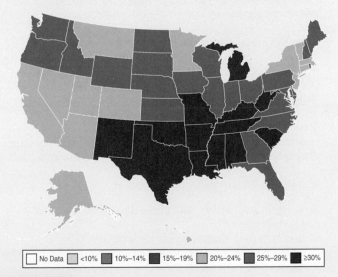

No Data | <10% | 10%–14% | 15%–19% | 20%–24% | 25%–29% | ≥30%

**Figure B**  Percentage of obesity (BMI ≥ 30) in U.S. adults, 2010.

**Source:** Centers for Disease Control and Prevention. Overweight and obesity: data and statistics. Trends by state, 1985–2010. http://www.cdc.gov/obesity/data/trends.html. Accessed 11/24/11.

**built environment** Any human-formed, developed, or structured areas, including the urban environment that consists of buildings, roads, fixtures, parks, and all other human developments that form its physical character.

Education is another factor associated with body weight. For both men and women, obesity prevalence was lowest among those with a college education; overall, prevalence was highest among those who did not graduate from high school.[77]

**The Built Environment**  Our immediate surroundings influence our behaviors, and researchers have begun to link aspects of the **built environment** with obesity. The built environment, which can be defined as "human formed, developed, or structured areas," includes buildings, roads, parks, and transportation systems.[78] These environments in which we live and work can either encourage or hinder physical activity and healthful eating.[79]

People who live in neighborhoods with sidewalks and safe streets are more physically active. But, when neighborhoods have low "walkability," BMIs tend to be higher. Socioeconomic factors are at work, too—lower-income neighborhoods have fewer recreational facilities and healthful eating options. Fast-food restaurants and convenience stores are more prevalent in low-income neighborhoods; the number of supermarkets triples in wealthier neighborhoods.[80]

**Social Factors**  Social factors also influence the development of obesity. Abundant high-calorie, highly palatable foods, pervasive advertising promoting their consumption, and the social enjoyment of eating all create pressures to overeat. At the same time, our culture tells us that we should be thin, and we may feel unhealthy pressures to diet. Table 8.6 summarizes social characteristics that are key predictors of obesity. The social network phenomena

| Table 8.6 | **Sociocultural Influences on Obesity** |

| *Social Contexts* | |
|---|---|
| Culture | People in developed societies have more body fat than those in developing societies. |
| History | Fatness is increasing in the United States, but idealized weights are decreasing. |
| *Social Characteristics* | |
| Age and lifestyle | Fatness increases during adulthood and declines in older adults. |
| Gender | Obesity is more prevalent in women than in men. |
| Race and ethnicity | Obesity is more prevalent in African American, Hispanic, Native American, and Pacific Islander women. |
| *Socioeconomic Status* | |
| Income | Obesity is more prevalent in lower-income women. |
| Education | Less-educated women have a higher incidence of obesity. |
| Occupational prestige | Obesity is more prevalent in women in less prestigious jobs. |
| Employment | Women who are unemployed have a higher incidence of obesity. |
| Household composition | Older adults who live with others have a higher incidence of obesity. |
| Marriage | Married men have a higher incidence of obesity. |
| Residence | Rural women have a higher incidence of obesity. |
| Region | People residing in the South have a higher incidence of obesity. |

**Source:** Adapted from Dalton S. Body weight terminology, definitions, and measurements. In: Dalton S, ed. *Overweight and Weight Management: The Health Professional's Guide to Understanding and Practice.* Gaithersburg, MD: Aspen; 1997:314.

is larger among females and adolescents with high body mass index.[82] There is consistent evidence that school friends are significantly similar in terms of their body mass index, and friends with the highest body mass index appear to be most similar. Frequency of fast-food consumption has also been found to cluster within groups of boys, as have body image concerns, dieting, and eating disorder among girls.[83] School friends may be critical in shaping young people's eating behaviors and bodyweight, thus suggesting the potential of social network–based health promotion interventions in schools.[84]

### Lifestyle and Behavior Factors

**Physical Activity**  Lack of exercise is a major contributing factor to weight gain and obesity. Reports from the Centers for Disease Control and Prevention indicate that, in 2009, 55 percent of adults never participated in any type of vigorous leisure-time physical activity.[85] Inactivity is more common among women, older adults, less affluent adults, and black and Hispanic adults.[86] Children are also getting less exercise. In both children and adults, research links excessive television viewing and computer use to overweight and obesity.[87] For all ages, obesity itself may lead to physical inactivity, although the strength of this relationship is unclear.

**Psychological Factors**  Some people adopt eating as a strategy for dealing with the stresses and challenges of life. (Others use drugs, alcohol, smoking, shopping, gambling, and so on.) Eating also can provide entertainment and alleviate boredom. Some people use eating as a pick-me-up when fatigued, and some use eating to distract themselves from difficult problems or as a means of punishing themselves or others for real or imagined transgressions.

Certain obese people may be more prone to emotional eating than others. These subgroups include **restrained eaters** and **binge eaters**.[88] Restrained eaters try to reduce their calorie intake by fasting or avoiding food as long as possible. They skip meals, delay eating, or severely restrict the types of food they eat. Then, like a dam that bursts, they overeat when environmental or emotional stress triggers a complete release of inhibitions toward eating. Although not all obese binge eaters follow this pattern, the "fast, then binge" behavior is common in obese people who chronically attempt to lose weight.[89] This pattern also occurs in women of normal weight who perceive themselves as fat. These restrained eating patterns appear to be passed on from mother to daughter.[90] In adolescents, dieting predicts binge eating, decreased physical activity, decreased breakfast consumption, and is also associated with increased BMI.[91] Therefore, in part, dieting during adolescence may lead to weight gain.

People with a healthy lifestyle have more effective ways to meet their needs. They communicate assertively and manage interpersonal conflict effectively, so they don't shrink from problems or overreact. The person with a healthy lifestyle knows how to create and maintain relationships with others and has a solid network of friends and loved ones. Food is used appropriately—to fuel life's activities and gain personal satisfaction, not to manage stress.

**Key Concepts**  *Obesity tends to run in families. Sex, age, and environmental factors such as socioeconomic status and employment status are related to weight. Lifestyle choices and behavioral factors also affect weight. Overly restrained eating may result in episodes of overeating and weight gain. Binge eating is common among people in weight-loss programs.*

**restrained eaters**  Individuals who routinely avoid food as long as possible, and then gorge on food.

**binge eaters**  Individuals who routinely consume a very large amount of food in a brief period of time (e.g., two hours) and lose control over how much and what is eaten.

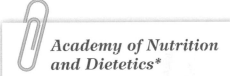

*Academy of Nutrition and Dietetics\**

**The Role of Dietetics Professionals in Health Promotion and Disease Prevention**

It is the position of the American Dietetic Association that primary prevention is the most effective, affordable course of action for preventing and reducing risk for chronic disease. Registered dietitians and dietetic technicians, registered, are leaders in delivering preventive services in both clinical and community settings, including advocating for funding and inclusion of these services in programs and policy initiatives at local, state, and federal levels. In addition, registered dietitians are leaders in facilitating and participating in research in chronic disease prevention and health promotion.

**Source:** Reproduced from Stitzel KF. Position of the Academy of Nutrition and Dietetics: the roles of registered dietitians and dietetic technicians registered in health promotion and disease promotion. *J Am Diet Assoc.* 2006;106(11):1875–1884.

\* Formerly the American Dietetic Association

## Health Risks of Overweight and Obesity

Overweight and obesity are major public health challenges. Obese people are at higher risk for heart disease, the leading cause of death in the United States and Canada, and for stroke, diabetes, hypertension, metabolic syndrome, some forms of cancer, gallbladder and joint diseases,[92] and psychosocial problems. The longer obesity persists, the higher the risks. Table 8.7 lists the effects that excess weight could have on your health. Scientists speculate that rising rates of obesity will soon reverse the increases in life expectancy that occurred throughout the twentieth century as a result of improved living conditions, advances in public health, and medical interventions.[93] The costs of obesity-related diseases are staggering. In the United States and Canada, estimates for the total economic cost of overweight and obesity was approximately $300 million for 2009. These costs included excess mortality, disability, and medical costs.[94]

The blood lipid levels that typically accompany obesity—high serum triglycerides, low HDL, and a high LDL/HDL ratio—increase the risk for atherosclerosis.[95] A person who is only mildly to moderately obese has an elevated risk of coronary heart disease. However, even modest weight loss (about 10 percent of body weight) reduces risk.

Type 2 diabetes, the most common form of diabetes in the United States and Canada, is three times more likely to develop in people who are obese, especially if they have abdominal ("apple") obesity. Obesity increases insulin

---

**Table 8.7    What Are the Risks of Being Overweight?**

**Hypertension**
Overweight people are more likely to have high blood pressure, a major risk factor for heart disease and stroke, than people who are not overweight.

**Heart Disease and Stroke**
Hypertension and very high blood levels of cholesterol and triglycerides (blood fats) can lead to heart disease and often are linked to being overweight. Being overweight also contributes to angina (chest pain caused by decreased oxygen to the heart) and sudden death from heart disease or stroke without any signs or symptoms.

**Diabetes**
Overweight people are twice as likely to develop type 2 diabetes as people who are not overweight. Type 2 diabetes is a major cause of early death, heart disease, kidney disease, stroke, and blindness.

**Cancer**
Several types of cancer are associated with being overweight. In women, these include cancer of the uterus, gallbladder, cervix, ovary, breast, and colon. Overweight men are at greater risk for developing cancer of the colon, rectum, and prostate. For some types of cancer, such as colon or breast, it is not clear whether the increased risk is due to the extra weight or a high-fat and high-calorie diet.

**Sleep Apnea**
Sleep apnea is a serious condition that is closely associated with being overweight. Sleep apnea can cause a person to stop breathing for short periods during sleep and to snore heavily. Sleep apnea may cause daytime sleepiness and even heart failure. The risk for sleep apnea increases with higher body weights. Weight loss usually improves sleep apnea.

**Osteoarthritis**
Extra weight appears to increase the risk of osteoarthritis by placing extra pressure on weight-bearing joints and wearing away the cartilage (tissue that cushions the joints) that normally protects them. Weight loss can decrease stress on the knees, hips, and lower back and may improve the symptoms of osteoarthritis.

**Gout**
Gout is a joint disease caused by high levels of uric acid in the blood. Uric acid sometimes forms into solid stone or crystal masses that become deposited in the joints. Gout is more common in overweight people, and the risk of developing the disorder increases with higher body weights. *Note:* Over the short term, some weight-loss diets may lead to an attack of gout in people who have high levels of uric acid or who have had gout before. People who have a history of gout should check with their doctors or other health professionals before trying to lose weight.

**Gallbladder Disease**
Gallbladder disease and gallstones are more common if you are overweight. Your risk of disease increases as your weight increases. It is not clear how being overweight may cause gallbladder disease. Weight loss itself, particularly rapid weight loss or loss of a large amount of weight, can actually increase your chances of developing gallstones. Modest, slow weight loss of about one pound a week is less likely to cause gallstones.

Source: NIH Publication No. 98-4098; May 1998.

resistance and compromises the ability of body cells to take up glucose. Diabetes, in turn, is a risk factor for heart disease, kidney disease, and vascular problems. Again, even modest levels of weight reduction can improve glucose tolerance.[96]

Overweight people are two to six times more likely to develop hypertension,[97] probably due to increased resistance in the peripheral blood vessels, changes in the way the kidneys handle sodium, and other changes in kidney function. Weight loss lowers blood pressure in overweight people with hypertension.

Metabolic syndrome has become increasingly common and is linked to the rising incidence of obesity.[98] Metabolic syndrome is characterized by the combination of three or more metabolic risk factors that include elevated triglycerides, low levels of HDL ("good") cholesterol, elevated blood pressure, insulin resistance, and abdominal obesity. Although the exact reason is unknown, obesity also appears to increase the risk of certain types of cancer. The same food pattern that contributes to obesity (a diet high in calories and fat as well as low in fiber, fruits, and vegetables) also may be a cancer risk. Inactivity not only encourages obesity but also increases cancer risk. For example, women who are physically active have a lower risk of breast cancer than sedentary women.[99] People who are obese have increased levels of hormones that influence development of some cancers. Obese women, for example, have more endometrial, gallbladder, cervical, and ovarian cancers than their lean counterparts.[100]

Obese people are more likely to have obstructive **sleep apnea**, in which the airway collapses during sleep and breathing stops for a short spell. As the body struggles for air, blood pressure spikes upward. Typically, the individual wakes up, gasps for air, begins breathing again, and then falls asleep until the airway collapses again and the cycle repeats. This pattern not only interrupts and prevents a good night's sleep, it also increases the risk of heart attack and stroke. Modest weight loss can alleviate sleep apnea, improve sleep quality, and reduce daytime drowsiness.[101]

### Weight Cycling

**Weight cycling**, also known as *yo-yo dieting*, is a pattern of losing and regaining weight, over and over again. In national surveys, approximately 10 to 40 percent of adult women have a history of weight cycling.[102] The pattern of weight cycling often results when a person has success with rapid weight loss but regains the weight. This up-and-down pattern of weight changes over time has negative effects on health risks, body composition, body fat distribution, and energy expenditure.[103] In addition, weight cycling has been associated with increased risk for metabolic syndrome, coronary heart disease, all-cause mortality, and with reduced quality of life, even if BMI is at a healthy range.[104] Obese individuals with large fluctuations in body weight have greater taste preference for sugar and fat and are prone to future weight gain.[105]

**Key Concepts** *Obesity is a risk factor for many chronic diseases, including heart disease, cancer, hypertension, and diabetes. In many cases, a modest amount of weight loss (about 10 percent) can improve symptoms and disease management.*

## Weight Management

Each person has a unique set of interrelated factors that lead to weight gain. Approaches to weight management are just as complex, and, to be effective, they must be tailored to the individual. As you continue reading, keep in mind the following definition of **weight management** from the Academy

**sleep apnea** Periods of absence of breathing during sleep.

**weight cycling** Repeated periods of gaining and losing weight. Also called *yo-yo dieting*.

**weight management** The adoption of healthful and sustainable eating and exercise behaviors that reduce disease risk and improve well-being.

of Nutrition and Dietetics (note that there is no mention of weight loss or ideal weight):

> Weight management is the adoption of healthful and sustainable eating and exercise behaviors indicated for reduced disease risk and improved feelings of energy and well-being.[106]

## The Perception of Weight

The weights of celebrity models often mold popular notions about desirable weight. In the early 1960s, as today, thin was "in." At that time, the trendsetter was supermodel Twiggy, who, at 5 feet 7 inches, weighed only 98 pounds; her BMI was a mere 15.4 kg/m$^2$. Since then, the number of diet and exercise articles in women's magazines has escalated, and diet books have become bestsellers. Dieting has become an institution with its own magazines, television shows, camps and resorts, and weight-loss gurus. The images in **Figure 8.13** show that beauty has not always been associated with thinness.

Despite obesity's link to health risks, a backlash against dieting has emerged. The antidiet advocates' rallying cry is "Diets don't work!" While acknowledging that severe obesity is dangerous, they argue for size acceptance and challenge the notion that mild obesity is unhealthful. In fact, data from the Centers for Disease Control and Prevention show that people who are overweight (BMI 25 to 30 kg/m$^2$) had no higher risk of mortality than people of normal weight.[107]

Health professionals now treat obesity as a complex disorder with multiple contributing factors. (See **Figure 8.14**.) They emphasize overall health and fitness rather than a number on the bathroom scale. Dietary recommendations emphasize moderation and a balanced diet that is low in fat and high in healthful foods such as fruits, vegetables, and whole grains. Behavior change is still an important part of weight management, but change is seen as an ongoing process that requires new skills for maintaining a healthy lifestyle over the

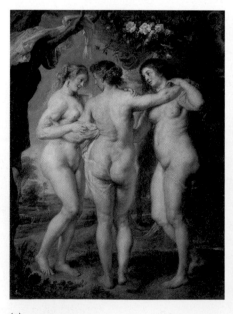

(a)

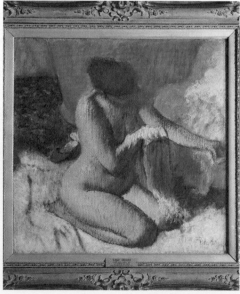

(b)

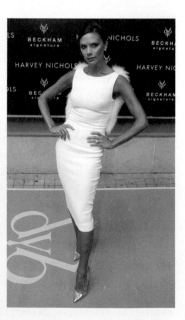

(c)

**Figure 8.13**   **Society's changing standards of beauty.** Over time, society has increasingly valued thinness. (a) Ruben's The Three Graces, 1639. (b) Degas's After the Bath, 1896. (c) Victoria Beckham, 2008.

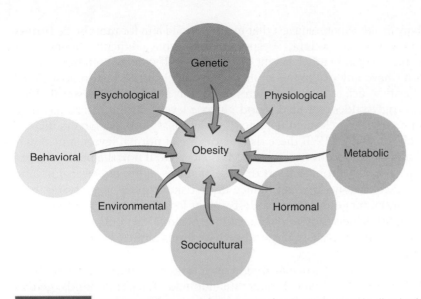

**Figure 8.14**   **Multiple factors contribute to obesity.** Obesity is a complex disorder that is not easy to treat.

long run. Although vigorous exercise isn't required, substantial increases in moderate exercise are needed for long-term weight management, and physical activity appears to be crucial in the prevention of weight regain.[108]

There are limitations as to what each of us can look like or what we can weigh. Although we shouldn't abandon efforts to achieve good health, we should balance our desire to lose weight with self-acceptance. If we engage in futile attempts to achieve an "ideal" body shape and weight, we may undermine our self-esteem and be harmed emotionally or even physically.

**Key Concepts** *Many factors contribute to the complex disorder of obesity. Currently, experts suggest that the best way to manage weight is to improve health by establishing healthful eating and exercise patterns and accepting the limitations of heredity.*

## What Goals Should I Set?

What are reasonable goals for weight management? Key recommendations of the *Dietary Guidelines for Americans, 2010* suggest targeting the following behavior changes to manage body weight:

1. Prevent and /or reduce overweight and obesity through improved eating and physical behavior.
2. Control total calorie intake to manage body weight.
3. Increase physical activity and reduce time spent in sedentary behaviors.
4. Maintain appropriate calorie balance during each stage of life.[109]

If you are overweight, it doesn't take major weight loss to improve health; a modest weight loss of roughly 10 percent of initial body weight (e.g., a 20-pound weight loss if you weighed 200 pounds) is enough to produce health benefits and perhaps to encourage continued success. A key initial goal is to prevent or stop weight gain. An estimated 100 kilocalories per day change in energy balance (produced by any combination of decreases in energy intake and increases in energy expenditure) could theoretically prevent weight gain in 90 percent of the U.S. adult population.[110] Goals must be realistic and attainable. (See **Figure 8.15**.)

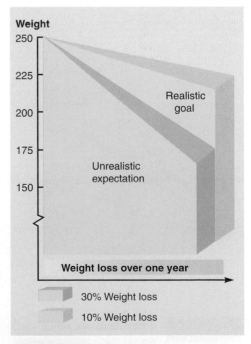

**Figure 8.15**   **Expectations and reasonable weight goals.** People who establish moderate rather than aggressive goals are more likely to succeed in their weight-loss program.

**metabolic fitness** The absence of all metabolic and biochemical risk factors associated with obesity.

Many health experts suggest that people should aim for **metabolic fitness** rather than a specific weight,[111] especially if they have difficulty achieving or maintaining recommended weight or BMI levels. If you are metabolically fit, you don't have any of the metabolic or biochemical risk factors associated with obesity—such as high cholesterol (especially low HDL cholesterol), high levels of triglycerides, elevated blood glucose levels, insulin resistance, high blood pressure, and elevated fatty acids synthesis. Other risk factors include excess abdominal fat.[112] If these risk factors are at normal levels, a person is considered metabolically fit, even if BMI is elevated. If not, the person has an increased risk for coronary heart disease, diabetes, gout, hypertension, and associated conditions. You can reduce these risk factors or even bring them within normal ranges through modest weight loss (5 to 10 percent of initial body weight) achieved by a low-fat, reduced-calorie diet and an increase in physical activity. Increasing physical activity levels alone can improve metabolic fitness.[113]

THINK
About It
**3**

Don't focus on a particular weight as your goal. Instead, focus on living a lifestyle that includes eating moderate amounts of healthful foods, getting plenty of exercise, thinking positively, and learning to cope with stress. Learn to use your body's hunger and satiation signals to regulate eating and then let the pounds fall where they may. Most people who follow this advice will approach the healthy BMI ranges discussed earlier. Some will still weigh more than societal standards call for—but their weight will be right for them. By letting a healthy lifestyle determine your weight, you can avoid developing unhealthy patterns of eating and a negative body image.

THINK
About It
**4**

## Adopting a Healthy Weight-Management Lifestyle

Most weight problems are lifestyle problems. Even though more and more young people are developing weight problems, most arrive at early adulthood with the advantage of having a "normal" body weight—neither too fat nor too thin. In fact, many young adults get away with terrible eating and exercise habits and don't develop a weight problem. But as the rapid growth of adolescence slows and family and career obligations increase, maintaining a healthy weight becomes a greater challenge. If you develop a lifestyle for successful weight management during early adulthood, healthy behavior patterns have a better chance of taking firm hold.

Permanent weight management is not something you start and stop. You need to adopt healthy behaviors that you can maintain throughout your life. People who have long-term success share common behavioral strategies that include eating a diet low in fat, frequent self-monitoring of body weight and food intake, and high levels of regular physical activity.[114] To maintain your weight over the long term, focus on healthy behaviors and develop coping strategies to deal with the stresses and challenges in your life. **Figure 8.16** shows the necessary components of an effective weight-management program.

**Key Concepts**  *Healthy weight management means focusing on metabolic fitness—healthy levels of blood lipids and blood pressure—rather than on achieving a specific weight. Permanent healthy behaviors are necessary for a long-term weight-management lifestyle.*

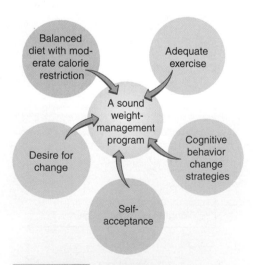

Figure 8.16    **Components of a sound weight-management program.**
Recognizing the need for change, establishing reasonable goals, adopting goal-directed activities and self-monitoring, and rewarding goal attainment can help successfully implement the components of a sound weight-management program.

## Diet and Eating Habits

In contrast to "dieting," which involves some form of food restriction, "diet" refers to your daily food choices. Everyone has a diet, but not everyone is dieting. You need to develop a balanced diet of moderate caloric intake that includes foods you enjoy and that enables you to maintain a healthy body composition.

### Total Calories

If you want to lose weight, you must take in fewer calories than you expend. Over the long term, you are more likely to control your weight successfully by cutting 200 to 300 kilocalories per day rather than drastically restricting your diet to only 1,000 to 1,200 kilocalories per day. Simply eliminating one can of regular soda from your daily routine would reduce your energy intake by about 150 kilocalories. Eating a half-serving of fries instead of a whole serving would save another 100 kilocalories. You don't need to make major diet changes; just make small, sustainable changes and focus on the balance of food groups suggested by MyPlate. The MyPlate website has interactive tools (http://www.choosemyplate.gov/tools.html) that can help you evaluate your intake and find small changes you can make.

Overconsumption of total calories is closely tied to portion sizes. Most of us significantly underestimate the amount of food we eat. Limiting portion sizes to those recommended in MyPlate is critical for weight management. You'll probably find it easier to monitor and manage your total food intake if you concentrate on portion sizes rather than counting calories.

### Crash Diets Don't Work

Don't go on a "crash diet" that contains only minimal calories. You need to consume enough food to meet your need for essential nutrients. Once you lose weight, you probably won't maintain it unless you continue some degree of calorie restriction, so it is important that you adopt a level of food intake that you can live with. A highly restricted diet just won't work long term.

### Balancing Energy Sources: Fat

In addition to balancing energy intake with energy output, achieving a balanced intake of energy sources is important for successful weight management. We all need some dietary fat, but, because fat is the most concentrated source of calories, limiting fat in the diet can help you limit your total calories. Research suggests that fat calories are more easily converted to body fat than calories from protein or carbohydrate.[115] Fat should supply about 20 to 35 percent of your average total daily calories, which translates into 45 to 75 grams of fat each day in a 2,000-kilocalorie diet.

High-fat, low-fiber diets tend to delay satiation and encourage overeating. If you eat a diet with lots of whole grains and fresh fruits and vegetables and reduce your reliance on meats and processed foods, you will reduce fat consumption and increase dietary fiber. Watch out for processed foods labeled "fat-free" or "reduced fat"; they can be high in calories and sugar despite their lower fat content.

A low-fat diet may aid in weight loss, but adopting a healthy lifestyle that can be maintained also is important, which translates into eating the correct types of fat. Studies show that eating unsaturated fats (from plant sources) and staying away from saturated fats (from animal sources) and *trans* fats will be beneficial for your heart. Include foods such as olive oil, nuts, and cold-water fish, which all contain modest amounts of unsaturated fats in your diet.

What about fat substitutes? The chemical structure of fake fats (such as olestra) is not digestible, so these compounds pass through the GI tract without providing any energy. They produce the mouthfeel of real fat without the calories but often with unwanted side effects. Snack products that contain olestra can cause abdominal cramps and diarrhea.

### Balancing Energy Sources: Carbohydrates

To lose weight, dieters often cut back on carbohydrate-rich foods such as bread, pasta, and potatoes. But these foods, along with vegetables, legumes,

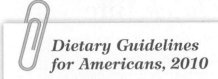

*Quick* Bite

**Double-Checking Your Dietary Recall**
When researchers checked the validity of food diaries and self-reports, they found that obese people underreport their energy intake by 20 to 50 percent and lean people underreport by 10 to 30 percent. Energy expenditure in the obese subjects was normal relative to their body size.

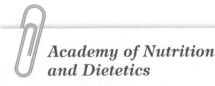

**Academy of Nutrition and Dietetics**

**Weight Management**
It is the position of the Academy of Nutrition and Dietetics that successful weight management to improve overall health for adults requires a lifelong commitment to healthful lifestyle behaviors emphasizing sustainable and enjoyable eating practices and daily physical activity.

**Source:** Reproduced from Seagle HM, et al. Position of the American Dietetic Association: weight management. *J Am Diet Assoc.* 2009;109:330–346.

## Quick Bite

**The Fletcherism Fad: Chew Until You . . .**
At the turn of the twentieth century, a retired businessman named Horace Fletcher started a dietary craze known as "Fletcherism." Calling the mouth "Nature's Food Filter," he believed that the sense of taste and the urge to swallow are perfect guides to nutrition. Although he recommended chewing food at least 50 times before swallowing, preferably until tasteless, he far exceeded this by once chewing a piece of onion 722 times. His philosophy did lead to some weight loss; people adhering to Fletcherism cut back on energy intake due to the additional mechanical effort of chewing.

## Quick Bite

**The Beverly Hills Diet**
The Beverly Hills Diet, introduced in 1980, begins with 10 days of fruit and water only. Many dieters reported an unpleasant side effect—diarrhea.

and whole grains, provide important nutrients and are rich in dietary fiber that can help you achieve and maintain a healthy body weight. Fiber-rich foods help provide a feeling of satiation, or fullness, that can keep you from overeating. Carbohydrates should make up about 45 to 65 percent of your total daily calories. Watch portion sizes and limit the high-fat accompaniments (e.g., sauces, toppings). Experiment with lower-fat alternatives. Instead of sour cream on your baked potato, try plain yogurt or even salsa! Rather than cream sauces on your pasta, use tomato-based sauces.

High-sugar foods usually provide calories but few nutrients. You should consume them sparingly, so choose fresh fruits and whole grains instead of candy, soft drinks, and sugary cereals. A good guide for choosing cereals is looking at the food label to pick ones with little added sugar and a moderate amount of fiber (at least 3 grams per serving).

### Balancing Energy Sources: Protein

Many popular diet books promote a high-protein, low-carbohydrate intake pattern. They often proclaim their plan to be a "scientific breakthrough," although most contain speculations that have been recycled since the 1800s!

Even though they promise "all you can eat," such diets typically severely restrict the number of food groups or types of foods you can eat, thereby indirectly lowering your energy intake (if you are not allowed to eat any carbohydrate-rich foods, this leaves you with little in the way of dietary choices). This lower overall energy intake is what actually causes any weight loss that occurs. A high-protein, low-carbohydrate, low-calorie diet is difficult to maintain and does not conform to the *Dietary Guidelines for Americans, 2010* recommendations. Most authorities recommend diets high in complex carbohydrates and moderate in protein consumption. (See the FYI feature "Learning Weight Management from Some of the 'Biggest' Weight Experts: Sumo Wrestlers.")

Although protein promotes a sense of fullness, animal foods high in protein often are high in saturated fat. Vegetarian sources of protein (such as tofu, soymilk, beans, and lentils) and plant-based fats are healthier choices. Including some protein in each meal is a good idea, but stick to the recommended intake: 10 to 35 percent of total daily calories.

### Eating Habits

Equally important to weight management is eating regularly. If you skip meals, you are apt to feel excessively hungry and deprived, and you will be more likely to snack or binge on high-calorie, high-fat, or sugary foods. A person who eats on a regular schedule is more likely to reduce total energy intake and improve lipid levels than a person who eats irregularly.[116] Also, a regular meal pattern usually includes breakfast—a benefit when trying to manage weight. Research shows that morning intake is much more satiating than late-night eating and will help reduce overall energy intake.[117] In a study of healthy, lean women, skipping breakfast lowered insulin sensitivity, raised LDL and total cholesterol, and led to higher energy intake.[118]

If you follow a regular pattern of eating and set up some "decision rules" that govern your food choices, you will be able to handle the many details that go into a healthful diet. Decision rules governing breakfast, for example, might be:

- Most of the time, choose a low-sugar, high-fiber cereal with nonfat milk or oatmeal with nonfat milk and fruit.
- Once in a while, have an egg that's prepared without added fat (e.g., hard boiled, scrambled) and a piece of whole-wheat toast.

- Sometimes have whole-grain pancakes and waffles topped with fruit.
- Occasionally have a donut or bagel with full-fat cream cheese.

When you proclaim some foods "off limits," you are setting up a rule to be broken. Instead, adopt the principle of "everything in moderation." Troublesome foods might be placed off limits temporarily until you regain control. If you can learn to eat in moderation, you can achieve a healthful diet and manage your weight successfully; no foods need to be entirely off limits, though some should be eaten prudently. Making the healthier choice more often than not is the essence of moderation.

**Key Concepts** *Balancing energy sources and controlling portion sizes can help reduce overall energy consumption. Reducing fat intake is a major step toward lowering calorie intake. Fiber-rich foods provide a feeling of fullness that can help prevent overeating. When planning a diet, aim for a caloric intake of 20 to 35 percent or less fat, 10 to 35 percent protein, and 45 to 65 percent carbohydrate.*

### Physical Activity

Regular physical activity is a vital component of weight management and promotes fitness and good health. At the same time, it discourages overeating by reducing stress, it produces positive feelings that reinforce self-worth and a sense of accomplishment, and it often includes pleasant socialization.

Look for ways to incorporate more physical activity into your daily life. (See **Figure 8.17**.) To prevent weight gain and maximize health benefits, adults should aim for 60 minutes of moderate-intensity physical activity each day,

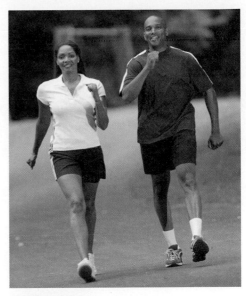

**Figure 8.17**    **Weight management through lifetime habits.** To achieve long-term weight management, healthy habits must become part of one's daily routine.

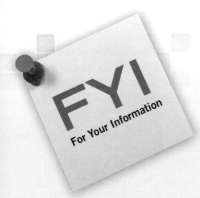

FYI
*For Your Information*

## Learning Weight Management from Some of the "Biggest" Weight Experts: Sumo Wrestlers

Is it possible to work out three to five hours a day, seven days a week, eat a relatively low-fat diet, and still gain weight? Yes! This is the how Sumo wrestlers train, a life that allows them to pack on the pounds. The world's biggest people are experts at putting on fat, which means that the lessons they've learned can help teach us how to keep the weight off. If you do not want to gain weight, follow these tips. The wrestlers, of course, will be doing just the opposite:[1]

- *Make your workouts slow and steady, not fast and frantic.* Sustained moderate workouts lasting 30 to 60 minutes are more helpful at burning calories than exerting yourself in a brief, intense burst of exercise. Sumo wrestlers train to win at a sport whose rules are simple: A wrestler loses when he is forced out of the wrestling ring or if anything other than his feet touch the mat. The average sumo wrestler stands about 6 feet tall and weighs 336 pounds. Sumo wrestler training is focused on being powerful enough to push over something the size of a refrigerator. Going for a 3-mile run or riding a bicycle for 60 minutes is not a priority for sumo wrestler workouts.

- *Don't skip breakfast.* Try not to go longer than four to five hours without eating. Your body will adapt to the threat of starvation and decrease your metabolism so you can survive on fewer calories. Most sumo wrestlers eat only twice a day.
- *Eat small meals and snacks throughout the day.* Split up your daily calories among breakfast, lunch, dinner, and a couple of snacks. You're less likely to put on weight eating small meals and never overeating, rather than letting yourself get too hungry and then eating too much. Sumo wrestlers eat about one-half of their overall daily food calories at one meal. For a person the size

of a sumo wrestler, that can be over 3,000 calories every day just for lunch!
- *Choose a well-balanced diet with a lot of variety.* Remember that balance, variety, and moderation are cornerstones of good nutrition. Sumo wrestlers eat a relatively low-fat diet but tend to have a diet heavy in complex carbohydrates, protein, and vegetables, with little fruit.

1   Anderson J, Christensen N, Hoffman E, et al. *Eat Right! Healthy Eating in College and Beyond.* San Francisco: Pearson Benjamin Cummings, 2007:67–79.

**positive self-talk** Constructive mental or verbal statements made to one's self to change a belief or behavior.

**negative self-talk** Mental or verbal statements made to one's self that reinforce negative or destructive self-perceptions.

but this doesn't have to be done all at once. Just walking more is beneficial. In many studies it has been shown that people who walk more tend to be thinner than those who do not walk as much. So, walk the dog for an extra half hour daily, for example. Use a stairway instead of an elevator. Walk briskly instead of using transportation. Take up an active hobby like bicycling, or if you live near the mountains, try hiking or skiing.

Increasing your activity level by just a small amount can help you maintain your current weight or lose a moderate amount of weight. "Going for the burn" and "no pain, no gain" were the mottoes of the aerobics movement during the 1970s and 1980s, but such intense activity is neither necessary nor desirable. Instead, regular exercise of moderate intensity—any activity that expends 4 to 7 kilocalories per minute (240 to 420 kilocalories per hour; see Table 8.2)—provides substantial health benefits.

Once you have increased your everyday activity level, consider beginning a formal exercise program that includes cardiorespiratory endurance exercise, resistance training, and stretching exercises. Regular, moderate cardiorespiratory endurance exercise, sustained for 45 minutes to 1 hour, can help trim body fat permanently. Strength training helps increase fat-free mass, which results in more calorie burning even outside of exercise periods.

One thing is clear: Regular exercise, maintained throughout life, makes weight management easier. The sooner you establish good habits, the better. You will succeed in maintaining your weight if you make exercise an integral part of the lifestyle you enjoy now and will enjoy in the future.

**Key Concepts** *Successful weight management involves regular physical activity as well as healthful food choices. Small increases in activity have significant health benefits and help weight loss and maintenance. To prevent weight gain and maximize health benefits, you should include at least 60 minutes of moderate physical activity in your daily routine.*

## Thinking and Emotions

What goes on in your head is another factor in a healthy lifestyle and successful weight management. The way you think about yourself and your world influences, and is influenced by, how you feel and how you act. Certain kinds of thinking produce negative emotions, which can undermine a healthy lifestyle.

When we compare ourselves to an internally held picture of an "ideal self," we are more likely to have low self-esteem and feel negative emotions. The "ideal self" we envision is often the result of having adopted perfectionistic goals and beliefs about how we and others "should" be. You might know someone who believes, "If I don't do things perfectly, I'm a failure" or "It's terrible if I'm not thin." When we accept these irrational beliefs, we may actually cause ourselves stress and emotional conflict. The remedy is to challenge such beliefs and replace them with more realistic ones.

The beliefs and attitudes you hold give rise to self-talk, an internal dialogue you carry on with yourself about events that happen to and around you. When you talk yourself through the steps of a job and then praise yourself when it's successfully completed, you are engaging in **positive self-talk**. When you make self-deprecating remarks or angry and guilt-producing comments and when you blame yourself unnecessarily, you are engaging in **negative self-talk**. Negative self-talk can undermine efforts at self-control and lead to feelings of anxiety and depression.

Your beliefs and attitudes influence how you interpret what happens to you and what you can expect in the future, as well as how you feel and react. Realistic beliefs and goals combined with positive self-talk and problem-solving efforts support a healthy lifestyle.

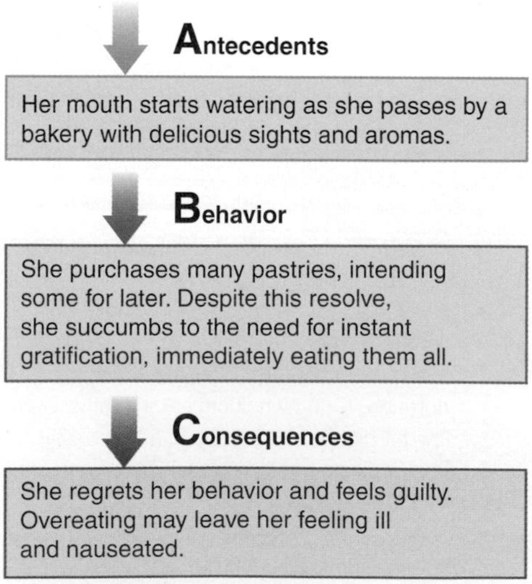

**A**ntecedents

Her mouth starts watering as she passes by a bakery with delicious sights and aromas.

**B**ehavior

She purchases many pastries, intending some for later. Despite this resolve, she succumbs to the need for instant gratification, immediately eating them all.

**C**onsequences

She regrets her behavior and feels guilty. Overeating may leave her feeling ill and nauseated.

**Figure 8.18** **The ABC model of eating behavior.** Conquering overeating often requires a psychological strategy for changing ingrained habits and other behaviors.

## Stress Management

Stress management can be an important part of weight management.[119] You can use the **ABC model of behavior** (**Figure 8.18**) to help you cope with daily stresses and their impacts on eating behavior.

The ABC model helps you manage events that trigger behaviors and factors that reinforce them. Antecedents, the "A" part of the model, are the events that precede the behavior and trigger it. Overeating is one possible behavior, the "B" part of the model. The consequences, or "C," follow and reinforce the "B." The "C" may be desirable, such as relief from stress, or undesirable, such as guilt or weight gain. The consequences may be immediate or like weight gain occur in the future; consequences that occur immediately have the greatest influence.

Identifying the cues (A) that trigger overeating is the first step to changing or avoiding these triggers. You might remove problem foods from the house or avoid the grocery store's candy aisle. You can sometimes manipulate antecedents to trigger positive behaviors (e.g., putting exercise clothes by the door to prompt exercise).

You can change the behavior of overeating (B) by using positive self-talk to encourage a new behavior and by avoiding excuses and rationalizations to eat something inappropriate.

Positive consequences (C) help to reinforce new behaviors. You could sign a contract with a friend that rewards you for deciding not to overeat. Rewards such as time for physical activity not only reinforce behavior but also develop fitness. Table 8.8 summarizes cognitive-behavioral tools for changing habits and behavior patterns.

> **ABC model of behavior** A behavioral model that includes the external and internal events that precede and follow the behavior. The "A" stands for antecedents, the events that precede the behavior ("B"), which is followed by consequences ("C") that positively or negatively reinforce the behavior.

### Table 8.8 — Cognitive-Behavioral Tools for Changing Behavior

**Self-Monitoring**

Prospectively recording information about behavior to identify the antecedents (what precedes and elicits a particular action), the behaviors of interest (usually eating behavior), and the consequences (the thoughts, feelings, and reactions that accompany the behavior of interest).

**Environmental Management**

Avoiding or changing cues that trigger undesirable behavior (e.g., not driving by the doughnut shop, putting the cookie jar out of sight), or instituting new cues to elicit new behaviors (e.g., putting your walking shoes by the door as a reminder to exercise); also called *stimulus control*.

**Alternate Behaviors**

Learning new ways of responding to old cues or circumstances that can't be changed or avoided (e.g., taking a walk when you get upset instead of getting something to eat).

**Reward**

Giving yourself, or arranging to be given, rewards for engaging in desired behaviors. Do not use food as a reward.

**Negative Reinforcement**

Arranging to give up something desirable (e.g., money) or to endure something undesirable (e.g., wash your friend's car) for engaging in unwanted behaviors.

**Social Support**

Getting others to participate in or otherwise provide emotional and physical support of your weight-management efforts.

**Cognitive Coping**

Reducing negative self-talk, increasing positive self-talk, and challenging beliefs that undermine your resolve and contribute to negative emotions; setting reasonable goals and avoiding "thinking traps."

**Managing Emotions**

Using reframing, disengagement, imagery, and self-soothing to reduce or manage negative emotions.

**Relapse Prevention and Recovery**

Identifying high-risk situations that pose a hazard for relapsing, and learning to recover from small indiscretions before they become major relapses.

**Source:** Adapted from Nash JD. *The New Maximize Your Body Potential.* Palo Alto, CA: Bull Publishing Company; 1997. Used with permission from Bull Publishing Company.

| Table 8.9 | Basic Tenets of Size Acceptance |
|---|---|

Human beings come in a variety of sizes and shapes. We celebrate this diversity as a positive characteristic of the human race.

There is no ideal body size, shape, or weight that every individual should strive to achieve.

Every body is a good body, whatever its size or shape.

Self-esteem and body image are strongly linked. Helping people feel good about their bodies and about who they are can help motivate and maintain healthy behaviors.

Appearance stereotyping is inherently unfair to the individual because it is based on superficial factors which the individual has little or no control over.

We respect the bodies of others even though they might be quite different from our own.

Each person is responsible for taking care of his/her body.

Good health is not defined by body size; it is a state of physical, mental, and social well-being.

People of all sizes and shapes can reduce their risk of poor health by adopting a healthy lifestyle.

Source: Data from Basic Tenets of Health at Every Size, developed by dietitians and nutritionists who are advocates of size acceptance; their efforts coordinated by Joanne P. Ikeda, MA, RD, Nutrition Education Specialist, Department of Nutritional Sciences, University of California, Berkeley.

## *Quick* Bite

### Diet Revolution?
The *Diet Revolution*, first promoted by Dr. Atkins in 1972, centered on putting dieters into a state of ketosis by consuming few carbohydrates. In 1973, the American Medical Association called the diet dangerous, and Atkins was required to testify before the U.S. Senate Select Committee on Nutrition.

### Balancing Acceptance and Change

It's not enough to change your behavior to manage obesity. Self-acceptance is equally necessary. (See Table 8.9.) Accepting yourself as you are will help your self-esteem and improve your general satisfaction with life. It is destructive to be overly concerned with the importance of body weight and shape or to have unattainable goals of idealized physical appearance. But don't confuse self-acceptance with complacency or a do-nothing attitude that ignores health risks.

If you must diet, do so in combination with exercise, and avoid very-low-calorie diets. Don't try to lose more than ½ to 1 pound per week. Realize that most low-calorie diets cause a rapid loss of body water at first. When this phase passes, weight loss declines. As a result, dieters often are misled into believing that their efforts are not working. They then give up, not realizing that smaller losses later in the diet actually are better than the initial big losses. In fact, the later loss is mostly fat loss, whereas the initial loss was primarily fluid loss.

**Key Concepts**  *Identifying cues that precede overeating can help a person make behavior changes. Long-term weight management should include self-acceptance and enhanced self-esteem. Goals of idealized body size and shape should be replaced with goals that promote good health and a lifetime of fitness.*

## Weight-Management Approaches

Do certain weight-loss diets have adverse health consequences? Is it unhealthy to lose weight quickly? Will the weight stay off? What motivates people to lose weight and to maintain weight? What are the barriers to losing weight and/or to maintaining weight?

In a study of popular weight-loss diets, 160 participants with an average BMI of 35 kg/m$^2$ were randomly assigned to one of four weight-loss diets: Weight Watchers (restriction of portion sizes and calories; 1,200 to 1,600 kilocalories daily), Atkins (low carbohydrate—less than 20 grams daily at onset, gradual increase to 50 grams), Zone (40-30-30 balance of percentage calories from carbohydrate, fat, and protein, respectively), and Ornish (vegetarian, less than 10 percent of calories from fat).[120] Subjects lost weight on all four diets, but no one diet was more effective than any of the others. Compliance was a key factor—only about 25 percent of subjects in each group maintained the diet at a level of 6 on a 10-point scale (1 = no adherence, 10 = perfect adherence), but dietary adherence was strongly associated with weight loss. Those who stuck to the diets best lost on average 7 percent of body weight, a meaningful start in reducing health risks.

A wide range of weight-management approaches is available to the consumer. It's important to investigate your options thoroughly to find the approach best suited to your personal needs.

### Self-Help Books and Manuals

Some people respond well to simple information provided in an easy-to-understand format. By referring to good, well-researched self-help manuals and books, they work to improve their eating and lifestyle behaviors. Although positive changes are desirable, few people achieve lasting weight loss.

The proliferation of diet books is nothing short of phenomenal, and each year dozens of dubious weight-loss diet books reach the market. When evaluating a diet book, be alert to the following warning flags:

1.  Unbalanced diet patterns. The recommended pattern should not stray too far from that of MyPlate.

2.  Claims of a "scientific breakthrough" or promises of "quick and easy" weight loss. There is no quick fix when it comes to weight management.
3.  Irrational food instructions: food restrictions (e.g., no fruits), illogical overemphasis of some foods (e.g., five grapefruits daily) or supplements, and irrational food patterns (e.g., don't eat meat and bread at the same meal). Such restrictions set the stage for feelings of deprivation and binge eating.
4.  The promise of a cure for some disease along with weight loss. That's not only a waste of money but also potentially dangerous.
5.  Lack of an exercise plan or suggestions for physical activity throughout the day.

Should you decide on the do-it-yourself route, develop specific goals for your diet, exercise, and maintenance plans. (See the FYI feature "Behaviors That Will Help You Manage Your Weight.") Keep tabs on your habits and become more involved in activities other than eating, especially fitness activities. Long-term success depends on maintaining the lifestyle changes that helped you lose the weight in the first place.

## Meal Replacements

Some people turn to meal replacements—shakes and bars, for example—to help lose weight. Meal replacements are convenient, often contain added vitamins and minerals, and reduce the choices and temptations available at mealtime. They also are highly processed and not as healthful as fresh, more natural foods. When compared with traditional, reduced-calorie diet programs, people using meal replacements lost slightly more weight and were less likely to stop the program.[121] The challenge is to learn long-term eating strategies that will allow weight management without reliance on special products.

## Self-Help Groups

Self-help groups, often led by laypeople, help many people cope with their weight. Such groups can share experiences, reduce the isolation and alienation felt by many obese people, and provide an understanding and accepting community.

## Commercial Programs

Commercial weight-loss programs provide group or individual counseling and group support. Some sell prepackaged foods or nutritional supplements. Some companies employ dietitians, health educators, psychologists, or physicians to develop and guide the program at the corporate level. The Federal Trade Commission (FTC) encourages commercial programs to release the following information to potential clients:

*   Staff training and education
*   Risks of overweight and obesity
*   Risks of their products or program
*   Cost
*   Program outcomes: success and failure rates

Be sure to obtain this information before you register for a weight-loss program, and think twice about any program that does not willingly provide it.

Several commercial programs, such as Optifast and Health Management Resources (HMR), use **very-low-calorie diets (VLCD)** containing only 400 to 800 kilocalories per day as the initial phase of treatment. When such diets were first introduced in the 1970s, several deaths resulted from cardiac

*Quick* Bite

**Letter on Corpulence**
Published in the early 1800s, *Bantry's Letter on Corpulence* was the first popular diet book in the United States. The book advocated restricting intake of carbohydrates.

**very-low-calorie diets (VLCD)** Diets supplying 400 to 800 kilocalories per day, which include adequate high-quality protein, little or no fat, and little carbohydrate.

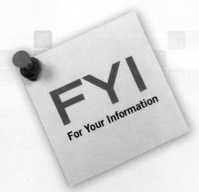

# Behaviors That Will Help You Manage Your Weight

The following behaviors have been shown to be helpful in managing your weight.[1]

## Set the Right Goals

Setting the right goals is an important first step. Most people trying to lose weight focus just on weight loss. However, you'll be more successful if you focus on dietary and exercise changes that lead to long-term weight change. Successful weight managers select no more than two or three goals at a time.

Effective goals are (1) specific, (2) attainable, and (3) forgiving. "Exercise more" is a commendable ideal, but it's not specific. "Walk 5 miles every day" is specific and measurable, but is it attainable if you're just starting out? "Walk 30 minutes every day" is more attainable, but what happens if you're held up at work or there's a thunderstorm? "Walk 30 minutes, five days each week" is specific, attainable, and forgiving. In short, a great goal!

## Nothing Succeeds Like Success

Select a series of short-term goals that get you closer and closer to the ultimate goal (e.g., consider reducing fat intake from 40 percent of calories to 35 percent and later to 30 percent). Nothing succeeds like success. This strategy employs two important behavioral principles: (1) consecutive goals that move you ahead in small steps are the best way to reach a distant point and (2) consecutive rewards keep the overall effort invigorated.

## Reward Success (But Not with Food)

You're more likely to keep working toward your goal if you are rewarded—especially when goals are difficult to reach. An effective reward is something that is desirable, timely, and contingent on meeting your goal. Your rewards may be tangible (e.g., a movie, payment toward buying a more costly item) or intangible (e.g., an afternoon off from studying, an hour of quiet time away from the daily demands of school). As you meet small goals, give yourself numerous small rewards; don't wait to meet your ultimate goal for a large reward. The long, difficult effort might lead you to give up.

## Balance Your (Food) Checkbook

Keeping track of your behavior—observing and recording calorie intake, servings of fruits and vegetables, exercise frequency and duration, or any other wellness behavior—can help alter that behavior. Self-monitoring usually changes a behavior in the desired direction and can produce "real-time" records for you and your health care provider. For example, you can track your exercise progress. A record of increasing exercise encourages you to keep up the good work. If the record shows little or no progress, you know that a change of strategy is needed. Some people find that specific self-monitoring forms make it easier, whereas others prefer to use their own recording system.

Although you don't need to step on the scale every day, monitoring your weight regularly (once a week) can help you maintain your lower weight. Use a graph rather than a list or calendar notations so you have a picture of cumulative progress. Changes in your body's water content, rather than fat content, are responsible for most of the up and down fluctuations from day to day. A long-term downward trend reflects fat losses.

## Avoid a Chain Reaction

Identify the social or environmental cues that seem to encourage undesirable eating, and then change those cues. For example, you may learn from reflection or self-monitoring that you're more likely to overeat while watching television, when treats are on display at the campus cafe, or when you're around a certain friend. You might then try to break the association between eating and the cue (don't eat while watching television), avoid or eliminate the cue (avoid sitting near the display counter), or change the circumstances surrounding the cue (plan to meet with your friend in non-food settings). In general, visible and accessible food items often are cues for unplanned eating.

## Get the (Fullness) Message

Changing the way you go about eating can make it easier to eat less without feeling deprived. It takes 15 or more minutes for your brain to get the message you've been fed. Slowing the rate of eating can allow satiation (fullness) signals to begin by the end of the meal. Eating lots of vegetables also can make you feel fuller. Another trick is to use smaller plates so moderate portions do not appear meager. Changing your eating schedule, or setting one, can be helpful, especially if you tend to skip or delay meals and overeat later.

## The Backsliding Phenomenon

You've just signed a contract with yourself to avoid high-fat desserts for one month when you're presented with an array of your favorite "to die for" desserts. You say to yourself, "just this once" and satisfy your craving. Most of us have experienced the "backsliding phenomenon" in which we have lost our resolve and slipped back into a former bad habit. When it happens, be prepared for it and move on with your resolve. You're most apt to backslide when you're tempted by something unexpected and your self-control is threatened. You can remove high-fat snacks from your home but not from other places you eat. Imagine tempting situations in your mind's eye and practice coping with them successfully. If you do slip, don't waste time with self-blame. Learn from the experience and get back on track.

1   National Heart, Lung, and Blood Institute. Guide to behavior change. http://www.nhlbi.nih.gov/health/public/heart/obesity/lose_wt/behavior.htm. Accessed 6/20/11.

abnormalities. As a result, VLCD should be undertaken only with close medical supervision.

### Professional Private Counselors

Private counselors can be physicians, psychotherapists, nutritionists, or registered dietitians. They provide individualized weight management and the support and attention that some obese people may need. Some programs use the Internet rather than face-to-face counseling sessions and have seen positive results. The Internet has shown potential for use in many areas of health behavior, including increased self-motivation and weight loss.[122] Although Internet-based weight loss programs are popular, a comparison of a commercial Internet-based weight-loss program to a self-help weight-loss manual found higher weight loss at one year in the self-help group (4 percent of initial body weight versus 1 percent).[123] This may be due to social influences and the addition of social networking to online weight loss programs may close the gap.

Carefully scrutinize the training and credentials of private counselors before committing to any program. Effective weight-loss counselors should do the following:[124]

1. Assess obesity risk.
2. Ask about readiness to lose weight.
3. Advise in designing a weight-control program.
4. Assist in establishing appropriate intervention.
5. Arrange for follow-up.

### Food and Drug Administration–Approved Weight-Loss Medications

The pharmaceutical industry has long searched for a "magic bullet" to battle obesity, but a cure has failed to emerge. With the recognition that obesity involves multiple factors, the focus is shifting to drugs with multiple mechanisms and drugs to be used in conjunction with proper diet and exercise.[125] Antiobesity medications generally fall into one of two categories: appetite suppressants and lipase inhibitors.

Most FDA-approved weight-loss medications are appetite suppressants and are approved for short-term use (a few weeks) only. Examples include phentermine (Adipex-P, Fastin, Obenix, Oby-Trim), phendimetrazine (Bontril, Melfiat, Flegine), and diethylpropion (Durad, Tenuate, Tepanil). Appetite suppressants work by limiting the desire for food either through decreasing appetite or increasing the feeling of fullness following eating. These medications make you feel less hungry by increasing one or more brain chemicals that affect mood and appetite.[126] Phentermine is the most commonly prescribed appetite-suppressant in the United States.

Only one weight-loss medication is approved by the FDA for long-term use (up to 2 years). This medication, Xenical (orlistat), is a lipase inhibitor, which works by reducing the body's ability to absorb dietary fat by about one-third.[127] It blocks the enzyme lipase, which is responsible for breaking down dietary fat.[128] Because the body cannot absorb fat that has not been broken down, the body eliminates it along with its calories. Orlistat must be accompanied by a low-fat diet, or the unabsorbed fat can produce diarrhea and flatulence. The drug also blocks fat-soluble nutrient absorption, so it's necessary to take a vitamin supplement as well.[129]

The FDA has approved the use of antiobesity drugs only in combination with calorie-restricted diets and regular physical activity. Aside from orlistat, antiobesity drugs can be addictive and have the potential for abuse. Antiobesity agents shouldn't be used in combination with each other or with other drugs for appetite control because the safety of such combinations has not

**Gastric Banding**

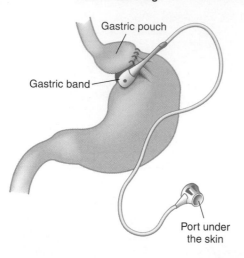

**Gastric Bypass**

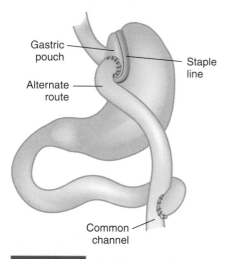

| Figure 8.19 | **Gastric surgery in obesity treatment.** In gastric banding, |

surgery reduces the size of the stomach. The band can be adjusted by an infusion of saline through a port that lies just beneath the skin. In gastric bypass, an alternate route carries food to the jejunum, bypassing the duodenum and most of the stomach.

**Source:** Reprinted with permission from Steinbrook R. Surgery for severe obesity. *New England Journal of Medicine.* 2004;350(11):1075–1079. © 2004 Massachusetts Medical Society. All rights reserved

**extreme obesity** Obesity characterized by body weight exceeding 100 percent of normal; a condition so severe it often requires surgery.

**morbid obesity** See *extreme obesity.*

been evaluated. The drugs should be used only in people who are obese—not people looking to lose just a few pounds. Are they effective? A review of numerous clinical trials suggests that the benefits of drug therapy over behavioral interventions are modest at best.[130]

### Over-the-Counter Drugs and Dietary Supplements Used for Weight Loss

Dietary supplement use is common among adults trying to lose weight. A recent study reported that one-third of those making a conscious effort to lose weight are using weight-loss supplements. It was also found that both the users and nonusers of these dietary supplements had misperceptions about their safety and usefulness.[131]

Nonprescription (over-the-counter, or OTC) weight-loss pills may contain caffeine, benzocaine, or fiber. Caffeine is a stimulant and diuretic. Benzocaine numbs the tongue, which reduces taste sensations and discourages eating. Pills with fiber are designed to fill the stomach and provide a feeling of fullness. Although moderately effective, fiber pills can lead to dehydration; much of the lost weight is water, which is easily regained when the pills are stopped.

Numerous dietary supplements are marketed for weight loss, with names like "Weight Away." Common ingredients include chromium picolinate, chitosan, hydroxycitric acid (HCA), glucomannan, green tea, and pyruvate. Few peer-reviewed scientific studies have evaluated these products for weight loss, and what little evidence exists is not convincing enough to recommend their use.[132]

Consumers should be cautious of dietary supplements marketed for weight loss and investigate the ingredients they contain. Generally, manufacturers do not need to register their products with FDA nor get FDA approval before selling dietary supplements.[133]

### Surgery

Sometimes surgery can successfully treat **extreme obesity** (also called **morbid obesity**)—a BMI of 40 kg/m² or higher. Surgery should be a last-ditch effort, taken only when all legitimate, less-invasive methods have failed. The two most common procedures are gastric banding and gastric bypass. Gastric banding reduces stomach size by creating a smaller upper stomach, or "pouch," thus limiting intake to only a few calories at one time.[134] Gastric bypass also creates a smaller stomach pouch and then connects that pouch to a shortened section of small intestine. (See **Figure 8.19**.) Reducing the size of the stomach reduces food intake, and bypassing the upper part of the small intestine reduces digestion and absorption of caloric foods. The absorption of some micronutrients also is reduced—an obvious drawback. The dramatic increase in the incidence of obesity has produced an unprecedented increase in the number of bariatric surgery procedures.[135]

The results of surgery are impressive; however, long-term success is highly variable. Surgical patients lose substantially more weight initially than those who try diet and exercise or weight-loss medications. Although weight loss tends to plateau by 18 to 24 months after surgery, it is not unusual for patients to have maintained a 50-percent loss of initial body weight after five years.[136]

The long-term effectiveness of gastric surgery depends on how patients manage and adhere to lifetime dietary and physical activity. Additionally, success with this procedure is more likely if the underlying cause of obesity is addressed prior to having the surgery. The initial weight loss results can be defeated by consuming high-calorie drinks or semisolid foods that overcome stomach size. With time the pouch stretches, allowing more solid foods, but by then doctors hope that the patient has established healthy eating habits. Also, RMR can decline significantly after gastric surgery, along with reductions in lean body mass, so exercise is important.[137] These patients are likely to need lifelong medical supervision.

Liposuction is a cosmetic surgical procedure that reshapes the body by removing fat. Although the procedure removes some fat cells, the body still has billions of other fat cells ready to store extra fat. Thus, liposuction is not effective for significant or long-term weight loss. It should not be undertaken casually. Risks include blood clots, perforation injuries, skin and nerve damage, and unfavorable drug reactions.

### Summary of Weight-Management Strategies

For best effect, weight-management strategies need to be individualized. Until the science of nutrigenomics advances far enough to match an individual's genetics to the right diet plan, dietary strategies should focus on the reduction of chronic disease risks (more fruits and vegetables, whole grains, and fish)[138] and be combined with physical activity to achieve a modest but persistent, reduction in calories.[139] For individuals who are morbidly obese, consultation with a physician is essential to determine the right approach for managing weight and improving health.

**Key Concepts** *Books, Internet resources, and commercial programs can help some individuals lose weight. However, consumers should always proceed with caution before spending money. Prescription and over-the-counter drugs to lose weight have varying effectiveness. Drugs have potential side effects and must be used with caution and medical supervision. For those who are morbidly obese, surgical intervention is an aggressive, last-resort approach to weight management. Liposuction removes fat cells from specific parts of the body, but it is not considered an effective approach to weight control.*

## Underweight

From a public health standpoint, underweight is much less of a problem than obesity, but those who are underweight can find it troublesome and frustrating. When underweight is simply an inherited pattern, there is no need to worry about health risks as long as diet and other health behaviors are appropriate. But your health is at risk if underweight results from undernutrition; deficits in protein, vitamins, and minerals, as well as energy, can cause health problems ranging from fatigue to compromised immune function.

## Causes and Assessment

The causes of underweight are as diverse as those of overweight and include:

- Altered response to hunger, appetite, satiation, satiety, and external cues (described earlier in this chapter)
- Factors in eating disorders, such as distorted body image, compulsive dieting, and compulsive overexercising
- Metabolic and hereditary factors
- Prolonged psychological and emotional stress
- Addiction to alcohol and street drugs
- Bizarre diet patterns or otherwise inadequate diets

Underweight can be a sign of underlying disease, such as cancer. Illness can speed up metabolic rate, spoil the appetite, or interfere with digestion. Correcting underweight helps improve the quality of life.

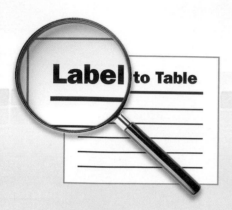

**Label to Table**

Do you believe that by choosing cookies or chips labeled "low-fat" or sticking with certain brand names associated with "diet foods" you are automatically making the right decisions? It may surprise you to know that many low-fat or fat-free products have nearly the same amount of calories as the full-fat versions! After reading this chapter you now know that when it comes to weight loss, total calories are just as important as calories from fat. If you eat a fat-free food but eat so much of it that your calories are excessive, you

will still gain weight. To illustrate this point, let's compare the nutrition labels from some leading cookie manufacturers. The lower fat cookies (on right) claim they are "better for you" and have "50% less fat" compared with regular cookies. Here are the labels:

| Regular Cookie | Lower Fat Cookie |
|---|---|
| Serving, 2 cookies (29 g) | Serving, 2 cookies (26 g) |
| Calories, 140 | Calories, 110 |
| Calories from fat, 50 | Calories from fat, 25 |
| Total fat, 6 g | Total fat, 3 g |

True, there is a 50 percent reduction in fat content (6 g vs. 3 g), which is an important part of the picture. However, take a look at the total calories. The lower fat cookies only have 30 fewer kilocalories than the regular cookies, which may be a surprise to those who think they are saving more.

There is another interesting piece of information on these labels—the serving size.

At first glance, you may think the serving sizes of the cookies are the same—two cookies. However, after further inspection you can see that the lower-fat cookies are slightly smaller. A 10 percent reduction in size/weight is certainly worth noting when you are trying to explain how a product can have fewer calories.

The next time you are in the cookie aisle debating whether you should settle a craving with a low-fat product or its full-fat version, be a smart consumer and read the label before you buy!

**Nutrition Facts**

Serving Size: 2 cookies (26g)
Servings Per Container: 18

**Amount Per Serving**

**Calories** 110   Calories from fat 25

|  | % Daily Value* |
|---|---|
| **Total Fat** 3g | 5% |
| Saturated Fat 0.5g | 3% |
| Polyunsaturated Fat 0g | |
| Monounsaturated Fat 1g | |
| Trans Fat 0g | |
| **Cholesterol** 0mg | 0% |
| **Sodium** 130mg | 5% |
| **Total Carbohydrate** 20g | 7% |
| Dietary Fiber 0g | 0% |
| Sugars 10g | |
| **Protein** 1g | |

| Vitamin A 0% | • | Vitamin C 0% |
|---|---|---|
| Calcium 0% | • | Iron 2% |

* Percent Daily Values are based on a 2,000 calorie diet. Your daily values may be higher or lower depending on your calorie needs:

| | | Calories: | 2000 | 2,500 |
|---|---|---|---|---|
| Total Fat | Less Than | | 65g | 80g |
| Sat Fat | Less Than | | 20g | 25g |
| Cholesterol | Less Than | | 300mg | 300mg |
| Sodium | Less Than | | 2,400mg | 2,400mg |
| Total Carbohydrate | | | 300g | 375g |
| Dietary Fiber | | | 25g | 30g |

Lower fat cookie

**Nutrition Facts**

Serving Size: 2 cookies (29g)
Servings Per Container about 16

**Amount Per Serving**

**Calories** 140   Calories from fat 50

|  | % Daily Value* |
|---|---|
| **Total Fat** 6g | 9% |
| Saturated Fat 1.5g | 8% |
| Trans Fat 0.5g | |
| **Cholesterol** 0mg | 0% |
| **Sodium** 105mg | 4% |
| **Total Carbohydrate** 21g | 7% |
| Dietary Fiber less than 1g | 3% |
| Sugars 8g | |
| **Protein** 2g | |

| Vitamin A 0% | • | Vitamin C 0% |
|---|---|---|
| Calcium 0% | • | Iron 4% |

* Percent Daily Values are based on a 2,000 calorie diet. Your daily values may be higher or lower depending on your calorie needs:

| | | Calories: | 2000 | 2,500 |
|---|---|---|---|---|
| Total Fat | Less Than | | 65g | 80g |
| Sat Fat | Less Than | | 20g | 25g |
| Cholesterol | Less Than | | 300mg | 300mg |
| Sodium | Less Than | | 2,400mg | 2,400mg |
| Total Carbohydrate | | | 300g | 375g |
| Dietary Fiber | | | 25g | 30g |

Regular cookie

## Weight-Gain Strategies

The way to gain weight is to create a positive energy balance. Here are some strategies:

- Have small, frequent meals consisting of nutrient-dense and energy-dense foods and beverages.
- Drink fluids at the end of the meal or, better yet, between meals to avoid filling the stomach with liquids of low nutrient density.
- Try high-calorie weight-gain beverages and foods, such as milkshakes made with ice cream or whole milk, adding peanut butter to snacks, and fruit juices.
- Use timers or other cues (similar to the ABC model discussed earlier but with a different goal) to prompt eating.
- Take a balanced vitamin/mineral supplement to ensure that poor appetite isn't a result of nutritional deficiency.

Sometimes prescription drugs, such as appetite stimulants, are helpful. Medication also can speed stomach emptying, improving appetite for the next meal. Digestive enzyme replacements help people who are underweight due to poor digestion or absorption.

Exercise has a role in weight gain as well. Simple anaerobic or isometric exercise encourages weight gain as lean body mass rather than fat.

**Key Concepts** *Underweight is not as common as overweight. Gaining weight can be difficult, but the basic concepts of energy balance apply. Changes in diet along with regular exercise are important strategies for gaining weight.*

# Learning Portfolio

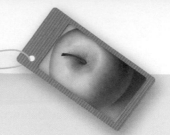

## Key Terms

## Study Points

- Energy balance is the relationship between energy intake and energy output.

- Food intake is regulated by hunger, satiation, satiety, and appetite, which are influenced by complex factors. Hunger is the physiological need to eat. Satiation is the feeling of fullness that leads to termination of a meal. Satiety is the feeling of satisfaction and lack of hunger that determines the interval until the next meal. Appetite is a desire to eat that is influenced by external factors such as flavors and smells, environmental factors, and cultural factors.

- Gastrointestinal stimulation, circulating nutrients, neurotransmitters, and hormones signal the brain to regulate food intake.

- The major components of energy expenditure are resting energy expenditure, the thermic effect of food, and energy for physical activity.

- Estimated Energy Requirements (EER) for adults predict total energy expenditure from age, height, weight, gender, and physical activity level.

- Body composition, age, gender, genetics, and hormonal activity affect the amount of energy used for resting metabolism.

- The energy cost of physical activity is affected by a person's size and the intensity and duration of the activity.

- Body composition, the relative amounts of fat and lean body mass, has a major influence on energy expenditure and risk of chronic disease.

- Body mass index—a ratio related to total body fatness and risk of chronic disease—is calculated with height and weight measurements.

- The prevalence of obesity and overweight is escalating worldwide, contributing to chronic disease.

- Health risks associated with obesity are more pronounced when excess body fat is located in the abdominal region of the body.

- The factors that cause obesity are not completely understood, but a complex interaction of hormonal and metabolic factors is believed to play a role, along with genetic, sociocultural, and psychological factors.

- Rather than focus on ideal body weight, many professionals now promote health and fitness goals.

- Physical activity improves fitness and helps achieve the negative energy balance needed for weight reduction.

- Abandoning unrealistic ideas of thinness and accepting body weight and shape are important elements in weight management.
- Long-term weight management includes a balanced diet of moderately restricted calorie intake, adequate exercise, cognitive-behavioral strategies for changing habits and behavior patterns, and attention to balancing self-acceptance and the desire for change.
- Surgical approaches to weight control should be considered only as a last resort for the morbidly obese.
- If the cause is not hereditary, being underweight can pose health problems.
- Gaining weight can be difficult for individuals who are underweight.

## Study Questions

1. Explain the concept of energy balance.
2. Define *hunger*, *satiation*, *satiety*, and *appetite*.
3. List and describe the three main components of energy expenditure.
4. Explain the three main factors that determine energy expenditure in activity.
5. What body mass index (BMI) values are associated with being underweight, overweight, and obese? Do these vary for men and women?
6. Obesity is seen as a complex disorder with multiple contributing factors. List the general types of factors involved in the development and maintenance of obesity.
7. What is the difference between hyperplastic and hypertrophic obesity?
8. Describe the concept of metabolic fitness.
9. What are the four components of a sound approach to weight management?
10. Explain how the ABCs of behavior modification can assist with weight control.
11. Define *underweight*.

## Try This

### A One-Week Energy Balance Check

The purpose of this exercise is to see if you're in energy balance by monitoring your body weight for one week. Measure your weight on a Monday morning soon after you wake up. Record your weight. Don't change your normal routine of exercise and food intake. One week later weigh yourself again (on a Monday morning just after waking). Did your weight change? If not, your energy intake closely matched your energy output. If so, did you gain or lose weight? What factors do you think contributed to your body weight change? Try repeating this exercise over a longer period of time. Measure and record your weight every Monday morning for six months. What happens?

### Increasing Your Energy Output

Physical activity is the part of your energy output that varies the most. The purpose of this exercise is to increase your energy expenditure by committing to daily exercise for one week. Make each exercise session about 30 minutes long, and remember that the longer the duration, the harder the intensity, and the larger the muscle groups involved, the greater the energy expenditure. Choose an exercise you enjoy—such as walking, jogging, cycling, swimming, or rollerblading. Once your week is complete, ask yourself these questions: How did this week's daily exercise affect my energy balance? Have I gained or lost weight during the week? Did I compensate for the extra energy expenditure by increasing my calorie intake?

### Changing Your Energy Input

Would you like to change your weight by a pound or two? The purpose of this exercise is to increase or decrease your energy input (calorie intake) so you gain or lose 1 pound by the end of a week. How? Make only minor adjustments in your usual diet but try to change the energy content for each of your meals by a small amount. Keep a food log and use the EatRight Analysis Software or Nutritionist Pro Software to estimate your calorie total for each of the days. Your goal is to change your calorie total by approximately 500 kilocalories per day. You should not consume fewer than 1,500 kilocalories (for women) or 1,800 kilocalories (for men) per day. Weigh yourself at the start of your week and at the end. What change, if any, do you see?

## What About Bobbie?

Remember, Bobbie is a 20-year-old college sophomore who weighs 155 pounds and is 5'4". She gained 10 pounds her freshman year and would like to lose it because she feels healthier when her weight is closer to 145 pounds. She exercises infrequently but likes to walk with her friends and occasionally goes to an aerobics class. How would you suggest she lose the extra 10 pounds? First, let's start by reducing her calorie intake slightly. Here is Bobbie's typical day of eating and some small changes in portion sizes that will save calories.

As you can see, small changes in Bobbie's diet can result in a 500-kilocalorie deficit, which will translate to approximately 1 pound per week of weight loss. This doesn't take into account any extra exercise she might do. If she starts to work out more regularly, she can make fewer changes in her calorie intake and still lose 1 pound per week.

| Typical Day | Alternative | Kcalories |
|---|---|---|
| **Breakfast** | | |
| 1 cinnamon-raisin bagel with 3 tablespoons light cream cheese Coffee, 2 tablespoons 2% milk and 2 teaspoons sugar | 1 tablespoon light cream cheese | 70 saved |
| **Snack** | | |
| Banana | | |
| **Lunch** | | |
| 2 slices sourdough bread 2 oz turkey lunch meat, 2 teaspoons regular mayo, 2 teaspoons mustard, 2 slices tomato, 2 slices dill pickle, shredded lettuce 12 oz diet cola Chocolate chip cookie | Salad with 2 cups iceberg lettuce with 2 tablespoons each of shredded carrot, chopped egg, croutons, kidney beans 1 tablespoon Italian dressing | 55 saved |
| **Snack** | | |
| 1½ oz tortilla chips with ½ cup salsa 16 oz water | 1 oz. tortilla chips | 70 saved |
| **Dinner** | | |
| 1½ cup pasta 3 oz meatballs with spaghetti sauce, 2 tablespoons Parmesan cheese | 1 cup pasta | 100 saved |
| 3 slices garlic bread | Delete garlic bread | 185 saved |
| ½ cup green beans | 1 cup green beans | 25 added |
| 1 teaspoon butter | Delete butter | 30 saved |
| 12 oz. diet cola | | |
| **Snack** | | |
| 1 slice cheese pizza | | |

**Total saved: ~500 calories**

# References

1   Wang GJ, Tomasi D, Backus W, et al. Gastric distention activates satiety circuitry in the human brain. *Neuroimage*. 2008;39(4):1824–1831.

2   Kalafatakis K, Triantafyllou K. Contribution of neurotensin in the immune and neuroendocrine modulation of normal and abnormal enteric function. *Regul Pept*. 2011;170(1–3):7–17.

3   Bartness TJ, Keen-Rinehart E, Dalley MJ, Teubner BJ. Neural and hormonal control of food hoarding. *Am J Physiol Regul Integr Comp Physiol*. 2011;301(3):R641–R655.

4   Karatas Z, Durmus Aydogdu S, Dinleyici EC, Colak O, Dogruel N. Breastmilk ghrelin, leptin, and fat levels changing foremilk to hindmilk: is that important for self-control of feeding? *Eur J Pediatr*. 2011;170(10):1273–1280.

5   Rosenbaum M, Leibel RL. Adaptive thermogenesis in humans. *Int J Obes*. 2010;34(suppl):S47–S55.

6   Monti V, Carlson JJ, Hunt SC, Adams TD. Relationship of ghrelin and leptin hormones with body mass index and waist circumference in a random sample of adults. *J Am Diet Assoc*. 2006;106(6):822–828.

7   Spruijt-Metz D, Belcher B, Anderson D, et al. A high-sugar/low-fiber meal compared with a low-sugar/high-fiber meal leads to higher leptin and physical activity levels in overweight Latina females. *J Am Diet Assoc*. 2009;109(6):1058–1063.

8   Ibid.

9   Blatt AD, Roe LS, Rolls BJ. Increasing the protein content of meals and its effect on daily energy intake. *J Am Diet Assoc*. 2011;111(2):290–294.

10  Perrigue MM, Monsivais P, Drewnowski A. Added soluble fiber enhances the satiating power of low-energy-density liquid yogurts. *J Am Diet Assoc*. 2009;109(11):1862–1868.

11  Wills HJ, Eldridge AL, Beiseigel J, et al. Greater satiety response with resistance starch and corn bran in human subjects. *Nutr Res*. 2009;29:100–105.

12  Maurao DM, Bressan J, Campell WW, Mattes RD. Effects of food form on appetite and energy intake in lean and obese young adults. *Int J Obes*. 2007;31:1688–1695.

13  Drewnowski A, Bellisle F. Liquid calories, sugar, and body weight. *Am J Clin Nutr*. 2007;85:651–661.

14  Dubois L, Farmer A, Girard M. Regular sugar-sweetened beverage consumption between meals increase risk of overweight among preschool-aged children. *J Am Diet Assoc*. 2007;107:924–934.

15  Spahn JM, Reeves RS, Keim KS, et al. State of the evidence regarding behavior change theories and strategies in nutrition counseling to facilitate health and food behavior change. *J Am Diet Assoc*. 2010;110(6):879–891.

16  Steenhuis IH, Vermeer WM. Portion size: review and framework for interventions. *Int J Behav Nutr Phys Act*. 2009;6:58.

17  Schwartz J, Byrd-Bredbenner C. Portion distortion: typical portion sizes selected by young adults. *J Am Diet Assoc*. 2006;106(9):1412–1418.

18  Rolls BJ, Morris EL, Roe LS. Portion size of food affects energy intake in normal-weight and overweight men and women. *Am J Clin Nutr*. 2002;76:1207–1213.

19  Marchiori D, Waroquier L, Klein O. Smaller food item sizes of snack foods influence reduced portions and caloric intake in young adults. *J Am Diet Assoc*. 2011;111(5):727–731.

20  Wansink B, Cheney MM. Super bowls: serving bowl size and food consumption. *JAMA*. 2005;293:1727–1728.

21  Orlet Fisher J, Rolls BJ, Birch LL. Children's bite size and intake of an entrée are greater with large portions than with age-appropriate or self-selected portions. *Am J Clin Nutr*. 2003;77(5):1164–1170.

22  Wansink B, Painter JE, North J. Bottomless bowls: why visual cues of portion size may influence intake. *Obes Res*. 2005;13:93–100.

23  Vermeer WM, Steenhuis IH, Seidell JC. Portion size: a qualitative study of consumers' attitudes toward point-of-purchase interventions aimed at portion size. *Health Educ Res*. 2010;25(1):109–120.

24  Wansink B, Van Ittersum K. Portion size me: downsizing our consumption norms. *J Am Diet Assoc*. 2007;107:1103–1106.

25  Hall JE, Guyton AC. *Guyton and Hall Textbook of Medical Physiology*. 12th ed. Philadelphia: Saunders Elsevier; 2011.

26  Wansink B. From mindless eating to mindlessly eating better. *Physiol Behav*. 2010;100(5):454–463.

27  Ibid.

28  Stroebele N, de Castro JM. Influence of physiological and subjective arousal on food intake in humans. *Nutrition*. 2006;22:996–1004.

29  Wilmore JH, Costill DL. *Physiology of Sports and Exercise*. 4th ed. Champaign, IL: Human Kinetics; 2008.

30  Fink HH, Burgoon LA, Mikesky AE. *Practical Applications in Sports Nutrition*. 2nd ed. Burlington, MA: Jones & Bartlett Learning; 2009.

31  Mahan LK, Escott-Stump S. *Krause's Food, Nutrition, and Diet Therapy*. 12th ed. Philadelphia: Saunders; 2007.

32  Wilmore JH, Costill DL. Op. cit.

33  Alahmadi MA, Hills AP, King NA, Byrne NM. Exercise intensity influences nonexercise activity thermogenesis in overweight and obese adults. *Med Sci Sports Exerc*. 2011;43(4):624–631.

34  Wilmore JH, Costill DL. Op. cit.

35  Granata GP, Brandon LJ. The thermic effect of food and obesity: discrepant results and methodological variations. *Nutr Rev*. 2002;60:223–233; and de

Jonge L, Bray GA. The thermic effect of food is reduced in obesity. *Nutr Rev.* 2002;60:295–297.

36  Farshchi HR, Taylor MA, Macdonald IA. Decreased thermic effect of food after an irregular compared with a regular meal pattern in healthy lean women. *Int J Obesity.* 2004;28:653–660.

37  Institute of Medicine, Food and Nutrition Board. *Dietary Reference Intakes for Energy, Carbohydrate, Fiber, Fat, Fatty Acids, Cholesterol, Protein, and Amino Acids.* Washington, DC: National Academies Press; 2005.

38  Houston D, Nicklas B, Zizza C. Weighty concerns: the growing prevalence of obesity among older adults. *J Am Diet Assoc.* 2009;109(11):1886–1895.

39  National Heart, Lung, and Blood Institute. *The Practical Guide: Identification, Evaluation and Treatment of Overweight and Obesity in Adults.* Washington, DC: US Department of Health and Human Services; 2000. NIH publication 00-4084. http://www.nhlbi.nih.gov/guidelines/obesity/prctgd_c.pdf. Accessed 6/20/11.

40  Flegal KM, Graubard BI, Williamson DF, Gail MH. Excess deaths associated with underweight, overweight, and obesity. *JAMA.* 2005;293:1861–1867.

41  National Heart Lung and Blood Institute, National Institute of Health. Assessing your weight and health risk. Body mass index (BMI). http://www.nhlbi.nih.gov/health/public/heart/obesity/lose_wt/risk.htm. Accessed 6/20/11.

42  National Center for Health Statistics. CDC growth charts: United States. http://www.cdc.gov/growthcharts. Accessed 6/20/11.

43  Barlow SE, Dietz WH. Obesity evaluation and treatment: expert committee recommendations. *Pediatrics.* 1998;102:E29. http://pediatrics.aappublications.org. Accessed 6/20/11.

44  Nana A, Slater GR, Hopkins WG, Burke LM. Effects of daily activities on DXA measurements of body composition in active people. *Med Sci Sports Exerc.* 2011 Jun 16.

45  Kishida K, Funahashi T, Matsuzawa Y. Visceral adiposity as a target for the management of the metabolic syndrome. *Ann Med.* 2011 May 25.

46  Yoshikawa K, Shimada M, Kurita N, et al. Visceral fat area is superior to body mass index as a predictive factor for risk with laparoscopy-assisted gastrectomy for gastric cancer. *Surg Endosc.* 2011;18(6):1–6.

47  Tybor DJ, Lichtenstein AH, Dallal GE, et al. Independent effects of age-related changes in waist circumference and BMI z scores in predicting cardiovascular disease risk factors in a prospective cohort of adolescent females. *Am J Clin Nutr.* 2011;93(2):392–401.

48  Lavizzo-Mourey R. Building the evidence to reverse an epidemic. *Am J Prev Med.* 2007;33(4):S162–S164.

49  Kopelman PG. Obesity as a medical problem. *Nature.* 2000;404:635–643.

50  Lien N, Henriksen HB, Nymoen LL, et al. Availability of data assessing the prevalence and trends of overweight and obesity among European adolescents. *Public Health Nutr.* 2010;13(10A):1680–1687.

51  Ujcic-Voortman JK, Box G, Baan CA, et al. Obesity and body fat distribution: ethnic differences and the role of socio-economic status. *Obes Facts.* 2011;4(1):53–60.

52  Mirmiran P, Sherafat-Kazemzadeh R, Jalali-Farahani S, Azizi F. Childhood obesity in the Middle East: a review. *East Mediterr Health J.* 2010;16(9):1009–1017.

53  Merchant A, Vatanparast H, Barlas S, et al. Carbohydrate intake and overweight and obesity among healthy adults. *J Am Diet Assoc.* 2009;109(7):1165–1172.

54  Manios Y, Maschonis G, Grammatikaki E, et al. Determinants of childhood obesity and association with maternal perceptions of their children's weight status: the "GENESIS" study. *J Am Diet Assoc.* 2010;110(10):1527–1531.

55  *Healthy People 2020.* Objectives—weight status. http://www.healthypeople.gov/2020/topicsobjectives2020/objectiveslist.aspx?topicId=29. Accessed 6/20/11.

56  Marketdata Enterprises, Inc. *The US Weight Loss & Diet Control Market.* 11th ed. May 1, 2011. http://www.marketresearch.com/Marketdata-Enterprises-Inc-v416/Weight-Loss-Diet-Control-11th-6314539. Accessed 8/14/11.

57  Gallup Consulting. In U.S., more would like to lose weight than are trying to. Gallup Health and Healthcare Poll. http://www.gallup.com. Accessed 6/20/11; and Bruke L, Steenkiste A, Music E, Styn M. A descriptive study of past experiences with weight-loss treatment. *J Am Diet Assoc.* 2008;108(4):640–647.

58  DeVault N, Kennedy T, Hermannm J, et al. It's all about kids: preventing overweight in elementary school children in Tulsa, OK. *J Am Diet Assoc.* 2009;109(4):680–687.

59  Bruke L, Steenkiste A, Music E, Styn M. Op. cit.

60  Dube L. *Obesity Prevention: The Role of Brain and Society on Individual Behavior.* Boston: Elsevier/Academic Press; 2010.

61  Abu-Rmeileh NM, Hart CL, McConnachie A, et al. Contribution of midparental BMI and other determinants of obesity in adult offspring. *Obesity.* 2008;16(6):1388–1393.

62  Hasselbalch AL. Genetics of dietary habits and obesity—a twin study. *Danish Med Bull.* 2010;57(9):B4182.

63  Barsh GS, Faroogi S, O'Rahilly S. Genetics of body-weight regulation. *Nature.* 2000;404:644–651.

64  Flegal K, Carroll M, Odgen C, Curtin L. Prevalence and trends in obesity among US adults. *JAMA.* 2010;303(3):235–241.

65  McArthur LH, Howard AB. Dietetics majors' weight-reduction beliefs, behaviors, and information sources. *J Am Coll Health.* 2001;49:175–181.

66  Cortese S, Falissard B, Pigaiani Y, et al. The relationship between body mass index and body size dissatisfaction in young adolescents: spline function analysis. *J Am Diet Assoc.* 2010;110(7):1098–1102.

67  Houston D, Nicklas B, Zizza C. Op. cit.

68  Montgomery K, Schubart K. Health promotion in culturally diverse and vulnerable populations. *Home Health Care Manage Prac.* 2010;22(2):131–139.

69  James W. The epidemiology of obesity. In: Chadwick D, Cardew G, eds. *The Origins and Consequences of Obesity.* Chichester, England: Wiley; 1996:1–16.

70  Holben DH, Pheley AM. Diabetes risk and obesity in food-insecure households in rural Appalachian Ohio. Preventing chronic disease. *Publ Health Res Pract Policy.* 2006;3(3):1–9.

71  Ibid.

72  Ibid.

73  Centers for Disease Control and Prevention. Overweight and obesity: data and statistics. Obesity rates among all children in the United States. http://www.cdc.gov/obesity/childhood/data.html. Accessed 6/20/11.

74  Boeckner L, Pullen C, Noble Walker S, et al. Eating behaviors and health history of rural midlife to older women in the Midwestern United States. *J Am Diet Assoc.* 2007;107(2):306–310.

75  Centers for Disease Control and Prevention. Overweight and obesity: data and statistics. Trends by state, 1985–2010. http://www.cdc.gov/obesity/data/trends.html. Accessed 11/24/11.

76  Akil L, Ahmad HA. Effects of socioeconomic factors on obesity rates in four southern states and Colorado. *Ethn Dis.* 2011;21(1):58–62.

77  National Center for Health Statistics. Prevalence of overweight and obesity among adults in the United States. http://www.cdc.gov/nchs/products/hestats.htm. Accessed 6/20/11.

78  Durand CP, Andalib M, Dunton GF, et al. A systematic review of built environment factors related to physical activity and obesity risk: implications for smart growth urban planning. *Obes Rev.* 2011;12(5):e173–182.

79  Kapinos KA, Yakusheva O. Environmental influences on young adult weight gain: evidence from a natural experiment. *J Adolesc Health.* 2011;48(1):52–58.

80  Safron M, Cislak A, Gasper T, Luszczynska A. Micro-environmental characteristics related to body weight, diet, and physical activity of children and adolescents: a systematic umbrella review. *Int J Environ Health Res.* 2011;27:1–25.

81  Christakis NA, Fowler JH. The spread of obesity in a large social network over 32 years. *N Engl J Med.* 2007;26;357(4):370–379.

82  Trogdon JG, Nonnemaker J, Pais J. Peer effects in adolescent overweight. *J Health Econ.* 2008;27(5):1388–1399.

83  Fletcher A, Bonell C, Sorhaindo A. You are what your friends eat: systematic review of social network analysis of young people's eating behaviours and bodyweight. *J Epidemiol Community Health.* 2011;65(6):548–555.

84  Ibid.

85  US Department of Health and Human Services and Centers for Disease Control and Prevention. Summary Health Statistics for US Adults: National Health Interview Survey, 2009. Series 10: No 249.

86  Keim NL, Blanton CA, Kretsch MJ. America's obesity epidemic: measuring physical activity to promote an active lifestyle. *J Am Diet Assoc.* 2004;104:1398–1409.

87  Fulton JE, Wang X, Yore MM, et al. Television viewing, computer use, and BMI among US children and adolescents. *J Phys Act Health.* 2009;6(suppl 1):S28–S35.

88 Faith MS, Allison DB, Geliebter A. Emotional eating and obesity. In: Dalton S, ed. Op. cit., 439–465.

89 Thomas JG, Butryn ML, Stice E, Lowe MR. A prospective test of the relation between weight change and risk for bulimia nervosa. *Int J Eat Disord.* 2011;44(4):295–303.

90 Nickelson J, Bryant C, Buhi E, DeBate R. A modified obesity proneness model describes how mother may influence the development of disordered eating behaviors and obesity. *J Am Diet Assoc.* 2008;108(9, suppl):A115.

91 Neumark-Sztainer D, Wall M, Haines J, Story M, Eiseberg ME. Why does dieting predict weight gain in adolescents? Findings from Project EAT-II: a 5-year longitudinal study. *J Am Diet Assoc.* 2007;107(3):448–455.

92 Houston D, Nicklas B, Zizza C. Op. cit.

93 Olshansky SJ, Passaro DJ, Hershow RC. A potential decline in life expectancy in the United States in the 21st century. *N Engl J Med.* 2005;352:1138–1145.

94 Behan D, Cox S. Obesity and its relation to mortality and morbidity costs. Society of Actuaries. December 2010. http://www.soa.org/files/pdf/research-2011-obesity-relation-mortality.pdf. Accessed 6/20/11.

95 Kuller L. The great fat debate: reducing cholesterol. *J Am Diet Assoc.* 2011;111(5):663–664.

96 Franz M, Powers M, Leontos C, et al. The evidence for medical nutrition therapy for type 1 and type 2 diabetes in adults. *J Am Diet Assoc.* 2010;110(12):1852–1889.

97 Gill CE, Cook EA, Smith CL, et al. Dietary Approaches to Stop Hypertension diet compliance decreases coronary heart disease risk in overweight and obese college-aged women. *J Am Diet Assoc.* 2010;110(suppl 9):A116.

98 Tung A. Anaesthetic considerations with the metabolic syndrome. *Br J Anaesthesia.* 2010;105(suppl 1):i24–i33.

99 Maitre C. Importance of physical activity in the prevention of breast cancer. *Bull Cancer.* 2009;96(5):543–551.

100 Schlienger JL, Luca F, Vinzio S, Pradignac A. Obesity and cancer. *Rev Med Intern.* 2009;30(9):776–782.

101 Carter R 3rd, Watenpaugh DE. Obesity and obstructive sleep apnea: or is it OBA and obesity? *Pathophysiology.* 2008;15(2):71–77.

102 Strycharm I, Lavoie M-E, Messier L. Anthropometric, metabolic, psychosocial, and dietary characteristics of overweight/obese postmenopausal women with a history of weight cycling: A MONET (Montreal Ottawa New Emerging Team) study. *J Am Diet Assoc.* 2009;109(4):718–724.

103 Ibid.

104 Ibid.

105 Ibid.

106 Academy of Nutrition and Dietetics. Position of the Academy of Nutrition and Dietetics: weight management. *J Am Diet Assoc.* 2009;109(2):330–346.

107 Flegal K, Graubard B, Williamson D, Gail M. Excess deaths associated with underweight, overweight, and obesity. *JAMA.* 2005;293:1861–1867.

108 Position of the Academy of Nutrition and Dietetics: weight management. Op. cit.

109 US Department of Agriculture and US Department of Health and Human Services. *Dietary Guidelines for Americans, 2010.* 7th ed. Washington, DC: US Government Printing Office; 2010.

110 Hill JO, Peters JC, Wyatt HR. Using the energy gap to address obesity: a commentary. *J Am Diet Assoc.* 2009;109(11):1848–1853.

111 Benson AC, Torode ME, Fiatarone Singh MA. Effects of resistance training on metabolic fitness in children and adolescents: a systematic review. *Obes Rev.* 2008;9(1):43–66.

112 Grundy SM, Cleeman JI, Daniels SR, et al. American Heart Association and National Heart, Lung, and Blood Institute scientific statement: diagnosis and management of metabolic syndrome. *Circulation.* 2005;112:e-pub.

113 Bluher M, Zimmer P. Metabolic and cardiovascular effects of physical activity, exercise and fitness I patients with type 2 diabetes. *Dtsch Med Wochenschr.* 2010;135(18):930–934.

114 National Weight Control Registry. NECR facts. http://www.nwcr.ws/Research/default.htm. Accessed 6/20/11.

115 Fink HH, Burgoon LA, Mikesky AE. Op. cit.

116 Larso NI, Neumark-Sztainer D, Hannan PJ, Story M. Family meals during adolescence are associated with higher diet quality and healthful meal patterns during young adulthood. *J Am Diet Assoc.* 2007;107(9):1502–1510.

117 Deshmukh-Taskar PR, Nicklas TA, O'Neil CE, et al. The relationship of breakfast skipping and type of breakfast consumption with nutrient intake and weight status in children and adolescents: The National Health and Nutrition Examination Survey, 1999–2006. *J Am Diet Assoc.* 2010;110(6):869–878.

118 Ibid.

119 Spahn J, Reeves R, Keim K. State of the evidence regarding behavior change theories and strategies in nutrition counseling to facilitate health and food behavior change. *J Am Diet Assoc.* 2010;110(6):879–891.

120 Dansinger ML, Gleason JA, Griffith JL, Selker HP, Schaefer EJ. Comparison of the Atkins, Ornish, Weight Watchers, and Zone diets for weight loss and heart disease risk reduction: a randomized trial. *JAMA.* 2005;293:43–53.

121 Smith TJ, Sigrist LD, Bathalon GP, et al. Efficacy of a meal-replacement program for promoting blood lipid changes and weight and body fat loss in US Army soldiers. *J Am Diet Assoc.* 2010;111(2):268–273.

122 Webber KH, Tate DF, Quintilliani LM. Motivational interviewing in Internet groups: a pilot study for weight loss. *J Am Diet Assoc.* 2008;108(6):1029–1032.

123 Womble LG, Wadden TA, McGuckin BG, et al. A randomized controlled trial of a commercial Internet weight loss program. *Obes Res.* 2004;12:1011–1018.

124 Serdula MK, Kahn LK, Dietz WH. Weight loss counseling revisited. *JAMA.* 2003;289(14):1747–1750.

125 Campfield LA. The role of pharmacological agents in the treatment of obesity. In: Dalton S, ed. Op. cit., 466–485.

126 US Department of Health and Human Services and Weight-Control Information Network (WIN). Prescription Medications for the Treatment of Obesity. http://win.niddk.nih.gov/Publications/prescription.htm#fdameds. Accessed 6/20/11.

127 Ibid.

128 Ibid.

129 Lucas KH, Kaplan-Machlis B. Orlistat—a novel weight loss therapy. *Ann Pharmacother.* 2001;35:314–328.

130 Mauro M, Taylor V, Wharton S, Sharma AM. Barriers to obesity treatment. *Eur J Inter Med.* 2008;19(3):173–180.

131 Pillitteri JL, Shiffman S, Rohay JM, et al. Use of dietary supplements for weight loss in the United States: results of a national survey. *Obesity.* 2008;16(4):790–796.

132 Pittler MH, Ernst E. Dietary supplements for body-weight reduction: a systematic review. *Am J Clin Nutr.* 2004;79:529–536; and Dwyer JT, Allison DB, Coates PM. Dietary supplements in weight reduction. *J Am Diet Assoc.* 2005;105:S80–S86.

133 US Food and Drug Administration. Dietary supplements. http://www.fda.gov/food/dietarysupplements/default.htm. Accessed 6/20/11.

134 Kulick D, Hark L, Deen D. The bariatric surgery patient: a growing role for registered dietitians. *J Am Diet Assoc.* 2010;110(4):593–599.

135 Ibid.

136 Steinbrook R. Surgery for severe obesity. *N Engl J Med.* 2004;350:1075–1079.

137 Carey DG, Pliego GJ, Raymond RC, Skau KB. Body composition and metabolic changes following bariatric surgery: effects on fat mass, lean mass and basal metabolic rate. *Obes Surg.* 2006;6:469–477.

138 Post RE, Mainous AG, Diaz VA, Matheson EM, Everett CJ. Use of the Nutrition Facts label in chronic disease management: results from the National Health and Nutrition Examination Survey. *J Am Diet Assoc.* 2010;110(4):628–632.

139 Kreider RB, Serra M, Beavers KM, et al. A structured diet and exercise program promotes favorable changes in weight loss, body composition, and weight maintenance. *J Am Diet Assoc.* 2011;111(6):828–843.

# CHAPTER 9

# Vitamins: Vital Keys to Health

## THINK About It

1   What food group, if any, supplies most of your vitamin needs?

2   When cooking vegetables, how often do you think about vitamin loss?

3   From a well-lighted area, you step into a dark room. Over time, you see details. What's going on?

4   You decide to follow a strict vegan lifestyle. What vitamin deficiencies should you watch out for?

5   Do you know anyone who takes vitamin C to prevent colds? What do you think of this strategy?

**Visit go.jblearning.com/inseldisco4e**

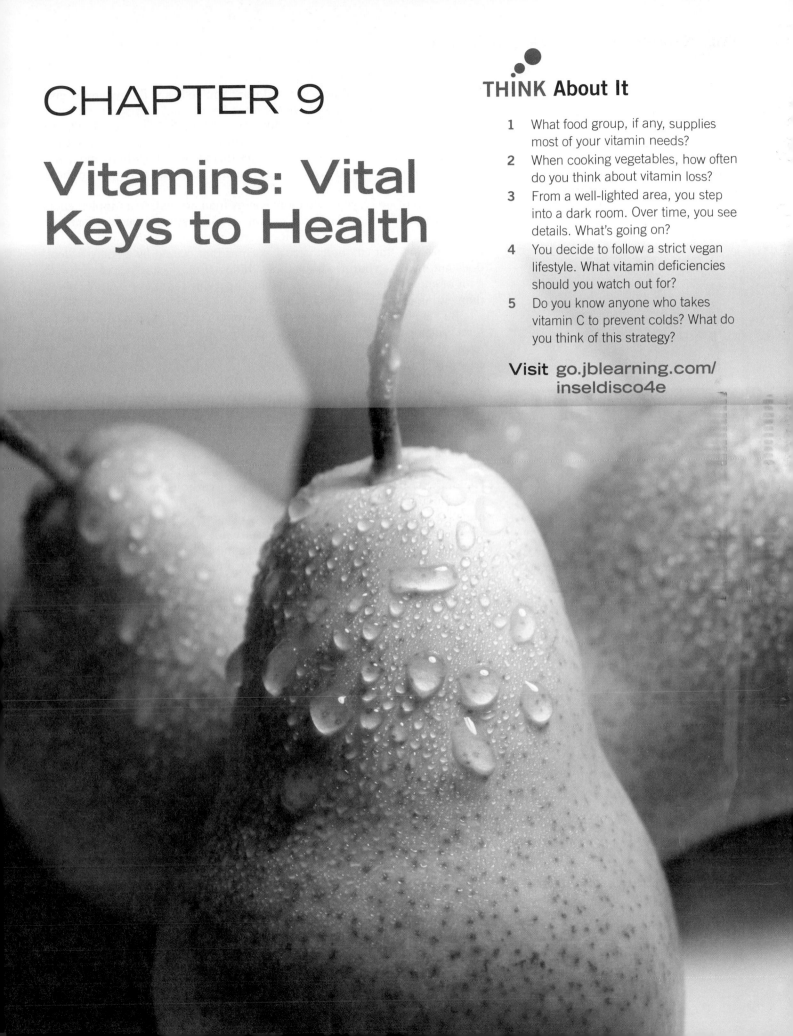

## *Quick* Bite

Feeling tired, run down, stressed out? You've heard that vitamins give you energy. So a lack of energy must be a signal that you need more vitamins, right? Well, probably not. Although many people like to think of vitamins as energy boosters, in truth, vitamins do not supply calories for the body—a fact that distinguishes them from fat, carbohydrate, and protein. However, you do need certain vitamins to obtain energy from those nutrients.

In times of stress, you need more energy than normal, so a supplement is in order, right? Well, yes and no. Certainly physical stresses, such as injury or illness, increase your body's need for energy, protein, vitamins, and minerals to aid healing. But emotional stress, such as that caused by anxiety or fear, does not increase your needs for those things. It may seem that you expend a lot of energy worrying about finals, but worrying requires no more energy than sitting and chatting with friends.

But surely if you do more physical exercise, you should take a vitamin, right? Again, not necessarily. Physical activity requires energy and the vitamins to metabolize it. But the extra food you eat to meet your greater energy needs contains vitamins, too—unless your diet consists mostly of chips, sodas, and the like. In most cases, adding fruits, vegetables, and grains as energy sources provides all the vitamins you need. So, check out your diet before you check out the vitamin supplements!

## Understanding Vitamins

Vitamins differ from fat, protein, and carbohydrate in many important ways. For one, the body requires large amounts of carbohydrates, proteins, and fats—amounts measured in grams. By comparison, the daily needs for vitamins are small—a mere microgram or two in some cases. In addition, unlike fat, protein, and carbohydrate, vitamins are not an energy source. However, many vitamins play crucial roles in extracting energy from those nutrients. Another difference is structural: Vitamins are individual units rather than long chains of smaller units.

Like fat, carbohydrate, and protein, however, vitamins are organic (carbon-containing) compounds essential for normal functioning, growth, and maintenance of the body. Vitamins often work together to get their jobs done (see **Figure 9.1**), so a deficiency of just one can cause profound health problems.

## Fat-Soluble Versus Water-Soluble Vitamins

Scientists classify vitamins as "fat-soluble" and "water-soluble." Vitamins A, D, E, and K are fat-soluble vitamins. The B vitamins and vitamin C, in contrast, dissolve in water. This difference in solubility affects the way our body absorbs, transports, and stores vitamins. (See **Figure 9.2**.)

Intestinal cells absorb fat-soluble vitamins along with dietary fat and package them into lipoproteins, which are released to the lymph system. Fat-soluble vitamins travel through the lymph system, and eventually the bloodstream, until they reach the liver.

Suppose you eat more fat-soluble vitamins than you need. As vitamin intake rises above the body's needs, the amount absorbed generally falls. Excess fat-soluble vitamins accumulate in your liver and fatty tissues, building up reserves that can tide you over for weeks or months.

Water-soluble vitamins are dissolved in the watery compartments of foods, and intestinal cells absorb water-soluble vitamins directly into the bloodstream. Although small variations in daily intake of water-soluble vitamins typically do not cause problems, they should be part of your daily diet.

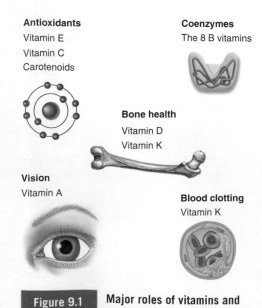

**Antioxidants**
Vitamin E
Vitamin C
Carotenoids

**Coenzymes**
The 8 B vitamins

**Bone health**
Vitamin D
Vitamin K

**Vision**
Vitamin A

**Blood clotting**
Vitamin K

**Figure 9.1**  **Major roles of vitamins and carotenoids.** Vitamins are crucial for normal functioning, growth, and maintenance of body tissues. Compared with carbohydrate, fat, and protein, the body needs tiny amounts of vitamins.

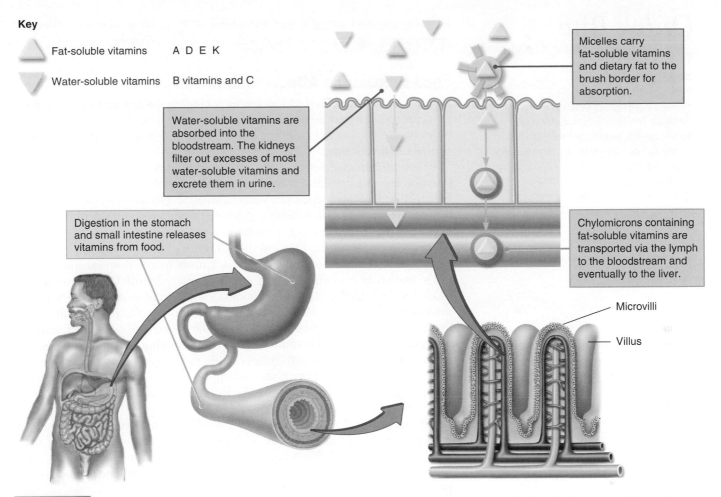

**Key**

△ Fat-soluble vitamins     A D E K

▽ Water-soluble vitamins     B vitamins and C

Micelles carry fat-soluble vitamins and dietary fat to the brush border for absorption.

Water-soluble vitamins are absorbed into the bloodstream. The kidneys filter out excesses of most water-soluble vitamins and excrete them in urine.

Digestion in the stomach and small intestine releases vitamins from food.

Chylomicrons containing fat-soluble vitamins are transported via the lymph to the bloodstream and eventually to the liver.

Microvilli

Villus

**Figure 9.2**   **Absorption of vitamins.** Water-soluble vitamins are absorbed by intestinal cells and delivered directly to the bloodstream. Fat-soluble vitamins are absorbed with fat into the lymphatic system.

Because your body does not store most water-soluble vitamins in appreciable amounts, it needs a regular supply from your diet. After 20 to 40 days of a diet deficient in vitamin C, for example, painful symptoms of vitamin C deficiency will emerge.

In general, excess fat-soluble vitamins, which tend to be stored in the body, are more likely to cause adverse effects than water-soluble vitamins. The kidneys filter out excess amounts of most water-soluble vitamins and excrete them in urine. But there are exceptions. For example, vitamin $B_{12}$ is stored in the liver in large amounts. Fat-soluble vitamins E and K are unlikely to be toxic. And large amounts of some water-soluble vitamins—vitamin $B_6$, folate, niacin, even vitamin C—can be problematic, often seriously so.

Vitamin toxicity is rarely linked to high vitamin intakes from food or to the use of supplements that contain even 100 to 150 percent of the recommended amounts. However, people who take megadoses of one or more vitamins risk consuming toxic amounts.

**Key Concepts** *Vitamins are organic substances needed in minuscule amounts to help regulate body processes. Vitamins can be classified as fat-soluble (vitamins A, D, E, and K) or water-soluble (the B vitamins and vitamin C). Fat-soluble vitamins, which are stored in the liver and fatty tissues of the body, are excreted more slowly than water-soluble*

## Quick Bite

*vitamins, and reserves last longer. Fat-soluble vitamins, when consumed in excess, generally pose a greater risk of toxicity than water-soluble vitamins.*

## Food Preparation Affects Vitamins in Foods

Vitamins are found in every food group, including the fats and oils that many of us are trying to reduce in our diets. This is one more reason to eat a variety of foods. No single food group or single choice within a food group is a good source of all vitamins.

THINK About It 1

Several factors determine the amounts of specific vitamins in a food. Because animals store and concentrate vitamins in their tissues, animal products tend to have fairly constant vitamin levels. Fruits and vegetables can be a different story. Sunlight, moisture, growing conditions, and the plant's maturity at harvest all affect vitamin content. Fortunately, our foods are grown in diverse locales, so eating a varied diet supplies plenty of vitamins.

In general, water-soluble vitamins are more fragile than fat-soluble vitamins, and some cooking practices are particularly harmful. Many cooks add baking soda, which is alkaline, to cooking water to reduce cooking time and intensify a vegetable's color. Both alkalinity and heat destroy vitamin C and the B vitamins thiamin and riboflavin. When vegetables are boiled, cooking water easily leaches water-soluble vitamins. Yet cooking only partially destroys a food's vitamin content, and some cooking methods are less destructive than others. The best cooking methods—steaming, stir-frying, and microwaving—use minimal amounts of water. (See the FYI feature "Fresh, Frozen, or Canned? Raw, Dried, or Cooked?")

THINK About It 2

Packaging and storage can affect a food's vitamin content. Exposure to light damages vitamin A and the B vitamin riboflavin. Exposure to air damages vitamins C and E. Most food processing (e.g., refining oils, milling grain, canning vegetables, drying fruit) reduces vitamin content. The more a food is processed or refined, the more it tends to lose vitamins.

### Enrichment and Fortification

Milling or refining grains removes the bran and germ to make white flour, white rice, refined cornmeal, flour for pasta, and most breakfast cereals. Processing grains also removes most B vitamins, vitamin E, and minerals such as iron, magnesium, and zinc. The loss of these nutrients from such staple foods could be devastating. In fact, during the nineteenth and early twentieth centuries, widespread adoption of these milling techniques left a wake of vitamin deficiency diseases like beriberi and pellagra.

To prevent overt deficiencies, processors now return iron and three B vitamins to the grains they process. Replacing lost nutrients is called "enrichment." Most countries now require food processors to enrich their staple grain products.

Food processors also "fortify" foods. Fortification is the process of adding extra nutrients to foods where they wouldn't be found naturally in consistently significant amounts. Iodized table salt (salt with added iodine) is a fortified food. Read the labels on some breakfast cereals—the ones with the long list of added vitamins and minerals are fortified foods. Because most breakfast cereals are fortified, they usually are good sources of vitamins and minerals. Fortification is sometimes required by law, as in the addition of vitamins A and D to milk and, most recently, the addition of folic acid to enriched cereal and grain products.

Enrichment and mandatory fortification programs helped eliminate most overt deficiency diseases in the United States and many other countries. However, mandatory enrichment replaces only some of the many nutrients

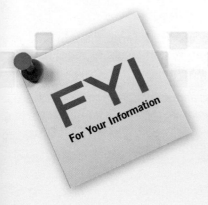

# Fresh, Frozen, or Canned? Raw, Dried, or Cooked?

## Selecting and Preparing Foods to Maximize Vitamin Content

Wouldn't it be great if we could all shop daily for fresh fruits and vegetables? When picked at their peak ripeness, fresh fruits and vegetables contain many different vitamins. Remember that light, heat, air, acid, and alkali can destroy many vitamins, and cooking liquids can leach them out. Even if you can't buy fresh foods daily, you can still minimize nutrient loss after purchase. Start by choosing clean, undamaged produce on your regular shopping trips. Then store foods with minimal exposure to light and air. Many fruits, most vegetables, and all animal products require refrigeration. Get them cold right away, and keep them cold. Because vitamin content can decrease with time, plan on using fruits and vegetables soon after purchase. The vitamin C of fresh green beans, for example, drops by half after six days at home.

What about frozen and canned foods? Their vitamin content is much better than you might guess. When vegetables are frozen immediately after they are picked, they can be more healthful choices than fresh vegetables that lose nutrients during shipping and storage.[1] Although canning uses destructive heat, the processor typically uses fresh-picked produce, which is higher in vitamins than fresh food transported to faraway markets. When using canned vegetables, incorporate the liquid in soups and stews to get the benefit of any vitamins that end up in the liquid. Recipes prepared with canned foods have similar nutritional values to those prepared with fresh or frozen ingredients.[2]

Carotenoids are stable during the canning process. In fact, research suggests the lycopene in processed tomato products is better absorbed into the body than that from raw tomatoes.[3] Unfortunately, vitamin C is lost from fruits and vegetables during canning, but much of the lost vitamin remains in the canning liquid or juice. Ready-to-drink orange juice loses about 2 percent of its vitamin C content each day once opened.[4]

Dried fruits are also a good way to eat your daily fruit. The biggest concern is portion size because when fruits are dried their nutrient, calorie, and sugar content becomes concentrated, and it is easy to eat too much. Dried fruits have a low to moderate glycemic index and a glycemic response that's comparable to that of fresh fruits. They are a

good source of nutrients such as potassium and fiber.[5] Data from the National Health and Nutrition Examination Survey (NHANES) showed that dried fruit consumption is associated with lower body mass index (BMI); reduced waist circumference; reduced abdominal obesity; improved nutrient intake (higher vitamin A, vitamin K, potassium, iron, magnesium, and fiber intake); more fruit servings per day; and healthier overall diets for both adults and children.[6]

What is the best way to cook vegetables? To maximize vitamin content, think minimal—minimal heat, minimal cooking water, and minimal exposure to air. A good rule of thumb: "minimize to maximize." Try to minimize handling the food before and during cooking. Dicing a food such as a potato reduces cooking time but also exposes more surface area to vitamin destruction. So, cut if you must, but not too small.

Because steaming, stir-frying, and microwaving minimize cooking time and water use, they are the best cooking methods for preserving vitamin content. If you boil foods, use the cooking water for sauces, stews, or soups to salvage lost water-soluble vitamins. And do not add baking soda to beans or vegetables (some folks do that to intensify color and tenderize). Baking soda destroys some vitamins.

Remember, to retain the most vitamins in your food, be gentle with storage, kind with cooking, and "minimize to maximize"!

1   Academy of Nutrition and Dietetics. Are fresh fruits and veggies better than frozen? http://www.eatright.org/Public/content.aspx?id=6442451896&terms=fresh+or+frozen. Accessed 7/12/11.

2   Fruit and Veggies—More Matters. Fresh, frozen canned, dried and 100% juice: all forms of fruits and vegetables matter! http://www.fruitsandveggiesmorematters.org/?page_id=47. Accessed 7/12/11.

3   Carlsen MH, Halvorsen BL, Holte K, et al. The total antioxidant content of more than 3,100 foods, beverages, spices, herbs, and supplements used worldwide. *Nutr J.* 2010;9:3.

4   Johnston CS, Bowling DL. Stability of ascorbic acid in commercially available orange juices. *J Am Diet Assoc.* 2002;102:525–529.

5   Fruit and Veggies—More Matters. About the buzz: fresh fruit is much healthier than dried fruit? Updated 7/6/11. http://www.fruitsandveggiesmorematters.org/?page_id=18744. Accessed 7/12/11.

6   Fruit and Veggies—More Matters. About the buzz: fresh fruit is much healthier than dried fruit? Op. cit.; and Keast D, Jones J. Dried fruit consumption associated with reduced improved overweight or obesity in adults: NHANES, 1999–2004. *Fed Am Soc Exp Bio J.* 2009;23:LB511.

lost in milling. Moreover, the American diet contains lots of highly refined foods that are not fortified or enriched, foods that have calories but almost no micronutrients.

## Provitamins

Some vitamins in foods are in inactive forms, called **provitamins** or **vitamin precursors**. The body must change them to an active form. One familiar provitamin is beta-carotene, found in many fruits and vegetables. Your body

**provitamins** Inactive forms of vitamins that the body can convert into active usable forms. Also referred to as vitamin precursors.

**vitamin precursors** See *provitamins*.

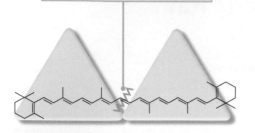

Once beta-carotene is absorbed, it can be cleaved in the middle to yield two molecules of vitamin A.

**Figure 9.3** **Beta-carotene.** Beta-carotene may be cleaved at different locations, so it may yield less than two molecules of vitamin A. Other provitamin A carotenoids yield less vitamin A than does beta-carotene.

converts much of the beta-carotene you eat to its active form, vitamin A. (See **Figure 9.3**.) When experts calculate vitamin requirements or monitor consumption, they must take provitamins into account.

**Key Concepts** *Growing conditions, storage, processing, and cooking affect the amounts of vitamins in foods. Enrichment and fortification programs replace some vitamins and minerals lost in processing and add other nutrients to foods. Provitamins are vitamin precursors that can be converted to an active vitamin form.*

# Fat-Soluble Vitamins A, D, E, K, and the Carotenoids

Despite their common property of dissolving in fat, the fat-soluble vitamins have diverse roles. Vitamin A is crucial for vision and renewing cells. Vitamin D helps regulate blood levels of calcium and is essential for bone health. Vitamin E and the carotenoids are antioxidants that help protect cells from damage. Vitamin K is known for its role in blood clotting, but it also is crucial for bone health along with vitamin D.

## Vitamin A: The Retinoids

Vitamin A's best known effects are in the eye. You need vitamin A to change incoming light to visual images and to keep the eye's surface healthy. Vitamin A also helps direct development of the body's cells—how and when they grow and divide and what form they take. As such, this vitamin is essential to proper growth and reproduction. It plays a role in immune function, both as a cell regulator and by helping maintain the skin and mucous membranes. In fact, vitamin A plays a crucial role in maintaining or regulating many tissues throughout the body.

The liver holds over 90 percent of the body's vitamin A reserves, with the rest deposited in fat tissue, lungs, and kidneys.[1] A healthy liver can store up to a year's supply of vitamin A, releasing it in just the right amounts to maintain normal vitamin A blood levels—a nice benefit, but one with a drawback: Large doses of vitamin A can exceed storage capacity and cause toxicity.

### Forms of Vitamin A

The body uses three active forms of vitamin A—**retinol**, **retinal**, and **retinoic acid**—known collectively as the **retinoids**. (See **Figure 9.4**.) Although all three forms are essential, retinol is the key player in the vitamin A family.[2]

Colorful plant pigments called **carotenoids** are precursors of vitamin A. There are several hundred carotenoids found in nature, but your body converts only a handful of them to vitamin A. Of the carotenoids, beta-carotene supplies the most vitamin A.

**retinol** The alcohol form of vitamin A; one of the retinoids; the main physiologically active form of vitamin A; interconvertible with retinal.

**retinal** The aldehyde form of vitamin A; one of the retinoids; the active form of vitamin A in the retina; interconvertible with retinol.

**retinoic acid** The acid form of vitamin A; one of the retinoids; formed from retinal but not interconvertible; helps growth, cell differentiation, and the immune system; does not have a role in vision or reproduction.

**retinoids** Compounds in foods that have chemical structures similar to vitamin A. Retinoids include the active forms of vitamin A (retinol, retinal, and retinoic acid) and the main storage forms of retinol (retinyl esters).

**carotenoids** A group of yellow, orange, and red pigments in plants. Some of these compounds are precursors of vitamin A.

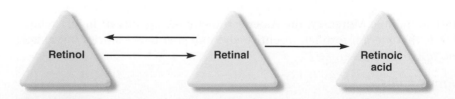

**Figure 9.4** **Forms of vitamin A.** Whereas retinol and retinal are interconvertible, the reaction that forms retinoic acid is irreversible.

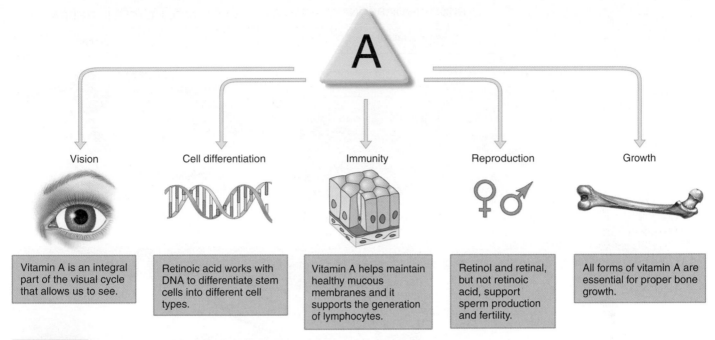

**Figure 9.5**   **Major functions of vitamin A.** Vitamin A plays a crucial role in vision and is essential for proper cell synthesis, reproduction, and bone growth.

## Functions of Vitamin A

Vitamin A is crucial for vision, for maintaining healthy cells (particularly skin cells) for fighting infections and bolstering immune function, and for promoting growth and development. (See **Figure 9.5**.)

### Vision: Night and Day

Vitamin A allows night vision and color vision, by actually becoming a functioning part of the retina. The **retina** is the paper-thin tissue lining the back of the eye, where light images are received and relayed to the brain, resulting in vision. **Rod cells**, the cells in the retina that react to dim light, are rich in a purple pigment called **rhodopsin**, or "visual purple." Rhodopsin is composed of a protein, **opsin**, plus vitamin A.

Light entering the eye and striking the retina splits rhodopsin, causing it to lose color as it releases opsin and vitamin A. (See **Figure 9.6**.) This **bleaching process** triggers electric impulses that the brain interprets as black-and-white visual images. In well-nourished people, vitamin A recombines with opsin, forming new rhodopsin that again can respond to light. If vitamin A levels are low, the body cannot re-form rhodopsin, and **night blindness** results. Although the eyes contain only 0.01 percent of the body's vitamin A, they are so sensitive to vitamin A levels that one injection of the vitamin can relieve this type of night blindness within minutes.[3]

If you awaken in the middle of the night and turn on a bright light, the light level is blinding until your eyes adjust. Rhodopsin breaks down quickly in bright light, and the reduced supply makes the rod cells less light sensitive. Conversely, when you enter a dark room, not only do your eyes dilate, but they also produce rhodopsin to increase their sensitivity to light. Known as **dark adaptation**, the speed of adjustment to dim light is related directly to the amount of vitamin A available to regenerate rhodopsin. People with night blindness cannot adjust to dim light or regain vision quickly after exposure to a flash of bright light.

THINK About It

3

**retina**  A paper-thin tissue that lines the back of the eye and contains cells called rods and cones.

**rod cells**  Light-sensitive cells in the retina that react to dim light and transmit black-and-white images.

**rhodopsin**  Found in rod cells, this light-sensitive pigment molecule consists of a protein called opsin combined with retinal.

**opsin**  A protein that combines with retinal to form rhodopsin in rod cells.

**bleaching process**  A complex light-stimulated reaction in which rod cells lose color as rhodopsin is split into vitamin A (retinal) and opsin.

**night blindness**  The inability of the eyes to adjust to dim light or to regain vision quickly after exposure to a flash of bright light.

**dark adaptation**  The process that increases the rhodopsin concentration in your eyes, allowing them to detect images in the dark better.

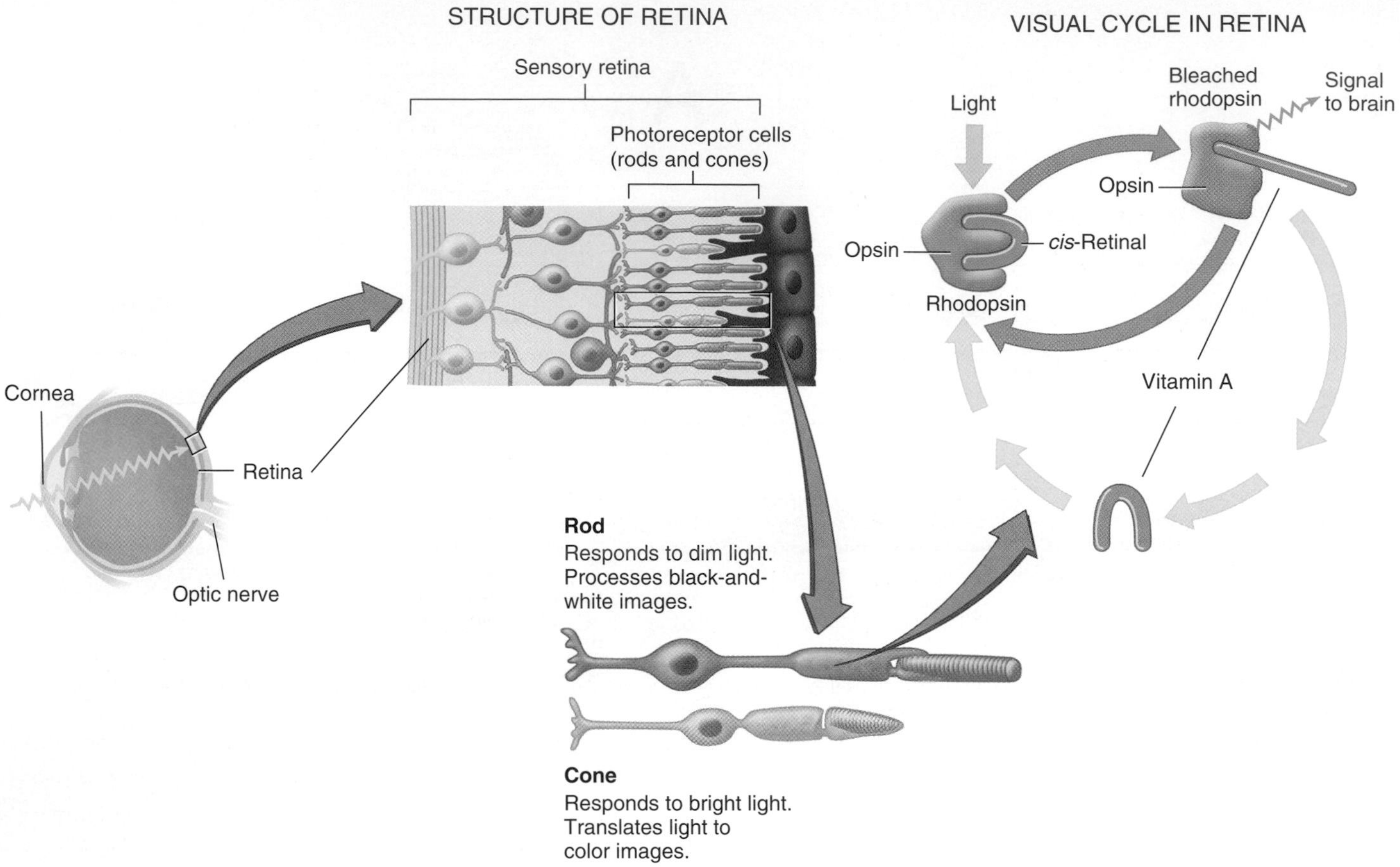

STRUCTURE OF RETINA

VISUAL CYCLE IN RETINA

**Figure 9.6** **Vitamin A and the visual cycle.** Rhodopsin is the combination of the protein opsin and vitamin A (retinal). When stimulated by light, both opsin and vitamin A change shape. This sends a signal to the brain, and you see an image in black and white. A similar process using a different protein called iodopsin provides color.

Color vision also requires vitamin A. **Cone cells**, which are responsible for color vision, are rich in the pigment **iodopsin**. The iodopsin cycle is similar to the rhodopsin cycle, with vitamin A playing a crucial role. A prolonged lack of vitamin A impairs color vision, but because it affects rod cells before cone cells, night blindness emerges first.

### Vitamin A in Cell Production and Differentiation

When your body needs to make the proteins that form new cells or other protein compounds, vitamin A plays a role in directing protein production. It helps regulate production of enzymes; blood carrier proteins; structural proteins, such as those in skin; and more.

Vitamin A works in cell differentiation, the process that causes immature, characterless cells (undifferentiated cells called **stem cells**) to mature into specific kinds of cells. For example, if you cut your hand, the new cells produced to repair the cut are specifically suited to the job; stomach cells or lung cells would not do.

With these very basic, crucially important biological functions, vitamin A plays a role in building and maintaining tissues throughout the body.

### Vitamin A and Skin

Skin, mucous membranes, and other lining materials in the body are all **epithelial tissues**. Together they cover us on the outside, act as a lining

**cone cells** Cells in the retina that are sensitive to bright light and translate it into color images.

**iodopsin** Color-sensitive pigment molecules in cone cells that consist of opsinlike proteins combined with retinal.

**stem cells** Formative cells whose daughter cells may differentiate into other cell types.

**epithelial tissues** Closely packed layers of epithelial cells that cover the body and line its cavities.

or covering on the inside, and provide lubrication where it's needed—for example, along bronchial tubes and the digestive tract. **Epithelial cells** are on the front line protecting your body, and they are destroyed and replaced relatively quickly. Replacing these cells requires vitamin A. Because the turnover of skin cells is rapid, signs of vitamin A deficiency show up early in the skin and mucous membranes.

### Vitamin A and Immune Function

Epithelial tissue is your body's first line of defense against bacterial, parasitic, and viral attack. But if dangerous microorganisms successfully breach these barriers, your body's defense system mobilizes immune cells to attack the invaders. To produce these immune cells, your body needs vitamin A.

### Vitamin A and Reproduction

Vitamin A aids reproduction, probably by keeping the secretion-producing linings of the reproductive tract healthy. In women, vitamin A helps maintain fertility. In men, it is needed for sperm production. Vitamin A's role in cell production and differentiation also makes it crucial to the proper development of an embryo.

### Vitamin A and Bones

Vitamin A helps produce bone cells needed for growth and is required for bone "remodeling." As children grow, their bones get longer. But simply adding length would produce some strange-looking bones. Therefore during normal growth, the bone ends are actually broken down and then lengthened; that is, they are remodeled. A lack of vitamin A in the growing child disrupts bone remodeling and interferes with the development of immature bone cells. The result is weak, poorly formed bones. On the other end of the spectrum, too much vitamin A has been linked to bone loss and an increased risk of fracture. Excessive amounts of vitamin A may interfere with the ability of vitamin D to promote calcium absorption and can trigger an increase in cellular activity that breaks down bone.[4]

## Dietary Recommendations for Vitamin A

Remember, vitamin A includes retinoids—retinol, retinoic acid, and retinal—and is formed from precursor carotenoids. Similar amounts of dietary retinoids and carotenoids do not provide the same amount of vitamin A. To reconcile the differences, scientists use a measure called **retinol activity equivalent (RAE)**. One retinol activity equivalent equals the activity of 1 microgram (1/1,000,000 of a gram) of retinol. On average, 12 micrograms of beta-carotene from food produce 1 microgram of retinol. Other provitamin carotenoids like alpha-carotene are converted even less efficiently: It takes 24 micrograms to produce 1 microgram of retinol.[5] (See **Figure 9.7**.)

You may read about the outdated measure "retinol equivalents," or RE, in older texts. You also may see another outdated measure, **International Units (IU)**, on vitamin labels. One IU equals about 0.3 microgram of retinol from animal foods and 3.6 micrograms of beta-carotene from plant foods.

Most Americans take in adequate amounts of vitamin A and have large stores of the vitamin in their livers. The RDA for vitamin A for males aged 14 years and older is 900 micrograms RAE per day. For females aged 14 years and older, the vitamin A RDA is 700 micrograms RAE per day. Pregnant women should consume slightly more vitamin A (770 micrograms), and women who are breastfeeding their children are advised to consume 1,300 micrograms RAE.[6]

**epithelial cells** The millions of cells that line and protect the external and internal surfaces of the body. Epithelial cells form epithelial tissues such as skin and mucous membranes.

**retinol activity equivalent (RAE)** A unit of measurement of the vitamin A content of a food. One RAE equals 1 microgram of retinol.

**International Units (IU)** An outdated system to measure vitamin activity, this measurement does not consider differences in bioavailability.

*Quick* Bite

**Vitamin A Isn't Just for Eyes**
A study conducted in Nepal showed that women who took vitamin A supplements during pregnancy had a much lower risk of maternal mortality than those who took a placebo. The researchers concluded that regular and adequate intake of vitamin A or beta-carotene can reduce the risk of pregnancy-related death in areas where vitamin A deficiency is common.

1 retinol activity equivalent (RAE) = 1 μg retinol

= 2 μg supplemental beta-carotene

= 12 μg dietary beta-carotene

= 24 mg dietary carotenoids

**Figure 9.7** Retinol activity equivalent conversion.

**provitamin A** Carotenoid precursors of vitamin A in foods of plant origin, primarily deeply colored fruits and vegetables.

## Sources of Vitamin A

Only foods of animal origin contain retinoids. Plant foods, especially yellow-orange vegetables and fruits, contain **provitamin A** carotenoids such as beta-carotene. (Read more under "The Carotenoids" later in this chapter.) On average, we get about one-quarter to one-third of our vitamin A as carotenoids, mainly beta-carotene, but that figure varies widely.

Liver is the richest source of vitamin A, just as you would expect, knowing that the liver stores vitamin A. Historically, people consumed fish liver oils, such as cod liver oil, for their vitamin A (and vitamin D) content, and cod liver oil remains a popular supplement today. Other good sources include butter, butterfat-containing dairy foods, and egg yolk. (See **Figure 9.8**.)

Because low-fat milk is fortified, it is a good vitamin A source, despite having little or no butterfat. Producers also fortify some foods of plant origin, including margarine, some breakfast cereals, and some special dietary foods like "nutrition bars."

**Key Concepts** *Vitamin A occurs in three forms in the body: retinol, retinal, and retinoic acid. Retinol is found in a few animal-derived foods. Vitamin A is also formed from precursors called carotenoids. Intake recommendations for vitamin A are expressed in RAEs (retinol activity equivalents) to account for differences between retinoids and carotenoids. Most vitamin A is processed and stored in the liver and is released as needed. Vitamin A in the cells of the retina plays a crucial role in vision. It is also involved in cell differentiation, reproduction, maintaining epithelial tissue, supporting other immune functions, and bone health.*

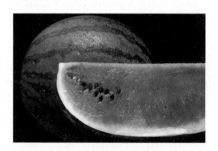

**Exceptionally high sources**
Beef liver
Carrots
Sweet potato
Chicken liver

**High sources**
Spinach
Mango
Cantaloupe
Collards
Romaine lettuce
Oatmeal, instant, fortified
Broccoli
Tomato juice
Wheat bran flakes cereal
Watermelon
Apricot

**Good sources**
Dried plums
All Bran cereal
Corn flakes cereal
Blackeyed peas
Green beans
Milk

**Figure 9.8**    **Food sources of vitamin A.** Vitamin A is found as retinol in animal foods and as beta-carotene and other carotenoids in plant foods. Some of the best sources are liver, orange and deep-yellow vegetables, and dark-green leafy vegetables.

## Vitamin A Deficiency

Although dietary deficiency of vitamin A is rare in North America and Western Europe, it is the leading cause of childhood blindness worldwide, especially in Southeast Asia, parts of Africa, and Central and South America. In these regions, vitamin A deficiency typically occurs alongside general protein-energy malnutrition in infants and young children. Protein deficiency reduces levels of retinol-binding protein, the blood carrier protein that transports vitamin A in the blood. Vitamin A deficiency interacts with other nutrient deficiencies and with infection, worsening respiratory infections or diarrhea and causing countless deaths. (See **Figure 9.9**.)

Certain North American groups are at risk for vitamin A deficiency. Premature infants do not have vitamin A reserves in their livers. People with alcoholism or liver disease may have damaged livers that cannot store much vitamin A. Fat malabsorption diseases and medicines that inhibit fat absorption also impair vitamin A absorption. Because the body needs zinc to use vitamin A efficiently, inadequate zinc intake can cause vitamin A deficiency symptoms.

### The Eyes

Early treatment can rapidly correct night blindness, an early symptom of vitamin A deficiency. But a worsening and prolonged deficiency threatens eyesight. Cells in the **cornea** (part of the eye's covering) stop reproducing, and the deficiency damages mucous membranes that provide lubrication. Without adequate moisture, dirt and bacteria accumulate as the eye dries out. As the cornea deteriorates, foamy white patches called Bitot's spots appear on the eye. In extreme cases, the cornea eventually develops sores and scars and may even liquefy, causing total blindness. Collectively, these are the symptoms of **xerophthalmia**, an irreversible condition.

### The Skin and Other Epithelial Cells

Hard, bumpy, scaly skin—"goose flesh" that doesn't go away—is an early symptom of vitamin A deficiency. The deficiency disrupts epithelial cell production, and the skin's hair follicles become plugged with **keratin**. Vitamin A deficiency also impairs normal secretions, blocking perspiration and mucus. The lack of mucus damages the linings of the mouth, respiratory tract, and urinary and genital tracts. Sperm production slows, and female fertility declines.

### Immune Function

Vitamin A deficiency leaves a person especially vulnerable to infection. Damaged epithelium allows microorganisms to breach this first line of defense. Under ordinary circumstances, entry of these enemy invaders would then trigger protective immune cells to quickly multiply. But immune cells need vitamin A to multiply. With too few immune cells to mount an effective attack, the invading microorganisms can cause severe, even fatal, diarrhea or respiratory infection. When a child is deficient in vitamin A, a relatively harmless infection such as measles can be fatal.[7]

### Other Effects

Because vitamin A is essential to cell growth and differentiation, a deficiency causes a variety of problems that include growth retardation, bone deformities, defective teeth, and kidney stones.

## Vitamin A Toxicity

Although it is difficult to overdo vitamin A from natural foods, consumption of large amounts of fish liver has been found to cause vitamin A toxicity in

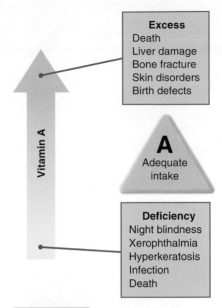

**Excess**
Death
Liver damage
Bone fracture
Skin disorders
Birth defects

**A**
Adequate intake

**Deficiency**
Night blindness
Xerophthalmia
Hyperkeratosis
Infection
Death

Vitamin A

**Figure 9.9**   **Vitamin A deficiency and toxicity.** A broad range of vitamin A intake is adequate and provides for normal function. Too little or too much vitamin A can have serious consequences.

**cornea** The transparent outer surface of the eye.

**xerophthalmia** A condition caused by vitamin A deficiency that dries the cornea and mucous membranes of the eye.

**keratin** A water-soluble fibrous protein that is the primary constituent of hair, nails, and the outer layer of skin.

**teratogen** Any substance that causes birth defects.

children.[8] In addition, the enthusiasm for megadose vitamin supplementation has increased the potential for toxic dosing. Vitamin A toxicity has a wide range of symptoms, both subtle and overt, including fatigue, vomiting, abdominal pain, bone and joint pain, loss of appetite, skin disorders, headache, blurred or double vision, hip fracture, and liver damage. (See Figure 9.9.). Vitamin A toxicity can be acute, but more often it develops gradually over months or years. Toxicity symptoms can often be corrected when intake levels are lowered.

Excess retinol is a known **teratogen** (causes birth defects). The birth defects it causes include cleft palate, heart abnormalities, and brain malfunction.[9] It is most dangerous during the first three months of pregnancy, when cell differentiation is most intense. Pregnant women should get the approval of their doctor before taking retinol-containing supplements.

The Tolerable Upper Intake Level (UL) for vitamin A for men and women, including women who are pregnant or breastfeeding, is 3,000 micrograms of retinol per day. Check out some vitamin A supplement labels. Those that contain 10,000 IU of retinol (not from carotenoids) are providing the UL of vitamin A. You may be surprised to see supplements with 25,000 IU—far above safe levels.

You may know people who consumed so much carrot juice that their skin acquired a yellowish-orange cast. Dark-skinned people may notice a yellowing of the palms and soles of their feet. Accumulation of excess beta-carotene in the blood is responsible for this harmless condition.

### Acne Treatment

Some "close cousins" (or analogs) of vitamin A are given in therapeutic doses to treat skin problems. Two commercially available forms of retinoic acid, Retin-A and Accutane, are widely used for acne. But, like vitamin A, these retinoids cause birth defects. Any woman who may become pregnant should not use these medicines. In fact, because these medications accumulate in fat stores, even when applied on the skin, women should discontinue them at least two years before pregnancy.

**Key Concepts**   *Vitamin A deficiency causes blindness; damages skin, bone, and other tissues; and limits immune function, leaving a person vulnerable to infection. Excessive vitamin A supplementation can cause toxicity, even with doses just a few times higher than the RDA. Vitamin A toxicity during pregnancy could be devastating; pregnant women should be wary of retinol-containing supplements and avoid retinoid-containing medicines.*

*Quick* Bite

**Avoid Polar Bear Liver**
Liver and onions may be your favorite meal, but do not use polar bear liver. Polar bear liver is so rich in vitamin A that a single serving can be toxic for humans.

## The Carotenoids

Carotenoids are plant pigments that give the deep yellow, orange, and red colors to fruits and vegetables such as apricots, carrots, and tomatoes. The major carotenoids are alpha-carotene, beta-carotene, lutein, zeaxanthin, cryptoxanthin, and lycopene. Among them, beta-carotene, the yellow-orange pigment in cantaloupe, carrots, and squash, is the most common. Alpha-carotene, beta-carotene, and beta-cryptoxanthin can be converted to vitamin A. Lycopene and lutein have no vitamin A activity.

## Functions of Carotenoids

Aside from conversion to vitamin A, the carotenoids do not appear to be essential in the technical sense; a carotenoid-free diet does not cause deficiency disease. Therefore, the Food and Nutrition Board has not established DRIs for them.[10] Yet people who eat generous amounts of foods rich in carotenoids

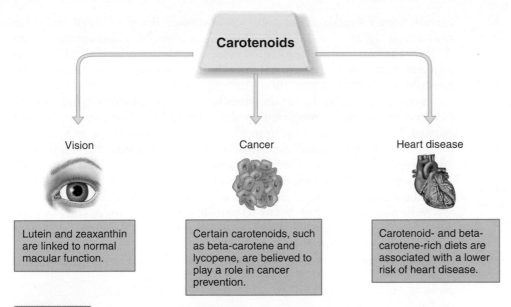

**Figure 9.10** **Major functions of carotenoids.** Independent of vitamin A activity, carotenoids may be involved in normal macular function and reduced risk of cancer and heart disease.

reduce their risk of many major degenerative diseases. Carotenoids are potent antioxidants, which may explain their beneficial effects. (See **Figure 9.10**.) (For more information on antioxidants, see the FYI feature "Antioxidants and Free Radicals.")

### Carotenoids and Vision

Lutein and zeaxanthin are found in the macula of the eye, the central portion of the retina responsible for sharp, detailed vision. Scientists believe that carotenoids may protect the eyes by inhibiting the oxidative damage that contributes to age-related blindness.[11] Research has demonstrated that a supplement containing carotenoids and other antioxidants can slow the progression of age-related macular degeneration.[12]

### Carotenoids and Cancer

People with the highest intakes of carotenoid-rich fruits and vegetables and/or high levels of specific carotenoids tend to have the lowest risk for certain cancers. Although preliminary research implied that eating tomato products like tomato sauce (yes, even ketchup), for example, was associated with reduced risk of prostate cancer,[13] more recent evidence suggests that neither dietary nor supplemental intakes of the carotenoid lycopene are significant for prostate cancer prevention.[14] Tomato products are excellent sources of lycopene, and research does suggest that a diet rich in lycopene reduces the risk of heart disease, osteoporosis, and several cancers.[15]

The beneficial effects of carotenoids on health generally reflect food intake, not supplement use. To date, trials of beta-carotene supplements for cancer prevention have been disappointing; paradoxically, megadose supplements are associated with increased lung cancer among smokers or those exposed to asbestos.[16]

## Food Sources, Absorption, and Storage of Carotenoids

Orange and yellow fruits and vegetables generally contain beta-carotene, alpha-carotene, and cryptoxanthin. Good sources of beta-carotene include

*Quick* Bite

**And They Called It Cantaloupe**
The word *cantaloupe* comes from a papal garden in a small town near Rome named Cantaloupo. One-half of a medium cantaloupe has 466 RAE as beta-carotene.

## *Quick* Bite

carrots, winter squash, sweet potatoes, and some orange-colored fruits like cantaloupe, apricots, and mango. Dark-green vegetables also contain abundant carotenoids, but the carotenoid colors are hidden by the plentiful green pigment chlorophyll. Carotenoids from dark-green leafy vegetables, however, produce less vitamin A than those from ripe orange-colored fruit.[17]

Surprisingly oranges and tangerines have little beta-carotene, but they are rich in cryptoxanthin. Cryptoxanthin also is found in mangos, nectarines, and papaya.[18] Lycopene has a more reddish color; you will see it in tomatoes, pink grapefruit, guava, and watermelon. Lutein and zeaxanthin are in leafy green vegetables, pumpkin, and red pepper. Because all major carotenoids are important, and they are difficult to identify in food just by looking, you should eat a wide variety of fruits and vegetables to ensure a good intake.

Your body absorbs only 20 to 40 percent of the carotenoids you eat, even less if your intake is high. Dietary fat increases absorption. Factors that limit fat absorption limit carotenoid absorption as well. That includes olestra, the fat substitute in some snack foods. Although manufacturers fortify olestra

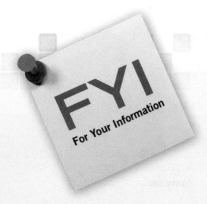

## Antioxidants and Free Radicals

An antioxidant prevents the damaging effects of oxygen. Say, wait a minute. Oxygen's a good thing, isn't it? Certainly, you couldn't live long without it!

But some forms of oxygen are very unstable. We call these unstable molecules "free radicals." They are extremely active and, when out of control, can attack or react with healthy body cells, damaging fragile cell membranes and genetic material and changing the character of fats and proteins. Antioxidants "neutralize" or "quench" free radicals, keeping them from becoming excessive or getting out of control. Several vitamins act as antioxidants.

Free radicals are generated during normal metabolism and they are normal substances. We put their destructive capabilities to good use. Their oxidizing action kills harmful microorganisms. They even destroy our body's own damaged cells, thus preventing cancerous growth.

Household bleach, a familiar oxidizing agent, is a good example of the "good guy–bad guy" nature of free radicals. Add it to dirty clothes, and it cleans them well, even killing germs. But add too much, and your clothes get holes. The sun's oxidizing rays are also bleaching agents, very helpful for white fabrics, but damaging to colors. Other examples of oxidative damage are the rusting of iron and the rancidity of fats.

Outside agents, such as tobacco smoke, toxic chemicals, excessive sunshine, and even some medical treatments, form free radicals in our bodies. In the presence of these agents, our antioxidants are depleted more quickly.

Excessive oxidation in the body is problematic. Chronic, excessive exposure to sunshine, for example, is associated with age-related macular degeneration and cataracts, two conditions that cause blindness. Researchers believe oxidative damage plays a role in these conditions; there's evidence that the antioxidants vitamin C, vitamin E, beta-carotene, and zinc can reduce the risk of developing advanced age-related macular

degeneration (AMD) by about 25 percent.[1] The oxidizing rays of the sun also accelerate skin wrinkling and, worse, cause skin cancer, due in part to oxidative damage of skin cells. Other cancers may originate when cellular DNA is damaged by free radicals; foods rich in antioxidants may prevent this damage.[2]

There is good evidence that oxidation has a pivotal role in initiating atherosclerosis. Free radicals oxidize blood lipids such as cholesterol; the damaged lipids are then deposited on the inside surface of artery walls, the beginning of atherosclerotic plaques. Vitamin E, our major fat-soluble antioxidant, may help block this process.[3]

Vitamin C and, under some circumstances, riboflavin are other antioxidants. Some minerals such as selenium function in antioxidant systems as well. The antioxidants often work in cooperation with each other. Vitamin C, a water-soluble antioxidant, restores vitamin E that is altered by its antioxidant activity. Selenium also works with vitamin E. In fact, to a certain extent, a selenium-rich diet can help treat a vitamin E deficiency.

Vitamins and minerals are only part of your antioxidant defense. Your body makes many of its own antioxidants. Examples are glutathione, coenzyme $Q_{10}$ (ubiquinone), and superoxide dismutase. Several of these have now been put into supplements. To have an effect, however, they

must survive digestion, be absorbed, and reach their site of activity in the body. Their value in supplement form remains largely unproved.

In addition to vitamins, fruits and vegetables contain many other antioxidants, which protect the plants from sunshine and other oxidants. These substances, along with other plant-produced chemicals, are sometimes called phytonutrients, phytochemicals, or nutraceuticals. Ingesting them probably gives us the same protection they give the plant. Supplement manufacturers also put these substances—examples are the bioflavonoids—in pills and add them to beverages marketed as "health-promoting." In these forms, neither their value nor their safety has been proved.

1    National Eye Institute, National Institutes of Health. The AREDS formulation and age-related macular degeneration. Updated 7/11. http://www.nei.nih.gov/amd/summary.asp#10. Accessed 7/12/11.

2    Institute of Medicine, Food and Nutrition Board. *Dietary Reference Intakes for Vitamin C, Vitamin E, Selenium, and Carotenoids.* Washington, DC: National Academies Press; 2000.

3    Ibid.

with retinol, they do not add carotenoids—a practice that concerns some nutritionists.

It's now known that cell walls of carotenoid-rich plants inhibit absorption. Cooking vegetables for a few minutes breaks the cell walls, releasing the carotenoids and improving their absorption.

## Carotenoid Supplementation

Carotenoid supplements have become popular in recent years. However, the Food and Nutrition Board advises against them for the general population, recommending carotenoid-rich fruits and vegetables instead.[19] A UL has not been set for the carotenoids.

# Vitamin D

This fat-soluble nutrient is called the sunshine vitamin. When the ultraviolet rays of the sun strike your skin, they convert cholesterol to vitamin D. Vitamin D is unique because, given sufficient sunlight, your body can make all that it needs—dietary vitamin D is unnecessary. However, when coupled with too little sun exposure, a lack of dietary vitamin D does cause a vitamin deficiency.

Vitamin D is essential for bone health, and it protects against certain cancers and other chronic diseases. In children, it promotes bone development and growth. In adults, it is necessary for bone maintenance. In older adults, vitamin D helps prevent bone loss and fractures. In addition, supplemental vitamin D can reduce the rate of falls in the elderly.[20] Vitamin D is currently under investigation for its role in the prevention of cardiovascular disease, type 2 diabetes,[21] and cancer.[22]

## Forms and Formation of Vitamin D

Vitamin D is a group of about 10 related compounds. The most important of these are vitamin $D_2$ (ergocalciferol), found in a few plant foods, and vitamin $D_3$ (cholecalciferol), found naturally only in a few animal-derived foods.

In the skin, UV radiation converts a form of cholesterol to cholecalciferol, which travels to the liver. The liver converts both synthesized and dietary vitamin D to an intermediate form, which it sends to the kidneys. The kidneys perform the final step—conversion to the active form of vitamin D, known as **25-hydroxyvitamin D [25(OH)D]**, or **calcitriol**.

## Functions of Vitamin D

Many simply regard vitamin D as a vitamin that keeps bones healthy. But it is first and foremost a regulator. (See **Figure 9.11.**) Because vitamin D made in one part of the body regulates activities in other parts, scientists consider it a hormone. Vitamin D has a role in preventing cancer cells from dividing and has anti-inflammatory properties, and as such it may play a role in preventing cancer and cardiovascular disease, an area of considerable research activity.[23] Vitamin D also is involved in the regulation of insulin formation and secretion, which suggests a role in blood sugar maintenance and the development of type 2 diabetes mellitus—another area of current research interest.[24]

### Regulation of Blood Calcium Levels

The primary regulatory role of 25(OH)D is to maintain blood calcium and phosphorus levels within a normal range. 25(OH)D acts in concert with two other hormones: **parathyroid hormone (PTH)** from the parathyroid glands and **calcitonin** from the thyroid gland. Together, levels of these three

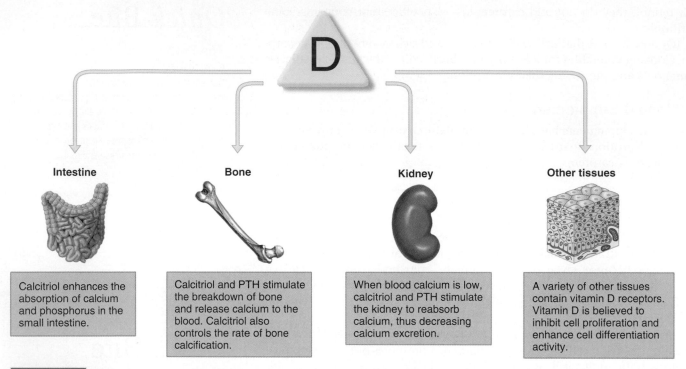

**Figure 9.11** **Major functions of vitamin D.** Vitamin D and calcium are essential to bone health. To regulate blood calcium levels, vitamin D works with parathyroid hormone (PTH) to stimulate the body to move calcium back and forth between the blood and the reservoir of calcium in bone.

hormones continually rise and fall, adjusting blood calcium levels by changing urinary calcium excretion, intestinal calcium absorption, and the flow of calcium in and out of bone.

Here's how it works. Much like a thermostat monitoring temperature, the parathyroid glands monitor blood calcium levels, releasing PTH when calcium levels drop. PTH signals specific bone cells to break down bone tissue and release calcium into the bloodstream. In addition, PTH signals the kidneys to slow calcium excretion and increase 25(OH)D production. In turn, 25(OH)D stimulates the small intestine to absorb more calcium from food, thereby raising blood calcium levels further.

When blood calcium levels become too high, the thyroid gland releases calcitonin and the parathyroid glands slow their release of PTH. Calcitonin inhibits factors causing bone breakdown, allowing bone-forming activities to prevail. Bone-forming cells remove calcium from the blood and deposit it in bone. Lower PTH levels allow the kidneys to continue excreting calcium and decrease 25(OH)D production. In turn, low 25(OH)D levels cause the small intestine to reduce calcium absorption from food, thereby lowering blood calcium levels further.

## Dietary Recommendations for Vitamin D

Despite our ability to synthesize vitamin D, it is an essential nutrient. The recently updated Dietary Reference Intakes for vitamin D are based on skeletal health and assumed only minimal sunlight exposure. When updating the recommendations, the Food and Nutrition Board recognized that sunlight availability varies throughout the year and that some people have limited exposure.[25] The expert panel considered the role of vitamin D in conditions such as cancer, cardiovascular disease, diabetes, infections, and autoimmune

*Quick* Bite

**A Fishy Cure**
Cod liver oil was well known in the early nineteenth century as a treatment for rickets, a bone disease common in children. It wasn't until the early 1900s, however, that vitamin D was identified as the "antirachitic" (antirickets) substance in cod liver oil.

disorders, but the evidence was insufficient to make additional intake recommendations.[26] The panel also cautioned against exceeding recommendations for calcium and vitamin D: "Higher levels of both nutrients have not been shown to confer greater benefits, and in fact, they have been linked to other health problems, challenging the concept that 'more is better.'"[27]

Because infants and children have inadequate vitamin D intakes and limited direct sun exposure, the panel recommended that all infants, children, and adolescents consume a minimum of 400 IU of daily vitamin D beginning soon after birth.[28] For people between the ages of 1 and 70 years, the RDA for vitamin D is 600 IU per day.[29] Because vitamin D skin synthesis decreases markedly with age, RDA recommendations increase to 800 IU per day for men and women over the age of 70.[30] In some journal articles and older textbooks, you may see vitamin D amounts stated as micrograms instead of IU. One microgram of vitamin D equals 40 IU.

## Sources of Vitamin D

We get vitamin D from exposure to sunlight, our diets, and from dietary supplements. Sensible sun exposure can provide an adequate amount of vitamin D, which is stored in body fat during the winter, when vitamin D production is low. How much exposure to the sun is needed for an adequate supply of vitamin D? Exposure of arms and legs for 5 to 30 minutes between the hours of 10 A.M. and 3 P.M. twice per week generally is adequate.[31] The exact amount of sun exposure depends on several factors, including time of day, season, location, sunscreen use, and skin type. The sun's rays are more intense at latitudes closer to the equator and during midday and summertime. Topical sunscreens (those with sun protection factor [SPF] of 8 or greater) block UV light. People with dark skin do not absorb UV rays as well as light-skinned people do. Pollution and smog can reduce UV rays. The major dietary sources of vitamin D are fortified foods, mainly fortified milk and fortified breakfast cereals. Other fortified foods, such as orange juice, margarine, yogurt, grains, and breads have become available in the United States. The few foods that naturally contain vitamin D include oily fish (e.g., salmon, sardines), egg yolk, butter, and liver, with amounts dependent on the animal's diet. (See **Figure 9.12**.) A diet high in oily fish prevents vitamin D deficiency. More concentrated vitamin D is available in cod liver or other fish liver oils. Plants are poor sources, so strict vegetarians must get their vitamin D through exposure to sunlight, fortified foods, or supplements.

## Vitamin D Deficiency

Vitamin D deficiency damages bones. Babies with vitamin D deficiency have soft, weak bones, which bend and bow under their weight as they start to walk. The condition is called **rickets** and is characterized by "bow legs," "knock-knees," and other skeletal deformities. In the United States and Canada, nutritional rickets was all but eliminated by vitamin D–fortified milk, infant vitamin supplements, and vitamin supplements for children with fat malabsorption conditions. Still, rickets from inadequate vitamin D intake and decreased sunlight exposure continues to occur in infants who are exclusively breastfed and infants with darker skin.[32]

Cases of rickets caused by a nutritional deficiency of vitamin D also have been reported in children and adolescents.[33] In a large, nationally representative sample, about 9 percent (7.6 million) of U.S. children and adolescents were found to be vitamin D deficient, which predisposes them to the development of rickets. These children and teens also were more likely to have hypertension and lower calcium and HDL cholesterol levels. Lower vitamin

*Quick* Bite

**"Children's Disease of the English"**
In the seventeenth century, vitamin D deficiency was so common in British children that rickets was called the "children's disease of the English." Diets provided little vitamin D, and the lack of sun during many months of the year inhibited vitamin D synthesis in the skin.

**rickets** A bone disease in children that results from vitamin D deficiency.

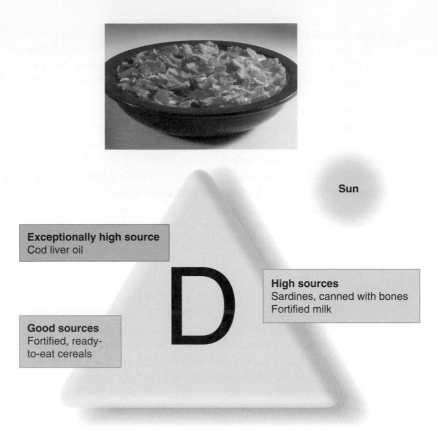

**Sun**

**Exceptionally high source**
Cod liver oil

**High sources**
Sardines, canned with bones
Fortified milk

**Good sources**
Fortified, ready-
to-eat cereals

| | |
|---|---|
| **Figure 9.12** | **Sources of vitamin D.** Given sufficient sunlight, your body can make all the vitamin D it needs. Only a few foods are naturally good sources of vitamin D. |

Therefore, fortified foods such as milk and ready-to-eat cereals are important dietary sources, especially for people with limited exposure to the sun.

**osteomalacia** A disease in adults that results from vitamin D deficiency; it is marked by softening of the bones, leading to bending of the spine, bowing of the legs, and increased risk for fractures.

**osteoporosis** A bone disease characterized by a decrease in bone mineral density and the appearance of small holes in bones due to loss of minerals.

D levels were found more often in older children, girls, non-Hispanic blacks, Mexican Americans, those living in low-income households, obese children, and those who spent more time watching television, playing video games, or using computers. In comparison, children who drank milk daily and/or took vitamin D supplements were less likely to be deficient.[34]

In adults, vitamin D deficiency causes **osteomalacia**, or "soft bones." The condition reduces calcium absorption and increases calcium loss from bone, increasing the risk of bone fractures. People with diseases that affect organs responsible for absorption or activation of vitamin D have a high risk of osteomalacia. Vitamin D deficiency worsens **osteoporosis**, a disease closely related to osteomalacia, with similar symptoms of bone loss and increased risk of fractures. Vitamin D deficiency causes muscle weakness and increases the risk of bone fractures.

Do we get optimal amounts of vitamin D? Unless a person frequently eats oily fish, it is difficult to obtain sufficient vitamin D from the diet, and increased sun exposure increases the risk of cancer. Factors contributing to low levels of vitamin D include excessive use of sunscreen, living in northern latitudes (see **Figure 9.13**), old age, and diets that exclude milk or other fortified foods.

## Vitamin D and Other Conditions

Researchers are currently investigating vitamin D's role in the prevention of numerous cancers, including colorectal cancer. They are also examining the potential role of vitamin D in the prevention and treatment of auto-immune diseases, such as diabetes, multiple sclerosis, and rheumatoid arthritis as well as hypertension and other medical conditions.[35]

## Vitamin D Toxicity

Although sun exposure does not cause vitamin D toxicity, supplement megadoses are highly toxic. The daily UL for adults over 19 years of age is 4,000 IU.[36] Because some people are adversely affected by elevated levels of vitamin D, high-dose supplementation should be used only after careful consideration and consultation with a knowledgeable medical professional.[37]

The hallmark of vitamin D toxicity is a high concentration of calcium in the blood. Initially, this increases urination and thirst. If prolonged, the body deposits excess calcium in soft tissues, causing pain and organ damage. Other symptoms include severe depression, nausea, vomiting, and loss of appetite. Ironically, excess vitamin D also causes loss of bone mass.

**Key Concepts** *The active form of vitamin D is 25(OH)D. Its best-understood function is regulation of blood calcium levels. Along with two other hormones, it regulates urinary calcium excretion, intestinal calcium absorption, and the amount of calcium in bone. Dietary needs increase with age, as the ability of skin to synthesize vitamin D declines. Most dietary vitamin D is from fortified milk and other fortified foods. Vitamin D deficiency in children causes rickets; in adults it leads to osteomalacia and contributes to osteoporosis. In excess, vitamin D causes loss of bone and deposits of calcium in soft tissue.*

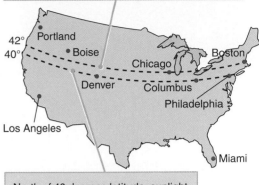

North of 42 degrees latitude, sunlight is too weak to synthesize vitamin D from late October through early March. The same effect occurs during the winter in the southern hemisphere south of 42 degrees latitude.

North of 40 degrees latitude, sunlight is too weak to synthesize vitamin D during January and February.

**Figure 9.13** **Mapping vitamin D synthesis.** Vitamin D synthesis halts for part of the winter if sunlight is too weak. In Los Angeles and Miami, the sunlight is strong enough to synthesize vitamin D year round, even in January.

# Vitamin E

Consumers have long embraced the practice of taking large amounts of vitamin E. Since its discovery in 1922 and the finding that its deficiency made laboratory rats sterile, vitamin E has been a reputed aphrodisiac. Vitamin E supplements also have been promoted for "antiaging," with the ability to prevent everything from gray hair and wrinkles to cancer and heart disease. Although science does not support most rumored benefits, a growing body of research suggests vitamin E may be important in defending against chronic diseases associated with aging.

## Forms of Vitamin E

Vitamin E is actually a family of eight similar compounds: alpha-, beta-, gamma-, and delta-**tocopherol** and alpha-, beta-, gamma-, and delta-**tocotrienol**. Although all are absorbed, only alpha-tocopherol is considered for the human vitamin E requirement, and milligrams of alpha-tocopherol are the standard measure of vitamin E.

Unlike the fat-soluble vitamins A and D, vitamin E is not stored primarily in the liver. Body fat holds about 90 percent of the vitamin E reserves. Virtually every tissue has some vitamin E providing protection within every cell membrane.

## Functions of Vitamin E

Vitamin E is our body's major fat-soluble antioxidant. It protects vulnerable polyunsaturated lipids in cell membranes, in the blood, and elsewhere throughout the body. (See **Figure 9.14**.) Like carotenoids, it works by countering, or "scavenging," free radicals. (For more on antioxidants, see the FYI feature "Antioxidants and Free Radicals.")

*Quick* **Bite**

**Too Much Cover**
In some Middle Eastern countries, many Arab women are clothed so that only their eyes are exposed to sunlight. Even though these women live in sunny climates near the equator, they often have low levels of vitamin D.

**tocopherol** The chemical name for vitamin E. There are four tocopherols (alpha, beta, gamma, and delta), but only alpha-tocopherol is active in the body.

**tocotrienol** Four compounds (alpha, beta, gamma, and delta) chemically related to tocopherols. The tocotrienols and tocopherols are collectively known as vitamin E.

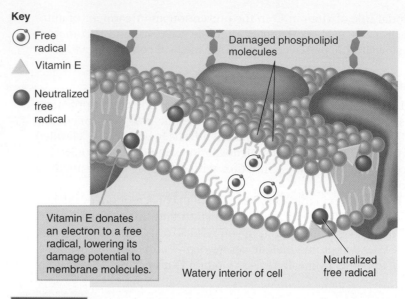

Key

- Free radical
- Vitamin E
- Neutralized free radical

Damaged phospholipid molecules

Vitamin E donates an electron to a free radical, lowering its damage potential to membrane molecules.

Watery interior of cell

Neutralized free radical

**Figure 9.14**    **Free radical damage.** Vitamin E helps prevent free radical damage to polyunsaturated fatty acids in cell membranes.

Numerous studies have suggested that dietary factors such as high intakes of antioxidant vitamins, including vitamin E, may lower the risk of some chronic diseases, especially heart disease.[38] However, results from large clinical trials generally do not support routine use of vitamin E supplementation for the prevention of cardiovascular disease or reduction in related morbidity and mortality.[39] Although antioxidant food sources, especially plant foods, whole grains, and vegetable oils, are recommended, current evidence is insufficient to recommend supplemental vitamin E for heart disease prevention in the general population.[40]

What about other age-related diseases? Nutritionists have investigated a possible preventive role for vitamin E and have found promising results in numerous conditions, including cancer; eye disorders, such as age-related macular degeneration and cataracts; immune function; cognitive declines; and Alzheimer's disease.[41] In general, however, research does not support large-scale supplementation with vitamin E for the prevention or treatment of these conditions. See **Figure 9.15** for the major functions of vitamin E.

## Dietary Recommendations for Vitamin E

Vitamin E needs are related to the intake of polyunsaturated fatty acids (PUFA), which are especially vulnerable to destructive oxidation. When you eat minimal amounts of PUFA, you need smaller amounts of protective vitamin E. When you eat more vegetable oils, the major PUFA source, you need more vitamin E. Because the vitamin E in vegetable oils tends to be proportional to their PUFA content, to some extent these oils help provide extra vitamin E as needed.

The RDA for vitamin E accommodates generous PUFA intake. It is set at 15 milligrams per day of alpha-tocopherol for adults (including pregnant women) and 19 milligrams per day for women who are breastfeeding. Supplement labels may still list vitamin E content in the outdated International Units. If the vitamin E in the supplement is from natural sources, 1 IU equals 0.67 milligrams alpha-tocopherol. If synthetic vitamin E is used, the conversion is 1 IU equals 0.45 milligrams alpha-tocopherol.

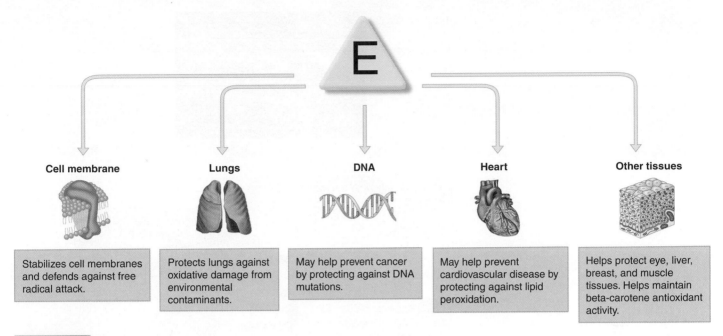

| Cell membrane | Lungs | DNA | Heart | Other tissues |
|---|---|---|---|---|
| Stabilizes cell membranes and defends against free radical attack. | Protects lungs against oxidative damage from environmental contaminants. | May help prevent cancer by protecting against DNA mutations. | May help prevent cardiovascular disease by protecting against lipid peroxidation. | Helps protect eye, liver, breast, and muscle tissues. Helps maintain beta-carotene antioxidant activity. |

**Figure 9.15**    **Major functions of vitamin E.** The antioxidant activity of vitamin E helps stabilize cell membranes, protects tissues from oxidative damage, and may reduce the risk of cancer and heart disease.

## Sources of Vitamin E

Alpha-tocopherol is present in appreciable amounts only in foods such as nuts (e.g., almonds), some seeds (e.g., sunflower), and vegetable oils (e.g., soybean, safflower, corn, canola). Whole-grain products provide vitamin E, and wheat germ oil has one of the highest vitamin E concentrations. Most fruits and vegetables contribute only small amounts, and animal-derived products are inconsistent sources, depending on the animal's diet. (See **Figure 9.16**.)

Although most Americans eat a diet relatively rich in soybean oil, only about 10 percent is alpha-tocopherol, the active form of vitamin E.[42] Foods made from vegetable oils, such as margarine and salad dressings, as well as nuts and seeds, also are good sources. Cooking, processing, and storage can reduce the vitamin E content of foods substantially. (See Table 9.1.) Light and heat accelerate vitamin E's destruction. Safflower oils stored at room temperature for three months lose more than half of their vitamin E. Roasting destroys 80 percent of the vitamin E in almonds. Consuming sufficient vitamin E to meet requirements appears to be challenging for most Americans, and estimates of dietary vitamin E intakes suggest that fewer than 10 percent of Americans consume recommended amounts.[43]

## Vitamin E Deficiency

Overt vitamin E deficiency is so rare in humans that the Food and Nutrition Board could not use signs of deficiency (e.g., neurological abnormalities) as a basis for estimating dietary requirements. Vitamin E deficiency occurs mostly in people with fat malabsorption or rare genetic disorders. In adults, it takes 5 to 10 years of a deficiency before symptoms emerge.

## Vitamin E Toxicity

For a fat-soluble vitamin, vitamin E is surprisingly nontoxic and adverse effects have not been found from consuming foods rich in vitamin E. However, it is

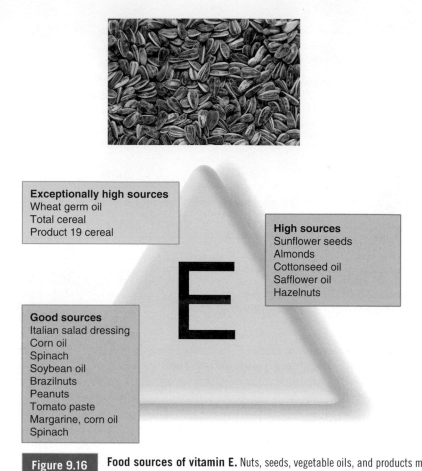

**Exceptionally high sources**
Wheat germ oil
Total cereal
Product 19 cereal

**High sources**
Sunflower seeds
Almonds
Cottonseed oil
Safflower oil
Hazelnuts

**Good sources**
Italian salad dressing
Corn oil
Spinach
Soybean oil
Brazilnuts
Peanuts
Tomato paste
Margarine, corn oil
Spinach

**Figure 9.16**    **Food sources of vitamin E.** Nuts, seeds, vegetable oils, and products made from vegetable oil, such as margarine, are among the best sources of vitamin E.

not totally safe, and large supplement amounts may cause an increased risk of bleeding, especially in people with vitamin K deficiency and in those taking anticoagulant medication or aspirin.[44] For adults, therefore, the UL is 1,000 milligrams per day of supplemental alpha-tocopherol. Despite some large studies that found that vitamin E supplementation led to a small increase in the risk of death, other evidence does not support those findings.[45]

**Table 9.1**    Reported Storage and Processing Losses of Vitamin E

| Food | Test Conditions | Vitamin E Losses |
|---|---|---|
| Peanut oil | Frying at 347°F (175°C), 30 minutes | 32% |
| Safflower oil | Storing at room temperature, 3 months | 55% |
| Tortillas | Storing at room temperature, 12 months | 95% |
| Almonds | Roasting | 80% |
| Wheat germ | Storing at 39°F (4°C), 6 months | 10% |
| Wheat | Processing to white flour | 92% |
| Bread | Baking | 5–50% |

**Source:** *Vitamin E Factbook.* LaGrange, IL: VERIS; 1999. Reprinted with permission from Veris Research Information Services.

**Key Concepts** *Alpha-tocopherol is the only form of vitamin E that meets the vitamin E requirements. It is an antioxidant, protecting cell membranes from the damaging effects of oxidation. Some evidence suggests that vitamin E might delay degenerative diseases such as heart disease and cancer. Vitamin E is found mainly in vegetable oils and products made from them. Considerable vitamin E is lost in food processing, cooking, and storage. Vitamin E deficiency is rare. Vitamin E is relatively nontoxic, though large doses interfere with blood clotting.*

## Vitamin K

Vitamin K was named for the Danish word *koagulation*. The name says it all. Vitamin K is essential for blood clotting. Without it, you would bleed to death from a single cut.

Vitamin K is actually a family of compounds known as quinones. It includes **phylloquinone** from plant sources, **menaquinones** from animal sources and synthesized by our intestinal bacteria, and **menadione**, a synthetic form. The liver holds most of the body's vitamin K reserve. Unlike other fat-soluble vitamins, the liver rapidly breaks down vitamin K and eliminates it, and thus reserves can be depleted quickly.

### Functions of Vitamin K

When you bleed from a cut, your body starts a chain of reactions that forms a clot and stops the flow of blood. Many reactions in this coagulation cascade require vitamin K and calcium. Megadoses of vitamin E interfere with vitamin K's clotting activities. Vitamin K also helps with bone formation.[46] (See **Figure 9.17**.) It increases bone strength and decreases fractures.[47]

### Dietary Recommendations for Vitamin K

Typical diets easily meet the dietary recommendations for vitamin K. The AI for vitamin K for adult men is 120 micrograms daily and for women, including those pregnant or breastfeeding, it is 90 micrograms.[48]

**phylloquinone** The form of vitamin K that comes from plant sources. Also known as *vitamin K₁*.

**menaquinones** The form of vitamin K that comes from animal sources or is produced by intestinal bacteria. Also known as *vitamin K₂*.

**menadione** A medicinal form of vitamin K. Also known as *vitamin K₃*.

## *Quick* Bite

**Does Blocking Vitamin K Cure or Kill?**
The medication warfarin (Coumadin) prevents undesired blood clotting by blocking vitamin K. Warfarin in very large amounts also is used in common rat poison to cause internal hemorrhage and death.

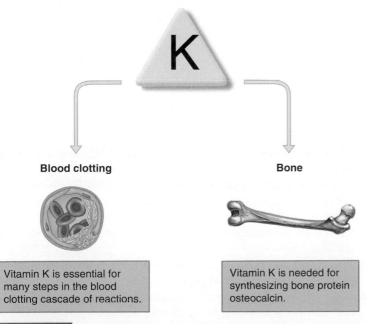

**Blood clotting**

Vitamin K is essential for many steps in the blood clotting cascade of reactions.

**Bone**

Vitamin K is needed for synthesizing bone protein osteocalcin.

**Figure 9.17**   **Major functions of vitamin K.** Without vitamin K, our blood would not clot and our bones would become weak.

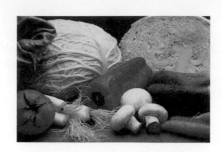

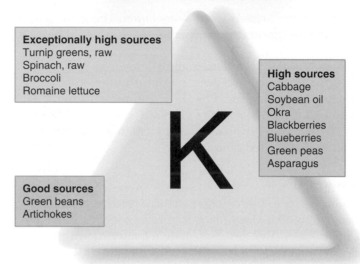

**Exceptionally high sources**
Turnip greens, raw
Spinach, raw
Broccoli
Romaine lettuce

**High sources**
Cabbage
Soybean oil
Okra
Blackberries
Blueberries
Green peas
Asparagus

**Good sources**
Green beans
Artichokes

**Figure 9.18** **Food sources of vitamin K.** The best sources of vitamin K are vegetables, especially those in the cabbage family.

## Sources of Vitamin K

Plant foods, especially green leafy vegetables, such as spinach, turnip greens, broccoli, and Brussels sprouts, are our primary sources of vitamin K. Certain plant oils and margarine, spreads, and salad dressings also are important sources.[49] (See **Figure 9.18.**)

Intestinal bacteria in the lower bowel also produce vitamin K. Although it is a widely held belief that intestinal bacteria supply roughly half the vitamin K requirement, experimental evidence to support this conviction is insufficient.[50]

## Vitamin K Deficiency

In adults, vitamin K deficiency is rare and usually occurs in people with fat malabsorption problems. However, newborn babies lack vitamin K–producing intestinal bacteria, so they are at risk of vitamin K deficiency. Because breast milk has little vitamin K, breastfed babies are especially vulnerable. Physicians routinely give newborns a vitamin K injection. This usually meets the infant's needs for several weeks, until vitamin K–producing bacteria establish themselves in the intestine.

Broad-spectrum antibiotic use is often blamed for vitamin K deficiency, presumably because it reduces bacterial production of vitamin K in the intestines. Although certain antibiotics weakly inhibit vitamin K metabolism in people with poor vitamin K status, among people with adequate vitamin K intake direct effects by antibiotics remain controversial.[51]

## Vitamin K Toxicity

Because the body excretes vitamin K much more rapidly than other fat-soluble vitamins, vitamin K toxicity from food is rare. The Food and Nutrition Board has not set a UL for vitamin K.

**Key Concepts** *Vitamin K is required for blood clotting and bone health. It is found primarily in green vegetables and in some vegetable oils. Newborns are routinely given injections of vitamin K. Deficiencies are very rare. Because vitamin K is readily excreted, especially compared with other fat-soluble vitamins, toxicity also is rare.*

## The Water-Soluble Vitamins: Eight Bs and a C

The scientists who first discovered vitamin B believed "it" was a single compound. As they learned more, they realized "it" was actually several vitamins. In fact there are eight B vitamins. Initially, to differentiate them, numbers were added to the letter B—vitamins $B_6$ and $B_{12}$, for example. Today, with the exception of $B_6$ and $B_{12}$, we usually refer to the B vitamins by their names: thiamin ($B_1$), riboflavin ($B_2$), niacin ($B_3$), pantothenic acid, biotin, and folate.

B vitamins act primarily as coenzymes (or parts of coenzymes)—the keys that unlock the action of enzymes. Enzymes regulate countless life-sustaining chemical reactions. They hurry reactions along or slow them down, as needed, even allowing them to proceed when it would otherwise be impossible. But many enzymes cannot work until the body supplies a missing component—a coenzyme.

Let's use an analogy to clarify how vitamins function as coenzymes. Suppose you had an appointment in 15 minutes and 10 miles away. You could walk there, but you would be too late. You could drive your car, but you cannot find your key. Now you find your key (the coenzyme), turn on your car (the enzyme), and quickly drive to your destination (the reaction taking place in your body). (See **Figure 9.19**.)

Vitamin C is an antioxidant, but unlike the antioxidant vitamin E, it is water-soluble. Despite differences in solubility, vitamin C and vitamin E work together. When vitamin E quenches a free radical, vitamin E in turn becomes a free radical, although a less reactive one. Vitamin C can stabilize it, restoring vitamin E's antioxidant abilities.

## Thiamin

The thiamin-deficiency disease **beriberi** was first described in Chinese writings over 4,000 years ago. But it was not widespread until the nineteenth century, when highly milled or "polished" white rice became popular. In 1885, Dr. K. Takaki of the Japanese Naval Medical Services first demonstrated beriberi's dietary origins. He cured sailors sick with beriberi by adding meat, milk, and whole grains to their diets. Years later, Christian Eijkman, a Dutch medical officer, fed birds only white rice until they had beriberi and then cured them by adding bran to their diet. This led to the discovery of an "anti-beriberi" factor—thiamin.

### Functions of Thiamin

Thiamin works as a coenzyme in reactions that produce energy. Deprive your body of thiamin, and you deprive every cell of its ability to use energy. As the vitamin component of the coenzyme **thiamin pyrophosphate (TPP)**, thiamin helps reactions that break down glucose, make RNA and DNA, or produce energy-rich molecules that power protein synthesis. TPP also helps

**beriberi** Thiamin-deficiency disease. Symptoms include muscle weakness, loss of appetite, nerve degeneration, and edema in some cases.

**thiamin pyrophosphate (TPP)** A coenzyme of which the vitamin thiamin is a part. It plays a key role in removing carboxyl groups in chemical reactions and helps drive the reaction that forms acetyl CoA from pyruvate during metabolism.

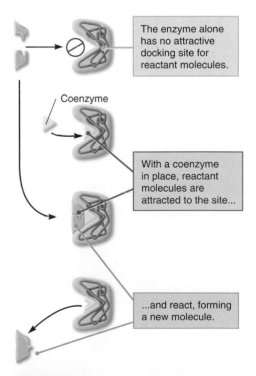

The enzyme alone has no attractive docking site for reactant molecules.

Coenzyme

With a coenzyme in place, reactant molecules are attracted to the site...

...and react, forming a new molecule.

**Figure 9.19** **The coenzyme–enzyme partnership.** The B vitamins form coenzymes that enable specific enzymes to catalyze reactions.

synthesize and regulate neurotransmitters—chemicals that act as messengers between nerve cells.

## Dietary Recommendations and Sources of Thiamin

Because thiamin needs are related to energy requirements and carbohydrate intake, they are slightly greater for men than women. The RDA for adult men aged 19 years and older is 1.2 milligrams per day; for adult women, it is 1.1 milligrams. Pregnancy and breastfeeding increase energy requirements, so thiamin RDA rises to 1.4 milligrams per day during pregnancy and 1.5 milligrams when a woman is breastfeeding.[52] If a person's diet supplies adequate energy and includes thiamin-rich foods, it generally contains enough thiamin.

Because thiamin is found in small amounts throughout the food supply, eating a wide variety of foods is the best way to ensure a good intake. Pork is one of the richest sources. Legumes (mature beans and peas), some nuts and seeds (e.g., sunflower seeds), and some types of fish and seafood are good sources. (See **Figure 9.20.**) Other meats, dairy products, and most fruits contain little thiamin. Most thiamin we eat comes from enriched grain products: bread, pasta, rice, and ready-to-eat cereals.[53] Heat and alkaline cooking water easily destroy thiamin, so cooking reduces a food's thiamin content.

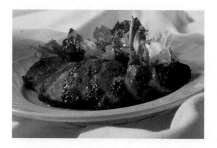

**Exceptionally high source**
Total cereal

**High sources**
Pork, loin roast
Oatmeal, instant, fortified
Ham
Corn flakes cereal
Fiber One cereal
Cheerios cereal
Bagel, enriched, plain
Tuna
White bread, enriched
Navy beans

# Thiamin

**Good sources**
Spaghetti, enriched
Orange juice
Grits, corn, enriched
Sesame seeds
Rice, white, enriched
Soybeans
Black beans
Baked beans
Wheat germ
Soy milk
Pecans
Salmon
Whole wheat bread
Oysters
Lentils

**Figure 9.20**    **Food sources of thiamin.** Pork, whole and enriched grains, and fortified cereals are rich in thiamin. Most animal foods contain little thiamin.

## Thiamin Deficiency

*Beriberi* means "I can't, I can't," in one of the languages of Southeast Asia. The phrase describes how doctors long ago diagnosed the disease: Their patients were unable to rise from a squatting position. In fact, overall profound muscle weakness combined with nerve destruction ultimately leaves the victim of beriberi almost unable to move.

Milder symptoms of thiamin deficiency can appear after only 10 days on a thiamin-free diet. These include headache, irritability, depression, and loss of appetite—signs of nervous system disturbance—and contribute to a worsening food intake, causing further muscle weakness and nerve degeneration.

Those body systems with high energy needs deteriorate first. Digestive damage causes diarrhea, muscle damage causes muscle wasting and pain, and nerve damage disrupts coordination and causes "pins and needles" sensations in hands and feet. Death, however, most often comes from damage to the heart. As the heart muscle fails, feet and legs fill with fluid (edema), the so-called wet beriberi. (See **Figure 9.21**.) Outbreaks of beriberi commonly occur in refugee and displaced populations dependent on international food aid. They often must subsist on milled white cereals, including polished rice and white flour, all poor sources of thiamin when not enriched.

In industrialized countries, thiamin deficiency usually is related to chronic alcoholism coupled with a poor diet. Alcohol interferes with B vitamin absorption. Alcohol-induced thiamin deficiency produces Wernicke-Korsakoff syndrome; symptoms include mental confusion and memory loss, staggered gait, and constant rapid eye movement. Although the syndrome most often is associated with the stereotypical "Skid Row" alcoholic, it can occur in any heavy drinker, especially an aging alcoholic.

## Thiamin Toxicity

Thiamin supplements, which are cheap to produce, often include up to 200 times the Daily Value for thiamin, but, to date, there have been no reports of thiamin toxicity. Following doses of 5 milligrams or more, thiamin absorption declines rapidly, and the kidneys quickly excrete the excess.[54]

# Riboflavin

At first, riboflavin and thiamin were considered the same vitamin. When riboflavin was finally isolated from the "anti-beriberi factor," it was dubbed vitamin $B_2$, and later "riboflavin" for its yellowish-green color (*flavin* means "yellow" in Latin). In foods, though, it may give a green or bluish cast. You'll notice the color in uncooked egg whites and some brands of fat-free milk.

## Functions of Riboflavin

Riboflavin is a part of two coenzymes, flavin mononucleotide and flavin adenine dinucleotide. Both coenzymes are required in reactions that extract energy from glucose, fatty acids, and amino acids. Riboflavin also supports the antioxidant activity of the enzyme **glutathione peroxidase**.

## Dietary Recommendations and Sources of Riboflavin

As with thiamin, riboflavin requirements increase along with increasing energy needs. For adults aged 19 and older, the RDA is 1.3 milligrams per day for men and 1.1 milligrams for women, reflecting the higher energy needs of men. Pregnancy increases the riboflavin RDA to 1.4 milligrams per day; breastfeeding increases it to 1.6 milligrams.

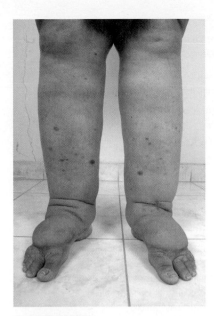

**Figure 9.21**   Edema, especially in the feet and legs, is a symptom of wet beriberi.

**glutathione peroxidase** A selenium-containing enzyme that reduces toxic hydrogen peroxide formed within cells; works with vitamin E to reduce free radical damage.

**ariboflavinosis** Riboflavin deficiency.

**glossitis** Inflammation of the tongue; a symptom of riboflavin deficiency.

**angular stomatitis** Inflammation and cracking at the corners of the mouth; a symptom of riboflavin deficiency.

**cheilosis** Inflammation and cracking of the lips; a symptom of riboflavin deficiency.

**seborrheic dermatitis** Disease of the oil-producing glands of the skin; a symptom of riboflavin deficiency.

**anemia** Abnormally low concentration of hemoglobin in the bloodstream; can be caused by impaired synthesis of red blood cells, increased destruction of red blood cells, or significant loss of blood.

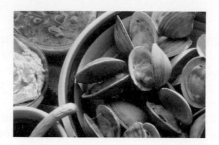

# Riboflavin

**Exceptionally high sources**
Beef liver
Wheat bran flakes cereal
Chicken liver

**High sources**
Yogurt, plain
Cheerios cereal
Fiber One cereal
Corn flakes cereal
Milk
Squid
Buttermilk
Oatmeal, instant, fortified
Clams
Pork, loin chops

**Good sources**
Eggs
Mushrooms
Herring
Almonds
Turkey, dark meat
Cottage cheese
Chicken, dark meat
Beef, porterhouse steak
Ham
White bread, enriched

**Figure 9.22**  **Food sources of riboflavin.** The best sources of riboflavin include milk, liver, whole and enriched grains, and fortified cereals.

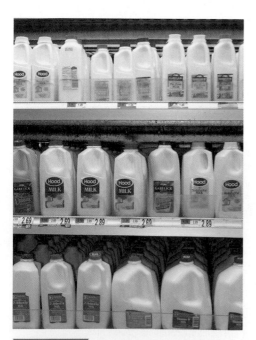

**Figure 9.23**  **Packaging affects riboflavin content in milk.** Light breaks down riboflavin easily, so foods high in riboflavin (e.g., milk) are best stored in opaque containers.

Milk and milk-containing beverages, cottage cheese, and yogurt are excellent riboflavin sources. Enriched grain products, eggs, and organ meats also are good sources. (See **Figure 9.22**.) Riboflavin generally is more stable than thiamin, but light can destroy it. Riboflavin-rich foods should be stored in opaque packages. For example, packaging milk in paper or plastic cartons rather than clear glass better protects milk's riboflavin content.[55] (See **Figure 9.23**.)

## Riboflavin Deficiency

Overt riboflavin deficiency (**ariboflavinosis**) is now rare, and like thiamin deficiency, occurs most often in chronic alcoholism. Long-term use of sedatives and other barbiturates accelerates liver breakdown of riboflavin and contributes to deficiency.

Riboflavin deficiency shows up first around the mouth. The tongue gets shiny, smooth, and inflamed (**glossitis**); the mouth becomes painful and sore; the skin at the corners of the mouth cracks (**angular stomatitis**); and the lips become inflamed and split (**cheilosis**). The oil-producing glands of the skin become clogged (**seborrheic dermatitis**); and as the deficiency becomes severe, a characteristic **anemia** develops. Riboflavin deficiency usually exists along with other nutrient deficiencies. In fact, because riboflavin is involved in the metabolism of other B vitamins, such as vitamin $B_6$, folate, and niacin, severe riboflavin deficiency may even make other deficiencies worse.

## Riboflavin Toxicity

Excess riboflavin is readily excreted, and even large doses don't appear harmful. There are no reported cases of toxicity. A UL has not been set for riboflavin.

# Niacin

Niacin is the name for two similar compounds: nicotinic acid and nicotinamide (also known as niacinamide). Ironically, this healthful substance got its name from a singularly unhealthful substance. In 1867, nicotinic acid was produced from nicotine in tobacco. Understand clearly, though, that nicotinic acid is not the same as or even closely related to nicotine. In the early 1940s, with its role as a vitamin established, it was renamed "niacin" so people wouldn't confuse it with nicotine.

## Functions of Niacin

Niacin forms a part of crucially important coenzymes that participate in at least 200 metabolic pathways. As such, it plays a key role in energy metabolism, both under normal conditions and during times of vigorous activity when energy use swings into high gear. The body also needs niacin to synthesize fatty acids.

## Dietary Recommendations and Sources of Niacin

Niacin is unique among the B vitamins—your body can make it from the amino acid **tryptophan** as well as obtain it from foods. Intake recommendations are expressed as **niacin equivalents (NE)**, a measure that includes both niacin and tryptophan. The RDA is 16 milligrams of NE per day for adult men and 14 milligrams per day for adult women, increasing to 18 milligrams during pregnancy and 17 milligrams during breastfeeding.

Most niacin in the American diet comes from meat, poultry, fish, nuts and peanuts, and enriched and whole-grain products.[51] (See **Figure 9.24**.) Niacin is stable when heated, so little is lost during cooking.

The niacin precursor tryptophan supplies about half of our niacin intake. Tryptophan is an essential amino acid and is an integral part of dietary protein. It is in almost all protein foods but is notably low in the protein of corn. Sixty milligrams of tryptophan yield about 1 milligram of niacin, or 1 niacin equivalent (NE). Because the body needs other nutrients (riboflavin, vitamin $B_6$, and iron) to convert tryptophan to niacin, a deficit of any of them can worsen a niacin deficiency.

## Niacin Deficiency

Pellagra is the disease of severe niacin deficiency. The word *pellagra* means "rough skin" in Italian and describes the dermatitis—a rough, darkened rash—that occurs where the victim's skin is exposed to sunlight. However, because niacin coenzymes are involved in just about every metabolic pathway, deficiency devastates the entire body. The hallmarks of pellagra are "the four Ds": dermatitis, diarrhea, dementia, and, ultimately, death. Deficiencies of other nutrients such as iron, riboflavin, and vitamin $B_6$ can contribute to the damage.

Descriptions of pellagra were first documented in 1735. But the great pellagra epidemic in America's South did not emerge until the early twentieth century. The rural poor began subsisting on a diet of corn (maize), molasses, and fatty salt pork, all poor sources of niacin and tryptophan. Although corn

*Quick* Bite

**Are You Smoking That Bread?**
In the 1940s, antitobacco forces were confused about the differences between niacin and nicotine. They mistakenly warned that niacin-enriched bread could cause an addiction to cigarettes!

**tryptophan** An amino acid that serves as a niacin precursor in the body. In the body, 60 milligrams of tryptophan yield about 1 milligram of niacin, or 1 niacin equivalent (NE).

**niacin equivalents (NE)** A measure that includes preformed dietary niacin as well as niacin derived from tryptophan; 60 milligrams of tryptophan yield about 1 milligram of niacin.

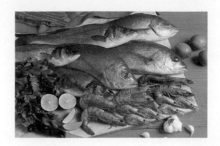

# Niacin

**Good sources**
Mushrooms
Salmon, canned, with bones
Beef, porterhouse steak
Beef, T-bone steak
Turkey, dark meat
Barley
Sardines, canned, with bones
Clams
Spaghetti, enriched
Shrimp
Cod
White bread, enriched
Rice, white, enriched

**High sources**
Beef liver
Chicken
Tuna
Oatmeal, instant, fortified
Halibut
Turkey, light meat
Salmon
All Bran cereal
Corn flakes cereal
Fiber One cereal
Pork, loin roast
Peanut butter
Beef, ground
Chicken liver
Ham

**Figure 9.24**  **Food sources of niacin.** Niacin is found mainly in meats and grains. Enrichment adds niacin as well as thiamin, riboflavin, folic acid, and iron to processed grains.

contains niacin, the niacin is bound to a protein, which impairs absorption. We now know that soaking corn in a solution of lime (calcium hydroxide) helps release niacin, which much improves absorption. (See **Figure 9.25.**)

Widespread pellagra began to decline during World War II after the federal government mandated enrichment of bread flour and other cereal grains with niacin. Today, pellagra has virtually disappeared in industrialized countries, except in some people with chronic alcoholism or disorders that disrupt synthesis from tryptophan. Pellagra continues to plague people living in Southeast Asia and Africa, however, whose diets lack sufficient niacin and protein.

## Niacin Toxicity and Medicinal Uses of Niacin

For adults, the UL for niacin is 35 milligrams per day from fortified foods, supplements, and medications. Although niacin has shown little severe toxicity, its side effects discourage widespread use.[56] The principal side effects are flushing (a feeling of prickly heat on the face and upper body), related itching, and tingling. Niacin's side effects usually are reversible with drug discontinuation or dose reduction.

Although serious liver toxicity has been reported, it is largely confined to the use of slow-release formulations taken as unregulated nutritional sup-

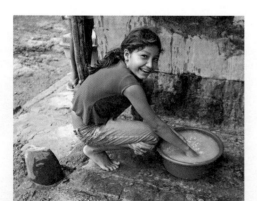

**Figure 9.25**  **Soaking corn in a solution of lime (calcium hydroxide) releases bound niacin.**

plements.[57] Because megadoses of niacin lower LDL cholesterol and raise HDL cholesterol, physicians may prescribe it. However, a recent study by the National Institutes of Health was stopped early when researchers discovered that the high dose, extended-release niacin plus statin treatment in people with heart and vascular disease did not reduce the risk of cardiovascular events, including heart attacks and stroke, and that there was a small and unexplained increase in stroke rates.[58] Note that these results cannot be applied to everyone. People considering or currently taking niacin supplementation should seek the advice of their physician.

**Key Concepts** *Thiamin, riboflavin, and niacin are all incorporated into coenzymes that metabolize carbohydrate, protein, and fat. Enriched grains are a major source of these B vitamins, with pork ranking as a good source of thiamin, milk as a major source of riboflavin, and high-protein foods as sources of niacin. Overt deficiencies of these vitamins are rare in North America. High doses of thiamin and riboflavin appear to be harmless, but megadoses of niacin should be taken only under medical supervision.*

# Vitamin B$_6$

Vitamin B$_6$ (also known as pyridoxine) is a group of six compounds, three with a phosphate group and three without. Digestion strips the phosphate group and sends the remaining compounds to the liver, which converts them to pyridoxal phosphate (PLP), the primary active coenzyme form.[59]

## Functions of Vitamin B$_6$

PLP is a coenzyme for more than 100 different enzymes. Its better-known roles involve protein and amino acid metabolism. Enzymes that require PLP help change one amino acid into another and enable us to make the nonessential amino acids. Without adequate vitamin B$_6$, all amino acids become essential—the body cannot make them and must get them from food. Vitamin B$_6$ also helps make glucose from amino acids (a process called gluconeogenesis) and helps release glucose from glycogen.

PLP supports white blood cell synthesis and a healthy immune system. Healthy red blood cells also need PLP. The coenzyme helps synthesize their oxygen-carrying hemoglobin and helps bind oxygen. PLP also helps produce a number of major neurotransmitters.

Vitamin B$_6$, folate, and vitamin B$_{12}$ work in concert to lower blood levels of the amino acid homocysteine. Each vitamin forms a coenzyme that helps convert homocysteine to other amino acids—cysteine and methionine. (See **Figure 9.26**.) Low intake of B$_6$ or folate can increase homocysteine levels, and high homocysteine levels may be a marker for heart disease.[60]

## Dietary Recommendations and Sources of Vitamin B$_6$

The vitamin B$_6$ RDA for men and women 19 to 50 years old is 1.3 milligrams per day. Because requirements appear to increase with age, the RDA is set at 1.7 milligrams for older men and 1.5 milligrams for older women.[61]

Good sources of vitamin B$_6$ include meat (especially organ meats like liver), fish, or poultry; potatoes and other starchy vegetables; and fortified soy-based meat substitutes.[62] Whole grains contain vitamin B$_6$, but it is lost in refining and is not replaced by enrichment. However, it is added to some fortified breakfast cereals. Vitamin B$_6$ also pops up in unexpected places, like bananas and sunflower seeds. (See **Figure 9.27**.)

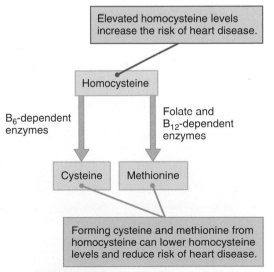

**Figure 9.26** **Homocysteine and heart disease.** Elevated homocysteine levels are linked to an increased risk of heart disease. Enzymes dependent on B$_6$, B$_{12}$, and folate help lower the amount of homocysteine by converting it to cysteine and methionine.

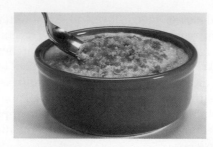

**Exceptionally high sources**
Wheat bran flakes cereal
All Bran cereal

**High sources**
Beef liver
Banana, fresh
Garbanzo beans
Chicken, light meat
Corn flakes cereal
Fiber One cereal
Cheerios cereal
Chicken liver
Turkey, light meat
Beef, ground
Ham
Pork, loin roast

**Good sources**
Halibut
Potato
Turkey, dark meat
Chicken, dark meat
Beef, porterhouse steak
Herring
Tomato juice
Sweet potato
Sesame seeds
Sunflower seeds

$B_6$

**Figure 9.27**  **Food sources of vitamin B$_6$.** Meats are generally good sources of vitamin B$_6$, along with certain fruits (e.g., bananas) and vegetables (e.g., potatoes).

Vitamin B$_6$ is not particularly stable and is especially sensitive to temperature. Heat can destroy up to half of a food's vitamin B$_6$.

## Vitamin B$_6$ Deficiency

Overt vitamin B$_6$ deficiency is rare, although some medications can cause deficiency. Excessive alcohol interferes with the vitamin's absorption and its coenzyme activities, worsening B$_6$ deficits created by the alcoholic's typically poor diet.

Overt vitamin B$_6$ deficiency produces a skin rash and anemia and also disrupts nervous system activity. Inadequate vitamin B$_6$ disrupts the synthesis of red blood cells and their oxygen-binding ability, causing an anemia in which red blood cells are small and pale (**microcytic hypochromic anemia**). The pale color reflects their lack of adequate hemoglobin to carry sufficient oxygen. Vitamin B$_6$ deficiency also damages the nervous system, causing depression, headaches, confusion, and convulsions.

Subtle deficits of vitamin B$_6$ disrupt homocysteine metabolism, leading to increased levels of homocysteine, which may be a marker for heart disease.

## Vitamin B$_6$ Toxicity and Medicinal Uses of Vitamin B$_6$

Vitamin B$_6$ megadoses are not without risk and can cause subtle neurological damage. Other side effects include upset stomach, headache, sleepiness, and a tingling, prickling, or burning sensation. Some women self-prescribe large doses of vitamin B$_6$ to treat premenstrual syndrome (PMS)—the headache,

**microcytic hypochromic anemia** Anemia characterized by small, pale red blood cells that lack adequate hemoglobin to carry oxygen; can be caused by deficiency of iron or vitamin B$_6$.

bloating, irritability, and depression that may occur during the week or so before the onset of menstruation. Although vitamin B$_6$ has long been reputed to be an antidote for PMS, research has failed to prove its effectiveness.[63] Women also have taken vitamin B$_6$ to reduce symptoms of morning sickness during pregnancy, depression, and side effects of oral contraceptive medications; however, current scientific evidence of these benefits is unclear.

High-dose vitamin B$_6$ has also been used for carpal tunnel syndrome—a wrist injury that causes painful tingling in hands and fingers. Most well-designed scientific studies have found no evidence that vitamin B$_6$ improves carpal tunnel syndrome, however.[64] The UL for vitamin B$_6$ intake is 100 milligrams per day. Unfortunately, over-the-counter supplements often contain this amount or more. Doses above the UL should be taken only under medical supervision.

## Folate

Folate is named for its best natural source: green leafy vegetables (foliage). The term *folate* actually refers to a group of several closely related folate forms. Folic acid is the most stable form and is used for supplementation and fortification.

### Functions of Folate

As a coenzyme, folate is crucial to DNA synthesis and cell division, amino acid metabolism, and the maturation of red blood cells and other cells. This involvement in basic cell reproduction and growth makes folate essential for healthy embryonic development. Good folate status in early pregnancy greatly reduces the risk of birth defects called **neural tube defects (NTD)**.[65] However, many women do not realize they have become pregnant or don't seek prenatal care until it's too late. That is why experts recommend folic acid supplements before pregnancy to all women who may become pregnant—and it is why the government mandated folic acid fortification. Folate functions in close cooperation with vitamins B$_6$ and B$_{12}$. All three support red blood cell synthesis and help control homocysteine levels.

Although not uniformly consistent, a large body of epidemiological studies generally indicates that a diet high in folate offers protection against various forms of cancer and colorectal cancer in particular.[66] However, the precise roles of folate and the effects of folate supplementation in cancer prevention remain unclear.[67]

### Dietary Recommendations and Sources of Folate

The body absorbs nearly 100 percent of folic acid in supplements and fortified foods, but only about half to two-thirds of the folate naturally present in food.[68] To account for these differences, RDA values are expressed as **dietary folate equivalents (DFE)**. For men and women aged 19 years and older, the RDA for folate is 400 micrograms of DFE per day. Requirements increase to 600 micrograms during pregnancy and 500 micrograms while breastfeeding. Because most U.S. women are not eating enough foods fortified with folic acid to optimally reduce the risk of birth defects, the U.S. Preventive Services Task Force recommends that all women who are capable of becoming pregnant take a daily supplement containing 400 to 800 micrograms of folic acid.[69]

Fortified breakfast cereals supply most dietary folate. Some even provide 400 micrograms in a moderate-size serving. Since 1998, folic acid fortification of enriched flour (including that used by commercial bakers) and enriched grain products has been mandatory in the United States and Canada.[70] A

**neural tube defects (NTD)** Birth defects resulting from failure of the neural tube to develop properly during early fetal development.

**dietary folate equivalents (DFE)** A measure of folate intake used to account for the high bioavailability of folic acid taken as a supplement compared with the lower bioavailability of the folate found in foods.

**DRI Values and Bioavailability of Folate**

1 µg DFE = 1 µg food folate

= 0.5 µg folic acid taken on an empty stomach

= 0.6 µg folic acid consumed with meals

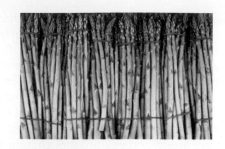

**Exceptionally high sources**
Chicken liver
All Bran cereal
Wheat bran flakes cereal
Product 19 cereal

# Folate

**High sources**
Beef liver
Spinach
Lentils
Pinto beans
Black beans
Oatmeal, instant, fortified
Asparagus
Romaine lettuce
Blackeyed peas
Corn flakes cereal
Turnip greens
Cheerios cereal
Soybeans
Spaghetti, enriched
Rice, white, enriched
Broccoli
White bread, enriched

**Good sources**
Collards
Sunflower seeds
Beets
Kidney beans
Artichokes
Mustard greens
Wheat germ
Tomato juice
Orange juice
Crab, Alaska king
Orange

**Figure 9.28** **Food sources of folate.** Good sources of folate are a diverse collection of foods: liver, legumes, leafy greens, and orange juice. Enriched grains and fortified cereals are other ways to include folic acid in the diet.

serving of enriched pasta, for example, typically provides 30 percent of the folate RDA. Dark-green leafy vegetables, asparagus, broccoli, orange juice, wheat germ, liver, sunflower seeds, and legumes are other good sources. (See **Figure 9.28**.)

Folate is extremely vulnerable to heat, ultraviolet light, and oxygen. Cooking and other food-processing and preparation techniques can destroy up to 90 percent of a food's folate. Experts recommend eating folate-rich fruits and vegetables raw or cooking them quickly in minimal amounts of water via steaming, stir-frying, or microwaving. Vitamin C in foods also helps protect folate from oxidation.

## Folate Deficiency

Our understanding of the role of folate in human health and disease has been expanding rapidly. Folate deficiency appears to play an important pathogenetic role in the development of anemia, atherosclerosis, neural tube defects, adverse pregnancy outcomes, and neuropsychiatric disorders. Mandatory fortification is important, and folic acid fortification is credited with reducing the number of neural tube defects by 50 to 70 percent.[71]

In developed countries, folate deficiency has been associated with people who have poor nutrition, such as the elderly or those with alcoholism. Others may have increased risk due to intestinal malabsorption, certain anemias, and the use of medications that interfere with folate absorption or activity.

When your folate reserves are good, your body normally can store enough folate to last two to four months without additional intake. Abnormal cell reproduction due to folate deficiency can be corrected within 24 hours by vitamin replacement.

### Anemia and Diarrhea

Both folate and vitamin $B_{12}$ are required for DNA synthesis and normal cell growth. A deficiency shows up soonest in cells that are reproducing the fastest. Red blood cells are rapidly dividing cells that must be replaced about every 120 days; they are among the first cells to be damaged by deficiency. The immature red blood cells cannot grow normally and cannot mature normally. Instead, these fragile blood cells grow into large bizarre shapes and have greatly shortened life spans. These abnormal cells replace normal red blood cells, leading to a type of anemia called **megaloblastic anemia.** (See **Figure 9.29.**) A lack of folate also impairs the synthesis of white blood cells, which are vital to the immune response.

Like blood cells, cells lining the gastrointestinal tract also divide rapidly and need frequent replacement. And, like blood cells, impaired DNA synthesis prevents gastrointestinal cells from maturing normally. Large, immature cells accumulate along the digestive tract. In the intestine, they interfere with absorption, causing diarrhea. In the mouth, the defective cells make the tongue sore and "beefy red."

### Birth Defects

Low folate levels during the early stages of pregnancy dramatically increase risk of neural tube defects. These defects in the central nervous system occur within the first 30 days after conception.[72] Most common is **spina bifida**, in which a protective covering fails to form over part or all of the fragile spinal cord. (See **Figure 9.30.**) Other neural tube defects include an abnormally small brain (**microencephaly**) or no brain at all (**anencephaly**).

### Heart Disease

Poor folate status can lead to elevated homocysteine levels, which were a primary factor in setting the folate RDA. Recommended folate intakes help maintain homocysteine at reduced levels.

## Folate Toxicity

Deficiency of either folate or vitamin $B_{12}$ produces the same type of anemia, but $B_{12}$ deficiency also causes nerve damage. Taking folate supplements can mask the symptoms of $B_{12}$ deficiency anemia until nerve damage becomes irreversible. (See the section "Vitamin $B_{12}$ Deficiency.")

**Normal red blood cell precursor**

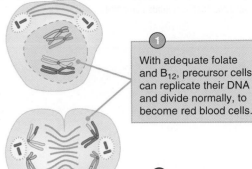

1. With adequate folate and $B_{12}$, precursor cells can replicate their DNA and divide normally, to become red blood cells.

**Megaloblast**

2. When deficient in folate or $B_{12}$, red blood cell precursors cannot form new DNA, and cannot divide.

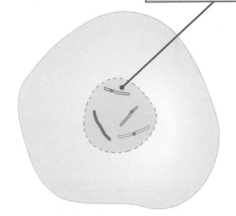

**Figure 9.29**   **Megaloblastic anemia.** When red blood cell precursors in the bone marrow cannot form new DNA, they cannot divide normally. These precursor cells continue to grow and become large, fragile, immature cells called megaloblasts. Megaloblasts displace red blood cells, resulting in megaloblastic anemia.

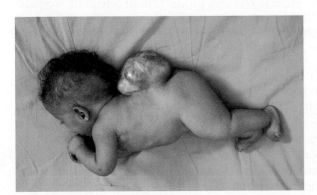

**Figure 9.30**   **Neural tube defects.** Poor folate status during the early stages of pregnancy, even before a woman may realize she is pregnant, increases the risk of a neural tube defect.

**megaloblastic anemia** Excess amounts of megaloblasts (immature red blood cells) in the blood caused by deficiency of folate or vitamin $B_{12}$.

**spina bifida** A type of neural tube birth defect.

**microencephaly** A type of neural tube birth defect in which the brain is abnormally small.

**anencephaly** A type of neural tube birth defect in which part or all of the brain is missing.

**myelin sheath** The protective coating that surrounds nerve fibers.

Although rare, hypersensitive people who take folic acid supplements may suffer hives or respiratory distress. The UL for adults is 1,000 micrograms per day of folic acid from supplements and fortified foods.

# Vitamin B$_{12}$

Vitamin B$_{12}$ is unlike other B vitamins. Plants do not provide it, and your body stores large amounts. Vitamin B$_{12}$ is a group of cobalt-containing compounds, known collectively as cobalamin. In the United States, cyanocobalamin is the only form of vitamin B$_{12}$ commercially available in supplements.

## Functions of Vitamin B$_{12}$

Vitamin B$_{12}$ is essential to the conversion of folate to an activated form. Without vitamin B$_{12}$, folate cannot function in DNA synthesis or blood cell synthesis, nor can it metabolize homocysteine. All folate functions are blocked. Thus, a deficiency of vitamin B$_{12}$ will produce folate deficiency symptoms, even though folate levels might be adequate.

Vitamin B$_{12}$ has another essential job. It helps maintain the **myelin sheath**, a protective coating that surrounds nerve fibers. A vitamin B$_{12}$ deficiency ultimately destroys nerve cells.

## Dietary Recommendations and Sources of Vitamin B$_{12}$

For healthy adults, the RDA for vitamin B$_{12}$ is 2.4 micrograms per day. Because up to 30 percent of people older than 50 may not absorb vitamin B$_{12}$ well, experts advise them to increase their intake by consuming B$_{12}$-fortified foods or supplements. Our bodies more efficiently absorb vitamin B$_{12}$ from these sources.[73] All naturally occurring vitamin B$_{12}$ originates with bacteria. Bacteria produce it, and animals obtain it from bacteria on their food or from their intestinal bacteria. Animals concentrate and store B$_{12}$, mainly in the liver. Consequently animal-derived foods are our only good natural source of vitamin B$_{12}$, and liver is the richest source.

Blue-green algae (cyanobacteria) are sometimes promoted as a B$_{12}$ plant source, but their cobalamin is an inactive form. For vegans (vegetarians who avoid eggs and dairy, as well as meats), the most reliable food sources are fortified breakfast cereals, fortified soy products, and other foods fortified with B$_{12}$. (See **Figure 9.31**.)

## Absorption of Vitamin B$_{12}$

Unless you're a vegan, it's easy to get enough vitamin B$_{12}$ from your diet. But absorbing it is another matter. Readying B$_{12}$ for absorption is a complex multistep digestive process, starting in the mouth and ending with absorption in the small intestine. The process requires production of adequate stomach acid and a substance called intrinsic factor. (See **Figure 9.32**.) A defect in any step can cause B$_{12}$ deficiency.

## Vitamin B$_{12}$ Deficiency

We can store enough vitamin B$_{12}$ in the liver to last more than 2 years, and symptoms of deficiency may not appear for up to 12 years. A vitamin B$_{12}$ deficiency is almost always due to impaired absorption, especially in older persons. Vegans who do not eat fortified cereals regularly or do not take vitamin B$_{12}$ supplements also risk vitamin B$_{12}$ deficiency. Vegan mothers who breastfeed but do not take supplemental vitamin B$_{12}$ may put their infants at risk of long-term neurologic problems.

THINK
About It

4

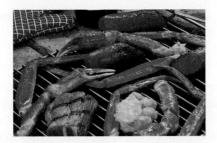

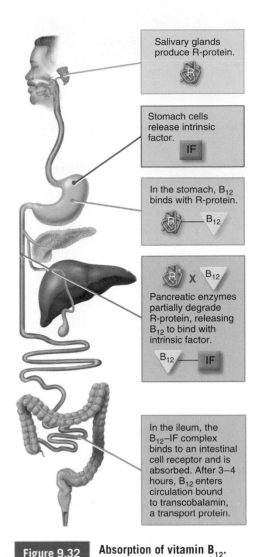

**Exceptionally high sources**
Beef liver
Clams
Oysters
Chicken liver
Herring
Crab
Wheat bran flakes cereal
All Bran cereal

# B$_{12}$

**High sources**
Salmon
Sardines
Lobster
Beef, ground
Beef, T-bone steak
Tuna
Yogurt, plain
Shrimp
Halibut
Soymilk, fortified

**Good sources**
Squid
Milk
Cod
Cottage cheese
Bologna, beef
Frankfurter, beef
Pork, loin chops

**Figure 9.31** | **Food sources of vitamin B$_{12}$.** Vitamin B$_{12}$ is found naturally only in foods of animal origin, such as liver, meats, and milk. Some cereals are fortified with vitamin B$_{12}$.

Salivary glands produce R-protein.

Stomach cells release intrinsic factor. IF

In the stomach, B$_{12}$ binds with R-protein.

Pancreatic enzymes partially degrade R-protein, releasing B$_{12}$ to bind with intrinsic factor.

In the ileum, the B$_{12}$–IF complex binds to an intestinal cell receptor and is absorbed. After 3–4 hours, B$_{12}$ enters circulation bound to transcobalamin, a transport protein.

**Figure 9.32** | **Absorption of vitamin B$_{12}$.** Absorption of B$_{12}$ is a complex process that involves many factors and sites in the GI tract. Defects in this process, especially a lack of intrinsic factor, impair B$_{12}$ absorption and can lead to B$_{12}$ deficiency.

**Pernicious anemia** is a major cause of vitamin B$_{12}$ deficiency. In this disease, an inappropriate immune response may attack and destroy certain cells lining the stomach. This, in turn, reduces the production of factors that are needed for B$_{12}$ absorption, and deficiency develops. In this type of anemia, red blood cells are large, fragile, and strangely shaped, just like in folate deficiency anemia. But, when a B$_{12}$ deficiency causes the anemia, nerve cells are irreversibly destroyed. This is the crucial difference between B$_{12}$ deficiency anemia and folate deficiency anemia—folate deficiency does not destroy nerves. If B$_{12}$ deficiency anemia is incorrectly treated with folic acid, anemia symptoms may disappear as nerve degeneration continues. The mistake may not become apparent until the damage is irreversible. Proper treatment of B$_{12}$ deficiency anemia includes B$_{12}$ injections, nasal spray, or megadose supplement.

## Vitamin B$_{12}$ Toxicity

Large vitamin B$_{12}$ doses have no apparent ill effect. Doses of 1,000 micrograms are used routinely in medical situations. A UL for vitamin B$_{12}$ has not been determined.

**Key Concepts** *Vitamin B$_6$, folate, and vitamin B$_{12}$ work closely together. Deficiency of folate increases risk for birth defects. Deficiency of B$_{12}$ causes irreversible nerve damage. All three deficiencies cause anemia. All three deficiencies compromise homocysteine metabolism. Fortified grains have become an important folate source. Only animal-derived*

**pernicious anemia** A form of anemia that results from an autoimmune disorder that damages cells lining the stomach and inhibits vitamin B$_{12}$ absorption; causes vitamin B$_{12}$ deficiency.

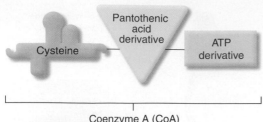

**Figure 9.33** **Pantothenic acid and coenzyme A.** Pantothenic acid forms part of coenzyme A, which, in turn, is a component of acetyl CoA. Through coenzyme A, pantothenic acid is involved in many metabolic reactions that extract energy from nutrients and other reactions that build fatty acids.

*or fortified foods contain significant amounts of vitamin* $B_{12}$. *Megadoses of vitamin* $B_6$ *can cause nerve damage.*

# Pantothenic Acid

Pantothenic acid is widespread in the food supply; in fact, its name comes from the Greek word *pantothen*, meaning "from every side." Although marketers have promoted pantothenic acid supplements as an "antistress" vitamin, there is no evidence from controlled studies to suggest it reduces feelings of anxiety or stress.[74]

## Functions of Pantothenic Acid

Pantothenic acid is a component of coenzyme A (CoA), which in turn is part of acetyl CoA, a compound that sits at the crossroads of energy-generating and biosynthetic pathways. (See **Figure 9.33**.) It is critical for extracting energy from nutrients and for building new fatty acids.

## Dietary Recommendations and Sources of Pantothenic Acid

There are few data upon which to base dietary recommendations for pantothenic acid, so an Adequate Intake level has been set instead. For adults aged 19 to 50, the AI is 5 milligrams per day. Mother Nature must have known the importance of this vitamin because it is found throughout the food supply. Pantothenic acid is in foods as diverse as meat, mushrooms, and oats.[75] Pantothenic acid is easily damaged. Freezing and canning appear to decrease the pantothenic acid content, and refining grains destroys nearly 75 percent.[76]

## Pantothenic Acid Deficiency

Pantothenic acid deficiencies are virtually nonexistent. In research settings, deficiency-induced symptoms include irritability and restlessness, fatigue, digestive disturbance, sleep disturbance, numbness and tingling, muscle cramps, staggered gait, and low blood glucose levels.

## Pantothenic Acid Toxicity

High intakes of pantothenic acid have no apparent adverse effects. Therefore a UL has not been established.

# Biotin

In 1924, researchers thought they had identified three growth factors—"bios II," "vitamin H," and "coenzyme R." But it soon became clear that there was only one substance at work—the B vitamin biotin.

## Functions of Biotin

Like the other B vitamins, biotin acts as a coenzyme in dozens of reactions. Among these reactions are amino acid metabolism, including the conversion of amino acids to glucose (gluconeogenesis); fatty acid synthesis; release of energy from fatty acids; and DNA synthesis.

## Dietary Recommendations and Sources of Biotin

We know so little about biotin requirements that the AI for adults is mathematically determined from the infant AI, which in turn is based on the biotin levels of human milk.[77] The AI for biotin for adults is 30 micrograms daily.

*Quick* Bite

**Busy Bacteria**
You may be aware that bacteria in the colon synthesize vitamin K, but did you know that these bacteria also make some biotin? However, in synthesizing this B vitamin these busy microbes may be undertaking a futile effort. Because the colon is downstream from the small intestine, the site of most biotin absorption, the bacteria's biotin may not be absorbed efficiently. Bacterial synthesis of biotin probably does not make an important contribution to your body's supply of biotin.

We also have little information on the biotin content of foods. We do know that some good sources are cauliflower, liver, peanuts, and cheese, whereas most fruits and meats are poor sources.

In raw egg white, a protein called **avidin** binds biotin and prevents its absorption. Cooking denatures avidin, preventing it from binding to biotin. Egg yolks are a good biotin source, as long as eggs are cooked.

**avidin** A protein in raw egg whites that binds biotin, preventing its absorption. Avidin is denatured by heat.

## Biotin Deficiency

Deficiency is rare, but it can occur. Eating raw egg whites—about a dozen or more daily over months or years—could produce biotin deficiency, but this scenario is unlikely. Some anticonvulsant drugs break down biotin, increasing risk of deficiency.

A rare genetic defect can lead to biotin depletion in infants. Symptoms progress from initial hair loss, rash, and delayed growth and development to convulsions and other neurological problems. Early diagnosis and daily biotin supplements usually clear up symptoms. If untreated, biotin deficiency can lead to coma and death.

## Biotin Toxicity

High doses of biotin do not appear toxic, and no UL for biotin has been established.

**Key Concepts** *Pantothenic acid and biotin are widespread in the food supply, and deficiencies are rare. Like the other B vitamins, they are parts of coenzymes involved in the metabolism of fat, carbohydrate, and protein.*

# Vitamin C

For centuries, the treacherous disease scurvy dogged humankind. Explorers and seafaring men especially feared this mysterious ailment that inflicted aching pain and made each journey a gamble with death. Writings dating back as far as 1500 B.C.E. describe their suffering in detail.

In 1747, James Lind, a Scottish physician, proved that eating lemons and oranges cured the disease. But scientists did not isolate the substance responsible for curing scurvy and name it vitamin C until 1930. The chemical name for vitamin C is ascorbic acid. This name comes from the fact that vitamin C is antiscorbutic (antiscurvy).

Most animals manufacture their own vitamin C, but humans cannot, sharing this dubious distinction with fruit-eating bats, guinea pigs, and a few other isolated species.

## Functions of Vitamin C

Unlike the B vitamins, vitamin C does not act as a coenzyme, yet it is an important participant in many reactions and is known for its antioxidant activities.

### Antioxidant Activity

Like vitamin E, vitamin C is an antioxidant and helps protect cells from oxidative damage But unlike vitamin E, vitamin C is water-soluble rather than fat-soluble. (See the FYI feature "Antioxidants and Free Radicals.") Eating foods rich in vitamin C may reduce the risk of chronic diseases such as heart disease, certain forms of cancer, and cataracts. It remains unclear whether the protective effects are due to vitamin C or to fruit and vegetable consumption in general. Study results for vitamin C supplements are contradictory.[78]

**connective tissues** Tissues composed primarily of fibrous proteins, such as collagen, and that contain few cells. Their primary function is to bind together and support various body structures.

### Collagen Synthesis

We need vitamin C to form collagen, a fibrous protein that helps reinforce the **connective tissues** that hold together the structures of the body. Collagen is made up of individual, linear proteins that wrap around one another like a cord of rope, forming a triple helix that imparts strength and flexibility. It is the most abundant protein in our bodies and the main fibrous component of skin, bone, tendons, cartilage, and teeth.

### Other Vital Roles

Your body needs vitamin C to make many other essential compounds, among them thyroid hormone, steroid hormones, bile salts, the neurotransmitter serotonin, and parts of the DNA molecule. Also, vitamin C enhances the absorption of iron from plant foods.

Vitamin C enables cells in our immune system to function effectively. Based in part on the vitamin's importance to immunity, vitamin C has been reputed to prevent or cure the common cold. However, studies show that, at best, vitamin C may slightly reduce the duration of a cold in people exposed to brief periods of severe physical exercise or cold environments.[79]

THINK About It
5

## Dietary Recommendations and Sources of Vitamin C

The RDA for vitamin C is 90 milligrams per day for men and 75 milligrams per day for women, increasing to 85 milligrams per day during pregnancy and 120 milligrams during breastfeeding (levels far above the 5 or 10 milligrams required daily to prevent scurvy). Cigarette smoking increases the need for vitamin C by 35 milligrams per day.[80]

Many, but not all, fruits and vegetables are high in vitamin C. Good sources include citrus fruits, tomatoes, fortified juice drinks, broccoli, strawberries, kiwifruit, cabbage, leafy greens, peppers, and potatoes. (See **Figure 9.34**.) Because vitamin C is highly vulnerable to heat and oxygen, fresh fruits and vegetables are best. Frozen orange juice concentrate preserves vitamin C content better than cartons of ready-to-drink orange juice. For more information about frozen foods, see the FYI feature "Fresh, Frozen, or Canned? Raw, Dried, or Cooked?"

The more vitamin C you consume, the less efficiently your intestines absorb the vitamin. If your intake is under 30 milligrams daily, you absorb nearly all of it. Between 30 and 120 milligrams, you absorb about 80 to 90 percent. As intake increases further, the efficiency of absorption continues to decline, falling to about 20 percent at 6,000 milligrams. Any excess vitamin C that is absorbed is excreted in urine.

## Quick Bite

**Chili Peppers Are Hot Stuff**

An estimated one-quarter of the world's adults eat chili peppers every day. By weight, chili peppers are one of the richest sources of vitamins A and C. In addition, capsaicin, the substance that causes your mouth to burn, jump-starts the digestive process by stimulating salivation, gastric secretions, and gut motility.

## Vitamin C Deficiency

After about a month on a diet without vitamin C, symptoms of scurvy start to surface. As the body loses its ability to synthesize collagen, connective tissue starts breaking down. Gums and joints begin to bleed. Small blood vessels break, and tiny hemorrhages appear just under the skin. Mild bruising produces exaggerated "black-and-blue marks." As the disease progresses, previously healed wounds reopen. Teeth are lost. Bone pain, fractures, diarrhea, and psychological problems such as depression appear. Left untreated, scurvy is fatal.

Scurvy is rare in developed countries, except among alcoholics or those on severely restricted diets.[81] Marginal vitamin C deficiency is more common; its symptoms include sore, inflamed gums and fatigue.

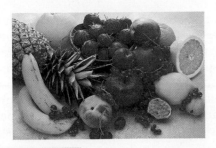

**Exceptionally high sources**
Orange juice
Strawberries
Oranges
Wheat bran flakes cereal

**High sources**
Cantaloupe
Tomato juice
Mango
Cauliflower
Broccoli
Watermelon
Spinach, raw
Pineapple
Mustard greens
Romaine lettuce
Sweet potato
Clams
Blueberries
Cabbage
Collards
Soybeans
Swiss chard
Banana
Okra

**Good sources**
Spinach, cooked
Peach
Acorn squash
Asparagus
Green beans
Potato
Corn flakes cereal
Cheerios cereal

**Figure 9.34** **Food sources of vitamin C.** Vitamin C is found mainly in fruits and vegetables. Although citrus fruits are notoriously good sources, many other popular fruits and vegetables are rich in vitamin C.

## Vitamin C Toxicity

Megadoses greater than 2,000 milligrams daily may cause abdominal cramps and diarrhea. In certain kidney conditions, excess vitamin C may cause kidney stones.[82] High vitamin C increases iron absorption—useful for some people, but problematic for those who already have too much body iron. At megadose levels, vitamin C may switch from its antioxidant role to a pro-oxidant role, encouraging oxidation.[83] The UL for vitamin C is 2,000 milligrams per day.

**Key Concepts**  *Vitamin C is found in many fruits and vegetables. It functions in collagen synthesis, acts as an antioxidant, helps boost iron absorption, plays a role in immunity, and helps synthesize many essential substances. Deficiency causes scurvy. Megadoses can cause digestive disturbance.*

## Choline: A Vitamin-Like Substance

Choline is a vitamin-like substance, but differs from a true vitamin. You can synthesize most, but probably not all, of the choline you need. Men who stay on a choline-free diet develop a deficiency over time. For this reason dietary recommendations are now made for choline.

Along with vitamins $B_{12}$, $B_6$, and folate, choline helps metabolize homocysteine. But unlike most vitamins, choline is more than a catalyst or coenzyme. Most choline in your body is actually a component of other substances, such as the neurotransmitter acetylcholine. It is also a component of phospholipids. You may recall that a phospholipid has two fatty acids (responsible for solubility in fat) and a phosphate–nitrogen group (responsible for solubility in water). Choline is the phosphate–nitrogen group in many phospholipids. In cell membranes phospholipids help protect the cell, allowing only certain substances to enter and leave, and they help maintain the cell's shape. Throughout the body, phospholipids act as emulsifiers, enabling fatty substances to mix with water-soluble ones.

The AI for choline is 550 milligrams per day for adult men and 425 milligrams for women.[84] Milk, liver, egg yolk, and peanuts are good sources, but overall it is abundant in the food supply. Deficiency in healthy people is unlikely. A deficiency produces fat accumulation in the liver and then liver damage. High doses of choline can cause diarrhea, falling blood pressure, and a disconcerting fishy body odor. The UL for choline is 3,500 milligrams per day.

## Conditional Nutrients

Relatively speaking, there are few substances we need for life that our bodies cannot make. These substances are nutrients such as vitamins that we must get from food. Our bodies routinely make countless other essential substances. However, under some circumstances—illnesses or inherited metabolic errors—we cannot make enough, so we must obtain them from our diets. These substances are "conditional nutrients." Inositol, carnitine, taurine, and lipoic acid are examples of nutrients that probably are conditional. Inositol helps form cell membrane phospholipids and precursors of eicosanoids, substances that work like hormones. Carnitine transports fatty acids to sites in the cell where your body can break them down. Taurine, derived from the amino acids methionine and cysteine, seems to play a role in such diverse functions as vision, insulin activity, and cell growth. Lipoic acid is a potent antioxidant and a necessary cofactor in many energy-releasing reactions. You may see conditional nutrients in dietary supplements, and they may be prescribed medically.

## Bogus Vitamins

Some supplements contain clearly unnecessary substances. Yet hucksters often call them "vitamins" and tout their supposed benefits: "health boosters," "youth-enhancers," "physical performance enhancers," and the like. Other products are subtly and unethically promoted to cure disease, despite ample scientific evidence to the contrary. Some supplements contain hesperidin, para-aminobenzoic acid (PABA), pangamic acid, or rutin, even though these substances are not essential for human health. Think twice before you buy them.

**Key Concepts**　*The vitamin-like substance choline is a component of phospholipids and neurotransmitters. A conditional nutrient is not ordinarily required from our diet. People with certain medical conditions may benefit from supplements of some conditional nutrients.*

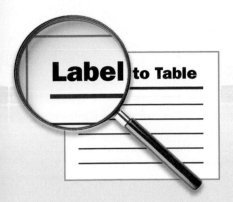

You've probably heard that milk is an excellent source of calcium, but did you know that milk also contains three of the four fat-soluble vitamins and contains a significant amount of some of the water-soluble vitamins? Let's take a look at the Nutrition Facts from a carton of nonfat milk:

| | |
|---|---|
| Calories | 90 |
| Total Fat | 0 |
| Cholesterol | less than 5 mg |
| Sodium | 130 mg |
| Total Carbohydrate | 13 g |
| Dietary Fiber | 0 g |
| Sugars | 12 g |
| Protein | 9 g |
| Vitamin A | 10% DV |
| Vitamin C | 4% DV |
| Calcium | 30% DV |
| Iron | 0% DV |
| Vitamin D | 25% DV |
| Vitamin $B_6$ | 5% DV |
| Vitamin $B_{12}$ | 15% DV |
| Riboflavin | 18% DV |

Milk contains the fat-soluble vitamins A and D. Vitamin A is found naturally in whole milk, but all milk is fortified with this vitamin. That includes whole, reduced-fat, evaporated, powdered, lactose-free, and fat-free milks. (But yogurt, cheese, and ice cream are not generally fortified.) Fortification provides 10 percent of the Daily Value for vitamin A in 1 cup. Drink 3 cups in a day, and you'll get about one-third of your recommended vitamin A. That's good news because dietary vitamin A is not always easy to obtain.

Keep in mind when selecting milk that nonfat (skim) milk contains vitamins A and D just like whole milk. Don't let the large banner "Vitamin A and D" printed on containers of whole milk trick you into thinking it contains more. It doesn't!

Vitamin D is important for bone health because it helps with absorption of calcium and phosphorus. Fortifying milk with vitamin D ensures that growing children will have the vitamin D they need, even if they don't get much sunlight or eat foods naturally rich in vitamin D such as sardines. As shown on the nutrition label here, just 1 cup of milk gives you one-quarter of the vitamin D Daily Value, or 2.5 micrograms.

Let's take a look at a few of the water-soluble vitamins now since milk is a good source of those too. The vitamin C Daily Value is always required on food labels, but riboflavin and vitamins $B_6$ and $B_{12}$ are not. They've been added here to emphasize that 1 cup of milk contributes 15 percent of your vitamin $B_{12}$ and 18 percent of your riboflavin needs for the day. Notice that vitamins C and $B_6$ are also found in milk at 4 percent and 5 percent of their Daily Value, respectively. This means drinking milk not only helps you grow and maintain a healthy skeleton but also provides B vitamins for other key body functions.

## Nutrition Facts

Serving Size: 1/2 cup (56g)
Servings Per Container: 8

**Amount Per Serving**

**Calories 200**                    Calories from fat 10

| | % Daily Value* |
|---|---|
| Total Fat 1g | 2% |
| Saturated Fat 0g | 0% |
| Trans Fat 0g | |
| Cholesterol 0mg | 0% |
| **Sodium** 0mg | 0% |
| **Total Carbohydrate** 41g | 14% |
| Dietary Fiber 2g | 8% |
| Sugars 1g | |
| **Protein** 7g | |

| | | |
|---|---|---|
| Vitamin A 0% | · | Vitamin C 0% |
| Calcium 0% | · | Iron 10% |
| Thiamin 35% | · | Riboflavin 15% |
| Niacin 20% | · | Folic acid 30% |

* Percent Daily Values are based on a 2,000 calorie diet. Your daily values may be higher or lower depending on your calorie needs:

| | | Calories: | 2000 | 2,500 |
|---|---|---|---|---|
| Total Fat | Less Than | | 65g | 80g |
| Sat Fat | Less Than | | 20g | 25g |
| Cholesterol | Less Than | | 300mg | 300mg |
| Sodium | Less Than | | 2,400mg | 2,400mg |
| Total Carbohydrate | | | 300g | 375g |
| Dietary Fiber | | | 25g | 30g |

Calories per gram:
Fat 9  Carbohydrate 4  Protein 4

# Learning Portfolio

## Key Terms

## Study Points

- There are two classes of vitamins: fat-soluble vitamins (A, D, E, and K) and water-soluble vitamins (eight B vitamins and vitamin C).

- Vitamin A comes from preformed retinoids and the precursor carotenoids. Sources include butterfat, liver, green leafy and yellow-orange vegetables, and yellow-orange fruits.

- Vitamin A is essential to vision, cell differentiation, growth and development, and immune function. Night blindness is an early symptom of vitamin A deficiency that, if not treated, can result in permanent blindness.

- In large doses, vitamin A is toxic. When taken during pregnancy, excess vitamin A may cause birth defects.

- Because UV light hitting the skin converts a cholesterol precursor to vitamin D, vitamin D is known as the "sunshine vitamin." Ultimately, the kidney converts this to the active form of vitamin D—25(OH)D.

- Vitamin D in foods is available mainly from fortified milk and other fortified products.

- The primary function of vitamin D is the regulation of blood levels of calcium. Vitamin D deficiency contributes to skeletal problems. Vitamin D can be toxic at doses just a few times larger than the AI level.

- Vitamin E is an important antioxidant in the body and may help reduce the risk of chronic diseases such as heart disease and cancer.

- Vitamin E is found in vegetable oils and foods made from those oils. Deficiency and toxicity of vitamin E are relatively rare.

- Vitamin K is an important factor in blood coagulation and bone health.

- Although synthesized by intestinal bacteria, most of the vitamin K in the body comes from dietary sources, especially green vegetables. Vitamin K deficiency is rare, but newborns are susceptible if not given an injection of vitamin K at birth. Because the body excretes vitamin K easily, toxicity is unlikely.

- All B vitamins function as coenzymes.

- Thiamin deficiency results in the classic disease beriberi. In industrialized countries, thiamin deficiency most often is associated with alcoholism. High doses of thiamin do not appear to be toxic.

- Milk is a good source of riboflavin, but light can destroy the vitamin. Packaging milk in paper or plastic cartons rather than in clear glass better protects milk's riboflavin content.

- Niacin deficiency results in pellagra, a disease characterized by diarrhea, dermatitis, dementia, and death. High doses of niacin, such as in the treatment of high blood cholesterol, can have toxic side effects, including liver damage.

- Vitamin $B_6$, folate, and vitamin $B_{12}$ work together to control blood levels of homocysteine.

- A deficiency of vitamin $B_6$ can lead to microcytic anemia—small, pale red blood cells.

- Poor folate status is associated with development of neural tube defects during pregnancy. Therefore, women of childbearing age need folic acid from supplements in addition to fortified foods and other dietary folate.

- Deficiency of either folate or vitamin $B_{12}$ can lead to megaloblastic anemia, but vitamin $B_{12}$ deficiency also causes irreversible nerve damage.
- Pantothenic acid is widespread in the food supply, and deficiency is virtually nonexistent. In the body, pantothenic acid is part of coenzyme A.
- Biotin deficiency is rare but may be induced by regularly consuming large quantities of raw egg whites.
- Vitamin C (ascorbic acid) functions in the synthesis of collagen and other vital compounds and also works as an antioxidant. Vitamin C deficiency causes scurvy.
- Choline is a vitamin-like substance that the body makes but which, under some circumstances, must be supplied by diet.

## Study Questions

1. Describe two differences between fat-soluble and water-soluble vitamins.
2. What are the main roles of vitamin A in the body? What is an early sign of vitamin A deficiency?
3. What is vitamin D's nickname? Why? Why is vitamin D also considered a hormone?
4. What is vitamin E's primary function? What are the best sources of vitamin E?
5. What is the best-known function of vitamin K?
6. Which two fat-soluble vitamins potentially are the most toxic? Which two are the least toxic?
7. List the nine water-soluble vitamins and one main function for each.
8. Name the diseases and/or characteristic symptoms of deficiencies of each water-soluble vitamin.
9. List the water-soluble vitamins demonstrated to be toxic in large doses. What signs indicate toxic levels of each vitamin?

## Try This

### The PUFA Protection Challenge: Vitamin E vs. Oxygen

The object of this experiment is to see if vitamin E protects polyunsaturated fats (PUFA) from oxidation. You'll need two glasses, one bottle of either safflower or corn oil, and some liquid vitamin E gel caps (can be purchased at any pharmacy). Pour equal amounts of oil into each glass. Bite a hole in 10 of the vitamin E gel caps, squeeze their contents into one of the glasses, and stir. Mark this glass with tape and write the letter E on it. Let the glasses sit uncovered on a countertop for several days or weeks. Check the freshness or rancidity of the oils by smelling them and noting whether they look clear or cloudy. Over time, one will become more rancid than the other. Which glass container won the challenge—the one with or without vitamin E? Why?

### Supplemental Income

The object of this exercise is to critically review vitamin supplements. Go to the drug store and look at a few multivitamin supplements and "stress" formulas. Look at the %DV for the water-soluble vitamins. Do you see any that have more than 1,000 percent of the DV? Compare prices. Is it more expensive to buy supplements with more of these vitamins? Considering what you learned in this chapter, would it benefit you to take supplements that contain such a high amount of these vitamins? Why do you think supplements contain such large quantities of these vitamins?

## What About Bobbie?

Let's take a look at Bobbie's intake of fat-soluble vitamin A and five water-soluble vitamins: thiamin, riboflavin, niacin, vitamin $B_{12}$, and vitamin C. Let's examine her day of eating (see the "Food Choices: Nutrients and Nourishment" chapter) using the guidelines you've learned in this chapter. How did Bobbie do in terms of these vitamins?

She did well: she consumed ample amounts of most vitamins due to her varied food choices. Here is a summary of each vitamin.

### Vitamin A

Bobbie's intake of 493 micrograms RAE is about 70 percent of the RDA of 700 micrograms RAE, so Bobbie is likely meeting her needs for vitamin A. Her best sources of vitamin A were both preformed vitamin A sources (foods of animal origin such as cream cheese and pizza cheese) and foods with vitamin A precursors (e.g., beta-carotene from carrots). Here are some ways she could improve her vitamin A intake:

- Use spinach greens as the base of her salad instead of iceberg lettuce.
- Continue adding shredded carrots to her salad, and consider adding them to her sandwich, too.
- Add a slice or two of tomato on top of the bagel with cream cheese.
- Alternate bagels (not high in vitamin A) and fortified cereals (high in vitamin A) for breakfast. This change also would add some milk to her

diet, which would further increase her vitamin A intake (approximately 140 micrograms RAE per cup).

## Thiamin

Bobbie consumed 2.0 milligrams of thiamin, which is more than the RDA of 1.1 milligrams. Most foods Bobbie ate this day contributed to her thiamin intake, but the ones that contributed the most were the enriched grains from the bread, bagel, and spaghetti.

## Riboflavin

Bobbie consumed 2.2 milligrams of riboflavin on this day, or more than the RDA of 1.1 milligrams. As with thiamin, a variety of foods contributed to her riboflavin intake, but the enriched grains (bread, bagel, and pasta) were among the best contributors. The meatballs Bobbie ate at dinner also contributed riboflavin.

## Niacin

Bobbie's intake of niacin also was above her RDA. She consumed 27.5 milligrams this day compared to her RDA of 14 milligrams. If you remember from the protein chapter that Bobbie's intake of protein was quite high, it shouldn't surprise you that her niacin intake is high, too. Meat, poultry, fish, and other protein-containing foods, along with enriched grains, are some of the best sources of niacin. In this case, Bobbie's turkey sandwich, spaghetti with meatballs, and cheese pizza contributed niacin.

## Vitamin $B_{12}$

Bobbie's intake of vitamin $B_{12}$ (3.7 micrograms), like her intake of the other B vitamins, was above the RDA (2.4 micrograms). The foods that contributed to Bobbie's vitamin $B_{12}$ intake were the animal products (turkey, egg, meatballs, Parmesan cheese, and cheese pizza).

## Vitamin C

Although Bobbie enjoys tomato products such as salsa, spaghetti sauce, and pizza sauce, her intake of vitamin C (42 milligrams) was less than the RDA of 75 milligrams. Here are some other ways Bobbie could include more vitamin C in her diet:

- Have some orange or grapefruit juice with breakfast.
- Choose spinach, broccoli, or Brussels sprouts instead of green beans for dinner.
- Use spinach as the base of her salad instead of iceberg lettuce.
- Add some sliced red pepper to her salad at lunch.
- Have an orange as a snack instead of tortilla chips.

# References

1 Mahan KL, Escott-Stump S, eds. *Krause's Food, Nutrition, and Diet Therapy.* 12th ed. Philadelphia: W.B. Saunders; 2008.

2 Institute of Medicine, Food and Nutrition Board. *Dietary Reference Intakes for Vitamin A, Vitamin K, Arsenic, Boron, Chromium, Copper, Iron, Manganese, Molybdenum, Nickel, Silicon, Vanadium, and Zinc.* Washington, DC: National Academies Press; 2001.

3 Guyton AC, Hall JE. *Textbook of Medical Physiology.* 12th ed. Philadelphia: Saunders; 2010.

4 National Institutes of Health Osteoporosis and Related Bone Diseases National Resource Center. Vitamin A and bone health. http://www.niams.nih.gov/Health_Info/Bone/Bone_Health/Nutrition/vitamin_a.asp. Accessed 7/6/11.

5 Institute of Medicine, Food and Nutrition Board. 2001. Op. cit.

6 Ibid.

7 Gropper SS, Smith JL, Groff JL. *Advanced Nutrition and Human Metabolism.* 5th ed. Belmont, CA: Cengage Learning; 2009.

8 Hayman RM, Dalziel SR. Acute vitamin A toxicity: a report of three paediatric cases. *J Paediatr Child Health.* 2011 Jun 17.

9 Institute of Medicine, Food and Nutrition Board. 2001. Op. cit.

10 Institute of Medicine, Food and Nutrition Board. *Dietary Reference Intakes for Vitamin C, Vitamin E, Selenium, and Carotenoids.* Washington, DC: National Academies Press; 2000.

11 Gropper SS, Smith JL, Groff JL. Op cit.

12 Olson JH, Erie JC, Bakri SJ. Nutritional supplementation and age-related macular degeneration. *Semin Ophthalmol.* 2011;26(3):131–136.

13 Rao AV, Rao LG. Carotenoids and human health. *Pharmacol Res.* 2007;55:207–216.

14 Kristal AR, Arnold KB, Neuhouser ML, et al. Diet, supplement use, and prostate cancer risk: results from the Prostate Cancer Prevention Trial. *Am J Epidemiol.* 2010;172 (5):566–577.

15 Rao AV, Rao LG. Op. cit.

16 Institute of Medicine, Food and Nutrition Board. 2000. Op. cit.

17 Institute of Medicine, Food and Nutrition Board. 2001. Op. cit.

18 US Department of Agriculture, Agricultural Research Service. USDA National Nutrient Database for Standard Reference, Release 23. 2010. Nutrient Data Laboratory Home Page. http://www.ars.usda.gov/ba/bhnrc/ndl. Accessed 7/6/11.

19 Institute of Medicine, Food and Nutrition Board. 2001. Op. cit.

20 Cameron ID, Murray GR, Gillespie LD, et al. Interventions for preventing falls in older people in nursing care facilities and hospitals. *Cochrane Database Syst Rev.* 2010;20(1):CD005465.

21 Wang L, Manson JE, Song Y, Sesso HD. Systematic review: vitamin D and calcium supplementation in prevention of cardiovascular events. *Ann Intern Med.* 2010;2;152(5):315–323; and Shapses SA, Manson JE. Vitamin D and prevention of cardiovascular disease and diabetes: why the evidence falls short. *JAMA.* 2011;305(24):2565–2566.

22 Manson JE, Mayne ST, Clinton SK. Vitamin D and prevention of cancer—ready for prime time? *N Engl J Med.* 2011;14;364(15):1385–1387; and Toner CD, Davis CD, Milner JA. The vitamin D and cancer conundrum: aiming at a moving target. *J Am Diet Assoc.* 2010;110(10):1492–1500.

23 Manson JE, Mayne ST, Clinton SK. Op cit.

24 Shapses SA, Manson JE. Op cit.

25 Institute of Medicine, Food and Nutrition Board. *Dietary Reference Intakes for Calcium and Vitamin D.* Washington, DC: National Academies Press; 2010.

26 Ibid.

27 Institute of Medicine. *Dietary Reference Intakes for Calcium and Vitamin D.* Report Brief. November 2010. http://www.iom.edu/~/media/Files/Report%20Files/2010/Dietary-Reference-Intakes-for-Calcium-and-Vitamin-D/Vitamin%20D%20and%20Calcium%202010%20Report%20Brief.pdf. Accessed 6/7/11.

28 Wagner CL, Greer FR, and the Section on Breastfeeding and Committee on Nutrition Clinical Report. Prevention of rickets and vitamin D deficiency in infants, children, and adolescents. *Pediatrics.* 2008;122(5):1142–1152.

29  Institute of Medicine, Food and Nutrition Board. 2010. Op. cit.

30  Ibid.

31  Holick MF. Vitamin D deficiency. *New Engl J Med.* 2007;357:266–281.

32  Wagner CL, Greer FR, and the Section on Breastfeeding and Committee on Nutrition Clinical Report. Op. cit.

33  Ibid.

34  Kumar J, Muntner P, Kaskel FJ, et al. Prevalence and associations of 25-hydroxyvitamin D deficiency in US children: NHANES 2001–2004. *Pediatrics.* Published online August 3, 2009. DOI: 10.1542/peds.2009-0051. Available at http://www.natap.org/2009/HIV/peds.pdf. Accessed 7/6/11.

35  The Linus Pauling Institute Micronutrient Information Center. Vitamin D. Updated 6/22/11. http://lpi.oregonstate.edu/infocenter/vitamins/vitaminD/index.html#lpi_recommend. Accessed 7/7/11.

36  Institute of Medicine, Food and Nutrition Board. 2010. Op. cit.

37  Toner CD, Davis CD, Milner JA. Op. cit.

38  Mente A, de Koning L, Shannon HS, Anand SS. A systematic review of the evidence supporting a causal link between dietary factors and coronary heart disease. *Arch Intern Med.* 2009;13;169(7):659–669.

39  National Institutes of Health Office of Dietary Supplements. Dietary supplement fact sheet. Vitamin E. http://ods.od.nih.gov/factsheets/vitamine. Accessed 7/8/11.

40  American Heart Association. Vitamin and mineral supplements. AHA scientific position. Updated 11/23/10. http://www.heart.org/HEARTORG/GettingHealthy/NutritionCenter/Vitamin-and-Mineral-Supplements_UCM_306033_Article.jsp. Accessed 7/8/11.

41  Huang HY, Caballero B, Chang S, et al. Multivitamin/mineral supplements and prevention of chronic disease: executive summary. *Am J Clin Nutr.* 2007;85(1):265S–268S.

42  Institute of Medicine, Food and Nutrition Board. 2000. Op. cit.

43  Moshfegh A, Goldman J, Cleveland L. *What We Eat in America, NHANES 2001–2002: Usual Nutrient Intakes from Food Compared to Dietary Reference Intakes.* Washington, DC: US Department of Agriculture, Agriculture Research Service; 2005.

44  Mayo Clinic. Vitamin E. Updated 7/1/11. http://www.mayoclinic.com/health/vitamin-e/NS_patient-vitamine. Accessed 7/7/11.

45  National Institutes of Health Office of Dietary Supplements. Op. cit.

46  Pearson DA. Bone health and osteoporosis: the role of vitamin K and potential antagonism by anticoagulants. *Nutr Clin Pract.* 2007;22(5):517–544.

47  Iwamoto J, Sato Y, Takeda T, Matsumoto H. High-dose vitamin K supplementation reduces fracture incidence in postmenopausal women: a review of the literature. *Nutr Res.* 2009;29(4):221–228.

48  Institute of Medicine, Food and Nutrition Board. 2001. Op. cit.

49  Booth SL, Rajabi AA. Determinants of vitamin K status in humans. *Vitam Horm.* 2008;78:1–22.

50  Ibid.

51  Ibid.

52  Institute of Medicine, Food and Nutrition Board. *Dietary Reference Intakes for Thiamin, Riboflavin, Niacin, Vitamin B6, Folate, Vitamin B12, Pantothenic Acid, Biotin, and Choline.* Washington, DC: National Academies Press; 1998.

53  Larson Duyff R. *The American Dietetic Association Complete Food and Nutrition Guide.* Hoboken, NJ: John Wiley and Sons, 2006.

54  Institute of Medicine, Food and Nutrition Board. 1998. Op. cit.

55  Mestdagh F, DeMeulenaer B, De Clippeleer J, et al. Protective influence of several packaging materials on light oxidation of milk. *J Dairy Sci.* 2005;88:499–510.

56  Brown BG. Expert commentary: niacin safety. *Am J Cardiol.* 2007;99(6A):32C–34C.

57  Guyton JF, Bayes HE. Safety considerations with niacin therapy. *Am J Cardiol.* 2007;99(6A):22C–31C.

58  National Institutes of Health. NIH stops clinical trial on combination cholesterol treatment. Press release. 5/26/2011. http://www.nih.gov/news/health/may2011/nhlbi-26.htm. Accessed 7/10/11.

59  Gropper SS, Smith JL, Groff JL. Op. cit.

60  Ciaccio M, Bellia C. Hyperhomocysteinemia and cardiovascular risk: effect of vitamin supplementation in risk reduction. *Curr Clin Pharmacol.* 2010;5(1):30–36.

61  Institute of Medicine, Food and Nutrition Board. 1998. Op. cit.

62  US Department of Agriculture, Agricultural Research Service. USDA National Nutrient Database for Standard Reference, Release 23. 2010. Nutrient Data Laboratory Home Page. http://www.ars.usda.gov/ba/bhnrc/ndl. Accessed 10/29/11.

63  National Institutes of Health, Office of Dietary Supplements. Dietary supplement fact sheet. Vitamin B6. Updated 8/24/07. http://ods.od.nih.gov/factsheets/vitaminb6.asp. Accessed 7/11/11.

64  LeBlanc KE, Cestia W. Carpal tunnel syndrome. *Am Fam Physician.* 2011;83(8):952–958.

65  Centers for Disease Control and Prevention. Folic acid. Updated 3/10/11. http://www.cdc.gov/ncbddd/folicacid/index.html. Accessed 7/10/11.

66  Lee JE, Willett WC, Fuchs CS, et al. Folate intake and risk of colorectal cancer and adenoma: modification by time. *Am J Clin Nutr.* 2011;93(4):817–825; and Kennedy DA, Stern SJ, Moretti M, et al. Folate intake and the risk of colorectal cancer: a systematic review and meta-analysis. *Cancer Epidemiol.* 2011;35(1):2–10.

67  Mason JB. Folate, cancer risk, and the Greek god, Proteus: a tale of two chameleons. *Nutr Rev.* 2009; 67(4): 206–212.

68  Institute of Medicine, Food and Nutrition Board. 1998. Op. cit.; and Suitor CW, Bailey LB. Dietary folate equivalents: interpretation and application. *J Am Diet Assoc.* 2000;100:88–94.

69  US Preventive Services Task Force Folic Acid for the Prevention of Neural Tube Defects. US Preventive Services Task Force recommendation statement. *Ann Intern Med.* 2009;150(9): 626–631.

70  Crider KS, Bailey LB, Berry RJ. Folic acid food fortification: its history, effect, concerns, and future directions. *Nutrients.* 2011;3:370–384.

71  Centers for Disease Control and Prevention. Facts about folic acid. Updated 3/10/11. http://www.cdc.gov/ncbddd/folicacid/about.html. Accessed 7/10/11.

72  National Institute of Neurological Disorders and Stroke, National Institutes of Health. Spina bifida fact sheet. Updated 12/09. http://www.ninds.nih.gov/disorders/spina_bifida/detail_spina_bifida.htm. Accessed 7/10/11.

73  Watanabe F. Vitamin B12 sources and bioavailability. *Exp Biol Med.* 2007;232(10):1266–1274.

74  Sarubin Fragakis A. *The Health Professional's Guide to Popular Dietary Supplements.* 3rd ed. Chicago: The Academy of Nutrition and Dietetics; 2007.

75  Institute of Medicine, Food and Nutrition Board. 1998. Op. cit.

76  Ibid.

77  Ibid.

78  Lykkesfeldt J, Poulsen HE. Is vitamin C supplementation beneficial? Lessons learned from randomised controlled trials. *Br J Nutr.* 2010;103(9):1251–1259.

79  Douglas RM, Hemila H, Chalker E, Treacy B. Vitamin C for preventing and treating the common cold. *Cochrane Database Syst Rev.* 2007;18(3):CD000980.

80  Institute of Medicine, Food and Nutrition Board. 2000. Op. cit.

81  Ibid.

82  Ibid.

83  Gropper SS, Smith JL, Groff JL. Op cit.

84  Institute of Medicine, Food and Nutrition Board. 1998. Op. cit.

# CHAPTER 10

# Water and Minerals: The Ocean Within

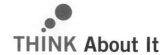

**THINK About It**

1 Do you ever feel dehydrated?

2 How often do you salt your food before tasting it?

3 You disclose to a friend that you tend to be low in iron. She knows you are a vegetarian and suggests you drink milk. What false assumption might she be making?

4 Some people argue that fluoridation is overdone. What is your position? Would you vote for fluoridating all water supplies?

**Visit go.jblearning.com/ inseldisco4e**

O n a coast-to-coast flight with your father and your older brother, you observe your father drinking water frequently throughout the flight, while your brother rejects the beverages offered. When you arrive at your destination, your brother complains of feeling utterly exhausted. In contrast, your father is lively and ready for a "night on the town"! How do you explain this?

First, it's important to know that the familiar beverage cart is not a random gesture of kindness by the airlines: regular fluid intake on flights is necessary for health! Although you may be unaware of it, water evaporates from the skin faster than usual in the low-humidity, high-altitude, pressurized cabin of an airplane, so drinking fluids during the flight helps prevent dehydration. But you must choose fluids carefully. Alcohol is a diuretic. This means that alcoholic beverages increase fluid loss as urine and therefore do not replace fluid losses as effectively as water, juice, and other caffeine-free beverages.

Your brother's lack of energy may be a symptom of mild dehydration. Dad had the right idea—plenty of water along the way.

## Water: Crucial to Life

Water is absolutely essential. You could probably survive weeks without food. But you can live only a few days without water. Humans have no capacity to store "spare" water, so we must quickly replace any that's lost.

Overall, water makes up between 45 and 75 percent of a person's weight. (See **Figure 10.1**.) About two-thirds of body water is intracellular fluid, the fluid inside cells. The remaining one-third is extracellular fluid, which is mainly between cells (interstitial) and in blood (the **plasma** portion). (See **Figure 10.2**.)

**plasma** The fluid portion of the blood that contains blood cells and other components.

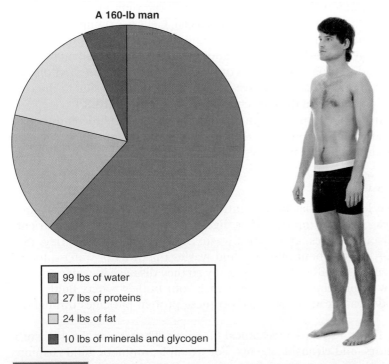

**A 160-lb man**

- ■ 99 lbs of water
- ■ 27 lbs of proteins
- □ 24 lbs of fat
- ■ 10 lbs of minerals and glycogen

**Figure 10.1** **Body composition.** The main constituent of the body is water. Generally, adult males have more lean tissue (and therefore more water) and less fat than adult females.

**salts** Compounds that result when the hydrogen of an acid is replaced with a metal or a group that acts like a metal.

**ions** Atoms or groups of atoms with an electrical charge resulting from the loss or gain of one or more electrons.

**electrolytes [ih-LEK-tro-lites]** Substances that separate into charged particles (ions) when dissolved in water or other solvents and thus become capable of conducting an electrical current. The terms *electrolyte* and *ion* often are used interchangeably.

**cations** Ions that carry a positive charge.

**anions** Ions that carry a negative charge.

**osmosis** The movement of a solvent, such as water, through a semipermeable membrane from the dilute to the concentrated side until the concentrations on both sides of the membrane are equal.

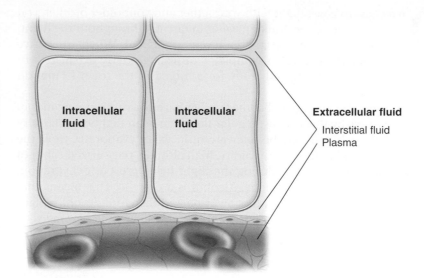

**Figure 10.2** **Intracellular and extracellular fluid.** Extracellular fluids and their dissolved substances (except for proteins) move across capillary membranes easily. Plasma (the fluid portion of the blood) has a higher concentration of proteins than interstitial fluid. Excluding protein, their compositions are roughly the same.

## Electrolytes and Water: A Delicate Balance

When minerals or **salts** dissolve in water, they form **ions** (**electrolytes**). Sodium and potassium, for example, form **cations** (positively charged ions), whereas chloride and phosphate form **anions** (negatively charged ions).

Your body precisely controls and balances the concentration of electrolytes dissolved in its watery fluids—there must be just the right mix of water and electrolytes, both within and outside of each cell. Cells use pumps embedded in their membranes to move electrolytes in and out. In concert with the movement of electrolytes, water flows back and forth through the cell membrane, a process called **osmosis**. When electrolytes are more concentrated on one side of the membrane, osmosis moves water from the dilute side to the concentrated side to equalize the concentrations. (See **Figure 10.3**.)

Cells must contain just the right amount of water. Too little and the cell will shrink and die. Too much and the cell will burst. Too much water in spaces surrounding cells causes swelling (edema).

## Functions of Water

Water is the highway that moves nutrients and wastes between cells and organs. It carries food through your digestive system, transports nutrients to your cells and tissues, and carries waste out of your body in urine. (See **Figure 10.4**.) What about nutrients and wastes that are not water-soluble? Your body either modifies them chemically so they dissolve in water or packages them with proteins (e.g., lipoproteins). Your body's watery fluids, such as the bloodstream, can easily transport these protein packages throughout the body.

Watery fluids also have mechanical functions. They act as shock absorbers, lubricators, and cleansing agents. For example, amniotic fluid cushions and protects the fetus, synovial fluid allows joints to move smoothly, tears lubricate and cleanse the eyes, and saliva moistens food and makes swallowing possible.

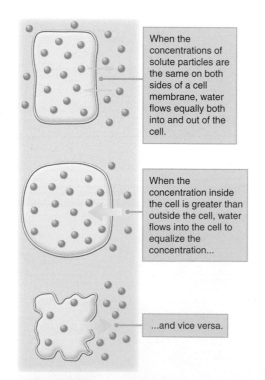

When the concentrations of solute particles are the same on both sides of a cell membrane, water flows equally both into and out of the cell.

When the concentration inside the cell is greater than outside the cell, water flows into the cell to equalize the concentration...

...and vice versa.

**Figure 10.3** **Osmosis.** Water moves across cell membranes to equalize concentrations of dissolved particles.

Water is an essential part of your body's chemistry. It helps break apart substances and is a by-product in many anabolic reactions (reactions that combine substances). Reactions involving water also help maintain the body's acid–base (pH) balance in the narrow range required for life.

Water has a high **heat capacity**, meaning a large amount of energy must be added or removed to raise or lower its temperature. When microwaving food, for example, you may have noticed that watery foods like soup heat much more slowly than foods like pizza that contain little water. Because your body is nearly two-thirds water, your body temperature remains relatively stable. Plus, water is the prime component of your body's cooling system. If you get too warm, blood vessels dilate and you begin to sweat. The perspiration on your skin evaporates and cools you off.

**Key Concepts** *Water is so essential that we cannot survive without it for more than a few days. We need water for temperature regulation, acid–base balance, lubrication, and protection. Water dissolves or carries vital substances throughout the body and participates in chemical reactions.*

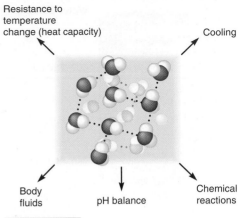

**Figure 10.4** **Functions of water.** Water is so critical to human body functioning that we can only live a few days without it.

## Intake Recommendations: How Much Water Is Enough?

There is no one answer to this question. We each need a different amount, depending on our size, body composition, and activity level, as well as the temperature and humidity of the environment.

The Adequate Intake (AI) for total water is 3.7 liters per day for men and 2.7 liters per day for women.[1] Intake recommendations are higher during pregnancy (3.0 liters per day) and lactation (3.8 liters per day). Activity and sweating increase water needs, so athletes and active people need much more water, especially if they work and train in warm, humid climates.

Water intake comes from a combination of drinking water, beverages, and the water in foods. Survey data suggest that about 75 to 80 percent of our total water intake comes from beverages, with the remaining 20 to 25 percent from foods. Some foods, such as fruits and vegetables, contain a substantial amount of water whereas others—grain products, for example—provide very little. (See **Figure 10.5**.) Our bodies also produce a small amount of water (about 250 to 350 milliliters per day) in metabolic reactions.

### Water Excretion: Where Does the Water Go?

We continuously lose water through various routes—exhaled air, perspiration, feces, and urine. (See water sources and water output in **Figure 10.6**.) **Insensible water loss**—the continuous evaporation of water from the lungs and skin—typically accounts for about one-fourth to one-half of daily fluid loss. These losses increase at high altitudes and during low humidity.

Each day, we typically lose about 1 to 2 liters of water in urine. If we eat the typical American diet containing excess protein and salt, our urine production increases to eliminate surplus urea (a breakdown product from protein) and sodium. Fever, coughing, rapid breathing, and watery nasal secretions all increase water loss significantly. This is one reason why doctors recommend increasing your fluid intake when you are sick.

**Key Concepts** *The AI for fluid intake is 3.7 liters per day for men and 2.7 liters per day for women. Water intake comes from a combination of foods, fluids, and water produced in normal metabolism. Fluid is lost mainly by urination. Additional losses occur through the skin and lungs and in feces. Water is critical in eliminating the body's waste products.*

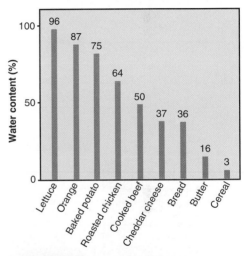

**Figure 10.5** **Water content of various foods.** As you might expect, crunchy vegetables contain more water than dry cereal. But did you know that potatoes contain a high percentage of water?

**heat capacity** The amount of energy required to raise the temperature of a substance 1°C.

**insensible water loss** The continual loss of body water by evaporation from the respiratory tract and diffusion through the skin.

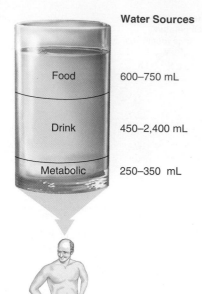

**Water Sources**

| | |
|---|---|
| Food | 600–750 mL |
| Drink | 450–2,400 mL |
| Metabolic | 250–350 mL |

**Water Output**

| | |
|---|---|
| Kidneys (urine) | 500–1,000 mL |
| Skin* | 450–1,900 mL |
| Lungs | 250–400 mL |
| Feces** | 100–200 mL |

\* (Insensible and perspiration)
The volume of perspiration is normally about 100 milliliters per day. In very hot weather or during heavy exercise, a person may lose 1 to 2 liters per hour.

\*\*People with severe diarrhea can lose several liters of water per day in feces.

**Figure 10.6** **Typical daily water intake and output.** To maintain water balance, your body regulates its fluid intake and output.

# Water Balance

Our bodies carefully maintain water balance by manipulating water intake and output. When water intake is low, the kidneys conserve water and only excrete a small volume of concentrated urine. When the body has an excess of water, the kidneys excrete a large volume of dilute urine.

How do the kidneys know when to conserve water? Special cells in the brain sense rising sodium levels in the body. These cells signal the pituitary gland to release **antidiuretic hormone (ADH)**, which in turn signals the kidneys to conserve water—effectively diluting sodium levels. Sensors in the kidneys themselves can detect a rapid loss of fluid through a drop in blood pressure. They trigger a complex process that includes the release of the hormone **aldosterone** by the adrenal glands. Aldosterone signals the kidneys to retain sodium. When sodium is retained, water follows to avoid an increased concentration of sodium.

## *Thirst*

Although taste, availability, cultural patterns, and personal habits influence our consumption of fluids, thirst remains our most important stimulus for drinking fluids. Yet thirst is not always a reliable guide to avoiding dehydration. In older adults, for example, sensitivity to thirst declines, placing them at higher risk for dehydration. Under normal circumstances, water losses in adults can range from 0.3 liters per hour in sedentary conditions to 2.0 liters per hour during high activity in the heat.[2] And, after you drink water, your body can take 30 to 60 minutes to absorb and distribute it throughout the body. For example, imagine you are rollerblading in the hot sun and after an hour you pause momentarily to quench your thirst with a ½-liter bottle of water. That's not enough! You still have a deficit of ½ to 1½ liters of water, and you'll continue to lose water while your body absorbs and distributes the water you just drank. To avoid dehydration in hot weather or when exercising, you need to drink fluids early and often.

THINK
About It

1

**Key Concepts** *The body uses complex mechanisms to precisely regulate water balance. Antidiuretic hormone (ADH) stimulates water reabsorption in the kidneys, and aldosterone stimulates the kidneys to reabsorb sodium and water. Although our sense of thirst usually reminds us to drink enough so that we don't become dehydrated, it is an unreliable signal during hot weather or heavy exercise, when fluid losses are high.*

# Alcohol, Caffeine, and Common Medications Affect Fluid Balance

Anyone who regularly consumes alcohol probably realizes that it is a diuretic—a substance that increases fluid loss through increased urination. Alcohol suppresses ADH production, and excessive alcohol consumption can cause dehydration with symptoms of thirst, weakness, dryness of mucous membranes, dizziness, and light-headedness—all common effects of a hangover.

A cup of coffee can provide a morning pick-me-up, but the caffeine is a diuretic. A typical pattern of many busy Americans is a few cups of coffee in the morning, a caffeinated soda with lunch, another in the afternoon, and maybe a glass of wine or a beer with dinner. Studies of the effects of caffeinated beverages on overall hydration status have produced inconsistent results, however.[3] Although some suggest that a fondness for caffeinated beverages can cause chronic mild dehydration, the DRI committee examining water and electrolyte requirements concluded that caffeinated beverages contribute to the total water intake in a manner similar to noncaffeinated beverages.[4]

Most Americans seem to consume a sufficient quantity and variety of fluids from foods and beverages to maintain fluid balance.[5]

Doctors often prescribe diuretic medications to help lower blood pressure or decrease swelling caused by fluid retention. Because these medications can disrupt sodium and potassium balance, doctors typically monitor the patient's blood electrolyte levels and may prescribe potassium supplements to maintain a proper balance.

## Dehydration

Any condition causing rapid water loss is dangerous: burns in which damaged skin cannot control water evaporation, the heat of fever, extreme environmental heat, or exertion without replenishing water. Early signs of dehydration include fatigue, dry mucous membranes, headache, and dark urine with a strong odor. Physical and mental performance slip. A water loss of 20 percent of body weight can cause coma and death. (See **Figure 10.7**.)

Chronic mild dehydration—a fluid deficit of as little as 1 to 2 percent of body weight—can cause declines in alertness and the ability to concentrate while increasing feelings of tiredness, reducing physical performance, and causing headache.[6] Such low levels of dehydration also impair decision making and reaction times. This may be important for tasks, such as driving a car, that involve judgment and skill. Chronic dehydration plays a role in the development of many conditions such as constipation, hypertension, coronary heart disease, glaucoma, and complications of diabetes.[7]

Seniors and infants are particularly vulnerable to dehydration. The sense of thirst often diminishes with age, and seniors often take diuretic medications. For a variety of reasons, seniors may eat and drink less. The resulting physical and mental deterioration creates a vicious cycle, with food and fluid intake continuing to worsen.

Because infants can lose water rapidly through their skin, they need ample fluid relative to their size. Breast milk or infant formula generally provides all the fluid a baby needs. Severe diarrhea can cause swift and deadly dehydration, especially in seniors and infants. Normally, the intestines reabsorb nearly all the fluid secreted by digestive organs. But when intestinal disease causes diarrhea or prolonged vomiting, dehydration can occur. With infection the underlying culprit, worldwide, dehydration is a major killer of babies and young children.

Water consumption, of course, is the primary treatment for dehydration. Often electrolytes also must be replaced, particularly in cases of diarrhea and vomiting. For moderate to severe dehydration, intravenous

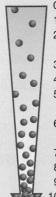

**% Body weight loss**

| | |
|---|---|
| 0 | |
| 1 | Thirst |
| 2 | Increased thirst, loss of appetite, discomfort |
| 3 | Impatience, decreased blood volume |
| 4 | Nausea, slowing of physical work |
| 5 | Difficulty concentrating, apathy, tingling extremities |
| 6 | Increasing body temperature, pulse and respiration rate |
| 7 | Stumbling, headache |
| 8 | Dizziness, labored breathing |
| 9 | Weakness, mental confusion |
| 10 | Muscle spasms, indistinct speech |
| 11 | Kidney failure, poor circulation due to decreased blood volume |

**Figure 10.7** **Effects of progressive dehydration.** Dehydration quickly diminishes physical and mental performance. Severe dehydration can be fatal.

## *Quick* Bite

### How Do Desert-Dwelling Animals Avoid Dehydration?

Some desert animals can concentrate their urine to nearly 100 times the maximum concentration of human urine. This allows such animals to survive on water obtained from food and their own metabolic reactions. Aquatic animals, in contrast, minimally concentrate their urine. Beavers concentrate their urine to only about half that of humans.

## *Quick* Bite

### Is Airline Drinking Water Tainted?

The tap water on airplanes may become unsanitary. This prompted the Environmental Protection Agency to launch the Airline Drinking Water Rule (ADWR) in 2009 to ensure that safe and reliable drinking water is available on aircrafts. The rule provides protection for the public against disease-causing organisms that are sometimes found in the tap water on airplanes. The ADWR requires airlines to sample for bacteria, follow best management practices, take corrective action, notify the public, train operators, and follow guidelines for reporting and recordkeeping to improve public health protection.

**Source:** Data from Environmental Protection Agency. Airline Drinking Water Rule (ADWR). http://water.epa.gov/lawsregs/rulesregs/sdwa/airlinewater. Accessed 7/20/11.

## Quick Bite

**Water, Water Everywhere and Not a Drop to Drink!**
When shipwrecked sailors drink seawater, they quickly become severely dehydrated. This is because the concentration of salt in seawater is about double the maximum concentration of salt in urine. Thus, it takes 2 liters of urine to rid the body of the solutes ingested by drinking 1 liter of seawater.

fluids and hospitalization may be necessary. In remote areas or developing countries, "rehydration packets"—a mix of potassium and sodium salts and sugar—dissolved in boiled water have saved countless lives. (See the FYI feature "Tap, Filtered, or Bottled: Which Water Is Best?")

## Water Intoxication

Because drinking fluids temporarily alleviates thirst, we rarely drink to the point of overhydration and dilution of body fluids. However, replacement of fluid losses following intensive or prolonged exercise with plain water (and no electrolytes) can result in overhydration and hyponatremia (low blood sodium) in athletes,[8] causing changes in mental status, difficulty breathing, seizures, coma, and death.[9] A fraternity hazing ritual, for example, caused fatal water intoxication in a California State University student who was forced to drink large quantities of water while exercising vigorously.[10]

Overhydration can occur in people with untreated glandular disorders that cause excessive water retention. Some mentally ill people have a compulsion to drink more water than their kidneys can handle (over 15 to 20 liters daily). Overhydration first causes headaches and then seizures. Several years ago,

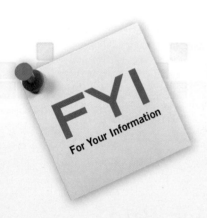

## Tap, Filtered, or Bottled: Which Water Is Best?

Everywhere you look, it seems as if more and more people are carrying and sipping from bottles of water. Theme parks even sell shoulder holsters to carry your bottle around with you. What's with the water craze? And what's wrong with the good old water fountain?

The popularity of bottled water exploded in the 1980s. Initially, bottled mineral waters, like Perrier, were associated with wealth and glamour. But like many trends adopted by the wealthy (white bread, for instance), bottled water soon became desirable to a wider range of people. It is estimated that Americans drink 8.5 billion gallons of bottled water each year![1] In 2009, U.S. per capita consumption of bottled water was 27.6 gallons.[2] Americans drink more

bottled water than any other beverage, except for carbonated soft drinks. Soft drink consumption, at 14 billion gallons per year, is just less than double that of bottled water consumption.[3] Both the major soft drink companies—Coca-Cola and PepsiCo—sell their own brands of bottled water.

Several factors have fueled the growth of the bottled water industry. Baby boomers are seeking natural, low-calorie beverages, and fitness consciousness has reemphasized the importance of hydration. Media reports of contaminated tap water in major metropolitan areas spark concerns about the safety and quality of tap water. Most Americans choose bottled water for what they think is not in it, rather than for what it contains.

From a nutritional perspective, it's important to drink plenty of fluids. Water is one of the best ways to replace lost fluids, and at the simplest level the source of the water doesn't really matter. Standards for municipal water systems are enforced by the Environmental Protection Agency (EPA), which requires regular testing and monitor-

ing. Tap water can be considered a safe, clean source of water. Many municipal water systems add fluoride to tap water, an important weapon in the prevention of tooth decay. However, home-installed filtration systems for removing chlorine also may remove added fluoride, and most bottled waters do not contain fluoride.

Some people don't like the taste of their local water supply and don't want to bother with maintaining a filtration system. In this case, or if you want your water "to go," bottled water may be the choice. The bottled water industry offers:

- High-volume, returnable containers from suppliers who stock the water coolers for offices or supermarkets
- The familiar brands (e.g., Evian, Zephyrhills, Dannon, Nala) that are sold as alternatives to soft drinks
- Bottled water in vending machines

The bottled water industry is regulated by the Food and Drug Administration (FDA), which in 1995 published Standards of Identity for bottled

water, set maximum allowable standards for contaminants, and established Current Good Manufacturing Practices (CGMP) for bottling plants. Keep in mind that the FDA regulates bottled waters that are sold interstate and not those sold only in a particular area or state. Individual states may have their own quality standards for locally distributed waters.

Look beyond the terms such as *artesian*, *mineral*, *spring*, or *purified* (see Table A). The labels on most bottled water list the source of the water. Some consumers may be surprised to find that their favorite brand of water is really from a municipal source, not an underground spring! Nutrition Facts labels are required if the manufacturer makes a claim (e.g., "sodium free") or adds minerals. These labels often do not show the natural mineral content of the water, which is really the only other nutritional aspect that could be expected.

The Academy of Nutrition and Dietetics suggests that consumers consider the following some dieters overenthusiastically followed a fad weight reduction diet calling for massive water intake and suffered seizures from overhydration.

**Key Concepts** *Diuretic medications increase urinary fluid losses. Alcohol and caffeine have mild diuretic effects. Dehydration is a potential consequence of gastrointestinal disease, burns, and heavy sweating. Treatment involves replacing fluids, along with electrolytes if the condition is severe. Although unlikely, water intoxication is possible.*

## Minerals

What distinguishes minerals from vitamins, carbohydrates, proteins, and fats? Minerals are elemental atoms or ions rather than organic compounds. Unlike vitamins, minerals are not destroyed by heat, light, acidity, or alkalinity. Calcium, for example, remains calcium, whether in seashells, milk, or bones. Iron remains iron, whether it is part of a cast-iron skillet or part of hemoglobin.

Like vitamins, however, minerals are "micronutrients." Compared with carbohydrates, proteins, and fats, they are needed in relatively small amounts—at most a few grams per day.

Minerals often are grouped as **major minerals** and **trace minerals**. The classification is arbitrarily based on the amount you need in your diet and

**major minerals** Major minerals are required in the diet and are present in the body in large amounts compared with trace minerals.

**trace minerals** Trace minerals are present in the body and required in the diet in relatively small amounts compared with major minerals. Also known as *microminerals*.

five factors when choosing between bottled and tap water: the environment, safety, cost, taste, and fluoride.[4] The bottom line, according to the Academy of Nutrition and Dietetics, is that both tap and bottled water are safe and that bottled water offers no nutritional advantages unless it is fortified. Bottled water may encourage fluid consumption by making water more accessible; however, this may come at an environmental cost by contributing to waste.[5] Drinking sufficient water is the primary objective, especially when it replaces high-calorie, low-nutrient beverages.

Once again, the choice is up to the consumer—and for water, no choice is clearly best.

1 Rodwan JR Jr. Bottled water 2009, challenging circumstances persist: future growth anticipated. US and international developments and statistics. International Bottled Water Association. http://www.bottledwater.org/files/2009BWstats.pdf. Accessed 7/20/11.

2 Ibid.

3 Ibid.

4 Academy of Nutrition and Dietetics. Bottled water: is bottled water a better choice than tap water? Updated 5/08. http://www.eatright.org/About/Content.aspx?id=7516. Accessed 7/20/11.

5 Ibid.

**Table A**  **Definitions of Bottled Water Terms**

*Mineral water* must contain at least 250 parts per million (ppm) of dissolved minerals and come from a geologically and physically protected underground water source.

*Purified water* is tap or ground water that has been treated by distillation, deionization, or reverse osmosis. This may be labeled "distilled water" if produced by steam distillation and condensation.

*Spring water* comes from an underground formation from which water flows naturally to the surface; it is collected either at the spring or from a bore hole to the underground formation.

*Artesian water* comes from tapping a confined underground aquifer that is below the natural water table. Generally the artesian well is located in a depression where the water table of the surrounding hills is higher. The "head" of pressure from the water table forces the water up through the tap line.

*Ground water* comes from a subsurface saturated zone and is not under the direct influence of surface water.

*Well water* comes from a drilled hole that taps the water of an aquifer and is pumped to the surface.

**Source:** Data from International Bottled Water Association. Labeling. http://www.bottledwater.org/content/labeling-0. Accessed 7/20/11.

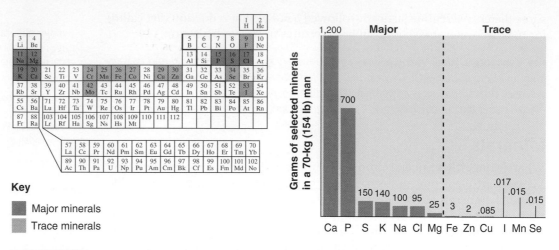

**Figure 10.8** **Minerals in the human body.** Dietary minerals also are elements in the periodic table. Based on the amount of a mineral needed in the diet and the amount in the body, nutritionists categorize a mineral as major or trace.

**Source:** Adapted from Gropper SS, Smith JL, Groff JL. *Advanced Nutrition and Human Metabolism.* 5th ed. Belmont, CA: Wadsworth/Cengage Learning; 2009; and Stipanuk MH. *Biochemical and Physiological Aspects of Human Nutrition.* 2nd ed. Philadelphia: WB Saunders; 2006.

the amount present in your body. You need more than 100 milligrams per day of each major mineral and less than 100 milligrams daily of each trace mineral. (See **Figure 10.8.**)

Compared with the major minerals, the total amount of each trace mineral present in your body is small. For example, your total body iron, a trace mineral, is 2 to 4 grams, or about the amount of iron in a small nail. Contrast that with your total body calcium, a major mineral. Most adult bodies contain over 1,000 grams.[11] Despite the amounts found in the body or required from diet, both major and trace minerals are important. Often a single mineral has several quite diverse functions. Some minerals, such as iodine, are components of hormones. Many are components of enzymes or enzyme cofactors. Others serve a structural function; for example, calcium and phosphorus are among the minerals that make bones hard.

## Minerals in Foods

Foods from both plants and animals are sources of minerals. Generally speaking, animal tissue contains minerals in the proportion that the animal needs, so animal-derived foods are more reliable mineral sources.

Plant foods can be excellent sources of several minerals, but the mineral content of plants can vary dramatically depending on the minerals in the soil where the plants are found. (See **Figure 10.9.**) Even the maturity of a vegetable, fruit, or grain can influence its mineral content. Because actual mineral content varies so much, the values published in food composition tables can be misleading. Often these values are omitted. Like plant foods, drinking water has variable mineral content, but it sometimes can be a significant source of minerals, such as sodium, magnesium, and fluoride.

## Bioavailability

Our GI tracts absorb a much smaller proportion of minerals than vitamins—and probably for good reason. Once absorbed, excess minerals often are difficult for the body to flush out. In many cases, the body adjusts mineral absorption to our needs. For example, a calcium-deficient person absorbs calcium more readily than does a person with normal calcium levels.

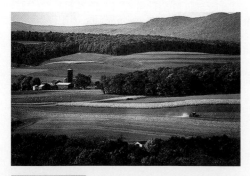

**Figure 10.9** **Growing conditions influence mineral content.** The mineral content of plants reflects the mineral content of the soil in which they are grown.

Megadosing with single-mineral supplements can hamper the absorption of other minerals. Minerals such as calcium, iron, zinc, and magnesium, for example, all have similar chemical properties and compete for absorption.

Fiber and other components of food also affect mineral bioavailability. (See **Figure 10.10**.) High-fiber diets reduce absorption of iron, calcium, zinc, and magnesium. **Phytate** (a component of whole grains) binds minerals and carries them out of the intestine unabsorbed. **Oxalate** (found in spinach and rhubarb) binds calcium, markedly reducing calcium absorption.

**Key Concepts** *Minerals are essential inorganic elements. They are found in a wide variety of foods, but their absorption is limited by several factors, among them our physiological need, presence of competing minerals, and presence of fiber.*

## Major Minerals and Health

The seven major minerals—sodium, potassium, chloride, calcium, phosphorus, magnesium, and sulfur—have significant roles, and when mineral status goes awry, your health can suffer. Two disorders in which major minerals play critical parts are hypertension and osteoporosis.

### Hypertension

Persistent high blood pressure (**hypertension**) often is called a "silent killer" because it usually presents no specific symptoms or early warning signs. Hypertension affects approximately one in three American adults and more than two-thirds of people older than 65.[12] Untreated hypertension may cause damage to vital organs, particularly the heart, the brain, the kidneys, and the eyes. It increases the risk of heart attack, congestive heart failure, stroke, and kidney failure. Even though the cause for most cases of hypertension is unknown, several factors clearly contribute to hypertension, including obesity, eating too much salt, lack of physical activity, and drinking too much alcohol. Heredity, race, and age are risk factors for hypertension that are beyond your control.

What role does diet play? Could changing our diets prevent or delay high blood pressure? And, for people who have hypertension, can changing their diet help control their blood pressure?

#### *Sodium and Hypertension*

Excessive sodium can hold excessive fluid in the body, at least temporarily. These excesses can burden the kidneys, heart, and blood vessels. The consensus among heart disease experts is that too much sodium, ingested routinely over the years, plays a role in the underlying causes of hypertension in genetically predisposed or "salt-sensitive" people. The more salt they eat, the higher their blood pressure.

THINK About It 2

Population studies appear to bear this out. Rates of hypertension are greater in countries with high sodium intakes. In contrast, primitive people, whose diets contain very little sodium, seldom have hypertension. Their blood pressure does not rise with age if they continue to eat their traditional diet. But if they adopt a "modern" (higher-sodium) diet, blood pressure tends to rise, and they are more likely to become hypertensive.[13]

The relation of dietary sodium to hypertension is one of the most heavily researched issues in nutrition. Unfortunately, study conclusions often differ. Among the most influential studies are the DASH (Dietary Approaches to Stop Hypertension) studies, two large, carefully controlled trials sponsored by the National Heart, Lung and Blood Institute (NHLBI). The DASH dietary recommendations have been endorsed by the NHLBI; the *Dietary Guidelines*

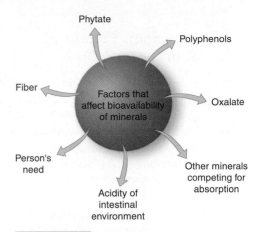

**Figure 10.10** **Factors that affect the bioavailability of minerals.** A person's need and the dietary components of a meal can enhance or inhibit the absorption of a mineral.

**phytate (phytic acid)** A phosphorus-containing compound in the outer husks of cereal grains that binds with minerals and inhibits their absorption.

**oxalate (oxalic acid)** An organic acid in some leafy green vegetables, such as spinach, that binds to calcium to form calcium oxalate, an insoluble compound the body cannot absorb.

**hypertension** Condition in which resting blood pressure persistently exceeds 140 mm Hg systolic or 90 mm Hg diastolic.

## *Quick* Bite

### Why Do Salty Foods Make You Thirsty?
The thirst mechanism is highly sensitive to extracellular sodium concentration. Even a tiny rise in sodium crosses the thirst threshold and triggers the desire to drink.

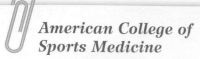

## American College of Sports Medicine

**Physical Activity and Bone Health**

Maintaining a vigorous level of physical activity across the lifespan should be viewed as an essential component of the prescription for achieving and maintaining optimal bone health. The following exercise prescription is recommended to help preserve bone health during adulthood:

- Mode: weight-bearing endurance activities (tennis; stair climbing; jogging, at least intermittently during walking), activities that involve jumping (volleyball, basketball), and resistance exercise (weight lifting)
- Intensity: moderate to high, in terms of bone-loading forces
- Frequency: weight-bearing endurance activities three to five times per week; resistance exercise two to three times per week
- Duration: 30–60 minutes per day of a combination of weight-bearing endurance activities, activities that involve jumping, and resistance exercise that targets all major muscle groups

**Source:** Kohrt WM, Bloomfield SA, Little KD, et al. American College of Sports Medicine stand: physical activity and bone health. *Med Sci Sports Exerc.* 2004;36:1985–1996. Reprinted by permission of Lippincott Williams & Wilkins, http://lww.com.

*for Americans, 2010*; the American Heart Association; and the U.S. dietary guidelines for the treatment of high blood pressure. Recent results indicate that following the DASH diet can reduce the risk of having a heart attack in the next 10 years by 18 percent and that African Americans benefit most from the dietary changes.[14] The combination of exercise and weight loss with the DASH diet has been found to result in even larger reductions in blood pressure for overweight or obese persons with above-normal blood pressure.[15]

In addition to being a low-salt (or low-sodium) plan, the DASH diet is based on fruits and vegetables, low-fat or nonfat dairy, and whole grains, making the overall eating plan high in fiber, low to moderate in fat, and rich in potassium, calcium, and magnesium.[16]

### Other Dietary Factors

Sodium is not the only dietary factor associated with hypertension. The carefully controlled DASH study also showed that foods low in fat and rich in calcium, magnesium, and potassium reduce blood pressure as well. Eating 10 servings of fruit and vegetables and 2 to 3 servings of low-fat dairy products daily, while limiting fat and saturated fat, brought systolic blood pressure down by 5.9 mm Hg, even at the highest sodium intake of 3,450 milligrams.[17] The DASH studies show that limiting sodium, fat, and cholesterol, as well as increasing fruits, vegetables, and low-fat dairy foods, can lower blood pressure. The NHLBI recommends that all Americans follow the DASH combination diet. The *Dietary Guidelines for Americans, 2010* echo the recommendations of the DASH eating plan.[18] Controlling weight, getting regular exercise, and reducing alcohol consumption also help reduce blood pressure.

**Key Concepts** *Hypertension is a risk factor for atherosclerosis, kidney disease, and stroke. Excess sodium intake raises blood pressure in those who are salt-sensitive. Inadequate levels of potassium, calcium, and possibly magnesium may also contribute to hypertension. Limiting sodium intake, along with eating lots of low-sodium vegetables, fruits, and low-fat dairy products, may help reduce hypertension and its side effects.*

## Osteoporosis

*Osteoporosis* means "porous bone." It's a good description. In osteoporosis, bone mass or density declines, and bone quality deteriorates, leaving the bones fragile and vulnerable to fracture. (See **Figure 10.11**.) Often called a "silent disease," osteoporosis develops over several years without outward symptoms or diagnosis. Eventually bone loss makes bones so weak they break with a mild strain, bump, or gentle fall. In fact, the break may occur first and cause the fall! Osteoporosis is the major cause of bone fracture in older adults, primarily postmenopausal women.

The U.S. Surgeon General estimates that by 2020, one in two Americans aged 50 years or older will be at risk for fractures from osteoporosis or low bone mass.[19] Although 80 percent of those with osteoporosis are women, by age 75 one-third of all men have osteoporosis. Table 10.1 lists the risk factors for osteoporosis.

### Calcium and Osteoporosis

Adequate calcium intake throughout life helps prevent osteoporosis. Good calcium intake during childhood and adolescence helps maximize peak bone mass at around age 30. Even in adulthood, adequate calcium slows bone loss, and it reduces fracture rates in postmenopausal women who are at increased risk of accelerating bone loss because of decreasing estrogen levels.

Calcium is clearly an important nutrient in bone health, but it's not the only one. Normal mineralization and maintenance of bone also require

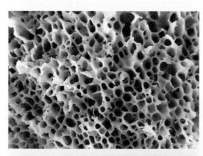

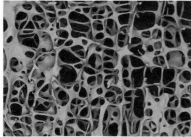

**Figure 10.11**    **Osteoporosis.** Normal bone (top) and osteoporotic bone (bottom). The osteoporotic bone is noticeably less dense.

vitamins D, A, and K; protein; and the minerals phosphorus, fluoride, and magnesium.

### Other Dietary and Lifestyle Factors

You need vitamin D for absorbing calcium and maintaining bone health. Vitamin D–fortified foods such as milk and vitamin D supplements help meet recommendations, especially for those with limited sunlight exposure. Phytate and oxalate, caffeine, and smoking can reduce calcium absorption or increase excretion rates. Regular weight-bearing exercise helps maximize bone mass when you're young and will slow bone loss during your later years. Suggestions to promote bone health and slow the development of osteoporosis are listed in Table 10.2.

In summary, the steps outlined in Table 10.2 can help reduce the risk of osteoporosis: Maintain adequate calcium and vitamin D intake throughout life; eat a healthful diet rich in other bone-building nutrients; perform weight-bearing exercise; and, in the case of postmenopausal women, consider estrogen supplements.

**Key Concepts** *Osteoporosis is the progressive loss of bone mass, resulting in fragile bones that break easily. Osteoporosis primarily affects postmenopausal women who have lower estrogen levels and accelerated rates of bone loss. Adequate calcium intake early in life helps maximize peak bone mass and reduces the risk of osteoporosis. Adequate amounts of vitamin D and regular exercise also are important for bone health.*

## Sodium

You probably know sodium best as a component of table salt. Table salt, or sodium chloride, is 40 percent sodium. And you've probably heard that we eat too much sodium. The *Dietary Guidelines* tell us to "Reduce daily sodium intake to less than 2,300 milligrams (mg), further reduce intake to 1,500 mg among persons who are 51 and older and those of any age who are African American or have hypertension, diabetes, or chronic kidney disease. The 1,500 mg recommendation applies to about half of the U.S. population, including children, and the majority of adults."[20]

Excess sodium in the human diet is a relatively recent problem. For centuries in many regions, salt was highly prized and hard to come by. Our language reflects that: "He's worth his salt" means he's a valuable person; the word *salary* is derived from the Latin word for salt. Sodium is, in fact, an essential nutrient of great importance.

Sodium is critical for regulating both cellular fluid and total body fluid. Although most sodium is in extracellular fluid, it acts in concert with other electrolytes both within and outside of cells to regulate fluid levels, blood pressure, and pH (acidity and alkalinity). The movement of sodium back and forth across cell membranes helps regulate the transit of other substances that tag along or travel in the opposite direction. Sodium, as well as other electrolytes, helps transmit nerve impulses and other electrical messages.

### Dietary Recommendations and Sources of Sodium

We rarely eat too little sodium; in fact, most of us eat substantially more than we need. Actual sodium requirements by the body are relatively small—only a few hundred milligrams daily. To make sure that the diet contains adequate amounts of all nutrients, however, the Food and Nutrition Board set the AI for sodium for adults at 1,500 milligrams per day (the amount in about ⅔ teaspoon of table salt).[21] This suggested AI level is similar to the American Heart Association's recommendation to limit sodium to less than 1,500 mil-

**Table 10.1    Risk Factors for Osteoporosis**

Advanced age
Female
Thin and/or small frame
Family history of osteoporosis
Early menopause, whether natural or surgically induced
Low testosterone levels in men
Abnormal absence of menstrual periods (amenorrhea)
Anorexia nervosa or bulimia nervosa
Medical conditions such as thyroid disease, rheumatoid arthritis, and problems that block intestinal absorption of calcium
Use of certain medications such as corticosteroids and anticonvulsants
Insufficient dietary calcium
Lack of weight-bearing exercise
Cigarette smoking
Excessive use of alcohol or caffeine

**Table 10.2    Promoting Bone Health**

To promote bone health and slow the development of osteoporosis, experts suggest the following:

- Eat foods rich in calcium and vitamin D.
- Eat foods that are high in calcium.
- Be physically active every day.
- Maintain a healthy body weight throughout your life.
- Protect yourself from falls.
- Avoid smoking and limit alcohol intake.
- Discuss increased risks with your doctor.

**Source:** Data from US Department of Health and Human Services. *Bone Health and Osteoporosis: A Report of the Surgeon General.* Rockville, MD: US Department of Health and Human Services, Office of the Surgeon General; 2004.

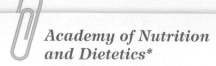

## Academy of Nutrition and Dietetics*

**Nutrition and Women's Health**
It is the position of the American Dietetic Association and Dietitians of Canada that women have specific nutritional needs and vulnerabilities and, as such, are at unique risk for various nutrition-related diseases and conditions. Therefore, the Academy of Nutrition and Dietetics and Dietitians of Canada strongly support research, health promotion activities, health services, and advocacy efforts that will enable women to adopt desirable nutrition practices for optimal health.

**Source:** Reproduced from Position of the Academy of Nutrition and Dietetics and Dietitians of Canada: nutrition and women's health. *J Am Diet Assoc.* 2004;104(6):984–1001.

* Formerly the American Dietetic Association

## *Quick* Bite

**Sacred Salt**
The physiological need for salt played an important role in shaping human history. Population groups tended to congregate where salt could be found, and civilizations in Africa, India, the Middle East, and China developed around rich salt deposits. At times, salt was traded at a value twice that of gold.

### Table 10.3  Sodium Content of Various Foods

| Food | Serving Size | Sodium (mg) |
|---|---|---|
| Cucumber, fresh | 1 large (8¼-inch) | 6 |
| Dill pickle | 1 large (4-inch) | 569 |
| Roast pork | 3 oz (85 g) | 54 |
| Ham, cured | 2 slices | 739[a] |
| Whole wheat bread | 1 slice | 132 |
| Biscuit from mix | 2½-inch biscuit | 292 |
| Fresh tomato | 1 medium | 6 |
| Tomato sauce, canned | 1 cup | 1,284 |
| Two-percent milk | 1 cup (240 mL) | 115 |
| American cheese | 1 slice (1 oz) | 356 |
| Baked potato | 1 medium | 20 |
| Potato chips | 1 oz | 149 |

[a] As food becomes more processed, the sodium content increases.

**Source:** US Department of Agriculture, Agricultural Research Service. USDA National Nutrient Database for Standard Reference, Release 23. 2010. http://www.ars.usda.gov/ba/bhnrc/ndl. Accessed 7/20/11.

ligrams per day.[22] Further, the Tolerable Upper Intake Level (UL) for sodium is 2,300 milligrams per day (the amount in about 1 teaspoon of table salt) and the level at which all Americans, regardless of risk factors, should try to stay below. The typical American diet contains 3,000 to 6,000 milligrams of sodium daily. Surprisingly, processed foods—not table salt—contribute the most sodium. (See Table 10.3.)

**Figure 10.12** shows a breakdown of the sources of sodium in our diets. Soy sauce and other sauces; pickled foods; salty or smoked meats, cheese, and fish; salted snack foods; bouillon cubes; and canned and instant soups are all high-sodium foods. Seasonings based on salt, such as "lemon salt" and "seasoning salt," and those containing the flavor enhancer monosodium glutamate (MSG) also are high in sodium. If your diet is based on Asian foods that contain liberal amounts of soy sauce and MSG, you could be taking in 12,000 to 16,000 milligrams of sodium per day.

## Dealing with Excess Sodium

Although some illnesses can drive down blood sodium to dangerously low levels, our bodies usually must deal with an excess of sodium. In some people, eating too much sodium over a long period of time can contribute to hypertension. (See the "Hypertension" section in this chapter.) Your intestinal tract absorbs nearly all dietary sodium, which travels throughout the body in the bloodstream. Your kidneys, those remarkable organs, retain the exact amount of sodium the body needs and excrete the excess sodium in the urine along with water.

Taking in too much sodium and not enough water can worsen dehydration. The old practice of giving athletes salt tablets before or after exercise is unnecessary and possibly harmful. However, radical sodium restriction is not a good idea, either. Even though most Americans consume too much sodium, severe sodium restriction can limit the availability of other essential nutrients such as vitamin $B_6$, calcium, iron, and magnesium.

**Key Concepts** *Sodium in the extracellular fluid plays a critical role in regulating water distribution and blood pressure. The American diet contains an overabundance of sodium—3,000 to 6,000 milligrams daily. The AI for sodium is 1,500 milligrams per day (the amount in about ⅔ teaspoon table salt), and the UL is 2,300 milligrams (the amount*

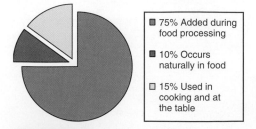

- ■ 75% Added during food processing
- ■ 10% Occurs naturally in food
- □ 15% Used in cooking and at the table

**Figure 10.12** Sources of dietary sodium.

*in about 1 teaspoon table salt). Processed foods supply most of the sodium in our diets. Extreme sodium restriction is unwise and may reduce the availability of some vitamins and minerals.*

## Potassium

Nearly all the body's potassium resides within cells, with the highest amount in muscle cells. The flow of potassium in and out of cells is coupled to the flow of sodium. Together, they help contract muscles, transmit nerve impulses, and regulate blood pressure and heartbeat. The central nervous system zealously protects its potassium, maintaining constant levels even when muscle and blood levels drop.

Like sodium, potassium affects blood pressure, but in a different way. When people with hypertension eat a diet low in sodium and rich in high-potassium foods (such as fruits and vegetables), their blood pressure often improves.[23]

## Dietary Recommendations and Sources of Potassium

Based on studies showing that potassium blunts the blood-pressure-raising effects of salt, the DRI committee suggested a target intake level (AI) of 4,700 milligrams of potassium per day for adults.[24] This amount is higher than the current Daily Value of 3,500 milligrams and substantially more than most Americans eat (2,000 to 3,000 milligrams per day).

Vegetables and fruits, especially potatoes, spinach, melons, and bananas, are important dietary potassium sources. Meat, fish, poultry, and dairy products are also good sources. (See **Figure 10.13**.) Many, but not all, salt substitutes contain potassium chloride. Generous intakes of fruits and vegetables, as recommended by the MyPlate food guidance system, will help increase potassium intake. African Americans may especially benefit from increased potassium intake—this population group typically has low intake of potassium and a high prevalence of hypertension and salt sensitivity.[25] Although food manufacturers often add sodium to processed foods, they do not routinely add potassium. So if a person's diet includes a lot of processed foods, it may fail to meet the potassium recommendations.

## When Potassium Balance Goes Awry

Moderate potassium deficiency is a likely factor in hypertension risk, especially when coupled with high sodium intakes. Results from a recent study suggest that U.S. adults who were eating more sodium and less potassium had a 50 percent higher risk of dying from any cause and more than twice the likelihood of dying from a heart attack over 15 years than adults who ate less sodium and more potassium.[26] These findings further emphasize current dietary recommendations to reduce sodium intake and eat more fruits and vegetables.

Low potassium intake can also disrupt acid–base balance in the body and contribute to bone loss and kidney stones.[27] Severe potassium deficiency usually results from excessive losses. Prolonged vomiting, chronic diarrhea, laxative abuse, and use of diuretics are the most common causes of low blood potassium.

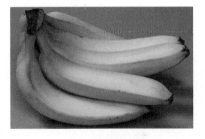
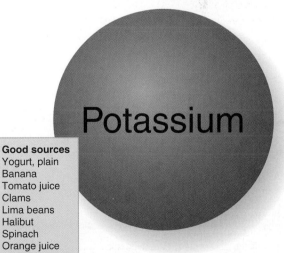

**Good sources**
Yogurt, plain
Banana
Tomato juice
Clams
Lima beans
Halibut
Spinach
Orange juice
Cantaloupe
Potato
Apricot
Baked beans
Milk
Acorn squash

**Figure 10.13** **Food sources of potassium.** The best food sources of potassium are fresh fruits and vegetables, certain dairy products, and fish.

## Quick Bite

**Versatile Potassium**
During the Middle Ages, saltpeter (potassium nitrate) was discovered to be a useful substance. It was used as a means of extracting other minerals from rock, as a fertilizer, and as an ingredient in gunpowder. It wasn't used to cure meat until the sixteenth or seventeenth century. Saltpeter was a major ingredient in the curing mixture until 1940, about the time that refrigeration emerged. Today, food manufacturers use small amounts of nitrites rather than saltpeter to preserve foods such as bacon, ham, and some sausages.

## Quick Bite

**Low-Calorie Chlorine?**
Sucralose is a low-calorie sweetener made from sugar. During manufacture, a multistep process substitutes three chlorine atoms for three hydrogen–oxygen groups on the sugar molecule. This creates an exceptionally stable molecular structure that is 600 times sweeter than sugar. The sucralose molecule is chemically and biologically inert, so it passes through the body without being digested and is eliminated after consumption.

Physicians monitor electrolyte blood levels of patients taking diuretics and recommend potassium supplements if needed. Symptoms of low blood potassium include muscle weakness, loss of appetite, and confusion. If potassium depletion is severe or rapid, heart rhythms may be disrupted—a potentially fatal problem.

Because the kidneys effectively remove excess potassium, in healthy people the risk of toxicity from dietary intake is low. Potassium supplements, available over the counter and sold in health food stores, should be taken only when recommended by a physician. Extremely high blood potassium levels can slow and eventually stop the heart.

**Key Concepts** *Potassium is found mainly in intracellular fluid. Along with sodium, it regulates muscle contractions and nerve impulse transmissions. For healthy adults, the AI for potassium is 4,700 milligrams per day, substantially more than most Americans consume. Vegetables and fruits are good potassium sources and are low in sodium. Extremely high or low blood potassium can cause heartbeat irregularities and death.*

## Chloride

Chloride is a component of table salt and other salts. (Do not confuse chloride with chlorine. Chlorine is a highly reactive gas used in water treatment plants to kill germs.)

Both sodium and chloride help maintain the body's fluid balance. You have probably noticed the salty taste that sodium chloride (NaCl) imparts to blood, sweat, and tears. Although chloride readily moves in and out of cells, it resides mainly in extracellular fluid. Chloride is crucial to transmitting nerve impulses and to maintaining acid–base balance. It also is a component of hydrochloric acid produced by the stomach. Hydrochloric acid is required for digestion; it also kills disease-causing bacteria ingested in food. White blood cells also use chloride ions to kill invading bacteria.[28]

### Dietary Recommendations and Sources of Chloride

Most of us consume much more chloride than the 2,300 milligrams per day that is the adult AI. The Daily Value for chloride is 3,400 milligrams, just under the adult UL for chloride, which is 3,600 milligrams per day. Most of our chloride intake comes from salt (for dietary sources, see the "Sodium" section earlier in this chapter). You usually can estimate the chloride content of processed foods from the sodium content with this simple formula:

$$\text{chloride content} = 1.5 \times \text{sodium content}$$

The average intake of chloride from salt alone is 4,500 milligrams per day (7.5 grams of salt), which is much more than recommended. Reducing the use of salt, as recommended in the *Dietary Guidelines for Americans, 2010* will reduce chloride intake. The kidneys excrete excess chloride, and some chloride also is lost in sweat. Severe dehydration is the only known cause of high blood chloride levels.

### Who Risks Chloride Deficiency?

Excessive chloride loss is the most common cause of chloride deficiency. Vomiting expels stomach acid (hydrochloric acid), which contains a lot of chloride. People with bulimia nervosa often use self-induced vomiting as a way to compensate for binge eating and thus may have low chloride levels. Low blood chloride slows blood flow to the brain and oxygen delivery to tissues. It also disrupts the body's acid–base balance and causes heartbeat irregularities. Untreated low blood chloride levels can be life threatening.

**Key Concepts** *In addition to its role as an electrolyte, chloride is a component of hydrochloric acid. The minimum chloride requirement for healthy adults is 750 milligrams per day, far below average intakes. People who frequently induce vomiting risk chloride deficiency.*

# Calcium

Although only 1.5 to 2 percent of our body weight, calcium is the most abundant mineral in our bodies. It's important to have adequate calcium throughout life so that bones and teeth can remain strong into old age. Getting enough calcium in your diet also may help prevent hypertension, decrease your odds of getting colon or breast cancer, improve weight control, and reduce the risk of developing kidney stones.

## Functions of Calcium

Over 99 percent of your body's calcium is found in bones and teeth, making them hard and strong. Although less than 1 percent of body calcium is in blood and soft tissue, that tiny amount has vitally important roles in muscle contraction, nerve impulse transmission, blood clotting, and cell metabolism. (See **Figure 10.14.**)

### Bone Structure

Think of bone as living tissue that responds to physical stresses. Most of the time, bone is able to withstand tremendous force without breaking. In fact, healthy bone has about the same strength as reinforced concrete.[29] By weight, bone is two-thirds mineral and one-third water and protein, primarily collagen. Most bone calcium is part of **hydroxyapatite**—a hard, crystalline complex of calcium and phosphorus that surrounds collagen fibers.

Our bones undergo constant remodeling by two types of bone cells— **osteoblasts** and **osteoclasts**. Osteoblasts are the construction team, and osteoclasts are the demolition team. Together they determine how bones grow and change over time. Bone **mineralization** is greatest while children are growing taller and for 5 to 10 years thereafter. Although we usually achieve our peak bone mass at around age 30, bone responds to physical activities throughout our lives. In areas under repeated stress, bone thickens and becomes denser. Even older adults can strengthen and rebuild their bones through weight-bearing exercise such as walking or weight lifting.[30]

Bone also is a reservoir of calcium and phosphorus. When needed, blood and soft tissues can draw upon this reserve. Blood calcium levels must be kept constant at all costs, even at the expense of bone strength, so that calcium's roles in nerve function, blood clotting, muscle contraction, and cellular metabolism can proceed without a hitch.

### Calcium, Muscles, and Metabolism

Calcium has a central role in muscle contractions, as the flow of calcium ions inside muscle cells causes muscles to contract or relax. During exercise, one cause of muscle fatigue is the impaired activity of calcium in muscle cells.

**Calmodulin** is a calcium-sensing protein found throughout the body. When it binds calcium, calmodulin helps regulate a number of cellular processes, including cell division, cell proliferation, **ciliary action**, and cell secretions.

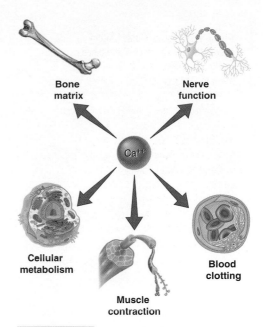

**Figure 10.14** **Functions of calcium.** In addition to its key role in bone health, calcium in blood and soft tissues is essential for such diverse functions as blood clotting, muscle contractions, and nerve impulse transmission.

**hydroxyapatite** A crystalline mineral compound of calcium and phosphorus that makes up bone.

**osteoblasts** Bone cells that synthesize and excrete the extracellular matrix that forms the structure of bone.

**osteoclasts** Bone cells that break down bone structure and release calcium and phosphate into the blood.

**mineralization** The addition of minerals, such as calcium and phosphate, to bones and teeth.

**calmodulin** A calcium-binding protein that regulates a variety of cellular activities, such as cell division and proliferation.

**ciliary action** Wavelike motion of small hairlike projections on some cells.

> **fibrin** A stringy, insoluble protein that is the final product of the blood-clotting process.

### *Other Functions of Calcium*

Blood cannot clot without calcium, but blood calcium levels seldom fall this low. Calcium participates in nearly every step in the production of **fibrin**, the protein that gives structure to blood clots. Nerve cells need calcium to transmit signals. In fact, the strength of a nerve signal is in direct proportion to the number of calcium ions crossing the nerve cell membrane.

## Regulation of Blood Calcium Levels

To prevent even minor dips in blood calcium levels, your body will demineralize bone. Even if calcium intake is very low, blood calcium levels remain steady. Three hormones—calcitriol (the active form of vitamin D), parathyroid hormone (PTH), and calcitonin—regulate calcium status.

When blood calcium levels are low, calcitriol increases intestinal absorption of calcium. PTH from the parathyroid glands activates osteoclasts that release bone calcium. PTH also signals the kidneys to conserve more calcium and to produce more calcitriol. When calcium levels become too high, the thyroid gland secretes calcitonin, which acts in opposition to PTH and causes blood calcium levels to return to normal.

## Dietary Recommendations for Calcium

During every life stage, optimal calcium intake is critical. If children and young adults fail to take in enough calcium, they are more likely to develop osteoporosis later in life. As we age, optimal calcium intake slows bone loss, helping preserve bone density.

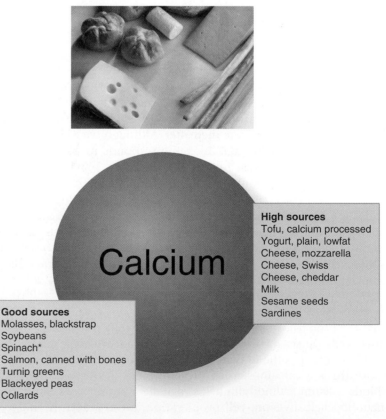

**High sources**
Tofu, calcium processed
Yogurt, plain, lowfat
Cheese, mozzarella
Cheese, Swiss
Cheese, cheddar
Milk
Sesame seeds
Sardines

**Good sources**
Molasses, blackstrap
Soybeans
Spinach*
Salmon, canned with bones
Turnip greens
Blackeyed peas
Collards

**Figure 10.15** **Food sources of calcium.** Calcium is found in milk and dairy products, certain green leafy vegetables, and canned fish with bones.

* In spinach, oxalate binds calcium and prevents absorption of all but about 5 percent of the plant's calcium.

Calcium recommendations are aimed at minimizing osteoporosis risk. The DRIs are 1,000 milligrams calcium per day for adults aged 19 to 50 years and men to age 70. For women 51 years and older and adults over the age of 70 years, this increases to 1,200 milligrams per day For children and teens aged 9 to 18 years, the DRI is 1,300 milligrams per day, a level meant to maximize peak bone mass.[31] Unfortunately, many of us fall far short of recommended calcium intakes. Most children and adolescents worldwide fail to meet calcium recommendations, making it difficult for them to achieve peak bone mass and leaving them vulnerable to osteoporosis as they age.[32] Excessive caffeine, alcohol, and sodium intake and misuse of diuretics—factors that increase urinary calcium—make bone loss worse.[33]

## Sources of Calcium

Dairy products are the best source of calcium in the American diet.[34] (See **Figure 10.15**.) Nonfat milk and yogurt are especially good, providing high calcium with minimal calories and little or no fat. Although ice cream and cheese are good sources, they are high in fat. Among dairy foods, cottage cheese and cream cheese contain the least calcium.

Other significant sources are green vegetables such as broccoli, Chinese cabbage, turnip greens and other "greens," and tofu processed with calcium. However, leafy vegetables in the spinach family are high in the mineral oxalate, which binds to calcium, thus preventing intestinal absorption. (See **Figure 10.16**.) If you eat the bones, canned fish with bones, such as sardines, provide lots of calcium.

Certain brands of soy milk, fruit juice, breakfast cereal, and bread are now fortified with calcium. These are convenient calcium sources for people who don't eat dairy foods. Check labels carefully because only a few products are fortified with calcium. Some dairies also add extra calcium or calcium-containing milk solids to their products.

People with limited dairy intake may need calcium supplements to ensure adequate intake. Flavored, chewable, calcium-containing antacids are an inexpensive and easy-to-take source of extra calcium. (See the FYI feature "Calcium Supplements: Are They Right for You?")

## Calcium Absorption

Calcium absorption is relatively inefficient, and we usually absorb only 25 to 35 percent of the calcium we eat.[35] Other dietary factors also affect absorption. Wheat bran, phytate (in whole grains, nuts, and seeds), and oxalate (in foods such as spinach) reduce calcium absorption. High supplement doses of phosphorus and magnesium may also interfere with calcium absorption. Because calcium depends on vitamin D to enter intestinal cells, calcium absorption drops dramatically if vitamin D status is poor.

Calcium absorption is particularly efficient during pregnancy and infancy and is least efficient in old age. If both a healthy child and a healthy adult eat exactly the same meal, all other things being equal, the growing child will absorb a much greater proportion of the dietary calcium than the adult. Low estrogen levels in postmenopausal women can lower calcium absorption to about 20 percent. Older women may take estrogen supplements, as well as calcium supplements, to maintain calcium absorption.

## When Calcium Balance Goes Awry

Because the body uses bone calcium to maintain normal blood calcium levels, low blood calcium is relatively uncommon in the absence of illness or vitamin D deficiency. Chronically low calcium intake can overtax this reserve and lead

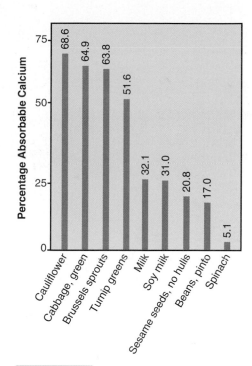

**Figure 10.16** **Bioavailability of calcium from different sources.** Your body can absorb more than two-thirds of the calcium in cauliflower, but only about 5 percent of the calcium in spinach. Oxalate in spinach binds calcium and inhibits its bioavailability.

**Source:** Adapted from Weaver CM, Plawecki KL. Dietary calcium: adequacy of a vegetarian diet. *Am J Clin Nutr.* 1994;59(suppl):1238S–1241S.

to suboptimal bone growth in childhood and adolescence or increased rate of bone loss after menopause. (See the "Osteoporosis" section in this chapter.) Studies also link low calcium intake to an increased risk of cardiovascular disease, hypertension, colon cancer, and obesity.[36]

Although certain illnesses can cause high blood calcium, dietary calcium intake does not. Of greater dietary concern is the interaction of calcium supplements with the absorption of iron, zinc, magnesium, and phosphorus. Although calcium supplements can dramatically affect absorption of other minerals, dietary calcium intake has not been shown to cause a deficiency for

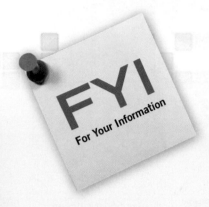

FYI
For Your Information

# Calcium Supplements: Are They Right for You?

After reading the section on calcium, you may be wondering whether you need a calcium supplement. After all, calcium is critical for so many bodily functions, and getting enough calcium reduces the risk of osteoporosis later in life.

Before you head to the supplement aisle at the grocery store, take a critical look at your diet, especially your intake of milk and other dairy products. In the United States and Canada, dairy foods are the major sources of dietary calcium; without them, it may be difficult to reach the AI for calcium. People who exclude dairy products, such as vegans and those with milk allergy, must choose foods carefully to find rich calcium sources.

Calcium sources vary widely in their bioavailability. Although labels are required to list the %DV for calcium, they don't indicate how much of that calcium the body will absorb. For example, ½ cup of spinach contains about 120 milligrams of calcium, but the body will absorb only 5 percent of that calcium! Intake recommendations are based on the mix of sources in the typical American diet. Other cultures manage on much lower intakes, in part because they do not consume the many food constituents that deplete calcium or reduce its absorption. Vegetarians may, in fact, need less calcium than meat eaters. If you are considering spinach as your sole source of calcium, however, check out Table A. It shows the amount of certain foods needed to equal the calcium available from 1 cup of milk (about 30 percent of the 300 milligrams of calcium in 1 cup of milk is bioavailable).

You can see from Table A that the amount of bioavailable calcium varies quite a bit among green leafy vegetables! If your diet is low in calcium, try adding some of the foods that are higher in calcium. Incorporating calcium-rich foods into the diet adds other important vitamins and minerals.

Even armed with more information about calcium in the diet, you may still decide to investigate the supplement market. Again, you have a variety of choices: calcium carbonate, calcium citrate, calcium lactate, calcium phosphate, coral calcium . . . how to decide? First, it's important to know that the absorption of calcium from most supplements is about equal—roughly 30 percent. The calcium citrate malate that is used in some

brands of fortified juice and a limited number of supplements is absorbed a little better—35 percent. However, a typical calcium citrate malate tablet has less calcium than a tablet of another type such as calcium carbonate. Calcium carbonate is usually the most concentrated per tablet, so taking fewer pills per day will supply enough; also, this type of supplement tends to be less expensive. Chelated calcium supplements can improve absorption a bit, but the extra expense probably is not worth it.

Other factors to consider are that, because minerals compete with each other for absorption, calcium supplements may be absorbed better if taken between meals. Also, you need to get plenty of vitamin D, either through casual exposure to the sun, in fortified milk, or as part of a supplement (many calcium supplements have added vitamin D). Vitamin D is important for the absorption of calcium. In addition, bones get stronger with regular, weight-bearing exercise, so make sure to include that in your healthful lifestyle.

### Table A — Foods That Provide the Calcium Equivalent of 1 Cup (8 fl oz) of Milk

| Food | Amount | Food | Amount |
|---|---|---|---|
| Almonds, dry roasted | 6 oz | Kohlrabi | 3½ cups |
| Beans, pinto | 6⅓ oz | Mustard greens | 1⅓ cups |
| Beans, red | 7 cups | Radish | 4½ cups |
| Beans, white | 2½ cups | Rutabaga | 2¼ cups |
| Broccoli | 2½ cups | Sesame seeds, no hulls | 12 oz |
| Brussels sprouts | 4 cups | Soy milk, unfortified | 30 cups |
| Cabbage, Chinese | 1 cup | Spinach | 7¾ cups |
| Cabbage, green | 3 cups | Tofu, calcium set | ½ cup |
| Calcium-fortified juices[a] | 5 fl oz | Turnip greens | 1 cup |
| Cauliflower | 4 cups | Watercress | 3½ cups |
| Kale | 1¾ cups | | |

[a] Fortified with calcium as calcium citrate malate.

**Source:** Adapted from Weaver CM, Plawecki KL. Dietary calcium: adequacy of a vegetarian diet. *Am J Clin Nutr.* 1994;59(suppl):1238S–1241S.

any of these minerals.[37] The Food and Nutrition Board has established a UL for calcium of 2,500 milligrams per day for adults aged 19 to 50 years.

**Key Concepts** *Calcium is a major component of bones and teeth. It is also required for muscle contraction, nerve impulse transmission, blood clotting, and regulation of cell metabolism. The body ensures adequate blood calcium levels by withdrawing it from bone if needed. Dairy foods and fortified foods are major dietary sources of calcium. Optimal calcium intake throughout life reduces chances of osteoporosis.*

## Phosphorus

Phosphorus, along with calcium, is a component of the mineral complex hydroxyapatite in bone. Bones are the major storehouse of phosphorus, holding nearly 85 percent of our supply. The remaining phosphorus is found in cells of soft tissues, with a little bit in extracellular fluid. Most of the body's phosphorus is in the form of phosphate ion (phosphorus joined to oxygen), our most abundant anion.

Phosphorus helps activate and deactivate enzymes during the final steps in the extraction of energy from carbohydrate, fat, and protein. It also is a component of ATP, the universal energy source, and of DNA and RNA. Phosphorus is also a component of phospholipids, found in cell membranes and lipoproteins.

### Dietary Recommendations and Sources of Phosphorus

The phosphorus RDA for adolescents is 1,250 milligrams per day to support growth. Although adults need only 700 milligrams per day, the average adult consumes much more, about 1,000 to 1,500 milligrams per day.

Phosphorus is abundant in our food supply. Foods rich in protein (milk, meat, and eggs) generally are rich in phosphorus. (See **Figure 10.17**.) Food additives, especially those in processed meat and soft drinks, supply up to 30 percent of our phosphorus. To improve moisture retention and smoothness, food processors often add phosphate salts to processed foods.

Because cow's milk contains more phosphorus than most foods, people with high dairy-product intakes have high-phosphorus diets. Soft drinks often contain phosphoric acid, although the phosphorus level is not high—about 50 milligrams in a 12-ounce cola, compared with 370 milligrams in 12 ounces of fat-free milk. However, among heavy cola drinkers, soda is an important contributor to phosphorus intake.[38] Dairy products have phosphorus plus calcium (460 milligrams in 12 ounces), whereas sodas have phosphorus but virtually no calcium (10 milligrams or less in a 12-ounce can)—an important distinction.

We absorb about 55 to 70 percent of the phosphorus we eat. Although phosphorus is part of phytate in plant seeds (beans, peas, cereals, and nuts), we can still absorb about 50 percent. Two familiar hormones, PTH (parathyroid hormone) and calcitriol (activated vitamin D), regulate intestinal absorption of phosphorus. When phosphorus levels are low, calcitriol enhances intestinal absorption of both calcium and phosphorus. When levels are high, PTH greatly increases urinary excretion of phosphorus.

### When Phosphate Balance Goes Awry

Phosphorus is so common in foods that only near total starvation causes deficiency. Some medical disorders, however, can cause low blood phosphate. Kidney disease is the most common cause of high blood phosphate. Other causes include overuse of vitamin D supplements, overuse of phosphate-containing laxatives, and diseases of the parathyroid gland. At the extreme, symptoms include muscle spasms and convulsions.

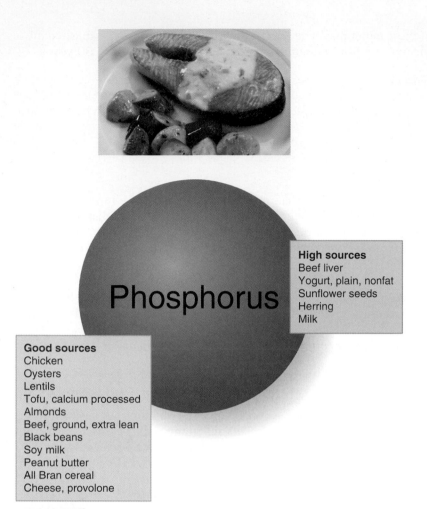

**High sources**
Beef liver
Yogurt, plain, nonfat
Sunflower seeds
Herring
Milk

**Good sources**
Chicken
Oysters
Lentils
Tofu, calcium processed
Almonds
Beef, ground, extra lean
Black beans
Soy milk
Peanut butter
All Bran cereal
Cheese, provolone

**Figure 10.17**  **Food sources of phosphorus.** Phosphorus is abundant in the food supply. Meats, legumes, nuts, dairy products, and grains tend to have more phosphorus than fruits and vegetables.

In the short run, high phosphorus intake is unlikely to produce problems in healthy people.[39] But over the long run, eating too much phosphorus, together with too little calcium, may increase bone loss. People who replace milk with cola increase their ratio of dietary phosphorus to calcium, possibly increasing their risk of osteoporosis later in life. The UL for phosphorus is 4,000 milligrams per day for people aged 9 to 70.

**Key Concepts** *Phosphorus is a component of bone, ATP, phospholipids, and genetic material. It acts as an electrolyte regulator as well. Milk, meat, and food additives are major sources of dietary phosphorus. Diets high in phosphorus and low in calcium can contribute to bone loss.*

## Magnesium

Magnesium is the fourth most abundant cation in our bodies. Bone holds about half the magnesium in our bodies, with the remainder distributed equally between muscle and other soft tissue. Like bone calcium, bone magnesium is a large reservoir that soft tissue can draw upon when needed. Most magnesium resides in cells, with only 1 percent in extracellular fluid.

Magnesium participates in more than 300 types of enzyme-driven reactions, including those in DNA and protein synthesis, blood clotting, muscle

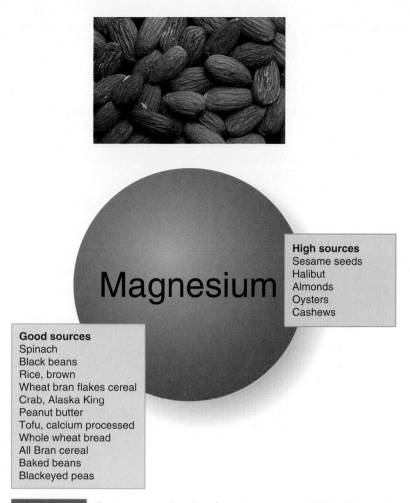

| Figure 10.18 | **Food sources of magnesium.** Most magnesium in the diet comes from plant foods such as grains, vegetables, and legumes. |

contraction, and ATP production. Because ATP is the universal energy source, an absence of magnesium would halt all cellular activity.

## Dietary Recommendations and Sources of Magnesium

The magnesium RDA is 400 milligrams per day for men aged 19 to 30 years, and 310 milligrams per day for women. The RDA rises for those 31 and older, to 420 milligrams for men and 320 milligrams for women. The average American gets only about three-fourths this level. Yet, overt symptoms of low magnesium are relatively uncommon in healthy people.[40]

Magnesium is found throughout the food supply. Our main sources are plant foods. Whole grains, many vegetables, legumes, tofu, and some seafood are good sources, and chocolate contains modest amounts. (See **Figure 10.18**.) In some communities, "hard" tap water has significant amounts of magnesium. Unfortunately, processing and refining removes much magnesium—up to 80 percent in refined grains—and enrichment does not replace it. In general, refined foods are low in magnesium.

We absorb about 50 percent of dietary magnesium. Although high-fiber diets often have a negative effect on mineral absorption, high-fiber foods containing fermentable carbohydrates (e.g., resistant starch, oligosaccharides, pectin) actually improve magnesium absorption. High calcium intake, usually

## Quick Bite

**Lost in Space**
Knowing that stress on bones maintains their strength, what would you guess happens in the gravity-free environment of outer space? Experience with prolonged space travel has made it clear that extensive bone and mineral loss are one health hazard of living without gravity's constant pull. Interestingly, changes in non-weight-bearing bones were not seen in studies of space travelers. As humans spend longer periods in space, scientists will be challenged to discover how to preserve bone strength without the constant stimulation of gravity on weight-bearing bones.

in the form of supplements, can interfere with magnesium absorption. People who must take calcium supplements should be sure to regularly eat foods with high magnesium content.

## When Magnesium Balance Goes Awry

Magnesium deficiency is often associated with alcoholism because alcohol increases urinary magnesium excretion. Poor magnesium intake typically goes hand in hand with poor intake of other nutrients, and magnesium deficiency by itself is unusual.[41] Poor magnesium status also may occur with certain chronic illnesses, such as diabetes mellitus, renal disease, or cardiovascular disease, and is worsened by diarrhea and vomiting.[42]

In research studies, healthy people on magnesium-deficient diets have no symptoms for several weeks. Once bone reserves are depleted, loss of appetite, nausea, and weakness gradually develop. Then muscle cramps, irritability, and confusion occur. Low magnesium disrupts heart rhythm; if the deficiency becomes extreme, heart abnormalities can lead to death. Magnesium toxicity causes diarrhea, nausea, weakness, paralysis, and cardiac and respiratory failure.[43] In the absence of kidney disease, an abnormally high blood level of magnesium is uncommon. The UL for supplemental magnesium is 350 milligrams per day.

**Key Concepts** *Magnesium participates in more than 300 reactions, including several in energy metabolism. It's required for cardiac and nerve function. Magnesium reserves are stored in bone. Whole grains and vegetables are good sources. People with chronic diarrhea, poor diet, and heavy alcohol use are at risk of deficiency. Because magnesium ions help regulate heartbeat, heart rhythm irregularities occur if blood levels are too low.*

## Sulfur

Unlike the other minerals discussed in this chapter, sulfur does not function alone. In the body, sulfur is primarily a component of organic (carbon-containing) nutrients, such as the vitamins biotin and thiamin, as well as the amino acids methionine and cysteine. The sulfur in amino acids helps stabilize the three-dimensional shapes of proteins such as those in skin, hair, and nails. The liver's detoxification pathways require sulfur, and sulfate (sulfur combined with oxygen) helps maintain acid–base balance. Typical diets contain ample sulfur, and deficiency is unknown in humans.

**Key Concepts** *Sulfur is a component of some amino acids and the vitamins biotin and thiamin. It helps proteins maintain their functional shapes. Sulfur is important in liver function and in maintaining acid–base balance. Human sulfur deficiency is unknown.*

## Quick Bite

**Do Onions Make You Cry?**
The cabbage and onion families have sulfur-based compounds that are transformed into odiferous compounds when their tissues are broken. Cutting into a raw onion mixes the contents of its cells, bringing enzymes into contact with an odorless precursor substance apparently derived from the sulfur-containing amino acid cysteine. The volatile result, a powerful sulfur-containing irritant, causes most people's eyes to water, apparently by dissolving in fluids that surround the eye and forming sulfuric acid.

## Trace Minerals

Despite the minute amounts in the body, trace minerals are crucial to many body functions. (See **Figure 10.19.**) Trace minerals serve as cofactors for enzymes, components of hormones, and participants in many chemical reactions. They are essential for growth and for normal functioning of the immune system. Deficiencies may cause delayed sexual maturation, poor growth, mediocre work performance, faulty immune function, tooth decay, and altered hormonal function.

Technological advances in recent years have triggered an explosion of exciting new research because scientists can now track trace minerals throughout the body more effectively. Working together, nutritionists, biochemists, biologists, immunologists, geneticists, and epidemiologists are uncovering the

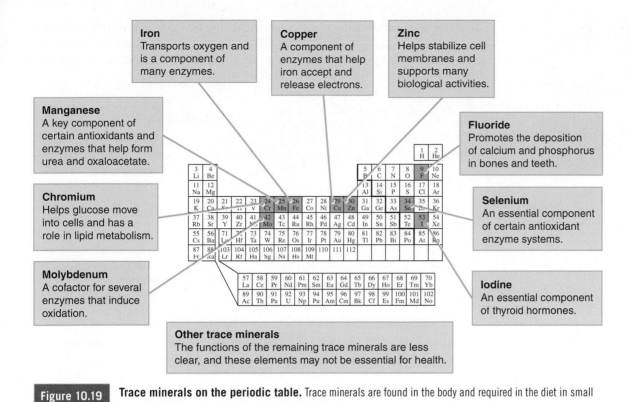

**Iron**
Transports oxygen and is a component of many enzymes.

**Copper**
A component of enzymes that help iron accept and release electrons.

**Zinc**
Helps stabilize cell membranes and supports many biological activities.

**Manganese**
A key component of certain antioxidants and enzymes that help form urea and oxaloacetate.

**Fluoride**
Promotes the deposition of calcium and phosphorus in bones and teeth.

**Chromium**
Helps glucose move into cells and has a role in lipid metabolism.

**Selenium**
An essential component of certain antioxidant enzyme systems.

**Molybdenum**
A cofactor for several enzymes that induce oxidation.

**Iodine**
An essential component of thyroid hormones.

**Other trace minerals**
The functions of the remaining trace minerals are less clear, and these elements may not be essential for health.

**Figure 10.19**  **Trace minerals on the periodic table.** Trace minerals are found in the body and required in the diet in small amounts, but they play important roles in the body.

mysteries behind many of these fascinating minerals and finding new links between trace minerals and a variety of diseases and genetic disorders.

# Iron

Iron is among the most abundant minerals in the earth's crust. Yet iron deficiency is the most common nutrient deficiency in the world. Not only does iron deficiency affect a large number of children and women in developing countries, it is the only nutrient deficiency that is significantly prevalent in industrialized countries.[44] Iron has a special property that allows it to easily transfer electrons to and from other atoms. This ability makes iron essential for numerous reactions and allows it to easily bind and release oxygen. Iron's abilities also endow it with a "dark side"—the ability to promote formation of destructive free radicals.

## Functions of Iron

Iron is well known for its role in transporting oxygen in the blood. Iron also is an essential component of hundreds of enzymes, many of which are involved in energy metabolism. In addition, iron plays a role in brain development and in the immune system. **Figure 10.20** shows the functions of iron.

### Oxygen Transport

Iron is vital to oxygen transport and sits at the center of **heme**—the iron-containing portion of hemoglobin and **myoglobin**. (See **Figure 10.21**.) Hemoglobin carries oxygen in the blood; myoglobin resides in muscle and moves oxygen into muscle cells.

As blood passes through the lungs, hemoglobin loads up on oxygen and turns bright red. It transports oxygen through arteries to tissues throughout

**heme**  A chemical complex with a central iron atom that forms the oxygen-binding part of hemoglobin and myoglobin.

**myoglobin**  The oxygen-transporting protein of muscle that resembles blood hemoglobin in function.

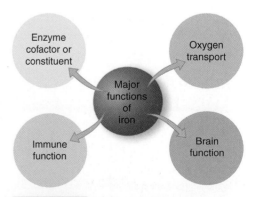

**Figure 10.20**  **Major functions of iron.** Well known for its role in transporting oxygen in the blood, iron also is essential for optimal immune function and nerve health. In addition, it is a cofactor in numerous reactions.

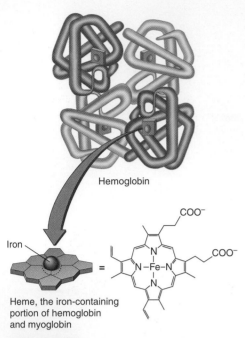

Hemoglobin

Iron

Heme, the iron-containing portion of hemoglobin and myoglobin

COO⁻

COO⁻

N—Fe—N

**Figure 10.21** **Heme in hemoglobin.** Iron in the heme portion of hemoglobin and myoglobin binds and releases oxygen easily. Hemoglobin in red blood cells transports oxygen in the blood and gives blood its red color.

the body. Upon reaching its destination, hemoglobin flows through tiny capillaries, crossing capillary walls and delivering its oxygen cargo to target cells. Depleted of oxygen, hemoglobin turns a dark bluish-red and travels through veins back to the lungs for another load of oxygen.

### Enzymes

Hundreds of enzymes contain iron or need iron as a cofactor. These enzymes drive reactions necessary for energy production, amino acid metabolism, and muscle function. Excess iron promotes the formation of highly reactive and destructive free radicals. Ironically, iron also is a cofactor of antioxidant enzymes that protect against free radical damage.

### Immune Function

Optimal immune function requires iron. However, in areas of the world with rampant disease and iron deficiency a dilemma arises. Iron nourishes certain bacteria, so iron supplementation can worsen an infection, particularly malaria.[45] In the absence of an infection, iron supplementation is appropriate for treating iron deficiency.

### Brain Function

Iron is essential for optimal brain and nervous system development and function. Children with iron-deficiency anemia often have learning and behavior problems.[46] How does a lack of iron affect the brain? We know that iron is involved in producing the protective covering, or myelin sheath, that surrounds nerve cells. Iron also is involved in producing neurotransmitters, chemicals that carry messages between nerve cells.

## Regulation of Iron in the Body

Total body iron averages about 4 grams in men and a little more than 2 grams in women.[47] Most of your body's iron is in hemoglobin, with the remainder in myoglobin and enzymes. If you're well nourished, you'll have good iron reserves stored as **ferritin** and **hemosiderin**.

But too much iron is toxic. So your body carefully performs a balancing act, adjusting iron absorption, transport, storage, and loss to optimize the amounts of actively functioning iron and iron reserves without exceeding safe levels.

### Iron Absorption

Intestinal cells act as gatekeepers, absorbing needed iron but turning away excess (and potentially harmful) iron. The actual amount absorbed depends on the body's iron status and need, normal GI function, the amount and type of iron in the diet, and dietary factors that enhance or inhibit iron absorption. Once intestinal cells admit iron, they can use it immediately, release it to the blood, or store it for later. During normal cell turnover, the GI tract sloughs intestinal cells. When excreted, these dead cells carry their stored iron out of the body.

**Effect of Iron Status on Iron Absorption** Iron status is the primary factor in determining how much iron a person will absorb from food.[48] Depending on need, iron absorption can vary from less than 1 percent to greater than 50 percent. On average, adult men absorb about 6 percent of dietary iron, and nonpregnant women of childbearing age absorb about 13 percent. Women absorb a higher proportion to make up for iron losses from menstruation.

Normally, absorption is more efficient when circulating iron and iron reserves are low. Absorption is highest among iron-deficient people, and it

**ferritin** A major storage form of iron.

**hemosiderin** An insoluble form of storage iron.

slows as iron reserves become filled. An increase in red blood cell production—during pregnancy, for example, or after blood loss—increases the body's need for iron and can trigger a severalfold increase in iron uptake.

**Effect of GI Function on Iron Absorption**  To prepare iron for intestinal absorption, you need adequate stomach acid. Because stomach acid generally declines with aging, iron absorption tends to be less efficient in seniors. Overuse of antacids also can affect iron bioavailability.

**Effect of the Amount and Form of Iron in Food**  All other factors being equal, the less iron in your diet, the greater the proportion you absorb. This ability to conserve dietary iron no doubt helped people survive when iron-rich foods were scarce. But it has its limits—if iron intake is routinely too low, anemia will emerge over time.

Food contains two types of iron: **heme iron** and **non-heme iron**. Heme iron is a part of hemoglobin and myoglobin, so it is found only in animal tissue. Meat, fish, and poultry contain about 40 percent heme iron and 60 percent non-heme iron. In contrast, plant foods and iron-fortified foods contain only non-heme iron. (See **Figure 10.22**.) Vegan diets, by definition, contain no heme iron.

Heme iron is much more bioavailable than non-heme iron.[49] Therefore, meats, poultry, fish, and seafood have the most efficiently absorbed iron. Vegetarians need more iron than do people who eat foods with heme iron.

**Dietary Factors That Enhance Iron Absorption**  You can improve the bioavailability of non-heme iron with vitamin C. (See Table 10.4.) Eating fruits and vegetables—good sources of vitamin C—along with iron-containing foods enhances non-heme iron absorption. Eating heme iron foods (called the meat factor) along with non-heme iron foods also improves non-heme iron absorption.

**Dietary Factors That Inhibit Iron Absorption**  Whole grains contain phytate, which inhibits iron absorption. However, whole-grain foods are healthy in other respects, so don't avoid them. Instead, include vitamin C–rich fruits and vegetables, which counter the inhibitory effects of phytate.

**Polyphenols**, found in tea, coffee, other beverages, and many plants, limit non-heme iron absorption. Foods from soybeans, foods containing oxalates, and high-fiber foods in general also tend to inhibit non-heme iron absorption.

Calcium, zinc, and iron compete for absorption, and each can inhibit absorption of another mineral.[50] Many women take calcium supplements to reduce their risk of osteoporosis. To minimize interference with iron absorption, they should take their calcium supplements alone at bedtime rather than with meals.

**heme iron**  The iron found in the hemoglobin and myoglobin of animal foods.

**non-heme iron**  The iron in plants and animal foods that is not part of hemoglobin or myoglobin.

**polyphenols**  Organic compounds that may produce bitterness in coffee and tea.

**MEAT**

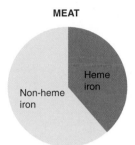

Beef, chicken, and fish contain about 40% heme and 60% non-heme iron. Eggs and dairy products contain no hemoglobin or myoglobin, so they contain only non-heme iron.

**LEGUMES AND VEGETABLES**

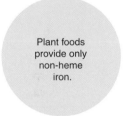

Beans, fortified cereals, soybeans, and green leafy vegetables are sources of non-heme iron.

**AVERAGE DAILY DIET**

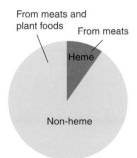

The average diet contains much more non-heme iron than heme iron.

| Figure 10.22 | **Sources of heme and non-heme iron.** Heme iron is found only in meats. Non-heme iron is found in both plant and animal foods. Eggs and dairy products contain small amounts of non-heme iron only. |

| Table 10.4 | **Factors That Affect Iron Absorption** |

| Inhibitors | Enhancers |
|---|---|
| Fiber and phytate | Vitamin C (ascorbic acid) |
| Calcium and phosphorus (milk/dairy) | Factor in meat, poultry, fish, and eggs |
| Tannins, found in tea | HCl secreted in the stomach |
| Polyphenols | Citric, malic, and lactic acid |
| Oxalate | |

> **transferrin** A protein synthesized in the liver that transports iron in the blood to the red blood cells for use in heme synthesis.

## Iron Transport and Storage

**Transferrin** is the carrier protein that ferries iron through the blood. It delivers iron from the intestines to the bone marrow for manufacture into hemoglobin, and it carries iron to all other body tissues as needed. (See **Figure 10.23**.)

The body stores surplus iron in two forms. Most iron is stored as ferritin, and smaller amounts are stored as hemosiderin. Although small amounts of ferritin circulate in blood, the liver, bone marrow, spleen, and skeletal muscle hold most iron reserves. Over time, a negative iron balance can deplete these reserves and iron deficiency ensues.

## Iron Turnover and Loss

The body is good at conserving iron, a trait probably acquired in ancient times when availability of high-iron foods was uncertain and irregular. The normal, routine destruction of old red blood cells releases iron, which the body recycles as it builds new red blood cells. A healthy adult man, for example, produces new red blood cells with about 95 percent recycled iron. Diet or iron stores must supply the remaining 5 percent. During periods of rapid growth and blood expansion, iron needs outstrip the supply of recycled and stored iron. Dietary iron makes up the difference. During infancy, for example, dietary iron supplies about 30 percent of iron for new red blood cells.

We lose small amounts of iron every day—a milligram or so in feces, sweat, and sloughed-off mucosal and skin cells. Women lose considerably more during menstruation. Pregnancy increases iron needs markedly to support growth of the fetus and expansion of the maternal blood supply. Blood loss with childbirth depletes iron; thus, women with repeated pregnancies close together are likely to have poor iron status and need extra iron.

Digestive disorders can increase blood and iron losses significantly. Any condition in which there is bleeding or accelerated destruction of intestinal cells—ulcer, cancer, inflammatory bowel disease, parasitic infection—can lead to iron-deficiency anemia.

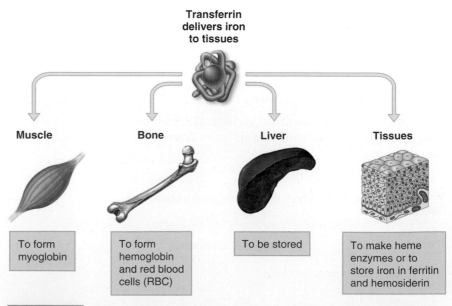

**Figure 10.23**　**Iron in the body.** Transferrin transports iron to tissues for the synthesis of heme or storage in ferritin and hemosiderin.

## Dietary Recommendations for Iron

The RDA for men and postmenopausal women is 8 milligrams per day. The RDA for women of childbearing age is 18 milligrams per day. Most men consume more than their RDA,[51] but many women fall well short of recommended amounts.

The iron needs of infants are a special concern. During the final weeks of pregnancy, babies ideally store enough iron in the liver, bone marrow, spleen, and hemoglobin-rich blood to see them through their first six months of life. However, if the mother's iron nutrition is poor or the baby is born early, the baby's iron stores are smaller and do not last. To help ensure that babies have adequate iron, pregnant women are urged to meet the RDA of 27 milligrams per day. Infant baby cereal and many infant formulas are fortified with iron.

## Sources of Iron

⦿ THINK About It 3

In terms of both amount and bioavailability, beef is an excellent dietary source of iron. Other excellent sources include clams, oysters, and liver. Poultry, fish, pork, lamb, tofu, and legumes are also good sources. (See **Figure 10.24**.) Whole-grain and enriched-grain products contain less bioavailable iron than does meat, but are significant sources of iron because they make up a major part of our diets. Fortified cereals also make an important contribution to iron intake in the United States and Canada. Dairy products are low in iron.

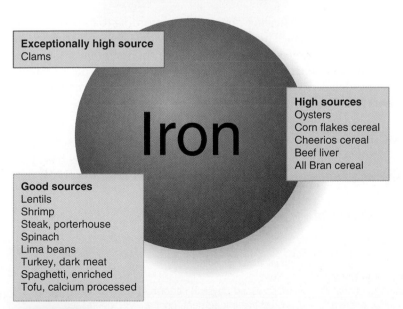

**Exceptionally high source**
Clams

# Iron

**High sources**
Oysters
Corn flakes cereal
Cheerios cereal
Beef liver
All Bran cereal

**Good sources**
Lentils
Shrimp
Steak, porterhouse
Spinach
Lima beans
Turkey, dark meat
Spaghetti, enriched
Tofu, calcium processed

**Figure 10.24**    **Food sources of iron.** Iron is found in red meats, certain seafoods, vegetables, and legumes and is added to enriched grains and breakfast cereals.

## Quick Bite

**Grandma's Cast-Iron Skillet Helped Her Avoid Iron Deficiency**

Iron deficiency is the most common form of malnutrition in the United States. However, this is a relatively recent phenomenon. Americans used to cook using cast-iron pots and pans. A study showed that using these utensils to cook acidic foods such as spaghetti sauce and apple butter increases the iron content of such foods by 30- to 100-fold. Our preference for stainless steel, aluminum, and enamelware eliminates this fortification.

A varied diet (adequate in calories, rich in fruits and vegetables, and with small amounts of lean animal flesh) generally provides adequate iron. Vegetarians who consume no animal tissue can maximize iron bioavailability from other sources by consuming vitamin C–rich fruits and vegetables with every meal.

## Iron Deficiency

Iron deficiency is the most common nutrient deficiency worldwide, especially in developing countries. Although less prevalent in the United States and Canada, it remains a public health concern. Infants and toddlers, adolescent girls, women of childbearing age, and pregnant women are particularly vulnerable.

Iron deficiency most commonly occurs in young children between 6 and 24 months old. Iron stores from fetal development have been depleted, and milk—a major source of energy in the young child's diet—is a poor source of iron. This is the age when cognitive and motor skills develop most rapidly, and inadequate iron during this critical time can cause irreversible developmental and intellectual deficits.

### Progression of Iron Deficiency

Iron deficiency progresses through three stages. (See Table 10.5.) During the first stage of iron deficiency, the body depletes iron stores, but there are no physiological impairments. During the second stage, the body depletes its supply of iron in circulating transferrin, and heme production starts to slip. Enzymes that need an iron cofactor cannot function properly, and energy metabolism starts to suffer; an iron-deficient person may not be able to work at full capacity. The third and most severe stage is iron-deficiency anemia. (See **Figure 10.25**.)

During iron-deficiency anemia, a lack of iron inhibits production of normal red blood cells, while normal cell turnover continues to deplete the red blood cell population. Red blood cell production falters, producing red blood cells that are small and pale and lack sufficient hemoglobin (microcytic hypochromic anemia). Inadequate vitamin $B_6$ also can cause this type of anemia.

The symptoms of iron-deficiency anemia vary according to its severity and the speed of its development. They include fatigue, pale skin, breathlessness with exertion, poor tolerance to cold temperature, poor immune function, behavioral changes, cognitive impairment, and decreased work performance. In children, iron deficiency causes impaired growth, apathy, short attention span, irritability, and reduced ability to learn.[52]

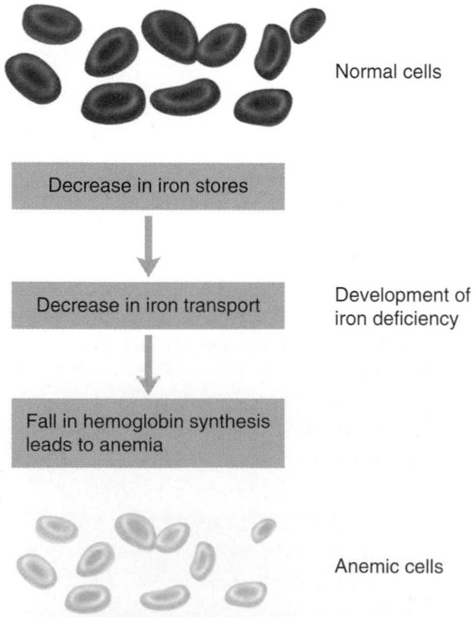

## Iron Toxicity

Iron pills can be hard on your digestive system. The UL for iron is based on the level that causes digestive distress. For adults, the UL for iron is 45 mil-

Normal cells

Decrease in iron stores

Development of iron deficiency

Decrease in iron transport

Fall in hemoglobin synthesis leads to anemia

Anemic cells

**Figure 10.25  Development of iron-deficiency anemia.** Iron deficiency can progress to iron-deficiency anemia, a severe form of iron deficiency that is accompanied by low hemoglobin levels.

**Table 10.5    Stages of Iron Deficiency**

| Stage | Functional Implications |
|---|---|
| Depletion of iron stores | None |
| Depletion of functional iron | Decreased physical performance |
| Iron-deficiency anemia | Cognitive impairment, poor growth, decreased performance, and decreased exercise tolerance |

ligrams per day, although physicians may prescribe supplements with larger amounts for treating iron-deficiency anemia.

### Iron Poisoning in Children

In the United States, accidental iron overdose is a leading cause of poisoning deaths in young children.[53] Even a few iron pills or a relatively moderate adult dose can cause the death of a small child. Parents often fail to appreciate the potential toxicity of iron and don't take precautions they would ordinarily use for other medicines. Symptoms of iron intoxication include nausea, vomiting, diarrhea, rapid heartbeat, dizziness, and confusion. Death can occur within hours of ingestion. If iron poisoning is suspected, the child must receive immediate emergency medical care.

### Hereditary Hemochromatosis

In hereditary **hemochromatosis**, a genetic defect causes excessive iron absorption and chronic **iron overload**. Although it was once believed to be rare, scientists now know that mild forms are quite common and are estimated to affect 1 to 6 people per 100 in the United States.[54] Iron buildup over the years leads to severe organ damage, causing diabetes, heart disease, arthritis, liver cirrhosis, and liver cancer.

Men are more vulnerable to hemochromatosis than women, who lose iron through menstruation and pregnancy. Early diagnosis and treatment control the condition and prevent organ damage. Treatment includes minimizing iron intake, avoiding excess vitamin C, and periodically removing some blood.

**Key Concepts** *Iron is a key component of the oxygen transporters hemoglobin and myoglobin and of many enzymes involved in energy metabolism. The body carefully regulates iron absorption, based on its iron needs. Heme iron is absorbed more efficiently than non-heme iron. Iron can be bound to transferrin for transport or stored as ferritin or hemosiderin. The best dietary sources of iron are organ meats and red meat. Plant foods contain only non-heme iron. Vitamin C–containing foods improve the bioavailability of non-heme iron. Iron deficiency develops gradually, and anemia is the most severe manifestation of deficiency. Iron poisoning, whether accidental or due to hemochromatosis, is potentially deadly.*

## Zinc

It's hard to believe that a nutrient so important to health could go unnoticed for so long. In fact, human zinc deficiency was not recognized until 1961.[55] A group of young men in Iran had a peculiar set of symptoms: severe growth retardation; poorly developed testicles (**hypogonadism**); anemia; and, among several, poor night vision. Their diet consisted mainly of wheat bread and was almost devoid of animal protein. They also ate clay (**geophagia**). Could their high-phytate, low-protein diet, along with geophagia, impair absorption of zinc and iron to such an extent? Six years later, a study in Egypt confirmed zinc's role; among a similar group of patients, zinc supplementation improved growth and genital development.[56]

### Functions of Zinc

Your body contains a small amount of zinc—1.5 to 2.5 grams, or about the amount of zinc that's in the thin zinc layer on a **galvanized** nail. Yet zinc is found in every body cell.

The functions of zinc fall into three categories: catalytic, structural, and regulatory. Zinc is a cofactor for nearly 100 enzymes, representing all the major enzyme types. In its structural role, zinc helps fold proteins into func-

**hemochromatosis** A hereditary disorder in which excessive absorption of iron results in abnormal iron deposits in the liver and other tissues.

**iron overload** Toxicity from excess iron.

**hypogonadism** Decreased functional activity of the gonads (ovaries or testes) with retardation of growth and sexual development.

**geophagia** Ingestion of clay or dirt.

**galvanized** Describes iron or steel with a thin layer of zinc plated onto it to protect against corrosion.

*Quick* Bite

**Bizarre Behavior or Nutritional Deficiency?**
In all cultures, races, and geographic regions, certain people have strange cravings for nonfood items. These cravings include ice (pagophagia), clay and dirt (geophagia), cornstarch (amylophagia), stone (lithophagia), paper, toilet tissue, soap, and foam. Pica, the compulsive consumption of nonfood items, often is associated with either iron or zinc deficiency, but it may also be the result of cultural beliefs or a response to family stresses. Whatever the cause, the behavior is not benign. It can injure teeth as well as cause constipation, intestinal obstruction or perforation, lead poisoning, pregnancy complications, poor growth in children, and mineral deficiencies.

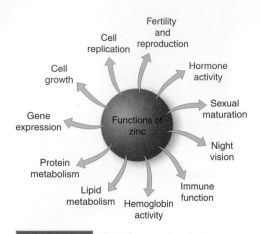

**Figure 10.26** **Functions of zinc in the body.** Because zinc is involved in so many different functions, it is fortunate that overt zinc deficiency is rare.

tional shapes. As a regulator, zinc helps control many diverse functions, including gene expression, cell death, and nerve transmission.[57] (See **Figure 10.26**.)

### Zinc and Enzymes

In many enzymes, zinc helps provide structural integrity or helps activate catalytic ability. For example, zinc performs a structural role in copper-zinc superoxide dismutase, an enzyme that speeds antioxidant reactions and helps protect cells from free radical damage. In the retina of the eye, the enzyme that activates vitamin A depends on zinc. Consequently, a lack of zinc can create a condition that resembles the night blindness caused by vitamin A deficiency.

### Zinc and Gene Regulation

As a component of certain small proteins, zinc enables those proteins to fold into a special form that interacts with DNA. This interaction "turns on" a gene, beginning the steps to protein production and cell multiplication.[58]

In severe zinc deficiency, cells fail to replicate. This may explain zinc's importance for normal growth of children and sexual maturation of adolescents. Furthermore, certain tissues with high turnover rates, such as the cells lining the GI tract, skin cells, immune cells, and blood cells, are particularly vulnerable to a zinc deficiency. As a result, zinc-deficient people often have diarrhea, dermatitis, and depressed immunity.

### Zinc and the Immune System

Zinc is vital to a vigorous immune response and is essential to the proper development and maintenance of the immune system. Without zinc, your body could not fight off invading viruses, bacteria, and fungi. Even mild deficiency may increase the risk of infection. (See the FYI feature "Zinc and the Common Cold.")

### Other Zinc Functions

Among zinc's many other functions, it interacts with hormones such as insulin and assists in linking oxygen to hemoglobin. Of special interest to nutritionists is zinc's role in the sense of taste. Zinc deficiency reduces taste perception, and poor appetite generally follows.

## Regulation of Zinc in the Body

When dietary zinc is low, our bodies have no long-term storehouse of zinc to draw upon. We maintain zinc balance, even when confronted with varying needs and dietary conditions, by adjusting absorption and excretion.

### Zinc Absorption

Much about absorption of dietary zinc is similar to that of iron. We absorb only about 10 to 35 percent of the zinc in our diets. The proportion that's absorbed depends on our zinc status, the zinc content of the meal, and the presence of competing minerals. People with zinc deficiency absorb zinc more efficiently than do people with optimal zinc status. Zinc absorption also increases during times of increased need, such as growth spurts, pregnancy, and lactation. As with iron, intestinal cells act as gatekeepers as they adjust their zinc absorption to maintain proper body levels.

Phytate from whole grains is the main dietary factor that inhibits zinc absorption.[59] For vegetarians whose diet consists of mainly phytate-rich unrefined grains and legumes, zinc requirements may exceed the RDAs.[60] Although calcium supplements may interfere in the absorption of zinc,[61] dietary calcium does not appear to reduce zinc absorption.[62] Non-heme iron in the form of iron supplements also depresses zinc absorption.[63] Iron from food, whether heme iron (from meat) or non-heme iron, does not have the same effect.[64]

### Zinc Transport, Distribution, and Excretion

Zinc circulates in the bloodstream bound to protein, traveling to the liver and tissues where it is most needed. Muscle and bone contain 90 percent of the body's zinc.

During digestion, the pancreas secretes a considerable amount of zinc in pancreatic juice. When needed, intestinal cells reabsorb most of this zinc. Otherwise, it is lost in feces, along with unabsorbed dietary zinc. Zinc is also

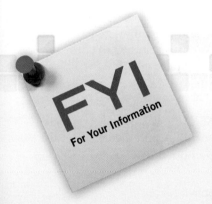

## Zinc and the Common Cold

The common cold, one of our most common illnesses, affects American adults 2 to 4 times per year and children 6 to 10 times per year.[1] Colds are even more frequent in young children in day-care settings and preschools. Because of missed work and decreased productivity, colds can be economically costly as well as a physical nuisance. A cure for the common cold would be of great benefit, and scientists have long pursued this goal.

Scientists have suggested several hypotheses, but the mechanism underlying a person's vulnerability to contracting a cold remains unclear. Zinc deficiency is known to impair immune function, but could all these people be zinc deficient? This is doubtful. Some speculate that zinc may reduce the severity and duration of cold symptoms by inhibiting viral replication. This is why products such as zinc lozenges and zinc syrups that "stick" are under investigation.

Although overall zinc supplementation may be beneficial under certain circumstances, studies of zinc and colds have produced conflicting results. One study with positive results gained considerable attention from the press and, as a result, zinc lozenges are on nearly every pharmacy shelf in the United States. In this study, colds resolved in an average of four days for participants in the zinc group, as compared to cold symptoms that persisted for seven days in the control group.[2] The same research group also studied children who took zinc gluconate lozenges at the first sign of cold symptoms, but found no difference between those who took zinc and those who did not for all cold symptoms to resolve—a median of nine days.[3]

Research continues to provide conflicting results, with some studies finding a benefit of lozenges[4] and others that zinc supplementation has no effect.[5] Review studies have also reported inconclusive findings.[6] However, a large systematic review of the scientific literature more recently concluded that "zinc (lozenges or syrup) is beneficial in reducing the duration and severity of the common cold in healthy people, when taken within 24 hours of onset of symptoms. People taking zinc are also less likely to have persistence of their cold symptoms beyond seven days of treatment."[7]

In addition to the mild side effects and the cost of the lozenges, such high doses of zinc could have harmful effects. People taking zinc lozenges (not syrup or tablet form) are more likely to experience adverse events, including bad taste and nausea.[8] Long-term use of high doses of zinc could also induce copper deficiency. In addition, loss of smell from the use of nasal zinc sprays prompted the FDA to issue a warning in 2009 instructing consumers to discontinue their use.[9]

Research to determine the effects of zinc for the treatment of the common cold is ongoing. Additional research is needed to determine the best zinc formulation, dose, and duration of treatment to provide a clinical benefit with minimal adverse effects before a general recommendation for zinc in the treatment of the common cold can be made.[10] Until there is more scientific agreement and standardized treatments, we should regard zinc as we would any other medical therapy and think twice before routinely giving children (and ourselves) zinc lozenges every time a cold strikes.

1    National Institute of Allergy and Infectious Diseases. Common cold. http://www3.niaid.nih.gov/healthscience/healthtopics/colds. Accessed 7/20/11.

2    Mossad SB, Macknin ML, Medendorp SV, Mason P. Zinc gluconate lozenges for treating the common cold: a randomized, double-blind placebo-controlled study. *Ann Intern Med.* 1996;125:81–88.

3    Macknin ML, Piedmonte M, Calendine C, et al. Zinc gluconate lozenges for treating the common cold in children: a randomized controlled trial. *JAMA.* 1998;279:1962–1967.

4    Prasad AS, Beck FW, Bao B, et al. Duration and severity of symptoms and levels of plasma interleukin-1 receptor antagonist, soluble tumor necrosis factor receptor, and adhesion molecules in patients with common cold treated with zinc acetate. *J Infect Dis.* 2008;197:795–802.

5    Eby GA, Halcomb WW. Ineffectiveness of zinc gluconate nasal spray and zinc orotate lozenges in common-cold treatment: a double-blind, placebo-controlled clinical trial. *Altern Ther Health Med.* 2006;12:34–38.

6    Caruso TJ, Prober CG, Gwaltney JM Jr. Treatment of naturally acquired common colds with zinc: a structured review. *Clin Infect Dis.* 2007;45:569–574.

7    Singh M, Das RR. Zinc for the common cold. *Cochrane Database Syst Rev.* 2011;16(2):CD001364.

8    Ibid.

9    US Department of Agriculture and US Food and Drug Administration. Warnings on three Zicam intranasal zinc products. Updated 6/16/09. http://www.fda.gov/ForConsumers/ConsumerUpdates/ucm166931.htm. Accessed 7/20/11.

10   Singh M, Das RR. Op. cit.

## Quick Bite

### Hair Analysis Is a Misguided Measure

Although its use has been discredited, hair analysis is promoted with the claim that it can reveal mineral deficiencies. However, this measure lacks sensitivity and is unreliable. The color, diameter, and rate of growth of a person's hair, the season of the year, the geographic location, and the person's age and gender can affect the levels of minerals in hair. It is possible for hair concentration of an element (zinc, for example) to be high even though deficiency exists in the body. Hair dyes, perming agents, and certain shampoos also alter the mineral content of hair.

lost from sloughed-off intestinal cells, skin, and hair; and minor amounts are excreted in urine, sweat, and other fluids.

## Dietary Recommendations for Zinc

The RDA for men is 11 milligrams per day, and for women over age 18, it is 8 milligrams per day, increasing to 11 milligrams during pregnancy and to 12 milligrams while breastfeeding.[65] Most people in the United States and Canada consume more than the RDA, but a significant number do not.

## Sources of Zinc

Zinc usually is abundant in foods that are good sources of protein, especially red meat and seafood such as oysters and clams. (See **Figure 10.27**.) For poultry, dark meat is a richer source than white meat. The zinc in animal foods is generally well absorbed. Conversely, whole grains have a relatively high amount of zinc, but it is poorly absorbed. Fruits and vegetables generally are poor zinc sources. Because diets that exclude meat are excluding the best zinc sources, adequate intake is a special concern for vegetarians.

## Zinc Deficiency

Zinc deficiency is uncommon in the United States and Canada. It usually occurs in people with illnesses that impair absorption. In other parts of the world, zinc deficiency is most prevalent in populations that subsist on cere-

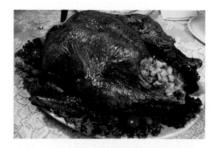

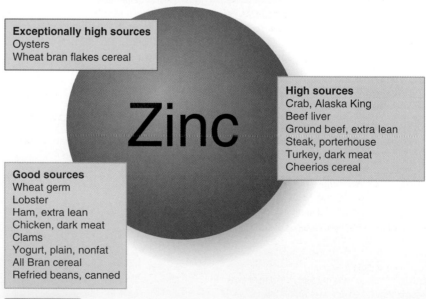

**Exceptionally high sources**
Oysters
Wheat bran flakes cereal

**High sources**
Crab, Alaska King
Beef liver
Ground beef, extra lean
Steak, porterhouse
Turkey, dark meat
Cheerios cereal

**Good sources**
Wheat germ
Lobster
Ham, extra lean
Chicken, dark meat
Clams
Yogurt, plain, nonfat
All Bran cereal
Refried beans, canned

**Figure 10.27**    **Food sources of zinc.** Meat, organ meats, and seafood are the best sources of zinc.

als and little else. Zinc from cereal grains is poorly absorbed. Among these populations, infections with pneumonia and diarrhea are commonplace and cause significant zinc losses. A downward spiral results: Zinc deficiency lowers immunity, and infection causes zinc loss, more infection, and more zinc loss. In some regions, zinc supplementation programs have cut the incidence of childhood respiratory infections and diarrhea.

Symptoms of moderate to severe zinc deficiency include poor growth, delayed or abnormal sexual development, diarrhea, severe skin rash and hair loss, impaired immune response, and impaired taste acuity. During pregnancy, zinc deficiency may contribute to complications and low birth weight.[66]

## Zinc Toxicity

The UL for zinc is set at 40 milligrams per day. Although toxicity from high dietary zinc intake is rare, chronic supplementation with too much zinc causes adverse effects. Chronic doses of zinc (100 to 150 milligrams per day) for prolonged periods can interfere with copper metabolism and cause low blood copper levels and impaired immunity.[67] Chronic high dosing of zinc relative to copper inhibits copper absorption and with time may induce a copper deficiency. But, for people with **Wilson's disease**, there's a benefit. Wilson's disease is a genetic disorder that causes excessive accumulation of copper in the body. For those who cannot tolerate drug treatment, zinc supplements of 150 milligrams daily can help prevent copper accumulation.[68]

**Key Concepts** *Zinc is important for normal growth and development, immune function, and the function of many enzymes. Zinc balance is maintained by regulating intestinal absorption. The best food sources are good protein sources, especially red meats and seafood. Zinc deficiency occurs most often among populations that subsist on cereals and grains.*

# Selenium

The story of selenium is a recent one and becomes more complex as scientists continue to explore its roles. Historically, because animals grazing on selenium-rich soils suffered selenium poisoning, scientists focused on its toxicity. This changed in 1957, when researchers first demonstrated selenium's nutritional benefits in vitamin E–deficient animals. But not until 1979 did evidence emerge that selenium is essential for humans. Chinese scientists reported an association between low selenium status and **Keshan disease**, a heart disorder that strikes children in the Keshan province of China. The Chinese scientists demonstrated that selenium supplements could prevent the disease. Although selenium deficiency does not cause the disease, it predisposes a child to heart damage after a particular type of viral infection. When selenium intake is adequate, the virus apparently does not cause Keshan disease.

## Functions of Selenium

In your body, most selenium joins up with one of two amino acids, methionine or cysteine, for storage or for its role as an antioxidant. Selenium is a component of a well-known family of antioxidants, the glutathione peroxidases. Like vitamin E, these enzymes work to prevent oxidative damage. In fact, to some extent selenium and vitamin E "spare" each other in this protection. A generous intake of one reduces the requirement for the other.

Selenium-containing enzymes are also involved in thyroid metabolism, converting thyroid hormone to its most active form. A deficiency of selenium worsens the **hypothyroidism** caused by iodine deficiency. (See the discussion of iodine later in this chapter.)

**Wilson's disease** Genetic disorder of increased copper absorption, which leads to toxic levels in the liver and heart.

**Keshan disease** Selenium-deficiency disease that impairs the structure and function of the heart.

**hypothyroidism** The result of a lowered level of circulating thyroid hormone, with slowing of mental and physical functions.

Selenium is important to immune function. As the Keshan studies showed, the body needs selenium to fight infections. Animals with depleted selenium get sicker from viral infections, and low selenium levels are associated with faster progression of viral disease in humans. Selenium may have some anti-cancer benefits, but more research is needed to clarify the relationship.[69] Selenium is also under investigation for its role in heart disease, arthritis, and HIV.[70]

## Absorption and Excretion of Selenium

Most selenium in food is bound to the amino acids methionine or cysteine, and in this form about 50 to 90 percent is bioavailable. Vitamins A, C, and E enhance selenium absorption, and phytate inhibits it. Excess selenium leaves the body mainly through feces and urine.

## Dietary Recommendations and Sources of Selenium

For both men and women, the selenium RDA is 55 micrograms per day.[71] U.S. and Canadian diets generally provide these levels. Selenium is found in both plant- and animal-derived foods. Selenium levels are quite variable in plant foods and generally reflect the selenium content of the soil in which the plant was grown. Brazil nuts are particularly high in selenium. The soil in Venezuela, where most Brazil nuts are harvested, is rich in selenium. As a result, a single Brazil nut provides more than the RDA for selenium. The selenium content of animal-derived foods is much more consistent. Organ meats, fish, seafood, and meats are consistently good sources. (See **Figure 10.28**.)

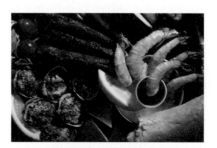

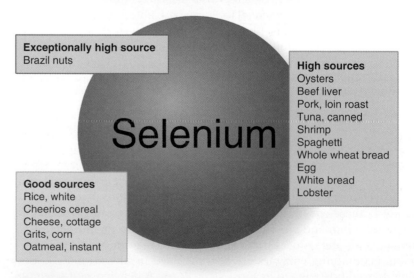

**Exceptionally high source**
Brazil nuts

**High sources**
Oysters
Beef liver
Pork, loin roast
Tuna, canned
Shrimp
Spaghetti
Whole wheat bread
Egg
White bread
Lobster

**Good sources**
Rice, white
Cheerios cereal
Cheese, cottage
Grits, corn
Oatmeal, instant

**Figure 10.28** **Food sources of selenium.** Selenium is found mainly in meats, organ meats, seafood, and grains.

## Selenium Deficiency and Toxicity

Selenium deficiency is rare, although it can be seen when soil selenium concentrations are low. Chronic selenium deficiency interferes with immune function. Three conditions have been associated with selenium deficiency: Keshan disease, which occurs in selenium-deficient children and results in an enlarged heart and poor heart function; Kashin-Beck disease, which results in diseases of the joints and bones; and **cretinism**, which results in mental retardation.[72]

There are isolated reports of selenium toxicity. Outward signs are brittle hair and nails and a garliclike body odor. Excessive intake may be accidental or the result of overenthusiastic supplementation. Chronic selenium toxicity also exists in isolated regions of the world where soil levels are very high. The UL is set at 400 micrograms per day for adults.

**Key Concepts**  *Selenium functions in antioxidant systems and spares vitamin E. It is involved in thyroid metabolism and immune function. Good dietary sources are Brazil nuts, organ meats, and seafood. Selenium deficiency is associated with Keshan disease, a rare heart ailment. Marginal deficiency may compromise immune function and increase cancer risk.*

## Iodine

Iodine deficiency has existed for centuries. The ancient Chinese wrote about it, and European artists of the Middle Ages included iodine-deficient people in their paintings.[73] Iodine deficiency existed in the American Midwest, too, until supplementation and fortification programs were begun around the mid-1920s. Prior to that, deficiency was so common the region was nicknamed "the goiter belt." Iodine deficiency remains a significant nutritional problem in some parts of the world, and its eradication is an important goal of the World Health Organization by encouraging universal salt iodization.[74]

Iodine is an essential component of thyroid hormones, which help regulate body temperature, basal metabolic rate, reproduction, and growth. Not surprisingly, most of the body's iodine is found in the thyroid gland. Selenium-dependent enzymes activate the major thyroid hormone, so a selenium deficiency can lead to inefficient use of iodine. In food, iodine is mostly in its ion form—iodide. Your intestines absorb nearly all dietary iodide. Raw vegetables in the cabbage family contain compounds known as **goitrogens**. These interfere with iodine absorption and can worsen deficiency. Cooking inactivates goitrogens. We excrete most excess iodine in urine, but also lose some in sweat, especially in hot, humid climates.

### Dietary Recommendations and Sources of Iodine

The iodine RDA for men and women is 150 micrograms per day, an amount that replaces iodine losses and provides a generous margin of safety.[75] Because the ocean is the best iodine source, the best food sources are ocean products: fish, seafood, and seaweed. (See **Figure 10.29.**) Saltwater fish have higher concentrations of iodine than do freshwater fish. Natural iodine levels in plants reflect soil iodine levels, and foods grown near the ocean are considerably richer in iodine than foods grown far inland. Because eons ago the Midwestern United States and Canada were covered by glaciers rather than the ocean, these regions have iodine-poor soils and produce food with little iodine.

The dairy industry adds iodine to cattle feed and uses sanitizing solutions that contain iodine. This substantially increases the iodine in milk and dairy products, which are now major contributors of iodine to the American diet. For many people, iodized salt is their primary iodine source. In the United

**cretinism**  A congenital condition often caused by severe iodine deficiency during gestation; characterized by arrested physical and mental development.

**goitrogens**  Compounds that interfere with iodine absorption and can induce goiter.

## *Quick* Bite

**Iodine or Iodide: What's in a Name?**
Although the terms *iodine* and *iodide* often are used interchangeably, chemically they are not identical. Iodine ($I_2$) is a bluish-black solid that gives off a purple vapor, which gives the element its name. Iodine stems from the Greek word *iôdêdes*, meaning "violet-colored." Iodide ($I^2$) is the colorless negative ion of iodine. Iodine circulates in the body either bound to protein or as free iodide ions. Sodium iodide and potassium iodide are iodide salts commonly used in medicines.

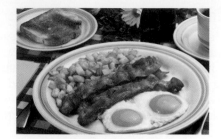

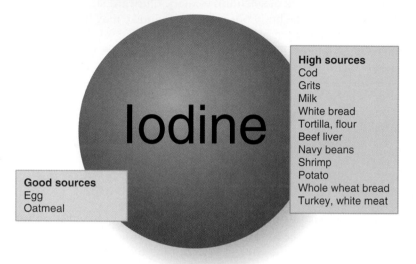

**Good sources**
Egg
Oatmeal

**High sources**
Cod
Grits
Milk
White bread
Tortilla, flour
Beef liver
Navy beans
Shrimp
Potato
Whole wheat bread
Turkey, white meat

**Figure 10.29** **Food sources of iodine.** Few foods are rich in iodine; it is found mainly in milk, seafood, and some grain products.

States, iodized salt contains an average of 76 micrograms of iodine per gram of salt.

## Iodine Deficiency

Iodine deficiency causes hypothyroidism, low levels of thyroid hormones. Its most apparent sign is **goiter**—an enlarged thyroid gland in the neck. (See **Figure 10.30**.)

Iodine deficiency inhibits thyroid hormone production. The body senses low levels of thyroid hormones and produces more and more **thyroid-stimulating hormone (TSH)**. The excessive TSH in turn stimulates the thyroid gland to grow, eventually causing a goiter. Other symptoms of hypothyroidism are intolerance to cold temperatures, decreased body temperature, weight gain, and sluggishness.

Mild or moderate iodine deficiency decreases IQ by about 10 to 15 points.[76] It also can decrease fertility and increase the risk of infant mortality. Severe iodine deficiency during early pregnancy causes cretinism in the baby. Symptoms of cretinism are mental retardation, stunted growth, deafness, and muteness.

Iodine deficiency has disappeared from the United States and Canada, but it still exists in the world's poor and isolated areas where the soils are low in iodine and little food from outside enters the local food supply. Deficiency may be worsened by diets low in selenium and high in goitrogenic vegetables.

**goiter** A chronic enlargement of the thyroid gland, visible as a swelling at the front of the neck; usually associated with iodine deficiency.

**thyroid-stimulating hormone (TSH)** Hormone secreted from the pituitary gland at the base of the brain; regulates synthesis of thyroid hormones.

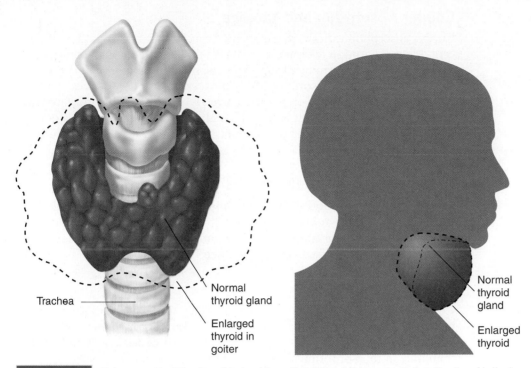

Trachea

Normal thyroid gland

Enlarged thyroid in goiter

Normal thyroid gland

Enlarged thyroid

**Figure 10.30** **Enlargement of the thyroid gland in goiter.** Iodine deficiency results in goiter. Use of iodized salt dramatically reduces goiter rates. This finding led to the widespread fortification of table salt with iodine.

## Iodine Toxicity

Large amounts of iodine inhibit synthesis of thyroid hormone, surprisingly, and stimulate thyroid growth and goiter. In other words, both too much and too little iodine cause goiter. Overzealous supplementation is the most common cause of iodine toxicity. The UL for iodine is 1,100 micrograms per day.

**Key Concepts** *Iodine is an essential component of thyroid hormones. Iodine deficiency causes overstimulation of the thyroid gland and eventual goiter. Deficiency during pregnancy can cause cretinism in the offspring. Important food sources include ocean fish and seafood, dairy products, and iodized salt. Worldwide, iodine deficiency continues to exist in some regions. Iodizing salt is a powerful preventive measure.*

## Copper

During the 1960s, researchers learned that copper was essential when they uncovered **Menkes' syndrome**, a rare genetic disease of copper deficiency. Dietary copper deficiency is not a significant public health concern, but excessive supplementation with other trace minerals can cause a secondary copper deficiency.

As a part of coenzymes, copper participates in dozens of reactions, among them energy release, skin pigment (melanin) production, and the production of the connective tissue proteins collagen and elastin. It plays a role in maintaining nerve health, immune function, and heart function. Copper is a component of the superoxide dismutases, enzymes involved in antioxidant reactions. Copper also is a component of **ceruloplasmin**, an enzyme required for iron transport. Without ceruloplasmin, iron accumulates in the liver, creating symptoms similar to hemochromatosis.

**Menkes' syndrome** A genetic disorder that results in copper deficiency.

**ceruloplasmin** A copper-dependent enzyme that enables iron to bind to transferrin. Also known as *ferroxidase I*.

albumin A protein that circulates in the blood and helps transport many minerals and some drugs.

## Copper Absorption and Storage

Copper absorption varies with dietary intake and can range from 20 to 50 percent. Most absorption takes place in the small intestine, though some occurs in the stomach. Some mineral supplements, most notably iron and zinc, can interfere with copper absorption. So can excessive use of antacids.

**Albumin** transports copper to the liver, where most is incorporated into ceruloplasmin. Little copper is stored. Unabsorbed copper, copper sloughed off in intestinal cells, and excess copper secreted in bile all leave the body via feces.

## Dietary Recommendations and Sources of Copper

The copper RDA for both men and women is 900 micrograms per day. It's not difficult to achieve because copper is widely distributed in foods. The richest food sources for copper include organ meats, shellfish, nuts and seeds, legumes, peanut butter, and chocolate. (See **Figure 10.31**.)

## Copper Deficiency

Copper deficiency is rare and occurs most often in infants born prematurely, who have low copper stores at birth and a very rapid growth rate. Cow's milk has little copper, so infants who are inappropriately fed cow's milk rather than human milk or formula could have low copper levels.

Copper deficiency reduces production of both red and white blood cells, causing anemia and poor immune function. Deficiency also causes bone

*Quick* Bite

**A Penny for Your . . .**
How do the amounts of zinc and copper in a U.S. penny compare with the amounts in your body? Today's penny is mostly zinc (2.4 grams), covered with some copper plating (62.5 milligrams). A penny's zinc is in the upper range of the body's zinc content, but the amount of copper falls short. It takes the copper in about 1½ pennies to equal the amount of copper in your body.

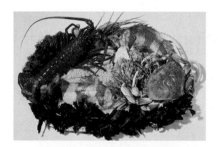

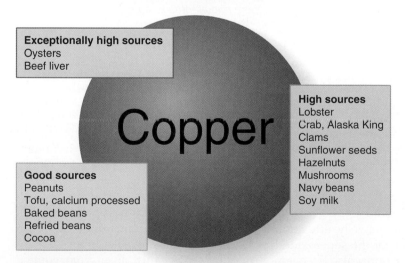

**Exceptionally high sources**
Oysters
Beef liver

# Copper

**High sources**
Lobster
Crab, Alaska King
Clams
Sunflower seeds
Hazelnuts
Mushrooms
Navy beans
Soy milk

**Good sources**
Peanuts
Tofu, calcium processed
Baked beans
Refried beans
Cocoa

**Figure 10.31**    **Food sources of copper.** Copper is found in a limited variety of foods. The best sources are seafood, legumes, and nuts.

abnormalities. Menkes' syndrome is an extremely rare (1 in 50,000 live births) genetic copper absorption disorder that usually is fatal in infancy or early childhood.[77]

## Copper Toxicity

Compared with other trace minerals, copper is relatively nontoxic. The UL for copper is 10 milligrams per day. However, in Wilson's disease, a rare (1 in 200,000) genetic disorder, excessive copper accumulates in the liver, brain, kidney, and eye. Like copper deficiency, copper excess causes anemia. People with Wilson's disease now avoid serious liver and neurologic problems with therapies that bind and remove copper. Zinc supplements, which inhibit copper absorption, also are used in treating Wilson's disease.

**Key Concepts** *Copper is a component of ceruloplasmin, superoxide dismutase, and many other enzymes. Good food sources include organ meats, shellfish, nuts and seeds, legumes, peanut butter, and chocolate. Copper deficiency and toxicity are rare.*

## Manganese

The body contains only 10 to 20 milligrams of manganese, yet manganese is a cofactor in reactions of key importance. It's involved in energy metabolism and in urea formation. Manganese-containing enzymes also are required for building cartilage. Like zinc and copper, manganese is a component of the antioxidant enzyme superoxide dismutase.

Absorption of manganese is very low, only 1 to 15 percent, probably a protection against toxicity. There is little storage, and any excess is excreted in bile and leaves via feces.

### Dietary Recommendations and Sources of Manganese

Adequate Intake (AI) for manganese is 2.3 milligrams per day for men and 1.8 milligrams per day for women. Tea, nuts, cereals, and some fruits are the best food sources of manganese. (See **Figure 10.32**.) Meat, dairy products, poultry, fish, and refined foods are poor sources.

### Manganese Deficiency and Toxicity

Most people are not at risk of manganese deficiency. However, some illnesses, such as **Lou Gehrig's disease** and **multiple sclerosis**, may cause suboptimal manganese status. In animal studies, manganese deficiency impairs growth, impairs energy metabolism, and produces bone abnormalities.

Manganese toxicity is a greater threat than manganese deficiency. However, incidents of toxicity have been due not to food, but to air pollutants. Foundry workers exposed to airborne manganese dust experience severe manganese toxicity. Their symptoms include irritability, hallucinations, and severe lack of coordination. Lower doses of airborne manganese can impair memory and motor coordination. The UL for manganese is 11 milligrams per day.

**Key Concepts** *Manganese is a cofactor in several enzyme systems. Food sources for manganese are tea, coffee, cereals, and some fruits. Toxicity from airborne manganese is a greater threat than deficiency.*

## Fluoride

Fluoride is a form of the element fluorine. Large-scale studies undertaken during the 1940s convincingly demonstrated that fluoride has the ability to

**Lou Gehrig's disease** A syndrome marked by muscular weakness and atrophy due to a degeneration of motor neurons of the spinal cord. Technically known as *amyotrophic lateral sclerosis (ALS)*.

**multiple sclerosis** A progressive disease that destroys the myelin sheath surrounding nerve fibers of the brain and spinal cord.

*Quick* Bite

### Egg Whites? Please Stand Up!

Although cooking food in a copper pot is inadvisable, copper mixing bowls can be a plus. Meringues made in ceramic or steel bowls tend to be snowy white and drier than those made in copper bowls. Making meringue in a copper bowl leads to a creamier, yellowish foam that is harder to overbeat into a lumpy liquid. The copper bowl contributes copper ions to conalbumin, a metal-binding protein, thus stabilizing the whipped egg whites.

## *Quick* Bite

**Highway Harvest**
Oil companies often add a type of manganese to modern gasoline as an antiknock compound to increase the octane rating for high-compression engines. It is now evident that plants along highways accumulate manganese from passing cars.

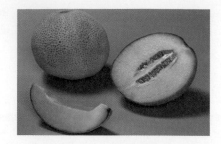

**Exceptionally high sources**
Wheat germ
Pineapple

## Manganese

**High sources**
Hazelnuts
Oatmeal
Whole wheat bread
Spinach
Tea
Sweet potato
Lima beans
Blackberries
Soybeans

**Good sources**
Turnip greens
Beets
Broccoli
Cocoa
Okra

**Figure 10.32**    **Food sources of manganese.** Manganese is found mainly in plant foods such as grains, legumes, vegetables, and some fruits.

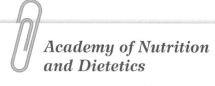

## *Academy of Nutrition and Dietetics*

**The Impact of Fluoride on Health**
The Academy of Nutrition and Dietetics reaffirms that fluoride is an important element for all mineralized tissues in the body. Appropriate fluoride exposure and usage is beneficial to bone and tooth integrity and, as such, has an important, positive impact on health throughout life.

**Source:** Reproduced from Palmer C, Wolfe SH. Position of the American Dietetic Association: the impact of fluoride on health. *J Am Diet Assoc.* 2005;105(10):1620–1628.

prevent dental caries. Since then, fluoride has been added to water supplies in many regions of the United States, and use of fluoridated toothpaste and mouthwash has become widespread.

### Functions of Fluoride

Nearly 99 percent of the body's fluoride is in bones and teeth, where it promotes deposition of calcium and phosphate. Every day there is a battle in your teeth between normal mineral loss and mineral deposition. When your mouth contains food, bacteria multiply and produce acids that eat away tooth enamel, especially beneath plaque. Fluoride inhibits bacterial activity and shifts the balance toward depositing minerals. This action in teeth helps counter normal mineral loss, a loss that acid-forming bacteria accelerate. Fluoride therefore inhibits tooth decay and loss of tooth enamel.

During infancy and childhood, while new teeth are being formed, fluoride acts systemically. In other words, it arrives via the bloodstream to the site of new tooth formation. There it is incorporated into the tooth structure. Throughout life, the fluoride in toothpaste and mouth rinses and other topically applied fluoride help strengthen tooth surfaces. Fluoride also may play a role in preventing bone loss.[78] Fluoride supplements have been used along with calcium and other medications to treat osteoporosis. Although the risk of fracture is reduced, optimal dosage is not clear, and fluoride is not an approved treatment for osteoporosis.

## Dietary Recommendations and Sources of Fluoride

Your body absorbs almost all fluoride extracted from water and other liquids, and about 50 to 80 percent of fluoride from food. Most excess fluoride is excreted in urine.

The fluoride AI for adults is 4 milligrams per day for men, and 3 milligrams for women. The AI is 0.01 milligram per day for infants up through 5 months and 0.5 milligram for those aged 6 to 11 months.[79] Dental caries is the most common chronic disease in children,[80] and the American Dental Association recommends fluoride supplements beginning with children 6 months of age whose drinking water supplies less than 0.3 milligrams fluoride per liter.[81]

Water is the main source of fluoride. Water naturally may contain fluoride, or fluoride may be added to produce fluoridated water. Fluoride naturally present in drinking water varies from less than 0.1 milligram to more than 10 milligrams per liter. Where naturally occurring fluoride levels are low, many water companies add fluoride. The Department of Health and Human Services recommends 0.7 milligrams of fluoride per liter of water, based on an assessment of the benefits versus side effects by the Environmental Protection Agency and the Department of Health and Human Services.[82] The Environmental Protection Agency requires public drinking water systems to remove excess fluoride so that it does not exceed 4.0 milligrams per liter.[83] The Centers for Disease Control and Prevention named the fluoridation of drinking water one of the 10 great public health achievements of the twentieth century.[84]

Other fluoride sources have emerged since we first began fluoridating water supplies. Today's fluoride sources include fluoride supplements, mouthwash, toothpaste, and some beverages. Almost one-quarter of U.S. children younger than 12 years of age and 30 percent of 2 year olds use supplemental vitamins, fluoride, and iron in a given week.[85]

## When Fluoride Balance Goes Awry

Low fluoride intake is associated with tooth decay. Adequate fluoride intake during infancy and childhood cuts the incidence of tooth decay by up to 30 to 60 percent. Prolonged excessive intake of fluoride causes **fluorosis**. (See Figure 10.33.) During tooth development, fluorosis damages teeth. In mild fluorosis, white specks form on the teeth. Severe fluorosis weakens teeth and produces permanent brownish stains. In adults, fluorosis is associated with hip fracture; weak, stiff joints; and chronic stomach inflammation.

> *Quick* Bite
>
> **Accidental Discovery**
> In the early 1900s, people noticed that inhabitants of towns with naturally high levels of fluoride in their water had healthier teeth. To test the correlation between fluoride and tooth decay, in 1945 four cities in the United States and one in Canada took part in a controlled study of water fluoridation. The results were impressive, establishing that fluoride helps to prevent tooth decay.

**fluorosis** Mottled discoloration and pitting of tooth enamel caused by prolonged ingestion of excess fluoride.

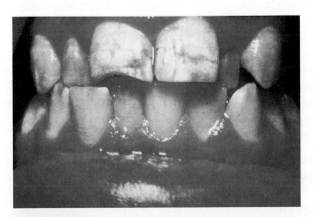

**Figure 10.33** **Tooth mottling in fluorosis.** During tooth development, prolonged excessive fluoride intake can cause fluorosis, which discolors and damages teeth.

## *Quick* Bite

**Conspiracy Theory**
Although the U.S. Public Health Service and the World Health Organization officially endorsed the fluoridation of water in the 1950s, some groups continue to oppose the practice. Objectors claim that water fluoridation violates civil rights, that fluoride is a "nerve poison," and that fluoride is unwanted compulsory medication that can have dangerous side effects. Some groups even claim that fluoridation is a component of a conspiracy for national destruction. So far, objectors have been unable to substantiate their claims, and the courts have upheld the constitutionality of fluoridation.

Fluorosis can occur in people living where water is naturally very high in fluoride, or in children who chronically swallow large amounts of fluoridated toothpaste. The UL for fluoride is 10 milligrams per day.

### The Fluoridation Debate

In some communities, water fluoridation programs have been in place for over 50 years. It is indisputable that these programs have substantially reduced tooth decay, and more than 90 professional health organizations endorse fluoridation of the public water supplies as the most effective dental public health measure.[86] However, opponents argue that fluoridation is involuntary: "If you administer fluoride by fluoridating the tap water in the community then you have no control of the dose an individual gets per day."[87]

THINK
About It
4

Some argue that availability of fluoride supplements and fluoride-containing dental products makes fluoridation unnecessary. Others fear fluorosis or a connection with cancer and other illnesses, although extensive reviews of the scientific literature have concluded that there is no relationship between fluoridation and cancer.[88]

Proponents cite the substantial evidence of improved dental health and lack of evidence showing harm.[89] Bone health also may benefit. The presence of fluoride in water is not unnatural, and levels in fluoridated water are far less than the amount that occurs naturally in some sources. To retain benefits yet avoid overconsumption, the American Dental Association recommends the fluoridation of all water supplies and regulation of other fluoride sources.

The AI levels for infants and children have been reduced to account for increased fluoride in the food supply. Fluoride supplements are available only by prescription.

**Key Concepts**  *Bones and teeth contain 99 percent of body fluoride. Fluoride supports mineralization of bones and teeth, and adequate intake reduces tooth decay. The main dietary source is water. The majority of municipal water supplies contain fluoride. Excess fluoride causes fluorosis with mottling of the teeth. Severe fluorosis causes weakened, brown-stained teeth.*

## Chromium

The best understood role of chromium is in glucose metabolism. Chromium appears to enhance the ability of insulin to move glucose into cells. Other functions of chromium involve nucleic acid metabolism, growth, and immune function. The amount of chromium in the body is exceedingly tiny—only about 4 to 6 milligrams.

Dietary chromium is poorly absorbed, and levels decrease with age. Chromium absorption appears to increase with need and decrease as dietary intake rises. Absorption improves when chromium is combined with an organic acid, as in chromium picolinate supplements. Excess chromium is excreted in urine.

### Dietary Recommendations and Sources of Chromium

The AI for adults 19 to 50 years of age is 35 micrograms per day for men and 25 micrograms per day for women; for older adults the daily AI decreases by 5 micrograms. The chromium content of foods varies widely. Good sources include brewer's yeast, processed meats, whole grains, green beans, broccoli, and spices. Cooking acidic foods in stainless steel containers leaches some chromium into the food.

## *Quick* Bite

**Chrome-Plated Cars**
The cars of the 1950s sported fins and loads of chrome. The chromium in your body is the same metal used for electroplating hard chrome. Using electric current, chromium molecules bind with the surface of the steel creating a bond between the metals so hard it will remain intact even when subjected to extreme force.

## Chromium Deficiency and Toxicity

It is difficult to detect chromium deficiency in the general population. In research settings, induced chromium deficiency inhibits glucose uptake by cells and raises blood glucose, insulin, and blood lipids. Patients who subsist on long-term intravenous feedings inadequate in chromium may suffer brain and nerve disorders.[90] The only known cases of chromium toxicity are from airborne chromium compounds in industrial settings. To date, no UL has been set for chromium, but up to 200 micrograms of inorganic chromium appears to be a safe supplement dose.

The role of chromium supplements remains controversial. Supplementation with chromium has been shown to reduce risk factors for type 2 diabetes[91] and cardiovascular disease.[92] However, the current body of evidence does not support chromium supplementation as a tool for diabetes management.[93] Based on perceived but unfounded beneficial effects on body composition, chromium supplements are popular among many athletes and bodybuilders. However, there is little evidence from well-designed studies that chromium increases lean body mass or decreases body fat.[94]

## Molybdenum

Molybdenum is essential to both plants and animals. In humans, molybdenum functions as a cofactor for several enzymes. Molybdenum is efficiently absorbed, and it's excreted rapidly in urine and bile. Dietary copper can inhibit molybdenum absorption, and vice versa. Doctors exploit the competition between copper and molybdenum by using a form of molybdenum to treat patients with Wilson's disease.

The RDA for molybdenum is 45 micrograms per day for adults. Peas, beans, and some breakfast cereals are the richest food sources, and organ meats also are good sources.

Molybdenum deficiency does not occur in people who eat a normal diet. Deficiency symptoms of weakness, mental confusion, and night blindness have occurred in people on long-term intravenous feeding or people with a rare genetic disorder.

Although molybdenum is unlikely to cause toxicity in humans, a UL for molybdenum has been set at 2,000 micrograms per day.

**Key Concepts**  *Chromium is involved in glucose metabolism and probably has other important roles as well. Molybdenum is required in several important enzyme systems. Deficiency or toxicity of chromium and molybdenum is very unlikely.*

## Other Trace Minerals and Ultratrace Minerals

Five of the minerals we have discussed—iodine, fluoride, manganese, molybdenum, and selenium—could be considered "ultratrace" minerals. They are found in the body in minuscule amounts, and, for most of these, we need less than 1 milligram daily. Although there is substantial research on these minerals, the functions of other trace and ultratrace minerals are less clear. Research and attention have focused on arsenic, boron, nickel, silicon, and vanadium. Although insufficient evidence exists to set an AI or RDA for these minerals, ULs have been established for boron, nickel, and vanadium.

### Arsenic

Although arsenic has been an infamous poison for centuries, inorganic arsenic may actually be an essential ultratrace element. Although no studies have

# Learning Portfolio

## Key Terms

## Study Points

- Water is the most essential nutrient; we can live much longer without food than without water.

- Water is important for chemical reactions, temperature regulation, maintaining acid–base balance, and transporting nutrients and waste. Fluids in the body lubricate and cushion joints, cleanse the eyes, and moisten the food we eat.

- Water is lost through exhaled air, perspiration, feces, and urine. Insensible water loss is the continuous evaporation of water from the lungs and skin. Diuretics increase fluid excretion. When fluid loss exceeds intake, resulting dehydration can seriously impair physical and mental performance.

- Minerals are inorganic elements and are categorized as major or trace depending on the amount in the body and the amount needed in the diet.

- The bioavailability of minerals may be affected by excess intake of single-mineral supplements; phytate, oxalate, and fiber in plant foods; and mineral status in the body.

- Sodium helps regulate water distribution and blood pressure. Most Americans eat too much dietary sodium, mainly from processed foods.

- Potassium is necessary for nerve and muscle function. Unprocessed foods, including fruits and vegetables, provide most dietary potassium. A diet high in potassium from fruits and vegetables may help to lower blood pressure. Chloride is a component of stomach acid. Chloride deficiency is most often associated with prolonged vomiting. Most Americans consume more chloride than recommended levels as part of salt (sodium chloride).

- Calcium, the most abundant mineral in the body, is found mainly in bones and teeth. It's required for blood clotting, nerve and muscle function, and cellular metabolism. Major dietary sources of calcium are dairy products and calcium-fortified foods.

- Phosphorus is a key component of ATP, DNA, RNA, phospholipids, and lipoproteins. Because phosphorus is widespread in foods, inadequate phosphorus intake is rare.

- Plant foods such as whole grains and vegetables are important sources of magnesium, which is a cofactor for hundreds of enzymes. Kidney disease, alcoholism, and overuse of diuretics may cause low magnesium levels.

- Sulfur does not function alone as a nutrient, but as a component of certain amino acids and the vitamins biotin and thiamin.

- Hypertension increases risk for heart disease, stroke, and kidney disease. Excessive sodium intake is linked to hypertension in people who are salt-sensitive. Other dietary factors linked to hypertension include low potassium, calcium, and magnesium intakes.

- Osteoporosis—weak, porous bones—results from excessive bone loss. Postmenopausal women are at highest risk for osteoporosis. Adequate dietary calcium, vitamin D, and physical activity throughout life reduce the risk for osteoporosis.

- Hemoglobin and myoglobin contain iron, which transports oxygen. Iron is also an enzyme cofactor, important for immune function and brain function.

- Due to menstruation, women of childbearing age need more iron than men do. Meats are the best source of iron, but enriched and whole grains are also significant sources in the American diet.

- Iron deficiency is the most common nutritional deficiency worldwide. Anemia is the most severe stage of deficiency, occurring after iron stores are depleted.

Iron toxicity can be acute or chronic. Accidental iron overdose is a leading cause of poisoning deaths of young children in the United States. Hemochromatosis is a disease of chronic excessive iron absorption.

■ Zinc is a cofactor for numerous enzymes and is crucial for normal growth, sexual development, and immune function. It is found in protein-rich foods, particularly meats. Deficiency results in poor growth, impaired taste, and impaired immune response.

■ Selenium is considered an antioxidant nutrient. It is also needed for thyroid function. Good sources of selenium are Brazil nuts, organ meats, and seafood. Deficiency of selenium in the Keshan region of China is associated with Keshan heart disease.

■ Iodine is required for thyroid function. Iodine deficiency causes enlarged thyroid or goiter. Severe deficiency during pregnancy can cause cretinism in the baby. Much of the iodine in the American diet comes from iodized salt.

■ Copper functions in many enzyme systems involved with antioxidant protection, iron utilization, and immune function. The richest food sources of copper include organ meats, shellfish, nuts and seeds, peanut butter, and chocolate. Copper deficiency is rare.

■ Manganese functions in many enzyme systems. The best food sources include tea, coffee, nuts, cereals, and some fruits. Manganese deficiency and toxicity are uncommon; toxicity is from manganese air pollutants.

■ Fluoride promotes mineralization of bones and teeth and protects teeth from decay. Water, which contains fluoride naturally or is fluoridated, is our main fluoride source. Excessive fluoride causes fluorosis, which mottles teeth.

■ Chromium is involved in glucose metabolism. Some good sources of chromium are mushrooms, dark chocolate, prunes, nuts, asparagus, and whole grains. Chromium toxicity is unlikely.

■ Molybdenum functions as an enzyme cofactor. Good food sources are peas, beans, and some breakfast cereals. Molybdenum deficiency and toxicity are both rare.

■ Ultratrace minerals are those required in extremely small amounts; the specific function of many of these nutrients is unknown. Some ultratrace minerals are arsenic, boron, nickel, silicon, and vanadium.

## Study Questions

1. List the biological functions of water.
2. Which major minerals affect blood pressure?
3. What are the major functions of calcium, other than its relation to bone health?
4. Explain the differences between "heme" and "non-heme" iron. Which is absorbed better?
5. List the three stages of iron deficiency.
6. What are the main functions of selenium?
7. What is goiter?
8. How does fluoride prevent tooth decay? Other than water, what sources supply fluoride?
9. What is chromium's best understood role in the body? Which foods are good sources of chromium?

## Try This

### Osmosis Experiment

Purchase some celery and let it sit for a week or two until it becomes limp. When the celery looks limp and lifeless, fill your sink with cold water and soak the celery. When it has soaked for several hours, take the celery out and examine its appearance. Notice anything different? Because the crispness of celery is due to osmotic pressure, when you soaked the limp celery, it absorbed water into its cells and became crisp again.

### A Simple Check on Your Zinc

Reported in *Lancet* in the early 1980s, this simple test can provide a rough signal of your zinc status. Buy some zinc sulfate at a health food store. Dissolve it in distilled water to make a 0.1 percent zinc sulfate solution. Refrain from eating, drinking, and smoking for at least an hour before the test. Then swish a teaspoon of the solution around your mouth for 10 seconds. If it tastes unpleasant or metallic, your level of zinc is probably adequate. However, if the solution tastes like water, you may be consuming less zinc than you need.

## What About Bobbie?

Let's take a look at Bobbie's intake of the minerals calcium, magnesium, sodium, iron, zinc, and selenium. Refer to the "Food Choices: Nutrients and Nourishment" chapter to refresh yourself regarding Bobbie's one-day intake. How do you think she did?

### Calcium

Bobbie's calcium intake was low on the day she recorded her food intake. She consumed 710 milligrams, but the RDA for a 20-year-old woman is 1,000 milligrams per day. If this day reflects her usual intake, then she is at risk of poor bone mineralization and lower than average peak bone mass. This increases her risk of osteoporosis.

## Magnesium

Bobbie's intake of magnesium was 310 milligrams, and the RDA for a woman her age is 320 milligrams per day. If this one-day record reflects her usual eating, she probably is consuming an adequate amount of magnesium and does not need to increase her intake of this mineral. Some of the best sources of magnesium in her diet were the banana, tortilla chips, and spaghetti noodles.

## Sodium

Bobbie's intake of 4,820 milligrams of sodium was much higher than the AI of 1,500 milligrams and twice the UL of 2,300 milligrams per day! This should not be a surprise because most of Bobbie's meals are either convenience items or prepared by someone else (e.g., the school's cafeteria), which makes it hard to control sodium content. The biggest contributors to her high intake of sodium were the sourdough bread, salad dressing, salsa, spaghetti sauce, and pizza. Bobbie should try to eat fewer convenience foods and more fresh foods. She would also benefit from drinking extra water because her intake of sodium is so high.

## Iron

Most of Bobbie's iron intake came from enriched grains and red meat. The spaghetti noodles, bagel, meatballs, and breads were the best iron sources in her diet. Overall, she consumed 20 milligrams of iron, compared with the RDA of 18 milligrams per day for women her age.

## Zinc

Bobbie's best source of zinc is red meat—the meatballs she had on her spaghetti. Other zinc sources were the turkey, spaghetti noodles, and pizza. Remember that zinc is much better absorbed from meats than from grains. Bobbie's intake of 12 milligrams of zinc was higher than the RDA of 8 milligrams per day.

## Selenium

Bobbie's best sources of selenium are grain products and meats. Again, the spaghetti noodles, bagel, bread, and meatballs were among the top sources in her day. Turkey also contributed a significant amount. Bobbie's overall selenium intake of 152 micrograms was well above the RDA of 55 micrograms per day for adults.

# References

1   Institute of Medicine, Food and Nutrition Board. *Dietary Reference Intakes for Water, Potassium, Sodium, Chloride, and Sulfate*. Washington, DC: National Academies Press; 2004.
2   Popkin BM, D'Anci KE, Rosenberg IH. Water, hydration, and health. *Nutr Rev*. 2010;68(8):439–458.
3   Institute of Medicine, Food and Nutrition Board. 2004. Op. cit.
4   Ibid.
5   Popkin BM, D'Anci KE, Rosenberg IH. Op. cit.
6   Shirreffs SM. Conference on "Multidisciplinary approaches to nutritional problems." Symposium on "Performance, exercise and health." Hydration, fluids, and performance. *Proc Nutr Soc*. 2009;68(1):17–22.
7   Manz F. Hydration and disease. *J Am Coll Nutr*. 2007;26(5):535S–541S.
8   Cosca DD, Navazio F. Common problems in endurance athletes. *Am Fam Physician*. 2007;76:237–244.
9   Stuempfle KJ. Exercise-associated hyponatremia during winter sports. *Phys Sportsmed*. 2010;38(1):101–106.
10  Nevius CW. In hazing, dumb stunts can be fatal. *San Francisco Chronicle*. 2/8/05. http://sfgate.com/cgi-bin/article.cgi?file=/c/a/2005/02/08/BAG61B7D341.DTL. Accessed 7/14/11.
11  Institute of Medicine, Food and Nutrition Board. *Dietary Reference Intakes for Calcium, Phosphorus, Magnesium, Vitamin D, and Fluoride*. Washington, DC: National Academies Press; 1997.
12  National Center for Health Statistics. *Health, United States, 2008*. Hyattsville, MD: National Center for Health Statistics; 2008.
13  Zemel MB. Dietary pattern and hypertension: the DASH study. *Nutr Rev*. 1997;55:303–308.
14  Chen ST, Maruthur NM, Appel LJ. The effect of dietary patterns of estimated coronary heart disease risk. Results from the Dietary Approaches to Stop Hypertension (DASH) trial. *Circ Cardiovasc Qual Outcomes*. 2010;3:484–489.
15  Blumenthal JA, Babyak MA, Hinderliter A, et al. Effects of the DASH diet alone and in combination with exercise and weight loss on blood pressure and cardiovascular biomarkers in men and women with high blood pressure: the ENCORE study. *Arch Intern Med*. 2010;170(2):126–135.
16  The DASH Diet Eating Plan. http://dashdiet.org/default.asp. Accessed 7/14/11.
17  Sacks FM, Svetkey LP, Vollmer WM, et al. Effects on blood pressure of reduced dietary sodium and the Dietary Approaches to Stop Hypertension (DASH) diet. *N Engl J Med*. 2001;344:3–10.
18  US Department of Health and Human Services and US Department of Agriculture. *Dietary Guidelines for Americans, 2010*. 7th ed. Washington, DC: US Government Printing Office; 2010.
19  Centers for Disease Control and Prevention. Nutrition for everyone. Calcium and bone health. Updated 4/6/11. http://www.cdc.gov/nutrition/everyone/basics/vitamins/calcium.html. Accessed 7/14/11; and US Department of Health and Human Services. *Bone Health and Osteoporosis: A Report of the Surgeon General*. Rockville, MD: US Department of Health and Human Services, Office of the Surgeon General; 2004.
20  US Department of Health and Human Services and US Department of Agriculture. Op. cit.
21  Institute of Medicine, Food and Nutrition Board. 2004. Op. cit.
22  American Heart Association. Diet and lifestyle recommendations. Updated 5/21/10. http://www.heart.org/HEARTORG/GettingHealthy/Diet-and-Lifestyle-Recommendations_UCM_305855_Article.jsp. Accessed 7/14/11.
23  Guyton AC, Hall JE. *Textbook of Medical Physiology*. 12th ed. Philadelphia: WB Saunders; 2010.
24  Institute of Medicine, Food and Nutrition Board. 2004. Op. cit
25  US Department of Health and Human Services and US Department of Agriculture. Op. cit.
26  Yang Q, Liu T, Kuklina EV, et al. Sodium and potassium intake and mortality among US adults. Prospective data from the Third National Health and Nutrition Examination Survey. *Arch Intern Med*. 2011;171(13):1183–1191.
27  Institute of Medicine, Food and Nutrition Board. 2004. Op. cit.
28  Guyton AC, Hall JE. Op. cit.
29  Ibid.
30  Howe TE, Shea B, Dawson LJ, et al. Exercise for preventing and treating osteoporosis in postmenopausal women. *Cochrane Database Syst Rev*. 2011;7:CD000333.
31  Institute of Medicine, Food and Nutrition Board. *Dietary Reference Intakes for Calcium and Vitamin D*. Washington, DC: National Academies Press; 2011.
32  Jung Yang Y, Martin BR, Boushey CJ. Development and evaluation of a brief calcium assessment tool for adolescents. *J Am Diet Assoc*. 2010;110:111–115.
33  National Institutes of Health, Office of Dietary Supplements. Dietary supplement fact sheet. Calcium. http://ods.od.nih.gov/factsheets/calcium. Accessed 7/18/11.

34  Institute of Medicine, Food and Nutrition Board. 2011. Op. cit.

35  Rafferty K, Heaney RP. Nutrient effects on the calcium economy: emphasizing the potassium controversy. *J Nutr*. 2008;138(1)(suppl):166S–171S.

36  National Institutes of Health, Office of Dietary Supplements. Op. cit.

37  Institute of Medicine, Food and Nutrition Board. 2011. Op. cit.

38  Institute of Medicine, Food and Nutrition Board. 1997. Op. cit.

39  Ibid.

40  Ibid.

41  Longo D, Fauci A, Kasper D, Hauser S, Jameson J, Loscalzo J. *Harrison's Principles of Internal Medicine*. 18th ed. New York: McGraw-Hill; 2011.

42  Gropper SS, Smith JL, Groff JL. *Advanced Nutrition and Human Metabolism*. 5th ed. Belmont, CA: Wadsworth/Cengage Learning; 2009.

43  Ibid.

44  World Health Organization. Micronutrient deficiencies: iron deficiency anemia. http://www.who.int/nutrition/topics/ida/en. Accessed 7/16/11.

45  Gleason G, Scrimshaw NS. An overview of the functional significance of iron deficiency. In: Kraemer K, Zimmermann MB. *Nutritional Anemia*. Basel, Switzerland: Sight and Life Press; 2007:45–58.

46  Ibid.

47  Institute of Medicine, Food and Nutrition Board. *Dietary Reference Intakes for Vitamin A, Vitamin K, Arsenic, Boron, Chromium, Copper, Iodine, Iron, Manganese, Molybdenum, Nickel, Silicon, Vanadium, and Zinc*. Washington, DC: National Academies Press; 2001.

48  Hurrell R, Egli I. Iron bioavailability and dietary reference values. *Am J Clin Nutr*. 2010;91(suppl):1461S–1467S.

49  Ibid.

50  Gropper SS, Smith JL, Groff JL. Op. cit.

51  Institute of Medicine, Food and Nutrition Board. 2001. Op. cit.

52  Ibid.

53  Spanierman CS. Iron toxicity in emergency medicine. Medscape. http://emedicine.medscape.com/article/815213-overview. Accessed 7/17/11.

54  Centers for Disease Control and Prevention. Hemochromatosis (iron storage disease). Updated 9/3/11. http://www.cdc.gov/ncbddd/hemochromatosis/training/epidemiology/prevalence.html. Accessed 7/17/11.

55  Prasad AS, Helstead JA, Nadami M. Syndrome of iron deficiency anaemia, hepatosplenomegaly, hypogonadism, dwarfism and geophagia. *Am J Med*. 1961;31:532–546.

56  Sandstead HH, Prasad AS, Schubert AR, et al. Human zinc deficiency endocrine manifestations and response to treatment. *Am J Clin Nutr*. 1967;20:422–442.

57  Institute of Medicine, Food and Nutrition Board. 2001. Op. cit.

58  Dibley MJ. Zinc. In: Bowman BA, Russell RM, eds. *Present Knowledge in Nutrition*. 9th ed. Washington, DC: ILSI Press; 2006.

59  Hambidge KM, Miller LV, Westcott JE, Sheng X, Krebs NF. Zinc bioavailability and homeostasis. *Am J Clin Nutr*. 2010;91(5):1478S–1483S.

60  Position of the Academy of Nutrition and Dietetics: vegetarian diets. *J Am Diet Assoc*. 2009;109(7):1266–1282.

61  Radak T. Zinc in vegetarian diets. Vegetarian Nutrition Dietetic Practice Group of the Academy of Nutrition and Dietetics. http://vegetariannutrition.net/docs/Zinc-Vegetarian-Nutrition.pdf. Accessed 7/18/11.

62  Hunt JR, Beiseigel JM. Dietary calcium does not exacerbate phytate inhibition of zinc absorption by women from conventional diets. *Am J Clin Nutr*. 2009;89:839–843.

63  Kannan S. Factors in vegetarian diets influencing iron and zinc bioavailability. Vegetarian Nutrition Dietetic Practice Group of the Academy of Nutrition and Dietetics. http://vndpg.org/articles/Iron-and-Zinc-Bioavailability-in-Vegetarian-Nutrition.php. Accessed 7/18/11.

64  Gropper SS, Smith JL, Groff JL. Op. cit.

65  Institute of Medicine, Food and Nutrition Board. 2001. Op. cit.

66  *The Merck Manual for Healthcare Professionals*. Zinc. Whitehouse Station, NJ: Merck & Co.; 2005. http://www.merck.com/mmpe/sec01/ch005/ch005j.html. Accessed 7/18/11.

67  Ibid.

68  *The Merck Manual for Healthcare Professionals*. Copper. Whitehouse Station, NJ: Merck & Co.; 2005. http://www.merck.com/mmpe/sec01/ch005/ch005c.html. Accessed 7/18/11.

69  Dennert G, Zwahlen M, Brinkman M, Vinceti M, Zeegers MP, Horneber M. Selenium for preventing cancer. *Cochrane Database Syst Rev*. 2011;5:CD005195.

70  National Institutes of Health, Office of Dietary Supplements. Dietary supplement fact sheet. Selenium. http://ods.od.nih.gov/factsheets/selenium. Accessed 7/18/11.

71  Institute of Medicine, Food and Nutrition Board. *Dietary Reference Intakes for Vitamin C, Vitamin E, Selenium, and Beta-Carotene, and Other Carotenoids*. Washington, DC: National Academies Press; 2000.

72  National Institutes of Health, Office of Dietary Supplements. Dietary supplement fact sheet. Selenium. Op. cit.

73  Hetzel BS. *The Story of Iodine Deficiency: An International Challenge in Nutrition*. Oxford: Oxford University Press; 1989.

74  World Health Organization. Micronutrient deficiencies: iodine deficiency disorders. http://www.who.int/nutrition/topics/idd/en/index.html. Accessed 7/18/11.

75  Institute of Medicine, Food and Nutrition Board. 2001. Op. cit.

76  *The Merck Manual for Healthcare Professionals*. Iodine. Whitehouse Station, NJ: Merck & Co.; 2005. http://www.merck.com/mmpe/sec01/ch005/ch005e.html. Accessed 7/19/11.

77  *The Merck Manual for Healthcare Professionals*. Copper. Whitehouse Station, NJ: Merck & Co.; 2005. http://www.merck.com/mmpe/sec01/ch005/ch005e.html. Accessed 7/19/11.

78  Everett ET. Fluoride's effects on the formation of teeth and bones, and the influence of genetics. *J Dent Res*. 2011;90(5):552–560.

79  Institute of Medicine, Food and Nutrition Board. Op. cit.

80  Benjamin RM. Oral health. The silent epidemic. *Public Health Rep*. 2010;125(2):158–159.

81  American Dental Association. Oral health topics. Fluoride supplements. Fluoride supplement dosing schedule, 2010. http://www.ada.org/3088.aspx#dosschedule. Accessed 7/19/11.

82  US Department of Health and Human Services. HHS and EPA announce new scientific assessments and actions on fluoride. 1/7/11. http://www.hhs.gov/news/press/2011pres/01/20110107a.html. Accessed 7/19/11.

83  Environmental Protection Agency. Basic information about fluoride in drinking water. Updated 5/20/11. http://water.epa.gov/drink/contaminants/basicinformation/fluoride.cfm. Accessed 7/19/11.

84  US Department of Health and Human Services. Op. cit.

85  Vernacchio L, Kelly JP, Kaufman DW, Mitchell AA. Vitamin, fluoride, and iron use among US children younger than 12 years of age: results from the Slone Survey, 1998–2007. *J Am Diet Assoc*. 2011;111(2):285–289.

86  Palmer C, Wolfe SH, Academy of Nutrition and Dietetics. Position of the Academy of Nutrition and Dietetics: the impact of fluoride on health. *J Am Diet Assoc*. 2005;105(10):1620–1628.

87  James Beck, Professor Emeritus of Medical Biophysics at the University of Calgary, as quoted in George C. Battle renewed over value of fluoridation. *CMAJ*. 2011;183(10):1173.

88  American Dental Association. Fluoridation facts. 2005. http://www.ada.org/sections/professionalResources/pdfs/fluoridation_facts.pdf. Accessed 7/19/11.

89  Ibid.

90  Hummel M, Standt E, Schnell O. Chromium in metabolic and cardiovascular disorders. *Horm Metab Res*. 2007;39:743–751.

91  Austin RP. Should I try chromium tablets? *Diabetes Forecast*. 7/11. http://forecast.diabetes.org/magazine/ask-experts/should-i-try-chromium-tablets. Accessed 7/19/11.

92  Sharma S, Agrawal RP, Choudhary M, Jain S, Goyal S, Agarwal V. Beneficial effect of chromium supplementation on glucose, HbA(1)C and lipid variables in individuals with newly onset type-2 diabetes. *J Trace Elem Med Biol*. 2011;25(3):149–153.

93  Chehade JM, Sheikh-Ali M, Mooradian AD. The role of micronutrients in managing diabetes. *Diabetes Spectr*. 2009;22(4):214–218.

94  Sarubin Fragakis A, Thomson C. *The Health Professional's Guide to Popular Dietary Supplements*. 3rd ed. Chicago: Academy of Nutrition and Dietetics; 2007.

95  Nielsen FH. Is boron nutritionally relevant? *Nutr Rev*. 2008;66(4):183–191.

# CHAPTER 11

# Sports Nutrition: Eating for Peak Performance

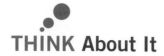

## THINK About It

1   How much importance do you place on being physically active?

2   How often do you suffer muscle fatigue? What do you think causes it?

3   How often do you think about food choices when you're planning a physical activity?

4   What kind of protein do you emphasize in your diet?

**Visit go.jblearning.com/ inseldisco4e**

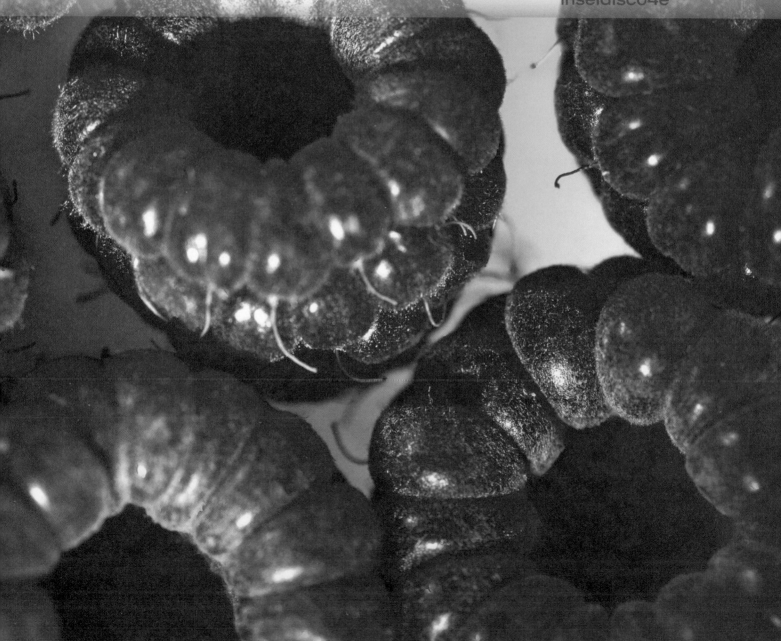

Today is the big 10,000-meter race. You've trained for months. Fans in the crowd shade their eyes as they watch you and your competitors walk onto the track. "Ready," shouts the starter. "Get set." You toe the starting line and adrenaline courses through your blood vessels, increasing your heart rate, diverting blood to your muscles, and mobilizing energy stores in your liver, muscles, and fat. "Go!" Within a fraction of a second, a torrent of calcium flows into your muscle cells, causing your muscles to contract and launch you away from the starting line.

How will you perform in this race? Will your breakfast help or hinder your performance? Will what you ate yesterday and the day before affect your stamina? Does it matter what you eat after you finish the race? Read on for the answers to these questions and to learn about the links between nutrition and sports performance.

## Nutrition and Physical Performance

**THINK About It**

**1**

Just how physically active do you need to be? (See **Figure 11.1**.) Both the National Institutes of Health (NIH) and Health Canada have found that just small to moderate amounts of physical activity can produce substantial health benefits. Physically active people have a lower risk of developing many chronic diseases, such as coronary heart disease, diabetes, hypertension, osteoporosis, and obesity. Active people also experience an increased sense of well-being and are much better equipped to cope with stress. Health Canada recommends choosing a variety of activities from three types of exercise: endurance, flexibility, and strength. (See **Figure 11.2**.)

The American College of Sports Medicine (ACSM) and the American Medical Association launched a program called "Exercise is Medicine" in 2007.[1] This program's vision is to make physical activity and exercise a standard part of disease prevention and treatment in the United States. The goals of this program include: (1) raising public awareness of the need for a physically active lifestyle; (2) emphasizing the medical importance of exercise to physicians and other healthcare workers; and (3) instructing physicians in writing prescriptions for exercise. The ACSM notes an important distinction between physical activity as it relates to health and exercise for physical fitness.[2] According to the ACSM, the level of physical activity that may reduce the risk of various chronic diseases may not be enough—in quantity or quality—to improve physical fitness. The Physical Activity Guidelines for Americans recommend that children and adolescents should do at least 60 minutes of physical activity daily, and all adults should avoid inactivity. For substantial health benefits, adults should do at least 2 hours and 30 minutes a week of moderate-intensity or 1 hour and 15 minutes a week of vigorous-intensity aerobic activity.[3]

What is physical fitness? Measures of fitness may include such factors as strength, endurance, flexibility, and breathing capacity. The ACSM defines physical fitness as "the ability to perform moderate to vigorous levels of physical activity without undue fatigue and the capability of maintaining this level of activity throughout life."[4] In other words, fitness is more than being able to run a long distance or lift a lot of weight at the gym. Being fit is not defined only by what kind of activity you do, how long you do it, or at what level of intensity. Although these are important measures of fitness, they only address single areas. Overall fitness is made up of five main components:

1. *Cardiorespiratory fitness:* The ability of the body's circulatory and respiratory systems to supply fuel during sustained physical activity.

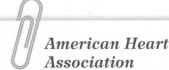

### American Heart Association

**Physical Activity**

Physical inactivity is a major risk factor for developing coronary artery disease. Even moderately intense physical activity such as brisk walking is beneficial when done regularly for a total of 30 minutes or longer on most days.

**Source:** American Heart Association, Inc.

# Develop an Active Lifestyle

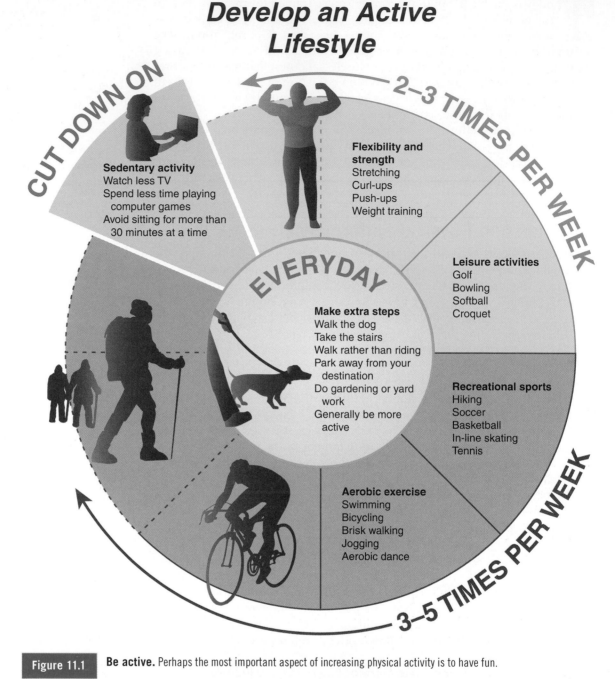

**CUT DOWN ON**

**Sedentary activity**
Watch less TV
Spend less time playing
   computer games
Avoid sitting for more than
   30 minutes at a time

**2–3 TIMES PER WEEK**

**Flexibility and strength**
Stretching
Curl-ups
Push-ups
Weight training

**Leisure activities**
Golf
Bowling
Softball
Croquet

**Recreational sports**
Hiking
Soccer
Basketball
In-line skating
Tennis

**3–5 TIMES PER WEEK**

**Aerobic exercise**
Swimming
Bicycling
Brisk walking
Jogging
Aerobic dance

**EVERYDAY**

**Make extra steps**
Walk the dog
Take the stairs
Walk rather than riding
Park away from your
   destination
Do gardening or yard
   work
Generally be more
   active

**Figure 11.1**   **Be active.** Perhaps the most important aspect of increasing physical activity is to have fun.

2. *Muscular strength:* The ability of the muscle to exert force during an activity.
3. *Muscular endurance:* The ability of the muscle to continue to perform without fatigue.
4. *Body composition:* The relative amounts of fat and lean body mass. Body composition is an important component to consider for health and weight management.
5. *Flexibility:* The range of motion around a joint. Good flexibility in the joints can help prevent injuries through all stages of life.

Table 11.1 shows guidelines for levels of physical activity to promote health and to achieve and maintain fitness.

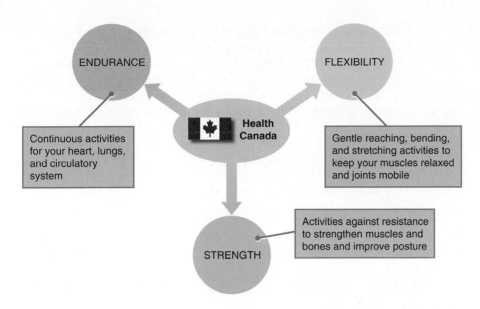

**Figure 11.2** **Variety is the spice of life.**
Health Canada recommends that you do a variety of activities from each group—endurance, flexibility, and strength—to receive the most health benefits.
**Source:** Data from *Canada's Physical Activity Guide to Healthy Active Living.*

**Table 11.1** **Guidelines for Physical Activity: Health and Fitness**

*Guidelines for Promoting Health*
**Frequency:** Daily activity
**Intensity:** Any level of intensity
**Duration:** Accumulation of a minimum of 30 minutes of total daily activity
**Mode:** Any activity
*Guidelines for Achieving and Maintaining Physical Fitness*
**Frequency:** 3 to 5 days per week
**Intensity:** 50 to 90 percent of maximum heart rate
**Duration:** 29 to 60 minutes of continuous or intermittent aerobic activity (minimum of 10-minute bouts accumulated during the day)
**Mode:** Activity using large muscle groups maintained continuously in a rhythmic and aerobic manner
**Resistance training:** 2 to 3 days per week to enhance strength and muscular endurance and to maintain fat-free mass
**Flexibility training:** Minimum of 2 days per week, incorporated into overall fitness program to develop and maintain range of motion
*Guidelines for Weight Loss and Prevention of Weight Regain*
*For overweight and obese adults to improve health*
**Frequency:** A minimum of 150 minutes per week
**Intensity:** Moderate
*For long-term weight loss*
**Frequency:** 200 to 300 minutes per week
**Intensity:** Moderate
*To prevent weight gain and provide modest weight loss*
**Frequency:** 150 to 250 minutes per week
**Intensity:** Moderate

**Sources:** Adapted from American College of Sports Medicine. Position stand: the recommended quantity and quality of exercise for developing and maintaining cardiorespiratory and muscular fitness and flexibility in healthy adults. *Med Sci Sports Exerc.* 1998;30:975–991; American College of Sports Medicine. Position stand: progression models in resistance training for healthy adults. *Med Sci Sports Exerc.* 2002;34:364–380. Reprinted by permission of Lippincott Williams & Wilkins, http://lww.com; and American College of Sports Medicine. Position stand: appropriate physical activity intervention strategies for weight loss and prevention of weight regain for adults. *Med Sci Sports Exerc.* 2009;41(2):459–471.

*Academy of Nutrition and Dietetics\**

**Nutrition and Athletic Performance**
It is the position of the American Dietetic Association, Dietitians of Canada, and the American College of Sports Medicine that physical activity, athletic performance, and recovery from exercise are enhanced by optimal nutrition. These organizations recommend appropriate selection of food and fluids, timing of intake, and supplement choices for optimal health and exercise performance.

**Source:** Reproduced from Rodriguez NR et al. Position of the Academy of Nutrition and Dietetics, Dietitians of Canada, and the American College of Sports Medicine: nutrition and athletic performance. *J Am Diet Assoc.* 2009;109(3):509–527.

\* Formerly the American Dietetic Association

Nutrition has taken its rightful place as a vital component of any program that seeks to enhance health, fitness, and athletic performance. In a joint position paper, the Academy of Nutrition and Dietetics, Dietitians of Canada, and the American College of Sports Medicine state that "physical activity, athletic performance, and recovery from exercise are enhanced by optimal nutrition."[5] But just what is "optimal nutrition"? Is it the same for a child who plays recreational softball and for a senior citizen who takes daily walks to reduce the risk of type 2 diabetes? What about the competitive athlete who strives to maximize athletic performance and uses nutrition to gain a competitive edge? To understand the relationship between physical activity and nutrition, you first need to appreciate how we use energy during exercise.

**Key Concepts**  *Exercise provides numerous health benefits, including reduced risk of chronic disease. Physical fitness includes strength, endurance, and flexibility. For optimal physical performance, nutrition is an essential part of all athletic training programs.*

## Energy Systems, Muscles, and Physical Performance

Let's return to your race. As you leave the starting line, your body immediately ramps up energy production to meet the increased demand. Just as a rocket uses different fuel systems and stages to power its leap into space, your body uses three different energy systems to launch, accelerate, and maintain exercise intensity.

### ATP–CP Energy System

As you launch yourself from the starting line, it takes less than a second for your contracting muscles to burn their entire reserve of adenosine triphosphate (ATP), the immediate energy source for cells. Luckily, your body has a small reservoir of **creatine phosphate** (also called **phosphocreatine**) that your muscles can convert quickly to ATP. (See **Figure 11.3**.) Muscle cells contain four to six times as much creatine phosphate as ATP.[6] Together, your available ATP and creatine phosphate, the **ATP–CP energy system**, can power an all-out effort for only 3 to 15 seconds.[7] To continue the race, you must enlist

**creatine phosphate**  An energy-rich compound that supplies energy and a phosphate group for the formation of ATP. Also called *phosphocreatine*.

**phosphocreatine**  See *creatine phosphate*.

**ATP–CP energy system**  A simple and immediate anaerobic energy system that maintains ATP levels. Creatine phosphate is broken down, releasing energy and a phosphate group, which is used to form ATP.

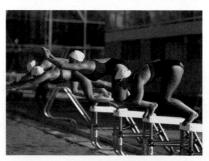

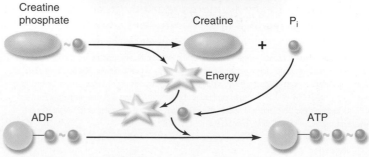

**Figure 11.3**  **ATP–CP energy system.** To maintain relatively constant ATP levels during an initial explosive burst of high-intensity activity, your body uses its ATP–CP energy system to generate ATP from creatine phosphate.

carbohydrate stored as glycogen in your muscles and liver. Your cells rapidly disassemble glycogen to glucose, from which they can extract ATP.

## Lactic Acid Energy System

For the next minute or two, the acceleration stage, your body uses the simplest and speediest chemical pathways to produce ATP from glucose—the **lactic acid energy system**. (See **Figure 11.4**.) Like the ATP–CP energy system, these pathways are anaerobic—they do not require oxygen. The raw material, glucose, is much more plentiful than creatine phosphate, but its breakdown also produces a by-product—lactate (lactic acid). Although research shows that cells can extract some energy from lactic acid aerobically,[8] most lactic acid accumulates in cells, making them more acidic. A rise in acidity impairs the breakdown of glucose and inhibits calcium binding. Without calcium, muscles cannot contract. For years, coaches and athletes have blamed lactic acid for muscle fatigue. But, it's the change in pH, rather than the lactic acid substance itself, that is the primary culprit.[9]

To continue running beyond the first few minutes, your body employs a sophisticated, oxygen-based system to process lactic acid and squeeze out much more ATP from glucose.

## Oxygen Energy System

For the endurance stage, cells can use lengthy, complex chemical pathways in their mitochondria—small units within cells that function as power-generating plants—to convert food and oxygen to ATP. (See **Figure 11.5**.) These reactions are aerobic—they require abundant oxygen. In contracting muscle, blood vessels dilate and deliver a 20-fold increase in oxygen-rich blood to muscle cells,[10] a sufficient supply for mitochondria to produce ATP. In contrast to the two anaerobic systems (ATP–CP system and lactic acid system), the **oxygen energy system** can produce a tremendous amount of ATP. Another advantage is that the oxygen energy system can extract energy from fat as well as from glucose. But, because the required oxygen must travel a long distance—from lungs to blood to muscle cells to mitochondria—the oxygen energy system produces ATP at a much slower rate than the anaerobic systems do.

## Teamwork in Energy Production

The energy systems work together to fuel athletic performance. (See **Figure 11.6**.) Although all three energy systems are always active, one system may be the primary fuel source for a particular activity or exercise intensity. As the first two minutes of your race elapse, the oxygen energy system is supplying about half of your muscles' energy needs. (See **Figure 11.7**.) By the time you pass the 30-minute mark, this aerobic system is supplying 95 percent; and at two hours or more, the oxygen energy system is supplying 98 percent of your muscles' energy needs.[11]

As long as ATP production by the mitochondria meets energy needs, you are exercising aerobically; highly trained athletes can sustain such exercise for hours. If the exercise rate exceeds your body's ability to supply oxygen to your muscles, you are exercising anaerobically, rapidly depleting your creatine phosphate and glycogen reserves. Once these are exhausted, if the available oxygen cannot support the oxygen energy system, performance plummets.

Carbohydrate stores are limited. A 68-kilogram (150-pound) man with 10 to 20 percent body fat, for example, has carbohydrate stores of 1,800 to 2,000 kilocalories in muscle glycogen, liver glycogen, and blood glucose. Compare this with the energy he stores in fat. His fat tissue holds roughly

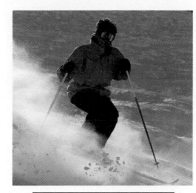
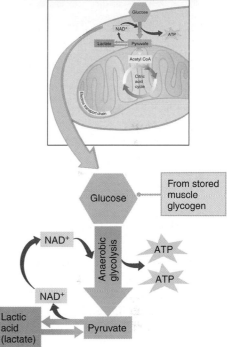

**Figure 11.4  Lactic acid energy system.** During short physical events requiring power and speed, the lactic acid energy system supplies much of the energy. Because the lactic acid system does not require oxygen, these events are anaerobic activities.

**lactic acid energy system** Anaerobic energy system; using glycolysis, the process rapidly produces energy (ATP) and lactate. Also called *anaerobic glycolysis*.

**oxygen energy system** A complex energy system that requires oxygen. To release ATP, it completes the breakdown of carbohydrate and fatty acids via the citric acid cycle and electron transport chain.

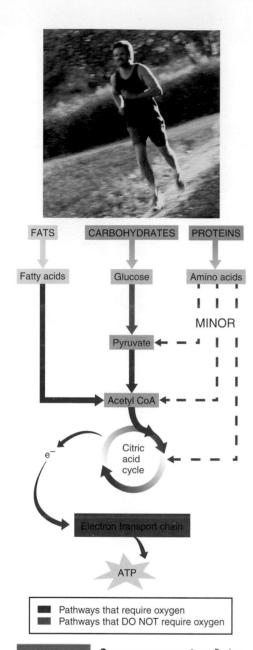

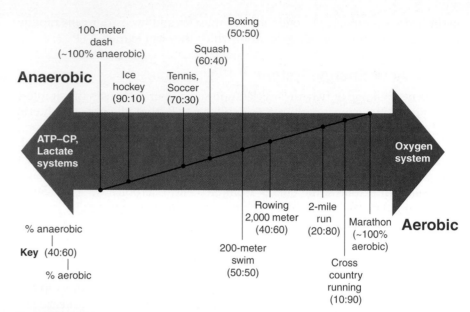

**Figure 11.6** **The anaerobic–aerobic continuum.** Most activities use ATP from both anaerobic and aerobic energy systems. However, the 100-meter dash is considered completely anaerobic, and the marathon is considered completely aerobic.

**Figure 11.5** **Oxygen energy system.** During longer endurance events (aerobic events), the oxygen energy system supplies most of the energy. This energy system requires oxygen and primarily relies on carbohydrate and fat as fuels.

63,000 to 120,000 kilocalories.[12] Although the body can burn protein for energy, in well-fed people protein probably provides no more than 5 percent of energy expended in exercise.[13]

## Glycogen Depletion

At the beginning of the race, your body rapidly uses muscle glycogen. But, as the race keeps going, the rate of glycogen use markedly slows. During the first one and a half hours, glycogen stores drop steadily to about one-third their starting levels. About three hours into the run, as glycogen stores become almost entirely depleted, you may "hit the wall." Your muscles become weak and heavy, your legs shake, and you become confused. Marathon runners commonly experience a sudden onset of exhaustive fatigue around the 18- to 20-mile mark. Drinking fluids that contain glucose can partially compensate for glycogen depletion and soften its effects. Dehydration can cause an even faster onset of fatigue, so drinking plenty of fluids is essential during endurance events.

As exercise intensity increases, glycogen depletion accelerates. Sprinting, for example, uses muscle glycogen 35 to 40 times faster than walking.[14] **Figure 11.8** illustrates how the sensation of fatigue relates to the depletion of muscle glycogen.

## Endurance Training

Have you ever trained for a long run only to realize that what started off to be a difficult distance gradually becomes a pretty easy run? Endurance training has effects on muscle capillaries that increase blood flow and produce marked improvement in endurance capacity.[15] Training enhances aerobic capacity by increasing the number of mitochondria and improving the body's ability to deliver oxygen to them. This decreases the reliance on anaerobic energy systems, extending the availability of glycogen reserves and delaying fatigue. Following weeks of endurance training, your long runs are much easier than before the start of your training cycle.

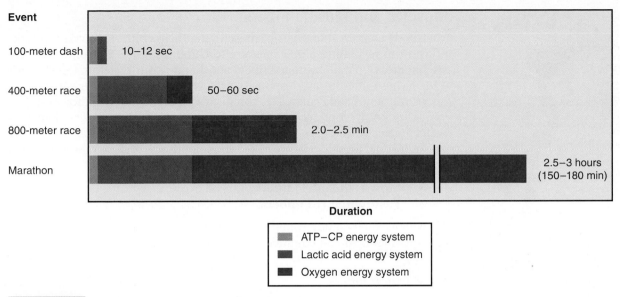

**Figure 11.7**  **Sports events and energy systems.** Short-term, explosive events rely upon the ATP–CP and lactic acid energy systems. For longer events, your body turns to the oxygen energy system. During endurance events, your body uses this system to burn fat as well as glucose.

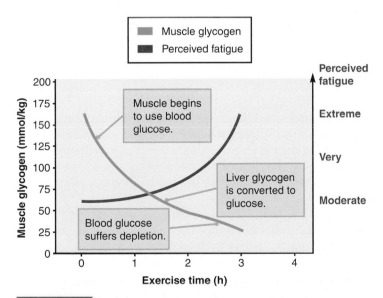

**Figure 11.8**  **Glycogen depletion and the sensation of fatigue.** As muscle glycogen levels decline, fatigue and eventually exhaustion set in.

**Key Concepts**  *Muscle cells use three different energy systems to produce ATP: the ATP–CP energy system, the lactic acid energy system, and the oxygen energy system. The ATP–CP and lactic acid energy systems rely on carbohydrate and do not require oxygen. The oxygen energy system requires oxygen and relies on carbohydrates and fats. During the early minutes of high-intensity exercise, the anaerobic systems are the predominant source of ATP. During lower-intensity endurance events, the third system supplies ATP, although at a much slower rate. Dehydration and depletion of glycogen stores are major factors in fatigue. Training increases the efficiency of oxygen delivery to muscle and increases the number of muscle mitochondria available for aerobic metabolism.*

## *Quick* Bite

### Use It or Lose It!
After only two weeks of inactivity, the benefits of training begin to disappear. Muscular endurance—the ability of a muscle to avoid fatigue—declines, and activities of certain oxidative enzymes drop by as much as 40 percent. By the fourth week, muscle glycogen levels also may drop by 40 percent. Flexibility is quickly lost, and inactivity can substantially decondition the heart muscle and cardiovascular system.

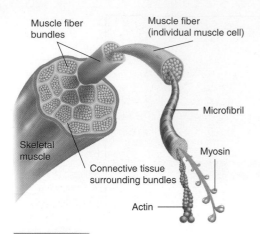

**Figure 11.9** **Basic structure of skeletal muscle.** A muscle fiber is an individual muscle cell that usually extends the entire length of the muscle. Each muscle fiber contains hundreds to thousands of microfibrils. Each microfibril contains thousands of actin and myosin filaments, large protein molecules responsible for muscle contractions.

## *Quick* Bite

**Pound for Pound?**
Women's muscles have smaller muscle fiber cross-sections and less muscle mass than men. For a given amount of muscle, however, there is no difference in strength between men and women.

**skeletal muscles** Muscles composed of bundles of parallel, striated muscle fibers under voluntary control. Also called *voluntary muscle* or *striated muscle*.

**muscle fibers** Individual muscle cells.

**slow-twitch (ST) fibers** Muscle fibers that develop tension more slowly and to a lesser extent than fast-twitch muscle fibers. ST fibers have high oxidative capacities and are slower to fatigue than fast-twitch fibers.

**fast-twitch (FT) fibers** Muscle fibers that can develop high tension rapidly. These fibers can fatigue quickly but are well suited to explosive movements in sprinting, jumping, and weight lifting.

**aerobic endurance** The ability of skeletal muscle to obtain a sufficient supply of oxygen from the heart and lungs to maintain muscular activity for a prolonged time.

## Muscles and Muscle Fibers

Your body contains hundreds of muscles that help control a myriad of functions, from regulating blood pressure to climbing stairs. **Skeletal muscles** are bundles of parallel, striated fibers attached to your skeleton. (See **Figure 11.9**.) These muscles are responsible for your physical movement and are under your conscious control. If you decide to bend your arm, for example, you consciously contract your biceps. Your body contains more than 600 skeletal muscles and uses 9 of them just to control your thumb!

Individual muscle cells are called **muscle fibers**; skeletal muscle has two primary types:

- **Slow-twitch (ST) fibers**
- **Fast-twitch (FT) fibers**

They derive their names from the difference in their speed of action. One type of fast-twitch fiber can contract 10 times faster than slow-twitch fibers.[16]

### Slow-Twitch Fibers

To power their activity, slow-twitch fibers efficiently produce energy by breaking down carbohydrate and fat via aerobic pathways—metabolic reactions that require oxygen. As long as the aerobic pathways are active, ST fibers can produce energy to sustain their movement. With a sufficient supply of oxygen, ST fibers can maintain muscular activity for a prolonged time. This ability is known as **aerobic endurance**.

Because ST fibers have high aerobic endurance, your body predominantly relies on them during low-intensity endurance events, such as a marathon, and during everyday activities, such as walking.

### Fast-Twitch Fibers

Compared with ST fibers, fast-twitch fibers have poor aerobic endurance. They are optimized to perform anaerobically (when the oxygen supply is limited). FT fibers can efficiently produce energy for their use via metabolic pathways that do not require oxygen. Bundles of FT fibers exert considerably more force than bundles of ST fibers; due to their limited endurance, however, FT fibers tire quickly.

The body recruits both ST and FT fibers during shorter, higher-intensity endurance events, such as the mile run or the 400-meter swim. During highly explosive events, such as the 100-meter dash and the 50-meter sprint swim, the body still recruits both types, but FT fibers contribute most of the muscle power.

### Fiber Type and the Athlete

Genes determine the relative proportion of muscle fiber types in athletes. Although distance runners who have a high percentage of ST fibers are well suited for endurance events, they will not become elite sprinters. Conversely, sprinters who have predominantly FT fibers are better equipped for explosive events, but they will not become competitive marathon runners. (See **Figure 11.10**.)

**Key Concepts** *A muscle cell is called a muscle fiber. The two main types of skeletal muscle fibers are slow-twitch and fast-twitch fibers. Slow-twitch fibers generate fuel through aerobic pathways, whereas fast-twitch fibers produce energy using anaerobic pathways. Fast-twitch fibers can exert more force but have limited endurance.*

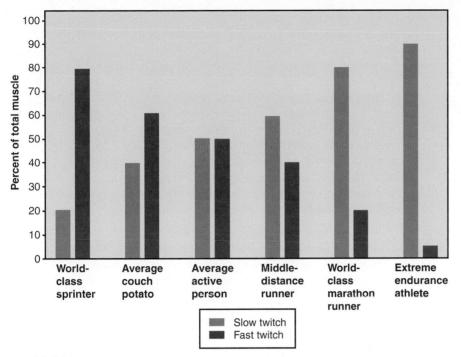

**Figure 11.10**     **What's your mix of muscle fibers?** If you are best at events requiring explosive movements, you may have a greater percentage of fast-twitch muscle fibers. If endurance events are your specialty, you may have more slow-twitch fibers.
**Source:** Adapted from Andersen JL, Scherling P, Saltin B. Muscle, genes and athletic performance. *Scientific American.* 2000;283(3):49.

## Optimal Nutrition for Athletic Performance

THINK
About It

**3**

The optimal diet for most physically active people—from the college student who plays intramural basketball to the 50-year-old woman who enjoys walking during her lunch break—includes a variety of nutrient-dense foods. Food choices should be high in carbohydrate (more than 60 percent of calories), low in fat (less than 30 percent of calories), and moderate in protein. When energy needs are met by eating a variety of foods, micronutrient (vitamins and minerals) needs are met as well.

Athletes, coaches, and scientists have long recognized that training and good nutrition go hand in hand when it comes to improving performance. An accumulating body of scientific evidence now confirms that nutrition can profoundly influence the molecular and cellular processes that occur in muscle during exercise and recovery.[17]

Optimal nutrition is an essential part of every athlete's training program and can make a difference when winning is measured in fractions of seconds or inches. General recommendations for competitive athletes include the following:[18]

- Consume adequate energy (calories) during periods of high-intensity and/or long-duration training to maintain body weight and health and to maximize training effects.
- Body weight and composition should not be the sole criterion for participation in sports; daily weigh-ins are discouraged.
- Carbohydrate recommendations for athletes range from 6 to 10 grams per kilogram body weight per day.

- Protein recommendations for endurance and strength-trained athletes range from 1.2 to 1.7 grams per kilogram body weight per day.
- Fat intake should range from 20 to 35 percent of total energy intake.
- At greatest risk of micronutrient deficiencies are athletes who restrict energy intake or use severe weight-loss practices, eliminate one or more food groups from their diet, or consume high- or low-carbohydrate diets of low micronutrient density.
- Adequate fluid intake before, during, and after exercise is important for health and optimal performance.
- In general, no vitamin and mineral supplements are required if an athlete is consuming adequate energy from a variety of foods to maintain body weight.

The underlying foundations of a training diet are similar to the basic principles incorporated in the *Dietary Guidelines for Americans* and Canada's Guidelines for Healthy Eating. The primary differences are increased fluid needs to cover an athlete's sweat losses and increased energy needs to fuel physical activity. Let's take a closer look at the nutritional needs of athletes.

## Energy Intake and Exercise

Adequate energy intake is the first nutrition priority for athletes. Meeting energy needs is critical for athletic performance and for maintaining or increasing lean body mass. Sports nutritionists recommend eating small, frequent meals to maintain energy metabolism, improve nutrient intake, achieve desired body composition, support a training schedule, and reduce injuries.[19] During times of high physical activity, energy and macronutrient needs—especially carbohydrate and protein intake—must be met in order to maintain body weight, replenish glycogen stores, and provide adequate protein for building and repairing tissues.[20]

World-class athletes who train strenuously three to four hours each day can almost double their energy needs. The energy demand can be so high that some athletes have trouble consuming enough calories.[21] In contrast, athletes who compete in sports where they are judged by build and in sports with weight classifications often restrict energy intake to avoid weight gain. Energy intakes that are too low can lead to a loss of muscle mass, menstrual dysfunction, lower bone density, and increased risk of fatigue, injury, and illness.[22]

## Carbohydrate and Exercise

Guidelines for athletes recommend high carbohydrate intakes during training.[23] A high-carbohydrate diet helps increase glycogen stores and extend endurance. (See **Figure 11.11**.) For endurance athletes, research suggests that carbohydrate should supply a minimum of 60 percent of total calories.[24] A high-carbohydrate diet also may prevent mental as well as physical fatigue and is important for stop-and-go sports such as basketball, football, and soccer.[25]

For all athletes, dietary carbohydrates should come mainly from complex carbohydrates, which provide many of the B vitamins necessary for energy metabolism, along with iron (if enriched) and fiber (if whole grain). Although added sugars should be minimized, some athletes may need to include more simple sugars to meet energy requirements.

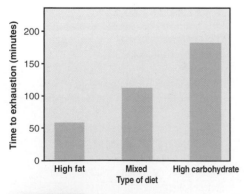

**Figure 11.11**   **Diet composition and endurance.** Athletes can exercise longer when eating a high-carbohydrate diet.

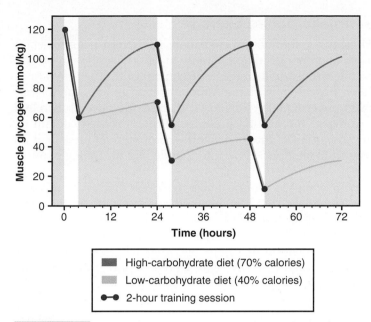

Legend:
- High-carbohydrate diet (70% calories)
- Low-carbohydrate diet (40% calories)
- 2-hour training session

**Figure 11.12** **Diet composition, training, and muscle glycogen.** A high-carbohydrate plus protein diet replenishes glycogen stores better than a low-carbohydrate diet does.

**Source:** Adapted from Ferguson-Stegall L, McCleave EL, Ding Z, et al. Postexercise carbohydrate-protein supplementation improves subsequent exercise performance and intracellular signaling for protein synthesis. *J Strength Cond Res.* 2011;24(5):1210–1224.

> **carbohydrate loading** Changes in dietary carbohydrate intake and exercise regimen before competition to maximize glycogen stores in the muscles. It is appropriate for endurance events lasting 60 to 90 consecutive minutes or longer. Also known as *glycogen loading.*
>
> **glycogen loading** See *carbohydrate loading.*

## Carbohydrate Loading

Just as you might top off the gas tank in a car before a long trip, athletes can fill their glycogen stores prior to training or competition. In a process called **carbohydrate loading**, or **glycogen loading**, athletes manipulate their carbohydrate intake and exercise regimen to maximize muscle glycogen stores. (See **Figure 11.12**.)

Current recommendations for carbohydrate loading include an intake of 60 to 70 percent of total calories from carbohydrate, along with a decrease in exercise intensity and duration prior to competition.[26] Table 11.2 is a training plan for endurance athletes that includes carbohydrate loading and exercise for the week before an event. The glycogen content of exercised muscles more than doubles in athletes who follow these recommendations, and this extends the duration of higher-intensity activity. For example, distance runners who carbohydrate-load may be able to keep a faster pace for a longer time and finish a race sooner.[27]

Even though "extra" glycogen prior to competition sounds like a perfect plan, there is a downside to carbohydrate loading. For each gram of glycogen stored in muscle tissue, the body also stores about 3 grams of water. Many athletes who carbohydrate-load complain about this weight gain and subsequent sluggishness. Some opt to train and compete without carbohydrate loading because, for them, the risk of physical discomfort outweighs the benefit of a greater carbohydrate store.

If you participate in an aerobic activity for fewer than 60 to 90 consecutive minutes, carbohydrate loading probably will provide no benefit. Instead, experts recommend that you taper your training program three to four days before competition and eat a diet that provides 70 percent of its calories from carbohydrate for one or two days before the event.[28]

**Table 11.2** **Carbohydrate-Loading Guidelines**

| Day | Training (70 percent of VO$_2$max) | Diet (g carbohydrate/ kg body weight) |
|---|---|---|
| 1 | 90 minutes | 5 |
| 2 | 40 minutes | 5 |
| 3 | 40 minutes | 5 |
| 4 | 20 minutes | 10 |
| 5 | 20 minutes | 10 |
| 6 | Rest | 10 |
| 7 | Competition | |

**Source:** Coleman EJ. Carbohydrate and exercise. In: Dunford M, ed. *Sports Nutrition: A Practice Manual for Professionals.* 4th ed. © 2006. Reprinted with permission from the Academy of Nutrition and Dietetics (formerly the American Dietetic Association).

## Carbohydrate Intake Before Exercise

Eating carbohydrate two to four hours before morning exercise helps replenish glycogen stores and improve endurance. Because many athletes have problems with GI distress, the carbohydrate and caloric content of the meal should be smaller when eaten closer to a workout. Although some athletes can tolerate solid foods, others prefer liquids to avoid GI distress. Because protein and fat take longer to digest and absorb, pre-exercise meals should contain no more than 10 to 15 percent of the total calories as protein and less than 20 percent of calories from fat. Table 11.3 offers guidelines for timing of meals before an event.

Many athletes are confused about whether to eat less than an hour before exercise. To decrease hunger, delay fatigue, and improve performance, athletes who cannot fully refuel several hours prior to a workout must rely on "last-minute" carbohydrate intake. Although early research suggested that consuming carbohydrate within one hour before activity could cause low blood glucose levels and early fatigue, later studies report no effect or no improved performance.[29]

| Table 11.3 | **Timing Meals Before Events** |

| | |
|---|---|
| **Time:** | 8 A.M. event, such as a road race or swim meet |
| **Meals:** | The night before, eat a high-carbohydrate dinner and drink extra water. The morning of the event, about 6:00 or 6:30, have a light 200- to 400-calorie meal (depending on your tolerance) such as yogurt and a banana, or one or two sports bars, and extra water. Eat familiar foods. If you want a bigger meal, you might want to get up and eat by 5:00 or 6:00. |
| **Time:** | 10 A.M. event, such as a bike race or soccer game |
| **Meals:** | The night before, eat a high-carbohydrate meal and drink extra water. The morning of the event, eat a familiar breakfast by 7:00 to allow three hours for the food to digest. This meal will prevent the fatigue that results from low blood sugar. If your body cannot handle any breakfast, eat a late snack before going to bed the night before. This will boost liver glycogen stores and prevent low blood sugar the next morning. |
| **Time:** | 2 P.M. event, such as a football or lacrosse game |
| **Meals:** | An afternoon game allows time for you to have either a big, high-carbohydrate breakfast and a light lunch, or a substantial brunch by 10:00, allowing four hours for digestion. As always, eat a high-carbohydrate dinner the night before, and drink extra fluids the day before and up to noontime. |
| **Time:** | 8 P.M. event, such as a basketball game |
| **Meals:** | A hefty, high-carbohydrate breakfast and lunch will be thoroughly digested by evening. Plan for dinner, as tolerated, by 5:00, or have a lighter meal between 6:00 and 7:00. Drink extra fluids all day. |
| **Time:** | All-day event, such as a 100-mile bike ride, triathlon training, or long, hard hike |
| **Meals:** | Two days before, cut back on your exercise; the day before, take a rest day to allow your muscles the chance to replace depleted glycogen stores. Eat carbohydrate-rich meals at breakfast, lunch, and dinner. Drink extra fluids. The day of the event, eat breakfast according to your tolerance—whatever you usually have before exercising. Throughout the day, plan to snack at least every 1.5 to 2 hours on wholesome carbohydrates to maintain a normal blood sugar. At lunchtime, eat a carbohydrate meal. Drink fluids before you get thirsty; you should need to urinate at least three times throughout the day. |

**Source:** Reprinted by permission from N. Clark, 2008, *Nancy Clark's sports nutrition guidebook*, 4th ed. (Champaign, IL: Human Kinetics), 173–175.

## *Pre-Exercise Meals and the Glycemic Index*

Independent of carbohydrate content individual foods have different effects on blood glucose levels. The glycemic index of foods is a measure of this effect and has attracted recent interest in relation to the diets of athletes. Current studies have produced mixed results, so it remains unclear whether the glycemic index of carbohydrate in pre-exercise meals affects performance.[30]

## Carbohydrate Intake During Exercise

During exercise, athletes can maintain their carbohydrate supply to exercising muscle by consuming beverages with low to moderate amounts of simple carbohydrate.[31] When an event lasts at least one hour, drinking fluids with 4 to 8 percent carbohydrate, the amount in sports drinks, enables athletes to exercise longer and sprint harder at the finish. Although sports drinks also are suitable during events lasting less than one hour, plain water is adequate for maintaining hydration during these shorter events.[32] Consuming carbohydrate before and during an event improves performance more than either strategy alone.

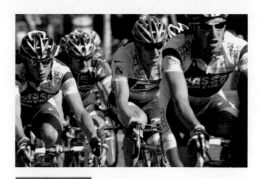

**Figure 11.13** | **Optimal nutrition.** Nutrition was an important part of Lance Armstrong's training regimen, allowing him to win the Tour de France a record seven times.

## Carbohydrate Intake Following Exercise

It can take 24 to 48 hours after an event to replenish glycogen stores, and the timing and type of carbohydrates are important factors in the refueling process. Athletes who ingest 1.5 grams of carbohydrate per kilogram body weight within 30 minutes after exercise have been shown to experience a greater rate of muscle glycogen resynthesis than when supplementation is delayed by two hours, largely due to a greater sensitivity of muscle to insulin.[33] Some research shows that the first 15 minutes are critical.[34]

The best way to replenish glycogen stores after intense exercise is to consume 1 to 1.5 grams of carbohydrate per kilogram of body weight within 30 minutes after a workout, followed by an additional 1 to 1.5 grams per kilogram two hours later.[35] A 70-kilogram (154-pound) athlete who exercises vigorously for 90 minutes or more, for example, would consume 70 to 100 grams of carbohydrate immediately after exercise, followed by another 70 to 100 grams two hours later. Consuming high-glycemic-index foods enhances glycogen synthesis.[36] Among simple sugars, glucose and sucrose appear equally effective in replenishing glycogen, but fructose alone is not as effective.[37] (See **Figure 11.13**.)

Carbohydrate intake after exercise also benefits protein metabolism. Several researchers have shown that these levels of carbohydrates taken immediately or one hour after resistance exercise decrease protein breakdown and enhance protein retention.[38]

**Key Concepts** *Energy intake is the most important element of the athlete's diet, and the major source of energy should be carbohydrates. Foods rich in complex carbohydrates, which also can provide fiber, iron, and B vitamins, are best. A high-carbohydrate diet prior to competition helps to maximize glycogen stores and endurance. Carbohydrate loading is a process of adjusting carbohydrate intake and training intensity to maximize glycogen stores just before an event. Consuming carbohydrates soon after exercise enhances the rebuilding of glycogen stores.*

# Dietary Fat and Exercise

During exercise, carbohydrates and fats are the two main fuel sources. Endurance (aerobic) training increases the capacity of your oxygen energy system, enhancing your body's ability to use fat as a fuel. Exercise intensity also affects

## Quick Bite

**The First Sports Trainers**
During the time of the ancient Olympic games, sports trainers demanded that their athletes follow strict training regimens: 10 months of regulated diet, bathing, exercise, rest, and massage. Until 480 B.C.E., Olympic athletes consumed a mostly vegetarian diet of cheese, porridge, figs, wine, and meal cakes. After twice winning the Olympic long race, however, Dromeus of Stymphalus revolutionized the ancient training diet by advocating mammoth amounts of meat and exercise.

fuel use. During low- to moderate-intensity exercise, fatty acids are the major fuel source. During high-intensity exercise, the predominant energy source is glucose.

This does not mean that endurance athletes should consume diets high in fat. High-fat diets usually are lower in carbohydrate, thus limiting muscles' ability to replenish glycogen stores. High-fat diets often are high in calories, saturated fat, and cholesterol; your body also digests fat more slowly than carbohydrate.

## Fat Intake and the Athlete

Fat intake should not be overly restricted. The acceptable macronutrient distribution range for fat intake is 20 to 35 percent of energy intake.[39] Extreme fat restriction limits food choices, especially sources of protein, iron, zinc, and essential fatty acids. In addition, athletes with high caloric needs (greater than 5,000 kilocalories per day) may find it difficult to eat enough food without consuming more than 20 to 35 percent of their calories from fat, the range recommended for the general population. Sports nutritionists recommend that any extra fat calories come from monounsaturated and polyunsaturated sources. Saturated fat intake should be limited to less than 10 percent of energy, and trans fats avoided as much as possible.

# Protein and Exercise

Historically, many athletes have believed that the best diets to help build muscle mass were based on foods from animal sources such as steak and eggs. The idea was that meat-eating athletes were stronger, more muscular, and more aggressive. Today, we know that strength and muscles are built with exercise (not extra protein) and that carbohydrates provide the fuel needed for muscle-building exercise.[40] Research suggests that athletes require only slightly higher protein intakes than sedentary people.[41]

## Protein Recommendations for Athletes

The adult Recommended Dietary Allowance (RDA) for protein is 0.8 gram of protein per kilogram of body weight per day.[42] People who regularly engage in low-intensity exercise do not need additional protein.[43]

Although the Food and Nutrition Board does not recommend a specific RDA for endurance or strength athletes, a position statement from the ASCM and the Academy of Nutrition and Dietetics recommends an upper limit of 1.7 grams of protein per kilogram per day to meet the needs of even the hardest-trained athletes.[44] Endurance athletes involved in heavy training may require 1.2 to 1.7 grams of protein per kilogram of body weight per day,[45] and resistance-trained athletes may need as much as 1.6 to 1.7 grams per kilogram of body weight.[46] Endurance athletes who are training for extreme events, such as the Tour de France, need up to 2 grams per kilogram.[47] Carbohydrate has a complementary role in muscle building. Pre-exercise ingestion of protein plus carbohydrates has been shown to produce significantly greater levels of muscle protein synthesis.[48]

An athlete's protein needs can be met easily through diet and without the use of supplements, provided that sound nutrition principles are followed and energy intake is adequate to maintain body weight.[49]

Increased protein synthesis during training is an indicator of muscle growth. Studies show that strength athletes consuming 1.4 grams of protein per kilogram of body weight per day synthesize more body protein than athletes consuming 0.9 grams. However, when protein intake was increased

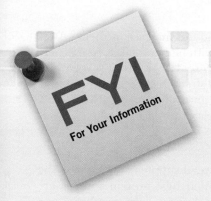

# Nutrition Periodization: Tailoring Nutrition Intake to Exercise Goals

Athletes, competitive as well as recreational, adjust their training schedules based on desired performance outcomes. Athletes are not constantly "in season," and their training during a 12-month period can be described as three phases: (1) preparation, (2) competition, and (3) transition. This concept is referred to as exercise periodization.[1]

Let's take a look at each training phase more closely:

- *Preparation:* Also called the *macrocycle*, this phase leads up to the competition phase. Training is both general and specific, with goals to improve aerobic endurance, strength, and flexibility.
- *Competition:* Also called the *mesocycle*, the performance goals during this phase are to improve strength and speed.
- *Transition:* Also called the *microcycle*, this phase is the time spent between competition and the next preparation cycle. Also referred to as the "off-season" or "active recovery," workouts in this phase are generally less structured and are intended for the athlete to improve his or her weaknesses.

During exercise periodization, an athlete's nutrition needs will change. Adjusting macronutrient (carbohydrate, fat, and protein) intake to enhance the training cycle enables athletes to provide the best combination of fuel for their bodies all year long.[2] This process is referred to as *nutrition periodization*, and it goes hand-in-hand with exercise periodization:

- *Preparation:* This is the one phase where, if needed, athletes should focus on changing their weight, body fat percentage, and/or building muscle. This is a time when habits regarding diet can be changed and an in-depth evaluation of regular dietary habits can occur. Adjustments are made within the diet to work toward a desired competition weight and/or body composition.
- *Competition:* During this phase, a routine for eating during the competition season should be well established. The focus should not be on changing weight or experimenting with different food choices. Recovery after exercise is an important focus.
- *Transition:* This is a time to focus on calorie-control and good nutrition. It is a time to experiment with and enjoy different types of foods.

Use the following as guidelines for successful nutrition periodization.[3]

### Daily Needs (No Weight Loss)

| Training Phase | Carbohydrate (g/kg) | Protein (g/kg) | Fat (g/kg) | Hydration (color of urine) |
|---|---|---|---|---|
| Preparation | 5–12+ | 1.2–1.7 | 0.8–1.0 | Lemonade |
| Pre-race | 7–13 | 1.4–2.0 | 0.8–2.0 | Lemonade |
| Race | 7–19 | 1.4–2.0 | 0.8–3.0 | Diluted lemonade |
| Transition | 5–6 | 1.2–1.4 | 0.8–1.0 | Lemonade |

### Daily Needs: Summary

| Training Phase | Daily Calorie Difference |
|---|---|
| Preparation | — |
| Pre-race | + 620–1,007 |
| Race | + 0–2,322 |
| Transition | – 620–5,101 |

### Example: 155-pound Male

| Training Phase | Carbohydrate (g)/Calories | Protein (g)/Calories | Fat (g)/Calories | Total Daily Calories |
|---|---|---|---|---|
| Preparation | 325–845+/1,408–3,380 | 85–120/340–480 | 56–70/504–630 | 2,252–4,490+ |
| Pre-race | 493–916/1,972–3,664 | 99–141/396–564 | 56–141/504–1,269 | 2,872–5,497 |
| Race | 493–1,339/1,972–5,356 | 99–151/396–564 | 56–211/504–1,899 | 2,872–7,819 |
| Transition | 352–453/340–396 | 85–99/340–396 | 56–70/504–630 | 2,252–2,718 |

1    Seebohar B. *Nutrition Periodization for Endurance Athletes.* Boulder, CO: Bull Publishing Co.; 2004. Reprinted with permission of Bull Publishing.

2    Block O, Kravitz L. Tailoring nutrient intake to exercise goals. *IDEA Fitness Journal.* 2006;3:48–55.

3    Seebohar B. *Nutrition Periodization for Endurance Athletes.* Boulder, CO: Bull Publishing Co.; 2004. Reprinted with permission of Bull Publishing.

Table 11.4 **Protein Requirements of Sedentary and Active People**

| Activity Level | Protein Requirements |
|---|---|
| Sedentary | 0.8 g/kg |
| Strength athlete | 1.6–1.7 g/kg |
| Endurance athlete | 1.2–1.4 g/kg |
| Maximum usable amount for adults | 2.0 g/kg |

**Source:** Adapted from Fink HH, Burgoon LA, Mikesky AE. *Practical Applications in Sports Nutrition.* 2nd ed. Burlington, MA: Jones & Bartlett Learning; 2009.

## *Quick* Bite

### Lost in Space
Vigorous weight training can double or triple a muscle's size, whereas the lack of use during space travel can shrink it by 20 percent in two weeks.

**diuresis** The formation and secretion of urine.

to 2.4 grams per kilogram, protein synthesis did not increase further.[50] After adjusting for higher levels of protein oxidation with higher intakes, researchers recommend that strength athletes consume 1.6 to 1.7 grams of protein per kilogram per day.[51] A 91-kilogram (200-pound) strength athlete who wants to build muscle mass would consume about 150 grams of protein. Table 11.4 shows the protein requirements of various levels of physical activity.

### Protein Intake and the Athlete

Athletes don't need protein powders or amino acid supplements to meet the protein demands of athletic performance.[52] Their best protein sources are high-quality protein foods, including legumes, low-fat dairy products, egg whites, lean beef and pork, chicken, turkey, and fish.

THINK
About It

4

Vegetarian athletes can achieve adequate protein intake and meet their energy needs by eating a variety of protein-rich foods from plant sources such as grains, nuts, beans, and seeds. Because plant proteins are less digestible than animal foods, the total amount of protein consumed may need to be somewhat higher.

### Protein Intake After Exercise

Protein combined with carbohydrate in a postexercise meal increases glycogen synthesis more than carbohydrate alone.[53] Researchers suggest athletes consume 4 grams of protein for every 10 grams of carbohydrate (grams protein = 40 percent grams carbohydrate).[54] For example, using postexercise recommendations of 1.5 grams of carbohydrate per kilogram of body weight, a 55-kilogram female athlete would need 82.5 grams of carbohydrate (55 g × 1.5 = 82.5 g) and 33 grams of protein (82.5 g × 0.40 = 33 g). How does this translate to food? A small bagel, 2 ounces of string cheese, and 8 ounces of low-fat yogurt would be a portable snack to enjoy after a hard workout (provides 86 grams of carbohydrate and 33 grams of protein). Another food that provides ample amounts of carbohydrate and protein is low-fat milk. Low-fat milk has been shown to be at least as effective as commercially available sports drinks as a rehydration beverage, if not more effective.[55] Milk is more nutrient dense than traditional sports drinks and, thus, can be a better beverage choice for individuals who partake in strength and endurance activities.

### Dangers of High Protein Intake

Excessive protein intake from food or supplements enhances **diuresis** (loss of body water) as the body attempts to excrete excess nitrogen through the urine. This increases the risk for dehydration and may contribute to mineral losses. High-protein diets often are high in saturated and total fat and may contribute to obesity, osteoporosis, heart disease, and certain types of cancer.

High intakes of single-amino-acid supplements may impair absorption of other amino acids. Further, the amount of amino acids contained in supplements is very small compared with the amount in food. For example, one pill may contain 500 milligrams of an amino acid, but 1 ounce of meat, poultry, or fish provides more than 7,000 milligrams of essential and nonessential amino acids! And, milligram for milligram, the cost of supplements is higher.

**Key Concepts** *Although fat is an important fuel for exercise, a high-fat diet is not necessary. General recommendations that fat not exceed 20 to 35 percent of total energy intake are appropriate for athletes. Dietary protein is a source of energy and also a source of amino acids for body protein synthesis. The protein requirements of athletes are slightly higher than those of sedentary adults but still within the normal range of protein consumption. High-protein diets are neither recommended nor necessary. Low-fat dairy* *products, egg whites, lean beef and pork, chicken, turkey, fish, and legumes are good sources of protein.*

# Vitamins, Minerals, and Athletic Performance

Many metabolic reactions that support exercise and physical activity require vitamins and minerals. They help extract energy from nutrients, transport oxygen, and repair tissues. Researchers have long debated whether physically active people have greater vitamin and mineral needs than sedentary people.

## B Vitamins

Because B vitamins are essential for energy metabolism, wouldn't athletes, with their high energy needs, require more B vitamins? There is no need to run to the supplement counter. B vitamins are needed for chemical reactions that release energy. But if athletes consume adequate calories and ample complex carbohydrates, fruits, and vegetables, they eat plenty of B vitamins. However, if athletes consume too few calories or eat mostly refined sugars in lieu of complex carbohydrates, they can compromise their B vitamin intake.

Vegan athletes who do not include fortified foods, such as some soy products and ready-to-eat cereals, may have a problem with vitamin $B_{12}$ intake. They should consult a medical advisor or registered dietitian to determine if they need $B_{12}$ supplements.

## Calcium

Calcium is essential for normal muscle function and strong bones. Adequate calcium intake coupled with regular exercise slows the deterioration of the skeleton with age and can reduce the risk of osteoporosis.

Inadequate calcium may increase the risk of stress fractures in athletes. This is of particular concern for the athlete suffering from amenorrhea. Athletes should strive to meet the Adequate Intake (AI) for calcium from a variety of low-fat dairy products and other calcium-rich foods. This is especially true for teens, whose calcium needs (1,300 milligrams per day) are higher than those of adults (1,000 milligrams per day).

## Iron

During endurance exercise iron is vital to oxygen delivery for aerobic energy production and may be the most critical mineral with implications for sports performance. As an essential part of hemoglobin and myoglobin, iron helps deliver oxygen to active muscle cells. It also is a key component of several enzymes vital to the production of ATP by the oxygen energy system.

Because of menstrual losses and lower dietary iron intakes, female athletes have a greater risk of iron deficiency than male athletes. In endurance athletes, the impact of running can cause mechanical trauma to capillaries in the feet and increase the breakdown of red blood cells. The increased breakdown may contribute to low iron status.[56] Some studies suggest that athletes involved in heavy training may need 30 to 70 percent more iron than nonathletes.[57] Endurance training also increases the volume of plasma in the blood without initially changing the amount of hemoglobin. This dilutes the hemoglobin, even though training typically maintains or increases the amount of total hemoglobin. This condition, called **sports anemia**, is a false anemia for most athletes and can be remedied with a few days of rest.

Although many elite athletes, especially females, have depleted iron stores (low serum ferritin), the incidence of iron-deficiency anemia in this population

**sports anemia** A lowered concentration of hemoglobin in the blood due to dilution. The increased plasma volume that dilutes the hemoglobin is a normal consequence of aerobic training.

is similar to that of the nonathletic female population.[58] In athletes with iron-deficiency anemia, supplementation has been reported to correct the anemia, which helps to improve exercise capacity.[59] Although anemia can seriously impair a person's capacity to perform activities, mild iron deficiency has little effect on athletic performance.[60]

## Other Trace Minerals

Strenuous exercise taxes the body's reserves of copper (essential for red blood cell synthesis) and zinc (vital to the work of many enzymes involved in energy production). During endurance events, increased fluid loss increases mineral losses—zinc in urine and relatively high amounts of both zinc and copper in sweat.

Although these losses may cause marginal deficiencies, supplementation is not necessarily recommended. High-dose supplements of iron, copper, or zinc can interfere with the normal absorption of these and other minerals, so an excess of one can cause a deficiency of the others. Table 11.5 is an example of a training diet that would meet an athlete's needs for vitamins and minerals through food, which is preferable to taking supplements.

**Key Concepts** *Vitamins and minerals are important components of athletes' diets. B vitamins are necessary for normal energy metabolism. Adequate calcium intake can help protect against stress fractures and, coupled with exercise, delays the onset of osteoporosis. Iron is needed to carry oxygen. Strenuous exercise can tax the body's reserves of both copper and zinc.*

## Table 11.5  A Sample Training Diet

Athlete performs prolonged daily training
Body weight = 70 kilograms
Energy intake = 3,400 kilocalories
*Macronutrients*

| Carbohydrate | Protein | Fat |
|---|---|---|
| 535 g | 128 g | 83 g |
| 63 percent kcal | 15 percent kcal | 22 percent kcal |
| 7.5 g/kg body weight[a] | 1.8 g/kg body weight[b] | |

*Breakfast*
8 oz orange juice
2 cup Cheerios cereal
8 oz 1% milk
1 large bran muffin
*Lunch*
2 slices whole wheat bread

2 oz turkey
2 slices tomato
Lettuce leaf
2 teaspoons mayonnaise

1 medium apple
12 oz cranberry juice
*Pre-exercise*
8 oz Gatorade
1 cereal bar

*Postexercise*
1 bagel
2 oz string cheese
16 oz apple juice
*Dinner*
3 oz chicken breast
1 large baked potato with 2 tablespoons low-fat sour cream
2 whole wheat dinner rolls
1 teaspoon margarine
1 cup cooked broccoli
1 cup salad greens with 2 tablespoons Italian salad dressing
8 oz 1% milk
1 cup low-fat frozen yogurt

[a] Recommended carbohydrate intake goals for prolonged daily training
[b] Recommended protein intake goals up to 2 g/kg body weight for extreme training loads

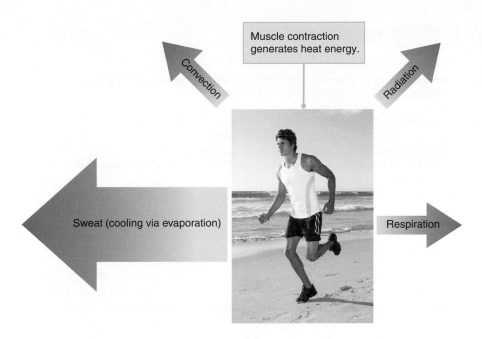

Muscle contraction generates heat energy.

Convection

Radiation

Sweat (cooling via evaporation)

Respiration

**Figure 11.14** **Dissipation of heat during exercise.** During exercise, radiation, convection, and respiration are responsible for some heat loss, but evaporation of sweat dissipates more than 80 percent of the heat generated by increased physical activity.

## Fluid Needs During Exercise

Exercise generates heat, and heavy exercise can increase heat production 15- to 20-fold. (See **Figure 11.14**.) The increase in body heat triggers sweating, and sweat cools your body as it evaporates on your skin. The body of a well-trained athlete begins to cool itself soon after exercise begins. Even before core body temperature rises, the athlete's body starts to produce sweat. Sweat rate is affected by environmental temperature (extreme heat or extreme cold), humidity (higher humidity increases the rate of sweat production but reduces efficiency of evaporation), type of clothing, fitness level, and initial fluid balance. During exercise in hot weather, the risk of dehydration and heat injury increases dramatically.[61] Normal sweat rates for athletes range from 0.5 to 2.0 liters per hour, depending on temperature, humidity, exercise intensity, and the individual's sweat response to exercise.[62]

To keep the body from overheating, blood must flow to the skin, where evaporating sweat can dissipate heat. During exercise, the cooling demand for blood flow to the skin may compete with the cardiovascular demand for blood to deliver "fuel" to working muscles. Dehydration stresses both systems, making each less efficient. Without fluid replacement during heavy exercise, athletes can become dehydrated quickly, and a water deficit of 2 percent of body weight degrades athletic performance.[63] Signs of dehydration include:

- Elevated heart rate at a given exercise intensity
- Increased rate of **perceived exertion** during activity
- Decreased performance
- Lethargy
- Concentrated urine
- Infrequent urination
- Loss of appetite

Drinking fluid during exercise helps offset fluid loss, minimize cardiovascular changes, reduce perception of effort, and maintain a supply of fuel to working muscles. When possible, athletes should drink fluid at rates that most closely match their sweat rates.[64] Because exercise inhibits the body's thirst signal, you probably won't take in enough fluid if you wait until you feel

**perceived exertion** The subjective experience of how difficult an effort is.

| Table 11.6 | **Typical Fluid Needs** |

| Activity Level | Environment | Fluid Requirements (liters per day) |
|---|---|---|
| Sedentary | Cool | 2–3 |
| Active | Cool | 3–6 |
| Sedentary | Warm | 3–5 |
| Active | Warm | 5–10+ |

**Note:** Fluid requirements include fluid from all sources—liquids, food, and metabolic water.

**Source:** Adapted from Murray R. Drink more! Advice from a world-class expert. *ACSM's Health and Fitness Journal.* 1997;1:19–23, 50.

thirsty to replenish your losses. Table 11.6 shows how much fluid a person should drink at various levels of physical activity.

## Hydration

Active people must train themselves to consume adequate amounts of fluid before, during, and after exercise. Each person will have different water electrolyte losses based on factors such as body weight, genetic makeup, and metabolism, so each person should customize his or her hydration strategies.[65] Specific formulas and calculations are available to guide individuals in assessing these factors.[66]

The goal of hydrating before exercise is to start the physical activity with normal plasma electrolyte levels.[67] When hydrating before exercise, individuals should slowly drink beverages at least four hours before the exercise task.[68] Consuming beverages with sodium can help to stimulate thirst and retain needed fluids.[69] Because even partial dehydration can compromise performance (see Table 11.7), athletes should maintain fluid balance during the event.

The goal of drinking during exercise is to prevent excessive dehydration (> 2 percent body weight loss) and excessive changes in electrolyte balance.[70] It is difficult to recommend a specific fluid and electrolyte replacement schedule because of the nature of different exercise tasks, weather conditions, and other factors. Individuals should develop customized fluid-replacement programs that prevent excessive dehydration. If time permits, consumption of

| Table 11.7 | **Adverse Effects of Dehydration on Exercise and Performance** |

| Percent Body Weight Loss | Adverse Effects on Performance |
|---|---|
| 1 | The thirst threshold. Leads to decrease in physical work capacity. |
| 2 | Stronger thirst, vague discomfort, loss of appetite. |
| 3 | Dry mouth, increasing hemoconcentration, reduction in urine output. |
| 4 | Decrease of 20–30 percent in physical work capacity. |
| 5 | Difficulty concentrating, headache, sleepiness. |
| 6 | Severe impairment in ability to regulate body temperature during exercise; increased respiratory rate, leading to tingling and numbness of extremities |
| 7 | Collapse is likely if combined with heat and exercise. |

## *Quick* Bite

**Sweating a World Record**
When Alberto Salazar ran the Olympic marathon in 1984, he went down in the record books for sweat production. He lost 12 pounds during the 26.2-mile race, despite drinking about 2 liters. His sweat rate was approximately 3.7 liters per hour.

normal meals and beverages will restore hydration status. Individuals who require rapid recovery from excessive dehydration can drink approximately 1.5 liters of fluid for each kilogram of body weight lost.[71] Consuming beverages and snacks that contain sodium will help expedite rapid and complete recovery by stimulating thirst and fluid retention.[72]

Should athletes choose water, sports drinks, or other beverages? During activities that last fewer than 60 continuous minutes, water can replace fluid lost in sweat and help offset the rise in core temperature.

During exercise that lasts longer than 60 continuous minutes, muscle and liver glycogen stores become depleted. Consuming fluids that contain carbohydrate and sodium can delay fatigue (see **Figure 11.15**), enhance palatability of fluids, and promote fluid retention.[73]

Optimal sports drinks provide energy (from glucose, glucose polymers, or sucrose) and electrolytes in a **palatable** solution that promotes rapid absorption (less than 10 percent carbohydrate concentration). (See Table 11.8.) The palatability of beverages containing electrolytes and 4 to 8 percent carbohydrate may increase the voluntary intake of fluid.[74] Beverages such as fruit juices and soft drinks are concentrated sources of carbohydrates (more than 10 percent) and may slow gastric emptying. In juices and many soft drinks, the main carbohydrate is fructose, which is associated with slower stomach emptying and abdominal cramps. Carbonated soft drinks may decrease the volume of fluid consumed and delay stomach emptying.

Athletes should avoid beverages that contain alcohol. Some athletes use alcohol for psychological benefits—calming nerves, improving self-confidence, and reducing anxiety, pain, and muscle tremor. This misguided effort fails to recognize alcohol's negative influence on physical performance. Alcohol slows reaction time, impairs coordination, and upsets balance. Its diuretic action contributes to dehydration and may impair regulation of body temperature.

For endurance events that last longer than four to five hours (or shorter events in high heat and humidity), athletes who do not replace electrolytes put themselves at risk for abnormally low levels of blood sodium. This life-threatening condition is associated with an excessive loss of electrolytes in sweat and with the excessive consumption of fluid, such as plain water, that does not replace electrolytes. See Table 11.9 for a summary of the American College of Sports Medicine's position on the amount and type of fluid to consume before, during, and after activity.

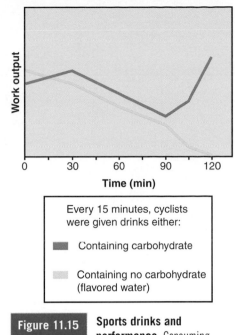

Every 15 minutes, cyclists were given drinks either:

■ Containing carbohydrate

■ Containing no carbohydrate (flavored water)

**Figure 11.15** **Sports drinks and performance.** Consuming carbohydrate drinks dramatically increases power output after 90 minutes.

**Table 11.8**  **Desirable Composition of Sports Beverages**

| Characteristic | Comment |
| --- | --- |
| Fuel source | Contains carbohydrate: glucose, sucrose, and glucose polymers (maltodextrin). Goal intake is 60–70 g/hr (approximately 1 liter of a 6–8 percent carbohydrate drink). |
| Electrolytes | Contains sodium (70–165 mg per 240 mL) and potassium (30–75 mg per 240 mL) to replace sweat electrolyte loss when exercise is longer than 3–4 hours. Electrolytes also enhance palatability. |
| Rapid absorption | Contains 6–8 percent carbohydrate. Higher carbohydrate concentration slows gastric emptying and intestinal absorption. |
| Palatability | Flavored beverages enhance consumption. Electrolytes enhance flavor. Carbonation may decrease amount of fluid consumed. |

**palatable** Pleasant tasting.

| Table 11.9 | American College of Sports Medicine Position on Fluid Replacement |
|---|---|

**Before Activity or Competition**
- Drink adequate fluids during the 24 hours before an event, especially during the meal before exercise, to promote proper hydration before exercise or competition.
- Drink about 500 milliliters (~17 ounces) of fluid about two hours before exercise to promote adequate hydration and allow time for excretion of excess ingested water.

**During Activity or Competition**
- Start drinking early and at regular intervals to consume fluids at a rate sufficient to replace all the water lost through sweating or consume the maximal amount that can be tolerated.
- Fluids should be cooler than ambient temperature and flavored to enhance palatability and promote fluid replacement.

**During Competition That Lasts More Than One Hour**
- To maintain blood glucose concentration and delay the onset of fatigue, the fluid replacement should contain 4 to 8 percent carbohydrate. Electrolytes (primarily salt) are added to make the solution taste better and reduce the risk of low blood levels of sodium. About 0.5 to 0.7 grams of sodium per liter of water replaces sodium lost by sweating.

**Following Activity or Competition**
- Complete restoration of the extracellular fluid compartment cannot be sustained without replacement of lost sodium.
- For each pound (0.45 kilograms) of body weight lost, consume at least 2 cups (0.47 liters) of fluid.
- Thirst sensation is not an adequate gauge of dehydration, and postexercise consumption stimulates obligatory urine losses. Research shows that drinking an amount of liquid that is 125 to 150 percent of fluid loss is usually enough to promote complete rehydration.

Source: Adapted from American College of Sports Medicine position stand. Exercise and fluid replacement. *Med Sci Sports Exerc.* 2007;39:377–390.

## Nutrition Needs of Youth in Sport

Young athletes (younger than 19 years) should place a higher priority on nutritional needs for growth and development than on athletic performance.[75] Studies indicate that young athletes' diets are often marginal or inadequate with regard to energy intake.[76] The consequences of chronic low energy intake include:[77]

- Short stature and delayed puberty
- Nutrient deficiencies and dehydration
- Menstrual irregularities
- Poor bone health
- Increased incidence of injuries
- Increased risk of developing eating disorders

Parents and youth need to understand the energy and nutrient demands of growth and training, and many need help in planning meals and snacks to meet those needs. Many sport activities for this age group take place after school, and some schools serve lunch as early as 10:45 A.M. To provide energy for the activity and nutrients for recovery, young people should have meals and snacks before and after exercise. Easily portable snacks include fruit, pretzels, dry cereal, cereal bars, yogurt, sports drinks, sandwiches, and milk. Young athletes must drink adequate fluids during the day as well as at practice and competition. This is especially important because youths have

*Quick* Bite

**Training: Young at Heart or Skeletal Old Age?**
With endurance training, younger athletes largely achieve improvements as a result of increased cardiac output. Older athletes show greater improvement in the activities of the oxidative enzymes in their skeletal muscles.

a high tolerance for exercising in heat, which puts them at increased risk for heat exhaustion and heatstroke.

**Key Concepts** *Exercise of any type increases fluid losses through sweat. Evaporation of sweat from the skin allows the body to cool itself. Fluid losses must be replaced to avoid dehydration. Athletes need to drink plenty of fluid before, during, and after exercise. Fluid choices depend on the duration of activity and the preferences of the athlete. Optimal sports drinks provide energy and electrolytes in a solution that promotes rapid absorption. Nutrient intakes by young athletes must support both competition and continued growth.*

## Nutrition Supplements and Ergogenic Aids

The pressure to win contributes to athletes' search for a competitive edge. Supplement use (i.e., for the purpose of enhancing athletic performance) is increasing among adolescent and collegiate athletes, and the average age for first time use is decreasing.[78] More than 75 percent of recreational and elite athletes use nutritional supplements and **ergogenic aids** with the expectation of improved performance,[79] and more than 30 percent of American male and female adolescents are reported to use high-energy drinks and capsules on a regular basis.[80] Nutrition supplements and ergogenic aids include products and practices that:

- Provide calories (e.g., liquid supplements, energy bars)
- Provide vitamins and minerals (including multivitamin supplements)
- Contribute to performance during exercise and enhance recovery after exercise (e.g., sports drinks, carbohydrate supplements)
- Are believed to stimulate and maintain muscle growth (e.g., purified amino acids)[81]
- Contain micronutrients, herbal, and/or cellular components that are promoted as ergogenic aids to enhance performance (e.g., caffeine, chromium picolinate, creatine)[82]
- Are used for nutritional, physiological, psychological, biomechanical, or pharmacological reasons (see Table 11.10)

Most nutritional supplements are unnecessary for athletes who select a variety of foods and meet their energy needs. However, iron and calcium

**ergogenic aids** Substances that can enhance athletic performance.

| Table 11.10 | **Types of Ergogenic Aids** |

| Type | Description | Examples |
|---|---|---|
| Nutritional | Any supplement, food product, manipulation that enhances work capacity or athletic performance | Carbohydrate loading; amino or dietary acid or vitamin supplements |
| Physiological | Any practice or substance that enhances the functioning of the body's various systems (e.g., cardiovascular, muscular) and, thus, improves athletic performance | Any type of physical training (e.g., endurance, strength), blood doping via transfusions, warming up and/or stretching |
| Psychological | Any practice or treatment that changes mental state and, thereby, enhances sport performance | Visualization, hypnosis, pep talks, relaxation techniques |
| Biomechanical | Any device, piece of equipment, or external product that can be used to improve athletic performance during practice or competition | Weight belts, knee wraps, oversize tennis rackets, body suits (swimming/track) |
| Pharmacological | Any substance or compound classified as a drug or hormonal agent that is used to improve output and/or sport performance | Hormones (e.g., growth hormones, anabolic steroids), caffeine output, and/or sport performance |

supplements may be recommended for female athletes if their diets are low in these nutrients. Liquid supplements and sports bars that contain carbohydrates, proteins, and fats can provide an easy way to increase energy intake. Sports drinks, gels, and recovery drinks also can contribute to needed fluids and carbohydrates before, during, and after exercise.

Dietary supplements marketed as performance enhancers are another matter. Herbals, glandulars, enzymes, hormones, and other compounds aimed at athletes carry many attractive claims. Although some products have been well researched, most lack vigorous clinical trials to evaluate efficacy, apply to only one gender (usually males), or are relevant to only one sport (e.g., weight lifting).

## Regulation and Concerns of Dietary and Herbal Supplements

All prescription and over-the-counter drugs and food additives must meet the Food and Drug Administration's (FDA) safety and effectiveness requirements. Dietary supplements, however, bypass these regulations. Before 1994, when the Dietary Supplement Health and Education Act (DSHEA) was signed into law, dietary supplements were regulated in the same manner as other foods. Prior to the DSHEA, many people felt that the FDA was too restrictive in regulating dietary supplements. As a result, the DSHEA was passed and dietary supplements were placed in a special category of "foods."[83] To market a supplement, the manufacturer must have evidence that the ingredients sold in their supplements are generally safe if required to do so by the FDA, and they must follow Good Manufacturing Practice Guidelines.

Manufacturers themselves have the responsibility to determine and communicate product safety, as well as defend any representations or claims made about the product and show that the claims are not false or misleading.[84] DSHEA requires supplement manufacturers to include the following information on the label: "This statement has not been evaluated by the FDA. This product is not intended to diagnose, treat, cure, or prevent any disease."[85] Over the last 10 to 15 years, in an effort to abide by the DSHEA requirements and to follow the Good Manufacturing Practice Guidelines, a number of supplement companies have employed teams of researchers (many of whom are MS- or PhD-prepared exercise physiologists or sports nutrition specialists) who help educate the public about nutrition and exercise, provide input on product development, conduct preliminary research on products, or assist in coordinating research trials conducted by independent research teams.[86]

Although laws exist to ensure product safety and reliability, there is still room for discrepancy between the actual content of supplements and what is reported on the label. Results of an extensive survey conducted in a laboratory in Germany looked at the prevalence of supplements contaminated with products not listed on their product labels. A total of 634 different product samples were purchased from 13 countries around the world. These were analyzed for the presence of steroid hormones and their precursors. Ninety-four supplements (14.8 percent of the total) were shown to contain prohibited substances. For another 10 percent, the analysis was inconclusive, but steroids may have been present. That is close to a one-in-four risk! Substantial numbers of positive tests were obtained from products bought in the Netherlands (26 percent), the United States (19 percent), United Kingdom (19 percent), and elsewhere. The names of the prohibited supplements have not been published, but they included vitamins and minerals, protein supplements, creatine, and many others.[87]

Two important conclusions can be drawn from the preceding information: (1) many supplements that people purchase online or in health food stores are produced in countries where product contamination has been found and where industry quality control points are often minimal, and (2) dietary supplements may contain substances not shown on the package label that may be harmful or can lead to a positive doping test in sport competitions.

Given the documented widespread contamination of nutritional supplements,[88] high-performing athletes are generally advised to stay away from supplements. This recommendation should not, however, be confused with responsible and educated use of supplements, if and when indicated. In fact, the Academy of Nutrition and Dietetics, the Dieticians of Canada, and the American College of Sports Medicine issued a joint position statement, published in 2009, regarding nutrition and athletic performance.[89] This position indicates that physical performance and recovery are enhanced by optimal nutrition, and even though athletes with an adequate diet normally do not need supplementation, it may be needed if energy intake is restricted or groups of food are eliminated from their diet.

A 2009 federal report addressed growing concerns about the supplement industry and underreporting of adverse events resulting from supplement use.[90] As a result, new changes to the industry's self-regulation may be on the horizon.

## Convenience Supplements

Convenience supplements are meal replacement powders, ready-to-drink supplements, energy bars, and energy gels. They represent the largest segment of the nutrition industry, claiming 50 to 75 percent of most company's sales.[91] They typically are fortified with 33 to 50 percent of the RDA for vitamins and minerals and generally differ on the amount of carbohydrate, protein, and fat they contain.[92] For use in sports nutrition, convenience supplements are best suited to provide carbohydrate, protein, and other nutrients prior to or following exercise in situations in which the athlete does not have time to choose, prepare, and eat a regular meal. They are most appropriately used to improve availability of macronutrients, not as a replacement for a day of good eating.

## Weight-Gain Powders

One common way athletes try to increase muscle mass is to add extra calories from protein to their diet. Studies have consistently shown that adding an extra 500 to 1,000 calories per day to your diet will promote significant weight gain,[93] and protein powders are a relatively easy way to do just that. However, only about 30 to 50 percent of the weight gained on high-calorie diets is muscle, while the remaining amount of weight gained is fat.[94] There is no evidence that increasing protein intake above recommended levels improves muscle growth; however, protein supplements may be useful to meet body needs for athletes whose protein intake is inadequate in their overall diet.[95] Remember, it is adequate resistance training fueled by sufficient calorie intake, along with adequate rest between training sessions, that promotes muscle formation, not protein intake alone. Because the extra calories in high-protein intake may increase body fat rather than muscle mass, caution should be used with this approach to weight gain.

## Amino Acids

Researchers have studied the use of individual amino acids to enhance performance and have not found obvious benefits. *Branched-chain amino acids*

## *Quick* Bite

(BCAAs) often are used as an anticatabolic compound in an effort to decrease the breakdown of body tissue. The BCAAs leucine, isoleucine, and valine are reported to aid in endurance exercise by counteracting central fatigue, possibly by interfering with tryptophan kinetics or other mechanisms, thus improving performance.[96] Supplements containing BCAAs may prove to be helpful for sports such as tennis, soccer, distance running, cycling, and swimming. The research has been conflicting, and further study is needed.[97] Because safety and effectiveness have not been established, BCAA supplements are not recommended.

*HMB*, also known as hydroxymethylbutyrate, beta-hydroxyisovalerate, and 3-hydroxyisovalerate, is a metabolite of the essential branched-chain amino acid leucine. It is found in foods such as catfish, citrus fruits, and breast milk.[98] HMB is promoted as an "anticatabolic" agent that suppresses protein breakdown and cellular damage after intense exercise, thereby allowing quicker recovery and increased lean body mass and strength.[99]

*Glutamine*, a dispensable amino acid, is a popular supplement for strength athletes. Proponents of glutamine supplements suggest that intense weight training produces catabolic effects on muscle protein and therefore would increase glutamine requirements. However, supplementation studies have not supported an ergogenic effect of glutamine supplementation.[100] Glutamine is also known to be used by immune cells, and some athletes use supplements enriched with glutamine in an attempt to optimize immune function.[101]

## Creatine

**Creatine**, a nitrogenous compound in meats and fish, is synthesized by the liver, pancreas, and kidney. Muscles store creatine mainly as creatine phosphate, which functions as part of the ATP–CP energy system. Creatine has become a popular supplement based on the theory that increasing muscle creatine would prolong short-term energy availability and, thus, improve performance in short-term, high-intensity activities (such as weight lifting).[102] Several well-controlled studies have shown improvements in muscle strength when creatine supplementation was added to a strength training regimen.[103] Creatine supplements also may improve the explosive power needed for sprints.[104] However, creatine supplements appear to have no benefit for aerobic training.

The main side effect seems to be immediate weight gain attributable to water retention. Anecdotal reports frequently cite gastrointestinal side effects, including nausea, diarrhea, dyspepsia, and abdominal pain, possibly due to malabsorption of high doses of creatine.[105] Other reported adverse effects include rash, dyspnea, anxiety, headache, and fatigue.[106] The *Physician's Desk Reference* states that contraindications to creatine use include kidney failure and other kidney disorders, and that creatine should be avoided in children, adolescents, pregnant women, nursing mothers, diabetics, and other persons at risk for kidney disease.[107]

Increases in muscle mass are probably a response to the increased stress that an athlete can put on muscle tissue by maximal exercise bursts—the supplement without weight training will have no effect. Also, the ability to store more CP may vary widely among people, so supplements may not be effective for everyone.

With the increasing popularity of creatine supplementation, long-term safety has been questioned. Anecdotal reports of muscle cramps, muscle strains, kidney dysfunction, and GI distress have raised concerns. However, college football players who have used creatine for as long as five years have not shown any negative health effects, including no detrimental effects on liver

**creatine** An important nitrogenous compound found in meats and fish and synthesized in the body from amino acids (glycine, arginine, and methionine).

or kidney function.[108] In another study of college football players, creatine supplementation during training did not increase the risk of muscle cramping or injury.[109] Nevertheless, the FDA has advised consumers to consult a physician before they use creatine.

## Antioxidants

As we exercise, our muscles consume more oxygen than when we are at rest. Increased oxygen consumption leads to increased production of free radicals. Free radicals can damage cell membranes and DNA, leading to conditions such as cancer, aging, and a number of degenerative diseases. So, exercise promotes health, but it may also increase cell damage.

Antioxidants, which are compounds that seek out and neutralize free radicals, may protect muscles and cells from the damage that can result from exercise.[110] Antioxidants come in different forms, such as vitamins, minerals, enzyme complexes, and herbs. Vitamin C, vitamin E, and beta-carotene are well-known antioxidants. Antioxidants can be obtained via food or supplements. Examples of good food sources of antioxidants include deep orange- and green colored vegetables, citrus fruits, whole grains, and green tea.

People who exercise infrequently or sporadically, as well as those who exercise intensely and for long periods of time, have higher risk for damage than those who exercise regularly and on a more moderate schedule. Studies show that regular, moderate exercise enhances the antioxidant defense system and protects against exercise-induced free radical damage. In contrast, intense exercise in untrained individuals overwhelms the body's defenses, resulting in increased free radical damage.

Does supplementing with antioxidants or eating foods rich in antioxidants repair free radical damage after exercise? The answer is complex. Nutrition deficiencies can create difficulties in training and recovery (possibly due to free radical damage); however, the role of antioxidant supplementation in a well-nourished athlete is controversial. It is not necessary, or advisable, for a well-nourished athlete to take antioxidant supplements.[111]

Regarding antioxidants and exercise, the best recommendation goes back to the basics: follow a balanced training program that emphasizes regular exercise, and eat five servings of fruits or vegetables each day. These practices will ensure that you are developing your antioxidant systems and that your diet is providing the necessary components.

## Caffeine

Caffeine is a natural stimulant. Research suggests that caffeine may affect athletic performance by facilitating signals between the nervous system and the muscles as well as by decreasing an athlete's perceived effort during exercise. Caffeine also may increase the body's ability to break down fat for energy. Evidence suggests that caffeine enhances endurance and provides a small, but worthwhile, enhancement of performance over a range of exercise protocols, from short-duration, high-intensity events to ultra-endurance events.[112] In studies that examined prolonged exercise lasting 60 minutes or longer, the beneficial effects from caffeine intake occurred at small to moderate levels of intake (1–3 milligrams per kilogram body weight or a total of 70 to 150 milligrams caffeine) and when caffeine was ingested at a variety of times (before and/or throughout exercise or toward the end of exercise when the athlete was becoming fatigued).[113]

Caffeine may produce ergogenic effects at doses as low as 250 milligrams (3.0 to 3.5 milligrams per kilogram body weight).[114] Most studies showing benefit used doses of around 400 to 600 milligrams,[115] and, on a bodyweight basis, a reasonable dose would be 5 milligrams per kilogram.[116] In the past, caffeine was banned by the World Anti-Doping Agency (WADA) above a threshold urinary concentration, but in 2007 the WADA declared it legal at any level.[117] However, the National Collegiate Athletic Association (NCAA) has set an upper legal limit of 15 micrograms per milliliter in urine.[118] The ergogenic benefits of caffeine use may depend on abstinence for several days before,[119] and its effect is more pronounced in relative nonusers (< 50 milligrams per day) than in regular users (> 300 milligrams per day).[120] A 100-milligram dose of caffeine increases urine levels by approximately 1.5 milligrams per milliliter; therefore, 800 to 1,000 milligrams would need to be ingested to approach the legal limit.[121]

Caution should be taken when consuming beverages that contain caffeine. At high levels of intake, caffeine has the potential to increase heart rate, impair or alter fine-motor control and technique, interfere with sleep patterns, and affect recovery between training sessions. It is important to find the lowest effective dose of caffeine that can be used to achieve performance enhancement.[122] No evidence suggests that performance increases with increases in caffeine intake, and long-term intake of large amounts of caffeine (> 500 milligrams per day) is generally discouraged.[123]

## Ephedrine

Ephedrine was a popular ergogenic supplement until its sale in the United States was prohibited by the FDA.[124] Despite its previous ban by the NFL, NCAA, and IOC, athletes continued to use ephedrine, either as a weight-loss aid or to gain a performance edge. Ephedrine stimulates the central nervous system and is an effective bronchodilator. In addition, it raises both heart rate and blood pressure. Athletes hoped its stimulatory effects would improve performance, suppress appetite, and promote weight loss. Some studies support these purported benefits, especially when ephedrine is combined with caffeine.[125]

Ephedrine became one of the most controversial supplements on the market. Found in many products as either the herbal ma huang (ephedra) or the synthetic ephedrine, serious side effects such as hypertension, insomnia, anxiety, tremors, headache, dependence, psychosis, nephrolithiasis, seizures, arrhythmias, strokes, myocardial infarction, and even death have been attributed to this supplement.[126] When the 2003 heatstroke-related death of Major League Baseball pitcher Steve Bechler was linked to ephedra use, sports organizations and other groups began to pay more attention. A government-sponsored review of safety and efficacy concluded that the use of ephedrine, ephedra-containing dietary supplements, or ephedrine plus caffeine is associated with two to three times the risk of nausea, vomiting, psychiatric symptoms such as anxiety and change in mood, autonomic hyperactivity, and palpitations.[127] Studies such as this led to the FDA's conclusion that ephedrine posed an unreasonable risk of illness and injury. Although prohibited by the FDA, ephedrine is still available to athletes via the Internet. Ephedra's risks clearly outweigh its benefits, however.

## Sodium Bicarbonate

**soda loading** Consumption of bicarbonate (baking soda) to raise blood pH. The intent is to increase the capacity to buffer acids, thus delaying fatigue. Also known as *bicarbonate loading*.

Some athletes consume sodium bicarbonate (baking soda) in the belief that it will help neutralize the buildup of lactic acid in muscles. Whether **soda loading** actually produces an ergogenic effect is controversial. Sodium bicarbonate ingestion has been shown to improve performance in single-bout, high-intensity events, probably due to an increase in buffering capacity.[128]

Likewise, studies that have evaluated events lasting from 2 to 10 minutes, where lactic acid buildup is most likely, have shown some positive results related to interval-training performance.[129]

Bicarbonate loading can also produce negative effects. Athletes who follow this regimen report side effects such as intestinal discomfort, stomach distress, nausea, cramping, diarrhea, and water retention. Although bicarbonate loading is not banned, it does have serious health-related consequences. Bicarbonate loading increases blood alkalinity and influences blood pressure. Anyone with high blood pressure (hypertension) should not bicarbonate-load.

## Chromium

The trace mineral chromium is vital to the movement of glucose into cells. Because of the link between chromium, glucose use, and insulin, chromium has become a popular supplement (typically in the form of chromium picolinate) for both weight loss and athletic performance. The theory is that by enhancing insulin action, chromium increases amino acid uptake, which then increases protein synthesis and promotes a gain in muscle mass.

Although the developers of the chromium picolinate supplements had promising results in several studies, a review of 24 studies found no significant reduction in body fat or increase in lean muscle mass.[130] Chromium supplementation does not appear to enhance body composition or performance in well-trained individuals.[131] Given these results and the potential risks from chromium picolinate supplementation, this supplement cannot be recommended.

## Iron

Iron supplements are used commonly by athletes for performance enhancement, a practice that can be helpful or harmful. In the presence of iron-deficiency anemia, which is more common in young athletes than in the general population, supplementation is clearly beneficial for performance.[132] In athletes, however, the diagnosis can be difficult to establish. The reason is that in response to training, hemoglobin concentration decreases as the plasma volume expands to a greater degree than does red cell mass, resulting in sports anemia. An elevated serum transferrin receptor level is an indicator of iron deficiency in athletes. Studies of iron supplementation showed objective performance improvement only in athletes who had iron-deficiency anemia or untrained individuals with low ferritin levels.[133] Athletes with normal or low ferritin levels do not benefit from supplementation.[134] Iron supplementation does not come without risks. Complications of iron overload include hemochromatosis.[135]

## Green Tea Extract

Because of claims that it can assist weight loss, green tea is more commonly used as an herbal supplement.[136] Caffeine is naturally present in green tea, and it is theorized that it is the combination of caffeine and green tea catechin that increases energy expenditure and promotes fat oxidation.[137] One study demonstrated that green tea catechin consumption enhanced exercise-induced changes in abdominal fat.[138] However, it must be noted that both human and animal studies have not supported these findings and have reported that supplementation of these extracts does not affect weight loss.[139] More research is necessary to determine if green tea extract contributes to improved exercise performance.

**anabolic steroids** Several compounds derived from testosterone or prepared synthetically. They promote body growth and masculinization and oppose the effects of estrogen.

**Key Concepts** *Numerous dietary supplements, such as those containing caffeine, chromium, creatine, and antioxidants, are marketed for performance-enhancing effects. However, few have been subjected to rigorous clinical trials or long-term safety evaluation. Athletes should consult a physician before adding dietary supplements to their training regimen.*

## Weight and Body Composition

Pete, a bodybuilder, wants to bulk up by gaining 15 pounds of muscle and not fat. Sarah, on the other hand, wants to compete as a lightweight rower and needs to lose 7 pounds. Some athletes struggle to lose weight, but others find it nearly impossible to gain weight and muscle mass. Whether intentionally gaining or losing weight, weight change should be accomplished slowly—during the off-season or at the beginning of the season before competition starts.

Body composition and body weight are just two of many factors that affect exercise performance. Body composition can affect strength, agility, and appearance. Body weight can influence speed, endurance, and power. Because body fat adds weight without adding strength, many sports emphasize low body fat percentages. Yet, by themselves, body composition and body weight do not accurately predict athletic performance.[140]

### Weight Gain: Build Muscle, Lose Fat

Weight gain is influenced by genetics, stage of adolescent development, gender, body mass, diet, training program, prior resistance training, motivation, and use of supplements and **anabolic steroids**, among other factors. Complex interactions among these factors make it difficult to predict an athlete's ability to meet a weight goal. However, experience tells us the following:

- Untrained male athletes can gain approximately 3 to 4 pounds of lean body mass per month in the early stages of a rigorous resistance-training program.[141] Because of their smaller muscle mass and lean tissue, young women can achieve only 50 to 75 percent of the gains seen in male counterparts but with the same relative strength.
- Approximately 20 percent of the increase in lean body mass occurs in the first year of resistance training, tapering to 1 to 3 percent in subsequent years. Scientists believe that the rate declines as muscle mass approaches the maximum potential amount determined by genetics.
- Some male athletes of high school age have difficulty gaining muscle mass. These athletes may be in the early stages of the adolescent growth spurt and may lack sufficient levels of the male hormones to stimulate muscle development.

Nutrition plays an important role in increasing lean body mass. Athletes must consume enough calories, along with adequate carbohydrate and protein, to gain the desired muscle mass.[142]

**Key Concepts** *Athletes often seek to improve their power and strength by increasing muscle mass. Weight gain as muscle requires increased dietary calories, primarily as carbohydrate, combined with strength training.*

### Weight Loss: The Panacea for Optimal Performance?

As the pressure to win increases, many coaches and athletes come to believe that weight loss and lower body fat composition will provide that competitive

*Quick* Bite

**What's the Best "Fat-Burning" Exercise?**
It's a common misconception that low-intensity exercise is superior for "fat burning." Aerobic activities do use a greater percentage of fat as fuel, but it is the total amount of calories expended during exercise that supports increased mobilization of fat in response to a caloric deficit. In terms of actual energy expenditure, higher-intensity exercise requires more calories for a given time period than exercise at a lower intensity. Thus, to lose body fat, the fuel (source of calories) is not as important as the amount of energy expended.

edge. Athletes strive for lower body weight and lower body fat for three reasons: (1) to improve appearance, especially in aesthetic sports (e.g., diving, figure skating, gymnastics); (2) to enhance performance where lower body weight may increase speed (e.g., race walking, running, pole vaulting, jumping, cross-country skiing); or (3) to qualify in a lower weight category (e.g., wrestling, boxing, and rowing).[143] **Figure 11.16** illustrates the key factors in a successful weight-loss program.

As healthy young adults, men average 15 percent body fat and women average 25 percent.[144] Although these averages provide starting points, recommendations for individual athletes must account for genetic background, age, gender, sport, health, and weight history. Male athletes should not go below 5 to 7 percent body fat. For female athletes, current research data suggest a minimum 13 to 17 percent body fat to maintain normal menstrual function, which in turn is important for maintaining bone health.[145]

Keeping accurate food and training records provides information on energy intake and expenditure. The best way for athletes to sustain a safe and sensible loss of body fat is to reduce calorie intake moderately and modify the training program. A combination of resistance training and aerobic activity is best for weight loss because it helps maintain or even increase lean body mass while simultaneously decreasing fat mass.

Beware of "fad" weight-loss methods such as ketogenic diets, high-protein diets, and semistarvation diets. These practices can compromise energy reserves, body composition, and psychological well-being, leading to decreased performance and increased health risks. Athletes often are alert to the latest supplements to hit the market. Many claim to accelerate the burning of body fat and augment weight loss. In reality, studies show that most "fat burners" are ineffective or associated with only very modest weight loss in obese subjects.[146]

**Key Concepts** *Before embarking on a weight-loss program, athletes should carefully evaluate their goals and set a realistic plan for weight loss and maintenance. Safe weight-loss practices include modest changes in food intake accompanied by gradual increases in aerobic activity.*

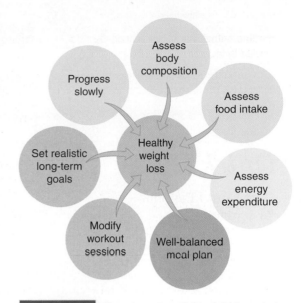

**Figure 11.16**   **Keys to successful weight loss.** Just as athletes focus on proper training techniques to avoid injury and improve performance, they should focus on proper weight-loss strategies to lose weight and maintain health.

## Weight Loss: Negative Consequences for the Competitive Athlete?

Changing body size and shape can have detrimental effects. An unrealistic perception of optimal body weight and a belief that weight loss is necessary for improved performance can contribute to unhealthy weight-loss practices.[147] Athletes risk medical problems when dieting goes awry.

### Making Weight

Wrestlers, weight lifters, boxers, jockeys, rowers, and coxswains face competitive pressures to "make weight" to compete or to be certified in a lower weight classification. Such athletes often resort to the **pathogenic** weight-control behaviors summarized in Table 11.11. Repeated cycles of rapid weight loss and subsequent regain increase risk of disordered eating, fatigue, psychological distress (e.g., anger, anxiety, depression), dehydration, and sudden death.

Studies show that wrestlers, in attempts to gain a competitive advantage, will try to reduce weight a few days before or on the day of competition.[148] Athletes can achieve weight loss of up to 22 pounds (10 kilograms) of body water in one day by fasting, restricting fluids, using diuretics, sitting in a sauna, and exercising in a hot environment using rubber suits. A fluid loss of only

**pathogenic** Capable of causing disease.

**cardiac output** The amount of blood expelled by the heart.

**hyperthermia** A much higher than normal body temperature.

## *Quick* Bite

### Ouch! But I Felt Fine Yesterday . . .

After a bout of heavy exercise, a person may not feel muscle soreness for a day or two. We do not fully understand this painful phenomenon, which is called *delayed-onset muscle soreness*. Activities that lengthen muscles seem to be the primary cause. The muscles suffer damage with micro-tears in their structure. This leads to an inflammatory response, causing localized muscle pain, swelling, and tenderness.

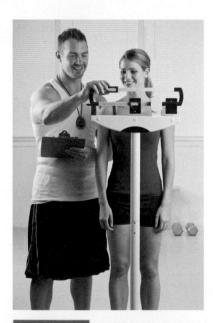

**Figure 11.17**    **Weighing in.** The NCAA discourages athletes from reducing their weight through intentional dehydration, a dangerous and potentially deadly practice.

| Table 11.11 | Pathogenic Weight-Loss Practices |
| --- | --- |

| Behavior | Consequence |
| --- | --- |
| Fasting | Loss of lean body mass and decreased metabolic rate |
| Diet pills | Medical side effects and weight regained when discontinued |
| Fat-free diets | Deficient in macronutrients and micronutrients; difficult to maintain |
| Diuretics | Dehydration and electrolyte imbalance; no fat loss |
| Laxatives | Dehydration; no fat loss; may be addicting |
| Sweating | Dehydration; heat injury; no fat loss |
| Excessive exercise | Risk of injury and overtraining; no fat loss |
| Enemas | Dehydration and GI problems; no fat loss |
| Fluid restriction | Dehydration; heat injury; no fat loss |
| Self-induced vomiting | Dehydration; acid–base and electrolyte imbalances; esophageal tears and GI bleeding; erosion of dental enamel and swollen parotid glands |

**Source:** Modified from Otis CL. Too slim, amenorrheic, fracture-prone: the female athlete triad. *ACSM's Health and Fitness.* 1998;2:2–25. Reprinted by permission of Lippincott Williams & Wilkins, http://lww.com.

2 percent of initial body weight (3 pounds for a 150-pound individual) can decrease athletic performance by elevating heart rate and lowering **cardiac output**. Moderate to severe dehydration (more than 3 to 5 percent of body weight) can be dangerous because of increased core body temperature, electrolyte imbalances, and cardiac and kidney changes. These conditions may result in heat illness, including heat cramps, heat exhaustion, or heatstroke.

Rapid weight loss can have serious health consequences. During one month in 1998, three previously healthy collegiate wrestlers died trying to make weight.[149] These athletes had not only dropped significant weight preseason—more than 20 pounds (9 kilograms)—but also lost between 3.5 and 9 pounds (1.6 and 4 kilograms) in the one to nine hours before their deaths. The wrestlers restricted food and fluid intake. To maximize sweat losses, they wore vapor-impermeable suits under cotton warm-up suits and exercised vigorously in hot environments. Dehydration and **hyperthermia** (elevated body temperature) led to their demise. Since 1998, the NCAA has revised the guidelines for monitoring weight-loss practices and weigh-in procedures. (See **Figure 11.17.**) This includes educating coaches and athletic trainers about healthy weight-control strategies and limiting the amount of preseason and precompetition weight loss.[150] More recently, the NCAA has adopted a new weigh-in format that requires athletes to have a season minimum weight established at the start of the year. This format attempts to prevent use of techniques and tools that have been used in the past for rapid dehydration resulting in rapid weight loss.[151]

**Key Concepts**  *Pathogenic weight-control practices increase risk of dehydration and compromise performance; they may have long-term serious consequences for athletes.*

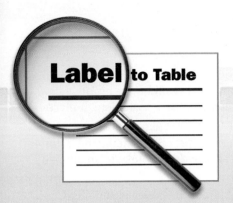

**Label** to Table

Sports drinks often are recommended instead of plain water for those who engage in vigorous physical activity. Their proponents claim that they quickly replenish the body's supply of nutrients, particularly electrolytes. Let's take a look at the Nutrition Facts panel from a popular sports drink, Gatorade.

First, look closely at the serving size—it's not the whole container. This is worth noting because many people might drink the whole container and assume they were getting 50 calories. Not true! The whole container has 200 calories (50 × 4 servings). It's always a good idea to look at the serving size when you are studying a nutrition label.

So, what makes this sports drink different from plain (and inexpensive) water? This one has added carbohydrate, sodium, and potassium. Replacing carbohydrate during long workouts prevents complete depletion of glycogen stores. Most sports drinks have between 5 and 8 percent simple sugar. Higher amounts would limit water absorption, and replacement of water is more critical than replacement of glucose.

Sodium and potassium are added to sports drinks to improve taste and help replace electrolytes that are lost during exercise. Gatorade con-tains 110 milligrams of sodium and 30 milligrams of potassium. For many athletes, and certainly for recreational exercisers, water really is the best fluid replacer. Although both sodium and potassium are lost in sweat, water is lost in greater quantities. Sports drinks have been shown to benefit only athletes who are strenuously exercising for longer than an hour. With prolonged exercise and sweat losses, large losses of electrolytes can make a person dizzy and weak, and may even lead to heat exhaustion or heatstroke.

The next time you head out for a bike ride, consider how long you'll be gone and how strenuous your ride will be, and then consider whether you'll need a sports drink. Also consider your personal taste—if a flavored sports drink will encourage you to replace fluids more than plain water will, that may be an important advantage. Just don't forget to read the label!

**Nutrition Facts**

Serving Size 8 fl oz (240mL)

Servings Per Container 4

**Amount Per Serving**

**Calories** 50

|  | % Daily Value* |
|---|---|
| **Total Fat** 0g |  |
| Trans Fat 0g | 0% |
| **Sodium** 110mg | 5% |
| **Potassium** 30mg | 1% |
| **Total Carbohydrate** 14g | 5% |
| Sugars 14g |  |
| **Protein** 0g |  |

Not a significant source of Calories from Fat, Saturated Fat, Trans Fat, Cholesterol, Dietary Fiber, Vitamin A, Vitamin C, Calcium, Iron.
* Percent Daily Values are based on a 2,000 calorie diet.

# *Learning* Portfolio

## Key Terms

## Study Points

- Exercise promotes health and reduces risk of chronic diseases.

- The ACSM defines physical fitness as "the ability to perform moderate to vigorous levels of physical activity without undue fatigue and the capability of maintaining this level of activity throughout life."

- The muscular system contains three types of muscles: smooth, cardiac, and skeletal. There are two types of muscle fibers: slow-twitch (ST) and fast-twitch (FT). ST fibers have high aerobic endurance; FT fibers are optimized to perform anaerobically. Your body depends predominantly on ST fibers for low-intensity events and FT fibers for highly explosive events.

- The body uses three systems to produce energy for physical activity: (1) the ATP–CP energy system (anaerobic), (2) the lactic acid energy system (anaerobic), and (3) the oxygen energy system (aerobic).

- Anaerobic and aerobic metabolism work together to fuel all types of exercise. During the early minutes of high-intensity exercise, the ATP–CP energy system and the lactic acid energy system provide most of the energy. Endurance activities are fueled primarily by the metabolism of glucose and fatty acids in the oxygen energy system.

- Training improves use of fat as a fuel by enhancing oxygen delivery and increasing the number of mitochondria in muscle.

- Carbohydrates should be the major source of energy in the athlete's diet and should come from complex carbohydrates, which can provide fiber, iron, and B vitamins. Athletes need carbohydrates so muscle glycogen stores and blood glucose concentrations will be adequate for training and competitive events. Likewise, carbohydrates are necessary to replenish glycogen stores after intense exercise.

- Carbohydrate loading is a process of reducing activity while increasing carbohydrate intake to maximize glycogen stores.

- Fat is a major fuel source for exercise, but high fat intake is neither required nor recommended.

- Protein needs of athletes are higher than for sedentary individuals, but generally athletes who consume adequate amounts of energy get enough protein. High-protein foods include low-fat dairy products, egg whites, lean beef and pork, chicken, turkey, fish, and legumes.

- Other nutrients important to the athlete's diet include B vitamins, iron, zinc, and calcium.

- Water is the most essential nutrient and is easily lost from the body with heavy sweating. Replacing fluid with water or sports drinks is important to prevent dehydration. Optimal sports drinks provide energy and electrolytes in a palatable solution that is rapidly absorbed.

- Athletes who are still growing have even higher energy and nutrient needs to support both physical activity and normal growth.

- Many dietary supplements are promoted as ergogenic aids—substances that enhance performance. Few well-controlled studies on their efficacy and safety have been done, however.

- Many athletes strive to either gain or lose weight so as to improve performance. In both cases, realistic goals and gradual changes are necessary for long-term success. Gains in muscle mass require increased calorie intake and weight training. Successful weight loss requires modest reductions in energy intake and increases in aerobic activity.

- Weight-control efforts that involve fasting, excessive sweating, purging, diuretics, or laxatives are detrimental to health.

## Study Questions

1. List the three different energy systems that your body uses to generate energy during exercise. When is each active during exercise?

2. What are muscle fibers, and what are the two major types?

3. What are the general recommendations for the balance of carbohydrate, fat, and protein in an athlete's diet?

4. What is carbohydrate loading?

5. How do protein recommendations for athletes vary from those for nonathletes?

6. Name three minerals that are of concern for athletes because they may not consume enough.

7. What is sports anemia and why does it happen? How does it compare with other anemias?

8. Define the term *ergogenic aid*. Is there a clear, research-based answer to whether ergogenic supplements work?

# Try This

## The Popularity of Ergogenic Aids

Take a trip to a health food store to see just how popular (and expensive!) ergogenic aids are. Try to locate each supplement listed in this chapter. Are they all available? What are their prices? Ask a salesperson what he or she knows about each of them. Do their answers match what you read in the text?

## Commit to Get Fit

Do you meet the American College of Sports Medicine's (ACSM) definition of fitness? Answer the questions below with a yes or no.

1. Do you exercise consistently three to five days per week?

2. When you exercise, does it include 20 to 60 minutes (20 minutes for intense activity and 60 minutes for less intense activity) of continuous aerobic activity?

3. Does your type of exercise use large muscle groups? Can you maintain it? Is it rhythmical and aerobic?

4. Does part of your activity include strength training of a moderate intensity (a minimum of one set of 8 to 12 repetitions of 8 to 10 exercises) at least two days per week?

If you answer *no* to any of these questions, you are not following the ACSM's suggestions to develop and maintain cardiorespiratory and muscular fitness. Choose a question to which you answered *no* and set a specific goal to include that factor in your exercise routine.

# What About Bobbie?

Imagine that Bobbie is training to compete in a marathon at the end of the semester. She has been exercising consistently and increasing her endurance and mileage times. She hasn't spent much time focusing on her diet, though, and wants to know what changes she could make to improve her nutrition and, therefore, performance. Assume that her current diet meets her calorie needs (see the "Food Choices: Nutrients and Nourishment" chapter). How would you compare Bobbie's diet to the guidelines you read about in this chapter?

## Macronutrient Contributions

Start with her overall contribution of carbohydrates, proteins, and fats. Compare Bobbie's macronutrient intake to the general sports nutrition recommendations.

|  | Bobbie's | Recommendations |
|---|---|---|
| Carbohydrates | 51 percent | 60 to 70 percent |
| Proteins | 17 percent | ~ 5 percent |
| Fats | 34 percent | ~ 20 percent |

As you can see, Bobbie's diet is higher in fat and lower in carbohydrates than is recommended for an athlete. If she were to reduce her intake of cream cheese, mayonnaise, cookies, and salad dressing and increase her fruits, vegetables, and whole grains, her diet would come closer to the recommendations for sports nutrition.

## Protein

Now let's calculate her protein need based on the athlete's guideline and see if she's consuming enough to maintain lean muscle mass and recover well from exercise.

The protein recommendation for an athlete is approximately 1.2 to 1.4 grams per kilogram of body weight. Bobbie weighs 155 pounds, so her recommended intake is as follows:

$$155 \text{ lb} \div 2.2 \text{ kg per lb} = 70.45 \text{ kg}$$

$$70.45 \text{ kg} \times 1.3 \text{ g/kg} = 91.6 \text{ g protein}$$

Bobbie's protein intake was 96 grams, which makes her protein intake a near perfect match for her needs.

## Minerals

Look at the two primary minerals that might be inadequate in diets of athletes, especially female athletes. Here is a comparison of Bobbie's calcium and iron intake and her daily recommendations.

|  | Bobbie's | Recommendations |
|---|---|---|
| Calcium | 710 mg | 1,000 mg |
| Iron | 20 mg | 8 mg |

As you can see, Bobbie did a very good job of consuming iron, but she is short of her calcium need. If she were to replace the diet soda she had at lunch with 1 cup of nonfat or 1% milk, her intake of calcium would rise to just about 1,000 milligrams. Or, she could change her afternoon snack of chips and salsa to a cup of yogurt to accomplish the same thing.

## Hydration

Check out Bobbie's intake of fluids in the "Food Choices: Nutrients and Nourishment" chapter. Although her overall fluid intake is consistent with the AI, how many ounces of plain water did she consume? That's right, she had only 16 ounces! Bobbie is making the same mistake that many athletes do—she's not drinking enough water. Poor hydration status will probably affect her performance adversely. Bobbie's biggest change should be to increase her fluid intake. She'd be smart to drink at least 12 to 16 ounces of caffeine-free fluids at all meals and snacks. This way she'll stay hydrated and be able to perform at an optimal level!

# References

1   American College of Sports Medicine (ACSM) and American Medical Association. ACSM and AMA launch "Exercise is Medicine" program. ACSM press release. 11/7/07. http://exerciseismedicine.org. Accessed 6/23/11.

2   Jonas S, Phillips E. *ACSM's Exercise Is Medicine: A Clinician's Guide to Exercise Prescription.* Philadelphia: Lippincott Williams & Wilkins; 2009.

3   US Department of Health and Human Services. 2008 Physical Activity Guidelines for Americans. http://www.health.gov/paguidelines/guidelines/summary.aspx. Accessed 6/23/11.

4   Jonas S, Phillips E. Op. cit.

5   Position of the American Dietetic Association, Dietitians of Canada, and the American College of Sports Medicine: nutrition and athletic performance. *J Am Diet Assoc.* 2009;109(3):509–527.

6   Connolly-Schoonen J. Physiology of anaerobic and aerobic exercise. In: Dunford M, ed. *Sports Nutrition: A Practice Manual for Professionals.* 4th ed. Chicago: Academy of Nutrition and Dietetics; 2006.

7   Fink HH, Burgoon LA, Mikesky AE. *Practical Applications in Sports Nutrition.* 2nd ed. Burlington, MA: Jones & Bartlett Learning; 2009.

8   Hashimoto T, Hussien R, Brooks GA. Colocalization of MCT1, CD147, and LDH in mitochondrial inner membrane of L6 muscle cells: evidence of a mitochondrial lactate oxidation complex. *Am J Physiol Endocrinol Metab.* 2006;290(6):E1237–E1244.

9   McArdle WD, Katch FI, Katch VL. *Exercise Physiology: Nutrition, Energy, and Human Performance.* Philadelphia: Lippincott Williams & Williams; 2009.

10  Brown GC. Speed limits. *The Sciences.* 2000;40(5):32–37.

11  McArdle WD, Katch FI, Katch VL. Op. cit.

12  Ibid.

13  Position of the American Dietetic Association, Dietitians of Canada, and the American College of Sports Medicine: nutrition and athletic performance. Op. cit.

14  Wilmore JH, Costill D, Kenney WL. *Physiology of Sport and Exercise.* 4th ed. Champaign, IL: Human Kinetics; 2008.

15  Jeukendrup A, Gleeson M. *Sport Nutrition: An Introduction to Energy Production and Performance.* 2nd ed. Champaign, IL: Human Kinetics; 2010.

16  Ibid.

17  Hawley, JA, Tipton KD, Millard-Stafford, ML. Promoting training adaptations through nutritional manipulations. *J Sports Sci.* 2006;24:709–721.

18  Position of the American Dietetic Association, Dietitians of Canada, and the American College of Sports Medicine: nutrition and athletic performance. Op. cit.

19  Mota J, Fidalgo F, Silva R, Ribeiro JC, Santos R, et al. Relationships between physical activity, obesity, and meal frequency in adolescents. *Ann Hum Biol.* 2008;35(1):1–10.

20  Position of the American Dietetic Association, Dietitians of Canada, and the American College of Sports Medicine: nutrition and athletic performance. Op. cit.

21  Sundgot-Borg J, Garthe I. Elite athletes in aesthetic and Olympic weight-class sports and the challenges of body weight and body composition. *J Sports Sci.* 2011;1–14.

22  Position of the American Dietetic Association, Dietitians of Canada, and the American College of Sports Medicine: nutrition and athletic performance. Op. cit.

23  Ibid.

24  Donaldson DM, Perry TL, Ross MC. Glycemic index and endurance performance. *Int J Sport Nutr Exer Metab.* 2010;20(2):154–165.

25  Dunford M. *Fundamentals of Sport and Exercise Nutrition.* Champaign, IL: Human Kinetics; 2010.

26  Sedlock DA. The latest on carbohydrate loading: a practical approach. *Curr Sports Med Rep.* 2008;7(4):209–213.

27  Coleman EJ. Carbohydrate and exercise. In: Dunford M, ed. *Sports Nutrition: A Practice Manual for Professionals.* 4th ed. Chicago: Academy of Nutrition and Dietetics; 2006.

28  Sedlock DA. Op. cit.

29  Position of the American Dietetic Association, Dietitians of Canada, and the American College of Sports Medicine: nutrition and athletic performance. Op. cit.

30  Ibid.

31  O'Reilly J, Wong S, Chen Y. Glycaemic index, glycaemic load, and exercise performance. *Sports Med.* 2010;40(1):27–39.

32  Position of the American Dietetic Association, Dietitians of Canada, and the American College of Sports Medicine: nutrition and athletic performance. Op. cit.

33  Kirksick C, Harvey T, Stout J, et al. International Society of Sports Nutrition position stand; nutrient timing. *J Int Soc Sports Nutr.* 2008;5–17.

34  Coleman EJ. Op. cit.

35  Ibid.

36  Hawley J, Burke L. *Peak Performance: Training and Nutritional Strategies for Sport.* Leonards, Australia: Allen & Unwin; 1998.

37  Position of the American Dietetic Association, Dietitians of Canada, and the American College of Sports Medicine: nutrition and athletic performance. Op. cit.

38  Gilson SF, Sounders MF, Moran CW, et al. Effects of chocolate milk consumption on markers of muscle recovery following soccer training: a randomized cross-over study. *J Int Soc Sports Nutr.* 2010;7:19.

39  Position of the American Dietetic Association, Dietitians of Canada, and the American College of Sports Medicine: nutrition and athletic performance. Op. cit.

40  Clark N. Nutrition: the power of protein. *The Physician and Sports Medicine. ASCA News.* vol. 96-4.

41  Campbell B, Kreider RB, Ziegenfuss T, et al. International Society of Sports Nutrition position stand: protein and exercise. *J Int Soc Sports Nutr.* 2007;4:8.

42  US Department of Health and Human Services and US Department of Agriculture. *Dietary Guidelines for Americans, 2010.* 7th ed. Washington, DC: US Government Printing Office; 2010.

43  Carroll C. Protein and exercise. In: Dunford M, ed. *Sports Nutrition: A Practice Manual for Professionals.* 4th ed. Chicago: Academy of Nutrition and Dietetics; 2006.

44  Phillips SM. Dietary protein for athletes: from requirements to metabolic advantages. *Appl Physiol Nutr Metab.* 2006;31:647–654.

45  Ibid.

46  Rodriguez NR, Di Marco NM, Langley S. American College of Sports Medicine position stand: nutrition and athletic performance. *Med Sci Sports Exerc.* 2009;41:709–731.

47  Fink HH, Burgoon LA, Mikesky AE. Op. cit.

48  Tipton KD, Elliott TA, Cree MG, et al. Ingestion of casein and whey protein results in muscle anabolism after resistance exercise. *Med Sci Sports Exerc.* 2004;36:2073–2081.

49  Position of the American Dietetic Association, Dietitians of Canada, and the American College of Sports Medicine: nutrition and athletic performance. Op. cit.

50  Tarnopolosky MA, Atkinson SA, MacDougall JD, et al. Evaluation of protein requirements for trained strength athletes. *J Appl Physiol.* 1992;73:1986.

51  Gibala MJ. Dietary protein, amino acid supplements, and recovery from exercise. *GSSI Sports Science Exchange.* 2002;15(4):1–4.

52  Position of the American Dietetic Association, Dietitians of Canada, and the American College of Sports Medicine: nutrition and athletic performance. Op. cit.

53  Stellingwerff T, Boit MK, Res PT. Nutritional strategies to optimize training and racing in middle-distance athletes. *J Sports Sci.* 2007;25(suppl 1):S17–S28.

54  Storlie J. From fork to muscle. *Training & Conditioning.* 1998;8:26, 28–29, 32–33.

55  Roy B. Milk: the new sports drink? A review. *J Int Soc Sports Nutr.* 2008;5:15.

56  Munoz M, Villar I, Garcia-Erce JA. An update on iron physiology. *World J Gastroenterol.* 2009;15(37):461–426.

57  Position of the American Dietetic Association, Dietitians of Canada, and the American College of Sports Medicine: nutrition and athletic performance. Op. cit.

58  Ibid.

59  Kreider RB, Wilborn CD, Taylor L, et al. ISSN exercise and sport nutrition review: research and recommendations. *J Int Soc Sports Nutr.* 2010;7:7.

60  Zhu YI, Haas JD. Iron depletion without anemia and physical performance in young women. *Am J Clin Nutr.* 1997;66:334–341.

61  Position of the American Dietetic Association, Dietitians of Canada, American College of Sports Medicine: nutrition and athletic performance. *Med Sci Sports Exerc.* 2009;41(3):709–731.

62  Kreider RB, Wilborn DC, Taylor L, Campbell B. Exercise and sport nutrition review: research and recommendations. *J Int Soc Sports Nutr.* 2010;7:7.

63  Position of the American Dietetic Association, Dietitians of Canada, and the American College of Sports Medicine: nutrition and athletic performance. Op. cit.

64  Williams MH. *Nutrition for Health, Fitness, and Sport.* 9th ed. Boston: McGraw-Hill; 2009.

65  Position of the American Dietetic Association, Dietitians of Canada, and the American College of Sports Medicine: nutrition and athletic performance. Op. cit.

66  American College of Sports Medicine, Sawka MN, Burke LM, et al. American College of Sports Medicine position stand. Exercise and fluid replacement. *Med Sci Sports Exerc.* 2007;39:377–390.

67  Ibid.

68  Ibid.

69  Ibid.

70  Ibid.

71  Ibid.

72  Ibid.

73  Pase DH, Stofan JR, Rowe CL, Horswill CA, Murray R. Exercise condition affects hedonic responses to sodium in a sport drink. *Appetite.* 2009;52(3):561–567.

74  Ibid.

75  Willet KL, Koszewski WM, Scheer J, Rudy J, Fischer JA. A descriptive study of the nutrition knowledge, attitudes, and behaviors of youth athletes and coaches. *J Am Diet Assoc.* 2010;110(suppl 9):A107.

76  Hunt SK, Colvin R. Nutritional practices and dietary habits of school children in a national youth sports program. *J Am Diet Assoc.* 2008;108(suppl 9):A96.

77  Brown JE. *Nutrition Through the Life Cycle.* 4th ed. Belmont, CA: Wadsworth Cengage Learning; 2011.

78  Castillo EM, Comstock RD. Prevalence of use of performance-enhancing substances among United States adolescents. *Pediatr Clin North Am.* 2007;54(4):663–675.

79  Petroczi A, Naughton D, Mazanov J, et al. Performance enhancement with supplements: incongruence between rational and practice. *Int Soc Sports Nutr.* 2007:4–19.

80  Hoffman J, Kang J, Ratamess N, et al. Examination of a pre-exercise, high energy supplement on exercise performance. *J Int Soc Sports Nutr.* 2009;6:2.

81  Ibid.

82  Dunford M, Smith M. Dietary supplement and ergogenic aids. In: Dunform M, *Sports Nutrition: A Practice Manual for Professionals.* 4th ed. Chicago: Academy of Nutrition and Dietetics; 2006.

83  Kreider RB, Almada AL, Antonia J, et al. Op. cit.

84  US Food and Drug Administration. Overview of dietary supplements: what is a dietary supplement? http://www.fda.gov/Food/DietarySupplements/ConsumerInformation/ucm110417.htm#regulate. Accessed 6/22/09.

85  Ibid.

86  Ibid.

87  Maughan R. Supplement contamination: is the risk real? Gatorade Sport Science Library. 2008. http://www.gssiweb.com/Article_Detail.aspx?articleid=613. Accessed 6/24/09.

88  Baume N, Mahler N, Kamber M, et al. Research of stimulants and anabolic steroids in dietary supplements. *Scand J Med Sci Sports.* 2006;16:41–48.

89  Position of the American Dietetic Association, Dietitians of Canada, and the American College of Sports Medicine: nutrition and athletic performance. Op. cit.

90  Sullivan M. FDA urged to step up regulation of supplements: adverse events are largely underreported. *Family Practice News.* 2009;29(6):1–2.

91  Kreider RB, Almada AL, Antonia J, et al. Op. cit.

92  Ibid.

93  Ibid.

94  Ibid.

95  Ciocca M. Medication and supplement use by athletes. *Clin Sports Med.* 2005;24:719–738.

96  Newsholme EA, Blomstrand E. Branched-chain amino acids and central fatigue. *J Nutr.* 2006;136:274S–276S.

97  Ibid.

98  Armsey TD, Hosey RG. Medical aspects of sports: epidemiology of injuries preparticipation physical examination, and drugs in sports. *Clin Sports Med.* 2004;23(2):255–279.

99  Tokish JM, Kocher MS, Hawkins RJ. Ergogenic aids: a review of basic science, performance, side effects, and status in sports. *Am J Sports Med.* 2004;32(6):1543–1553.

100  Antonio J, Sanders MS, Kalman D, et al. The effects of high-dose glutamine ingestion on weightlifting performance. *J Strength Cond Res.* 2002;16:157–160; and Haub MD, Potteiger JA, Nau KL, et al. Acute l-glutamine ingestion does not improve maximal effort exercise. *J Sports Med Phys Fitness.* 1998;38:240–244.

101  Ciocca M. Op. cit.

102  Buford T, Kreider R, Stout J, et al. International Society of Sports Nutrition position stand: creatine supplementation and exercise. *J Int Soc Sports Nutr.* 2007;4:6.

103  Cribb PJ, Williams AD, Hayes A. A creatine-protein-carbohydrate supplement enhances responses to resistance training. *Med Sci Sports Exerc.* 2007;39:1960–1968.

104  Skare OC, Skalberg AR. Creatine supplementation improves sprint performance in male sprinters. *Scand J Med Sci Sports.* 2001;11:96–102.

105  Lattavo A, Kopperud A, Rogers P. Creatine and other supplements. *Pediatr Clin North Am.* 2007;54(4):735–760.

106  PDR Health. Creatine. http://www.pdrhealth.com/durg_info/nmdrugprofiles/cre_0086.shtml. Accessed 7/2/09.

107  Buford T, Kreider R, Stout J, et al. Op. cit.

108  Kreider RB, Melton C, Rasmussen CI, et al. Long-term creatine supplementation does not significantly affect clinical markers of health in athletes. *Mol Cell Biochem.* 2003;244:95–104; and Mayhew DL, Mayhew JL, Ware JS. Effects of long-term creatine supplementation on liver and kidney functions in American college football players. *Int J Sport Nutr Exerc Metab.* 2003;12:453–460.

109  Greenwood M, Kreider RB, Melton C, et al. Creatine supplementation during college football training does not increase the incidence of cramping or injury. *Mol Cell Biochem.* 2003;244:83–88.

110  Position of the American Dietetic Association, Dietitians of Canada, and the American College of Sports Medicine: nutrition and athletic performance. Op. cit.

111  Jenkins RR. Exercise and oxidative stress methodology: a critique. *Am J Clin Nutr*. 2000;72(suppl):670S–674S.

112  Australian Sports Commission, Australian Institute of Sports. Fact sheet: caffeine. http://www.ausport.gov.au/ais/nutrition/supplements/supplement_fact_sheets/group_a_supplements/caffeine. Accessed 7/17/08.

113  Ibid.

114  Lattavo A, Kopperud A, Rogers P. Op. cit.

115  Keisler BD, Armsey TD. Caffeine as an ergogenic aid. *Curr Sports Med Rep*. 2006;5(4):215–219.

116  Lattavo A, Kopperud A, Rogers P. Op. cit.

117  World Anti-Doping Agency. Prohibited list. 2011. http://www.wada-ama.org/en/World-Anti-Doping-Program/Sports-and-Anti-Doping-Organizations/International-Standards/Prohibited-List/The-2011-Prohibited-List. Accessed 6/23/11.

118  National Collegiate Athletic Association. NCAA banned substance list. http://www.ncaa.org/wps/wcm/connect/53e6f4804e0b8a129949f91ad6fc8b25/2009-10+Banned+Drug+Classes.pdf?MOD=AJPERES&CACHEID=53e6f4804e0b8a129949f91ad6fc8b25. Accessed 6/23/11.

119  Lattavo A, Kopperud A, Rogers P. Op. cit.

120  Ibid.

121  World Anti-Doping Agency. Op. cit.

122  Keisler BD, Armsey TD. Op. cit.

123  Ibid.

124  US Food and Drug Administration. FDA issues regulation prohibiting sale of dietary supplements containing ephedrine alkaloids and reiterates its advice that consumers stop using these products. *FDA News*. 2/6/2004. http://www.cfsan.fda.gov/~lrd/fpephed6.html. Accessed 1/31/09.

125  Bell DG, McLellan TM, Sabiston CM. Effect of ingesting caffeine and ephedrine on 10-km run performance. *Med Sci Sports Exerc*. 2002;34:344–349; Jacobs I, Pasternak H, Bell DG. Effects of ephedrine, caffeine, and their combination on muscular endurance. *Med Sci Sports Exerc*. 2003;35:987–994; and Shekelle PG, Hardy ML, Morton SG, et al. Efficacy and safety of ephedra and ephedrine for weight loss and athletic performance: a meta-analysis. *JAMA*. 2003;289:1537–1545.

126  Lattavo A, Kopperud A, Rogers P. Op. cit.

127  Shekelle PG, Hardy ML, Morton SG, et al. Op. cit.

128  Lattavo A, Kopperud A, Rogers P. Op. cit.

129  Joyce S, Minahan C, Anderson M, Osborne M. Acute and chronic loading of sodium bicarbonate in highly trained swimmers. *Eur J Appl Physiol*. 2011 May 17.

130  Vincent JB. The potential value of chromium picolinate as a nutritional supplement, weight loss agent, and muscle development agent. *Sports Med*. 2003;33:213–230.

131  Kreider RB, Wilborn CD, Taylor L, et al. Op. cit.

132  Ciocca M. Medication and supplement use by athletes. *Clin Sports Med*. 2005:24;719–738.

133  Lattavo A, Kopperud A, Rogers P. Op. cit.

134  Ibid.

135  Zoller U, Vogel W. Iron supplementation in athletes: first do no harm. *Nutrition*. 2004;20:615–619.

136  Sarma DN, Barrett ML, Chavez ML, et al. Safety of green tea extracts: a systematic review by the US Pharmacopeia. *Drug Safety*. 2008;31(6):469–484.

137  Rains TM, Agarwal S, Maki KC. Antiobesity effects of green tea catechins: a mechanistic review. *J Nutr Biochem*. 2011;22(1):1–7.

138  Maki KC, Reeves MS, Farmer M, Yasunaga K, et al. Green tea catechin consumption enhances exercise-induced abdominal fat loss in overweight and obese adults. *J Nutr*. 2009;139(2):264–270.

139  Kreider R, Wilborn C, Taylor L, et al. Op. cit.

140  Williams MH. Op. cit.

141  Cormie P, McGuigan MR, Newton FU. Adaptations in athletic performance after ballistic power versus strength training. *Med Sci Sports Exerc*. 2010;42(8):1582–1598.

142  Williams MH. Op. cit.

143  McArdle WD, Katch FI, Katch VL. *Essentials of Exercise Physiology*. 4th ed. Philadelphia: Lippincott Williams & Wilkins; 2010.

144  Ibid.

145  Williams MH. Op. cit.

146  Michels Blanck H, Serdula MK, Gillespie C, et al. Use of nonprescription dietary supplements for weight loss is common among Americans. *J Am Diet Assoc*. 2007;107(12):441–447.

147  Ranby KW, Aiken LS, MacKinnon DP, et al. A mediation analysis of the ATHENA intervention for female athletes: prevention of athletic-enhancing substance use and unhealthy weight loss behaviors. *J Pediatr Psychol*. 2009;34(10):1069–1083.

148  Lingor RJ, Olson A. Fluid and diet patterns associated with weight cycling and changes in body composition assessed by continuous monitoring throughout a college wrestling season. *J Strength Cond Res*. 2010;24(7):1763–1772.

149  Rapid weight loss in wrestlers results in death. *MMWR*. 1998;47(6):105–108.

150  Kundrat S. Sport nutrition for coaches. *J Nutr Educ Behav*. 2010;42(6):430.

151  Center for Nutrition in Sport and Human Performance. Taking it to the mat: the wrestler's guide to optimal performance. http://www.ncaa.org/wps/wcm/connect/e0d12b804e0bbaf1a21df21ad6fc8b25/mat.pdf?MOD=AJPERES&CACHEID=e0d12b804e0bbaf1a21df21ad6fc8b25. Accessed 6/23/11.

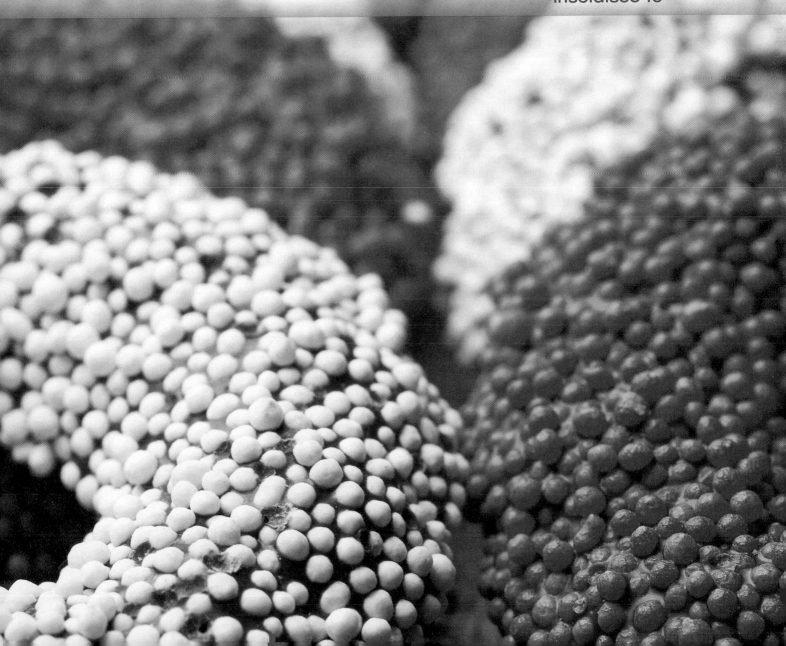

# Spotlight on Eating Disorders

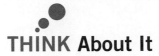

## THINK About It

1  What's your view of the ideal female body?

2  When should you be concerned that you—or someone you know—is dieting obsessively?

3  Given the right situation, what foods are you likely to binge on?

4  How many magazines do you read that promote dieting or encourage thinness?

**Visit go.jblearning.com/ inseldisco4e**

**eating disorders** A spectrum of abnormal eating patterns that eventually may endanger a person's health or increase the risk for other diseases. Generally, psychological factors play a key role.

**disordered eating** An abnormal change in eating pattern related to an illness, a stressful event, or a desire to improve one's health or appearance. If it persists it may lead to an eating disorder.

**anorexia nervosa [an-or-EX-ee-uh ner-VOH-sah]** An eating disorder marked by prolonged decrease of appetite and refusal to eat, leading to self-starvation and excessive weight loss. It results in part from a distorted body image and intense fear of becoming fat, often linked to social pressures.

**body image** A person's mental concept of his or her physical appearance, constructed from many different influences.

A gaunt, hollow-cheeked college freshman confides to her roommate that she feels chubby. After an enormous lunch, a secretary works her way through a bag of cookies, and polishes off a box of chocolates. A swimming champion who obsesses over every calorie becomes concerned that she hasn't had a period in two months. Disordered eating? Very likely! Eating disorder? Possibly!

**Eating disorders** and **disordered eating** are not the same. An eating disorder such as anorexia nervosa or bulimia nervosa is an illness that can seriously interfere with daily activities. Disordered eating is usually a temporary or mild change in eating patterns. Although it can occur after an illness or stressful event, it often is related to a dietary change intended to improve one's health or appearance. Unless disordered eating persists, it rarely requires professional intervention. Disordered eating, however, can become an eating disorder.

Most of us take much pleasure in eating. For people with an eating disorder, however, food is a source of continual stress and anxiety. (See **Figure SED.1**.) Eating disorders include a spectrum of emotional illnesses ranging from self-imposed starvation to chronic binge eating. These illnesses stem from severe distortions of the eating process and produce physical consequences that often threaten life and require professional intervention.[1]

On particular occasions most of us have eaten to the point of discomfort. (Thanksgiving dinner comes to mind.) And, many of us have cut out desserts at one time or another, hoping to fit into a special outfit or to lose weight for an athletic event or job interview. But stuffing yourself at a holiday meal or going on an occasional diet does not constitute an eating disorder. According to the *Manual of Clinical Dietetics*, a defining characteristic of an eating disorder is a persistent inability to eat in moderation.[2]

## The Eating Disorder Continuum

The American Psychiatric Association's *Diagnostic and Statistical Manual of Mental Disorders* (DSM-IV) assigns eating disorders to one of three categories, with small but significant areas of overlap. These categories form a continuum, with self-starvation at one end and compulsive overeating at the other. (See **Figure SED.2**.) **Anorexia nervosa** occurs at the self-starvation end of the continuum. Anorexia is a self-imposed starvation syndrome that is triggered by a severely distorted **body image**.

What is perceived as beautiful can vary with cultural and individual preferences. Fashion designers, for example, view beauty as sinewy women who line the fashion catwalks and fill fashion magazines and appear in stark contrast to the majority of U.S. women, whose average dress size has grown to size 14. In contrast to the Western preference for bony beauty, some cultures do not view obesity negatively but instead prize large, corpulent bodies. People

**Figure SED.1** **Can you spot the person with the eating disorder?** Some people with eating disorders have normal body weights and are difficult to spot.

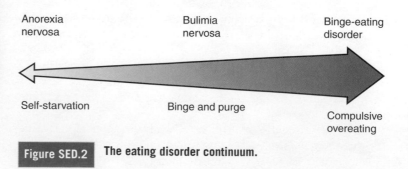

| Anorexia nervosa | Bulimia nervosa | Binge-eating disorder |
|---|---|---|
| Self-starvation | Binge and purge | Compulsive overeating |

**Figure SED.2** The eating disorder continuum.

with anorexia are at war with their bodies. Even when they are dangerously underweight, people with anorexia typically see themselves as fat. Severely restricting food intake is another symptom of anorexia nervosa. It may also involve purging (self-induced vomiting) and exercising excessively. Anorexia is most prevalent among adolescent females.

At the opposite end of the continuum is **binge-eating disorder**, formerly known as **compulsive overeating**. People with this disorder chronically consume massive quantities of food. Sufferers are typically obese; however, not all obese people binge eat. Diagnosis of binge-eating disorder is based on a person having an average of two binge-eating episodes per week for six months. Such episodes often are triggered by emotions such as frustration, anger, depression, and anxiety.[3]

In the middle of the continuum is **bulimia nervosa**. Like those with binge-eating disorder, people with bulimia nervosa compulsively gorge themselves. Like those with anorexia, people with bulimia desperately want to be thin and resort to purging to reach this goal. After gorging, people with bulimia often become disgusted with themselves and terrified of getting fat. To compensate, bulimic people make themselves vomit, use laxatives, exercise excessively, and take other action to avoid gaining weight.

Few people who suffer from eating disorders are purely anorexic, bulimic, or binge eaters. Many swing from one disordered eating pattern to another, alternately starving and gorging themselves. People may suffer from binge-eating disorder at one point in their lives, and anorexia or bulimia at another.[4] Studies also find that disordered eating behaviors during adolescence are at increased risk for dieting and disordered eating behaviors 10 years later.[5] Table SED.1 shows the diagnostic criteria for these eating disorders.

## History of a Modern Malady

The first formal report of anorexia nervosa appeared in the medical literature in the 1870s.[6] Informal reports of a "voluntary starvation syndrome" were published as early as 1694.[7] Some nutritional anthropologists argue that eating disorders can be traced to even more ancient times. During the Middle Ages, for instance, early Christian ascetics, who led lives of contemplation and rigorous self-denial, shunned worldly pleasures, including food, to show obedience and become closer to God. These people alternated periods of semistarvation with frequent fasts. Was this anorexia disguised as religious devotion? Some scholars think so, and current studies have found relationships among religious affiliations and disordered eating even today.[8]

Early Greeks and Romans, in contrast, exhibited exaggerated bingeing and purging behavior at banquets that lasted for days. Guests gorged to the point of physical pain, then tickled their throats with feathers to induce vomiting. Once their stomachs were empty, they returned to the table. Rather than finding this behavior repulsive or shameful, the ancient Romans glorified it. They even built areas known as vomitoriums into their banquet halls.[9]

Some scholars contend these ancient Romans had bulimia. Others disagree, arguing that the Roman men ate for pleasure in the company of others and purged only so they could rejoin the feast. In contrast, modern bulimia sufferers are usually females who gorge and purge in isolation—and in hopes of achieving an unrealistic cultural standard of beauty. Furthermore, today's bulimia sufferers invariably feel shame, low self-esteem, and even self-hate connected with their eating habits.

Although eating disorders are not an exclusively modern malady, it's clear that eating disorders have become increasingly common in the past four decades. A British model named Twiggy, nicknamed for her sticklike appear-

**binge-eating disorder** An eating disorder marked by repeated episodes of binge eating and a feeling of loss of control. The diagnosis is based on a person's having an average of at least two binge-eating episodes per week for six months.

**compulsive overeating** See *binge-eating disorder*.

**bulimia nervosa [bull-EEM-ee-uh]** An eating disorder marked by consumption of large amounts of food at one time (binge eating) followed by a behavior such as self-induced vomiting, use of laxatives, excessive exercise, fasting, or other practices to avoid weight gain.

**Table SED.1    Diagnostic Criteria for Eating Disorders**

*Anorexia Nervosa*
- Body weight < 85 percent of expected weight (or BMI ≤ 17.5 kg/m²)
- Intense fear of weight gain
- Inaccurate perception of one's own body size, weight, or shape
- Amenorrhea (in females after menarche)

*Bulimia Nervosa*
- Recurrent binge eating (at least two times per week for three months)
- Recurrent purging, excessive exercise, or fasting (at least two times per week for three months)
- Excessive concern about body weight or shape
- Absence of anorexia nervosa

*Binge-Eating Disorder*
- Recurrent binge eating (at least two times per week for six months)
- Marked distress with at least three of the following:
- Eating very rapidly
- Eating until uncomfortably full
- Eating when not hungry
- Eating alone
- Feeling disgusted or guilty after a binge
- No recurrent purging, no excessive exercising, and no fasting
- Absence of anorexia nervosa

**Source:** Reprinted with permission from *Diagnostic and Statistical Manual of Mental Disorders*, 4th ed. Text Revision. Copyright © 2000. American Psychiatric Association.

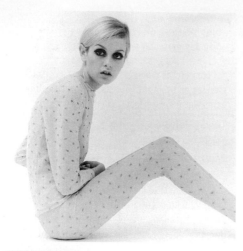

**Figure SED.3** **Eye of the beholder.** In the 1960s, Twiggy became the new role model for young women who wanted to be thin and glamorous.

ance, ushered in the epidemic in the early 1960s. Fashion magazine stories reported that she subsisted on water, lettuce, and a single daily serving of steak and that she had learned to suppress her hunger pangs. Rather than condemn these clearly dangerous eating habits, the magazines held Twiggy up as a model of self-control for girls and young women. (See **Figure SED.3**.)

Our national denial regarding the dangers of semistarvation ended abruptly and dramatically in 1983 with the highly publicized death of 32-year-old pop singer Karen Carpenter from complications of anorexia. Widespread media coverage of her death highlighted the lethal potential of eating disorders and made the terms *anorexia* and *bulimia* household words. Other stars of film, television, sports, and the fashion world—Princess Diana, Jane Fonda, Janet Jackson, Ally Sheedy, Calista Flockhart, Cathy Rigby, Zina Garrison, Felicity Huffman, Lindsay Lohan, Mary-Kate Olsen, and Kate Beckinsale, to mention a few—have spoken about their eating disorders. Some have described the physical, emotional, and social damage these diseases caused in their own lives. But, ironically, increased visibility and knowledge have not stemmed the tide of eating disorders. To the contrary, the prevalence of eating disorders and disordered eating continues to increase,[10] and the age of onset of anorexia nervosa and bulimia nervosa is decreasing.[11]

**Key Concepts** *Eating disorders are unhealthy behavioral conditions known to exist from ancient times. Today, they have become alarmingly common in industrialized countries, particularly the United States. Eating disorders range from the self-starvation of anorexia nervosa to the compulsive overeating of binge-eating disorder.*

## No Simple Causes

Certain people appear to have a predisposition to eating disorders that may be rooted in psychological, biological, or cultural causes. A person who suffers from depression or **obsessive-compulsive disorder**, for example, may have an increased risk of developing an eating disorder. The vulnerability also may be biological. Indeed, some evidence suggests that genetic factors may create an increased risk for eating disorders. Another important factor in the development of eating disorders is society's emphasis on extreme thinness. It is clear that eating disorders are complex problems, with multiple causes. Social, psychological, and biological factors all play roles.

Eating disorders can develop when people, especially women, feel social pressure to achieve an unrealistic standard of thinness. Modern Western culture would have women weigh less than what is considered healthy. This means that most women cannot attain what society considers the "ideal" female form without significant food deprivation. These pressures affect even very young girls, starting with their first Barbie doll and her attenuated, unnatural shape (see **Figure SED.4**), if not before.[12]

THINK
About It

1

Psychological factors are important as well. These encompass everything from peer relationships to relationships with parents. Studies have shown that adolescent girls who were teased about their weight by peers had a more negative image of their bodies and lower self-esteem, regardless of their actual weight.[13] In addition, children who were subjected to weight-based teasing did not perform as well in school as those who had not suffered such teasing.[14] Findings were similar for adolescent boys and for teens of varied racial and ethnic backgrounds. Studies have also linked more severe forms of emotional trauma to disordered eating. For example, trauma exposure and distress have been linked to eating for psychological reasons, and ultimately to binge eating.[15] One study found that more than 50 percent of bulimic and anorexic patients suffered from **post-traumatic stress disorder (PTSD)**.[16]

**obsessive-compulsive disorder** A disorder in which a person attempts to relieve anxiety by ritualistic behavior and continuous repetition of certain acts.

**post-traumatic stress disorder (PTSD)** An anxiety disorder characterized by an emotional response to a traumatic event or situation involving severe external stress.

PTSD occurs in people who have endured a significant trauma, such as child abuse or rape. Eating disorders also may be associated with dysfunctional family relationships. Some psychologists believe that people with anorexia and bulimia are trying to fulfill unrealistic parental expectations of perfection, in part by succumbing to societal pressure to be very thin.

Scientists have made major advances in understanding the biological foundation of eating disorders, and studies have linked abnormal levels of neurotransmitters, especially serotonin, in people to their eating disorders.[17] Researchers, for example, have shown that bulimia patients experience spontaneous improvement in eating habits from antidepressant medication that increases brain levels of serotonin.[18] Many antiobesity drugs also affect serotonin levels.[19]

Neurotransmitters are just one focus of research into the biology of eating disorders. Another line of investigation focuses on genes. Recently, researchers have confirmed that eating disorders run in families. For some women, social characteristics within the family, such as having highly educated parents and grandparents, as well as achieving higher grades in school have been found to increase the risk for developing an eating disorder.[20] In addition, eating disorders occur most frequently in families with a history of obsessive-compulsive disorders, anxiety disorders, and depression.[21] Both depression and obsessive-compulsive behavior have been linked to atypical levels of serotonin and norepinephrine in the brain.[22]

It's likely that a number of genes are involved in the development of eating disorders. Two genes in particular—leptin and **orexin**—have gained a lot of attention for their possible contribution to body weight. The leptin gene regulates the body's production of leptin, a hormone that causes rapid weight loss in genetically obese mice. (Unfortunately, leptin has not stimulated the same reaction in humans.) The orexin gene regulates production of two appetite-stimulating hormones: orexin A and orexin B (after the Greek word *orexis*, meaning "appetite"). Rodents injected with either hormone have been shown to increase their food consumption 8- to 10-fold.[23]

The discoveries of leptin and orexin genes significantly advance our understanding of brain chemistry and eating disorders and may eventually lead to new classes of more effective drugs. Drugs that mimic orexins, for example, might help patients with anorexia or other wasting syndromes by increasing their appetites. Conversely, drugs that block orexins might help patients struggling with obesity and binge eating. Or a leptinlike drug may eventually be used to stimulate weight loss. At the very least, discovery of these genes supports the idea that biological factors probably contribute to the development of eating disorders in vulnerable people.

**Key Concepts** *The precise causes of eating disorders remain obscure. Researchers have debated whether eating disorders are primarily psychological or genetic in origin. The current view is that eating disorders are a result of the complex interaction of social, biological, and psychological factors. In other words, eating disorders occur in biologically susceptible individuals exposed to particular types of environmental stimuli.*

## Anorexia Nervosa

Although they learned about the condition in medical school, until the 1960s few doctors saw a case of anorexia nervosa. By the mid-1970s, however, physicians were reporting many cases of anorexia, particularly among young women. Today this serious disorder occurs in about 1 in 200 women, usually starting in adolescence. More than 90 percent of cases occur in women, and the death rate from anorexia nervosa is about 10 times the death rate of women without anorexia.[24]

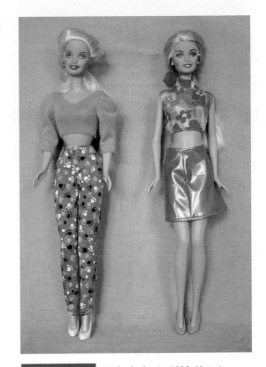

**Figure SED.4**  **Thin is in.** In 1998, Mattel overhauled Barbie's look for the millennium, giving her slimmer hips, a wider waist, and smaller breasts. Barbie's periodic overhauls are meant to fit the fashion of the times. Does the new Barbie (right) represent a realistic role model for today's young girls?

**orexin** A class of hormones in the brain that may affect human food consumption.

## *Quick* Bite

**Magazine Manipulations**
When researchers studied fifth-through twelfth-grade girls in a working-class suburb in the Northeast United States, nearly 50 percent reported that they wanted to lose weight because of pictures in magazines. Frequent readers of fashion magazines were two to three times more likely to be influenced to diet or exercise to lose weight. Seventy percent of the girls reported that magazine pictures influenced their conception of the perfect body.

# *Quick* Bite

## A Skinny Trend

In 1970, the average Playboy Playmate weighed 11 percent below the national average. Only 8 years later, in 1978, the average weight of Playboy Playmates was 17 percent below average. Today, the average model is 22 to 23 percent leaner than the average American woman.

# *Quick* Bite

## Fashion Designers and Weight Guidelines for Models

The fashion industry sells women an ideal of beauty embodied in the models who walk the runways and appear in fashion magazines. Spurred by the deaths of several South American models—one reportedly trying to live on lettuce and Diet Coke—fashion designers in Spain and Italy issued regulations in late 2006 to raise weight limits for fashion models. They require a BMI of at least 18, which means that models must weigh at least 56 kilograms (123 pounds) if their height is greater than or equal to 1.75 meters (5 feet, 9 inches). These figures are in sync with World Health Organization (WHO) standards of the minimum healthy weight. Designers excluded super-skinny models who did not meet the minimum requirements from performing in a Madrid fashion show.

The U.S. fashion industry has not followed suit. It has no plans to require models to achieve an objective measure of health, such as a height-to-weight ratio, despite a poll on *Elle* magazine's website in which two-thirds of respondents indicated they wished that American designers would follow the examples of fashion show organizers in Milan and Madrid in banning overly skinny models. However, at a meeting of the Council of Fashion Designers of America the industry introduced guidelines for designers, aimed at promoting healthier behavior among its models and at educating designers on how to recognize disorders.

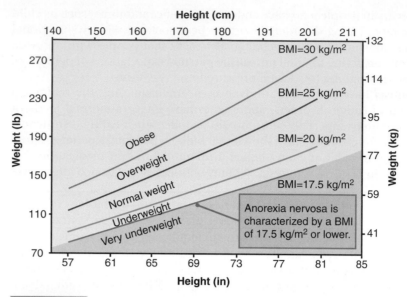

**Figure SED.5**  **BMI and underweight.** When managing eating disorders, BMI can help guide decisions about nutrition, medications, and psychotherapy.

**Source:** Reprinted with permission from *Diagnostic and Statistical Manual of Mental Disorders*, 4th ed. Text Revision. Copyright © 2000. American Psychiatric Association.

The term *anorexia nervosa*, which translates to "nervous loss of appetite," is misleading. People diagnosed with anorexia don't lose their appetite except in the final stages of the disorder. Instead, they are obsessed with food. But their obsession with thinness is even greater. The German term for the disorder, *pubertätsmagersucht*, or "mania for leanness," more accurately reflects the nature of the disease. The hallmark of anorexia nervosa is dramatic loss of weight, usually to less than 85 percent of the expected weight for height or a BMI of less than or equal to 17.5 kg/m². (See **Figure SED.5**.)

Anorexia is more prevalent in industrialized societies that have an abundance of food and an attitude that equates beauty, particularly feminine beauty, with thinness. Nine of 10 anorexia sufferers are female—probably because Western society emphasizes thinness more for women than for men.[25] Studies show that the peak age of onset is between 15 and 19 years old,[26] and the typical anorexia sufferer has been an upper-class Caucasian female adolescent. Unfortunately, during the past decade, anorexia has become more of an equal-opportunity disorder. Physicians have reported cases of the disorder in young women from all social and ethnic backgrounds; it is especially prevalent in women who participate in activities that emphasize leanness, including modeling, ballet, and gymnastics. In addition, anorexia has increased significantly among African American women.[27]

## Causes of Anorexia Nervosa

On the surface, anorexia nervosa usually seems to result from a weight-loss program gone awry. A high school freshman may go on a diet after her boyfriend or gymnastics coach tells her she is too heavy. An eighth-grader may want to lose weight to be more popular at a new school. The diet may start out just fine, but it never stops.

Beneath the surface, psychological issues are typically at work. Because most cases of anorexia begin around the age of puberty, some psychologists theorize that anorexic behavior is an attempt to prevent or delay sexual maturation. By maintaining a childlike body, a young girl may hope to avoid the pressures of the teen years and the responsibilities of adulthood. In addition, psychologists report that anorexia sufferers tend to be rigid, perfectionistic, all-or-nothing thinkers. Sufferers tend to lack a sense of independence and control over their own destiny. They may attempt to compensate for this through acts of intense self-discipline. Parents may facilitate this syndrome by being overly protective or rigid or by holding a child to excessively high standards of achievement.[28] Additional risk factors commonly associated with onset of anorexia include extremely high levels of exercise, distorted body image, obsessive-compulsive disorders, and negative self-esteem.[29] In addition, it has been suggested that a person with both a high punishment sensitivity and low reward reactivity/sensitivity might form a personality cluster associated with the risk of developing an eating disorder.[30]

## Warning Signs

Parents and friends of people with anorexia often miss early signs of the disease. Avoidance of particular foods, unconventional food choices, or a rigorous exercise routine can easily be mistaken as determination to lose a few pounds, rather than the underlying issue, an obsession with food and dieting. Many eating disorders start with a simple diet. Stress and a lack of appropriate coping mechanisms, dysfunctional family relationships, and drug abuse may cause dieting to get out of control.[31]

Initially, someone with anorexia has a feeling of power. Sufferers enjoy a feeling of control as they learn to deny their hunger and limit their food intake. Early warning signs include obsessively counting calories; developing lists of "safe" foods and foods to avoid; cutting foods, even peas, into small pieces; and spending a great deal of time rearranging food on a plate. To suppress hunger, a person with anorexia may drink up to 30 cups of water or diet soda a day. Anorexia sufferers also may channel their obsessions with food into the preparation of elaborate meals for others without eating any of the food themselves.[32] Table SED.2 shows the warning signs of anorexia.

THINK
About It
2

As the disease progresses, anorexia sufferers become increasingly disillusioned, withdrawn, and hostile. Success always seems beyond their grasp. No matter how thin they are, they see themselves as overweight. (See **Figure SED.6**.) When they eat more than they think they should, they may induce vomiting or use **emetics**, **enemas**, **diuretics**, or **laxatives**. Or, they may exercise relentlessly. Eventually, their efforts to avoid obesity take over their lives. They start to avoid social situations that may expose their behaviors and so withdraw more and more from friends and family. Groggy and irritable from food deprivation and sleep disturbances, people with advanced anorexia spend so little time on their schoolwork or jobs that their performance deteriorates. Yet when confronted with their obsessive dieting or deteriorating behavior, they will deny that anything is unusual.[33]

## Treatment

Just as there is no one cause for anorexia nervosa, there is no single way to cure it. Successful treatment of anorexia nervosa requires a collaborative approach by an interdisciplinary team of psychological, nutritional, and medical specialists.[34] Research suggests that with intensive therapy most patients can achieve normal weight. However, they may struggle all their lives with a moderate to severe preoccupation with food and body weight, poor social relationships, and depression. The longer someone suffers from anorexia nervosa before they receive treatment, the poorer the chances are for complete recovery; therefore, the earlier a patient begins treatment, the better the prognosis.

---

**Table SED.2** **Warning Signs of Anorexia**

Anorexia nervosa is a disorder in which preoccupation with dieting and thinness leads to excessive weight loss. The person with anorexia may not acknowledge that weight loss and restricted eating are problems. Family and friends can help by recognizing that the following are warning signs:

- Loss of a significant amount of weight
- Continuing to diet (although thin)
- Feeling fat, even after losing weight
- Fear of weight gain
- Cessation of monthly menstrual periods
- Preoccupation with food, calories, nutrition, and/or cooking
- Preferring to eat in isolation
- Exercising compulsively
- Bingeing and purging

---

**emetics** Agents that induce vomiting.

**enemas** Infusions of fluid into the rectum, usually for cleansing or other therapeutic purposes.

**diuretics [dye-u-RET-iks]** Drugs or other substances that promote the formation and release of urine. Diuretics are given to reduce body fluid volume in treating such disorders as high blood pressure, congestive heart disease, and edema. Both alcohol and caffeine act as diuretics.

**laxatives** Substances that promote evacuation of the bowel by increasing the bulk of the feces, lubricating the intestinal wall, or softening the stool.

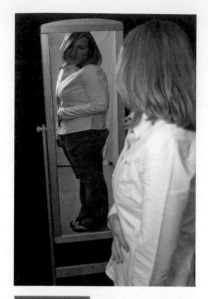

**Figure SED.6**    Distorted body image.

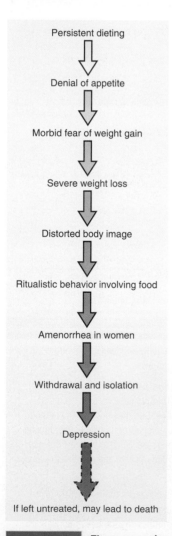

Persistent dieting

Denial of appetite

Morbid fear of weight gain

Severe weight loss

Distorted body image

Ritualistic behavior involving food

Amenorrhea in women

Withdrawal and isolation

Depression

If left untreated, may lead to death

**Figure SED.7**    The progression of anorexia.

The course of anorexia varies greatly. In rare instances, a sufferer recovers spontaneously without treatment. More typically, a patient recovers only after a variety of treatments or enters a cyclical pattern of weight gain and relapse. Thirty to 50 percent of anorexia patients also have symptoms of bulimia, which can complicate diagnosis and treatment.[35] Tragically, in 6 to 18 percent of cases, the disease proves fatal. (See **Figure SED.7**.) Patients who have other emotional disorders, such as major depression or substance abuse, are the most likely to die from complications of the disease. Potentially fatal complications of anorexia include starvation and suicide.[36]

As with many other behavioral disorders, people with anorexia usually deny the danger of their situation. And so family and friends must intervene to get sufferers to treatment—often by getting together and supportively confronting the person with evidence that something is seriously wrong. This common technique helps people accept the need for at least an initial medical screening. The complex and multifaceted nature of anorexia requires a team of experienced healthcare professionals, including physicians, clinical dietitians, and psychotherapists so both the physical and psychological aspects of the disorder can be addressed. One of the best places to find an experienced team of therapists is at an eating disorder clinic associated with a major medical facility.[37] The first goal of treatment is to stabilize the patient's physical condition. The second is to convert the patient, who is typically reluctant, into a willing participant in the treatment plan. A combination of hospitalization, psychotherapy, and pharmacotherapy is often necessary.

Restoring the patient's nutritional status is of prime importance. Otherwise, dehydration, starvation, and electrolyte imbalances can lead to serious health problems and even death. (See Table SED.3.) If a patient has lost more than 30 percent of body weight over a three-month period or weighs 70 percent or less of the standard weight considered healthy for height, hospitalization is essential. (See Table SED.4.) Restoration of body weight and return of menses are primary therapeutic goals for treatment.[38] Once the patient's physical condition has stabilized and some physical symptoms of starvation have disappeared, psychotherapy can begin in earnest. Many therapists use a cognitive behavioral approach to help the patient challenge irrational beliefs and establish healthy attitudes and behaviors for gaining and maintaining weight.

The early phases of weight gain are fraught with challenges for both patient and clinician. Patients must gain a certain amount of weight to prevent death or permanent damage while the psychotherapeutic portion of their treatment is still in the very early phases. At first, the patient is encouraged to simply eat enough food to minimize or stop weight loss. Next, the patient is started on a very slow process of weight gain, all the while receiving intensive psychotherapy. The first sign of weight gain can precipitate a crisis. Phobia of obesity may return with renewed vengeance. Many patients refuse to eat. Others resist treatment in covert ways. If not restricted to bed and closely supervised, they may try to burn off calories through relentless exercise or by purging. To avoid detection, they adopt a series of behaviors to conceal their lack of weight gain. These include wearing concealing clothes or "bulking up" before weigh-ins by filling their pockets with coins or drinking large amounts of water or diet soda.[39]

Psychologists use a variety of psychotherapeutic techniques to help the patient deal with underlying emotional issues such as depression. Treatment programs generally use a combination of behavioral therapy, individual psychotherapy, patient education, family education, and family therapy. Frequently, therapists find family conflicts at the heart of the eating disorder. Ongoing therapy for the patient and family is key to successful recovery.

As the patient's symptoms resolve, she or he must find new ways to relate to and communicate with family members. Family members must remain open and willing to change their behavior toward the person with the eating disorder.

Dietitians work closely with the psychotherapist to help patients develop a realistic view of food and to reshape their food selection and eating behaviors. Although no pharmaceutical agent has been developed specifically to treat anorexia, some antidepressants have proved useful.

Most patients with anorexia nervosa require continued intervention after discharge from the hospital or treatment program. Support groups for people with eating disorders and their families can be an important link in the recovery process. Support groups also can be a useful technique for easing a resistant patient into treatment. With expert help and ongoing therapy, patients with anorexia can develop new mechanisms for coping with life's stresses, eventually replacing their disordered relationship with food with new, healthier interpersonal relationships.

**Key Concepts** *The hallmark symptoms of anorexia nervosa are a mania for thinness and self-imposed starvation. Sufferers manifest a body weight as much as 15 percent below normal, a severely distorted body image, withdrawal from family and friends, and various physical and psychological changes related to starvation.*

## Bulimia Nervosa

The behavior we now call bulimia was practiced as long ago as Greek and Roman times. Gerald Russell, a British psychiatrist, first coined the term *bulimia nervosa* in 1979 to describe a syndrome of bingeing and purging in young Caucasian women. The average patient with bulimia is an unmarried Caucasian woman in her twenties or thirties with a normal or near-normal body weight. (See **Figure SED.8.**) People with bulimia are more likely to be sexually active than are those with anorexia and often are involved in destructive relationships. Almost anyone can be affected, however.

The relationships among dieting, bingeing severity, and alcohol use have been studied in samples of college-age women. Researchers have found a relationship among binge drinking, dieting, and maladaptive coping patterns, such as using substances and/or denial as coping mechanisms.[40] It has also been shown that girls who engage in binge eating, alcohol use, or both have higher levels of negative urgency, or the tendency to act rashly when distressed.[41]

People with bulimia nervosa tend to feel very disorganized. They report suffering from depression and low self-esteem. Many were sexually abused as children. Food was often a source of comfort, and eating gradually evolved

| Table SED.3 | Side Effects of Excessive Weight Loss in Anorexia Nervosa |

**Emaciation**
- Loss of fat stores and muscle mass
- Reduced thyroid metabolism
- Cold intolerance
- Difficulty maintaining core body temperature

**Hematological**
- Leukopenia (abnormal decrease of white blood cells)
- Iron-deficiency anemia

**Other**
- Growth of lanugo (fine, babylike hairs) over the trunk
- Osteopenia (mineral depletion in bone)
- Premature osteoporosis

**Neuropsychiatric**
- Abnormal taste sensation
- Depression
- Impaired thought processes

**Cardiac**
- Loss of cardiac muscle, resulting in a smaller heart
- Abnormal heart rhythm
- Increased risk of sudden death

**Gastrointestinal**
- Delayed gastric emptying
- Bloating
- Constipation
- Abdominal pain

| Table SED.4 | When Hospitalization Is Needed |

Suggested criteria for hospitalization for individuals with anorexia nervosa include:
- Weight loss of greater than 30 percent over three months
- Severe metabolic disturbance
- Severe depression or suicide risk
- Severe bingeing and purging
- Failure to maintain outpatient weight contract
- Psychosis
- Family crisis

**Source:** Reprinted with permission from *Diagnostic and Statistical Manual of Mental Disorders*, 4th ed. Text Revision. Copyright © 2000. American Psychiatric Association.

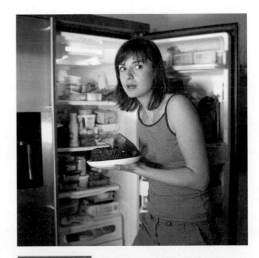

**Figure SED.8** **Bulimia nervosa.** The typical person suffering from bulimia is an unmarried Caucasian woman in her twenties or thirties.

# *Quick* Bite

**binge** Consumption of a very large amount of food in a brief time (e.g., two hours) accompanied by a loss of control over how much and what is eaten.

**purge** Emptying of the GI tract by self-induced vomiting and/or misuse of laxatives, diuretics, or enemas.

**Table SED.5  Warning Signs of Bulimia**

Bulimia nervosa involves frequent episodes of binge eating, almost always followed by purging and intense feelings of guilt or shame. The sufferer feels out of control and recognizes that the behavior is not normal. The signs that a person may have bulimia include:

- Bingeing or eating uncontrollably
- Compensating for binges by strict dieting, fasting, vigorous exercise, vomiting, or abusing laxatives or diuretics in an attempt to lose weight
- Using the bathroom frequently after meals
- Preoccupation with body weight
- Depression or mood swings
- Irregular menstrual periods
- Dental problems, swollen cheeks or glands, heartburn, or bloating
- Personal or family problems with drugs or alcohol

into a tool for dealing with every unpleasant event, from boredom to major life crises.

It is estimated that between 1 and 3 percent of American adolescent and young adult females have bulimia. But bulimia, particularly in its milder forms, often goes undetected. This is because people with bulimia are very secretive about their behaviors, typically limiting their binge-and-purge episodes to the middle of the night or times when they are assured of privacy. Also, unlike patients with anorexia or binge-eating disorder, whose body weights may hint at their underlying psychiatric disorder, the body weight of a patient with bulimia is usually average or only slightly above average. Several studies have found that as many as 40 percent of college-age women occasionally binge and purge—often enough to raise concern but too infrequently for an official diagnosis of bulimia.[42]

The college environment itself may be conducive to overconsumption due to factors such as readily available energy-dense foods and academic pressures leading to sedentary activities, such as reading, studying, and sitting at a computer, while at the same time devaluing exercise and organized sports participation.[43] For example, a survey of college students found their priorities, in order of most to least important, to be going to class, studying, hanging out with friends, sleeping, exercising, dating or meeting partners, eating healthy foods, work, having an ideal body, surfing the Internet, and going to a great party.[44] Before entering college, healthful meals and regular exercise are generally part of a regular routine, but these positive health behaviors appear to decline in the transition from high school to college, an environment vulnerable to unhealthy eating patterns, which may start with occasional food binges.[45] Table SED.5 lists the warning signs of bulimia.

## Causes of Bulimia

Bulimia seems to occur most often in people who have an intense desire to nurture themselves with food but who are also strongly influenced by our societal obsession with thinness. One description of people with bulimia characterizes them as being obsessed with food but repulsed by fat. In contrast to people with anorexia, people with bulimia focus more on food than on thinness.

Psychologists who have treated patients with bulimia have found that they typically did not receive sufficient nurturing during their formative years. Whereas families of anorexic patients tend to have a lot of rigidly defined roles and rules, families of bulimic patients tend to lack structure. Roles may be loosely defined. Parents are often described as distant and judgmental. Significant family conflict usually exists. Patients often feel that their families failed to provide an adequate sense of security and protection.

## Obsessed by Thoughts of Food

A person with bulimia chronically **binges** and **purges**. To meet the official definition of the disorder, bingeing and purging occurs at least twice a week for at least three months. Purging may be accompanied or replaced by fasting, excessive exercise, or other behaviors that compensate for the binge episode. Between binges, people with bulimia typically restrict their dietary intake to a limited number of low-calorie foods they consider "safe." This dietary control is an illusion, however. The average bulimic sufferer is obsessed by thoughts of food and spends a great deal of time both planning the next binge and trying to resist the urge to binge.[46] **Figure SED.9** illustrates the binge-and-purge pattern of bulimia.

Just what triggers a binge is not clear. People with bulimia tend to be all-or-nothing thinkers. If they eat a single piece of food from their forbidden list, such as a cookie, they feel driven to consume the entire box. Some researchers believe that hunger caused by very restrictive dieting, combined with a buildup of everyday stresses, overwhelms the person's resolve and precipitates a binge.

During a binge, individuals with bulimia typically consume massive quantities of highly palatable "forbidden" foods such as pastry, ice cream, and candy. This gorging takes place over a relatively short time span—say, an hour or two. Binges may contain up to 10,000 kilocalories. Afterward, feeling physically ill from overindulgence, sufferers use a variety of purging techniques, such as self-induced vomiting or excessive quantities of laxatives, to rid themselves of the food. Or they may follow a binge with a period of very strict fasting and heightened exercise.

Purging leads to a variety of physical symptoms. Over time, gastric acid in vomit burns the lining of the pharynx, esophagus, and mouth, erodes tooth enamel, and may even result in loss of teeth. Repeated vomiting also can enlarge the salivary glands and erode the lining of the stomach and esophagus.

Excessive self-induced vomiting and diarrhea can upset the body's delicate biochemical balance through loss of electrolytes and body water. Among other dangers, changes in electrolyte balance can trigger an irregular heartbeat and precipitate a life-threatening medical crisis.

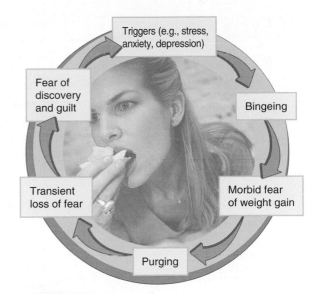

**Figure SED.9**    **The binge-and-purge cycle of bulimia.**

## Diary of an Eating Disorder

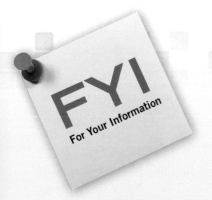

Every time I leave one of my sessions I feel better. We talk about stuff; I feel, express, and even cry. Today was the third time since I left her office to come home and throw up. I think things are getting better despite the fact that my mind focuses 80 percent of the time on food during the 55 minutes. But, it's like the kitchen is a refuge for my mind. I always know it will be there, waiting to embrace me when I get home.

Alone is how I hope to find it. I have been thinking of what I will sink my teeth into first. Usually I go for the fat-free chocolate cake, then to the frozen yogurt (which makes it all come up much smoother). I don't think this is normal, though I am not really concerned. I feel like a million-pound weight has been swept away by the effortless flush of the toilet. The hardest thing is to look in the mirror after I have thrown up. Sometimes I wipe my face before I look. Other times I leave the spit, bile, and food on my mouth and hands. I just stand there holding my hands up, with my shoulders slumped over. I produce this expression of absolute helplessness—then I laugh. I guess I am amazed by the act I've just committed. I can't explain why; I can't believe that it is really me doing this. Why would I do something like throw up? I really have no reason to torture myself. Bulimia was always them—I can't possibly be like that. I throw up, but I am not a bulimic. I sure as hell don't have an eating disorder.

I am totally for this whole counseling thing because I feel sad a lot and I want to feel better. But I can't leave there and not feel that I have to get this crap out. All this stuff that we talk about.

Today, Dr. Tant asked me when this all began. My first thought was, "Oh this throwing up thing? I can't remember." But, I do recall one time when my ex-boyfriend Matt and I had gone to a really nice dinner. My recollection of the evening was that it was perfect. I remember thinking about how this food was really fattening, though, and how it would make me fat if I kept it down. I didn't know or have the willpower to just not eat it. Over and over, I tortured and berated myself about the effects this dinner would have on my body. I couldn't bear it. This dinner was no longer one meal; it was going to ruin my body and make me fat. I couldn't stand that food being inside me another moment. Looking back I can't imagine how I could have thrown up right there on the

side of the road. It was like I had no couth. I told Matt to pull over, and I just stuck my hand down my throat. Rationalizing the act while engaging in it, I then jumped back in the truck to carry on with the night. We never discussed my vile act, other than Matt saying, "I can't believe you just did that."

"I know," I responded, "but it just was making me feel so sick. I mean, my stomach was really nauseous [sic]." Basically I don't know when I began this war with myself, but I know it caused me to fear myself. The rest is a blur—its beginning, its incentive. I heard Dr. Tant's question. I just didn't have the answer.

—Chelsea Browning Smith

**Source:** Smith CB. *Diary of an Eating Disorder*. Dallas, TX: Taylor Publishing Company; 1998. Reprinted by permission of Taylor Trade Publishing, an imprint of Rowman & Littlefield Publishing Group.

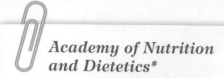

### *Academy of Nutrition and Dietetics\**

**Nutrition Intervention in the Treatment of Anorexia Nervosa, Bulimia Nervosa, and Other Eating Disorders**

It is the position of the American Dietetic Association that nutrition intervention, including nutritional counseling, by a registered dietitian is an essential component of the team treatment of patients with anorexia nervosa, bulimia nervosa, and other eating disorders during assessment and treatment across the continuum of care.

**Source:** Reproduced from Position of the Academy of Nutrition and Dietetics: nutrition intervention in the treatment of anorexia nervosa, bulimia nervosa, and other eating disorders. *J Am Diet Assoc.* 2006;106:(12):2073–2082.

\* Formerly the American Dietetic Association

---

**Table SED.6    Side Effects of Purging in Bulimia Nervosa**

*Metabolic Effects*
- Electrolyte abnormalities
- Low blood magnesium

*Gastrointestinal*
- Inflammation of the salivary glands
- Pancreatic inflammation and enlargement
- Esophageal inflammation or ulcers
- Gastric erosion
- Dysfunctional bowel

*Dental*
- Erosion of dental enamel, particularly of front teeth, with corresponding decay

*Neuropsychiatric*
- Fatigue
- Weakness
- Impaired thought processes
- Seizures (related to large fluid shifts and electrolyte disturbances)
- Mild inflammation of peripheral nerves

---

Excessive use of emetics (drugs to induce vomiting) and laxatives carries its own risks. Repeated use of emetics is toxic to the liver and kidneys, and abuse of laxatives can damage the lining of the large intestine. Table SED.6 shows the side effects of bulimic purging.

## Treatment

Little research has been done on the long-term course of bulimia. It appears, however, that bulimia is easier to treat than anorexia, perhaps because bulimic patients tend to recognize that their behavior is abnormal. Following treatment, more than half of patients report an improvement in their binge-eating and coping behaviors. About 30 percent of patients eventually become symptom-free. The rest, however, struggle with the disorder to some degree throughout their lives. To reduce the risk of relapse, therapists encourage patients to stay involved in support groups after completing formal therapy.

Cognitive behavior therapy is key to helping patients reshape their attitudes about food and identify situations that trigger bingeing. The therapist's goal is to help patients let go of their need to categorize foods as safe or dangerous, good or bad. Patients must learn techniques for dealing with stress and uncomfortable or painful memories and feelings. Depression, which typically accompanies this disorder, must be treated as well. Many patients with bulimia also require treatment for substance abuse. A patient is hospitalized only when severely depressed or when purging is so frequent that physical damage has occurred or is imminent.

Medication can be an effective adjunct to psychotherapy. Serotonin-enhancing antidepressants have been used successfully to treat bulimia.

**Key Concepts** *Key symptoms of bulimia nervosa are binge-eating episodes at least twice a week for three months, followed by behaviors that compensate for the binges, such as severe dieting, purging, or a combination of dieting and purging. The body weights of people with bulimia are typically close to or slightly above that considered healthy for their heights.*

## Binge-Eating Disorder

Binge eating is the most common eating disorder in industrialized nations. It differs from bulimia in that the person with binge disorder does not attempt to compensate for his or her binge by purging or other means. Overeating has been reported in the medical literature since scribes first put stylus to tablet. And over past generations, societies, including our own, have considered obesity a sign of good health, wealth, and even fertility. But modern Western society is not among these. Binge eating is now recognized as an eating disorder not otherwise specified (EDNOS). This term is used to describe those conditions that meet the definition for eating disorders but not the criteria for anorexia or bulimia.[47] EDNOS comprises the largest category of eating disorders. Its precise causes are unclear, but binge eating seems to be related to an intense desire to nurture oneself with food or to reduce stress by eating.[48] In 1994, the American Psychiatric Association recognized binge-eating disorder as an emotional illness.[49] (See Table SED.7.)

### Stress and Conflict Often Trigger Binge Eating

A person with binge-eating disorder consumes excessive quantities of food in a relatively short period of time at least twice a week. Unlike the bulimia sufferer, however, the person with binge-eating disorder does not attempt to compensate by purging or other means. In some instances, binge eaters adopt a grazing pattern. "Grazers" eat constantly for extended periods of time, eventually consuming an exceptionally large quantity of food. This pattern of overindulgence may be seen in people who restrict their food intake at work or school but seek solace in food at home.

Many binge eaters begin dieting in grade school and start bingeing during adolescence or in their early twenties. Typically, they try numerous weight-loss programs without long-term success. Research suggests that dieting during adolescence does not predict weight loss or even weight maintenance but rather predicts weight gain and overweight status over time. In Project EAT (Eating Among Teens), a five-year longitudinal study of eating and weight in adolescents, adolescents who reported dieting were at nearly twice the risk for being overweight five years later.[50]

Binge eaters exhibit many of the same characteristics as bulimic patients. More than 50 percent have clinical depression. Feelings of depression, loneliness, anxiety, or stress can precipitate a binge. Like other patients with eating disorders, those with binge-eating disorder are all-or-nothing thinkers. They tend to categorize foods as safe or dangerous. Eating even a small serving of a forbidden food can trigger a binge. Typical binge foods include sweets, pastries, ice cream, and high-fat snacks such as nuts and chips. However, if junk foods aren't handy, binge eaters may eat large quantities of starchy foods such as potatoes, bread, and pasta. **Figure SED.10** illustrates some factors that trigger binge eating.

Most binge eaters are people who have not learned to express or even acknowledge their feelings. During therapy sessions, many binge eaters report feeling helpless to influence the course of events or behaviors of others around them. Rather than acknowledge their feelings, they swallow them—aided by large quantities of food. They become addicted to the behavior itself because it is the only way they can get relief from stress. (See **Figure SED.11**.)

Binge eating often is a learned response to stress or conflict, passed down from one generation to the next. Parents may use food rather than affection and discussion to shape their children's behavior. Food is used for celebration and consolation, for reward and punishment. Children growing up in such environments learn to eat in response to emotions rather than hunger. As adults, they turn to food to satisfy all their emotional needs.

## Treatment

Little is known about the course and prognosis of binge-eating disorder. However, people who become obese as a result of this disorder are at risk of developing weight-related health problems, including type 2 diabetes, hypertension, degenerative joint disease, heart disease, and even certain cancers.

People who have binge-eating disorder are rarely able to control the condition themselves. They usually require therapy to help them identify their long-buried emotions and learn techniques for giving voice to their feelings. Therapists experienced in treating this disorder discourage patients from trying to lose weight initially. Any attempts to restrict food intake can backfire by creating anxiety and provoking a binge. The major focus of therapy is to help patients identify their emotions and separate true biological hunger from emotional hunger. Once significant progress is made in these areas, the patient is better equipped psychologically to address weight issues.

Long-term support is key to keeping binge eaters from relapsing. Self-help groups such as Overeaters Anonymous are one source of support. These groups are organized according to the 12-step philosophy of Alcoholics Anonymous. In addition, many hospitals in large urban areas have support groups led by trained therapists.

Many patients with binge-eating disorder benefit from antidepressant medications. These drugs reduce the urge to binge, most likely by altering the

THINK
About It
3

*Quick* Bite

**When Plumpness Was Valued**
In centuries past, extra pounds displayed one's wealth and prosperity. The wealthy could afford abundant food and didn't perform physical labor.

Table SED.7    **Warning Signs of Binge-Eating Disorder**

Binge eaters, like bulimia sufferers, experience periods of uncontrolled eating that they usually keep secret. Binge eaters often are depressed and sometimes have other psychological problems. Signs that a person may have a binge-eating disorder include:
- Episodes of binge eating
- Eating when not physically hungry
- Frequent dieting
- Feeling unable to stop eating voluntarily
- Awareness that eating patterns are abnormal
- Weight fluctuations
- Depressed mood
- Attribution of social and professional successes and failures to weight

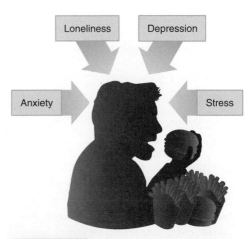

Figure SED.10    **Emotions.** Feelings of loneliness, depression, anxiety, or stress can trigger a binge-eating episode.

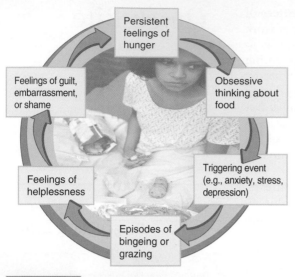

Figure SED.11 **The vicious cycle of binge eating.**
Binge-eating disorder is the most common eating disorder.

brain's serotonin level. Various weight-management medications are now in development. These also may curb the urge to binge.

**Key Concepts** *Binge-eating disorder is the most common eating disorder seen in people of all ages and backgrounds. Like people with bulimia, those with binge-eating disorder consume significantly more food than is typically eaten in a given period of time. Unlike bulimia, those with binge-eating disorder do not purge or fast. Not all binge eaters are obese, although many obese people binge.*

## Body Dysmorphic Disorder

People with **body dysmorphic disorder (BDD)** are preoccupied with an imagined or slight defect in appearance, worrying, for example, that their skin is scarred, that they are balding, or their nose is too big. Such people may engage in long rituals of grooming, repeatedly combing hair, applying makeup, or picking at their skin. The condition's severity varies. Whereas some people can manage it, for others the preoccupation causes significant distress and impairment: They may have few friends, avoid dating, miss school or work, and feel very self-conscious in social situations.

Many patients affected with BDD have coexisting conditions, such as obsessive-compulsive disorder (OCD), major depression, delusions, or social phobia. Approximately 2 to 7 percent of patients who undergo plastic surgery have BDD and are generally unhappy with the results.

BDD affects 1 to 2 percent of the general population; however, BDD frequently goes undiagnosed. Sufferers are ashamed of their problem and fail to report it to their physicians. Even though it is a serious and distressing condition, it is easily trivialized. In addition, even many health professionals are unaware that BDD is a psychiatric disorder that often responds to psychiatric treatment. Many people seek treatment from dermatologists, plastic surgeons, and other physicians, but these professionals often are ignorant of this disorder and thus are unhelpful.

Psychiatric treatment, including medication and cognitive-behavior therapy, can effectively decrease symptoms and suffering. The therapist helps the person with BDD resist compulsive BDD behaviors (e.g., mirror checking), face avoided situations (e.g., social situations), and develop a more realistic view of his or her appearance. Medications, including selective serotonin reuptake inhibitors (SSRIs), can relieve obsession and decrease distress and depression.[51]

**Key Concepts** *Body dysmorphic disorder often coexists with other conditions such as obsessive-compulsive disorder, major depression, delusions, or social phobia. Patients with BDD magnify slight defects and are preoccupied with their appearance.*

## Night-Eating Syndrome

When a person grazes through the evening, finds herself plotting midnight refrigerator raids, and wakes at night to eat, she may have **night-eating syndrome (NES)**. A person with this disorder

- Eats more than half of daily calories during and after the evening meal
- Wakes up at least once a night to eat, especially high-carbohydrate snacks
- Feels tense, anxious, worried, or guilty while eating
- Lacks appetite for breakfast and postpones it for hours
- Persists in this behavior for at least three months

**body dysmorphic disorder (BDD)** An eating disorder in which a distressing and impairing preoccupation with an imagined or slight defect in appearance is the primary symptom.

**night-eating syndrome (NES)** An eating disorder in which a habitual pattern of interrupting sleep to eat is the primary symptom.

Night-eating syndrome is a fairly uncommon eating disorder in the general population—perhaps only 1 to 2 percent of adults in the general population have this problem—but it affects up to a quarter of obese people. Although underlying causes are not fully understood, the disorder may result from a combination of biologic, genetic, and emotional factors. Researchers have noted several hormonal imbalances among NES sufferers, such as low levels of both melatonin (a sleep-inducing hormone) and leptin (an appetite-suppressing hormone). Cortisol—the so-called stress hormone that kicks in when we feel tense—appears higher at night in night eaters, perhaps arousing them to wake up and head for the kitchen. Stress, depression, and anxiety commonly affect mood among those with the condition.

Night-eating syndrome involves a disturbed food-intake circadian rhythm, which may be out of sync by as much as four to five hours with a person's normal sleep rhythm. It is possibly the first clinical disorder to manifest differing circadian rhythms of two biological systems.

The heavy preference for carbohydrates, which triggers the brain to produce "feel-good" neurochemicals, suggests that night eating may be an attempt to self-medicate mood problems. A dietitian can help develop meal plans that distribute intake more evenly throughout the day so a person is not as vulnerable to caloric loading in the evening. Stress-reduction programs, including psychological therapy, can be helpful.

**Key Concepts** *Night-eating syndrome, though uncommon, affects up to a quarter of obese people. People with NES interrupt normal sleep to eat and often feel stressed, anxious, and depressed. They typically have hormonal imbalances. Psychotherapy and stress reduction therapy can be helpful.*

## Males: An Overlooked Population

As many as a million boys and men in the United States struggle with eating disorders.[52] Yet males with eating disorders have been "ignored, neglected or dismissed because of statistical infrequency of the disease, combined with the pervasive myth that eating disorders are a female disease," according to Arnold E. Andersen, former director of the Eating and Weight Disorders Clinic at Johns Hopkins University and scientific editor of the book *Males with Eating Disorders*.[53]

Women who develop eating disorders may feel fat, but they typically are near average weight. In contrast, most men who develop these diseases are overweight. Many were seriously teased about their weight as children. Whereas women are concerned primarily with weight, men are concerned with shape and muscle definition. Indeed, men often develop disordered eating habits while trying to improve their athletic performance. More men than women diet to prevent medical consequences associated with being overweight.

Why do fewer males than females develop full-blown eating disorders? Some researchers suggest that there is a "dose-response" relationship between the amount of sociocultural pressure to be thin and the probability of developing an eating disorder. The more people are believed to deviate from our culture's body ideals, the more likely they are to be perceived (by themselves and their peers) as personal failures.[54] Note that articles and advertisements that promote dieting usually are targeted at young women rather than young men. When men are exposed to activities that require leanness, such as wrestling, swimming, running, and horse racing, they exhibit a substantial increase in anorexic behavior. In fact, perceived pressure from social agents such as advertising, verbal messages, and social situations related to eating and dieting are strong predictors of eating disorders,[55] indicating that cultural

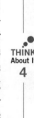

THINK
About It

4

## Table SED.8    Signs of an Undisclosed Eating Disorder

People with eating disorders usually exhibit several of the following signs.

*Physical*
- Arrested growth
- Marked change or frequent fluctuations in weight
- Inability to gain weight
- Fatigue
- Constipation or diarrhea
- Susceptibility to fractures
- Delayed menarche
- Calcium or phosphorus imbalances, abnormal blood pH, or high serum amylase levels

*Behavioral*
- Change in eating habits
- Difficulty in social settings

Source: Becker AE, Grinspoon SK, Klibanski A, Herzog DB. Eating disorders. *N Engl J Med.* 1999;340(14):1092–1098. Copyright © 1999 Massachusetts Medical Society. All rights reserved. Reprinted with permission.

---

**anorexia athletica** Eating disorder associated with competitive participation in athletic activity.

**female athlete triad** A syndrome in young female athletes that involves disordered eating, amenorrhea, and lowered bone density.

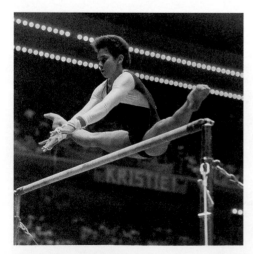

**Christy Henrich.** Christy, a top Olympic gymnast, weighed less than 60 pounds when she died in 1994 at age 22 of multiple organ failure, a complication resulting from anorexia and bulimia.

---

conditions, rather than gender, are the contributing factor for developing an eating disorder.

Furthermore, the degree of thinness held up as desirable for women is 15 percent below a healthy body weight whereas the degree of thinness held up as desirable for men is well within the healthy limits of normal weight. Thus, women are more likely than men to alter their eating habits to achieve the desired appearance.

## An Unrecognized Disorder

Like women, most men develop eating disorders during adolescence. But males can develop eating disorders during preadolescence and young adulthood as well. The diagnostic criteria for anorexia and bulimia in men and women are similar. But doctors are so conditioned to viewing eating disorders as a female phenomenon that they often miss eating disorders in males. Likewise, the patient, his family, and friends may not recognize disordered eating patterns. (See Table SED.8.) Because our culture accepts overeating among men more readily than in women, binge eating in particular may go unrecognized in men. In addition, anorexia may elude diagnosis in men more often than in women because malnourished men don't experience definitive symptoms, such as a woman's loss of menstrual periods, that can alert professionals and others to the problem. Men also tend to view an eating disorder as a "woman's disease," so they often are hesitant to seek medical attention.[56]

**Key Concepts**  *Men also suffer from eating disorders, although at rates much lower than those of women. Like women, men typically develop eating disorders during adolescence and young adulthood, but they are more often overweight and striving for a particular body shape and muscularity. Although the diagnostic criteria are the same, with the exception of amenorrhea, eating disorders in men are often undiagnosed due to societal conditioning that views eating disorders as "female" diseases.*

# Anorexia Athletica

Regardless of social or ethnic background, participation in competitive athletics seems to be a common link in the development of eating disorders among males and females. Sports-related eating disorders are known as **anorexia athletica**.[57] Among those who participate in sports, and particularly team sports, there is a correlation between eating disorders and the excessive physical activity demanded during sports training.[58] Participation in lean sports (i.e., those that emphasize leanness or body image), such as distance running, swimming, gymnastics, dance, and diving, increases the risk for developing an eating disorder.[59] Athletes who have anorexia athletica want to achieve an unrealistic body size that they consider desirable for competition. In many cases, athletes with mild eating disorders are able to disguise their disease as attention to fitness. People who are addicted to their exercise routine are at greater risk of developing eating disorders.[60]

Coaches and trainers play a significant role in the development of eating disorders among athletes.[61] "Get down to your fighting weight," reflects the prevailing concept that leanness equals performance.[62]

# The Female Athlete Triad

Although the majority of female athletes benefit from increased physical activity, there are those who go too far and risk developing a trio of medical problems. Female athletes who fall prey to the "thin-at-any-cost" philosophy are at risk of developing a condition known as the **female athlete triad**. (See

Figure SED.12.) This syndrome is characterized by problems with the inter-relationship among energy availability, menstrual function, and bone mineral density, which may have clinical consequences including eating disorders, **amenorrhea**, and premature osteoporosis.[63] Research is now exploring a possible fourth component—endothelial dysfunction. Consequences of this include imbalance between vasodilating and vasoconstricting substances produced by (or acting on) the endothelium, which affects electrolyte volume and content and mediates coagulation. Athletic-associated amenorrhea combined with endothelial dysfunction is a concern for future cardiovascular risk, public health issues, and athletic performance.[64]

Who is at the greatest risk of suffering from the female athlete triad? They tend to be female athletes who compete in endurance sports such as long-distance running; aesthetic sports, such as gymnastics; antigravitational sports, such as indoor rock climbing; and sports with weight classifications, such as karate or wrestling.[65]

## Triad Factor 1: Disordered Eating

Restrictive eating behaviors practiced by girls and women in sports or physical activities that emphasize leanness are of special concern. When these athletes try to lose weight as a way to improve their athletic performance, they may be putting themselves at risk for disordered eating. Research suggests that female athletes are at greater risk for disordered eating than females not involved with an athletics program.[66]

## Triad Factor 2: Amenorrhea

Once body fat falls below 20 percent, a woman's estrogen levels often drop significantly. As a result, women's bodies enter a menopause-like state years ahead of time. Their periods become irregular or cease altogether. Bone loss accelerates, just as it would after natural menopause. Many female athletes who suffer from this triad have the bone density of women in their fifties and sixties. Weakened bones are more likely to fracture during exercise or daily activities. Stress fractures can be a red flag for female athlete triad. Because much of this bone loss is irreversible, women who suffer from the female athlete triad are at increased risk of developing osteoporosis.[67]

In the general population, 2 to 5 percent of women have amenorrhea. However, the prevalence is much higher in athletes.[68] Research indicates that amenorrhea in athletic women is related to the combined effects of increased physical activity, weight loss, low body fat levels, and insufficient energy intake.

## Triad Factor 3: Premature Osteoporosis

Health consequences of amenorrhea often include premature osteoporosis. Research shows that amenorrheic athletes experience rapid loss of bone mineral density in the spine, which can spread to other parts of the skeleton if amenorrhea continues for a long time.

Treatment involves replacing estrogen, which is low in amenorrheic females. Calcium supplementation is also recommended. Although bone mineralization may never return to normal in amenorrheic athletes, studies indicate that reducing the intensity of training, improving dietary intake, and increasing body weight can help restore menstruation and increase bone density.[69]

To help combat this alarming trend, the American College of Sports Medicine and the National Collegiate Athletic Association (NCAA) have

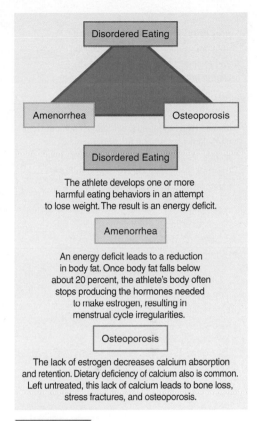

**Figure SED.12** **Female athlete triad.** Disordered eating that results in excessive weight loss can lead to amenorrhea, which, in turn, can lead to osteoporosis.

**amenorrhea [A-men-or-Ee-a]** Absence or abnormal stoppage of menses in a female; commonly indicated by the absence of three to six consecutive menstrual cycles.

**pregorexia** A term used to describe pregnant women who reduce calories and exercise in excess in an effort to control pregnancy weight gain.

**infantile anorexia** Severe feeding difficulties that begin with the introduction of solid foods to infants. Symptoms include persistent food refusal for more than one month, malnutrition, parental concern about the child's poor food intake, and significant caregiver–infant conflict during feeding.

established an eating disorders awareness campaign aimed at coaches and trainers. The NCAA also has a three-part video series, *Nutrition and Eating Disorders*, to acquaint coaches and trainers with the causes and effects of eating disorders as well as the steps to take when they suspect an athlete has an eating disorder.

Screening, referral, and education are keys to preventing the female athlete triad. Prevention and treatment are most successful when they are interdisciplinary efforts provided by a team of medical, athletic, nutrition, and mental health experts. Proactive sports education includes reducing the emphasis on body weight, eliminating group weigh-ins, treating each athlete individually, and facilitating healthy weight management.

**Key Concepts** *Athletics can be a gateway to eating disorders. Female athletes who develop restrictive eating habits are at risk for developing a severe syndrome known as the female athlete triad. Disordered eating, amenorrhea, and abnormally low bone density characterize this syndrome. If not corrected, the female athlete triad can hinder athletic performance and set the stage for lifelong health problems.*

## Pregorexia

In the summer of 2008, the mainstream media introduced us to a new term, **pregorexia**, to describe pregnant women who reduce calories and exercise in excess in an effort to control pregnancy weight gain.[70] However, many women gain too much weight while pregnant, which prompted the American College of Obstetricians and Gynecology to encourage physicians to discuss appropriate weight gain with their pregnant patients.[71] But what about those women with a history of eating disorders who become pregnant? Women who struggled with body image prior to becoming pregnant may need special attention, care, and recommendations. The good news is that research shows that some women with eating disorders experience a reduction in the severity of their symptoms during pregnancy.[72] However it is viewed, the term *pregorexia* has given healthcare professionals an avenue into talking about eating disorders with women who are or who are trying to become pregnant.

## Infantile Anorexia

Can unwitting parents create disordered eating in infants, perhaps setting the stage for eating disorders later in life? Do maternal feeding patterns play a role?[73] Childhood nutrition specialist Ellyn Satter has analyzed videotapes of infant feedings. Satter examined whether parents responded to—or ignored—their babies' nonverbal eating readiness cues. She concluded that many parents fail to recognize their babies' body language: They feed their babies too rapidly or too slowly, they offer foods the baby doesn't care for, or they persist in trying to feed a clearly full baby who is turning away from food. These well-meaning parents may inadvertently teach their babies to ignore hunger and satiety (fullness) cues and, instead, to eat in response to outside influences.[74]

**Infantile anorexia** is described as a feeding disorder of infancy characterized by extreme food refusal, growth deficiency, and an apparent lack of appetite.[75] It can result in acute and/or chronic malnutrition. In addition, the condition usually results in conflict in the mother–infant relationship over issues of autonomy, dependency, and control.[76] Symptoms include persistent food refusal for more than a month, malnutrition, parental concern about the child's poor food intake, and significant caregiver–infant conflict during feeding. The disorder typically starts or worsens during the transition from nursing to spoon-feeding and self-feeding, between ages 6 months and 3 years. Food refusal by the infant usually varies from meal to meal and among different caregivers, with the result being inadequate food intake in general.

Babies with infantile anorexia should not be confused with picky eaters. Picky eaters may initially refuse all foods but allow themselves to be coaxed into eating. Picky eaters have strong food likes and dislikes but are not malnourished. And the relationship between the picky eaters and their parents or caregivers lacks the element of frustration and conflict seen in infantile anorexia.

Infantile anorexia has many serious consequences. Malnutrition can impair the developing brain and adds special stress to the parent–infant relationship. Furthermore, early conflict around meals may herald a lifelong unhealthy relationship with food.

**Key Concepts** *Researchers are continuously recognizing associations between eating disorders and behaviors such as vegetarianism and smoking. Even babies and young children may suffer from disordered eating patterns.*

## Combating Eating Disorders

Eating disorders are extremely difficult to treat, although advances in neurochemistry and scientific understanding of the mind–body connection may provide new avenues of treatment. Most experts agree that emphasis should be placed on preventing eating disorders. (See Table SED.9.)

Preventing eating disorders depends on establishing appropriate mind–body–food relationships. Eating intuitively, an alternative approach to the diet mentality of our culture, suggests that we should trust ourselves and follow the body's signals. This approach might entail reframing our relationships

| Table SED.9 | **Combating Disordered Eating in Athletes** |

*De-emphasize Body Weight*
Do not view the athlete's weight as the primary contributor to, or detractor from, athletic performance. Research indicates that athletes can achieve appropriate weight and fitness when the focus is on physical conditioning and strength development, as well as the cognitive and emotional aspects of performance.

*Eliminate Group Weigh-ins*
Often viewed as a way to motivate the team, the practice of group weigh-ins can be destructive to people who are struggling with their body image and disordered eating. If there is a legitimate reason for weighing an athlete, explain the reason and weigh the athlete privately.

*Treat Each Athlete Individually*
Many athletes have an unrealistic perception of what an ideal body weight is, especially in sports for which leanness is considered important. Additionally, athletes may strive for weight and body composition that may be realistic in only a few genetically endowed people. It is important to understand that genetic and biological processes, rather than one's willpower to control food intake, affect a person's weight.

*Facilitate Healthy Weight Management*
Be sensitive to issues related to weight control and dieting. Because many athletes have limited knowledge of sports nutrition, they resort to pathogenic weight-loss practices. Athletes can benefit from nutrition counseling by a sports nutritionist or a registered dietitian who has experience in working with athletes and disordered eating.

Source: Thompson RA, Sherman RT. Reducing the risk of eating disorders in athletics. *Eating Disorders: Journal of Treatment and Prevention.* 1993;1:65–78. Reproduced by permission of Taylor & Francis Ltd, http://www.tandf.co.uk/journals.

to our body, for example, learning to distinguish physical from emotional feelings and gaining a sense of body wisdom. It's also a process of making peace with food and expunging constant "food worry" thoughts. One plan for learning to eat intuitively is presented in Table SED.10.

Although intuitive eating appears simple, it entails complex processes. For example, one basic principle of intuitive eating is the ability to respond to inner body cues. "Eat when you're hungry and stop when you're full" may sound like a no-brainer, but it requires developing sensitivity to your body's signals.

**Table SED.10** **Intuitive Eating**

The first six principles are positive steps to better nutrition and health. They are followed by your steps to rid yourself of false diet principles that we have been misled to believe and that have promoted eating disorders.

*1. Honor Your Hunger*

Feed your body with adequate energy and carbohydrates. Excessive hunger can trigger a primal drive to overeat. Intentions of moderate, conscious eating are fleeting and irrelevant. Learning to honor this first biological signal sets the stage for rebuilding trust with yourself and food.

*2. Respect Your Body Signals*

Your body will tell you that you are no longer hungry. Pause in the middle of a meal or food and ask yourself how the food tastes and what your current fullness level is.

*3. Discover the Satisfaction Factor*

When you eat what you really want, in an environment that is inviting and conducive, the pleasure you derive will be a powerful force in helping you feel satisfied and content. By providing this experience for yourself, you will find that it takes less food to decide you've had "enough."

*4. Respect Your Body*

Your have a genetic blueprint. Just as a size 8 foot does not squeeze into a size 6 shoe, it is equally futile (and uncomfortable) to aim for a body size unrelated to your genes. But mostly, respect your body so you can feel better about who you are. It's hard to reject the diet mentality if you are unrealistic and overly critical about your body shape.

*5. Exercise—Feel the Difference*

Mobilize yourself, but forget militant exercise. Shift your focus to how it feels to move your body, rather than the calorie-burning effect of exercise. If you focus on how you feel from working out, such as energized, it can make the difference between rolling out of bed for a brisk morning walk and hitting the snooze alarm.

*6. Honor Your Health—Gentle Nutrition*

Make food choices that honor your health and tastebuds while making you feel well. Remember that you don't have to eat a perfect diet to be healthy. You will not suddenly get a nutrient deficiency or gain weight from one snack, one meal, or one day of eating. It's what you eat consistently over time that matters; progress, not perfection, is what counts.

*7. Honor Your Feelings Without Using Food*

Find ways to comfort, nurture, distract, and resolve your issues without using food. Anxiety, loneliness, boredom, anger are emotions. Each has its own trigger, and each has its own appeasement. Food won't fix any of these feelings, although it may temporarily comfort, distract from pain, or even numb you into a food hangover. If anything, eating for an emotional hunger will complicate your problems.

*8. Reject the Diet Mentality*

Disregard diets that offer you false hopes of losing weight quickly, easily, and permanently. Reject lies that lead you to feel like a failure when each new diet stops working and you gain back the weight.

*9. Make Peace with Food*

Call a truce, stop the food fight! Give yourself unconditional permission to eat. Denying yourself a particular food can lead to feelings of deprivation that build into uncontrollable cravings, and often bingeing. No "last supper" overeating, and no overwhelming guilt.

*10. Challenge the Food Police*

Shout "no" to wrongheaded thoughts that declare you're "good" for eating less than 1,000 calories or "bad" because you're eating chocolate cake. The food police monitor the unreasonable rules that dieting has created. The police station is housed deep in your psyche, and its loudspeaker shouts negative barbs, hopeless phrases, and guilt-provoking indictments. Chasing the food police away is a critical step in returning to intuitive eating.

**Source:** Courtesy of Evelyn Tribole and Elyse Resch. http://www.intuitiveeating.com.

| Table SED.11 | **Preventing Eating Disorders** |

To join the effort to prevent eating disorders, follow these tips:

- Celebrate the diversity of human body shapes and sizes.
- Present accurate information about nutrition, weight management, and health.
- Discourage restrictive eating practices, including skipping meals.
- Encourage people to eat in response to hunger, not emotions.
- Reinforce messages about good eating and activity patterns at school and at home.
- Carefully phrase comments about a person's weight, body, or fitness level.
- Teach children and young people how to constructively express negative emotions.
- Encourage parents, teachers, coaches, and other professionals who work with children to do likewise.
- Encourage people of all ages to focus on personal qualities rather than physical appearance, of themselves and others.
- Find and promote images of fit people of all sizes and shapes.

**Quick Bite**

**Scary Statistics**
About 5 million Americans have anorexia nervosa, bulimia, or binge-eating disorders. Researchers estimate that 15 percent of young women have disordered eating attitudes and behaviors. Every year an estimated 1,000 people die from anorexia nervosa.

The NIH believes that healthcare professionals should lead the eating disorder prevention effort by learning to promote self-esteem in their patients and teaching patients that people can be healthy at every size. Ideally, this approach would have a ripple effect: Patients would transmit these beliefs to others. A variety of public information campaigns aimed at parents and people who work with children and adolescents have evolved over the past decade to help promote eating disorder awareness. One of the most prominent examples is the Body Size Acceptance campaign coordinated through the University of California, Berkeley, under the direction of Joanne Ikeda. (See Table SED.11.)

# *Learning* Portfolio

## Key Terms

## Study Points

- An eating disorder is a complex emotional illness, the primary symptom of which is significantly altered eating habits. Eating disorders occur in susceptible people exposed to particular types of environmental stimuli.

- Although eating disorders existed even in ancient times, they have become alarmingly common in industrialized countries.

- Eating disorders involve highly restrictive eating patterns (seen in anorexia nervosa), a combination of compulsive overeating and purging (seen in bulimia nervosa), or unrestricted binge eating.

- Eating disorders are common in people who participate in body-conscious activities such as dance, wrestling, gymnastics, and bodybuilding.

- From 1 to 5 percent of people with eating disorders are male.

- Anorexia nervosa is an obsession for thinness manifested in self-imposed starvation.

- The typical person with anorexia nervosa is a young Caucasian woman from an upper-class, achievement-oriented family.

- Victims of anorexia nervosa have a body weight at least 15 percent below normal, a distorted body image, and physical and psychological symptoms related to starvation.

- The body weight of people with bulimia nervosa is close to or even slightly above that considered healthy for their height.

- Key symptoms of bulimia nervosa are binge-eating episodes occurring at least twice a week for three months, followed by severe dieting, purging, or a combination of dieting and purging.

- Binge-eating disorder is the most common eating disorder.

- Like those with bulimia, people with binge-eating disorder consume more food than is typically eaten in a given period of time.

- People with body dysmorphic disorder (BDD) are preoccupied with an imagined or slight defect in appearance.

- In night-eating syndrome, the food intake rhythm may be out of sync with a person's normal sleep rhythm by as much as four to five hours.

- Many competitive athletes, both male and female, have disordered eating behaviors.

- Disordered eating, amenorrhea, and abnormally low bone density characterize the female athlete triad.

- The best treatment for eating disorders is prevention. Once an eating disorder has become entrenched, intensive and prolonged treatment is typically required. Many people require lifelong support to maintain healthful eating and lifestyle habits.

## Study Questions

1. List the diagnostic criteria for anorexia nervosa, bulimia nervosa, and binge-eating disorder.
2. What are the warning signs of anorexia nervosa?
3. What is the usual treatment for people with anorexia nervosa, and what do most experts say about their recovery?
4. What is the typical profile of a person with bulimia nervosa?
5. Describe an eating binge and all the behaviors that constitute purging.
6. How does binge-eating disorder differ from bulimia?

## Try This

### Is There Any Help Out There?

How much help is available in your community for people with eating disorders? Scan the telephone directory (Yellow Pages) and the Internet for eating disorder clinics, programs, and centers. Call them to inquire about their services. Do they have a psychologist, medical doctor, dietitian, nurse, and/or social worker on staff? Is it an inpatient or outpatient program? What is their philosophy of therapy? What is their success rate? What are their payment plans?

# What About Bobbie?

Bobbie's friend Janet has been struggling with anorexia nervosa for some time. Bobbie recently expressed concern again and asked Janet about her eating habits. Janet told Bobbie she eats the following foods in a typical day:

---

**"Breakfast"**
1 head of iceberg lettuce, with salt and pepper but no dressing (If she wakes up really hungry, she'll have another with vinegar on it.)

**"Snack"**
6 to 8 white mushrooms

**"Lunch"**
3 or 4 dill pickles

**"Dinner"**
1 12-ounce can artichoke hearts (rinsed)

**"Fluids"**
Fluids include mineral water, diet cola, and/or caffeinated tea.

---

Let's compare this intake with Bobbie's daily intake (see the "Food Choices: Nutrients and Nourishment" chapter to review Bobbie's one-day diet). First, Janet's daily intake is just under 300 kilocalories compared with Bobbie's 2,440. Not only is Janet at risk due to her lack of calories, but her intake of protein is approximately 0 grams. Her body has already used any glycogen it had as reserve fuel. In addition, at 5 feet 3 inches and 98 pounds, she has very little reserve fat tissue for future energy needs. Without intake of dietary protein, her organ and muscle tissues have become prime targets for degradation. Even though Janet takes a multivitamin and a mineral supplement, if she doesn't seek help soon, she may suffer the typical symptoms and effects of starvation and malnutrition.

# References

1    Academy of Nutrition and Dietetics. Position of the Academy of Nutrition and Dietetics: nutrition intervention in the treatment of anorexia nervosa, bulimia nervosa, and eating disorders not otherwise specified (EDNOS). *J Am Diet Assoc.* 2003;103:748–765.

2    Academy of Nutrition and Dietetics. *Manual of Clinical Dietetics.* 6th ed. Chicago: Academy of Nutrition and Dietetics; 2000.

3    Siegel M, Brisman J, Weinshel M. *Surviving an Eating Disorder, Strategies for Family and Friends.* 3rd ed. New York: Collins Living; 2009.

4    Neumark-Sztainer D, Wall M, Larson N, Eisenberg M, Loth K. Dieting and disordered eating behaviors from adolescence to young adulthood: findings from a 10-year longitudinal study. *J Am Diet Assoc.* 2011;111(7):1004–1011.

5    Ibid.

6    Pearce JM. Richard Morton: origins of anorexia nervosa. *Eur Neurol.* 2004;52:191–192.

7    Ibid.

8    Gates K, Pritchard M. The relationship among religious affiliation, religious angst, and disordered eating. *Eat Weight Disord.* 2009;14(1):e11–e15.

9    Reid TR. The world according to Rome. *National Geographic.* 1997;8:54–83.

10   Hudson JL, Hiripi E, Pope HG, Kessler RC. The prevalence and correlates of eating disorders in the national comorbidity survey replication. *Biol Psychiatry.* 2007;61:348–358.

11   Favaro A, Caregaro L, Tenconi E, Bosello R, Santonastaso P. Time trends in age at onset of anorexia nervosa and bulimia nervosa. *J Clin Psychiatry.* 2009;70(12):1715–1721.

12   Dittmar H, Halliwell E, Ive S. Does Barbie make girls want to be thin? The effect of experimental exposure to images of dolls on the body image of 5- to 8-year-old girls. *Dev Psychol.* 2006;42(2):283–292.

13   Yoo JJ, Jonson KK. Effects of appearance-related testing on ethnically diverse adolescent girls. *Adolescence.* 2007;42(166):353–380.

14   Krukowski RA, West S, Perez P, et al. Overweight children, weight-based teasing, and academic performance. *Int J Pediatr Obes.* 2009;4(4):274–280.

15   Harrington EF, Crowther JH, Shipherd JC. Trauma, binge eating, and the "strong Black woman." *J Consult Clin Psychol.* 2010;78(4):469–479.

16   Tagay S, Schlegl S, Senf W. Traumatic events, posttraumatic stress symptomatology and somatoform symptoms in eating disorder patients. *Eur Eat Disord Rev.* 2010;18(2):124–132.

17   Fitzpatrick KK, Lock J. Anorexia nervosa. *Clin Evid* (Online). 2011 Apr 11. pii:1011.

18   Flament MF, Bissada H, Spettigue W. Evidence-based pharmacotherapy of eating disorders. *Int J Neuropsychopharmacol.* 2011 Mar 18:1–19.

19   Redman LM, Ravussin E. Lorcaserin for the treatment of obesity. *Drugs Today* (Barc). 2010;46(12):901–910.

20   Ahren-Moonga J, Silverwood R, AF Klinteberg B, Koupil I. Association of higher parental and grandparental education and higher school grades with risk of hospitalization for eating disorders in females. The Uppsala Birth Cohort Multigenerational Study. *Am J Epidemiol.* 2009;170(5):566–575.

21   Perdereau F, Faucher S, Wallier J, Vibert S, Godart N. Family history of anxiety and mood disorders in anorexia nervosa: review of the literature. *Eat Weight Disord.* 2008;13(1):1–13.

22   Briley M, Moret C. Improvement of social adaptation in depression with serotonin and norepinephrine reuptake inhibitors. *Neuropsychiatr Dis Treat.* 2010;6:647–655.

23   Stice E, Yokum S, Zaid D, Dagher A. Dopamine-based reward circuitry responsivity, genetics, and overeating. *Curr Top Behav Neurosci.* 2011;6:81–93.

24   American Medical Association. JAMA patient page; anorexia nervosa. *JAMA.* 2006;295(22):2684.

25   Urquhart CS, Mihalynuk TV. Disordered eating in women: implications for the obesity pandemic. *Can J Diet Pract Res.* 2011;72(1):50.

26   Stice E, Marti CN, Shaw H, Jaconis M. An 8-year longitudinal study of the natural history of threshold, subthreshold, and partial eating disorders from a community sample of adolescents. *J Abnorm Psychol.* 2009;118(3):587–597.

27   Wood NA, Petrie TA. Body dissatisfaction, ethnic identity, and disordered eating among African American women. *J Couns Psychol.* 2010;57(2):141–153.

28   Ma JL. Eating disorders, parent–child conflicts, and family therapy in Shenzhen, China. *Qual Health Res.* 2008;18(6):803–810.

29   Academy of Nutrition and Dietetics. Position of the Academy of Nutrition and Dietetics: nutrition intervention in the treatment of anorexia nervosa, bulimia nervosa, and other eating disorders. *J Am Diet Assoc.* 2006;109:2073–2082.

30   Harrison A, Treasure J, Smillie LD. Approach and avoidance motivation in eating disorders. *Psychiatry Res.* 2011;188(3):396–401.

31   Byrd-Bredbenner C, Moe G, Beshgetoor D, Bernign J. *Wardlaw's Perspectives in Nutrition.* 8th ed. New York: McGraw-Hill; 2009.

32   Keel PK, Dorer DJ, Eddy KT, et al. Predictors of mortality in eating disorders. *Arch Gen Psych.* 2003;60:179–183.

33   Academy of Nutrition and Dietetics. 2006. Op. cit.

34  Ibid.

35  Monteleone P, Di Genio M, Monteleone AM, Di Filippo C, Maj M. Investigation of factors associated to crossover from anorexia nervosa restricting type (ANR) and anorexia nervosa binge-purging type (ANBP) to bulimia nervosa and comparison of bulimia nervosa patients with or without previous ANR or ANBP. *Compr Psychiatry*. 2011;52(1):56–62.

36  Mehler PS, Winkelman AB, Anderson DM, Gaudiani JL. Nutritional rehabilitation: practical guidelines for refeeding the anorectic patient. *J Nutr Metab*. 2010 Feb 7:pii:625782; and Forcano L, Alvarez E, Santamaria JJ, Jimenez-Murcia S, et al. Suicide attempts in anorexia nervosa subtypes. *Compr Psychiatry*. 2011;52(4):352–358.

37  Fitzpatrick KK, Lock J. Anorexia nervosa. *Clin Evid* (Online). 2011 Apr 11;pii:1011.

38  Gentile MG, Manna GM, Pastorelli P, Oitolini A. Resumption of menses after 32 years in anorexia nervosa. *Eat Weight Disord*. 2011 May 23.

39  Keel PK, Dorer DJ, Eddy KT, et al. Op. cit.

40  Khaylis A, Trockel M, Taylor CB. Binge drinking in women at risk for developing eating disorders. *Int J Eat Disord*. 2009;42(5):409–414.

41  Fischer S, Settles R, Collins B, Gunn R, Smith GT. The role of negative urgency and expectancies in problem drinking and disordered eating: Testing a model of comorbidity in pathological and at-risk samples. *Psychol Addict Behav*. 2011 May 23.

42  Greene GW, Schembre SM, White AA, et al. Identifying clusters of college students at elevated health risk based on eating and exercise behaviors and psychosocial determinants of body weight. *J Am Diet Assoc*. 2011;111(3):394–400.

43  Strong KA, Parks SL, Anderson E, Winett R, Davy BM. Weight gain prevention: identifying theory-based targets for health behavior change in young adults. *J Am Diet Assoc*. 2008;108(10):1708–1715.

44  Ibid.

45  Ibid.

46  French SA, Leffert N, Story M, et al. Adolescent binge/purge and weight loss behaviors: associations with developmental assets. *J Adolesc Health*. 2001;28:211–221.

47  Academy of Nutrition and Dietetics. 2006. Op. cit.

48  American Psychiatric Association. *Diagnostic and Statistical Manual of Mental Disorders, Fourth Edition, Text Revision (DSM–IV–TR)*. Washington, DC: American Psychiatric Association; 2000.

49  Allen KL, Fursland A, Watson H, Byrne SM. Eating disorder diagnosis in general practice settings: comparison with structured clinical interview and self-report questionnaires. *J Ment Health*. 2011;20(3):270–280.

50  Neumark-Sztainer D, Wall M, Haines J, Story M, Eisenberg ME. Why does dieting predict weight gain in adolescents? Findings from Project EAT-II: a 5-year longitudinal study. *J Am Diet Assoc*. 2007;107(3):448–455.

51  Fenske JN, Schwenk TL. Obsessive compulsive disorder: diagnosis and management. *Am Fam Physician*. 2009;80(3):239–245.

52  Hudson JI, Hiripi E, Pope HG, Kessler RC. The prevalence and correlates of eating disorders in the National Comorbidity Survey Replication. *Biol Psychiatry*. 2007;61:348–358.

53  National Institute of Mental Health. The numbers count: mental disorders in America. 2008. http://nimh.nih.gov.

54  Klczynski PA, Goold KW, Mudry JJ. Culture, obesity stereotypes, self-esteem and the "thin ideal": a social identity perspective. *J Youth Adolesc*. 2004;33(4):307–317.

55  Caqueo-Urizar A, Ferrer-Garcia M, Toro J, Gutierrez-Maldonado J, et al. Associations between sociocultural pressures to be thin, body distress, and eating disorder symptomatology among Chilean adolescent girls. *Body Image*. 2011;8(1):78–81.

56  Andersen AE, Cohn L, Holbrook T. *Making Weight: Men's Conflicts with Food, Weight, Shape, and Appearance*. Carlsbad, CA: Gurze Books; 2000.

57  Resch M. Eating disorders in sports—sport in eating disorders. *Orv Hetil*. 2007;148(40):1899–1902.

58  Ibid.

59  Sundgot-Borgen J, Torstveit MK. Aspects of disordered eating continuum in elite high-intensity sports. *Scand J Med Sci Sports*. 2010;20(suppl 2):112–121.

60  Schaal K, Tafflet M, Nassif H, et al. Psychological balance in high level athletes: gender-based differences and sport-specific patterns. *PLoS One*. 2011;6(5):e19007.

61  Nattiv A, Loucks AB, Manore MM, Sanborn CF, Sundgot-Borgen J, Warren MP. American College of Sports Medicine position stand. The female athlete triad. *Med Sci Sports Exerc*. 2007;39(10):1867–1882.

62  Otis CI, Drinkwater B, Johnson M, et al. American College of Sports Medicine position stand. The female athlete triad. *Med Sci Sports Exerc*. 2005;37(2):184–193.

63  Nattiv A, Loucks AB, Manore MM, Sanborn CF, Sundgot-Borgen J, Warren MP. Op. cit.

64  Zach KN, Smith Machin A, Hoch AZ. Advances in management of the female athlete triad and eating disorders. *Clin Sports Med*. 2011;30(3):551–573.

65  Nattiv A, Loucks AB, Manore MM, Sanborn CF, Sundgot-Borgen J, Warren MP. Op. cit.

66  Hoch AZ, Pajewski NM, Moraski L, et al. Prevalence of the female athlete triad in high school athletes and sedentary students. *Clin J Sport Med*. 2009;19(5):421–428.

67  Ackerman KE, Misra M. bone health and the female athlete triad in adolescent athletes. *Phys Sportsmed*. 2011;39(1):131–141.

68  Enea C, Boisseau N, Fargeas-Gluck MA, Diaz V, Dugue B. Circulating androgens in women: exercise-induced changes. *Sports Med*. 2011;41(1):1–15.

69  Ibid.

70  Mathieu J. What is pregorexia? *J Am Diet Assoc*. 2009;109(6):976–979.

71  Ibid.

72  Ibid.

73  Kroller K, Warschburger P. Problematic eating behavior in childhood: do maternal feeding patterns play a role? *Prax Kinderpsychol Kinderpsychiatr*. 2011;60(4):253–269.

74  Satter E. *Secrets of Feeding a Healthy Family: Orchestrating and Enjoying the Family Meal*. Madison, WI: Kelcy Press; 2008.

75  Ammaniti M, Lucarelli L, Cimino S, D'Olimpio F, Chatoor I. Feeding disorders of infancy: a longitudinal study to middle childhood. *Int J Eat Disord*. 2011 Apr 14.

76  Kroller K, Warschburger P. Op. cit.

# CHAPTER 12

# Life Cycle: Maternal and Infant Nutrition

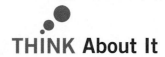

## THINK About It

1  Saying that she is "eating for two," your pregnant friend can't stop eating. What do you think about this?

2  Your best friend tells you she is pregnant. You know that she enjoys wine with dinner. What do you say to her?

3  Were you breastfed? Do you know of any benefits?

4  At a fast-food restaurant, you observe a man and woman giving a very young infant tiny pieces of french fries and a baby bottle filled with cola. Any thoughts?

**Visit go.jblearning.com/inseldisco4e**

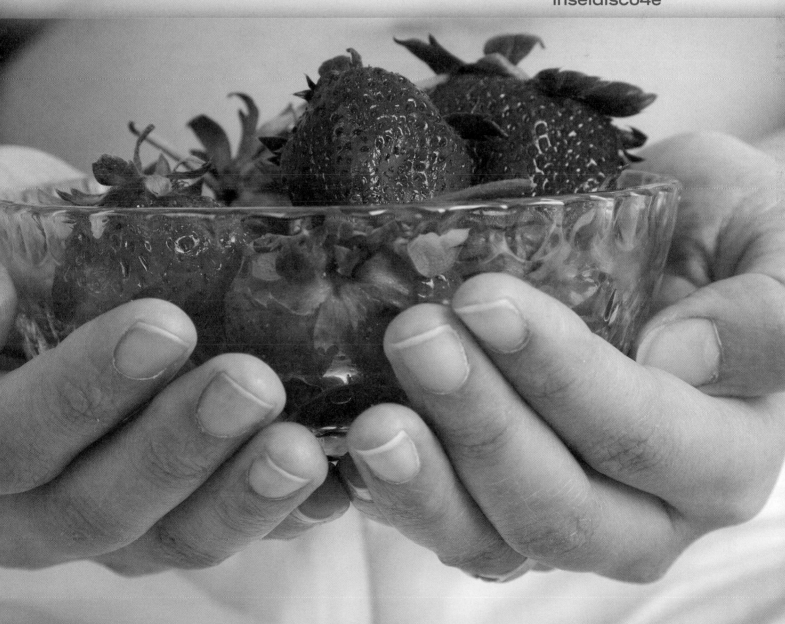

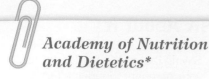

## Academy of Nutrition and Dietetics*

**Nutrition and Lifestyle for a Healthy Pregnancy Outcome**

It is the position of the American Dietetic Association that women of childbearing age should maintain good nutritional status through a lifestyle that optimizes maternal health and reduces the risk of birth defects, suboptimal fetal development, and chronic health problems in their children. The key components of a health-promoting lifestyle during pregnancy include appropriate weight gain; appropriate physical activity; consumption of a variety of foods in accordance with the *Dietary Guidelines for Americans 2005*; appropriate and timely vitamin and mineral supplementation; avoidance of alcohol, tobacco, and other harmful substances; and safe food handling. Pregnant women with inappropriate weight gain, hyperemesis, poor dietary patterns, phenylketonuria, certain chronic health problems, or a history of substance abuse should be referred to a registered dietitian for medical nutrition therapy.

**Source:** Reproduced from Kaiser L, Allen LH. Position of the Academy of Nutrition and Dietetics: nutrition and lifestyle for a healthy pregnancy outcome. *J Am Diet Assoc.* 2008;108(3):553–561.

\* Formerly the American Dietetic Association

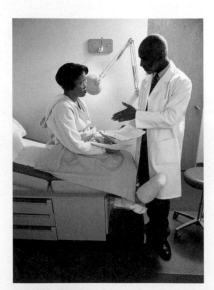

**Figure 12.1**   **Preconception care.** Planning and care before pregnancy are recommended for all prospective mothers.

Imagine waking up tomorrow and finding a newborn baby in the house! Play along for a moment with the idea that it's your baby. Would your current eating habits be sufficient to support the nutritional demands of pregnancy? If not, what changes would you need to make and why? What about other aspects of your lifestyle that you might need to modify before pregnancy, such as smoking, alcohol use, and exercise? How would you feed a new baby? Breastfeeding poses its own nutritional demands on the mother but benefits the infant in many ways. If you've never shopped for infant formula or baby food before, you may be surprised at the variety of choices and confused as to which is best. So, although the likelihood of waking up tomorrow and finding a newborn in the house is remote, it's never too early to learn about the nutritional implications of pregnancy, breastfeeding, and infant feeding.

## Pregnancy

For the mother, pregnancy is a time of tremendous physiological changes, and these changes demand healthful dietary and lifestyle choices. Energy and nutrient needs both increase, but the need for calories increases by a smaller percentage than for most vitamins and minerals. As a result, food choices during pregnancy must be nutrient-dense.

What about tobacco and alcohol? Research clearly shows that both substances produce damaging effects on a developing fetus, and it's essential for the mother to abstain from both tobacco and alcohol during pregnancy. Although research about the effects of caffeine is less conclusive, most healthcare professionals also recommend limiting caffeine intake during pregnancy.

### Nutrition Before Conception

Everyone knows a woman needs to eat healthfully once she becomes pregnant. But, her nutritional status at the moment of conception also is important. The mother's vitamin status at conception, for example, can mean the difference between producing a healthy baby and one with a devastating birth defect. In addition, a woman's weight from the embryo's conception can influence her pregnancy and delivery and the baby's health.

For these reasons, it's important for a woman to get health care and guidance before she gets pregnant. Many experts recommend extending prenatal care—the routine professional health care that a woman receives during her pregnancy—to include the preconception period as well. (See **Figure 12.1**.) Although extending prenatal healthcare is certainly a worthy goal, it is important to realize that about half the pregnancies in the United States are unplanned. Hence, good nutrition for all women of childbearing age is an important public health objective.

Preconception care can be defined as a set of interventions that identify and modify biomedical, behavioral, and social risks to a woman's health or pregnancy outcome through prevention and management.[1] The overall goal is to provide (1) screening for risks, (2) health promotion and education, and (3) interventions to address identified risks. Nutrition is an important aspect of all three goals. Risk screening includes an evaluation of a prospective mother's vitamin status and weight, as well as her health habits—including use of alcohol, tobacco, and other substances—and her overall medical condition. Health promotion and education provides the would-be mother information about what she can do to maximize her chances of a trouble-free pregnancy, an uneventful delivery, and a healthy, full-term baby. Intervention can be as simple as recommending a folic acid supplement or as complex as treating an eating disorder or a substance abuse problem. Before conception, the goal is to resolve the nutrition and health issues that could harm a mother or her baby. Table 12.1 lists 10 recommendations for preconception health developed by the Centers for Disease Control and Prevention (CDC).

## Weight

Although everyone should be concerned about maintaining a healthful weight, a woman contemplating pregnancy needs to pay especially careful attention to weight. Maternal obesity can complicate pregnancy and delivery and may compromise a baby's health. Similarly, being too thin carries its own risks.

Body mass index (BMI) is an indicator of a prospective mother's weight status. Lean women with a BMI less than 20 kg/m$^2$ have increased risks of **preterm delivery**.[2] At the other end of the spectrum, nearly two-thirds of U.S. women of childbearing age are overweight or obese, and one-fifth are obese at the start of pregnancy.[3] Overweight and obese women have increased risks of several problems, including preterm delivery and stillbirth.[4] In addition, obese women are at higher risk for the following:[5]

- High blood pressure
- Gestational diabetes—a form of diabetes that is associated with pregnancy; it often is controlled through diet alone
- **Preeclampsia**—a condition of late pregnancy marked by maternal high blood pressure and protein in the urine
- Prolonged labor
- Unplanned cesarean section
- Difficulty initiating and continuing breastfeeding

Of course, the time to lose or gain weight is well before a pregnancy begins. It is not a good idea for pregnant women, even obese pregnant women,

| Table 12.1 | Recommendations for Preconception Health |
| --- | --- |
| **Individual responsibility** | Each woman, man, and couple should be encouraged to have a reproductive life plan. |
| **Consumer awareness** | Increase public awareness of appropriate preconception health behaviors. |
| **Preventive visits** | Provide risk assessment and health promotion counseling to all women of childbearing age during primary care visits. |
| **Intervention for identified risks** | Provide interventions to women following risk identification. |
| **Interconception care** | Use the interconception period for intensive interventions. |
| **Pre-pregnancy check-ups** | Offer pre-pregnancy visits as a component of maternity care. |
| **Health insurance coverage** | Increase coverage to ensure access for low-income women. |
| **Public health programs** | Integrate preconception health into existing public health programs. |
| **Research** | Increase the evidence base for methods to improve preconception health. |
| **Monitoring** | Use public health surveillance mechanisms to monitor the effectiveness of preconception care. |

Source: Centers for Disease Control and Prevention. Recommendations to improve preconception health and health care—United States. *MMWR.* 2006;55(RR-06):1–23. http://www.cdc.gov/mmwr/preview/mmwrhtml/rr5506a1.htm. Accessed 8/3/11.

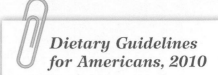

## Dietary Guidelines for Americans, 2010

**Key Recommendations**
- Maintain appropriate calorie balance during each stage of life—childhood, adolescence, adulthood, pregnancy and breastfeeding, and older age.

**Key Recommendations for Specific Population Groups**

Women Capable of Becoming Pregnant
- Choose foods that supply heme iron, which is more readily absorbed by the body, additional iron sources, and enhancers of iron absorption such as vitamin C–rich foods.
- Consume 400 micrograms (mcg) per day of synthetic folic acid (from fortified foods and/or supplements) in addition to food forms of folate from a varied diet.

**Women Who Are Pregnant or Breastfeeding**
- Consume 8 to 12 ounces of seafood per week from a variety of seafood types.
- Due to their high methyl mercury content, limit white (albacore) tuna to 6 ounces per week and do not eat the following four types of fish: tilefish, shark, swordfish, and king mackerel.
- If pregnant, take an iron supplement, as recommended by an obstetrician or other healthcare provider.

**preterm delivery** A delivery that occurs before the 37th week of gestation.

**preeclampsia** A condition of late pregnancy characterized by maternal hypertension, edema, and proteinuria.

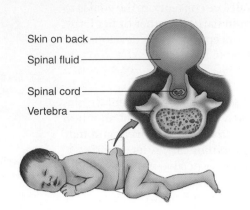

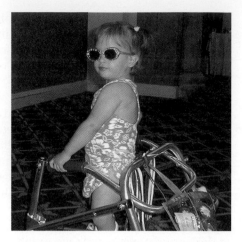

Skin on back
Spinal fluid
Spinal cord
Vertebra

**Figure 12.2** **Spina bifida is a neural tube defect.** Low maternal folate status during the early stages of pregnancy can cause embryonic neural tube defects.

**morning sickness** A persistent or recurring nausea that often occurs during early pregnancy, frequently—but not always—in the morning.

to try to lose weight or follow a restrictive diet during pregnancy. And a thin woman who finds it hard to put on weight under normal circumstances is unlikely to find it any easier when she's pregnant, especially if she experiences **morning sickness**.

### Vitamins

A good diet and healthy eating habits go a long way toward meeting the demands of pregnancy, but even a diet that includes all of the food groups may not contain enough of certain nutrients. This is especially true for folic acid, a nutrient needed to prevent neural tube defects, which are birth defects that involve the spinal column.[6] One of the most common neural tube defects is spina bifida, a birth defect in which part of the spinal cord protrudes through the spinal column, causing varying degrees of paralysis and lack of bowel and bladder control. (See **Figure 12.2.**)

The U.S. Preventive Services Task Force recommends that all women of childbearing age take a daily supplement of 400 to 800 micrograms of synthetic folic acid to reduce the risk of producing a fetal neural tube defect.[7] The CDC estimates that 50 to 70 percent of the birth defects spina bifida and anencephaly could be avoided if women consumed 400 micrograms of folic acid daily before and during pregnancy.[8]

This recommendation encompasses all women of childbearing age—not just pregnant women—because neural tube development occurs before the sixth week of fetal life. During this period, a woman may not know she is pregnant or may not have made appropriate dietary changes. This recommended intake of folic acid is in addition to folate (the natural form of the vitamin) consumed from other foods. Folic acid is added to all enriched grain products and many ready-to-eat cereals. Table 12.2 presents the folate content of selected grain products. The rate of neural tube defects has been declining in recent years, in part as a result of folic acid fortification.

Just as it's important to get enough folic acid, it also is crucial to avoid getting too much vitamin A (retinol) during pregnancy. Some vitamin A is good for you; too much may be teratogenic. A teratogen is a substance that causes birth defects—literally, the term means "monster-producing." The Institute of Medicine considered this link between excessive retinol intake and birth defects in setting the Tolerable Upper Intake Level (UL) of retinol

**Table 12.2** **Folate in Grain Products**

| Foods | Folate DFE (micrograms) |
|---|---|
| Ready-to-eat cereals, such as Cheerios, 1 cup | 493 |
| Egg noodles, cooked, 1 cup | 221 |
| Rice, enriched, cooked, 1 cup | 195 |
| Tortilla, flour, enriched, 1 | 54 |
| Bagel, enriched, 2 oz | 76 |
| Bread, white, enriched, 1 slice | 43 |

**Source:** Data from US Department of Agriculture, Agricultural Research Service. 2010. USDA National Nutrient Database for Standard Reference, Release 23. Nutrient Data Laboratory Home Page. http://www.ars.usda.gov/ba/bhnrc/ndl. Accessed 7/20/11.

for women of childbearing age. The UL is 3,000 micrograms (10,000 IU) of retinol from food and supplements for women over the age of 18. For teens, the UL is 2,800 micrograms (9,300 IU).

Any woman who might become pregnant must avoid using drugs that contain vitamin A or vitamin A analogs; examples are the acne medications isotretinoin (Accutane) and tretinoin (Retin-A). Because these medications are potent teratogens, doctors prescribe such drugs to women of childbearing age only if tests show a woman is not pregnant, and she practices birth control.

Pregnant women can—and should—eat as much as they like of fruits and vegetables rich in beta-carotene and other carotenoids. These foods pose no risk of birth defects and offer many health benefits.

### Substance Use

Many women plan to give up cigarettes, alcohol, or other drugs when they get pregnant. It is more important to give up these substances well before becoming pregnant, which emphasizes the need for preconception guidance.[9] (See **Figure 12.3**.) A woman who uses or abuses tobacco, alcohol, or illicit drugs during pregnancy is likely to have higher pregnancy-related complications and more infant health problems.

**Key Concepts** *Ideally, the time to prepare nutritionally for pregnancy is well before conceiving. A woman who has adequate nutrient stores, particularly of folic acid, and is at a healthy weight is reducing the risk for maternal and fetal complications during pregnancy. In addition to healthful diet selections, avoiding cigarettes, alcohol, and other drugs is important when contemplating pregnancy.*

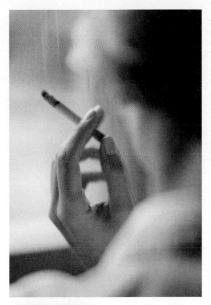

**Figure 12.3** **Substance use.** Using tobacco, alcohol, or illicit drugs before and during pregnancy puts the baby at risk. If you use these substances, stop before becoming pregnant.

## Physiology of Pregnancy

Pregnancy is an awe-inspiring process of growth and development that affects both mother and fetus. An understanding of the stages of growth and development of the fetus, along with the physiological changes that occur in the mother during pregnancy, will help to explain the nutrient needs of a pregnant woman.

### Stages of Human Fetal Growth

How long does pregnancy last? Nine months, right? Well, it depends on when you start counting. When a healthcare provider gives an expectant mother a due date, it is typically calculated as 40 weeks from the date of the start of her last menstrual period, roughly 10 to 14 days before the actual date of conception. This 40-week period often is described as three **trimesters** of 13 or 14 weeks each; however, this division does not reflect specific stages in fetal development.

**Figure 12.4** illustrates the early stages of pregnancy. Following fertilization of the egg (ovum) comes the **blastogenic stage**—a period of rapid cell division. As these cells divide, they begin to differentiate. The inner cells in this growing mass will form the fetus; the outer layer of cells will become the **placenta**. During this stage, which lasts about two weeks, the fertilized ovum implants itself in the wall of the mother's uterus.

The next period of pregnancy, the **embryonic stage**, extends from the end of the second week through the eighth week after conception. The placenta, a vital organ that serves as a conduit between mother and child, forms on the mother's uterine wall during this stage. Attached to the placenta by its umbilical cord, the embryo now receives nourishment from its mother: nearly everything the mother eats, drinks, or smokes reaches the embryo.

The embryonic stage also is a period of **organogenesis**. By the time the embryo is eight weeks old, all the main internal organs have formed, along

**trimesters** Three equal time periods of pregnancy, each lasting approximately 13 to 14 weeks.

**blastogenic stage** The first stage of embryonic gestation during which tissue proliferation by rapid cell division begins.

**placenta** The organ formed during pregnancy that produces hormones for the maintenance of pregnancy and across which oxygen and nutrients are transferred from mother to infant; it also allows waste materials to be transferred from infant to mother.

**embryonic stage** The developmental stage between the time of implantation (about two weeks after fertilization) through the seventh or eighth week; the stage of major organ system differentiation and development of main external features.

**organogenesis** The period when organ systems are developing in a growing fetus.

## *Quick* Bite

### Would It Be Healthier to Menstruate *Less* Often?

Women in industrialized countries, who start menstruating at an average age of 12.5 years, will go through 350 to 400 menstrual cycles in their lifetimes. In populations where birth control is not used, however, women spend the majority of their fertile years either pregnant or lactating. Menarche in these populations occurs at an average age of 16. In addition, because menstrual cycles do not occur during pregnancy and may not occur during lactation, women in natural-fertility populations, such as the Dogon of West Africa, experience only about 110 menstrual cycles in a lifetime. Women who go through fewer menstrual cycles are exposed to less estrogen and other steroid hormones. Researchers hypothesize that this may partly explain why nonindustrialized societies have lower cancer rates than industrialized societies.

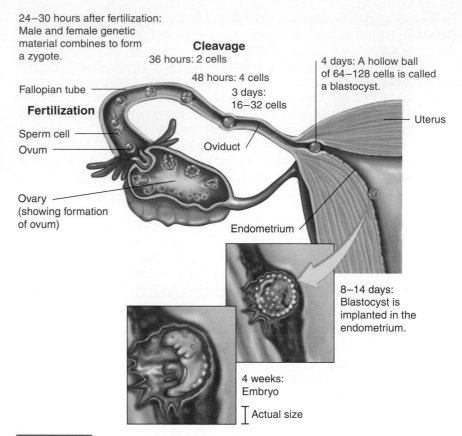

**Figure 12.4**  **Early stages of pregnancy.** The fertilized egg divides rapidly and begins to differentiate. The inner cells become the fetus, and the outer cells become the placenta.

with major external body structures. (See **Figure 12.5**.) Because nutrient deficiencies or excesses and intake of harmful substances can result in congenital abnormalities (birth defects) or spontaneous abortion (miscarriage), this stage is a **critical period of development**.

The longest period of gestation is the **fetal stage**, the period from the end of the embryonic period until the baby is born. During this time, the fetus is growing rapidly, with dramatic changes in body proportions. From the end of the third month of development until birth at full term, fetal weight increases nearly 500-fold. The typical newborn is about 20 inches (50 centimeters) long and weighs approximately 7 pounds, 7 ounces (3.4 kilograms).

**Key Concepts**  *From conception to full-term baby, the process of fetal development is typically described in three stages. The blastogenic stage involves rapid cell division of the fertilized ovum and its implantation in the mother's uterine wall. Cells differentiate and organ systems and body structures are formed during the embryonic stage. The fetal stage, the longest stage of pregnancy, is marked by growth in size and change in body proportions.*

### Maternal Physiological Changes and Nutrition

While the fertilized ovum is developing from a mass of dividing cells to an embryo to a fetus, changes are occurring in the mother's body as well. (See **Figure 12.6**.) These changes occur as the result of various hormones secreted mainly by the placenta.

**critical period of development**  Time during which the environment has the greatest impact on the developing embryo.

**fetal stage**  The period of rapid growth from the end of the embryonic stage until birth.

**Developing organs and structures –** ▨ = Critical period of development

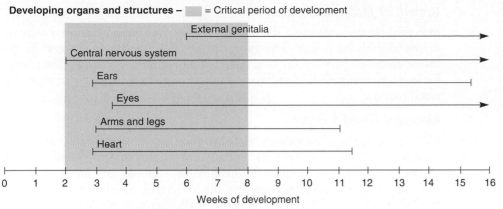

External genitalia

Central nervous system

Ears

Eyes

Arms and legs

Heart

0 1 2 3 4 5 6 7 8 9 10 11 12 13 14 15 16

Weeks of development

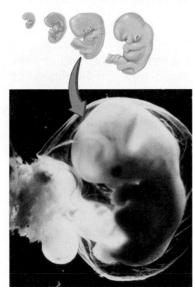

**Figure 12.5 Embryonic development.** During the embryonic stage—week 2 through week 8—all the major organ systems are forming. During this critical period of development, the embryo is highly vulnerable to nutrient deficiencies and toxicities as well as harmful substances, such as tobacco smoke.

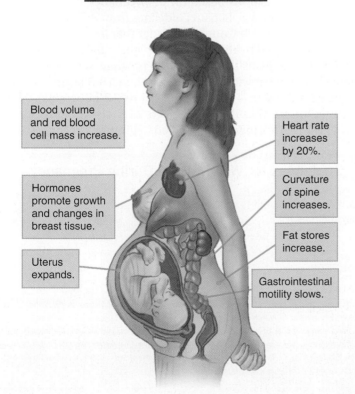

Blood volume and red blood cell mass increase.

Hormones promote growth and changes in breast tissue.

Uterus expands.

Heart rate increases by 20%.

Curvature of spine increases.

Fat stores increase.

Gastrointestinal motility slows.

**Figure 12.6 Maternal changes during pregnancy.** Hormones released throughout pregnancy influence the growth of the baby and alter the way the mother's organs function.

## *Quick* Bite

### Growth of Maternal Tissue

Maternal tissues, including the breasts, uterus, and adipose stores, increase in size during pregnancy. Hormones promote growth and changes in the breast tissue to prepare for lactation. Fat stores increase to provide energy for late pregnancy and for **lactation** and are a major component of maternal weight gain.

### Maternal Blood Volume

During the course of pregnancy, blood volume expands by nearly 50 percent. Production of red blood cells also increases. Iron, folate, and vitamin $B_{12}$ are all key nutrients in red blood cell production. Hemoglobin and hematocrit values increase during pregnancy, but this difference often is due to the dilution of the blood cells by an increase in plasma volume than to nutrient deficiency.

### Gastrointestinal Changes

During pregnancy, maternal gastrointestinal motility slows, and food moves more slowly through the intestinal tract. On the plus side, nutrient absorption is increased because nutrients spend more time in the small intestine. On the other hand, slower motility can contribute to the mother's nausea, heartburn, constipation, and hemorrhoids.

**Key Concepts** *The mother's body is undergoing various changes during pregnancy, guided by changing levels of hormones. Uterine, breast, and adipose tissues grow; blood volume expands; and gastrointestinal motility slows. All these changes have nutritional and dietary implications for pregnant women.*

## Maternal Weight Gain

How much weight should a woman gain during pregnancy? Doctors' recommendations have varied over the years from minimal weight gain to unlimited weight gain to recommendations based on prepregnancy BMI, as shown in Table 12.3. New pregnancy weight gain guidelines from the Institute of Medicine and the National Research Council consider that a woman's health and that of her infant are affected by the woman's weight at the start of pregnancy as well as how much she gains throughout the pregnancy.[10]

For underweight women with a BMI of less than 18.5 $kg/m^2$, the recommended weight gain is 28 to 40 pounds (12.5 to 18 kilograms). Normal-weight women with a starting BMI of 18.5 to 24.9 $kg/m^2$ should gain 25 to 35 pounds (11.5 to 16 kilograms). Women beginning pregnancy with an

### Table 12.3    Guidelines for Weight Gain During Pregnancy

| Prepregnancy BMI ($kg/m^2$) | Weight Gain[a] | |
| --- | --- | --- |
| | (lb) | (kg) |
| Underweight (< 18.5) | 28–40 | 12.5–18 |
| Normal (18.5–24.9) | 25–35 | 11.5–16 |
| Overweight (25.0–29.9) | 15–25 | 7.0–11.5 |
| Obese (> 30.0) | 11–20 | 5–9 |

[a] Young adolescents should strive for gains at the upper end of the recommended range. Short women (< 157 centimeters or 62 inches) should strive for gains at the lower end of the range.

**Source:** Modified from Lederman SA et al. Body fat and water changes during pregnancy in women with different body weight and weight gain. *Obstet Gynecol.* 1997;90(4):483–488. Reproduced with permission from *Dietary Reference Intakes for Energy, Carbohydrate, Fiber, Fat, Fatty Acids, Cholesterol, Protein, and Amino Acids (Macronutrients).* Copyright 2005 by the National Academy of Sciences, courtesy of the National Academies Press, Washington, DC.

**lactation** The process of synthesizing and secreting breast milk.

overweight BMI of 25.0 to 29.9 kg/m² are recommended to gain 15 to 25 pounds (7 to 11.5 kilograms). For the heaviest women—those with BMIs greater than 30.0 kg/m² at the start of pregnancy—a weight gain of 11 to 20 pounds (5 to 9 kilograms) is recommended.

When maternal weight gain is within these limits, infants are more likely to be born normal weight and at term. These guidelines reflect the greater number of overweight and obese women currently in the United States and advise women to choose a healthy diet and to exercise to achieve a normal BMI prior to getting pregnant. Although weight gain varies widely among women who give birth to healthy, full-term infants, pregnancy weight gain guidelines aim to lower risks associated with pregnancy weight change.[11]

Twin births account for one of every 34 live births in the United States. Of course, women who carry two or more fetuses need to gain more weight than women who carry just one. For normal-weight women the recommended weight gain for carrying twins is 37 to 54 pounds (17 to 25 kilograms). Overweight women should gain 31 to 50 pounds (14 to 23 kilograms), and obese women should gain 25 to 42 pounds (11 to 19 kilograms).[12] There is currently not enough information to establish weight gain guidelines for underweight women with multiple fetuses. However, a higher weight gain often is recommended for women who were underweight prior to pregnancy.

The pattern of weight gain is important to a healthy pregnancy outcome. During the first trimester, average weight gain is low, less than 5 pounds for most women. Over the second and third trimesters, the suggested weight gain is a little less than 1 pound (0.4 kilograms) per week, with more gain suggested for underweight women and those carrying twins and a lower gain for women who are overweight and obese.[13] Monitoring the amount and rate of weight gain is an important component of prenatal care.

The weight gained during pregnancy goes to the fetus and associated tissues and fluids and to maternal tissue growth. In a typical final weight gain of 27.5 pounds (12.5 kilograms), the fetus, placenta, and **amniotic fluid** account for nearly 40 percent of that weight. Maternal tissues (i.e., adipose stores, breast and uterine growth, and expanded blood and extracellular fluid volumes) account for the remaining 60 percent. (See **Figure 12.7**.)

**Key Concepts** *Weight gained during pregnancy is added to fetal and maternal tissues and fluids. Weight gain recommendations are based on BMI prior to pregnancy. Women of normal weight (BMI = 18.5–24.9 kg/m2) should gain 25 to 35 pounds over the course of pregnancy. Most of this weight gain occurs during the second and third trimesters.*

## Energy and Nutrition During Pregnancy

A pregnant woman requires added calories to grow and maintain not just her developing fetus but the support system as well—the placenta, increased breast tissue, and fat stores. Growth and development of the fetus also require protein, vitamins, and minerals.

### Energy

Resting energy expenditure (REE) increases during pregnancy because of the energy requirements of the fetus and placenta and the increased workload on the mother's heart and lungs.[14] Energy also is needed to support weight gain, primarily in the second and third trimesters. Using median energy expenditure as a guide, pregnant women need approximately 340 extra kilocalories per day during the second trimester and an extra 450 kilocalories per day during the third trimester.[15] Because actual energy expenditure varies widely, weight gain during pregnancy is probably the best indicator of adequate calorie intake.[16]

THINK
About It
1

> **amniotic fluid** The fluid that surrounds the fetus; contained in the amniotic sac inside the uterus.

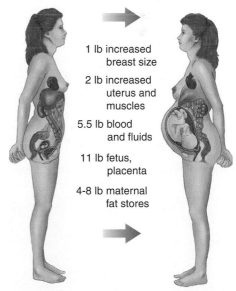

1 lb increased breast size

2 lb increased uterus and muscles

5.5 lb blood and fluids

11 lb fetus, placenta

4-8 lb maternal fat stores

(a) First trimester      (b) Third trimester

**Figure 12.7** **Components of maternal weight gain.** During the first trimester, most women gain less than 5 pounds. Over the second and third trimesters, the suggested weight gain is a little less than 1 pound per week for women who begin pregnancy at a normal weight.

### Nutrients to Support Pregnancy

Most healthy women who eat a well-balanced diet have no trouble meeting the majority of their nutrient requirements during pregnancy without vitamin and mineral supplements. However, despite even the best effort, many women have difficulty meeting increased recommendations during pregnancy for numerous nutrients, most often iron and folic acid. As a preventive measure, it is, therefore, recommended that all women planning to become pregnant take a multivitamin/mineral supplement containing folic acid.[17] Essential nutrients can be grouped into two broad categories: macronutrients (proteins, fats, and carbohydrates) and micronutrients (vitamins and minerals). Table 12.4 shows the nutrient recommendations for pregnant women compared with nonpregnant women. The USDA recently introduced the Daily Food Plan for Moms, an interactive website that uses the *Dietary Guidelines for*

**Table 12.4    Nutritional Recommendations for Pregnancy**

| | Nonpregnant | Pregnant | % Increase |
|---|---|---|---|
| Energy (kcal) | 2,400 | 2,740/2,852 | 14–18 |
| Protein (g) | 46 | 71 | 54 |
| Vitamin A (µg RAE) | 700 | 770 | 10 |
| Vitamin D (IU) | 600 | 600 | 0 |
| Vitamin E (mg) | 15 | 15 | 0 |
| Vitamin K (µg) | 90 | 90 | 0 |
| Thiamin (mg) | 1.1 | 1.4 | 27 |
| Riboflavin (mg) | 1.1 | 1.4 | 27 |
| Niacin (mg) | 14 | 18 | 29 |
| Vitamin $B_6$ (mg) | 1.3 | 1.9 | 46 |
| Folate (µg) | 400 | 600 | 50 |
| Vitamin $B_{12}$ (µg) | 2.4 | 2.6 | 8 |
| Pantothenic acid (mg) | 5 | 6 | 20 |
| Biotin (µg) | 30 | 30 | 0 |
| Choline (mg) | 425 | 450 | 6 |
| Vitamin C (mg) | 75 | 85 | 13 |
| Calcium (mg) | 1,000 | 1,000 | 0 |
| Phosphorus (mg) | 700 | 700 | 0 |
| Magnesium (mg) | 310 | 350 | 13 |
| Iron (mg) | 18 | 27 | 50 |
| Zinc (mg) | 8 | 11 | 38 |
| Selenium (µg) | 55 | 60 | 9 |
| Iodine (µg) | 150 | 220 | 47 |
| Fluoride (mg) | 3 | 3 | 0 |
| Copper (µg) | 900 | 1,000 | 11 |
| Chromium (µg) | 25 | 30 | 20 |
| Manganese (mg) | 1.8 | 2 | 11 |
| Molybdenum (µg) | 45 | 50 | 11 |
| Sodium (mg) | 1,500 | 1,500 | 0 |
| Chloride (mg) | 2,300 | 2,300 | 0 |
| Potassium (mg) | 4,700 | 4,700 | 0 |
| Water (mL) | 2,700 | 3,000 | 11 |

Needs for most nutrients increase during pregnancy. Generally, vitamin and mineral needs increase more than energy needs, which means that food choices should be nutrient-dense. Values for energy are based on Estimated Energy Requirements (EER) for a reference 19-year-old active woman. The first number for pregnancy represents the second trimester; the other number is for the third trimester. Values for protein, vitamins, minerals, and water are RDAs or AIs for ages 19 to 30.

*Americans, 2010* and MyPlate nutritional guidance to help pregnant and nursing mothers meet their individual nutritional requirements.[18]

### Macronutrients

Macronutrients supply energy and provide the building blocks for protein synthesis. The recommended balance of energy sources does not change during pregnancy. A low-fat, moderate-protein, high-carbohydrate diet is still appropriate.

**Protein** Extra protein is needed during pregnancy for the synthesis of new maternal, placental, and fetal tissues. A pregnant woman's RDA for protein is 1.1 grams per kilogram per day (an additional 25 grams per day over nonpregnant needs). Nonpregnant women typically consume this amount of protein. Thus, many women need not increase their protein intake to reach the levels recommended for pregnancy. Pregnant women who are vegetarians, including vegans, also should be able to meet their protein needs from food

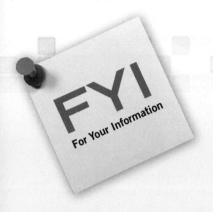

# Vegetarianism and Pregnancy

Can pregnant women meet all of their nutritional needs on a vegetarian diet? A fair question. A review of the scientific evidence suggests the answer is "yes," as a vegetarian diet can be nutritionally adequate in pregnancy and result in positive maternal and infant health outcomes.[1]

Common vegetarian practices include the avoidance of meat, poultry, and fish (lacto-ovo-vegetarian and lactovegetarian) and the avoidance of all animal foods (vegan). These foods are important sources of iron, zinc, calcium, vitamin $B_{12}$, *omega* fatty acids, and other nutrients. Although vegetarian diets can provide reasonable quantities of trace elements, animal-derived foods frequently contribute larger amounts that the body absorbs more easily. To meet the demands of pregnancy, supplementation may be in order.

Supplemental iron is generally recommended for all pregnant women. Supplemental vitamin $B_{12}$ (2.0 micrograms per day) is also recommended for vegan mothers. If their sun exposure is limited, they also may need daily supplementation of vitamin D.[2] Vegetarians with low calcium intake (< 600 milligrams per day) should consume a supplement that provides at least 500 milligrams per day. Some vegan foods, such as fortified soy milks, may contain these important nutrients. It is important to check the label to be sure.

The overall nutrient content of a vegetarian diet depends on both the energy content and the variety of the foods consumed. The sample meal plan in Table A provides an example of a vegan diet for pregnant women.

1    Craig WJ, Mangels AR. Position of the American Dietetic Association: vegetarian diets. *J Am Diet Assoc.* 2009;109(7):1266–1282.

2    Institute of Medicine, Food and Nutrition Board. *Dietary Reference Intakes for Calcium and Vitamin D.* Washington, DC: National Academies Press; 2011.

**Table A**  **Sample Meal Plan for a Vegan Pregnancy**

**Breakfast**
½ cup oatmeal with maple syrup
1 slice whole wheat toast with
   Fruit spread
1 cup fortified soymilk
½ cup calcium-fortified orange juice

**Morning Snack**
½ whole-wheat bagel with
   Margarine
1 banana

**Lunch**
Veggie burger on whole-wheat bun with
   Mustard
   Ketchup
1 cup steamed collard greens
Medium apple
1 cup fortified soymilk

**Afternoon Snack**
¾ cup ready-to-eat cereal with
   1 cup blueberries
   1 cup fortified soymilk

**Dinner**
¾ cup tofu stir-fried with
   1 cup vegetables
1 cup brown rice
1 medium orange

**Evening Snack**
Whole-grain crackers with
   2 tablespoons peanut butter
4 oz apple juice

**Note:** This sample meal plan provides approximately 2,200 calories, 100 grams of protein, 55 grams of fat (22 percent of calories), and 336 grams of carbohydrate. This sample meal plan meets the recommendations for calcium, zinc, vitamin $B_{12}$, folate, thiamin, riboflavin, and niacin. Supplemental iron and vitamin D may be needed.
**Source:** Reproduced from *Vegan Nutrition in Pregnancy and Childhood* by Reed Mangels, PhD, RD. Courtesy of The Vegetarian Resource Group, www.vrg.org.

sources alone—as long as they select a variety of protein sources and consume enough total calories. (See the FYI feature "Vegetarianism and Pregnancy.")

**Fats** Dietary fats provide vital fuel for the mother and for the development of placental tissues. Needs for essential fatty acids during pregnancy are slightly higher than those of nonpregnant women.[19] The pregnant woman's body also stores fats to support breastfeeding after childbirth. Very-low-fat diets (in which fewer than 10 percent of daily calories come from dietary fats) are not recommended for pregnancy. Such diets are unlikely to supply sufficient amounts of essential fatty acids, fat-soluble vitamins, or calories.

**Carbohydrates** Carbohydrates provide the main source of extra calories during pregnancy. Food choices should emphasize complex carbohydrates such as whole-grain breads, fortified cereals, rice, and pasta. In addition to supplying vitamins and minerals, these foods can increase fiber intake substantially. A fiber-rich diet is recommended during pregnancy to help prevent constipation and hemorrhoids. The AI for fiber increases from 25 to 28 grams per day during pregnancy.

**Key Concepts** *Most healthy women with well-balanced diets meet the majority of their nutrient requirements during pregnancy. The actual increase in energy needs varies substantially among women. The adequacy of energy intake can be measured by the amount of weight gained. Weight loss is not advised during pregnancy, even for obese women. As long as energy intake is adequate and a variety of foods is eaten, protein intake should be more than adequate to support prenatal growth and development.*

### Micronutrients

A pregnant woman has an increased need for many vitamins and minerals that support growth and development. In addition, her increased energy needs mean she requires higher amounts of nutrients such as the B vitamins thiamin, riboflavin, niacin, and pantothenic acid that are essential for energy metabolism.

Needs for the other B vitamins (except biotin) also increase. Folate and vitamin $B_{12}$ are used in synthesis of DNA and red blood cells, and vitamin $B_6$ is crucial for metabolism of amino acids. Of these vitamins, folate needs increase the most, from 400 micrograms per day to 600 micrograms per day during pregnancy. Vitamin C needs increase slightly during pregnancy, from 75 to 85 milligrams per day for women aged 19 to 50 years. For the fat-soluble vitamins, the RDA for vitamin A increases slightly during pregnancy while the recommended intake levels for vitamins D, E, and K are unchanged.

For most minerals, recommended intakes are higher during pregnancy—most dramatically for iron. The RDA for iron increases from 18 milligrams per day to 27 milligrams per day. Iron is necessary to make red blood cells and is important for normal growth and energy metabolism. Iron deficiency and its associated anemia is the most common nutrient deficiency in pregnancy. Table 12.5 lists the characteristics of women who are at particularly high risk for iron deficiency.

Because getting 27 milligrams of iron in the daily diet is not easy, experts recommend iron supplementation for the general population of pregnant women.[20] A woman can maximize absorption of an iron supplement by eating it on an empty stomach (between meals or at bedtime) and washing it down with liquids other than milk, tea, or coffee, which inhibit absorption.

**Key Concepts** *Needs for vitamins and minerals increase during pregnancy, some more than others. Extra vitamins and minerals are needed to support growth and development*

**Table 12.5** **Factors Associated with Increased Risk for Iron Deficiency During Pregnancy**

Young age (e.g., 15 to 19 years)
Twin or triplet pregnancy
Multiple pregnancies
Diets low in meat
Low socioeconomic status
Low level of education
Black or Hispanic ethnicity
Previous diagnosis of iron deficiency or iron-deficiency anemia

*as well as increased energy use. Recommended intake levels increase most dramatically for folate and iron.*

## Food Choices for Pregnant Women

You may be surprised to learn that the recommended diet for a pregnant woman does not differ much from that for adults in the general population. Variety is the key to a well-balanced diet. The extra calories needed for pregnancy are easy to obtain from an additional serving from each of the following food groups—grains, vegetables, fruits, and low-fat milk. Because the increased need for energy is proportionately less than the increased need for most nutrients, nutrient-dense foods are important. There is little room in the diet plan for high-calorie, high-fat, low-nutrient "extras."

### Supplementation

Other than iron and folate, a pregnant woman can get all the nutrients she needs by making healthful choices using the food intake patterns of the USDA's Daily Food Plan for Moms. In an ideal world, healthcare providers would evaluate the dietary intake of all prenatal women and recommend dietary changes to improve nutrition where needed. In reality, this seldom happens, and pregnant women in the United States and Canada routinely receive prescriptions for prenatal vitamin/mineral supplements. The amount and balance of nutrients in prenatal formulations is appropriate for pregnancy. Because toxic levels can be reached quickly, especially for vitamins A and D, pregnant women should avoid high doses and multiple supplements. In addition, because most herbal preparations have not been evaluated for safety during pregnancy, they are not recommended.

### Foods to Avoid

Alcohol is completely off limits to pregnant women. If a mother-to-be is experiencing problems with nausea and vomiting, she may want to abstain for a while from foods that aggravate these symptoms. Cultural traditions may dictate changes in diet during pregnancy, but these tend to reflect traditional beliefs and practices rather than health science.

The *Dietary Guidelines for Americans, 2010* advises that women who are pregnant or breastfeeding consume 8 to 12 ounces of a variety of seafood types weekly; however, due to high mercury content, it limits albacore tuna to 6 ounces per week and suggests avoiding tilefish, shark, swordfish, and king mackerel.[21] In addition, the Food and Drug Administration (FDA) and the Environmental Protection Agency (EPA) advise that women who may become pregnant, pregnant women, lactating mothers, and young children check local advisories about the safety of fish caught by family and friends in local lakes, rivers, and coastal areas.[22]

The question of whether to reduce or eliminate caffeine intake during pregnancy continues to be debated. High caffeine intake has been linked to delayed conception, spontaneous miscarriage, and low birth weight.[23] However, caffeine intake during pregnancy does not appear to be associated with birth defects[24] or preterm birth.[25] The Academy of Nutrition and Dietetics recommends that pregnant women consume less than 300 milligrams of caffeine per day.[26] Table 12.6 shows caffeine content of common beverages and foods.

**Key Concepts** *With the exception of iron and folate, a well-balanced, varied diet can easily meet all a pregnant woman's nutrient needs. Pregnant women should choose nutrient-dense foods in the proportions found in the USDA's Daily Food Plan for Moms. Although vitamin/mineral supplementation is common during pregnancy, it probably is*

**Table 12.6** **Caffeine Content of Common Beverages and Foods**

| Food | Serving Size (fluid ounces) | Caffeine (mg) |
|---|---|---|
| Coffee, regular, brewed | 8 | 130 |
| Coffee, Starbucks, brewed | 8 | 160 |
| Espresso, regular | 1 | 40 |
| Espresso, Starbucks | 1 | 75 |
| Frappuccino beverage, Starbucks | 9.5 | 115 |
| Tea, regular, brewed | 8 | 50 |
| Tea, fruited, Snapple | 8 | 20 |
| Tea, latte, Starbucks Tazo Chai | 8 | 50 |
| Vault | 12 | 70 |
| Mountain Dew | 12 | 55 |
| Coca-Cola/Pepsi, regular, flavored, diet | 12 | 35–45 |
| Sprite/7-Up | 12 | 0 |
| Red Bull | 8.3 | 80 |
| Ice cream, coffee | 8 | 50–80 |
| Milk chocolate, Hershey's | 1.55 ounces | 10 |
| Dark chocolate, Hershey's | 1.45 ounces | 20 |

Source: Adapted from Center for Science in the Public Interest. Caffeine content of food and drugs. http://www.cspinet.org/new/cafchart.htm. Accessed 8/4/11.

> **low-birth-weight infant** A newborn who weighs less than 2,500 grams (5.5 pounds) as a result of either premature birth or inadequate growth in utero.

*not needed other than for iron and folate. When supplements are used, they should be designed for pregnant women. Pregnant women should avoid alcohol, limit fish high in mercury, and moderate their intake of caffeine.*

## Substance Use and Pregnancy Outcome

When a pregnant woman eats, she eats for herself and her unborn baby. When she smokes, drinks, or uses drugs, she does so for her unborn baby as well. The consequences of these behaviors may be felt for generations.

### Tobacco and Alcohol

Smoking during pregnancy increases the risks of miscarrying, delivering a stillborn infant, giving birth prematurely, and delivering a **low-birth-weight infant**.[27] Women in lower socioeconomic groups have the highest rates of cigarette use before, during, and after pregnancy. Women in the highest socioeconomic groups, meanwhile, are the most likely to quit smoking during pregnancy but are just as likely as other women to take up the habit again after giving birth.

Fetal alcohol syndrome (FAS) describes a consistent pattern of physical, cognitive, and behavioral problems in infants born to women who use alcohol heavily during pregnancy. Children severely afflicted by the syndrome show marked growth deficiencies before and after birth: physical anomalies such as a small head, certain characteristic facial deformities (see **Figure 12.8**), heart defects, and joint and limb irregularities; mental retardation; and central nervous system disorders. The greater a mother's alcohol use during pregnancy, the more severe the symptoms of FAS tend to be in the child. There is no known safe threshold for alcohol use in pregnancy. The only way to avoid alcohol-related risks to a fetus is to avoid all alcohol during pregnancy.

THINK
About It

2

### Drugs

Approximately 4 percent of pregnant women use illicit drugs such as marijuana, cocaine, and heroin.[28] Drug use is higher among younger women and African American women.

Marijuana use increases the risk for premature delivery and low birth weight. In addition, maternal marijuana use may result in some of the same physical abnormalities seen in infants with FAS. Effects on the fetus vary depending on the mother's diet, frequency of marijuana use, and the use of other drugs. Marijuana use also reduces fertility in both women and men.

Cocaine use increases risks of stroke, prematurity, fetal growth retardation, miscarriage, and certain birth defects. Some of these problems may stem from nutritional deficiencies in the mother before and during pregnancy as well as from concurrent tobacco and alcohol use, which is common among cocaine users. **Figure 12.9** illustrates the possible effects of a woman's use of drugs, alcohol, or tobacco while she is pregnant.

**Key Concepts** *Smoking, alcohol, and illicit drug use during pregnancy can all have devastating effects on fetal development. Low birth weight, preterm delivery, and birth defects are some of the consequences. Fetal alcohol syndrome is a specific set of physical, mental, and behavioral defects caused by alcohol consumption during pregnancy. A pregnant woman should avoid all these substances.*

## Special Situations During Pregnancy

Most women progress through pregnancy with no more than a mild period of morning sickness or problems with constipation or heartburn. However, complications such as abnormal glucose tolerance or elevated blood pressure

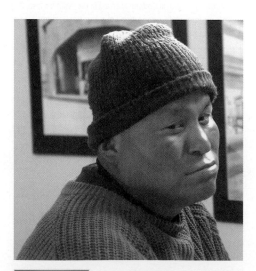

| Figure 12.8 | **Fetal alcohol syndrome.** The facial characteristics of a person with fetal alcohol syndrome include a short nose with a flattened bridge, eyelids with extra folds, and a thin upper lip with no groove below the nose.

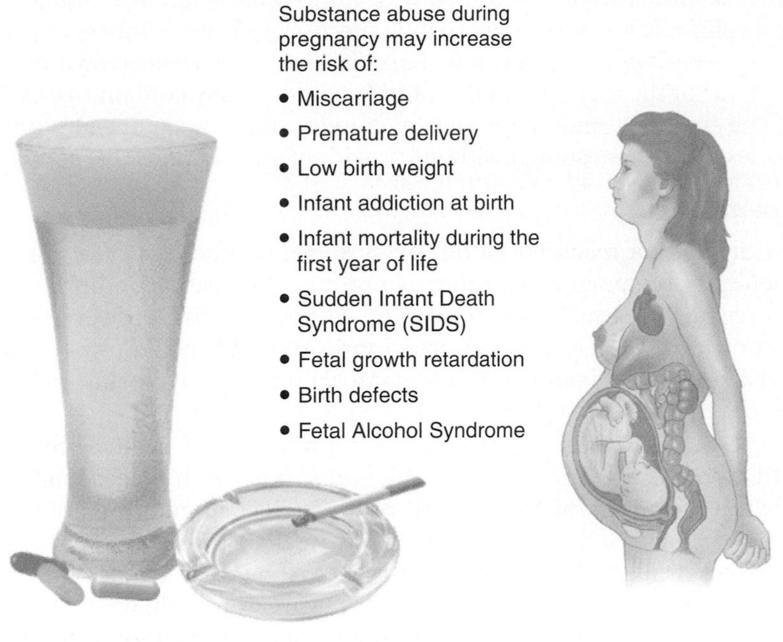

Substance abuse during pregnancy may increase the risk of:

- Miscarriage
- Premature delivery
- Low birth weight
- Infant addiction at birth
- Infant mortality during the first year of life
- Sudden Infant Death Syndrome (SIDS)
- Fetal growth retardation
- Birth defects
- Fetal Alcohol Syndrome

**Figure 12.9** **Substance use can lead to birth defects.** When a pregnant woman smokes, drinks, or uses drugs, so does her growing baby. The consequences of these behaviors may be felt for generations.

may affect dietary choices and nutritional status. In addition, some women have unique nutritional needs during pregnancy.

### Gastrointestinal Distress

Morning sickness, or nausea associated with pregnancy, is most common early in pregnancy as the mother's body adjusts to changes in hormone levels. Many pregnant women find they experience less and milder bouts of morning sickness if they eat dry cereal, toast, or crackers about half an hour before getting out of bed. (See **Figure 12.10**.) Keeping some food in the stomach throughout the day helps, too. This means eating smaller, more frequent meals and drinking liquids between meals instead of with food. Avoiding food aromas that trigger nausea is another useful tactic.

Heartburn and constipation are the result of slowed GI movement. Remaining upright for at least an hour after eating and having smaller, more frequent meals may prevent heartburn. Getting plenty of fiber and fluids in the diet and getting regular mild to moderate exercise can limit constipation. Of course, a pregnant woman should always consult her healthcare provider before using a prescription drug, over-the-counter medicine, herbal supplement, or home remedy for nausea, vomiting, heartburn, or constipation.

### Food Cravings and Aversions

Many pregnant women experience specific food cravings and/or aversions, and we often laugh at stories about unusual combinations such as pickles and ice cream. These changes in food preferences may be linked to taste and metabolic changes, but they rarely are based on a nutrient deficiency or other physiological condition. Most cravings and aversions do not affect the quality of the diet unless food choices become very narrow.

Some pregnant women crave nonfood items such as starch or clay. The term *pica* describes routine consumption of nonfood items such as dirt, clay, laundry starch, ice, or

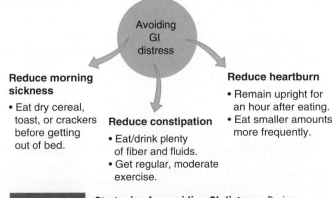

Avoiding GI distress

**Reduce morning sickness**
- Eat dry cereal, toast, or crackers before getting out of bed.

**Reduce constipation**
- Eat/drink plenty of fiber and fluids.
- Get regular, moderate exercise.

**Reduce heartburn**
- Remain upright for an hour after eating.
- Eat smaller amounts more frequently.

**Figure 12.10** **Strategies for avoiding GI distress.** During pregnancy, most women experience GI distress as morning sickness, constipation, or heartburn.

## Quick Bite

**eclampsia** The occurrence of seizures in a pregnant woman that are unrelated to brain conditions.

**gestational diabetes** A condition that results in high blood glucose levels during pregnancy.

Table 12.7 **Factors Associated with Risk for Gestational Diabetes**

Being older than 25 years
Obesity, at any age
Family history of diabetes mellitus
Previous poor pregnancy outcome
History of abnormal glucose tolerance
Ethnicity associated with high incidence of diabetes

burnt matches. Although this behavior may seem outlandish, in many cases it is a culturally accepted practice that affects significant numbers of pregnant women worldwide.[29] Pica can be harmful if nonfood items crowd nutritious foods out of the diet. In addition, nonfood items may contain toxins, bacteria, and parasites, and, in the case of laundry starch, a significant number of calories may be consumed without providing any vitamins and minerals.

### Hypertension

Measurement of maternal blood pressure is a routine part of prenatal care. When not accompanied by other symptoms, increased blood pressure during pregnancy is usually temporary and carries little risk. However, the combination of hypertension and proteinuria (protein in the urine) indicates preeclampsia in the mother. If preeclampsia progresses to **eclampsia**, it can threaten the lives of both mother and baby.

Preeclampsia during pregnancy is more common in first pregnancies, in adolescents, women older than 35, and women with preexisting diabetes or hypertension. In mild cases, bed rest and close monitoring are the treatments of choice. Sodium restriction and drug therapy are not recommended. Severe cases may require more aggressive treatment. Calcium supplementation may be useful for women with low calcium intake; however, conclusive links between nutrient intake and development or prevention of preeclampsia have not been found.[30] Early identification of preeclampsia through routine prenatal care is important for good maternal and fetal outcomes.

### Diabetes

A pregnant woman with diabetes faces special challenges. She has an increased risk of developing preeclampsia and a greater-than-average chance of problems that affect the fetus, including fetal death. However, with early prenatal intervention and careful control of blood glucose levels, these risks can be reduced to the same level as in nondiabetic pregnancies.[31]

Pregnancy may require frequent adjustments of both diet and insulin to keep blood glucose in check. Insulin requirements often decrease during the first half of pregnancy but then increase during the second half. Women who did not need insulin before they became pregnant and were able to control their blood glucose through diet alone may begin to need insulin during their pregnancy.

### Gestational Diabetes

**Gestational diabetes** is a condition in which abnormal glucose tolerance exists only during pregnancy and resolves after delivery. The hormones of pregnancy tend to counteract insulin, and in about 4 percent of pregnancies, this results in a rise in blood glucose. Table 12.7 lists factors associated with an increased risk of gestational diabetes. Gestational diabetes often can be controlled through diet, although some cases require insulin therapy.

### HIV/AIDS

Women with the HIV virus can potentially pass the virus to the baby during pregnancy, delivery, or breastfeeding. Medical treatments used routinely in the United States and other developed countries reduce the risk of transmission during pregnancy and delivery in the approximately 6,000 HIV-infected women that give birth each year.[32] More than 90 percent of all cases of childhood HIV infection is attributable to mother-to-child transmission of HIV, especially in countries where effective HIV/AIDS drugs are not available.[33] In developing countries where treatments are not available, women with HIV or AIDS are likely to have multiple nutrition problems, including protein-energy malnutrition, vitamin and mineral deficiencies, and inadequate weight gain, all of which pose risks to the fetus.

### Adolescence

Despite prevention efforts, almost 410,000 infants were born to teenagers in 2009; the majority of these pregnancies were unintended.[34] Pregnant adolescents are nutritionally at risk. Their own needs for growth and development are compromised by the extra demands posed by the growth and development of the fetus. Pregnant adolescents additionally are at greater risk for preeclampsia, anemia, premature birth, low-birth-weight babies, infant mortality, and sexually transmitted diseases.[35]

Even before becoming pregnant, many teenagers do not demonstrate healthful eating patterns. Their diets are likely to be inadequate in total calories, calcium, iron, zinc, riboflavin, folic acid, and vitamins A, D, and $B_6$. Poverty, smoking, and abuse of alcohol and other substances compound the negative effects of adolescent nutritional inadequacies.

Nutrition care for pregnant teens starts with determining daily energy needs. The Institute of Medicine recommends that pregnant adolescents be encouraged to strive for weight gains toward the upper end of the range recommended for adult mothers (see Table 12.3). The need for supplemental vitamins and minerals is also greater in this age group.

**Key Concepts**  *Numerous factors affect the dietary needs and choices of pregnant women. Routine prenatal care is important to identify unhealthful eating behaviors and potential complications such as preeclampsia and gestational diabetes. Pregnant women with diabetes or HIV/AIDS need special dietary intervention. Pregnant teens have especially high nutrient needs to fuel not only fetal growth but also their own adolescent growth.*

## Lactation

During pregnancy, physiological changes in breast tissue and fat stores prepare the woman's body for the demands of lactation. Preparation for lactation also involves education. Although breastfeeding is one of the most natural functions of a woman's body, knowledge about lactation can make breastfeeding a success for both mother and infant.

## Breastfeeding Trends

Public health goals since the late 1970s have been to increase the percentage of infants who are breastfed. The goal of Healthy People 2020 is to increase the proportion of newborns who are initially breastfed to almost 82 percent.[36] Efforts to promote breastfeeding have been successful; 74 percent of infants are now breastfed initially.[37] However, only 44 percent of infants are still being breastfed at 6 months of age,[38] which is a lower rate than the Healthy People 2020 goal of 60.6 percent.[39] What are the reasons for this trend? Lack of knowledge about the benefits of breastfeeding for both mother and baby surely plays a role. Societal attitudes regarding the acceptability of breastfeeding also are influential and vary across cultural and demographic groups. Some states have actually had to pass laws stating that breastfeeding in public is not indecent exposure! In addition, the decline in breastfeeding through the 1950s and 1960s affected the attitudes and knowledge base of today's grandmothers.

Parents should make decisions about feeding their infants based on accurate information, so providing information about the mechanics of breastfeeding as well as the benefits for both mother and baby should be an integral part of prenatal care.

---

*Quick* **Bite**

**Breastfeeding and Birth Control**
Does breastfeeding prevent pregnancy? No. But under certain conditions, breastfeeding can dramatically reduce the chances of becoming pregnant. During the first six months after giving birth, a woman who has not yet had a period and fully breastfeeds her baby (no other liquids or solids) has less than a 2 percent chance of pregnancy. Still, it's important to use a reliable method of birth control while breastfeeding.

---

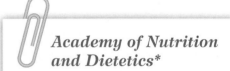

*Academy of Nutrition and Dietetics**

**Promoting and Supporting Breastfeeding**
It is the position of the American Dietetic Association that exclusive breastfeeding provides optimal nutrition and health protection for the first 6 months of life and breastfeeding with complementary foods from 6 months until at least 12 months of age is the ideal feeding pattern for infants. Breastfeeding is an important public health strategy for improving infant and child morbidity and mortality, improving maternal morbidity, and helping to control healthcare costs.

**Source:** Reproduced from James DC, Lessen R. Position of the Academy of Nutrition and Dietetics: promoting and supporting breastfeeding. *J Am Diet Assoc.* 2009;109(11): 1926–1942.

* Formerly the American Dietetic Association

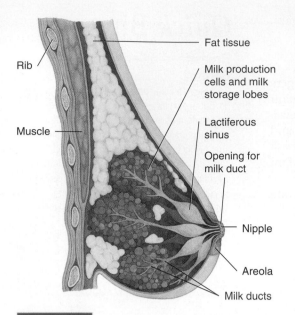

**Figure 12.11**    **Anatomy of the breast.** During pregnancy, breasts increase in size and undergo internal development. By the start of the third trimester, breasts are capable of producing milk.

## Physiology of Lactation

Virtually every woman who wants to breastfeed her newborn can do so. The size or shape of the breast has no impact on the lactation process. **Figure 12.11** shows the anatomy of a normal breast.

### Changes During Adolescence and Pregnancy

Although mammary tissue is present in newborns, that tissue does not grow and develop until the onset of puberty. Throughout adolescence, the amount of breast tissue grows and the mammary glands and ducts develop. An adolescent who becomes pregnant shortly after her first period or who has had only irregular periods prior to becoming pregnant may have underdeveloped mammary glands and insufficient breast tissue to support lactation. However, most teen mothers have no difficulty breastfeeding their babies.

During pregnancy, the breast tissue changes so milk production is possible. Not only does the breast change in size, but the structure of the glands and ducts also becomes more intricate, and secretory cells are formed. The mammary tissue is mature and capable of producing milk by the start of the third trimester.

### After Delivery

Although birth triggers a rapid increase in milk production and secretion, full lactation does not begin as soon as the baby is born. One of the best ways to establish lactation is to put the newborn to the breast as soon after delivery as possible. During the first two or three days after birth, a nursing infant receives **colostrum**, an immature milk that is quite high in protein and immunoglobulins (immunoprotective factors). If the newborn is fed regularly at the breast, lactation will be firmly established within two or three weeks after birth, and mature milk will be produced.

### Hormonal Controls

Maturation of breast tissue and the production and release of breast milk are controlled by several hormones. (See **Figure 12.12**.) During lactation, the pituitary gland produces two important hormones—**prolactin** and **oxytocin**. The infant suckling at the breast stimulates the release of prolactin from the mother's pituitary gland. In turn, prolactin stimulates the production of milk in the breast tissue. Giving water or infant formula to the baby reduces the time spent nursing at the breast, and milk production declines.

The second hormone, oxytocin, allows milk to be released from the mammary glands to the nipple and therefore to the hungry infant. It would be inconvenient and messy if milk were released from the breast as soon as it was produced! So, the infant suckling at the breast signals the mother's pituitary gland to release oxytocin, which in turn stimulates the release of milk. This process, often called the **let-down reflex**, may be accompanied by a tingling sensation in the breast that lets the mother know the infant is receiving milk. Let-down can be inhibited by anxiety, stress, and fatigue. It also can be stimulated by thoughts of the baby or hearing the baby cry.

**Key Concepts** *Increasing the proportion of infants who are breastfed is an important public health goal. Prenatal care should include information about the physiology of lactation and its benefits for mother and baby. Changes in breast tissue that allow lactation culminate at delivery. Breast milk changes composition in the two or three weeks following the infant's birth. The first milk, colostrum, is high in protein and immune factors. Key hormones that regulate milk production and release are prolactin and oxytocin.*

**colostrum**  A thick yellow fluid secreted by the breast during pregnancy and the first days after delivery.

**prolactin**  A pituitary hormone that stimulates the production of milk in breast tissue.

**oxytocin**  A pituitary hormone that stimulates the release of milk from the breast.

**let-down reflex**  The release of milk from the breast tissue in response to the stimulus of the hormone oxytocin. The major stimulus for oxytocin release is the infant suckling at the breast.

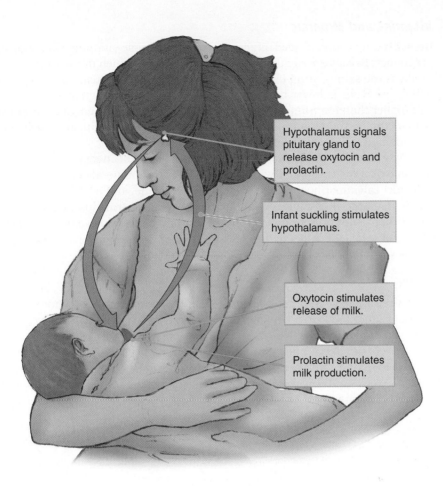

Hypothalamus signals pituitary gland to release oxytocin and prolactin.

Infant suckling stimulates hypothalamus.

Oxytocin stimulates release of milk.

Prolactin stimulates milk production.

**Figure 12.12** **Hormonal control of lactation.** When an infant nurses, the infant's suckling stimulates the nipple, which sends nerve signals to the hypothalamus. In turn, the hypothalamus signals the pituitary gland to release hormones that stimulate milk production and release.

## Nutrition for Breastfeeding Women

To provide adequate nutrition for her baby while protecting her own nutritional status, a breastfeeding mother must choose a varied, healthful, nutrient-dense diet. Her needs for energy and most nutrients are higher or the same as for pregnancy.

### Energy

The energy needed to support milk production is obtained in part by mobilization of fat stores, with the remaining kilocalories provided by the diet. On average, well-nourished breastfeeding women lose weight slowly, about 0.8 kilograms (approximately 1¾ pounds) per month, with weight stabilizing after about six months. Based on this rate of weight loss, a breastfeeding woman needs an extra intake of 330 kilocalories per day during the first six months of lactation and 400 extra kilocalories daily during the second six months.[40] This may be an overestimation of actual needs for many women, especially those who are sedentary. To ensure adequate milk production and avoid nutrient deficiencies, a nursing mother should consume at least 1,800 kilocalories per day.

### Protein

Adequate protein intake also is important while nursing. The RDA for protein is 1.3 grams per kilogram per day, or an additional 25 grams over the nonpregnant RDA. Unless calorie intake is very low, lack of dietary protein is uncommon among women in the United States and Canada.

**colic** Periodic inconsolable crying in an otherwise healthy infant that appears to result from abdominal cramping and discomfort.

## Vitamins and Minerals

Breastfeeding women need higher amounts of most vitamins than during pregnancy. Exceptions include vitamins D and K, for which the recommended intake is the same during lactation and pregnancy, and niacin and folate, for which the RDA is lower during lactation than during pregnancy (although still higher than for women in the general population). When vitamin intake is inadequate, the vitamin content of breast milk can diminish, which puts the infant at risk for deficiency.

For minerals, current RDA and AI values suggest increased needs during lactation (as compared with pregnancy) for all minerals except sodium, chloride, calcium, phosphorus, magnesium, fluoride, and molybdenum. Iron needs decrease below nonpregnant values because iron losses from menstruation are not present during the early months of exclusive breastfeeding. Maternal intake of minerals has less influence on levels in breast milk than is true for vitamins.

## Water

Breastfeeding women require plenty of fluids. A nursing mother should drink about 2 liters (~8 cups) of water per day and at least 1 cup of water each time she breastfeeds her baby. The AI for total water (beverages plus foods) is 3.8 liters per day. Coffee and other caffeinated beverages are acceptable if limited to 1 or 2 cups per day—if they do not replace other fluids. Because caffeine passes into the breast milk, caffeine can make some breastfed infants wakeful and jittery.

**Key Concepts** *Energy and nutrient needs are usually even higher during lactation than during pregnancy. Intake recommendations suggest an additional 330 to 400 kilocalories and 25 extra grams of protein each day above nonpregnant needs. Low vitamin intake affects the nutritional quality of breast milk. Recommended intake levels for minerals are generally higher during lactation than during pregnancy. Fluids also are important for adequate milk production.*

## Food Choices

Choosing a variety of foods from the USDA's Daily Food Plan for Moms is the best way to meet the nutritional demands of lactation. Following the food intake patterns of the Daily Food Plan for Moms, diets of 2,200 to 2,800 kilocalories per day easily can meet most nutrient needs. From each food group, nursing moms should choose foods that have the vitamins and minerals they need and make choices that are low in added sugar and solid fats.[41] Nursing mothers should eat plenty of vegetables, the source of many essential micronutrients. Although vegetables in the cabbage family, including broccoli, cauliflower, kale, and Brussels sprouts, have long been considered causes of **colic** symptoms in breastfed infants, these vegetables may have an unwarranted bad reputation. Scientific evidence that these vegetables cause distress for infants remains weak. Removal of numerous foods from the diet should be done only under the supervision of a registered dietitian.

## Supplementation

Some breastfeeding women may need routine vitamin/mineral supplementation.[42] This group would include, for example, those women who do not follow dietary guidelines and vegan women, who avoid all animal products. Vitamin $B_{12}$ is likely to be too low in the milk of nursing vegans, and they should take a $B_{12}$ supplement.[43] For breastfeeding women who do not get regular sun exposure and do not drink milk or other fortified products, a vitamin D supplement may be warranted.[44] For most nursing mothers, though,

*Quick* Bite

**Flavored Breast Milk**
When lactating mothers exercise vigorously, the amount of lactic acid in breast milk can increase. Some babies dislike the taste and tend to nurse less. Alcohol also can cause a taste that babies dislike. What flavors do babies like? When mothers consume vanilla, mint, or garlic, some babies nurse more.

dietary counseling to improve food choices is the preferred way to address nutrient imbalances.

## Practices to Avoid During Lactation

When a nursing mother smokes or uses alcohol or other drugs, these substances show up in her breast milk. Women who smoke are encouraged to quit smoking; however, breast milk remains the ideal food for their infants.[45] It is a myth that drinking alcohol enhances the let-down reflex, making it easier to nurse. Rather, alcohol inhibits the milk-ejection reflex so the baby gets less milk with a higher concentration of alcohol. An occasional drink is not harmful, but breastfeeding should be avoided for two hours after the drink.[46] Illicit drugs also show up in breast milk and can be transferred to the infant. If a new mother cannot abstain from using these drugs, she should not breastfeed.

**Key Concepts** *Food choices during lactation should follow the USDA Daily Food Plan for Moms and emphasize nutrient-dense foods. With good choices and adequate calories, a lactating woman may not need vitamin and mineral supplements. During pregnancy and lactation, a woman should avoid smoking, alcohol, and illicit drugs. She should consult a healthcare professional before taking medications or dietary supplements.*

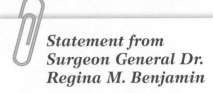

### *Statement from Surgeon General Dr. Regina M. Benjamin*

**Benefits of Breastfeeding**

One of the most highly effective preventive measures a mother can take to protect the health of her infant and herself is to breast-feed. It protects babies from many infections and illnesses, such as diarrhea and pneumonia. Children who have been breastfed have lower rates of childhood obesity. Mothers who breastfeed have a decreased risk of breast and ovarian cancers.

**Source:** Statement from Surgeon General Dr. Regina M. Benjamin on World Breastfeeding Week, August 1–7, 2011. Press release 8/1/11. http://www.hhs.gov/news/press/2011pres/08/20110801e.html. Accessed 8/3/11.

## Benefits of Breastfeeding

**THINK**
**About It**

**3**

Breast milk is the optimal food for the health, growth, and development of infants.[47] Both mother and infant benefit from breastfeeding; in fact, the larger society benefits through reduced infant illness and lower healthcare costs. It is estimated that $13 billion in U.S. healthcare costs could be saved annually if 90 percent of babies were breastfed exclusively for six months.[48]

### Benefits for Infants

Human milk provides optimal nutrition for babies, as you will see in the section "Energy and Nutrient Needs of Infancy." Breast milk provides more than nutrients, however, and the health-promoting factors in breast milk are difficult, if not impossible, to replicate in infant formula.

Breast milk has been shown to protect infants from infections and illnesses, including diarrhea, ear infections, pneumonia, and asthma,[49] leading to fewer healthcare visits, less prescription medication use, and fewer hospitalizations and resulting in decreased healthcare costs.[50] Breastfeeding also reduces an infant's risk of SIDS.[51] In addition, a baby's risk of obesity declines with each month of breastfeeding.[52] Babies who are breastfed for at least six months are less likely to develop obesity, and breastfeeding for nine months reduces a baby's chance of being overweight by more than 30 percent.[53] Evidence suggests that other health effects occur in a dose-response relationship as well, with the best outcomes for infants who are exclusively breastfed for at least six months.[54] Prolonged and exclusive breastfeeding also improves children's cognitive development.[55]

What makes breast milk so important for infant health? Colostrum contains substantial amounts of antibodies, including immunoglobulin A (IgA), the first line of defense against most infectious agents.[56] Breastfeeding also appears to stimulate development of the infant's own immune system.[57] Breastfeeding promotes a close bond between mother and infant that may be important to normal psychological development. It is important for mothers (and fathers) who bottle-feed to promote the same type of closeness while feeding.

As long as mother and baby are in reasonably close proximity, breast milk is always ready when the baby is ready to eat. There's nothing to pre-

Table 12.8 **Potential Benefits of Breastfeeding for Infants and Mothers**

| Benefits for Infants | Benefits for Mothers |
|---|---|
| Optimal nutrition for infant | Strong bonding with infant |
| Strong bonding with mother | Increased energy expenditure, which may lead to faster return to prepregnancy weight |
| Safe, fresh milk | |
| Enhanced immune system | |
| Reduced risk for acute otitis media, nonspecific gastroenteritis, severe lower respiratory tract infections, and asthma | Faster shrinking of the uterus |
| | Reduced postpartum bleeding and delayed the menstrual cycle |
| Protection against allergies and intolerances | Decreased risk for chronic diseases such as type 2 diabetes, breast and ovarian cancer |
| Promotion of correct development of jaw and teeth | |
| Association with higher intelligence quotient and school performance through adolescence | Improved bone density and decreased risk for hip fracture |
| | Decreased risk for postpartum depression |
| Reduced risk for chronic disease such as obesity, types 1 and 2 diabetes, heart disease, hypertension, hypercholesterolemia, and childhood leukemia | Enhanced self-esteem in the maternal role |
| | Time saved from preparing and mixing formula |
| Reduced risk for sudden infant death syndrome | Money saved from not buying formula and increased medical expenses associated with formula feeding |
| Reduced risk for infant morbidity and mortality | |

**Source:** Reproduced with permission from Position of the American Dietetic Association: promoting and supporting breastfeeding. *J Am Diet Assoc.* 2009;109:1926–1942.

pare, mix, or heat; and for a hungry infant, that's an important advantage! Breast milk is always the perfect temperature and is sterile. In addition, links between breastfeeding and reduced risk of disorders such as type 1 diabetes, cardiovascular diseases, childhood obesity, and Crohn's disease have been suggested; these need further study. Table 12.8 lists some of the possible protective benefits of human milk.

### Benefits for Mother

Breastfeeding stimulates uterine contractions, which help the uterus return to its normal size. If the baby is put to the breast immediately after delivery, these same contractions (an effect of oxytocin) also can help control blood loss. Although not an effective method of birth control, exclusive breastfeeding suppresses ovulation in many women. Breastfeeding may help some women return to their prepregnancy weight more quickly.[58]

Breastfeeding is as convenient for mother as it is for baby and is certainly less expensive than formula feeding. Although more comprehensive studies are needed, some evidence suggests that breastfeeding reduces a woman's risk of ovarian cancer, breast cancer, and osteoporosis[59] as well as postpartum depression.[60] If, as expected, a breastfed baby has fewer episodes of infectious illness, this saves healthcare costs and reduces employee absences and lost income for working mothers. In light of these benefits, government programs are now encouraging hospitals and workplaces to be more "baby friendly."[61] Additionally, communities are being encouraged to support breastfeeding mothers. As of 2011, 45 states have laws that allow women to breastfeed in any private or public location.[62]

## *Quick* Bite

### Breastfeeding to Control Blood Pressure?

Oxytocin, the hormone produced while breastfeeding, can lower the blood pressure of nursing mothers. Research shows that breastfeeding mothers have lower blood pressures after nursing than do bottle-feeding mothers. When asked to discuss stressful events, nursing mothers show smaller increases in blood pressure than the bottle-feeders. Mothers often claim that they feel relaxed during breastfeeding, which may account for the difference in blood pressure.

## Contraindications to Breastfeeding

Nearly all women who want to breastfeed can do so successfully, and breast-feeding rates are steadily increasing.[63] There are times, however, when breast-feeding is inappropriate because of infant or maternal disease or drug use. Depending on the specifics of the operation, breast enlargement or reduction surgery may or may not preclude breastfeeding.[64] The main concern is whether milk ducts and major nerves were cut or damaged.

In the case of infectious or chronic diseases, individual situations should be discussed with the healthcare provider. For example, a woman with untreated tuberculosis should not breastfeed because the illness may be transmitted to her child. In the United States and Canada, where safe feeding alterna-tives exist, women infected with the human immunodeficiency virus (HIV) are advised not to breastfeed because HIV can be transmitted to the baby through breast milk.

Some medications pass directly into human milk, and some prescribed medications may preclude breastfeeding. If the mother is using an illegal drug such as cocaine, she should not breastfeed. Women taking prescription or over-the-counter medicines or herbal supplements should discuss the effects of these products on breast milk with their healthcare providers.

**Key Concepts**  *Health benefits and convenience are key advantages of breastfeeding. For the infant, breastfeeding has been linked to reduced incidence of many infectious diseases as well as to other conditions. For a mother, breastfeeding speeds recovery of normal uterine size and may reduce her disease risk. Although breastfeeding is the pre-ferred method of infant feeding, there are times when breastfeeding is contraindicated. These situations should be identified and discussed as part of prenatal care.*

## Resources for Pregnant and Lactating Women and Their Children

Many agencies support research and education programs that promote the health of pregnant and breastfeeding women and their children. You may be familiar with the March of Dimes and its efforts to reduce birth defects and prematurity through optimal nutrition during pregnancy. La Leche League is a voluntary health and education organization that offers programs and educational materials to help breastfeeding mothers learn about the benefits and practice of breastfeeding.

The **Special Supplemental Nutrition Program for Women, Infants, and Children (WIC)** is a much-acclaimed program of the Food and Nutri-tion Service of the USDA. WIC provides food assistance, nutrition education, and referrals to healthcare services for low-income pregnant, postpartum, and breastfeeding women as well as for infants and children up to age 5.

Although WIC services include breastfeeding education and support, WIC participants are less likely to breastfeed their infants.[65] Continued promotion of breastfeeding by WIC and other public health programs can have both health and economic benefits. Participation in WIC improves household food security and reduces hunger.[66] Periodically, WIC participants are required to bring their infants into the local WIC office. These visits give WIC staff an opportunity to evaluate the infant's growth and provide the caregiver addi-tional nutrition education.

## Infancy

**Infancy** is the period of a child's life between birth and 1 year. Because of the rapid growth that occurs during this time, nutritional needs are higher

**Special Supplemental Nutrition Program for Women, Infants, and Children (WIC)**  A USDA program that provides federal grants to states for supplemental foods, healthcare referrals, and nutrition education for low-income pregnant, breastfeeding, and nonbreastfeeding postpartum women and/or infants and children at nutritional risk.

**infancy**  The period between birth and 12 months of age.

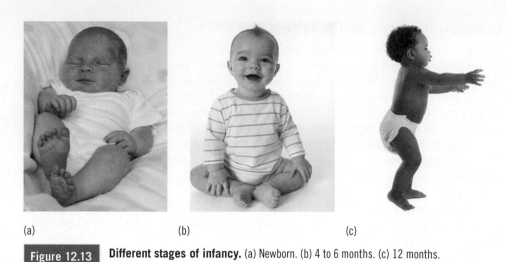

(a)                                    (b)                                    (c)

Figure 12.13    **Different stages of infancy.** (a) Newborn. (b) 4 to 6 months. (c) 12 months.

per unit of body weight than at any other time in the life cycle. Despite the critical importance of nutrition at this stage, feeding an infant is a fairly simple process. Human milk provides all nutrients an infant needs and is the model for infant formulas. By 4 to 6 months, the infant's physical development and physiological maturation signal readiness for the addition of "solid" foods to the diet.

Human infants need love as much as they need food. Without love and nurturing, a baby can fail to thrive even if she is offered all of the right nutrients. If an infant is not nourished emotionally, nutrition recommendations and requirements become meaningless.

## Infant Growth and Development

Birth weight is the best predictor of the child's health in the first year of life; however, it is important to correlate weight with length of development. The risk profile of an infant who has a low birth weight because of **prematurity** is different from that of a **full-term baby** with a low birth weight.

Immediately after birth, an infant loses about 6 percent of its body weight. This is normal and expected. By 10 to 14 days, the infant should return to his birth weight. Over the next 12 months, the infant's growth will be phenomenal. By the age of 4 to 6 months, a healthy infant will have doubled his birth weight. By his first birthday, the infant will have tripled his birth weight and increased his length by about 50 percent. The infant's body proportions change, too, so by age 1 he is looking less like a baby and more like a **toddler**. (See **Figure 12.13**.)

Length (used instead of height because infants can't stand) and **head circumference** are more sensitive measures than weight for assessing a baby's growth and nutritional status. Weight alone reflects just recent nutritional intake. Head circumference measures brain growth and development. Chronic malnutrition can limit this growth and is reflected in inadequate gains in head size. Regular measurements of head circumference, therefore, can verify proper growth. Head circumference measurements are useful in infants and children up to age 2.

### Growth Charts

During routine checkups throughout infancy (and during childhood and adolescence), healthcare practitioners measure weight, length or height, and head circumference and plot these values on **growth charts**. (See **Figure 12.14**.)

**prematurity** Birth before 37 weeks of gestation.

**full-term baby** A baby delivered during the normal period of human gestation, between 38 and 41 weeks.

**toddler** A child between 12 and 36 months of age.

**head circumference** Measurement of the largest part of the infant's head (just above the eyebrows and ears); used to determine brain growth.

**growth charts** Charts that plot the weight, length, and head circumference of infants and children as they grow.

Charts for weight-for-age, length- (or height-) for-age, head circumference-for-age, weight-for-length, and BMI-for-age are available for boys and girls and for two age ranges: birth to 36 months and 2 to 20 years. Healthcare practitioners use growth charts to show the growth of an individual child over time. These charts also allow comparison of one child's growth to that of children in the general population.

**Key Concepts**  *A typical infant doubles its birth weight by age 4 to 6 months and triples it by 12 months. Infant length increases about 50 percent during the first year. Healthcare practitioners use growth charts to follow and assess an infant's growth in weight, length, and head circumference.*

## Energy and Nutrient Needs During Infancy

How do scientists determine the nutrient needs of newborns and young infants? Studies with babies as subjects are rare—the logistical and ethical questions are daunting! So how else can we know what babies need? It's simple; we just look at breast milk—the food designed especially for babies. The composition of human milk is the gold standard by which infant nutrient needs are determined. Babies who are not breastfed are given infant formula. In the United States, most infant formulas have a base of modified cow's milk or soy protein. To ensure that formula meets all of an infant's nutrient needs, federal regulations require that the formula's composition complies with nutritional standards.

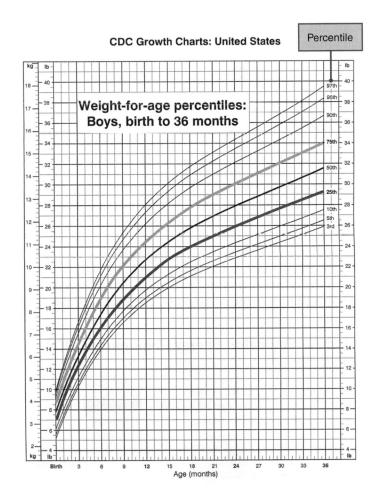

**Figure 12.14**  **Growth chart.** The Centers for Disease Control and Prevention (CDC) has complete sets of growth charts available on the Internet at http://www.cdc.gov/growthcharts.

**Source:** Developed by the National Center for Health Statistics in collaboration with the National Center for Chronic Disease Prevention and Health Promotion (2000).

**fluorosis** Condition caused by excessive intake of fluorides that is characterized in children by discoloration and pitting of the teeth.

If a breastfed baby does not get adequate sunlight exposure and if the baby's mother is deficient in vitamin D, the infant's risk is especially high. In 2008, the American Academy of Pediatrics (AAP) increased its recommendation for daily vitamin D to 400 IU per day for all infants, children, and adolescents, beginning the first few days after birth.[75]

**Vitamin K** Vitamin K is necessary for producing prothrombin, a substance needed for blood to clot. Although intestinal bacteria synthesize vitamin K, the gut is sterile at birth. Because babies are born with minimal stores of vitamin K, it is recommended that a single dose of vitamin K be given at birth. Both human milk and infant formula provide adequate vitamin K, and as feeding begins helpful bacteria begin to flourish in the infant's intestinal tract.

**Vitamin $B_{12}$** Vitamin $B_{12}$ is essential for cell division and normal folate metabolism. Mothers who regularly eat meat, fish, and dairy products produce milk that is adequate in vitamin $B_{12}$. This may not be true of strict vegetarians, whose diet—and milk—may be deficient in vitamin $B_{12}$. Breastfed infants of vegan mothers may need a vitamin $B_{12}$ supplement.

**Iron** Iron is essential for growth and development, and iron-deficiency anemia is the most common nutritional deficiency in the United States. Human milk is not a rich source of iron, but it does not need to be. Approximately 50 percent of the iron in breast milk is absorbed, compared with only 4 percent of the iron in infant formula. If the mother has consumed an iron-rich diet during pregnancy, the fetus builds up large enough iron stores during gestation to meet most of its iron needs for the first few months of life. These stores begin to diminish during the fourth month of life. By the age of 6 months, a breastfed infant needs an additional iron source. Iron-fortified infant cereals can meet this need. For formula-fed babies, iron supplementation is needed from birth. The AAP therefore recommends iron-fortified formula for all formula-fed babies.[76]

**Fluoride** Human milk is low in fluoride, a mineral important for dental health. Current research has led the American Dental Association and the AAP to recommend fluoride supplements for breastfed infants beginning at the age of 6 months, depending on fluoride content of the local water supply.[77] In a given week, almost one-quarter of U.S. children younger than 12 years and 30 percent of 2-year-olds use supplemental fluoride.[78] If the local water supply has adequate fluoride and the formula is mixed with tap water, formula-fed infants do not need fluoride supplements. If the water used to mix formula has inadequate fluoride, fluoride supplements are indicated. Fluoridation policies and the fluoride content of tap water vary among municipalities. Oversupplementation with fluoride in children has been associated with mild dental **fluorosis** in developing teeth; therefore, ingestion of higher than recommended levels is discouraged.[79]

**Key Concepts** *Energy and nutrient needs for infants are estimated based on the composition of human milk. Because of their rapid growth and development, infants have high energy and nutrient needs per kilogram of body weight. Caregivers must give special attention to vitamin D, iron, and fluoride to ensure that the infant obtains enough. If breast milk or formula (properly mixed) is meeting energy needs, the fluid needs of the infant also are being met.*

## Newborn Breastfeeding

The AAP has identified breastfeeding as the ideal method of feeding to achieve optimal growth and development[80] and recommends that breastfeeding begin as soon after birth as possible and continue at least through the first 12 months of life.[81] Feedings should occur at least every two to three hours, for a total of 8 to 12 feedings per day. Duration of feedings is guided by the infant's behavior and may last from 10 to 15 minutes per breast. Hospitals should provide every opportunity for breastfeeding to begin before the baby goes home. Nurses or **lactation consultants** should be available to offer professional breastfeeding support to new mothers. The AAP recommends that no supplements of formula or water be given to breastfed neonates unless medically indicated.

## Alternative Feeding: Infant Formula

Women may decide not to breastfeed or to breastfeed only briefly. Their infants need infant formulas designed to provide adequate nutrition.

### Standard Infant Formulas

Standard infant formulas use cow's milk as a base. In making infant formula, manufacturers first remove the milk fat and replace it with vegetable oils. Infant formula is fortified with all the essential vitamins and minerals according to guidelines established by the AAP and enforced by the Food and Drug Administration. Infant formulas are available with or without added iron, but, because of the decreased bioavailability of iron in infant formulas and the infant's high needs, the AAP recommends using only iron-fortified formulas.

Although formula manufacturers try to mimic the composition of human milk, formula remains an imperfect copy. Several brands of infant formula contain three fatty acids that are prevalent in human milk: arachidonic acid (ARA), eicosapentaenoic acid (EPA), and docosahexaenoic acid (DHA). Some studies show that supplemental ARA and EPA may benefit infants' visual function and cognitive development; however, a large review of studies found that most randomized controlled trials have not shown a beneficial effect of long-chain polyunsaturated fatty acid supplementation of formula milk on the neurodevelopmental, visual, and physical outcomes of full-term newborns.[82] Human milk also contains more cholesterol than infant formulas.

### Soy-Based Formulas

Formula-fed infants who develop vomiting, diarrhea, constipation, abdominal pain, or colic are frequently switched to soy-based formulas. In these formulas, soy is the source of protein. To compensate for the inferior digestibility of soy protein, soy formulas contain more protein than formulas based on cow's milk. Soy formulas are lactose-free and iron-fortified. Corn syrup and sucrose are the carbohydrate sources.

### Other Types of Formula

Special formulas are available for infants who are allergic to both cow's milk and soy protein, those who are premature, and those who have rare defects in metabolic pathways. These special formulas often have their protein content modified in either its digestibility or its amino acid composition. Many special formulas contain medium-chain triglycerides as the major fat source. This type of fat is very well digested and absorbed. These special formulas are expensive and often taste bad, but they are essential for many infants.

### Formula Preparation

Formulas come in three forms: ready-to-feed, concentrate, and powdered. Although the ready-to-feed version is most convenient, it is also the most

*Quick* Bite

**What's a Biberon?**
Many people consider Dr. Nils Rosen von Rosenstein to be the father of pediatrics. In his 1764 textbook, he describes a "biberon," a leather nipple used for artificial infant feeding. He also describes 14 types of infant diarrhea.

expensive. As the name implies, the formula can be poured directly from the can into a bottle and fed to the baby. Liquid concentrate formula is mixed with an equal amount of water before feeding. Powdered formula also is mixed with water and is the least expensive.

When using infant formulas, principles of food safety must be observed. Infants have immature immune systems and may develop infections from improperly prepared or stored formula. Prepared formula should be refrigerated immediately and kept in the refrigerator until needed. If formula is not used within 48 hours, it should be discarded. For at least the first few months, the AAP recommends sterilizing all equipment used for feeding.

Improperly mixed formula is another danger, whether a result of ignorance in following instructions or of economics. Some caregivers on limited budgets might purposely overdilute formula to make it last longer. This deprives the infant of necessary calories and protein and provides too much water. Other caregivers might overconcentrate the formula in the misguided belief that this might encourage faster growth. Overconcentrated formula provides too much protein and too little water and may cause problems with an infant's kidney function and hydration.

## Breast Milk or Formula: How Much Is Enough?

It is fairly simple to use DRI values and breast milk or formula composition to estimate an infant's needs based on body weight. For example, a newborn who weighs 7 pounds, 11 ounces (3.5 kilograms) requires approximately 390 kilocalories and 5 grams of protein each day. This amount is provided by approximately 600 milliliters (~20 fluid ounces) of breast milk or infant formula.

It's easy to keep track of how much formula an infant has consumed, but what about a breastfed baby? Although you can't see how much breast milk a nursing infant is consuming, there are other ways to tell that a baby is getting enough to eat. An adequately fed newborn will breastfeed 8 to 12 times, wet at least six diapers, and have at least three loose stools each day in the first week of life. The newborn also will regain his or her birth weight within the first two weeks. Normal growth, regular elimination patterns, and a satisfied demeanor are the best indicators that a baby is getting enough to eat.

## Feeding Technique

Feeding should take place in a loving and warm environment. A breastfeeding mother holds her baby close, at a distance that encourages mother–baby eye contact. (See **Figure 12.19**.) During bottle-feeding, the caregiver needs to hold the baby close and make eye contact. Propping the bottle against a pillow or other object so the baby can feed alone should be avoided.

Babies swallow air while feeding, whether at the breast or with a bottle, and they need to be burped. Babies generally need to be burped after 15 minutes or 2 to 3 ounces of formula. Just as the infant sends signals of readiness for feeding, she also signals fullness. Fullness cues include fussiness, playfulness, sleep, or just turning away. Parents need to learn these cues and respond to them.

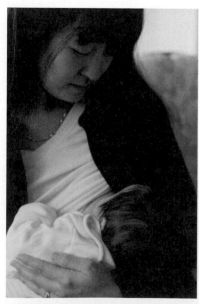

**Figure 12.19**   **Breastfeeding.** Breastfeeding nurtures an infant emotionally as well as physically. This intensely rewarding time helps to bond a mother and her child.

**Key Concepts**   *Human milk provides all necessary nutrients for growth and development and enhances the immune system of the maturing infant. Infants who are not breastfed receive infant formula, which should be fortified with iron. Careful preparation and storage of the formula ensures proper nutrient composition and food safety. Formula feedings should nourish the baby emotionally as well as nutritionally.*

## Introduction of Solid Foods into the Infant's Diet

Based on an infant's physiological needs (e.g., depletion of iron stores) and physical development (e.g., the ability to sit up), solid foods, also called **complementary foods**, are introduced. To say that we are introducing solid foods is a bit of a misnomer; we are really referring to pureed and liquefied cereals, fruits, vegetables, and meats that are added to the infant's diet of breast milk or infant formula. According to the American Academy of Pediatrics, solid foods should be introduced when infants are developmentally ready, around 4 to 6 months of age, to ensure they get adequate nutrition.[83]

### Physiological Indicators of Infant Readiness for Solid Foods

Before a baby reaches 6 months of age, solid food is not necessary for nutrition; in fact, early introduction of supplemental foods can be detrimental. By the age of 4 to 6 months, however, an infant is physiologically ready to expand his diet. For example, at this age a baby has increased levels of digestive enzymes so foods other than human milk or formula can be digested with ease. In addition, the infant is more able to maintain adequate hydration by the age of 6 months. Before this age, adding cereals or other solid foods to the diet can negatively affect an infant's hydration. It is probably no coincidence that the iron stores acquired in the mother's womb become depleted at the same time the baby is physiologically ready to expand his or her diet. However, solid food is a supplement to, not a replacement for, human milk or formula at this time.

### Developmental Readiness for Solid Foods

If you attempt to spoon-feed a very young infant, for example, at 3 weeks of age, the infant's tongue will push the spoon and food right back out. This **extrusion reflex** is a sign that the infant is not ready for solid foods. By 4 to 6 months of age, the infant will no longer push the food out and is capable of transferring food from the front of the mouth to the back, an ability necessary for swallowing solid foods. Also, the infant can purposefully bring her hand to her mouth, an ability necessary for self-feeding. In addition, if the baby is able to control her head and neck while sitting with minimal support, she is ready to be fed solids.

### Start Healthy Feeding Guidelines

The *Start Healthy Feeding Guidelines for Infants and Toddlers* are science-based, practical guidelines for feeding healthy babies for the first two years.[84] The *Start Healthy Feeding Guidelines* were designed to answer parents' and caregivers' questions, such as "When is my baby ready for complementary foods? What foods should I feed my baby? How do I feed these foods?"[85] The appropriate age for introduction of complementary foods balances physiological and developmental readiness with nutritional requirements for growth and development. **Figure 12.20** summarizes the *Start Healthy Feeding Guidelines*.

Signs of readiness for the introduction of infant cereals and thin, pureed foods include the ability to sit with support and the ability to take food from a spoon and move it forward and backward in the mouth with the tongue. As the infant's body control improves and she can sit independently, she also will develop the ability to pick up and hold objects in her hand. She will be able to take in thicker pureed foods and soft mashed foods without lumps.

Babies who can crawl also are likely to be ready to self-feed finger foods such as baby biscuits or crackers. Babies at this stage can hold small foods between the thumb and first finger and also hold a cup (preferably one with

THINK
About It
4

**complementary foods** Any foods or liquids other than breast milk or infant formula fed to an infant.

**extrusion reflex** A young infant's response when a spoon is put in its mouth; the tongue is thrust forward, indicating that the baby is not ready for spoon feeding.

| Development Stage | Newborn | Head Up | Supported Sitter | Independent Sitter | Crawler | Beginning to Walk | Independent Toddler |
|---|---|---|---|---|---|---|---|
| | | | | | | | |
| Physical Skills | • Needs head support | • More skillful head control with support emerging | • Sits with help or support<br>• On tummy, pushes up on arms with straight elbows | • Sits independently<br>• Can pick up and hold small object in hand<br>• Leans toward food or spoon | • Learns to crawl<br>• May pull self to stand | • Pulls self to stand<br>• Stands alone<br>• Takes early steps | • Walks well alone<br>• Runs |
| Eating Skills | • Baby establishes a suck-swallow-breathe pattern during breast or bottle feeding | • Breastfeeds or bottle feeds<br>• Tongue moves forward and back to suck | • May push food out of mouth with tongue, which gradually decreases with age<br>• Moves pureed food forward and backward in mouth with tongue to swallow<br>• Recognizes spoon and holds mouth open as spoon approaches | • Learns to keep thick purees in mouth<br>• Pulls head downward and presses upper lip to draw food from spoon<br>• Tries to rake foods toward self into fist<br>• Can transfer food from one hand to the other<br>• Can drink from a cup held by feeder | • Learns to move tongue from side to side to transfer food around mouth and push food to the side of the mouth so food can be mashed<br>• Begins to use jaw and tongue to mash food<br>• Plays with spoon at mealtime, may bring it to mouth, but does not use it for self-feeding yet<br>• Can feed self finger foods<br>• Holds cup independently<br>• Holds small foods between thumb and first finger | • Feeds self easily with fingers<br>• Can drink from a straw<br>• Can hold cup with two hands and take swallows<br>• More skillful at chewing<br>• Dips spoon in food rather than scooping<br>• Demands to spoon-feed self<br>• Bites through a variety of textures | • Chews and swallows firmer foods skillfully<br>• Learns to use a fork for spearing<br>• Uses spoon with less spilling<br>• Can hold cup in one hand and set it down skillfully |
| Baby's Hunger & Fullness Cues | • Cries or fusses to show hunger<br>• Gazes at caregiver, opens mouth during feeding indicating desire to continue<br>• Spits out nipple or falls asleep when full<br>• Stops sucking when full | • Cries or fusses to show hunger<br>• Smiles, gazes at caregiver, or coos during feeding to indicate desire to continue<br>• Spits out nipple or falls asleep when full<br>• Stops sucking when full | • Moves head forward to reach spoon when hungry<br>• May swipe the food toward the mouth when hungry<br>• Turns head away from spoon when full<br>• May be distracted or notice surroundings more when full | • Reaches for spoon or food when hungry<br>• Points to food when hungry<br>• Slows down in eating when full<br>• Clenches mouth shut or pushes food away when full | • Reaches for food when hungry<br>• Points to food when hungry<br>• Shows excitement when food is presented when hungry<br>• Pushes food away when full<br>• Slows down in eating when full | • Expresses desire for specific foods with words or sounds<br>• Shakes head to say "no more" when full | • Combines phrases with gestures, such as "want that" and pointing<br>• Can lead parent to refrigerator and point to a desired food or drink<br>• Uses words like "all done" and "get down"<br>• Plays with food or throws food when full |
| Appropriate Foods & Textures | • Breastmilk or infant formula | • Breastmilk or infant formula | • Breastmilk or infant formula<br>• Infant cereals<br>• Thin pureed foods | • Breastmilk or infant formula<br>• 100% Juice<br>• Thin pureed baby foods<br>• Thicker pureed baby foods<br>• Soft mashed foods without lumps<br>• 100% Juice | • Breastmilk or infant formula<br>• 100% Juice<br>• Infant cereals<br>• Pureed foods<br>• Ground or soft mashed foods with tiny soft noticeable lumps<br>• Foods with soft texture<br>• Crunchy foods that dissolve (such as baby biscuits or crackers)<br>• Increase variety of flavors offered | • Breastmilk or infant formula or whole milk<br>• 100% Juice<br>• Coarsely chopped foods, including foods with noticeable pieces<br>• Foods with soft to moderate texture<br>• Toddler foods<br>• Bite sized pieces of food<br>• Bites through a variety of textures | • Whole milk<br>• 100% Juice<br>• Coarsely chopped foods<br>• Toddler foods<br>• Bite-sized pieces of food<br>• Becomes efficient at eating foods of varying textures and taking controlled bites of soft solids, hard solids, or crunchy foods by 2 years |

**Figure 12.20** The *Start Healthy Feeding Guidelines.* Summary of physical and eating skills, hunger and fullness cues, and appropriate food textures for children 0 to 24 months of age.

**Source:** Reproduced from Butte N, Cobb K, Dwyer J, et al. The *Start Healthy Feeding Guidelines* for infants and toddlers. *J Am Diet Assoc.* 2004;104(3):442–454.

a cap and spout) independently. A baby is able to participate in the feeding process, and as his dexterity improves he will be able to pick up small pieces of food. It is important that caregivers monitor the child's eating to make sure the youngster does not choke on food or on nonfood items.

At the end of the first year, when a baby is standing alone and beginning to walk, his diet can expand even further with bite-size pieces of table foods and a wider variety of textures. Self-feeding with his fingers is much easier, and he desires to self-feed with a spoon as well—a messy but developmentally appropriate thing to do. Most table foods are appropriate for the child at this stage.

There is no scientific evidence to support introduction of complementary foods in any particular order; cultural practices play a large role in determining which foods are introduced first. Introducing a source of iron, such as an iron-fortified infant cereal or pureed meats, is necessary because iron stores developed in pregnancy are declining. No matter what food is introduced first, new foods should be introduced one at a time, at intervals of about one week, to see how well the infant tolerates each food and to be on the lookout for allergic reactions. Throughout the first year, breast milk or infant formula still forms the major portion of the infant's diet. Ideally, however, the child will have been introduced to a variety of foods by his or her first birthday.

Parents and caregivers should take care that complementary foods be soft in texture to avoid the risk of choking. Delaying—until age 1—the introduction of common food allergens, particularly cow's milk, egg whites, and wheat, can prevent food allergies for many infants. In addition to its allergic potential, whole cow's milk provides too much protein and too little iron, is low in essential fatty acids, may impair kidney function and lead to dehydration, and has been linked to development of type 1 diabetes.[86] In families with a strong history of allergies, introduction of eggs should be delayed until age 2, and peanuts, tree nuts, fish, and shellfish should not be introduced before age 3.

Along with observing the infant's developmental readiness for complementary foods, parents and caregivers need to be alert to an infant's hunger and satiety cues. The suggestions in Table 12.11 can help new parents establish a healthy feeding relationship with their child.

**Table 12.11**   **Suggestions for Establishing a Healthy Feeding Relationship with a Child**

| Do | Why |
|---|---|
| Wash the baby's hands before feeding. | To clean any dirt or germs off the hands to keep the baby's food clean |
| Use a small spoon or let the baby use his or her fingers. | To help the baby learn proper eating habits |
| Place food on the tip of the spoon and put food in the middle of the baby's tongue. | To make it easy for the baby to swallow |
| Remove food from the jar before feeding. Do not feed the baby food from the jar. | To prevent the saliva from the baby's mouth from spoiling the remainder of the food in the jar |
| Give only one new food at a time, and wait at least one week before giving another new food. | To give the baby time to get used to each new flavor and texture, and to see if the baby is allergic to the new food |

**Source:** US Department of Agriculture, Food and Nutrition Service. Feeding infants. A guide for use in the child nutrition programs. FNS-258. 2002. http://www.FNS.usda.gov/tn/resources/feeding_infants.html. Accessed 8/3/11.

**gastroesophageal reflux** A backflow of stomach contents into the esophagus, accompanied by a burning pain because of the acidity of the gastric juices.

**failure to thrive (FTT)** Abnormally low gains in length (height) and weight during infancy and childhood; may result from physical problems or poor feeding, but many affected children have no apparent disease or defect.

Various caregivers may be involved in a child's nutrition. In today's society, it is inappropriate to assume that the caregiver is solely the mother, father, grandparent, or even a relative of the child. Many children spend the majority of their feeding time in a child-care setting. Child-care staff have an important role in supporting healthy eating behaviors of young children.[87]

**Key Concepts** *An infant's physiological needs and developmental readiness usually indicate the appropriate time to introduce solid foods. Semisolid and solid foods should be introduced slowly to check for food intolerances and allergic reactions. The caregiver should choose foods that meet the child's nutritional needs and suit his or her developmental capabilities.*

## Feeding Problems During Infancy

### Colic

The term *colic* refers to continuous crying and distress in a healthy infant—apparently due to abdominal cramping and discomfort. Infants with colic usually cry for hours, despite efforts to comfort them. In some cases, a change in formula or a change in the breastfeeding mother's diet provides some relief, such as the mother's elimination of milk products or other allergenic foods from the diet; however, often there is no clearly effective treatment.[88] Most often, colic goes away on its own, usually by the age of 3 to 4 months.

### Early Childhood Caries

Decay in the primary teeth, known as *early childhood caries*, and sometimes called "baby-bottle tooth decay" (see **Figure 12.21**) can result if baby teeth are bathed too long in milk, formula, or juice, which nourish decay-producing bacteria. Other factors, such as inadequate development of tooth enamel, also contribute.[89] The problem is often associated with routinely putting a baby to bed with a bottle so the baby's teeth are awash in formula or juice for much or all of the night. Children with early childhood caries are more susceptible to caries in the permanent teeth and lifelong dental problems.[90]

### Iron-Deficiency Anemia: Milk Anemia

Human milk and cow's milk both are low in iron. As discussed earlier, this is usually not a problem—the iron in breast milk is well absorbed, and regular cow's milk is not recommended for babies younger than 1 year. Iron deficiency may develop in older infants who do not eat enough iron-rich foods.

### Gastroesophageal Reflux

**Gastroesophageal reflux** is the regurgitation of the stomach contents into the esophagus after a feeding. This type of spitting up occurs in 3 percent of newborns, usually males, and typically disappears within 12 to 18 months. Concern is warranted if reflux makes a child difficult to feed or results in coughing, choking, or frequent vomiting. Adding cereal to bottle feedings is not recommended for a baby who has reflux.

### Diarrhea

Stool patterns vary from infant to infant, as well as in the same infant over time. Healthy, thriving breastfed infants may have up to 12 stools per day—or only 1 per week. Formula-fed infants usually have one to seven bowel movements per day. Diarrhea—the frequent passage of loose, watery stools—can rapidly dehydrate an infant. Infants with diarrhea require increased fluids, and caregivers should consult the child's pediatrician for specific advice about how to meet this need.

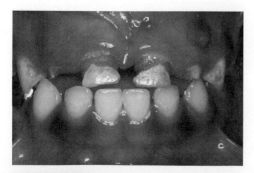

**Figure 12.21** **Early childhood caries.** A baby routinely put to bed with a bottle can develop extensive tooth decay.

## Failure to Thrive

Full-term infants who experience poor growth in the absence of disease or physical defect suffer from **failure to thrive (FTT)**. (See **Figure 12.22**.) Although this can occur at any age, in infancy it usually occurs in the second half of the first year. Common causes include poverty and a resulting shortage of food, inappropriate foods in an infant's diet, improper formula preparation, or excessive consumption of fruit juice or fruit drinks. (See the FYI feature "Fruit Juices and Drinks.") In addition, well-meaning parents may introduce low-fat or nonfat milk in an attempt to prevent obesity. Babies need a high-fat diet to support normal growth and brain development. As stated, regular cow's milk should not be introduced before age 1. Low-fat milks are inappropriate for children younger than 2 years.

Untreated, FTT can delay cognitive, motor, and language development. Studies indicate, however, that intensive intervention can correct FTT and allow the baby to resume a normal growth pattern. Intervention includes nutrition education for caregivers, maintenance of food records by the caregiver, frequent weight checks of the infant, and perhaps social service intervention for the family.

Although there is nothing complex about the nutrient needs and food choices appropriate for babies, it is important for caregivers to receive some education about proper feeding. Some practices we

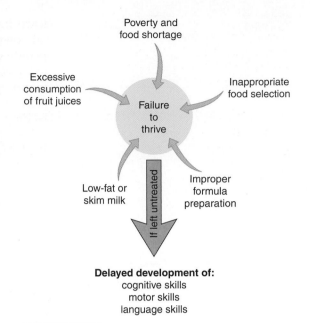

| **Figure 12.22** | **Failure to thrive.** Failure to thrive can result from many different causes. If untreated, the effects are lifelong. |

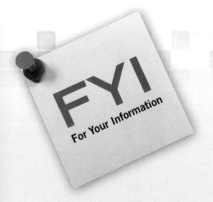

# Fruit Juices and Drinks

Fruit juices are popular beverages for children aged 6 months to 5 years. Juices do contribute benefits to the diet. They are refreshing and sweet; accessible and affordable; more healthful than soft drinks; and provide energy, water, and selected minerals and vitamins. A glass of 100-percent fruit juice counts as one fruit serving. If juice is being used as a source of vitamin C, drinking just 3 to 6 fluid ounces per day meets vitamin C intake recommendations.

High fruit juice consumption among young children has been implicated as a contributing factor to both failure to thrive and obesity. Failure to thrive may result if fruit juices replace other food sources (particularly milk) or if sorbitol and fructose, found in higher amounts in apple and pear juice, cause diarrhea and malabsorption.[1] Although the link between excessive juice consumption and obesity has not been proven,[2] studies suggest that it is more likely to be a factor in those children who are at risk for overweight and obesity.[3]

The vast array of juice drinks and fruit beverages available in the marketplace can make it difficult for parents to find nutritious choices. At best, these beverages contain added vitamin C and, in some cases, vitamin A and calcium. However, beverages that are less than 100-percent fruit juice are more like soft drinks than fruits and, as such, should be severely limited in the diets of young children.

To keep intake of fruit juices to a healthy level, the American Academy of Pediatrics recommends the following practices:[4]

- Wait until at least 6 months of age before introducing juice.
- Avoid giving infants juice in bottles or other containers that allow easy consumption throughout the day. Avoid giving juice at bedtime.
- Limit consumption of fruit juice to 4 to 6 fluid ounces per day for children 1 to 6 years old.
- Encourage caregivers to offer fruit rather than fruit juice to children.
- Determine the amount of juice being consumed when evaluating children with malnutrition (overnutrition and undernutrition) and in children with dental caries.
- Educate parents about the differences between fruit juice and fruit drinks.

1   Nobugrot T, Chasalow F, Lifshitz F. Carbohydrate absorption from one serving of fruit juice in young children: age and carbohydrate composition effects. *J Am Coll Nutr.* 1997;16:152–158.

2   O'Connor TM, Yang S, Nicklas TA. Beverage intake among preschool children and its effect on weight status. *Pediatrics.* 2006;188:1010–1018.

3   Faith MS, Dennison B, Edmunds LS, Stratton HH. Fruit juice intake predicts increased adiposity gain in children from low-income families: weight status-by-environment interaction. *Pediatrics.* 2006;118:2066–2075; and Nelson JA, Carpenter K, Chiasson MA. Diet, activity, and overweight among preschool-age children enrolled in the Special Supplemental Nutrition Program for Women, Infants, and Children (WIC). *Prev Chronic Dis.* 4/06. http://www.cdc.gov/pcd/issues/2006/apr/05_0135.htm. Accessed 8/3/11.

4   American Academy of Pediatrics Committee on Nutrition. Policy statement. The use and misuse of fruit juice in pediatrics. *Pediatrics.* 2001;107:1210–1213. Statement reaffirmed October 2006. *Pediatrics.* 2007;119:405.

learn from friends, parents, and other family members, or remember from our own childhood, are inappropriate for babies. Studies show that even people who receive nutrition education in the WIC program introduce solid foods much too early and feed infants sweetened tea, soft drinks, and other inappropriate foods.[91] Newborns don't come with instructions, but caregivers can always turn to a pediatrician or registered dietitian for answers to feeding questions.

**Key Concepts** *Feeding-related problems of infancy include colic, baby bottle tooth decay, iron-deficiency anemia, gastroesophageal reflux, diarrhea, and failure to thrive. Usually minor adjustments in food choices or feeding techniques solve these problems; however, caregivers may need the guidance of a pediatrician or registered dietitian.*

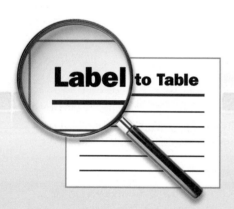

A pregnant woman requires more nutrients than usual. The RDA for both iron and folate increases by 50 percent during pregnancy. Iron, especially, is difficult to get in this quantity from the diet. Enriched grains and fortified foods, such as cereals, make it easier to obtain these essential nutrients. Let's look at the Nutrition Facts label from a popular breakfast cereal.

Take a look at how much folic acid a 1-cup serving of this breakfast cereal contains—50% DV (DV = 400 micrograms). The DV for folate is the same as the RDA for nonpregnant women; for pregnancy, the RDA increases to 600 micrograms. If orange juice accompanies the cereal, another 15% DV (60 milligrams) is added for a 1-cup serving. So, these two foods provide a substantial amount of the folate that a pregnant woman would need.

Iron also is extremely important for pregnancy because of its role in growth and its importance as blood volume increases during pregnancy. One serving of this breakfast cereal provides almost half of the Daily Value of 18 milligrams (45 percent of 18 milligrams equals 8 milligrams). However, during pregnancy, the RDA for iron is 27 milligrams. So, one serving of this cereal provides nearly one-third of the iron needed each day—a good start. Having orange juice with the cereal will enhance iron absorption.

## Nutrition Facts

Serving Size: 1 cup (30g)

Servings Per Container about 9

| Amount Per Serving | with 1/2 cup | |
|---|---|---|
| **Calories** | Cheerios | skim milk |
| Calories from Fat | 110 | 150 |
| % Daily Value** | 15 | 20 |
| **Total Fat** 2g* | | |
| Saturated Fat 0g | 3% | 3% |
| Trans Fat 0g | 0% | 3% |
| Polyunsaturated Fat 0.5g | | |
| Monounsaturated Fat 0.5g | | |
| **Cholesterol** 0g | 0% | 1% |
| **Sodium** 280mg | 12% | 15% |
| **Total Carbohydrate** 22g | 7% | 9% |
| Dietary Fiber 0g | 11% | 11% |
| Sugars 1g | | |
| **Protein** 3g | | |
| Vitamin A | 10% | 15% |
| Vitamin C | 10% | 10% |
| Calcium | 4% | 20% |
| Iron | 45% | 45% |
| Vitamin D | 10% | 25% |
| Thiamin | 25% | 30% |
| Riboflavin | 25% | 35% |
| Niacin | 25% | 25% |
| Vitamin B 6 | 25% | 25% |
| Folic Acid | 50% | 50% |
| Vitamin B 12 | 25% | 35% |
| Phosphorus | 10% | 25% |

# Learning Portfolio

## Key Terms

## Study Points

■ Nutritional status before pregnancy is an important consideration of having a healthy baby. Moreover, it is an integral part of all aspects of preconception care: risk assessment, health promotion, and intervention. Being either overweight or underweight prior to pregnancy increases risk of complications.

■ Folic acid supplementation before pregnancy has been shown to reduce the risk of neural tube defects such as spina bifida.

■ Excessive intake of some vitamins (vitamin A, in particular) and use of tobacco, alcohol, and drugs increase the risk of poor pregnancy outcomes; women should discontinue these practices before they become pregnant.

■ Gestation can be divided into three stages: blastogenic, embryonic, and fetal. In the blastogenic stage, the fertilized ovum begins rapid cell division and implants itself in the uterine wall. During the embryonic stage, organ systems and other body structures form. During the fetal stage, the longest period of gestation, the fetus grows in size and changes in proportions.

■ Women who enter pregnancy at a normal BMI should gain 25 to 35 pounds during pregnancy. Underweight women should gain more weight and overweight women less. Energy needs increase by 340 to 450 kilocalories per day for the second and third trimesters.

■ By using the USDA's Daily Food Plans for Moms to plan food intake, pregnant women who consume enough energy should be able to meet all their nutrient needs with the exception of iron and folate. They should get needed extra calories mainly from grains, fruits, and vegetables.

■ Limiting caffeine intake during pregnancy is recommended. Smoking during pregnancy increases the risk of preterm delivery and low birth weight. Alcohol and drug use can interfere with normal fetal development and should be avoided during pregnancy.

■ Gastrointestinal distress such as morning sickness, heartburn, and constipation are common during pregnancy and result from the action of various hormones on the GI tract. Although most food cravings or aversions present no problems, excessive consumption of nonfood items, known as pica, interferes with adequate nutrition.

■ During pregnancy, hormones control the development of breast tissue in preparation for milk production. Colostrum, the first milk, which is rich in protein and antibodies, is produced soon after delivery. By two to three weeks after delivery, lactation is well established, and mature milk is being produced.

■ The pituitary hormone prolactin stimulates milk production. Oxytocin, another pituitary hormone, stimulates milk release, which is known as the let-down reflex.

■ Unless they reduce their physical activity, breastfeeding women need 330 to 400 more kilocalories per day than they did when they were not pregnant. By obtaining adequate energy and using the USDA's Daily Food Plan for Moms to balance choices, most lactating women can obtain all the nutrients they need from their diet. Cigarettes, alcohol, and illicit drugs should not be used while breastfeeding.

■ Mothers benefit from breastfeeding through enhanced physiologic recovery, convenience, and emotional bonding. Contraindications to breastfeeding include infection with HIV or active tuberculosis and regular use of certain medications.

■ Infants receive optimal nutrition from human milk. Breastfeeding can reduce the incidence of infectious diseases, allergies, and other problems during infancy.

■ La Leche League, the March of Dimes, and the WIC program for low-income women are among the numerous resources for support and education of pregnant and breastfeeding women.

■ Infancy is the fastest growth stage in the life cycle; infants double their birth weight in 4 to 6 months and triple it by 1 year of age. The nutritional status of infants is assessed primarily through measurements of growth.

■ Infants' energy needs must be met through a high-fat diet, which provides the maximum calories in minimal volume. Infants' protein and fluid needs are also high.

■ Human milk is low in vitamin D; breastfed babies need regular sun exposure or supplemental vitamin D. For breastfed infants, iron-fortified foods need to be introduced by 6 months of age. Formula-fed infants should be given iron-fortified formula.

■ Infant formulas usually are based on either cow's milk or soy protein. Unmodified cow's milk is inappropriate for infants throughout the first year of life.

■ The FDA regulates the vitamin and mineral composition of infant formulas to ensure adequate infant nutrition. Formula is available in ready-to-feed, liquid concentrate, and powdered forms.

■ A nurturing environment is important to the feeding of infants, no matter what the milk source.

■ Solid foods are introduced to the infant one at a time, usually beginning with iron-fortified infant cereal. Potential allergens, such as cow's milk, egg whites, and wheat, should be delayed until the baby is at least 12 months old. Developmental markers, such as head and body control and the absence of the extrusion reflex, show readiness for solid foods.

■ Colic, although troublesome to infant and caregiver, is not usually caused by diet. Iron-deficiency anemia is common in infants who lack iron-rich foods. Infants are susceptible to dehydration, especially when diarrhea is prolonged. Failure to thrive describes an infant who is not growing well; intervention may be required to correct feeding practices of caregivers.

## Study Questions

1. Describe the three stages of fetal growth.
2. What are some of the physiological changes that occur in a woman during pregnancy?
3. How do the recommended intake values for calories, protein, folate, and iron change for pregnancy?
4. What contributes to morning sickness, and how can a woman minimize its effects?
5. What are some of the benefits of breastfeeding for the infant? For the mother?
6. Is it okay for an infant to experience weight loss immediately after birth? If an infant does lose weight, does it mean he or she is at nutritional risk?

7. How much water does a breastfed or formula-fed infant need each day?
8. Is it necessary to give breastfed infants supplements of vitamins and/or minerals? If so, which ones?
9. Describe the process for introducing solid foods into an infant's diet.
10. List the feeding problems that may occur during infancy.

## Try This

### For Just One Week, Can You Eat Like You're Expecting?

The purpose of this exercise is to see if you can follow the nutrition guidelines for pregnancy for just one week. Keep in mind that pregnant women attempt to do this for 38 to 40 weeks! Your goal is to reduce or eliminate caffeine, alcohol, and over-the-counter medications. Make an effort to eat according to MyPlate each day, selecting the most nutrient-dense choices from each group. You should also take a basic multivitamin/mineral tablet (in place of a woman's prenatal supplement) daily. This will ensure that you consume the amounts of protein, vitamins, and minerals recommended for pregnancy.

### Costs of Infant Formula

The purpose of this exercise is to find out how much it might cost to feed an infant. An average 3-month-old baby weighs about 13 pounds (6 kilograms) and would need about 650 kilocalories per day. Using standard infant formula, this baby would need about 32 ounces of formula each day. Now, go to a grocery store and find the infant formulas. If you were to purchase ready-to-feed formula, how much would it cost to feed this baby for one day? What if you were to use concentrated liquid formula? Powdered formula?

## What About Bobbie?

Let's pretend Bobbie is pregnant and in her second trimester. She wants to know whether she's meeting her basic nutrient needs by following her usual diet. Let's examine her day of eating (see the "Food Choices: Nutrients and Nourishment" chapter). How do you think she's doing? Let's compare Bobbie's intake of nutrients to the recommendations for pregnant women.

### Protein

You may recall that Bobbie's diet is quite high in protein. Her intake was 96 grams, and her nonpregnancy RDA (based on her weight) was 56 grams. During pregnancy, however, Bobbie needs extra protein to ensure her body can handle the demands of tissue growth. An extra 25 grams per day (for a total of 81 grams) is adequate to meet the needs of pregnancy. Bobbie's intake is higher than this and could be reduced.

## Folate

Bobbie's intake of folate was 650 micrograms, which is consistent with her pregnancy RDA of 600 micrograms. Her intake is mainly from enriched grains. By adding other folate-rich foods to her diet, such as spinach, legumes, and orange juice, she would obtain other vital nutrients. If Bobbie is adhering to proper prenatal care, then she is consuming a prenatal supplement with folic acid as well.

## Iron

Bobbie's intake of iron for one day was 20 milligrams. This is substantially lower than her pregnancy RDA of 27 milligrams. This places Bobbie at greater risk for iron-deficiency anemia, a common condition in pregnancy. In addition to taking a prenatal supplement that contains iron, Bobbie is advised to continue choosing iron-rich lean red meats, such as beef meatballs, for dinner. She also would benefit from adding more dark-green leafy vegetables to her diet, along with a squeeze of lemon (or other source of vitamin C) to increase the absorption of the non-heme iron. With these additions to her diet, Bobbie will lower her chances of having iron-deficiency anemia during her pregnancy.

# References

1   Centers for Disease Control and Prevention. Recommendations to improve preconception health and health care—United States. *MMWR*. 2006;55(RR-06):1–23.

2   Salihu HM, Mbah AK, Alio AP, et al. Low pre-pregnancy body mass index and risk of medically indicated versus spontaneous preterm singleton birth. *Eur J Obstet Gynecol Reprod Biol*. 2009;144(2):119–123.

3   Rasmussen KM, Yaktine AL, eds. *Weight Gain During Pregnancy: Reexamining the Guidelines*. Washington, DC: National Academies Press; 2009.

4   Ibid.

5   Ibid.

6   Centers for Disease Control and Prevention. Folic acid: what you should know. Updated 3/10/11. http://www.cdc.gov/ncbddd/folicacid/index.html. Accessed 8/2/11.

7   US Preventative Services Task Force. Folic Acid to Prevent Neural Tube Defects. 2009. http://www.uspreventiveservicestaskforce.org/uspstf/uspsnrfol.htm. Accessed 8/2/11.

8   Centers for Disease Control and Prevention. 2011. Op. cit.

9   Lum KJ, Sundaram R, Buck Louis GM. Women's lifestyle behaviors while trying to become pregnant: evidence supporting preconception guidance. *Am J Obstet Gynecol*. 2011;205(3):203.e1–203.e7.

10  Rasmussen KM, Yaktine AL, eds. Op. cit.

11  Ibid.

12  Ibid.

13  Ibid.

14  Institute of Medicine, Food and Nutrition Board. *Dietary Reference Intakes for Energy, Carbohydrate, Fiber, Fat, Fatty Acids, Cholesterol, Protein, and Amino Acids*. Washington, DC: National Academies Press; 2002.

15  Ibid.

16  Academy of Nutrition and Dietetics. Position of the American Dietetic Association: nutrition and lifestyle for a healthy pregnancy outcome. *J Am Diet Assoc*. 2008;108:553–561.

17  US Preventive Services Task Force. Folic acid for the prevention of neural tube defects: US Preventive Services Task Force recommendation statement. *Ann Intern Med*. 2009;150(9):626–631.

18  US Department of Agriculture. Choose MyPlate.gov daily food plans for pregnancy and breastfeeding. Updated 6/4/11. http://www.choosemyplate.gov/mypyramidmoms. Accessed 8/2/11.

19  Institute of Medicine, Food and Nutrition Board. 2002. Op. cit.

20  Academy of Nutrition and Dietetics. Op. cit.

21  US Department of Health and Human Services, US Department of Agriculture. *Dietary Guidelines for Americans, 2010*. 7th ed. Washington, DC: US Government Printing Office; 2010.

22  US Department of Health and Human Services, US Environmental Protection Agency. What you need to know about mercury in fish and shellfish. 3/04. http://www.cfsan.fda.gov/~dms/admehg3.html. Accessed 8/2/11.

23  Higdon JV, Frei B. Coffee and health: a review of recent human research. *Crit Rev Food Sci Nutr*. 2006;46:101–123; and Greenwood DC, Alwan N, Boylan S, et al. Caffeine intake during pregnancy, late miscarriage and stillbirth. *Eur J Epidemiol*. 2010;25(4):275–280.

24  Browne ML, Hoyt AT, Feldkamp ML, et al. Maternal caffeine intake and risk of selected birth defects in the National Birth Defects Prevention Study. *Birth Defects Res A Clin Mol Teratol*. 2011;91(2):93–101.

25  Maslova E, Bhattacharya S, Lin SW, Michels KB. Caffeine consumption during pregnancy and risk of preterm birth: a meta-analysis. *Am J Clin Nutr*. 2010;92(5):1120–1132.

26  Academy of Nutrition and Dietetics. Op. cit.

27  Raatikainen K, Huurinainen P, Heinonen S. Smoking in early gestation or through pregnancy: a decision crucial to pregnancy outcome. *Prev Med*. 2007;44:59–63.

28  March of Dimes. Illicit drug use during pregnancy. 1/08. http://www.marchofdimes.com/professionals/14332_1169.asp. Accessed 8/2/11.

29  Young SL. Pica in pregnancy: new ideas about an old condition. *Annu Rev Nutr*. 2010;21;30:403–422.

30  Turner RE. Nutrition during pregnancy. In: Shils ME, Ross AC, Shike M, et al., eds. *Modern Nutrition in Health and Disease*. 10th ed. Baltimore, MD: Lippincott Williams & Wilkins; 2006; and Rumbold AR, Crowther CA, Haslam RR, et al. Vitamins C and E and the risks of preeclampsia and perinatal complications. *N Engl J Med*. 2006;354(17):1796–1806.

31  Academy of Nutrition and Dietetics. Op. cit.

32  March of Dimes. HIV and AIDS in pregnancy. 5/09. http://www.marchofdimes.com/complications_hiv.html. Accessed 8/2/11.

33  US Department of Health and Human Services, National Institutes of Health, National Institute of Allergy and Infectious Disease. HIV/AIDS. Prevention of mother-to-child transmission. http://www.niaid.nih.gov/topics/HIVAIDS/Research/prevention/Pages/mtct.aspx. Accessed 8/2/11.

34  Centers for Disease Control and Prevention. Teen pregnancy. The importance of prevention. Updated 7/25/11. http://www.cdc.gov/TeenPregnancy/index.htm. Accessed 8/2/11.

35  March of Dimes. Quick references fact sheet: teenage pregnancy. 11/09. http://www.marchofdimes.com/professionals/14332_1159.asp. Accessed 8/1/11.

36  US Department of Health and Human Services. *Healthy People 2020*. Maternal, infant, and child health. http://www.healthypeople.gov/2020/topicsobjectives2020/objectiveslist.aspx?topicid=26/. Accessed 8/2/11.

37  Ibid.

38  US Department of Health and Human Services, Centers for Disease Control and Prevention. Breastfeeding report card—United States, 2011. 8/11. http://www.cdc.gov/breastfeeding/pdf/2011BreastfeedingReportCard.pdf. Accessed 8/2/11.

39  Ibid.

40  Institute of Medicine, Food and Nutrition Board. 2002. Op. cit.

41  US Department of Agriculture. Pregnancy and breastfeeding. Updated 6/4/11. http://www.choosemyplate.gov/mypyramidmoms/breastfeeding_nutrition_needs.html. Accessed 8/2/11.

42  Ibid.

43  National Institutes of Health, Office of Dietary Supplements. Dietary supplement fact sheet. Vitamin $B_{12}$. http://ods.od.nih.gov/factsheets/VitaminB12-HealthProfessional. Accessed 8/2/11.

44  American Academy of Pediatrics policy statement. Breastfeeding and the use of human milk. *Pediatrics*. 2005;115:496–506.

45  Centers for Disease Control and Prevention. Breastfeeding. Tobacco use. Should mothers who smoke breastfeed? Updated 10/20/09. http://www.cdc.gov/breastfeeding/disease/tobacco.htm. Accessed 8/3/11.

46  American Academy of Pediatrics policy statement. Breastfeeding and the use of human milk. Op. cit.

47  Ibid.; and Academy of Nutrition and Dietetics. Position of the American Dietetic Association: promoting and supporting breastfeeding. *J Am Diet Assoc*. 2005;105:810–843.

48  Bartick M, Reinhold A. The burden of suboptimal breastfeeding in the United States: a pediatric cost analysis. *Pediatrics*. 2010;125(5):e1048–e1056.

49  US Department of Health and Human Services. Everyone can help make breastfeeding easier, Surgeon General says in "call to action." Press release. 1/20/11. http://www.hhs.gov/news/press/2011pres/01/20110120a.html. Accessed 8/2/11.

50  National Conference of State Legislatures. Breastfeeding laws. 5/11. http://www.ncsl.org/default.aspx?tabid=14389. Accessed 8/2/11.

51  Academy of Nutrition and Dietetics. Position of the American Dietetic Association: promoting and supporting breastfeeding. Op. cit.; and The Surgeon General's call to action to support breastfeeding. Fact sheet. 1/20/11. http://www.surgeongeneral.gov/topics/breastfeeding/factsheet.html. Accessed 8/3/11.

52  Centers for Disease Control and Prevention. Vital signs. Hospital support for breastfeeding. Preventing obesity begins in hospitals. Updated 8/11. http://www.cdc.gov/vitalsigns/BreastFeeding/?s_cid=vitalsigns_081. Accessed 8/3/11.

53  Ibid.

54  American Academy of Pediatrics policy statement. Breastfeeding and the use of human milk. Op. cit.; and Academy of Nutrition and Dietetics. Position of the American Dietetic Association: promoting and supporting breastfeeding. Op. cit.

55  Kramer MS, Aboud F, Mironova E, et al. Breastfeeding and child cognitive development: new evidence from a large randomized trial. *Arch Gen Psychiatry*. 2008;65(5):578–584.

56  Niers L, Stasse-Wolthuis M, Rombouts FM, Rijkers GT. Nutritional support for the infant's immune system. *Nutr Rev*. 2007;65(8, Pt 1):347–360.

57  Walker A. Breast milk as the gold standard for protective nutrients. *J Pediatr*. 2010;156(2 suppl):S3–S7.

58  US Department of Agriculture. Pregnancy and breastfeeding. Weight loss during breastfeeding. http://www.choosemyplate.gov/mypyramidmoms/breastfeeding_weight_loss.html. Accessed 8/3/11.

59  American Academy of Pediatrics. Breastfeeding and the use of human milk. Op. cit.

60  Academy of Nutrition and Dietetics. Position of the American Dietetic Association: promoting and supporting breastfeeding. Op. cit.

61  National Conference of State Legislatures. Op. cit.

62  Ibid.

63  Centers for Disease Control and Prevention. 2008 Pediatric Nutrition Surveillance: national summary of trends in breastfeeding children aged < 5 years. http://www.cdc.gov/pednss/pednss_tables/pdf/national_table13.pdf. Accessed 8/3/11.

64  Riordan J, Wambach K. *Breastfeeding and Human Lactation*. 4th ed. Burlington, MA: Jones & Bartlett Learning; 2010.

65  Jacknowitz A, Novello D, Tiehen L. Special Supplemental Nutrition Program for Women, Infants, and Children and infant feeding practices. *Pediatrics*. 2007;119:281–289.

66  Metallinos-Katsaras E, Gorman KS, Wilde P, Kallio J. A longitudinal study of WIC participation on household food insecurity. *Matern Child Health J*. 2011;15(5):627–633.

67  Institute of Medicine, Food and Nutrition Board. 2002. Op. cit.

68  Ibid.

69  Ibid.

70  Ibid.

71  Institute of Medicine, Food and Nutrition Board. *Dietary Reference Intakes for Water, Potassium, Sodium, Chloride, and Sulfate*. Washington, DC: National Academies Press; 2004.

72  American Academy of Pediatrics policy statement. Breastfeeding and the use of human milk. Op. cit.

73  Wagner CL, Greer FR. Section on Breastfeeding and Committee on Nutrition. Prevention of rickets and vitamin D deficiency in infants, children, and adolescents. *Pediatrics*. 2008;122(5):1142–1152.

74  Institute of Medicine, Food and Nutrition Board. *Dietary Reference Intakes for Calcium and Vitamin D*. Washington, DC: National Academies Press; 2011.

75  Wagner, CL, Greer FR. Op. cit.

76  Kleinman RE, ed. *Pediatric Nutrition Handbook*. 6th ed. Elk Grove Village, IL: American Academy of Pediatrics; 2008.

77  American Dental Association. Fluoride supplements. Fluoride supplement dosage schedule—2011. http://www.ada.org/3088.aspx#dosschedule. Accessed 8/3/11.

78  Vernacchio L, Kelly JP, Kaufman DW, Mitchell AA. Vitamin, fluoride, and iron use among US children younger than 12 years of age: results from the Slone Survey, 1998–2007. *J Am Diet Assoc*. 2011;111:285–289.

79  Ibid.

80  American Academy of Pediatrics policy statement. Breastfeeding and the use of human milk. Op. cit.

81  Kleinman RE, ed. Op. cit.

82  Simmer K, Patole SK, Rao SC. Long-chain polyunsaturated fatty acid supplementation in infants born at term. *Cochrane Database Syst Rev*. 2008;1:CD000376.

83  American Academy of Pediatrics. Healthy children ages and stages. Switching to solid foods. Updated 1/7/11. http://www.healthychildren.org/english/ages-stages/baby/feeding-nutrition/pages/Switching-To-Solid-Foods.aspx. Accessed 8/3/11.

84  Pac S, McMahon K, Ripple M, et al. Development of the *Start Healthy Feeding Guidelines* for infants and toddlers. *J Am Diet Assoc*. 2004;104:455–467.

85  Butte N, Cobb K, Dwyer J, et al. The *Start Healthy Feeding Guidelines* for infants and toddlers. *J Am Diet Assoc*. 2004;104:442–454.

86  Goldfarb MF. Relation of time of introduction of cow milk protein to an infant and risk of type-1 diabetes mellitus. *J Proteome Res*. 2008;7:2165–2167.

87  Academy of Nutrition and Dietetics. Position of the American Dietetic Association: benchmarks for nutrition in child care. *J Am Diet Assoc*. 2011;111:607–615.

88  USDA Food and Nutrition Service. Special Supplemental Program for Women Infants and Children (WIC). Infant nutrition and feeding. Updated 3/09. http://www.nal.usda.gov/wicworks/Topics/FG/CompleteIFG.pdf. Accessed 8/3/11.

89  American Academy of Pediatric Dentistry. Policy on early childhood caries (ECC): unique challenges and treatment options. Revised 2008. http://www.aapd.org/media/Policies_Guidelines/P_ECCUniqueChallenges.pdf. Accessed 8/3/11.

90  National Maternal and Child Oral Health Resource Center. Promoting awareness, preventing pain: facts on early childhood caries (ECC). 2004. http://www.mchoralhealth.org/PDFs/ECCFactSheet.pdf. Accessed 8/3/11.

91  Jacknowitz A, Novello D, Tiehen L. Op. cit.

# CHAPTER 13

# Life Cycle: From Childhood Through Adulthood

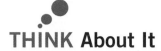

**THINK About It**

1   Were you a "picky" eater as a child? What about now?

2   What's your experience with acne and eating particular foods?

3   What behavior changes would you consider making now that would help you live longer?

4   Your grandfather lives by himself and relies on frozen foods for his nutritional needs. How do you feel about this strategy?

**Visit go.jblearning.com/ inseldisco4e**

**childhood** The period of life from age 1 to the onset of puberty.

**adolescence** The period between onset of puberty and adulthood.

It's the year 2050. Who are you? Where do you live? What is your life like? How healthy are you? If projections made earlier in the century were accurate, you are part of the largest segment of the population— in 2050 between one-third and one-fourth of Americans are older than 65. Perhaps you have retired recently, or maybe you continue to work in your profession. Think about how technology has changed in your lifetime; new methods of communication have developed that make e-mail and the Internet old-fashioned, so late twentieth century!

Consider how much you have changed over the years. Throughout childhood and adolescence you were growing, sometimes quite rapidly! Whether you fueled that growth with burgers and fries, black beans and rice, chips and soft drinks, or yogurt and salads will have determined a lot about your health status in 2050. Did you continue the eating habits you had in college, and did these allow you to control your weight, blood cholesterol, and blood pressure? Or, perhaps in the year 2050 these conditions are no longer of concern. Advances in genetics may have allowed gene therapy to replace diet therapy and medications for chronic diseases.

Now we will look at how continued growth in childhood and adolescence affects nutritional needs. In addition, we'll see how nutritional needs change as we age, and we'll consider feeding practices, meal planning, and obstacles to healthful eating for each age group.

## Childhood

**Childhood** refers to a period of life occurring from age 1 through the beginning of **adolescence**. Growth in childhood, although continuous, occurs at a significantly slower rate than in infancy. During the childhood years, a typical child will gain about 5 pounds and grow 2 to 3 inches each year. Children can be categorized in three groups based on their age and development: toddlers (ages 1–3), preschoolers (ages 4–5), and school-aged children (ages 6–10).

### Energy and Nutrient Needs During Childhood

An average 1-year-old requires about 850 to 1,000 kilocalories per day.[1] This daily energy requirement gradually increases until it almost doubles by around age 10.

#### Energy and Protein

Estimated Energy Requirements (EER) for children can be calculated based on sex, age, height, weight, and activity level (see Table 13.1). In contrast to the 175 kilocalories per day needed during early infancy, the added energy cost for growth during childhood is only 20 kilocalories per day.

Although total energy requirements increase, the kilocalories needed per kilogram of body weight slowly decrease as children move through childhood. The same is true for protein requirements (see Table 13.2).

#### Vitamins and Minerals

As long as a healthy child cooperates by eating a variety of healthful foods, a well-planned diet should provide most nutrients a child needs. One exception is iron. Children aged 4 to 8 years require 10 milligrams of iron per day but may not get that amount without careful meal planning. High consumption of milk, a poor source of iron, can displace iron-rich foods, contributing to inadequate iron intake, thus milk intake during childhood should be limited to 3 to 4 cups per day. This allows room in the diet for high-iron food sources such as lean meats, legumes, fish, poultry, and iron-enriched breads and cereals. (See Table 13.3.) Iron deficiency not only affects growth but

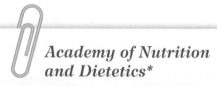

*Academy of Nutrition and Dietetics\**

**Dietary Guidance for Healthy Children Aged 2 to 11 Years**

It is the position of the American Dietetic Association that children ages 2 to 11 years should achieve optimal physical and cognitive development, attain a healthy weight, enjoy food, and reduce the risk of chronic disease through appropriate eating habits and participation in regular physical activity.

**Source:** Reproduced from Nicklas T, Hayes D. Position of the Academy of Nutrition and Dietetics: nutrition guidance for healthy children aged 2 to 11 years. *J Am Diet Assoc.* 2008;108(6):1038–1047.

\* Formerly the American Dietetic Association

| Table 13.1 | **Estimated Energy Requirement Equations for Children (Ages 3 Through 8)** |
|---|---|

*Males*
EER = 88.5 − 61.9 × age [y] + PA × (26.7 × weight [kg] + 903 × height [m]) − 20 kcal/day
Physical activity (PA)
   Sedentary = 1.00
   Low active = 1.13
   Active = 1.26
   Very active = 1.42
*Females*
EER = 135.3 − 30.8 × age [y] + PA × (10.0 × weight [kg] + 934 × height [m]) + 20 kcal/day
Physical activity (PA):
   Sedentary = 1.00
   Low active = 1.16
   Active = 1.31
   Very active = 1.56

**Source:** Reproduced with permission from *Dietary Reference Intakes for Energy, Carbohydrate, Fiber, Fat, Fatty Acids, Cholesterol, Protein, and Amino Acids (Macronutrients).* Copyright © 2005 by the National Academy of Sciences, courtesy of the National Academies Press, Washington, DC.

| Table 13.2 | **Protein RDAs for Childhood** |
|---|---|

| Age (y) | Protein (g/kg) | Reference Weight[a] (kg) | Protein (g/d) |
|---|---|---|---|
| 1–3 | 1.05 | 12 | 13 |
| 4–8 | 0.95 | 20 | 19 |

[a] Reference weights are based on median weights of children in that age group.

**Source:** Reproduced with permission from *Dietary Reference Intakes for Energy, Carbohydrate, Fiber, Fat, Fatty Acids, Cholesterol, Protein, and Amino Acids (Macronutrients).* Copyright © 2005 by the National Academy of Sciences, courtesy of the National Academies Press, Washington, DC.

| Table 13.3 | **Iron-Rich Foods and Snacks** |
|---|---|

*Iron-Rich Foods*
Ground beef
Poultry
Fish
Legumes
Dark-green vegetables
Enriched breads, cereals, rice, and pasta
*Iron-Rich Snacks*
Cream of Wheat
Cooked macaroni or pasta
Enriched cereals, either dry or with milk
Tortillas filled with refried beans
Dried apricots
Raisins (for older children)
Bean dip
Chili, mildly seasoned
Peanut butter on enriched bread or graham crackers
Sloppy Joe
Casseroles with meat (many children do not like plain meats)

also can impair the child's mood, attention span, focus, and ability to learn.[2] (See **Figure 13.1**.) American children do not consistently meet dietary recommendations for the fruit, grain, and dairy groups, which are important sources of these nutrients.

### Vitamin and Mineral Supplements

Many caregivers would rather give a child a vitamin/mineral pill than plan and prepare the meals necessary to ensure an adequate diet. However, the balanced diet a child needs is not much different from the diet an adult needs. In fact, MyPyramid for Kids (see **Figure 13.2**) shows the same balance of food groups as is recommended for adults. Caregivers who understand this may be less tempted to rely on supplements to achieve a balanced diet.

Some children should receive nutrient supplements. Among them are children whose diets are restricted for medical reasons, those with chronic diseases, those who are malnourished, and those with food allergies that require them to avoid multiple foods or food groups.[3] (For more on food allergies, see the FYI feature "Food Hypersensitivities and Allergies.") Caregivers need to be reminded that vitamin and mineral supplements for children are dangerous in large doses. Vitamin and mineral preparations must be treated

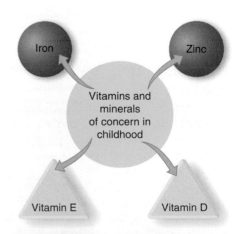

| Figure 13.1 | **Micronutrients of concern in childhood.** Milk is low in iron, |
|---|---|

and young children also may have low intakes of magnesium, potassium, calcium, and vitamin E.

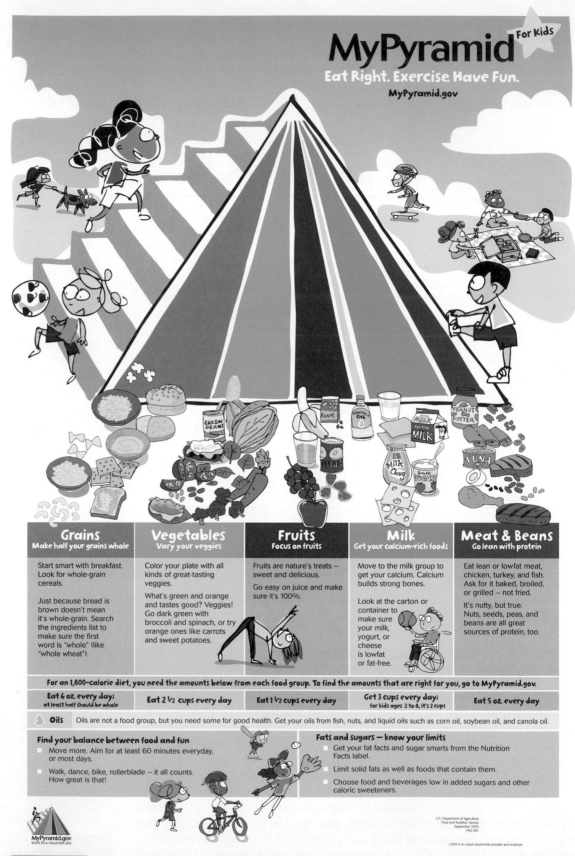

**Figure 13.2** **MyPyramid for kids and MyPyramid for preschoolers.** Children's needs for a variety of foods and regular physical activity are reflected in a Pyramid designed just for them.

**Source:** Courtesy of US Department of Agriculture.

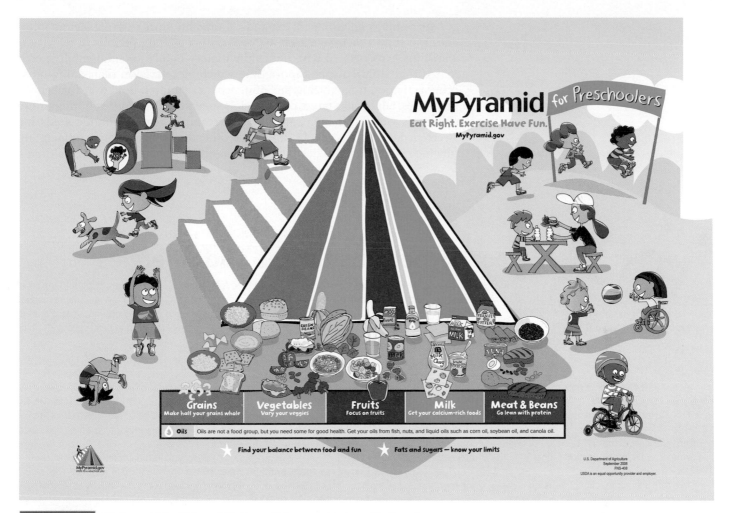

**Figure 13.2** **MyPyramid for kids and MyPyramid for preschoolers.** *(Continued)*

like all medicines and kept safely out of children's reach. Supplements containing iron in doses over 30 milligrams are especially dangerous to children. Accidental consumption of vitamin and mineral or iron supplements should be treated as a poisoning emergency.

## Influences on Childhood Food Habits and Intake

THINK
About It
1

Children develop food preferences at an early age. Toddlers start to exhibit unique feeding practices and styles. For some, this means that one food cannot touch another, or that foods cannot be green, or that all foods must be green. All these "preferences" are merely a toddler's way of exhibiting control over his or her environment while experimenting and exploring. Although it may seem like an eternity to even the most patient caregiver, these food habits are usually temporary. The wise caregiver allows this process to occur naturally rather than wage food battles that ultimately the child wins. Nutrition professionals advocate child-feeding practices where caregivers are responsible for positive structure, age-appropriate support, and healthful food and beverage choices, and children are responsible for whether and how much to eat. This division of responsibility promotes self-regulation of energy intake.[4] More and more children are spending time in organized day care settings. Child-care workers are playing an increasingly important role in the development of children's health and nutritional habits.[5]

*Academy of Nutrition and Dietetics\**

**Benchmarks for Nutrition in Child Care**
It is the position of the American Dietetic Association that child-care programs should achieve recommended benchmarks for meeting children's nutrition needs in a safe, sanitary, and supportive environment that promotes optimal growth and development. Use of child care has become increasingly common and is now the norm for the majority of families in the United States.

**Source:** Reproduced from Benjamin Neelon SE, Briley ME. Position of the Academy of Nutrition and Dietetics: benchmarks for nutrition in child care. *J Am Diet Assoc.* 2011;111:607–615.

\* Formerly the American Dietetic Association

As a child's environment expands, more and more external factors influence the child's diet. Sedentary behavior, such as long periods of television watching, is associated with unhealthy dietary habits in children.[6] It is estimated that children spend more time watching television than doing most other activities. Recognizing the influence that children hold over household purchases, advertisers target commercials specifically at children during prime children's viewing hours. Cartoons, for example, feature countless ads for sweetened cereals, fast foods, candy, and other foods high in sugar or fat, none of which is necessary or desirable. Television advertising influences children's

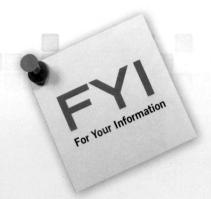

# Food Hypersensitivities and Allergies

Food allergies, or food hypersensitivities, are allergic reactions to food proteins. Allergies are different from food intolerances (such as lactose intolerance) that may involve digestive problems rather than an immune response. Allergies are less likely than intolerances to be transient and tend to have more serious consequences. Proteins that trigger allergies are known as allergens. The most common food allergens are found in milk, eggs, tree nuts, peanuts, soy, wheat, fish, and shellfish.

About 25 percent of people in the general population think they suffer from food allergies. In 2007, 3.9 percent of children younger than 18 years—that's 3 million, or 4 of every 100 children—were reported to have food or digestive allergies, a figure 18 percent higher than in 1997.[1]

In a true allergic reaction, the immune system responds to an allergen with a cascade of chemical reactions that can cause wheezing, difficulty breathing, and hives, as well as a host of other symptoms. (See Table A.) Food allergy symptoms often affect more than one body system and may change in severity from one reaction to the next.

Anaphylaxis, the most severe allergic reaction, usually takes place within the first hour after eating the offending food. Shock and respiratory failure can rapidly ensue. Anaphylaxis can be fatal, so immediate emergency care is essential.

Allergy symptoms that occur immediately after a food is eaten make detective work easier. If symptoms are slow to evolve, a child may suffer chronic diarrhea and even experience failure to thrive before the problem is identified.

When identification of the food culprit isn't so obvious, an elimination diet can shed light. All suspected foods are eliminated from the diet and slowly reintroduced, one by one, on a specific schedule. Both intake and reactions are carefully recorded. Prolonged or improper use of such a diet can have severe nutritional consequences. A registered dietitian can help with diet planning to ensure nutritional adequacy.

The double-blind, placebo-controlled food challenge is the gold standard of food allergy testing. Although definitive, it can be dangerous for people prone to anaphylactic reactions. In this test, under physician supervision, increasing amounts of a suspected food are given to the child, and allergy symptoms and signs are noted. This test must be done by trained personnel with emergency equipment handy.

The treatment for food allergy entails avoiding the offending allergen. Each child with a food allergy needs a nutrition assessment that tracks specific nutrients missing as a result of eliminating the offending foods. For example, if a toddler is avoiding milk and milk products due to a cow's milk allergy, the nutrients most at risk would be protein, vitamin D, and calcium. As a child's diet includes more and more foods, careful label reading is the key to identifying allergen-containing foods. Organizations such as the Food Allergy & Anaphylaxis Network (FAAN) provide materials for deciphering food labels.[2] FAAN also offers tips for successful traveling and dining with a child who has food allergies.

Many children naturally outgrow food allergies by the time they are 3 years old. Once outgrown, the food allergy is unlikely to return.[3]

1   Branum AM, Lukacs SL. *Food allergy among US children: trends in prevalence and hospitalizations.* 10/08. NCHS Data Brief 10. http://www.cdc.gov/nchs/data/databriefs/db10.htm. Accessed 8/8/11.

2   The Food Allergy & Anaphylaxis Network. http://www.foodallergy.org. Accessed 8/8/11.

3   Ibid.

| Table A | Symptoms of Food Allergies |
|---------|----------------------------|

| **Gastrointestinal Tract** | **Respiratory Tract** |
|---|---|
| Itching of the lips, mouth, and throat | Runny or stuffed-up nose, sneezing, and postnasal discharge |
| Swelling of the throat | Recurrent croup |
| Abdominal cramping and distention | Chronic pneumonia |
| Diarrhea | Middle-ear infections |
| Colic | **Systemic** |
| Gastrointestinal bleeding | Anaphylaxis |
| Protein-losing enteropathy | Heart rhythm irregularities |
| **Skin** | Low blood pressure |
| Hives | |
| Swelling | |
| Eczema, contact dermatitis | |

food preferences, purchasing requests, and consumption.[7] Ninety-one percent of food ads during Saturday morning television programming push foods of poor nutritional quality.[8] Children are more likely to eat an unhealthy diet if they watch a lot of television.[9] Studies show an association between young children watching morning television and eating a poor diet, including higher intakes of sugar-sweetened beverages, fast food, red and processed meat, total energy intake, and percent energy intake from *trans* fats and lower intakes of fruit and vegetables, calcium, and dietary fiber.[10]

Social events and parties often promote unhealthful eating habits. No matter what the occasion, the menu for children's parties rarely varies. The staples are pizza, ice cream, soft drinks, and candy. None of these foods alone is a problem, but the fact that these foods are offered at the majority of social gatherings is. Popular snacks and beverages also tend to be too high in sugar and fat. Serving more healthful but still child-friendly snacks, such as those in Table 13.4, breaks this tradition.

**Key Concepts** *Children grow at a slower rate than they did as infants but still gain 2 to 3 inches and about 5 pounds per year. They should be able to obtain adequate energy and nutrients from their meals and snacks. Iron-deficiency anemia is the most common nutritional deficiency among American children. Cow's milk is not an adequate source of iron and should be limited to 3 to 4 cups per day to allow for other, high-iron foods. Outside influences, such as television viewing, affect children's preferences for foods with low nutrient density.*

## Nutritional Concerns of Childhood

The major challenges to promoting healthful childhood nutrition are combating malnutrition and hunger, chronic disease, overweight and obesity, lead toxicity, and nutrition concerns for vegetarian practices.

### Malnutrition and Hunger in Childhood

Of all issues facing children with respect to growth and nutrition, none is so devastating as hunger and subsequent malnutrition. Throughout the world, 60 percent of deaths of young children can be attributed to undernutrition.[11] Deficiencies in vitamin A, zinc, iron, and protein also result in illness, stunted growth, limited development, and, in the case of vitamin A, possibly permanent blindness.

In the United States, 17 million children live in the more than 4 million households that experience **food insecurity**.[12] In many of these households, young children are protected from substantial reductions in food intake.

The U.S. Department of Agriculture (USDA) has 15 nutrition assistance programs that address hunger, including the **Supplemental Nutrition Assistance Program (SNAP)**—formerly the Food Stamp Program—the **School Breakfast Program**, the **National School Lunch Program**, the **Summer Food Service Program**, and the Special Supplemental Nutrition Program for Women, Infants, and Children (WIC). Federal programs help to create a safety net for these children. (See **Figure 13.3**.)

For many children, the meals provided through the National School Lunch, Breakfast, and Summer Food Service Programs are the major—and, in some cases, only—sources of calories and other nutrients. Those who plan and serve meals have the challenge of balancing popular foods that children will eat with foods that provide good nutrition. To ensure the nutritional needs of the more than 31 million children receiving meals through school lunch programs, the Child Nutrition Reauthorization Healthy Hunger-Free Kids Act of 2010 represents a national effort to provide children with healthier and more nutritious food choices.[13] The main objectives of the Healthy Hunger-

| Table 13.4 | **Healthy Snacks** |
| --- | --- |

Cereal and milk
Yogurt shake: plain yogurt, fresh fruit
Peanut butter on celery
Popcorn sprinkled with Parmesan cheese
Fresh vegetables and a yogurt dip
Bananas with peanut butter
Graham crackers and peanut butter
Sliced apples with cheese
Bagel and melted cheese
Bran muffins
Pumpkin, banana, or zucchini bread
Mini pizza on English muffin
Homemade pita pocket sandwiches
Yogurt with fresh fruit or granola
Vegetable soup
Fresh fruit
Colored peppers and hummus
Cucumbers with plain yogurt
Cheese and whole grain crackers

**food insecurity** People who take in enough calories but have diets of reduced quality that do not meet all daily nutritional requirements.

**Supplementary Nutrition Assistance Program (SNAP)** A USDA program that helps single people and families with little or no income to buy food. Formerly known as the *Food Stamp Program*.

**School Breakfast Program** A USDA program that assists schools in providing a nutritious morning meal to children nationwide.

**National School Lunch Program** A USDA program that provides nutritious lunches and the opportunity to practice skills learned in classroom nutrition education; enacted in 1946 to provide U.S. children with at least one healthful meal every school day.

**Summer Food Service Program** A USDA program that helps children in lower-income families to continue receiving nutritious meals during long school vacations when they do not have access to school lunch or breakfast.

## Quick Bite

| Figure 13.3 | **Federal safety net for children.** Because of nutritive |

needs during critical growth stages, children are more vulnerable than adults to the effects of malnutrition. For many children, these federal programs provide the major—and, in some cases, the only—sources of calories and other nutrients.

**hyperactivity** A maladaptive and abnormal increase in activity that is inconsistent with developmental levels. Includes frequent fidgeting, inappropriate running, excessive talking, and difficulty in engaging in quiet activities.

## Quick Bite

Free Kids Act focus on improving nutrition and reducing childhood obesity, increasing access to school meal programs, and improving the monitoring and the integrity of school meal programs.[14]

### Food and Behavior

The term **hyperactivity** usually is defined as an abnormal increase in activity that is maladaptive and inconsistent with developmental level. However, common usage has blurred its meaning. Parents often use this term to describe what they view as unruly behavior in children, particularly in classroom settings or structured home settings such as meal time. In social settings, children typically react to situations surrounding parties (where high-sugar foods are often served) in excitable ways. This is not proof of a cause-and-effect relationship between those foods and those behaviors.

Attention-deficit hyperactivity disorder (ADHD) is characterized by inattentive, hyperactive, and impulsive behavior that is unrestrained and frenetic. ADHD is estimated to affect 5 percent of children worldwide.[15] Genetic and environmental factors are both involved in the etiology of ADHD. Sugar and certain food additives, including preservatives and colorings, have all been thought to cause or exacerbate behavioral disorders. Many parents and caregivers often blame sugar for "hyper" behavior in children. However, this association has not been clearly demonstrated.[16] Although the cause remains controversial, studies do suggest that certain food colorings and additives may enhance hyperactive behaviors in some children; further research is needed.[17] For some children, ADHD can be triggered by various foods, and a diet that eliminates these foods can produce a favorable response in sensitive children.[18]

Caffeine products can make children jittery and interfere with their sleep. Because children have small body sizes, the effects of a caffeinated beverage are intensified. Many soft drinks are high in caffeine; examples include Mountain Dew (55 milligrams per 12-ounce can), Surge (51 milligrams per 12-ounce can), and Coca-Cola (37 milligrams per 12-ounce can). Popular energy drinks also can be substantial sources of caffeine.

### Childhood Overweight

In the United States, overweight in childhood is increasing at an alarming rate. (See the FYI feature "Childhood and Teenage Obesity: 'The First Generation That Does Not Outlive Their Parents.'") Approximately 32 percent of children ages 2 to 19 years are overweight (BMI from the 85th to 94th percentile) or obese (BMI greater than the 95th percentile).[19] An overweight child is likely to reach maturity earlier than a child of normal weight but perhaps at the expense of height. Some overweight children already deal with the cardiovascular consequences of obesity, such as lipid abnormalities and hypertension, and many overweight children develop type 2 diabetes prior to the teen years. Finally, overweight children are more likely to have social and academic difficulties[20] and experience the psychological trauma associated with obesity in our culture. Factors involved in the development of overweight in childhood include genetics, environment, behavior, and activity levels. (See **Figure 13.4**.)

Programs designed to treat childhood obesity generally provide behavior modification, exercise counseling, psychological support or therapy, family counseling, and family meal-planning advice. In some cases the goal is not weight loss but rather to allow the child's height to catch up with his or her weight. Instead of restricting caloric intake or food choices, the usual strategy is to increase activity and improve food choices.

To meet the challenge of childhood obesity and direct children toward healthy, active lifestyles, the White House Task Force on Childhood Obesity launched a comprehensive campaign, called Let's Move![21] (See **Figure 13.5**.) The primary goal of Let's Move! is to end childhood obesity within a generation. Comprehensive strategies of Let's Move! include providing parents with helpful information; creating environments that support healthy choices; providing healthier foods in schools; ensuring that every family has access to healthy, affordable foods; and helping children become more physically active.[22]

### Nutrition and Chronic Disease in Childhood

When is it appropriate to adopt adult dietary guidelines for children? It is well documented that early signs of chronic disease can appear in childhood. Evidence of early plaque development has been seen in the coronary arteries of adolescents and is associated with adult cardiovascular diseases. However, the low-fat, high-fiber diet advocated for adults may jeopardize a very young child's growth. Infants and toddlers younger than 2 years old need fat in their diets for growth, organ protection, and central nervous system development. Dietary restrictions at this age are not appropriate.

For children older than 2 years, however, efforts to lower fat, saturated fat, and cholesterol intake may reduce risks of chronic disease. Dietary choices in line with the *Dietary Guidelines for Americans* are recommended. But it's important that parents and caregivers not misinterpret the recommendations and instead restrict children's energy intake. During the preschool and school years, gradual changes can bring food choices in line with the *Dietary Guidelines for Americans*. Caregivers should offer children healthful choices and, as they grow, educate them about proper adult nutrition.

Because of the rising rates of childhood obesity and incidence of chronic diseases related to weight, the American Academy of Pediatrics (AAP) now recommends screening children who have a positive family history of abnormal blood lipids or premature cardiovascular disease for blood lipid abnormalities.[23] For those children with high levels of LDL cholesterol, lifestyle interventions such as changes in diet and physical activity are recommended. In some circumstances, medication may be warranted.

### Lead Toxicity

Reducing elevated blood levels among children is one of the objectives of Healthy People 2020.[24] During the period from 1999 to 2004, 1.4 percent of children in the United States aged 1 to 5 years had elevated blood lead levels, compared with 8.6 percent of children during the period from 1988 to 1991.[25] Lead toxicity can result in slow growth and iron-deficiency anemia and can damage the brain and central nervous system, leading to a host of learning disabilities and behavior problems. Increased blood lead levels are associated with reduced IQ, even at levels less than the Centers for Disease Control and Prevention/World Health Organization "level of concern" of 10 micrograms per deciliter.[26]

Lead is present in the plumbing of old homes; old paint; house dust in homes with cracked or peeling lead-based paint; and, in some areas, the soil. Children can ingest lead by drinking contaminated water, eating paint chips, or sucking their fingers after playing in or around lead-contaminated house dust or soil. Lead toxicity occurs more frequently in areas of poverty, where lead contamination is more common and where iron-deficiency anemia is present.

Low intakes of iron, calcium, and zinc tend to result in increased lead absorption. Children with an adequate intake of these micronutrients show less incidence of lead toxicity. Therefore, many programs established to reduce the incidence of lead toxicity in children also promote good nutrition, with an emphasis on adequate iron, calcium, and zinc consumption.

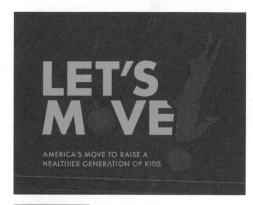

**Figure 13.4** **Factors that contribute to childhood obesity.** Childhood obesity is on the rise, and it predisposes children to health problems when they become adults.

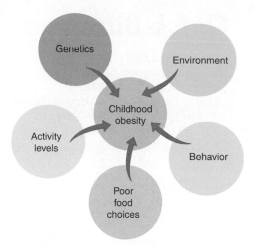

**Figure 13.5** **Let's Move!** **Source:** Courtesy of Let's Move!

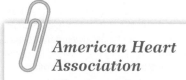

### *American Heart Association*

**Overweight in Children**

Overweight children are more likely to become overweight adults. Successfully preventing or treating overweight in childhood may reduce the risk of adult overweight. This may help reduce the risk of heart disease and other diseases.

**Source:** American Heart Association, Inc.

## Quick Bite

**Tragedy in Lead**
About 5 percent of American children demonstrate signs of lead toxicity, defined as a blood level of 10 micrograms of lead per deciliter. When children are exposed to lead on a continuous or regular basis, brain function is negatively affected.

## Vegetarianism in Childhood

Well-planned lacto-vegetarian, lacto-ovo-vegetarian, and vegan diets satisfy the nutrient needs of children.[27] Vegetarian children have lower intakes of total fat, saturated fat, and cholesterol and higher intakes of fruits, vegetables, and fiber. Sources of calcium, iron, zinc, vitamin $B_{12}$, and vitamin D need to be emphasized, especially for children following vegan diets. For a vegan child, legumes and nuts should be substituted for meats, and calcium- and vitamin $B_{12}$–fortified soy milk should be substituted for cow's milk. It is difficult to determine a safe level of sunlight exposure to synthesize vitamin D. Due to

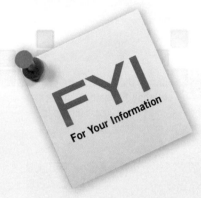

# Childhood and Teenage Obesity: "The First Generation That Does Not Outlive Their Parents"

The most recent data on childhood obesity are frightening. Obesity affects 18 percent of all children and adolescents (ages 2–19 years) in the United States, triple the rate from just about one generation ago.[1] To meet the objective of promoting high-quality and longer lives free of preventable disease, disability, injury, and premature death, the Healthy People 2020 agenda calls for a 10 percent reduction in the percentage of children and adolescents considered obese in the United States.[2]

Compared to their normal-weight counterparts, obese children and adolescents are more likely to have risk factors associated with cardiovascular disease (CVD), such as high blood pressure, high cholesterol, and dyslipidemia. Seventy percent of obese children have at least one CVD risk factor, and 39 percent have two or more risk factors.[3] Other health problems connected to overweight and obesity in children and adolescents include sleep apnea, asthma, liver damage, type 2 diabetes, and an increased risk for becoming obese in adulthood, thus compounding the risk for health problems through adulthood. In addition to the burden of physical health problems, overweight/obese children and adolescents are also likely to be plagued with teasing, harassment, and decreased self-esteem.

### What's Causing the Epidemic?

The causes of childhood obesity are numerous and far-reaching but can be narrowed down to a few main contributors:

- *Meals consumed away from home.* What used to be a weekly treat—"eating out"—has become an almost daily occurrence in this country. The number of meals consumed away from home has increased from 16 percent in 1978 to more than 30 percent in recent years. Intake of fruits, vegetables, and whole grains has decreased, whereas the quantity of saturated fat, sodium, and sugar has increased.[4] Americans spend approximately 42 percent of their food budget paying for foods consumed away from

home, which have been found to be less nutritious than foods prepared at home.[5]
- *Physical inactivity.* In 2009, only 18 percent of high school students met the *2008 Physical Activity Guidelines for Americans*, and only 33 percent attended physical education class every day. To make matters worse, physical activity drops as young people age.[6] Children and adolescents spend approximately 7.5 hours per day using entertainment media that promotes a sedentary lifestyle.[7] The *Dietary Guidelines for Americans, 2010* includes physical activity guidelines as part of the guidance provided to promote a healthy lifestyle.
- *"Competitive" foods.* In the United States, more than half of middle and high schools allow the advertisement of less healthy foods and offer access to sugary drinks throughout the day from vending machines, school canteens, fundraising events, and parties.[8] On any given day, 80 percent of all children and adolescents in the United States consume sugary beverages.[9] Although more than 12 million children attend day care on a regular basis, not all states have regulations to ensure healthy eating and physical activity in that setting.
- *Food deserts.* Many rural, unsafe, lower-income, and minority neighborhoods have inadequate access to stores and supermarkets that offer healthy, reasonably priced food items such as fruits and vegetables. Adding to the food problem is the reality

that, in some neighborhoods, children do not have a safe place to play outside. Fifty percent of U.S. children do not have parks, community centers, or sidewalks in their neighborhood.[10]
- *Acceptance of obesity in social circles.* Studies suggest that close friends and associates of obese people are at higher risk of becoming obese themselves. A person's risk of becoming obese increases by 57 percent if he or she has obese friends, 40 percent if he or she has an obese sibling, and 37 percent if he or she has an obese spouse. However, the same is not true amid neighbors in similar geographic areas, which indicates that obesity within a given social circle might influence overweight and obesity environments.[11]

### What Can Be Done?

The approach or solution to the childhood obesity epidemic in this country is not a simple one. This generation has been referred to as "the first generation not expected to outlive their parents."[12] The severity of the problem has increased over the past 30 years. Until now, the focus to reduce childhood overweight and obesity has concentrated mainly on school-age children, with only slight consideration to children under age 5. The Institute of Medicine now recommends that efforts be shifted to preventing childhood obesity before children enter the school system.[13]

During their first years of life, children develop the eating patterns that can influence

the risks associated with direct sunlight exposure, current AAP guidelines advocate decreasing sunlight exposure.[28] The new recommended daily intake of vitamin D is 400 IU/day for all infants, children, and adolescents beginning in the first few days of life. Children who do not get regular sunlight exposure or drink at least 32 ounces of vitamin D–fortified milk each day should take supplemental vitamin D daily.[29]

**Key Concepts** *Hunger and malnutrition affect a significant number of our nation's children. To combat the growing number of hungry children, programs such as the Special Supplemental Nutrition Program for Women, Infants, and Children (WIC), the National*

| Table A | **Health Problems That May Result from Childhood Obesity** |
|---|---|

Heart disease, caused by:
- High cholesterol and/or
- High blood pressure

Type 2 diabetes
Asthma
Sleep apnea
Social discrimination

**Source:** Reproduced from Centers for Disease Control and Prevention. Tips for Parents: Ideas to Help Children Maintain a Healthy Weight. http://www.cdc.gov/healthyweight/children. Accessed 8/8/11.

health and well-being throughout the lifecycle. Childhood obesity predisposes individuals to becoming obese adults and increases the risks for obesity-related diseases and conditions. (See Table A.) Healthcare agencies should encourage pediatricians and other healthcare providers to emphasize to parents and caregivers the risks to their children's health, especially when they notice a trend towards unhealthy weight status.

The complexity of childhood obesity requires states, communities, and parents to work together toward "helping children make the healthy choice the easy choice." The Centers for Disease Control and Prevention (CDC) offers the following recommendations for reducing obesity in children and adolescents:[14]

**States and communities:**
- Assess retail food environment to determine availability and accessibility to healthier foods.
- Develop incentive programs for supermarkets and farmers markets to establish and maintain their businesses in low-income areas and to sell healthier foods.
- Increase the number of programs that provide local fruits and vegetables and increase the number of salad bars in schools.
- Implement regulations/licensing requirements for child-care providers to decrease the availability of less healthy foodstuffs and sugary beverages and to limit screen time in support of daily physical activities.
- Encourage schools to partake in programs such as the USDA's HealthierUS School Challenge (HUSSC), increase free drinking water while limiting the sale of sugary beverages, support breastfeeding programs in schools and workplaces, and promote safe neighborhoods that encourage physical activity that improves access to parks and playgrounds.

**Parents:**
- Implement the American Academy of Pediatrics guideline and limit children's media and screen time to no more than one to two hours per day.
- Monitor the foods provided in schools and child-care setting to ensure healthier foods and beverages are provided and that physical activity is part of the curriculum.
- In the home, provide plenty of fruits and vegetables, limit foods high in fat and sugar (including sugary beverages), and promote physical activities.

1  Ogden C, Carroll M. Prevalence of obesity among children and adolescents: United States, trends 1963–1965 through 2007–2008. Division of Health and Nutrition Examination Surveys. NCHS Health E-Stat. 7/1/10. http://www.cdc.gov/nchs/data/hestat/obesity_child_07_08/obesity_child_07_08.htm. Accessed 11/8/11.

2  *Healthy People 2020.* http://www.healthypeople.gov/2020/about/default.aspx. Accessed 6/11/11.

3  Freedman DS, Mei Z, Srinivasan SR, Berenson GS, Dietz WH. Cardiovascular risk factors and excess adiposity among overweight children and adolescents: the Bogalusa Heart Study. *J Pediatr.* 2007:150(1):12–17.

4  Todd JE, Mancino L, Lin BH. The impact of food away from home on adult diet quality. US Department of Agriculture, Economic Research Center; 2010. http://www.ers.usda.gov/publications/err90/err90_reportsummary.pdf. Accessed 6/19/11.

5  Ibid.

6  Centers for Disease Control and Prevention. Healthy you. Physical activity. Updated 5/10. http://www.cdc.gov/healthyyouth/physicalactivity/index.htm. Accessed 6/19/11.

7  Centers for Disease Control and Prevention. Overweight and obesity: a growing problem. Updated 4/21/11. http://www.cdc.gov/obesity/childhood/problem.html. Accessed 11/28/11.

8  Ibid.

9  Ibid.

10  Ibid.

11  Christakis NA, Fowler JH. The spread of obesity in a large social network over 32 years. *N Engl J Med.* 2007;357:370–379.

12  Bost EM. Testimony of Eric M. Bost, Under Secretary, Food, Nutrition, and Consumer Services, Before the House Committee on Government Reform Subcommittee on Human Rights and Wellness. US Department of Agriculture. 9/24/04. http://www.fns.usda.gov/cga/speeches/ct091504.html. Accessed 6/26/11.

13  Birch LL, Parker L, Burns A. *Early Childhood Obesity Prevention Policies.* Washington, DC: National Academies Press; 2011.

14  Centers for Disease Control and Prevention. Overweight and obesity: strategies and solutions. 4/21/11. http://www.cdc.gov/obesity/childhood/solutions.html. Accessed 6/26/11.

**puberty** The period of life during which the secondary sex characteristics develop and the ability to reproduce is attained.

**menarche** First menstrual period.

**epiphyses** The heads of the long bones that are separated from the shaft of the bone until the bone stops growing.

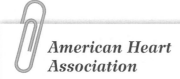

*American Heart Association*

**Fiber and Children's Diets**

Children older than 2 years should gradually adopt American Heart Association dietary recommendations. That means saturated fat intake should be less than 7 percent of total calories, *trans* fat intake should be less than 1 percent of total calories, and dietary cholesterol should be limited to no more than 300 milligrams daily. Children also should get the majority of calories from complex carbohydrates high in fiber.

Both children and adults should consume 14 grams of fiber per 1,000 calories consumed. Read the Nutrition Facts panel on the food label to determine how much fiber is in the food you are choosing.

**Source:** Reproduced with permission, www.heart.org, © 2011 American Heart Association, Inc.

*School Lunch Program, and the School Breakfast Program are vital. Other concerns common to childhood include overweight, lead toxicity, and chronic disease prevention. Infants and toddlers should not be given low-fat, high-fiber diets; when children reach the age of 3, caregivers should begin to adjust children's diets to follow appropriate dietary guidelines. For vegetarian children, dietary sources of calcium, iron, zinc, vitamin D, and vitamin B$_{12}$ require special attention.*

# Adolescence

Adolescents seem to add inches overnight. Many caregivers complain that they cannot keep enough food in the house to satisfy an adolescent's appetite! Adolescence is commonly defined as the time between the onset of **puberty** and adulthood. This maturation process involves both physical growth and emotional maturation.

## Physical Growth and Development

Hormones drive growth, which varies from child to child. In general, growth spurts begin between ages 10 and 12 for girls and between ages 12 and 14 for boys.[30] This spurt, or period of maximal growth, lasts about two years.

### Height

The first phase of adolescent physical growth is linear. On average, boys grow 8 inches and girls grow 6 inches during puberty. This growth is uneven. The hands and feet enlarge first. The calves and forearms lengthen next, followed by expansion of the hips, chest, shoulders, and trunk. As a result, adolescents often appear awkward or clumsy. After the main growth spurt, growth continues for two to three years but at a much slower rate.

For girls, peak growth occurs about one year before **menarche**, the onset of menstruation. A typical girl has achieved about 95 percent of her adult height by menarche and grows only 2 to 4 inches during the remainder of adolescence. Growth rates are closely related to sexual maturation, reflected in breast development (girls), change of voice (boys), development of sexual organs, and growth of pubic hair. When the growth plates at the ends of the long bones (**epiphyses**) close, skeletal growth is complete. This is a critical point in development. An adolescent who is malnourished and of small stature at the point of epiphyseal closure may not achieve his or her full potential height.

### Weight

The second physical growth phase of adolescence involves lateral growth. Here, the adolescent "fills out," or gains weight. External factors such as diet and exercise affect weight gain more than linear growth, so weight gain can vary widely among adolescents. However, a typical healthy girl will gain 35 pounds during adolescence; a typical boy will gain 45 pounds. In our weight-sensitive society, adolescents should be prepared for this normal, expected weight gain. Although the bulk of an adolescent's lateral growth occurs after the linear growth spurt, a significant portion of the two growth stages overlaps. For girls, for example, peak weight gain usually occurs around the time of menarche.

### Body Composition

Before puberty, the body compositions of boys and girls do not differ greatly. However, during adolescence, the changes are dramatic. Boys experience greater increases in lean body mass, resulting in more obvious muscle definition. Girls accumulate greater stores of body fat, specifically around the hips and buttocks, upper arms, breasts, and upper back.

### Emotional Maturity: Developmental Tasks

Adolescence is a time not only of great physical growth but also of tremendous emotional growth. This psychological development affects food choices, eating habits, and body image. Many teens become more interested in the healthful aspects of nutrition. Others experiment with unhealthful food choices as an exercise in independence or in an attempt to achieve an idealized body.

## Nutrient Needs of Adolescents

Although growth, not age, should be the ultimate indicator of nutrient needs, Daily Reference Intakes (DRIs) are established based on age. Separate recommendations for males and females reflect their differences in growth rates and body composition seen during adolescence.

### Energy and Protein

Energy needs, as total kilocalories per day, are greater during adolescence than at any other time of life, with the exception of pregnancy and lactation. Equations used to calculate Estimated Energy Requirements (EER) are the same as for children, except for the added energy factor for growth, which is higher for adolescents. (See Table 13.5.) Recommended energy intakes are guidelines only; adjustments often are needed to meet individual requirements.

To support growth, an adolescent's protein needs per unit body weight are higher than an adult's but less than a rapidly growing infant's. (See Table 13.6.) By age 14 to 18, the protein RDA has declined nearly to adult levels (as grams per kilogram body weight), reflecting the end of linear growth for most teens. American teens rarely have a problem getting adequate protein, but teen girls risk a lack of protein if they cut calories too drastically in attempts to control weight.

### Vitamins and Minerals

Along with increased needs for energy and protein, adolescents have higher vitamin and mineral needs compared with people at most other life stages. Three nutrients of particular concern for adolescents are vitamin A, calcium, and iron, each of which plays an important role in growth. (See **Figure 13.6**.)

Teens can improve their vitamin A intake by including more fruits and vegetables in their diets. If diets are deficient in vitamin A, then adequate calcium, which is essential for bone formation and maximal bone density, can be harder to obtain. Many teens, especially girls, actually reduce their calcium intake by replacing calcium-rich milk in their diets with soft drinks. During puberty, adolescents normally gain 15 percent of their full adult height and accumulate half their ultimate adult bone mass. Adolescents who do not

---

**Table 13.5** **Estimated Energy Requirement Equations for Adolescence (Ages 9 Through 18)**

*Males*
EER = 88.5 − 61.9 × age [y] + PA × (26.7 3 weight [kg] + 903 × height [m]) + 25 kcal/day
Physical activity (PA):
    Sedentary = 1.00
    Low active = 1.13
    Active = 1.26
    Very active = 1.42

*Females*
EER = 135.3 − 30.8 × age [y] + PA × (10.0 × weight [kg] + 934 × height [m]) + 25 kcal/day
Physical activity (PA):
    Sedentary = 1.0
    Low active = 1.16
    Active = 1.31
    Very active = 1.56

**Source:** Reproduced with permission from *Dietary Reference Intakes for Energy, Carbohydrate, Fiber, Fat, Fatty Acids, Cholesterol, Protein, and Amino Acids (Macronutrients).* Copyright © 2005 by the National Academy of Sciences, courtesy of the National Academies Press, Washington, DC.

---

**Table 13.6** **Protein RDAs for Adolescence**

| Age (y) | Protein (g/kg) | Reference Weight[a] (kg) | Protein (g/d) |
|---|---|---|---|
| 9–13, female and male | 0.95 | 36 | 34 |
| 14–18, female | 0.85 | 54 | 46 |
| 14–18, male | 0.85 | 61 | 52 |

[a] Reference weights are based on median weights for that sex and age group.

**Source:** Reproduced with permission from *Dietary Reference Intakes for Energy, Carbohydrate, Fiber, Fat, Fatty Acids, Cholesterol, Protein, and Amino Acids (Macronutrients).* Copyright © 2005 by the National Academy of Sciences, courtesy of the National Academies Press, Washington, DC.

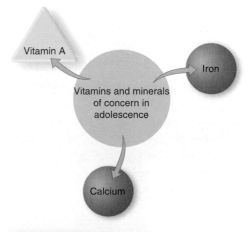

**Figure 13.6** **Micronutrients of concern in adolescence.** In human nutrition, vitamin A is important for growth, and calcium is essential for building strong bones. Teen girls especially need adequate iron intake to replace iron lost due to menstruation.

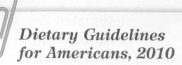

## Dietary Guidelines for Americans, 2010

**Key Recommendations**

- Prevent and/or reduce overweight and obesity through improved eating and physical activity behaviors.
- Control total calorie intake to manage body weight. For people who are overweight or obese, this will mean consuming fewer calories from foods and beverages.
- Increase physical activity and reduce time spent in sedentary behaviors.
- Maintain appropriate calorie balance during each stage of life—childhood, adolescence, adulthood, pregnancy and breastfeeding, and older age.

## *Quick* Bite

**Body Fat**
By adulthood, a typical woman's body composition is 23 percent fat. A typical man, in contrast, has 12 percent body fat.

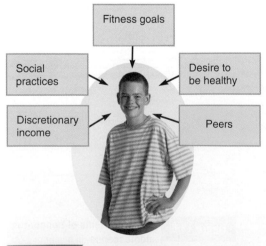

**Figure 13.7** **Factors that influence adolescent food choices.** Social, cultural, and psychological factors, especially peer pressure, strongly influence adolescent food choices.

achieve sufficient bone density have a greater risk of developing osteoporosis later in life. The RDA for calcium for adolescents, ages 9 to 18 years, is 1,300 milligrams a day, and the RDA for vitamin D is 600 IU a day.[31] Dairy products are rich in calcium (about 300 milligrams per cup of milk or yogurt) and vitamin D and convenient to eat; without these or calcium-fortified products, it is difficult to achieve the RDA. Adolescent boys need added iron to support growth of muscle and lean body mass.

Teenage girls need added iron to replace blood lost during menstruation. The recommended intake for boys aged 14 to 18 is 11 milligrams per day; for teen girls, it is 15 milligrams per day. As long as they take in enough calories, both groups should be able to obtain this iron from nutrient-dense foods. During adolescence, however, food selection often is less than optimal. Careful meal planning is required to maximize teenagers' iron consumption.

### Influences on Adolescent Food Intake

Teenagers want and need to make their own food choices and purchases and may want to take over their food preparation. Although the parent can set a good example, parental influence is much weaker now. Factors that influence an adolescent's food selection and consumption include the desire to be healthy, fitness goals, amount of discretionary income, social practices, and peers. (See **Figure 13.7**.)

Teens have more access to foods than children do. They also usually have their own money and may have access to independent transportation. Along with this increased freedom comes greater spending power. Teens enjoy spending money on food and making their own selections. The food industry responds accordingly by marketing directly to teens. The message is enjoyment and pleasure, and advertised products may not be nutritionally adequate.

Teens perceive benefits to eating healthful foods, such as enhanced physical and mental performance, increased energy, and psychological well-being. However, teens attending school are faced with more food choices than ever before. In addition to the standard school lunch or breakfast program outlined earlier, most middle schools and high schools have vending machines, snack carts, school stores, or even private vendors supplying foods such as pizza for cafeteria meals. Vending and other food sales can be a major source of revenue for many schools, supporting athletic programs and other after-school activities.

Although healthier choices may be available, the strongest risk factor for buying unhealthful snacks and beverages at school is simply the influential proximity of vending machines in schools.[32] Availability of these unhealthy snacks may affect students' weight through their increased consumption of these products.[33]

More than half of all middle and high schools offer sugary drinks and less healthful foods for their students to purchase.[34] Sugar-sweetened beverages (SSBs) are the largest source of added sugars in the diet of children and adolescents in the United States. The increased caloric intake resulting from SSBs is a leading dietary contributor to the prevalence of obesity among adolescents.[35]

Health professionals and others have expressed concern about the presence of low-nutrient-density "competitive" foods (e.g., snacks and soft drinks sold side by side with school lunches), and many states have pursued legislation to either remove vending machines or change the products available during the school day. The Healthy Hunger-Free Kids Act of 2010 gives the USDA the authority to establish national nutrition standards for all food and beverages sold and served in schools at any time of the school day.[36]

Despite efforts to provide healthier options in schools, vending machines continue to offer foods and beverages that are high in fat, sugar, and calories with minimal nutritional value.[37] The most frequently consumed competitive products are the foods and beverages that are energy dense and low in nutrients; such foods are consumed by over 40 percent of children daily while at school.[38]

Vending machines are widely available in U.S. schools, placing schools in a unique position to influence student diets.[39] Consistent with the *Dietary Guidelines for Americans, 2010* recommendation to reduce intake of calories from solid fats and added sugars, the AAP states that routine ingestion of sports drinks by children and adolescents should be avoided or restricted.[40] To reduce consumption of SSBs, the CDC is encouraging schools to improve access to free drinking water and to implement other strategies to reduce student consumption of SSBs through changes in school policies.[41] Also necessary is the involvement of families, media, and other institutions that interact with adolescents to discourage their consumption of SSBs and to increase their awareness of the potential detrimental health effects of a poor diet.[42]

**Key Concepts** *Humans need more calories and nutrients during adolescence than at any other stage of life, with the exception of pregnancy and lactation. During this stage boys grow about 8 inches, gain about 45 pounds, and increase their lean body mass. Girls grow about 6 inches, gain about 35 pounds, and increase their body fat. As at earlier ages, calcium, iron, and vitamin A often are lacking in adolescent diets. Factors that determine food selection and consumption include the desire to be healthy, fitness goals, amount of discretionary income, social practices, and peers.*

## Nutrition-Related Concerns for Adolescents

Adolescents are often preoccupied with weight, appearance, and eating habits. They need to know whether and how their eating practices can affect body image and development, fitness, acne, and obesity.

### Fitness and Sports

For many adolescents, an interest in fitness becomes the catalyst for learning about nutrition and improving dietary habits. Some teens, unfortunately, become obsessed with their athletic performance, food intake, and body appearance and go to extremes that can jeopardize not only their current athletic performance but also their long-term health.

### Acne

THINK
About It
2

Many teens blame certain foods for their **acne**. Myths surrounding acne and diet abound, but research has not found any correlation between acne and chocolate, greasy foods, soft drinks, nuts, or milk. Nevertheless, the difference in the incidence of acne between Westernized and non-Westernized societies is striking, and researchers are investigating the connections between diet and acne.[43] Specifically, dietary components such as dairy products, high glycemic–index foods, fat intake, and fatty acid composition have recently been investigated with regard to acne.[44] Preliminary research suggests that a low glycemic–load diet may be helpful, but further controlled testing is needed before specific recommendations can be made.[45]

Effective treatments for acne include topical benzoyl peroxide, low-dose oral antibiotics, and two medications derived from vitamin A—Retin-A and Accutane. Although both these medications are derivatives of vitamin A, there is no correlation between dietary vitamin A and acne.

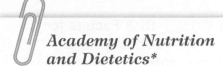

**Academy of Nutrition and Dietetics***

**Child and Adolescent Nutrition Assistance Programs**

It is the position of the American Dietetic Association that children and adolescents should have access to an adequate supply of healthful and safe foods that promote optimal physical, cognitive, and social growth and development. Nutrition assistance programs, such as food assistance and meal service programs and nutrition education initiatives, play a vital role in meeting this critical need.

**Source:** Reproduced from Stang J, Bayerl CT. Position of the Academy of Nutrition and Dietetics: child and adolescent nutrition assistance programs. *J Am Diet Assoc.* 2010;110:791–799.

* Formerly the American Dietetic Association

**acne** An inflammatory skin eruption that usually occurs in or near the sebaceous glands of the face, neck, shoulders, and upper back.

| Table 13.7 | Risk Factors for Obesity in Adolescents |
| --- | --- |

Genetics
Extent and duration of breastfeeding
Early menarche
Participation in high-risk behaviors such as smoking, alcohol use, and sexual experimentation
Family and parental dynamics
Food insecurity
Socioeconomic status
Lack of safe place for physical activity
Inconsistent access to healthful food choices
Low cognitive stimulation at home
Parental food choices
Parental food-related behaviors
Lack of regular family meals
Low level of physical activity—leisure time activities and activities of daily living, school physical activity programs

**Source:** Data from American Academy of Pediatrics. Prevention of pediatric overweight and obesity. *Pediatrics.* 2003;112(2):424–430.

## *Eating Disorders*

Eating disorders frequently begin during adolescence. Adolescents often become preoccupied with their weight, appearance, and eating habits. Although eating disorders are found more often in girls than in boys, they are increasing among males. Thus, eating disorders shouldn't be ignored or dismissed as only a "girl's problem."

## *Adolescent Obesity*

As in childhood, obesity rates in adolescence are climbing. One contributing factor is a decline in physical activity by many teens.[46] Obese adolescents have an increased risk of developing high blood pressure, abnormal glucose tolerance and type 2 diabetes, breathing problems, joint pain, and heart burn.[47] They also suffer psychologically from poor self-esteem, exacerbated by being teased and ostracized by peers, and from longing to be slimmer. In addition, adolescent obesity sets the stage for adult obesity, with all its attendant health consequences.[48] Finally, overweight adolescents, who spend on average 7.5 hours daily watching television or using other forms of entertainment media, could be spending some of that time in physical activity.[49] Nutrition education may positively influence the knowledge, attitudes, and eating behaviors of high school students, leading to a healthier lifestyle and reducing their risk of becoming overweight.[50] Table 13.7 lists the factors that can put an adolescent at risk for obesity.

## *Tobacco, Alcohol, and Recreational Drugs*

Developmentally, adolescence is a period of experimentation, and many adolescents experiment with smoking and/or prescription or illegal drugs. Although survey results from 2010 show a continuing gradual decline in alcohol use and binge drinking among teenagers, its use remains widespread in this group.[51] Marijuana is the most often used illegal drug and—along with tobacco, illicit drugs, and the nonmedical use of prescription medications—continues to be used at high rates.[52] Nearly one-fourth of high school seniors graduate as tobacco smokers, and many young females smoke in an attempt to control appetite and weight. An adolescent who smokes tobacco often has a lower energy intake and subsequently decreased nutrient intake.

Marijuana has the opposite effect on hunger. Many teens who smoke marijuana will experience "the munchies," a desire to snack and munch—usually on snacks high in calories but with low nutrient density. Smoking marijuana carries the same risks as smoking tobacco. In addition, marijuana sometimes is laced with other drugs, including LSD and amphetamines.

Adolescents who drink alcohol are at greater risk of harming themselves or others through violence and accidental injury.[53] In addition, teens who drink are replacing needed nutrients with empty alcohol calories. Finally, alcohol can interfere with the absorption and metabolism of necessary nutrients. Growing adolescents cannot afford to have nutrients replaced or poorly absorbed during growth.

Other drugs, such as cocaine, pose further risks. In using illegal drugs, the adolescent becomes preoccupied with both the acquisition and use of the drug; these activities take priority over food intake or selection. Teens who use drugs are usually underweight and report poor appetites.

**Key Concepts** *Adolescence can be an uncomfortable time for the teen who is concerned with body image, body changes, or athletic activities. Although many teens blame certain foods for their acne, research has not found a definite correlation between acne and diet. Many adolescents are preoccupied with their weight, appearance, and eating habits. Adolescent obesity is on the rise, and eating disorders frequently begin during*

## *Quick* Bite

### The Dangers of Teenage Smoking

The CDC estimates that nearly 4 million adolescents smoke regularly. Each day, about 6,000 young people try a cigarette, and more than 3,000 become regular smokers. The CDC predicts that of all young people currently under the age of 18, more than 5 million will die prematurely of a smoking-related disease. Research shows that the earlier a person begins to smoke, the greater the damage.

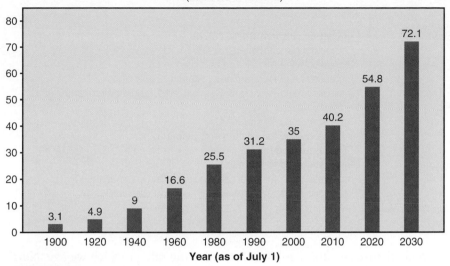

**Number of Persons 65+, 1900–2030**
(numbers in millions)

| Figure 13.8 | **The aging U.S. population.** The number of people over age 65 is growing rapidly. |
|---|---|

**Source:** Administration on Aging. A profile of older Americans: 2010 future growth. Updated 2/25/11. http://www.aoa.gov/aoaroot/aging_statistics/Profile/2010/4.aspx. Accessed 8/8/11.

*adolescence. Use of tobacco, alcohol, or recreational drugs can influence nutrient intake and interfere with good nutrition.*

## Staying Young While Growing Older

Just when does old age begin? The answer is increasingly elusive, as more people remain healthy and active well into their seventies, eighties, and even nineties. Today, older adults represent the fastest-growing segment of the U.S. population: since 1900, the percentage of Americans age 65 and older has more than tripled from 4.1 to 12.9 percent of the population in 2010.[54] (See **Figure 13.8.**) The Baby Boomers started turning 65 in 2011, and experts estimate that by 2030 nearly one in five Americans will be older than age 65. The population aged 85 and older is projected to increase from more than 5.7 million in 2010 to nearly 20 million by 2050.[55]

Age-related changes in body composition, sensory abilities, organ systems, and immune function are normal. (See **Figure 13.9.**) We age at different rates, and many age-related declines will have little impact on our day-to-day lives. Other changes affect our nutrient needs and nutrient status (see Table 13.8), so it becomes especially important to eat nutrient-dense food.

As we get older, many of us fear loss of mental function even more than loss of physical function. Yet, as the years advance, most people maintain cognitive function with only subtle changes. Staying physically and mentally active is a key factor in maintaining function and independence. In most cases, slight changes involving sensory acuity, secondary memory, and information-processing speed do not affect quality of life or lead to progressive or rapid declines in mental function. However, when depression or dementia is suspected, professional evaluation becomes necessary. Overmedication or drug interactions, rather than disease, may be responsible for the changes in behavior.

Although it is not possible to stop the aging process, we can control aspects of our lifestyle that contribute to a healthier old age. Many of our choices—food, exercise, smoking, and alcohol—affect not only our risk for

*Quick* Bite

**Longevity Champions**
In the United States, women live an average of five years longer than men do.

Saliva production
Digestive secretions
Lactase secretions
Gastrointestinal motility
Cardiac output
Blood volume
Kidney function
Liver function
Immune function
Vitamin absorption

Blood pressure
Body weight
Bone loss

| Figure 13.9 | **Age-related physiological changes.** As we age, most physiological changes emerge gradually. |
|---|---|

| Table 13.8 | Age-Related Changes and Nutrient Needs |
|---|---|

| Change in Body Composition or Physiologic Function | Impact on Nutrient Requirement |
|---|---|
| Decreased muscle mass | Decreased need for energy |
| Decreased bone density | Increased need for calcium and vitamin D |
| Decreased immune function | Increased need for vitamin $B_6$, vitamin E, and zinc |
| Increased gastric pH | Increased need for vitamin $B_{12}$, folic acid, calcium, iron, and zinc |
| Decreased skin capacity for cholecalciferol synthesis | Increased need for vitamin D |
| Increased wintertime parathyroid hormone production | Increased need for vitamin D |
| Decreased calcium bioavailability | Increased need for calcium and vitamin D |
| Decreased hepatic uptake of retinol | Decreased need for vitamin A |
| Decreased efficiency in metabolic use of vitamin $B_6$ | Increased need for vitamin $B_6$ |
| Increased oxidative stress status | Increased need for beta-carotene, vitamin C, and vitamin E |
| Increased levels of homocysteine | Increased need for folate, vitamin $B_6$, and vitamin $B_{12}$ |

**Source:** Adapted from Blumberg J. Nutritional needs of seniors. *J Am Coll Nutr.* 1997;16(6):517–523.

chronic disease (see **Figure 13.10**) but also the rate at which we age. Nutrition is a key factor in promoting health and ability to function at advanced ages. It also plays an important role in medical nutrition therapy for disease management. Eating is not only a necessity of everyday life, it is an important pleasure and social component at every age.

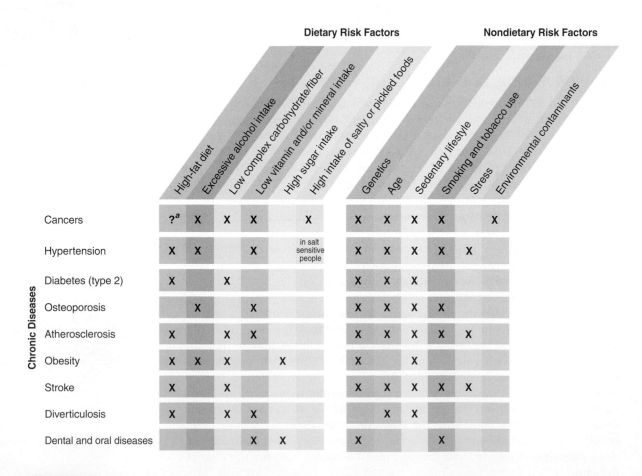

| Figure 13.10 | **Risk factors for disease.** Diet, lifestyle choices, and genetics interact to shape a person's risk profile. |
|---|---|

[a] The Nurses' Health Study, a large prospective study, found no evidence linking higher total fat intake with increased risk of breast cancer. These results call into question theories that link dietary fat to other cancers.

## Weight and Body Composition

Poor food choices and too many calories, combined with a sedentary lifestyle, have resulted in a growing number of overweight and obese older adults.[56] People who are overweight when they enter their later years or who gain weight with age have an increased risk of chronic diseases such as heart disease, diabetes, metabolic syndrome, and cancer.[57] In addition, many older adults who have an increase in body fat and loss of muscle mass decline physically and are unable to function independently in their normal activities of daily living.

**THINK**
About It
**3**

In contrast, people who enter their mature years on the lean side—and who remain lean due to a healthy, active lifestyle—increase their chances of enjoying a healthy old age. But thinness alone is not always a health advantage. Obviously, older adults who lose weight due to illness enjoy no health benefits from losing these pounds. Weight loss puts them at increased risk for further illness, including cardiovascular disease and osteoporosis—especially if the original illness also limits activity. And, of course, leanness due to tobacco use or alcoholism increases a person's vulnerability to a decline in health.

## Physical Activity

Lean body mass (muscle mass) and strength commonly decline with age. However, this may not be a simple physiological consequence of aging. Decreases in physical activity that accompany advancing age contribute to loss of lean mass and therefore strength.[58] Our posture begins to deteriorate in our fifties—from bad habits, bone loss, and a decrease in muscle tone. Poor posture can affect lung and cardiovascular function, mobility, and balance. Diseases such as stroke, heart disease, arthritis, and diabetes become more common and may cause severe physical disability. These conditions, however, do not automatically preclude us as older adults from participating in physical activity with qualified supervision. In fact, they may instead provide additional justification for appropriate exercises for the older adult.[59] Medications and nutritional deficiencies may lead to impaired motor function; therefore, older adults should be evaluated by their physician prior to beginning a new exercise program.

Although physical activity cannot stop biological aging, regular exercise can help to minimize the physiological effects of a sedentary lifestyle and limit the progression of disabling conditions and chronic diseases.[60] The U.S. Department of Health and Human Services' *2008 Physical Activity Guidelines for Americans* states that "regular physical activity is essential for healthy aging" and that all adults should avoid inactivity.[61] (See Table 13.9.) These recommendations for physical activity for older adults are included in the *Dietary Guidelines for Americans, 2010.* Canada also addresses this issue in its *Physical Activity Guide for Older Adults.* (See **Figure 13.11.**) The benefits of an individualized exercise prescription designed to increase physical activity—a program that includes aerobic activities, flexibility exercises, and progressive resistance strength training—may be most profound for those who are aging. Increased self-confidence, better balance and mobility, fewer falls and fractures, enhanced mental acuity, and improved appetite and nutrient intake are but a few of the physical and psychological benefits of exercise during our older years. (See **Figure 13.12.**) The bottom line is that all adults, even older adults, should

**Table 13.9** **2008 Physical Activity Guidelines for Americans Age 65 Years and Older**

- Older adults should follow these physical activity guidelines. When older adults cannot meet the adult guidelines, they should be as physically active as their abilities and conditions will allow.
- Older adults should do exercises that maintain or improve balance if they are at risk of falling.
- Older adults should determine their level of effort for physical activity relative to their level of fitness.
- Older adults with chronic conditions should understand whether and how their conditions affect their ability to do regular physical activity safely.

**Source:** Reproduced from *Dietary Guidelines for Americans, 2010.* 7th ed. US Government Printing Office; 2010. Courtesy of US Department of Agriculture and US Department of Health and Human Services.

### Canadian Physical Activity Guidelines

**FOR OLDER ADULTS - 65 YEARS & OLDER**

**Guidelines**

To achieve health benefits, and improve functional abilities, adults aged 65 years and older should accumulate at least 150 minutes of moderate- to vigorous-intensity aerobic physical activity per week, in bouts of 10 minutes or more.

It is also beneficial to add muscle and bone strengthening activities using major muscle groups, at least 2 days per week.

Those with poor mobility should perform physical activities to enhance balance and prevent falls.

More physical activity provides greater health benefits.

**Let's Talk Intensity!**

Moderate-intensity physical activities will cause older adults to sweat a little and to breathe harder. Activities like:
- Brisk walking
- Bicycling

Vigorous-intensity physical activities will cause older adults to sweat and be 'out of breath'. Activities like:
- Cross-country skiing
- Swimming

**Being active for at least 150 minutes per week can help reduce the risk of:**
- Chronic disease (such as high blood pressure and heart disease) and,
- Premature death

And also help to:
- Maintain functional independence
- Maintain mobility
- Improve fitness
- Improve or maintain body weight
- Maintain bone health and,
- Maintain mental health and feel better

**Pick a time. Pick a place. Make a plan and move more!**
- ☑ Join a community urban poling or mall walking group.
- ☑ Go for a brisk walk around the block after lunch.
- ☑ Take a dance class in the afternoon.
- ☑ Train for and participate in a run or walk for charity!
- ☑ Take up a favourite sport again.
- ☑ Be active with the family! Plan to have "active reunions".
- ☑ Go for a nature hike on the weekend.
- ☑ Take the dog for a walk after dinner.

*Now is the time. Walk, run, or wheel, and embrace life.*

PARTICIPaction    CSEP | SCPE
www.csep.ca/guidelines

**Figure 13.11** **Canada's *Physical Activity Guide for Older Adults.***

**Source:** Canadian Physical Activity Guidelines, © 2011. Used with permi[...] Canadian Society for Exercise Physiology, www.csep.ca/guidelines.

**Moderate Evidence**
Lower risk of hip fracture and increased bone density
Lower risk of lung and endometrial cancers
Weight maintenance after weight loss
Improved sleep quality

**Moderate to Strong Evidence**
Better functional health (for older adults)
Reduced abdominal obesity

**Strong Evidence**
Lower risk of early death
Lower risk of coronary heart disease, stroke, high
    blood pressure, type 2 diabetes, metabolic
    syndrome, colon cancer, and breast cancer
Prevention of weight gain
Weight loss, particularly when combined with reduced
    calorie intake
Improved cardiorespiratory and muscular fitness
Prevention of falls
Reduced depression
Better cognitive function (for older adults)

**Figure 13.12**    **Health benefits associated with regular physical activity for adults and older adults.** Physical activity helps adults maintain their health and independence as they age.

**Note:** The Advisory Committee rated the evidence of health benefits of physical activity as strong, moderate, or weak. To do so, the Advisory Committee considered the type, number, and quality of studies available, as well as consistency of findings across studies that addressed each outcome. The Advisory Committee also considered evidence for causality and dose response in assigning the strength-of-evidence rating.

**Source:** Adapted from US Department of Health and Human Services. *2008 Physical Activity Guidelines for Americans.* ODPHP Publication No. U0036. Washington, DC: US Department of Health and Human Services; 2008. http://www.health.gov/paguidelines/guidelines/chapter2.aspx. Accessed 8/8/11.

**urinary tract infection (UTI)**  An infection of one or more structures in the urinary tract; usually caused by bacteria.

**taste threshold**  The minimum amount of flavor that must be present for a taste to be detected.

*Quick* Bite

**ing Water**
    percent of the body is
    ter. By the time a
    e that number has
    to changes in body

avoid inactive lifestyles and regularly engage in various forms of physical activity.[62]

## Immunity

In the fifth decade of life (from age 40 to 50 years), the body's defense mechanisms begin to weaken. The immune system loses some of its ability to fight viruses, bacteria, and other foreign bodies. Older adults are more vulnerable to upper respiratory tract infections such as influenza and pneumonia, **urinary tract infections**, pressure sores, and foodborne illnesses. Physical barriers to infectious agents, foreign bodies, and chemicals weaken as well. These barriers include the skin, the acid environment in the stomach, and swallowing and coughing reflexes.

Inadequate consumption of protein can compromise immunity and health in older adults. Because of poor appetite, difficulty chewing, financial constraints, concerns about fat intake, or lactose intolerance, older people may reduce their intake of meat, dairy products, fresh fruits, and vegetables, making it difficult for them to get all the calories, protein (see **Figure 13.13**), and other essential nutrients they need. A poor diet can lead to suppressed immunity, decreased muscle mass, slowed wound healing, and osteoporosis.

**Key Concepts**  *Lifestyle choices, such as diet and exercise, affect how we age. Control of body weight can reduce our risk for many chronic diseases associated with aging. Adequate protein, vitamins, and minerals can protect our immune status. Regular physical activity not only helps us to maintain the ability to function in daily activities and enables our independence but also reduces disease risk and improves mental health.*

## Taste and Smell

In older adults, the **taste threshold**—the minimum amount of a flavor that must be present to detect the taste—is more than double that of college-aged adults. Sensitivity to sweet and salty tastes goes first, so older adults often increase their intake of foods high in sugar and sodium—increasing health problems that stem from overconsumption of these nutrients. Along with taste, our sense of smell diminishes with age, especially in the seventh decade of life (60 to 70 years old) and beyond. Medication use can also alter taste and flavor perception. Ideas that older people should be served bland foods are misguided. Intensifying flavors and aromas of food and varying temperature and textures are strategies older adults can use to compensate for diminished taste and smell of foods.[63] (See **Figure 13.14**.)

## Gastrointestinal Changes

Saliva production tends to decrease as we age, especially in people who take medications for conditions such as congestive heart failure. Lack of saliva negatively affects the preparation of food for digestion and contributes to gum disease—a breach in one of the immune system's first lines of defense against infection.

With age, digestive secretions decline. Most significant are reductions in the stomach secretions of hydrochloric acid and pepsin. These reductions can allow the development of atrophic gastritis—a chronic inflammation of the stomach lining that is common among older adults. Atrophic gastritis can interfere with normal absorption of vitamin $B_{12}$, leading to a deficiency of this vitamin.[64] Although reduced lactase production also is associated with aging, a complete intolerance to milk and dairy products is less common than older people often suspect. Most people with reduced lactase production can include some milk, cheese, and yogurt in their diets.

Constipation, gas, and bloating are common complaints of old age. These problems are due to a slowing of gastrointestinal motility with aging, along with decreased physical activity, a diet low in fiber, and low fluid intake. Feelings of fullness may cause older people to eat less. Reduced digestive secretions lower the amount of nutrients older adults absorb from the foods they do eat. Myths and misinformation about the gastrointestinal (GI) effects of various foods, even among the medical community, may steer a person away from nutrient-dense foods such as dairy products, legumes, broccoli, cauliflower, tomatoes, and citrus products. Although many older adults mistakenly blame these foods for causing problems with gas, others may be sensitive to lactose in dairy products or may have had an adverse reaction to members of the cabbage family or "acid"-containing foods. GI distress also may be caused by factors totally unrelated to the food itself—inappropriate food preparation, lack of adequate fluid, and physical inactivity. Regardless of the cause, once people have an adverse reaction, they may associate it with a recently consumed food and become reluctant to try it again.

**Key Concepts** *The perception of taste declines with age. To detect flavors, older adults need food with stronger flavors and odors. This loss of taste may contribute to loss of appetite and poor food intake. Age-related changes in the GI tract reduce nutrient absorption. Decreased motility contributes to constipation.*

## Nutrient Needs of the Mature Adult

To live life to its fullest, you need good nutrition. A lifestyle that incorporates the *Dietary Guidelines for Americans*, together with regular physical activity, is essential to a long and productive life. **Figure 13.15** shows the modified MyPyramid for older adults.

### Energy

Mainly because of reduced physical activity and loss of lean body mass, our energy requirements decline as we age. In other words, a 60-year-old man will need to increase his physical activity and/or decrease his caloric intake to maintain his weight as he ages. Physical activity increases energy requirements while also helping to delay some loss in lean mass, thus allowing us to eat more without gaining weight and increasing the likelihood that our diets will be adequate in essential nutrients.

The EER equations are the same for older adults as for younger adults. Individual energy needs depend on activity, lean body mass, and the presence of disease; a person who is bed- or chair-ridden, for example, usually requires fewer calories than a mobile person.

### Protein

Protein needs (as grams per kilogram of body weight) do not change as we age but may be somewhat harder for us to meet as our overall energy needs decrease and our tastes change. As our caloric needs decrease and our protein needs remain constant, an adequate diet must contain relatively more protein. For healthy older people, the RDA for protein is 0.8 grams per kilogram of body weight, or, on average, 46 grams per day for women and 56 grams for men. To meet their protein needs and maximize muscle protein synthesis, older adults should include 25 to 30 grams of high-quality protein with each meal.[65] Chronically ill individuals may need more protein than the average person to maintain nitrogen balance. Trauma, stress, and infection also may increase protein needs. However, there are risks associated with high protein

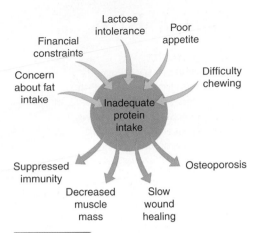

**Figure 13.13** **Protein malnutrition in older adults.** A combination of several factors can lead to inadequate protein intake, which compromises immunity and health.

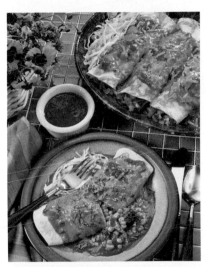

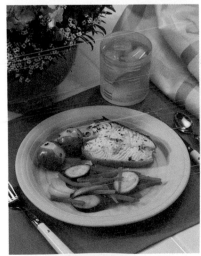

**Figure 13.14** **Older adults need stronger flavors.** More highly spiced m rather than bland ones may encourage an older to eat more.

## *Quick* Bite

### Hardy Hearts

By the end of a normal life span, the human heart has pumped more than 3 billion times. Despite this heavy use, heart failures are usually caused by problems with blood vessels and valves; the heart muscle itself rarely wears out.

## MyPlate for Older Adults

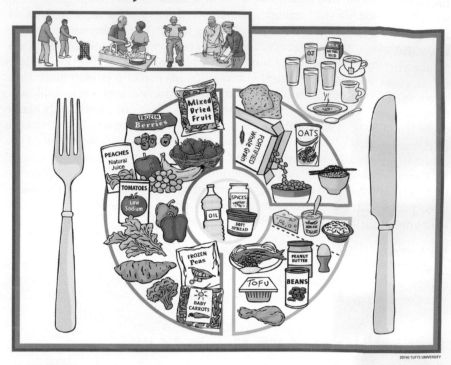

| Figure 13.15 | Modified MyPlate for older adults. |

**Source:** © 2011 Tufts University. For details about the MyPlate for Older Adults, please see http://nutrition.tufts.edu/research/myplate-older-adults.

intake, including dehydration, nitrogen overload, and adverse effects on the kidneys.

## Carbohydrate

After infancy, carbohydrates should make up 45 to 65 percent of calories in the diet. Because foods with primarily simple carbohydrates provide little nutrient value, the best choices are foods with complex carbohydrates.

Fiber, a complex carbohydrate, has many potential benefits, including preventing constipation and diverticulosis, helping to promote a healthy body weight, and reducing risk for diabetes. Because the Adequate Intake (AI) for fiber is based on calorie intake (14 grams per 1,000 kilocalories per day), and energy needs decline with age, the AI for fiber is 30 grams per day for men over age 50 and 21 grams per day for women. Fiber also can help to reduce blood cholesterol, making these recommendations especially important for those who are at risk for heart disease. Five or more servings of fruits and vegetables daily, accompanied by whole-grain breads or cereals high in bran, will supply this amount easily. To avoid abdominal discomfort, increase dietary fiber intake gradually. When increasing dietary fiber intake, it is essential to consume adequate fluids—ideally water—to avoid dehydration and constipation.

## Fat

Excess dietary fat can lead to obesity, which, in turn, increases the risk for diabetes, heart disease, and some types of cancer. Younger people should limit their dietary cholesterol and fat, but severe restrictions in older adults may be counterproductive. Extreme fat phobia may contribute to nutritional deficiencies among older people who are afraid to drink milk, eat red meat, or even eat poultry or fish. Too few animal products in the diet may contribute to a lack of dietary protein; deficiency of minerals such as calcium, iron, and zinc; and poor vitamin $B_{12}$ intake and absorption.

Healthy people who are at low risk for heart disease should obtain 20 to 35 percent of their daily calories from fat, with no more than 8 to 10 percent of the calories from saturated fat. They should limit their cholesterol intake to 300 milligrams per day. People at increased risk for heart disease should limit saturated fat and cholesterol even more, according to their physicians' advice.

## Water

Nutritionists often call water the forgotten nutrient. Water is essential to all body functions; if intake is inadequate, cellular metabolism becomes difficult, if not impossible. In older adults a decreased thirst response and a reduction in kidney function can increase the risk of dehydration.[66] Diuretic medications, alcohol, and caffeine all increase fluid excretion and can contribute to dehydration. Fluid recommendations for older adults are the same as for younger adults: 3,700 milliliters per day for men and 2,700 milliliters per day for women.[67] These fluids are obtained from both beverages and foods.

**Key Concepts** *Although caloric needs decline with loss of lean tissue and reduced physical activity, protein needs do not change for older adults. A high-carbohydrate, moderate-fat diet is still recommended. Water is important; because of their diminished thirst response, older adults may not drink enough.*

## Vitamins and Minerals

As we age, our micronutrient status changes, especially our needs for vitamin D, vitamin $B_{12}$, and calcium. (See **Figure 13.16**.) In many cases, our vitamin needs remain stable, while our energy needs decline. In other cases, age-related declines in absorption, use, or activation of nutrients lead to increased dietary vitamin and mineral needs. Therefore, it is especially important for older adults to eat nutrient-dense foods.

### Vitamin D

Vitamin D promotes bone health; too little dietary vitamin D can lead to brittle and porous bones that are susceptible to fracture. Recently, vitamin D has been investigated for its role in the prevention and treatment of cancer, type 1 and type 2 diabetes, hypertension, glucose metabolism, heart disease, arthritis, and multiple sclerosis.[68] Older adults often have low vitamin D status.[69] Not only are aging tissues less able to take up vitamin D from the blood, but aging skin also is less able to synthesize vitamin D when exposed to sunlight. In addition, many older adults spend more time indoors and have reduced exposure to sunlight. When they go outside, many avoid the sun and use sunscreens—a good strategy for skin cancer prevention but one that reduces vitamin D synthesis. Older adults with lactose intolerance often avoid dairy products, reducing their vitamin D intake and further compromising vitamin D status. The RDA for vitamin D for adults aged 51 through

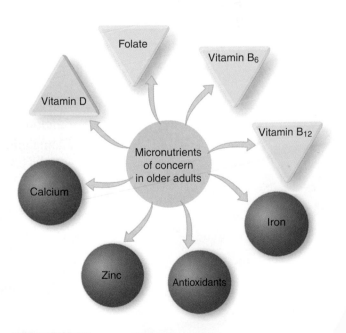

**Figure 13.16** **Micronutrients of particular concern for older people.** As we age, our energy needs decline, but our vitamin and mineral needs remain stable. This makes nutrient-dense fo' especially important for older adults.

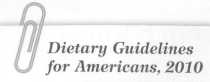

*Dietary Guidelines for Americans, 2010*

**Key Recommendations**

Reduce daily sodium intake to less than 2,300 milligrams (mg)—the amount in about 1 teaspoon of table salt—and further reduce intake to 1,500 mg among persons who are 51 and older and those of any age who are African American or have hypertension, diabetes, or chronic kidney disease. The 1,500 mg recommendation applies to about half the U.S. population, including children, and the majority of adults.

**Individuals ages 50 years and older:**

- Consume foods fortified with vitamin $B_{12}$ such as fortified cereals or dietary supplements.

70 is 600 IU per day. For adults 70 and older, the RDA is 800 IU per day. Younger adults also need 600 IU per day.[70]

## B Vitamins

The B vitamins deserve special consideration in adults and the aged. Extensive research links inadequate folate, vitamin $B_6$, and vitamin $B_{12}$ to elevated levels of plasma homocysteine, which is associated with an increased risk for cardiovascular disease and mortality.[71] High homocysteine levels have also been found to be an independent risk factor for cognitive impairment and dementia.[72] The prevalence of vitamin $B_{12}$ deficiency increases with age. Six percent of adults aged 60 or older are vitamin $B_{12}$ deficient, and close to 20 percent have marginal status.[73] Although most adults consume adequate amounts of dietary vitamin $B_{12}$, 10 to 30 percent of older adults lose their ability to absorb protein-bound vitamin $B_{12}$ from foods. An intake of 2.4 micrograms per day of vitamin $B_{12}$ is recommended for all adults older than 51 years. Because it is easier to absorb synthetic $B_{12}$ than food-bound $B_{12}$, scientists suggest that adults older than 50 use fortified foods or $B_{12}$-containing supplements to meet their vitamin $B_{12}$ requirements.

## Antioxidants

Antioxidants are substances that reduce cell damage caused by free radicals. Antioxidants such as those found in fruits and vegetables are desirable and important for reducing oxidative stress and degenerative diseases common in older adults. Cataracts and age-related macular degeneration (ARMD) are common conditions that affect the vision of older adults. Antioxidant supplements may have a beneficial effect in slowing the progression of ARMD[74] but do not prevent ARMD.[75] In addition, antioxidants may protect against damage to the brain that may lead to Alzheimer's disease and other declines in cognition that are common in older adults.[76]

**Key Concepts**  *Vitamin D, folate, vitamin $B_6$, vitamin $B_{12}$, and antioxidants are key nutrients for older adults. Vitamin D status can decline due to reduced intake, synthesis, and activation. Poor folate, $B_6$, and $B_{12}$ status may result in high homocysteine levels, a risk factor for heart disease. Vitamin $B_{12}$ absorption declines with age; $B_{12}$ is more easily absorbed from fortified foods and supplements, so these become important sources for older adults. Antioxidants help to lower the prevalence and progression of degenerative diseases such as ARMD and Alzheimer's.*

## Calcium

Maintaining adequate calcium intake reduces the rate of age-related bone loss and the incidence of fractures, especially of the hip.[77] For women ages 51 to 70 years, the RDA for calcium is 1,200 milligrams per day, 200 milligrams per day higher than the RDA for men of the same age. For both men and women over the age of 70, the RDA for calcium is 1,200 milligrams per day.[78] As we age, we are less able to absorb calcium, partly because of a loss of vitamin D receptors in the gut. Stomach inflammation also reduces calcium absorption, as does an increase in the consumption of fiber—a practice that doctors recommend for its laxative effects. Because of real or perceived lactose intolerance, many older people have a low intake of dairy foods and therefore of calcium.

## Zinc

Although clinical zinc deficiencies are uncommon, older adults frequently have marginal zinc intakes. Stress, especially in hospitalized older adults, appears to increase the risk of zinc deficiency and suppress immune function.

## Weight and Body Composition

Poor food choices and too many calories, combined with a sedentary lifestyle, have resulted in a growing number of overweight and obese older adults.[56] People who are overweight when they enter their later years or who gain weight with age have an increased risk of chronic diseases such as heart disease, diabetes, metabolic syndrome, and cancer.[57] In addition, many older adults who have an increase in body fat and loss of muscle mass decline physically and are unable to function independently in their normal activities of daily living.

**THINK**
**About It**
**3**

In contrast, people who enter their mature years on the lean side—and who remain lean due to a healthy, active lifestyle—increase their chances of enjoying a healthy old age. But thinness alone is not always a health advantage. Obviously, older adults who lose weight due to illness enjoy no health benefits from losing these pounds. Weight loss puts them at increased risk for further illness, including cardiovascular disease and osteoporosis— especially if the original illness also limits activity. And, of course, leanness due to tobacco use or alcoholism increases a person's vulnerability to a decline in health.

## Physical Activity

Lean body mass (muscle mass) and strength commonly decline with age. However, this may not be a simple physiological consequence of aging. Decreases in physical activity that accompany advancing age contribute to loss of lean mass and therefore strength.[58] Our posture begins to deteriorate in our fifties—from bad habits, bone loss, and a decrease in muscle tone. Poor posture can affect lung and cardiovascular function, mobility, and balance. Diseases such as stroke, heart disease, arthritis, and diabetes become more common and may cause severe physical disability. These conditions, however, do not automatically preclude us as older adults from participating in physical activity with qualified supervision. In fact, they may instead provide additional justification for appropriate exercises for the older adult.[59] Medications and nutritional deficiencies may lead to impaired motor function; therefore, older adults should be evaluated by their physician prior to beginning a new exercise program.

Although physical activity cannot stop biological aging, regular exercise can help to minimize the physiological effects of a sedentary lifestyle and limit the progression of disabling conditions and chronic diseases.[60] The U.S. Department of Health and Human Services' *2008 Physical Activity Guidelines for Americans* states that "regular physical activity is essential for healthy aging" and that all adults should avoid inactivity.[61] (See Table 13.9.) These recommendations for physical activity for older adults are included in the *Dietary Guidelines for Americans, 2010.* Canada also addresses this issue in its *Physical Activity Guide for Older Adults.* (See **Figure 13.11.**) The benefits of an individualized exercise prescription designed to increase physical activity—a program that includes aerobic activities, flexibility exercises, and progressive resistance strength training—may be most profound for those who are aging. Increased self-confidence, better balance and mobility, fewer falls and fractures, enhanced mental acuity, and improved appetite and nutrient intake are but a few of the physical and psychological benefits of exercise during our older years. (See **Figure 13.12.**) The bottom line is that all adults, even older adults, should

| Table 13.9 | 2008 Physical Activity Guidelines for Americans Age 65 Years and Older |
|---|---|

- Older adults should follow these physical activity guidelines. When older adults cannot meet the adult guidelines, they should be as physically active as their abilities and conditions will allow.
- Older adults should do exercises that maintain or improve balance if they are at risk of falling.
- Older adults should determine their level of effort for physical activity relative to their level of fitness.
- Older adults with chronic conditions should understand whether and how their conditions affect their ability to do regular physical activity safely.

**Source:** Reproduced from *Dietary Guidelines for Americans, 2010.* 7th ed. US Government Printing Office; 2010. Courtesy of US Department of Agriculture and US Department of Health and Human Services.

## Canadian Physical Activity Guidelines

FOR OLDER ADULTS - 65 YEARS & OLDER

### Guidelines

 To achieve health benefits, and improve functional abilities, adults aged 65 years and older should accumulate at least 150 minutes of moderate- to vigorous-intensity aerobic physical activity per week, in bouts of 10 minutes or more.

 It is also beneficial to add muscle and bone strengthening activities using major muscle groups, at least 2 days per week.

 Those with poor mobility should perform physical activities to enhance balance and prevent falls.

More physical activity provides greater health benefits.

**Let's Talk Intensity!**

Moderate-intensity physical activities will cause older adults to sweat a little and to breathe harder. Activities like:
- Brisk walking
- Bicycling

Vigorous-intensity physical activities will cause older adults to sweat and be 'out of breath'. Activities like:
- Cross-country skiing
- Swimming

**Being active for at least 150 minutes per week can help reduce the risk of:**
- Chronic disease (such as high blood pressure and heart disease) and,
- Premature death

And also help to:
- Maintain functional independence
- Maintain mobility
- Improve fitness
- Improve or maintain body weight
- Maintain bone health and,
- Maintain mental health and feel better

**Pick a time. Pick a place. Make a plan and move more!**

☑ Join a community urban poling or mail walking group.
☑ Go for a brisk walk around the block after lunch.
☑ Take a dance class in the afternoon.
☑ Train for and participate in a run or walk for charity!
☑ Take up a favourite sport again.
☑ Be active with the family! Plan to have "active reunions".
☑ Go for a nature hike on the weekend.
☑ Take the dog for a walk after dinner.

*Now is the time. Walk, run, or wheel, and embrace life.*

| Figure 13.11 | Canada's *Physical Activity Guide for Older Adults.* |
|---|---|

**Source:** Canadian Physical Activity Guidelines, © 2011. Used with permission from the Canadian Society for Exercise Physiology, www.csep.ca/guidelines.

**Moderate Evidence**
Lower risk of hip fracture and increased bone density
Lower risk of lung and endometrial cancers
Weight maintenance after weight loss
Improved sleep quality

**Moderate to Strong Evidence**
Better functional health (for older adults)
Reduced abdominal obesity

**Strong Evidence**
Lower risk of early death
Lower risk of coronary heart disease, stroke, high
    blood pressure, type 2 diabetes, metabolic
    syndrome, colon cancer, and breast cancer
Prevention of weight gain
Weight loss, particularly when combined with reduced
    calorie intake
Improved cardiorespiratory and muscular fitness
Prevention of falls
Reduced depression
Better cognitive function (for older adults)

**Figure 13.12** **Health benefits associated with regular physical activity for adults and older adults.** Physical activity helps adults maintain their health and independence as they age.

**Note:** The Advisory Committee rated the evidence of health benefits of physical activity as strong, moderate, or weak. To do so, the Advisory Committee considered the type, number, and quality of studies available, as well as consistency of findings across studies that addressed each outcome. The Advisory Committee also considered evidence for causality and dose response in assigning the strength-of-evidence rating.

**Source:** Adapted from US Department of Health and Human Services. *2008 Physical Activity Guidelines for Americans.* ODPHP Publication No. U0036. Washington, DC: US Department of Health and Human Services; 2008. http://www.health.gov/paguidelines/guidelines/chapter2.aspx. Accessed 8/8/11.

**urinary tract infection (UTI)** An infection of one or more structures in the urinary tract; usually caused by bacteria.

**taste threshold** The minimum amount of flavor that must be present for a taste to be detected.

## *Quick* Bite

**Losing Water**
At birth, 75 percent of the body is composed of water. By the time a person reaches old age that number has dwindled to 50 percent due to changes in body composition.

avoid inactive lifestyles and regularly engage in various forms of physical activity.[62]

## Immunity

In the fifth decade of life (from age 40 to 50 years), the body's defense mechanisms begin to weaken. The immune system loses some of its ability to fight viruses, bacteria, and other foreign bodies. Older adults are more vulnerable to upper respiratory tract infections such as influenza and pneumonia, **urinary tract infections**, pressure sores, and foodborne illnesses. Physical barriers to infectious agents, foreign bodies, and chemicals weaken as well. These barriers include the skin, the acid environment in the stomach, and swallowing and coughing reflexes.

Inadequate consumption of protein can compromise immunity and health in older adults. Because of poor appetite, difficulty chewing, financial constraints, concerns about fat intake, or lactose intolerance, older people may reduce their intake of meat, dairy products, fresh fruits, and vegetables, making it difficult for them to get all the calories, protein (see **Figure 13.13**), and other essential nutrients they need. A poor diet can lead to suppressed immunity, decreased muscle mass, slowed wound healing, and osteoporosis.

**Key Concepts** *Lifestyle choices, such as diet and exercise, affect how we age. Control of body weight can reduce our risk for many chronic diseases associated with aging. Adequate protein, vitamins, and minerals can protect our immune status. Regular physical activity not only helps us to maintain the ability to function in daily activities and enables our independence but also reduces disease risk and improves mental health.*

## Taste and Smell

In older adults, the **taste threshold**—the minimum amount of a flavor that must be present to detect the taste—is more than double that of college-aged adults. Sensitivity to sweet and salty tastes goes first, so older adults often increase their intake of foods high in sugar and sodium—increasing health problems that stem from overconsumption of these nutrients. Along with taste, our sense of smell diminishes with age, especially in the seventh decade of life (60 to 70 years old) and beyond. Medication use can also alter taste and flavor perception. Ideas that older people should be served bland foods are misguided. Intensifying flavors and aromas of food and varying temperature and textures are strategies older adults can use to compensate for diminished taste and smell of foods.[63] (See **Figure 13.14**.)

## Gastrointestinal Changes

Saliva production tends to decrease as we age, especially in people who take medications for conditions such as congestive heart failure. Lack of saliva negatively affects the preparation of food for digestion and contributes to gum disease—a breach in one of the immune system's first lines of defense against infection.

With age, digestive secretions decline. Most significant are reductions in the stomach secretions of hydrochloric acid and pepsin. These reductions can allow the development of atrophic gastritis—a chronic inflammation of the stomach lining that is common among older adults. Atrophic gastritis can interfere with normal absorption of vitamin $B_{12}$, leading to a deficiency of this vitamin.[64] Although reduced lactase production also is associated with aging, a complete intolerance to milk and dairy products is less common than older people often suspect. Most people with reduced lactase production can include some milk, cheese, and yogurt in their diets.

Constipation, gas, and bloating are common complaints of old age. These problems are due to a slowing of gastrointestinal motility with aging, along with decreased physical activity, a diet low in fiber, and low fluid intake. Feelings of fullness may cause older people to eat less. Reduced digestive secretions lower the amount of nutrients older adults absorb from the foods they do eat. Myths and misinformation about the gastrointestinal (GI) effects of various foods, even among the medical community, may steer a person away from nutrient-dense foods such as dairy products, legumes, broccoli, cauliflower, tomatoes, and citrus products. Although many older adults mistakenly blame these foods for causing problems with gas, others may be sensitive to lactose in dairy products or may have had an adverse reaction to members of the cabbage family or "acid"-containing foods. GI distress also may be caused by factors totally unrelated to the food itself—inappropriate food preparation, lack of adequate fluid, and physical inactivity. Regardless of the cause, once people have an adverse reaction, they may associate it with a recently consumed food and become reluctant to try it again.

**Key Concepts**  *The perception of taste declines with age. To detect flavors, older adults need food with stronger flavors and odors. This loss of taste may contribute to loss of appetite and poor food intake. Age-related changes in the GI tract reduce nutrient absorption. Decreased motility contributes to constipation.*

## Nutrient Needs of the Mature Adult

To live life to its fullest, you need good nutrition. A lifestyle that incorporates the *Dietary Guidelines for Americans*, together with regular physical activity, is essential to a long and productive life. **Figure 13.15** shows the modified MyPyramid for older adults.

### Energy

Mainly because of reduced physical activity and loss of lean body mass, our energy requirements decline as we age. In other words, a 60-year-old man will need to increase his physical activity and/or decrease his caloric intake to maintain his weight as he ages. Physical activity increases energy requirements while also helping to delay some loss in lean mass, thus allowing us to eat more without gaining weight and increasing the likelihood that our diets will be adequate in essential nutrients.

The EER equations are the same for older adults as for younger adults. Individual energy needs depend on activity, lean body mass, and the presence of disease; a person who is bed- or chair-ridden, for example, usually requires fewer calories than a mobile person.

### Protein

Protein needs (as grams per kilogram of body weight) do not change as we age but may be somewhat harder for us to meet as our overall energy needs decrease and our tastes change. As our caloric needs decrease and our protein needs remain constant, an adequate diet must contain relatively more protein. For healthy older people, the RDA for protein is 0.8 grams per kilogram of body weight, or, on average, 46 grams per day for women and 56 grams for men. To meet their protein needs and maximize muscle protein synthesis, older adults should include 25 to 30 grams of high-quality protein with each meal.[65] Chronically ill individuals may need more protein than the average person to maintain nitrogen balance. Trauma, stress, and infection also may increase protein needs. However, there are risks associated with high protein

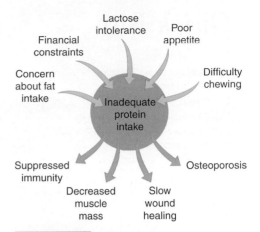

**Figure 13.13**  **Protein malnutrition in older adults.** A combination of several factors can lead to inadequate protein intake, which compromises immunity and health.

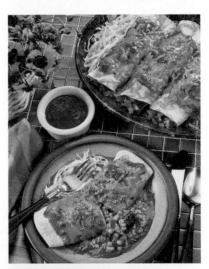

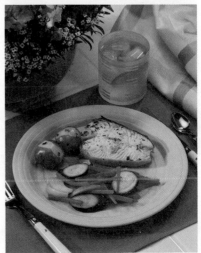

**Figure 13.14**  **Older adults need stronger flavors.** More highly spiced meals rather than bland ones may encourage an older adult to eat more.

## *Quick* Bite

**Hardy Hearts**
By the end of a normal life span, the human heart has pumped more than 3 billion times. Despite this heavy use, heart failures are usually caused by problems with blood vessels and valves; the heart muscle itself rarely wears out.

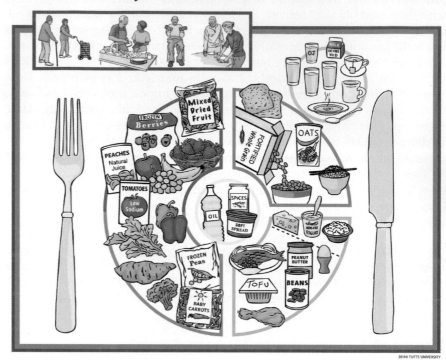

## MyPlate for Older Adults

| Figure 13.15 | **Modified MyPlate for older adults.** |
| --- | --- |

**Source:** © 2011 Tufts University. For details about the MyPlate for Older Adults, please see http://nutrition.tufts.edu/research/myplate-older-adults.

intake, including dehydration, nitrogen overload, and adverse effects on the kidneys.

## Carbohydrate

After infancy, carbohydrates should make up 45 to 65 percent of calories in the diet. Because foods with primarily simple carbohydrates provide little nutrient value, the best choices are foods with complex carbohydrates.

Fiber, a complex carbohydrate, has many potential benefits, including preventing constipation and diverticulosis, helping to promote a healthy body weight, and reducing risk for diabetes. Because the Adequate Intake (AI) for fiber is based on calorie intake (14 grams per 1,000 kilocalories per day), and energy needs decline with age, the AI for fiber is 30 grams per day for men over age 50 and 21 grams per day for women. Fiber also can help to reduce blood cholesterol, making these recommendations especially important for those who are at risk for heart disease. Five or more servings of fruits and vegetables daily, accompanied by whole-grain breads or cereals high in bran, will supply this amount easily. To avoid abdominal discomfort, increase dietary fiber intake gradually. When increasing dietary fiber intake, it is essential to consume adequate fluids—ideally water—to avoid dehydration and constipation.

## Fat

Excess dietary fat can lead to obesity, which, in turn, increases the risk for diabetes, heart disease, and some types of cancer. Younger people should limit their dietary cholesterol and fat, but severe restrictions in older adults may be counterproductive. Extreme fat phobia may contribute to nutritional deficiencies among older people who are afraid to drink milk, eat red meat, or even eat poultry or fish. Too few animal products in the diet may contribute to a lack of dietary protein; deficiency of minerals such as calcium, iron, and zinc; and poor vitamin $B_{12}$ intake and absorption.

Healthy people who are at low risk for heart disease should obtain 20 to 35 percent of their daily calories from fat, with no more than 8 to 10 percent of the calories from saturated fat. They should limit their cholesterol intake to 300 milligrams per day. People at increased risk for heart disease should limit saturated fat and cholesterol even more, according to their physicians' advice.

## Water

Nutritionists often call water the forgotten nutrient. Water is essential to all body functions; if intake is inadequate, cellular metabolism becomes difficult, if not impossible. In older adults a decreased thirst response and a reduction in kidney function can increase the risk of dehydration.[66] Diuretic medications, alcohol, and caffeine all increase fluid excretion and can contribute to dehydration. Fluid recommendations for older adults are the same as for younger adults: 3,700 milliliters per day for men and 2,700 milliliters per day for women.[67] These fluids are obtained from both beverages and foods.

**Key Concepts** *Although caloric needs decline with loss of lean tissue and reduced physical activity, protein needs do not change for older adults. A high-carbohydrate, moderate-fat diet is still recommended. Water is important; because of their diminished thirst response, older adults may not drink enough.*

## Vitamins and Minerals

As we age, our micronutrient status changes, especially our needs for vitamin D, vitamin $B_{12}$, and calcium. (See **Figure 13.16**.) In many cases, our vitamin needs remain stable, while our energy needs decline. In other cases, age-related declines in absorption, use, or activation of nutrients lead to increased dietary vitamin and mineral needs. Therefore, it is especially important for older adults to eat nutrient-dense foods.

### Vitamin D

Vitamin D promotes bone health; too little dietary vitamin D can lead to brittle and porous bones that are susceptible to fracture. Recently, vitamin D has been investigated for its role in the prevention and treatment of cancer, type 1 and type 2 diabetes, hypertension, glucose metabolism, heart disease, arthritis, and multiple sclerosis.[68] Older adults often have low vitamin D status.[69] Not only are aging tissues less able to take up vitamin D from the blood, but aging skin also is less able to synthesize vitamin D when exposed to sunlight. In addition, many older adults spend more time indoors and have reduced exposure to sunlight. When they go outside, many avoid the sun and use sunscreens—a good strategy for skin cancer prevention but one that reduces vitamin D synthesis. Older adults with lactose intolerance often avoid dairy products, reducing their vitamin D intake and further compromising vitamin D status. The RDA for vitamin D for adults aged 51 through

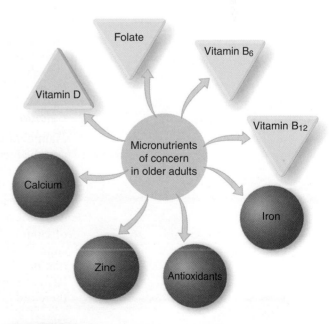

**Figure 13.16** **Micronutrients of particular concern for older people.** As we age, our energy needs decline, but our vitamin and mineral needs remain stable. This makes nutrient-dense foods especially important for older adults.

70 is 600 IU per day. For adults 70 and older, the RDA is 800 IU per day. Younger adults also need 600 IU per day.[70]

### B Vitamins

The B vitamins deserve special consideration in adults and the aged. Extensive research links inadequate folate, vitamin $B_6$, and vitamin $B_{12}$ to elevated levels of plasma homocysteine, which is associated with an increased risk for cardiovascular disease and mortality.[71] High homocysteine levels have also been found to be an independent risk factor for cognitive impairment and dementia.[72] The prevalence of vitamin $B_{12}$ deficiency increases with age. Six percent of adults aged 60 or older are vitamin $B_{12}$ deficient, and close to 20 percent have marginal status.[73] Although most adults consume adequate amounts of dietary vitamin $B_{12}$, 10 to 30 percent of older adults lose their ability to absorb protein-bound vitamin $B_{12}$ from foods. An intake of 2.4 micrograms per day of vitamin $B_{12}$ is recommended for all adults older than 51 years. Because it is easier to absorb synthetic $B_{12}$ than food-bound $B_{12}$, scientists suggest that adults older than 50 use fortified foods or $B_{12}$-containing supplements to meet their vitamin $B_{12}$ requirements.

### Antioxidants

Antioxidants are substances that reduce cell damage caused by free radicals. Antioxidants such as those found in fruits and vegetables are desirable and important for reducing oxidative stress and degenerative diseases common in older adults. Cataracts and age-related macular degeneration (ARMD) are common conditions that affect the vision of older adults. Antioxidant supplements may have a beneficial effect in slowing the progression of ARMD[74] but do not prevent ARMD.[75] In addition, antioxidants may protect against damage to the brain that may lead to Alzheimer's disease and other declines in cognition that are common in older adults.[76]

**Key Concepts** *Vitamin D, folate, vitamin $B_6$, vitamin $B_{12}$, and antioxidants are key nutrients for older adults. Vitamin D status can decline due to reduced intake, synthesis, and activation. Poor folate, $B_6$, and $B_{12}$ status may result in high homocysteine levels, a risk factor for heart disease. Vitamin $B_{12}$ absorption declines with age; $B_{12}$ is more easily absorbed from fortified foods and supplements, so these become important sources for older adults. Antioxidants help to lower the prevalence and progression of degenerative diseases such as ARMD and Alzheimer's.*

### Calcium

Maintaining adequate calcium intake reduces the rate of age-related bone loss and the incidence of fractures, especially of the hip.[77] For women ages 51 to 70 years, the RDA for calcium is 1,200 milligrams per day, 200 milligrams per day higher than the RDA for men of the same age. For both men and women over the age of 70, the RDA for calcium is 1,200 milligrams per day.[78] As we age, we are less able to absorb calcium, partly because of a loss of vitamin D receptors in the gut. Stomach inflammation also reduces calcium absorption, as does an increase in the consumption of fiber—a practice that doctors recommend for its laxative effects. Because of real or perceived lactose intolerance, many older people have a low intake of dairy foods and therefore of calcium.

### Zinc

Although clinical zinc deficiencies are uncommon, older adults frequently have marginal zinc intakes. Stress, especially in hospitalized older adults, appears to increase the risk of zinc deficiency and suppress immune function.

Studies show that zinc supplementation hastens wound healing but only in people who are zinc deficient. Because excess zinc may interfere with immune function and the absorption of other minerals and may work to lower HDL cholesterol, people of all ages should avoid excessive and continuous zinc supplementation.

### Iron

Iron remains an important nutrient throughout the life cycle. Following menopause, the RDA for women drops to the same level as for men, 8 milligrams per day. Iron deficiency is a concern for older adults who have limited intake of iron from the best sources—red meats, fish, and poultry. Reduced meat consumption may result from taste changes, economics, poor dentition, or a combination of factors.

## To Supplement or Not to Supplement

Increased use of dietary supplements, including vitamins, minerals, and herbal and botanical products, is widespread.[79] Although food is "the best medicine," some older adults may feel they need a supplement to meet their nutrient needs. Older adults take nutritional supplements for two main reasons: (1) to prevent deficiencies and (2) because of the potential health-promoting effects of these nutrients.[80] Food is more than the sum of its known nutrients, however, and replacing food with supplements may be a poor trade-off. In addition, some nutrients in large amounts can be toxic; they also can affect the absorption of other nutrients or interfere with the absorption and metabolism of prescription medications.

Excessive use of vitamin supplements by older adults may result in **hypervitaminosis**. The need for vitamin A decreases with age, increasing the chances that supplementation may lead to liver dysfunction, bone and joint pain, headaches, and other problems. Also, taking large amounts of vitamin C may increase the likelihood of kidney stones and gastric bleeding. Because we know that many older people use vitamin supplements and megadoses that may have negative effects on health, it is important to inform them of the ULs for micronutrients. The UL represents a level of intake from a combination of food and dietary supplements that should not be exceeded on a routine basis. (See Table 13.10.)

**Key Concepts** *Important minerals for older adults are calcium, zinc, and iron. Calcium is important to reduce the risk for osteoporosis. Marginal zinc deficiency has been suspected in many older adults and may be the result of reduced intake of red meats. Iron needs decline for women as they go through menopause. Excessive supplementation with certain vitamins or minerals can lead to health problems.*

## Nutrition-Related Concerns of Mature Adults

Many factors can interfere with intake or use of nutrients by older adults. Therefore, caretakers, healthcare practitioners, and seniors themselves must pay attention to nutritional status. To manage acute or chronic nutrition-related conditions, seniors may need to make specific dietary changes.

## Drug–Drug and Drug–Nutrient Interactions

Drugs not only affect the way the body uses nutrients, but they also can alter the activities of other drugs. In turn, foods and nutrients can enhance or interfere with the effects of drugs. (See Table 13.11.) Some drugs interfere with appetite; others cause dry mouth. Because many older adults take several

**Table 13.10** **The UL Values for Vitamins and Minerals for Adults**

| Nutrient | UL Value |
|---|---|
| Vitamin A (as retinol) | 3,000 μg/d |
| Vitamin C | 2,000 mg/d |
| Vitamin D | 4,000 IU |
| Vitamin E[a] | 1,000 mg/d |
| Niacin[a] | 35 mg/d |
| Vitamin B$_6$ | 100 mg/d |
| Folic acid | 1,000 μg/d |
| Choline | 3,500 mg/d |
| Boron | 20 mg/d |
| Calcium | 2,500 mg/d (19–50); 2,000 mg/d (51+ years) |
| Chloride | 3,600 mg/d |
| Copper | 10,000 μg/d |
| Fluoride | 10 mg/d |
| Iodine | 1,100 μg/d |
| Iron | 45 mg/d |
| Magnesium | 350 mg/d |
| Manganese | 11 mg/d |
| Molybdenum | 2,000 μg/d |
| Nickel | 1 mg/d |
| Phosphorus | 4,000 mg/d; 3,000 mg/d (for 70+ years) |
| Selenium | 400 μg/d |
| Sodium | 2,300 mg/d |
| Vanadium | 1.8 mg/d |
| Zinc | 40 mg/d |

[a] From fortified foods and supplements only.

**hypervitaminosis** High levels of vitamins in the blood, usually a result of excess supplement intake.

| Table 13.11 | Examples of Food–Drug Interactions |
|---|---|

| Drug | Food That Interacts | Effect of the Food | What to Do |
|---|---|---|---|
| **Analgesic** | | | |
| Acetaminophen (Tylenol) | Alcohol | Increases risk for liver toxicity | Avoid alcohol. |
| **Antibiotic** | | | |
| Tetracyclines | Dairy products; iron supplements | Decreases drug absorption | Do not take with milk. Take 1 hour before or 2 hours after food or milk. |
| Amoxicillin, penicillin | Food | Decreases drug absorption | Take 1 hour before or 2 hours after meals. |
| Azithromycin (Zithromax), erythromycin | Food | Decreases drug absorption | Take 1 hour before or 2 hours after meals. |
| Nitrofurantoin (Macrobid) | Food | Decreases GI distress, slows drug absorption | Take with food or milk. |
| **Anticoagulant** | | | |
| Warfarin (Coumadin) | Foods rich in vitamin K | Decreases drug effectiveness | Limit foods high in vitamin K: liver, broccoli, spinach, kale, cauliflower, and Brussels sprouts. |
| **Antifungal** | | | |
| Griseofulvin (Fulvicin) | High-fat meal | Increases drug absorption | Take with high-fat meal. |
| **Antihistamine** | | | |
| Diphenhydramine (Benadryl), chlorpheniramine (Chlor-Trimeton) | Alcohol | Increases drowsiness | Avoid alcohol. |
| **Antihypertensive** | | | |
| Felodipine (Plendil), nifedipine | Grapefruit juice | Increases drug absorption | Consult physician or pharmacist before changing diet. |
| **Anti-inflammatory** | | | |
| Naproxen (Aleve) | Food or milk | Decreases GI irritation | Take with food or milk. |
| Ibuprofen (Motrin) | Alcohol | Increases risk for liver damage or stomach bleeding | Avoid alcohol. |
| **Diuretic** | | | |
| Spironolactone (Aldactone) | Food | Decreases GI irritation | Take with food. |
| **Psychotherapeutic (MAO Inhibitors)** | | | |
| Tranylcypromine (Parnate) | Foods high in tyramine: aged cheeses, Chianti wine, pickled herring, brewer's yeast, fava beans | Risk for hypertensive crisis | Avoid foods high in tyramine. |

**Note:** Grapefruit juice contains a compound not found in other juices. This compound increases the absorption of some drugs and can enhance their effects. Talk with your pharmacist or doctor to see if your medicine is affected by grapefruit juice before changing your routine.

**Source:** Bobroff LB, Lentz A, Turner RE. *Food/Drug and Drug/Nutrient Interactions: What You Should Know About Your Medications.* Gainesville, FL: University of Florida; March 2009. Publication FCS 8092 in a series of the Department of Family, Youth and Community Sciences, Florida Cooperative Extension Service, Institute of Food and Agricultural Sciences. http://edis.ifas.ufl.edu/pdffiles/HE/HE77600.pdf. Accessed 8/8/11. Reprinted by permission.

medications or are on long-term drug therapy, they may find themselves at increased nutritional risk.

Herbal supplements and vitamins or minerals in high doses should be viewed as drugs, particularly when taken in conjunction with prescription or over-the-counter medications. Although herbal products almost certainly interact with other medicines, many interactions are not well documented. In addition to the health and safety issues, supplement therapies can be costly. It is critical that older adults tell their healthcare providers all the drugs and supplements that they take on a regular basis so possible interactions can be identified and avoided.

## Depression

Many studies report high levels of well-being among older adults, especially those who remain independent. Although depression is one of the most common psychological effects of aging, it is most common among institutionalized and low-income people.

In later life, life transitions and stressful events can become frequent companions that increase the likelihood and severity of depression. Among these stressors are the loss of loved ones, including spouse and friends; physical disability; perceived loss of physical attractiveness; inability to psychologically defend oneself from unpleasant events; inability to care for oneself, which forces one to depend upon caregivers and long-term care; social isolation; and, inevitably, the approach of death. In older adults, depression often leads to malnutrition and may manifest itself as either anorexia (loss of appetite) or obesity.

Alcoholism is prevalent among socially isolated or depressed older adults. People who consume excessive amounts of alcohol often have diets low in essential nutrients.

## Anorexia of Aging

Poor food intake that accompanies age can result from **anorexia of aging**. Reductions in appetite and food intake contribute to undernutrition in older adults.[81] Malnutrition, in turn, can contribute to numerous problems, including immune deficiencies, anemia, falls, and cognitive decline. It can be difficult to pinpoint treatment strategies for anorexia in older people. However, treating even one aspect of the problem can provide at least temporary improvement. Unfortunately, lifelong inappropriate food habits, social factors, living conditions, and fear of injury may interfere with a person's ability and desire to stay or become healthy.

**Key Concepts** *Among the problems older adults face are lack of appetite and the side effects and interactions of medications they use. Medicines have the potential to interact with food and nutrients in the diet, and a lack of knowledge of these possibilities increases the risk for harmful effects. Although many older adults have high levels of well-being, depression is common among institutionalized and low-income seniors.*

## Arthritis

*Arthritis* is a general term that describes more than 100 diseases that cause pain and swelling of joints and connective tissue. (See **Figure 13.17**.) Arthritis is a chronic, lifelong affliction that, at its worst, can make movement difficult or even impossible. Unfortunately, there is no proven cure for arthritis. At best, appropriate treatment programs reduce symptoms. In terms of nutrition, arthritis pain may impair appetite or make it hard to prepare meals, and some arthritis medications may interfere with nutrient absorption. These factors underscore the importance of a nutrient-dense diet for arthritis sufferers.

Weight management is important in treating arthritis. Excess weight puts undue pressure on the hips and knees. Weight loss by people who are overweight or obese may reduce the risk of developing osteoarthritis, particularly of the knee.[82]

## Bowel and Bladder Regulation

As a result of physiological and lifestyle changes, older adults are susceptible to problems with their bowels and bladder. Inadequate hydration not only affects the bladder, but it also makes constipation more likely. Age-related

**anorexia of aging** Loss of appetite and wasting associated with old age.

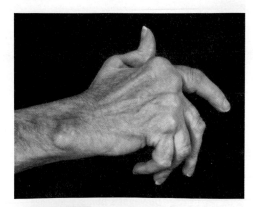

**Figure 13.17** **Arthritis.** Degeneration of the finger joints can cause a debilitating lack of function.

## *Quick* Bite

### Why Elephants Don't Need Dentures

Elephants are the only mammals with a built-in tooth replacement system. As they age, elephants go through six sets of teeth, changing about every 10 years. When elephants are around 70 years old, about the maximum life span, the last set of molars wears out.

decreases in intestinal motility and transit time, accompanied by poor food intake, may exacerbate the problem. In addition, lack of physical activity contributes to loss of muscle tone needed for regular elimination.

Chronic constipation is one of the most common health complaints among older adults. Excessive use of laxatives may cause nutritional deficiencies by decreasing transit time and preventing adequate absorption of nutrients. Decreased transit time also reduces water reabsorption by the GI tract and contributes to dehydration.

Increasing dietary fiber and fluid is one of the most effective treatments for bowel and bladder problems. Older adults should gradually switch to—and then maintain—a high-fiber diet. They also should be careful to maintain adequate fluid intake and exercise regularly. Supplementation with prebiotics, such as fructooligosaccharides, and probiotics, such as *Lactobacillus acidophilus*, also may improve the older adult's gastrointestinal health.[83]

**Key Concepts** *Arthritis and changes in bowel and bladder habits are common problems in older adults. Weight management is an important component of arthritis treatment. Because of increased risk of dehydration and constipation, older adults should be encouraged to follow a high-fiber diet and consume plenty of fluids.*

## Dental Health

The mouth is the gateway to the rest of the gastrointestinal system. Poor oral health can impair the ability to eat and obtain adequate nutrition. Missing teeth or poorly fitting dentures make some older adults self-conscious about eating, which leaves them unable to eat comfortably in public. Mouth pain and difficulty swallowing interfere with the process of eating, and tooth loss can alter choices and quality of food. Meats, fresh fruits, and fresh vegetables often are avoided. Oral infections affect the whole body and may increase the risk of other chronic diseases, including heart disease.

**macular degeneration** Progressive deterioration of the macula, an area in the center of the retina, that eventually leads to loss of central vision.

## Vision Problems

Poor vision and blindness interfere with the ability to buy and prepare food; visually impaired people cannot read food labels, cookbooks, or the settings on stoves or microwave ovens. **Macular degeneration** is a common disease of the eye that gradually leads to loss of vision. It affects about 6 percent of people between the ages of 65 and 74, and about 20 percent of those aged 75 to 85. Research has found that people with a higher intake of green leafy vegetables are less likely to develop this sight-robbing disorder. Greens, such as collards and spinach, show the most promise when consumed five or more times per week. By preventing free radical damage, antioxidants in these foods may protect the eye and the blood vessels that supply it. The National Eye Institute's Age-Related Eye Disease Study (AREDS) found that taking a specific high-dose formulation of antioxidants and zinc (beta-carotene; vitamins A, C, and E; copper; and zinc) significantly reduces the progression of advanced age-related macular degeneration and its associated vision loss.[84]

## Osteoporosis

Osteoporosis is the deterioration of bone structure (see **Figure 13.18**) until, often without warning, the fragile bone breaks upon the slightest impact. Although osteoporosis affects older adults of both genders, it is most common in postmenopausal women.

Nutritional factors, particularly early in life, are thought to play an important role in the development of osteoporosis. Although regular weight-bearing exercise helps prevent osteoporosis, inactivity increases osteoporosis risk.

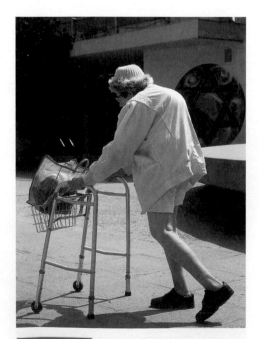

**Figure 13.18** **Dowager's hump.** A hunched back, sometimes called a dowager's hump, due to collapsed vertebrae, is a visible symptom of osteoporosis.

Long periods of inactivity, such as may be imposed by complete bed rest or illnesses that limit mobility, can promote the disease.

Although prevention is the best treatment for osteoporosis, many people enter later life with bad habits—poor nutrition and physical inactivity—that put them at risk. Adopting a diet that is rich in calcium and vitamin D and engaging in regular physical activity, particularly weight-bearing exercises, minimizes osteoporosis risks.

## Alzheimer's Disease

Among its other ravages, **Alzheimer's disease (AD)** eventually destroys a person's ability to obtain, prepare, and consume an optimal diet. Although much more research is needed to determine their effects, antioxidants may offer some protection from the disease.[85]

Most cases of Alzheimer's disease begin after age 70, but it can strike genetically predisposed people at a younger age. During the first stage of the disease, the afflicted person may gradually lose their sense of smell, but, because it begins to change gradually, it may not be readily noticed.

As the disease progresses, the person becomes unable to complete simple tasks that require learned motor movement, such as using a can opener. There is an increase in behavior problems, including wandering, and, if problems occur frequently, it can affect the person's ability to maintain weight and nutritional status.

In late stages of the disease about one-third of those with AD develop overactivity, which drains the nutritional reserve and increases calorie needs. At each stage, the caregiver must carefully plan the person's diet to meet psychological and physical needs, paying particular attention to optimum nutrition without excess weight gain.

**Key Concepts** *Oral health, vision, and bone health all decline with aging. Tooth loss and oral pain can reduce food intake and nutrient quality. Loss of vision can make food shopping and preparation difficult. Osteoporosis, most common in postmenopausal women, can cause debilitating fractures. Alzheimer's disease eventually destroys the ability to obtain, prepare, and consume an optimal diet. Management of these conditions depends first on their identification by healthcare professionals.*

# Meal Management for Mature Adults

Many older adults are at nutritional risk because of economics, social isolation, physical restrictions, inability to shop for or prepare food, and medical conditions. Fortunately, there are a number of ways that older people can remain independent and have access to an adequate diet.

## Managing Independently

Independent and assisted-living programs allow people to live relatively care-free yet independent lives. Senior citizen apartment buildings and retirement villages offer a variety of services, including balanced meals. Programs such as **Meals on Wheels** and the **Older Americans Act Nutrition Program** (formerly known as the Elderly Nutrition Program) provide meals to homebound people as well as those in congregate (group) settings. Most programs provide meals at least five times per week. The Older Americans Act Nutrition Program is supported primarily with federal funds; volunteer time, in-kind donations, and participant contributions make up the remainder. The Supplemental Nutrition Assistance Program (SNAP), formerly the *Food Stamp Program*, is another option that provides low-income elderly households with the means to purchase food. Unfortunately, because SNAP carries a "welfare"

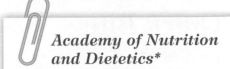

*Academy of Nutrition and Dietetics\**

**Nutrition Across the Spectrum of Aging**
It is the position of the American Dietetic Association that older Americans receive appropriate care; have broadened access to coordinated, comprehensive food and nutrition services; and receive the benefits of ongoing research to identify the most effective food and nutrition programs, interventions, and therapies across the spectrum of aging.

**Source:** Position of the Academy of Nutrition and Dietetics: nutrition across the spectrum of aging. *J Am Diet Assoc.* 2005;105(4):616–633.

\* Formerly the American Dietetic Association

**Alzheimer's disease (AD)** A presenile dementia characterized by accumulation of plaques in certain regions of the brain and degeneration of a certain class of neurons.

**Meals on Wheels** A voluntary, nonprofit organization established to provide nutritious meals to homebound people (regardless of age) so they may maintain their independence and quality of life.

**Older Americans Act Nutrition Program** A federally funded program (formerly known as the *Elderly Nutrition Program*) that provides older adults with nutritionally sound meals through meals-on-wheels programs or in senior citizen centers and similar congregate settings.

## Quick Bite

**Meno-What?**
Most animal species do not go through menopause.

**Table 13.12    Important Resources for Older Adults**

### Resource Directory for Older People
**http://www.aoa.gov**
The Resource Directory for Older People is a cooperative effort of the National Institute on Aging and the Administration on Aging. This directory provides resources for older adults, their caregivers and family members, and those in the legal and healthcare professions. Available via the Internet, it provides telephone numbers (some toll free), names, addresses, and fax numbers for organizations that work with older adults.

### The Eldercare Locator
**http://www.eldercare.gov**
**(800) 677-1116 (toll free)**
The National Association of Area Agencies on Aging and the National Association of State Units on Aging administer the Eldercare Locator, a public service of the Administration on Aging, U.S. Department of Health and Human Services. The Eldercare Locator is a nationwide directory-assistance service that helps older persons and their families identify resources for aging Americans.

stigma, some older adults are reluctant to use it. In addition, many people who need some help buying food do not meet the eligibility requirements. Participants in the Older Americans Act Nutrition Programs have improved food and nutrient intake levels compared to nonparticipants and have a higher number of regular social contacts—another important factor in eating well.[86] Participation in food assistance programs can also reduce the incidence of depression and overweight associated with food insecurity.[87]

## Wise Eating for One or Two

Preparing meals that are healthful and tasty is a challenge for those living alone or in small households. As discussed earlier in this chapter, our nutrition needs—with the exception of calories—do not decrease as we age, but our ability to meet them does. Reliance on convenience foods, fast foods, and eating out can adversely affect the nutritional status of older adults. Men who live alone are especially likely to eat out or skip meals rather than prepare food for themselves. For both men and women, physical disability or illness can quash the desire to prepare and eat meals.

Some simple changes in appliances and food-preparation techniques can help older adults overcome common obstacles to food preparation. Those who can't or won't cook can use microwave or toaster ovens and small appliances to prepare simple meals. A meal based on a lower-sodium, low-fat convenience entree can meet nutritional needs if accompanied by vegetables, whole-grain bread, milk, and fruit.

THINK
About It

4

## Finding Community Resources

An older person's need for community support typically changes from decade to decade. Sometimes identifying community resources can be challenging, and financial considerations may further limit access to resources that can assist older people in their own homes. Within local communities, area agencies on aging, social and rehabilitation services, cooperative extension services, churches, and extended-care facilities may have lists of resources and educational programs for older adults. Table 13.12 lists important resources for older adults.

**Key Concepts** *Older adults who obtain adequate food and nutrient intake while living independently may require assistance from time to time. This assistance may take the form of help with food shopping or preparation or identification of community resources that can stretch the food dollar. Numerous resources exist to assist older adults in maintaining a productive, high-quality life.*

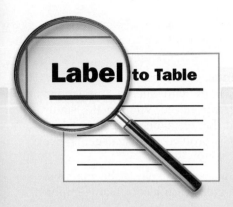

**Label to Table**

What is it about fruit snacks that attracts kids? The sweet flavors, bright colors, shapes, and logos of favorite movie or television characters? Probably all of these. Parents may be attracted by claims for vitamins. So are these nutritious snacks or little more than candy? Let's look at the label.

On the positive side, this is a fat-free snack and contains little sodium. However, most of the calories, 56 of 80, come from sugar (14 grams × 4 kilocalories per gram), and the remainder from starch and protein. The ingredient list shows that the first three ingredients are sugars: corn syrup, sucrose, and fruit juice from concentrate.

The vitamins added to fruit snacks are the only redeeming feature of the product, providing 25 percent of the DV for vitamins A, C, and E. But is there a better way to get these nutrients? One-half cup of orange juice provides two-thirds of the DV for vitamin C and significant amounts of thiamin, folate, and potassium as well. Just a handful of baby carrots provides more than 100% DV for vitamin A, along with some fiber. Vitamin E is widespread in the food supply—a small amount of salad dressing as a dip for the carrots would add vitamin E.

So, the fruit snacks are not as devoid of nutrients as candy, but they are not as nutrient-dense as fruits and vegetables. The fruit snacks may have some nutrient value, but they are high in sugar and, like all sugary snacks, should be limited.

## Nutrition Facts

Serving Size: 1 pouch (26g/0.9 oz)
Servings Per Container 10

Amount Per Serving

**Calories** 80

| | % Daily Value* |
|---|---|
| **Total Fat** 0g | |
| **Sodium** 15mg | 0% |
| **Total Carbohydrate** 19g | 1% |
| Sugars 14g | 6% |
| **Protein** 1g | |

Vitamin A    25%
(100% as beta carotene)
Vitamin C    25%
Vitamin E    25%

Not a significant source of calories from fat, saturated fat, trans fat, cholesterol, dietary fiber, calcium, or iron.

*Percent Daily Values are based on a 2,000 calorie diet. Your daily values may be higher or lower depending on your calorie needs:

| | | Calories: | 2,000 | 2,500 |
|---|---|---|---|---|
| Total Fat | Less Than | | 65g | 80g |
| Sat Fat | Less Than | | 20g | 25g |
| Cholesterol | Less Than | | 300mg | 300mg |
| Sodium | Less Than | | 2,400mg | 2,400mg |
| Total Carbohydrate | | | 300g | 375g |
| Dietary Fiber | | | 25g | 30g |

Calories per gram:
Fat 9   •   Carbohydrate 4   •   Protein 4

# *Learning* Portfolio

## Key Terms

## Study Points

- For children and adolescents, growth is the key determinant of nutrient needs. If diets are planned carefully, children do not need vitamin/mineral supplementation.

- Federally funded nutrition and feeding programs reduce malnutrition and hunger among American children.

- Adoption of adult-style diets to reduce risk of chronic disease should begin gradually after the age of 3.

- Obesity and eating disorders are increasing among American children and teens; treatment programs should address food choices and activity levels rather than impose strict calorie limits. Vegetarian diets for children need to be planned carefully to avoid nutrient deficiencies.

- Total energy and nutrient needs of adolescents are high to support growth and maturation. Girls need more iron than boys do to compensate for losses after the onset of menstruation. Active teens need more calories and nutrients than sedentary teens; fluid intake also is a priority.

- Nutrition and physical activity are two important, controllable components of a healthy life and healthful aging. Moreover, numerous physiological and psychological aspects of the aging process affect food intake and nutritional status.

- Energy needs decline with age, reflecting loss of lean body mass and reduced physical activity. The protein RDA and the recommended balance of carbohydrate and fat calories in the diet are similar for young and older adults. Fluid intake needs special attention due to the reduced thirst response that occurs with age.

- Because of reduced intake, synthesis, and activation, vitamin D status declines with age; recommended intake levels are therefore raised. Vitamin $B_{12}$ status may be compromised due to inadequate absorption. Antioxidants may help protect against degenerative diseases.

- Calcium and zinc intakes are likely to be marginal in the diets of older adults. Iron also remains important.

- Dietary supplements, both vitamin/mineral and herbal/botanical, should be used with caution, preferably with professional advice.

- Because many older adults take multiple medications, they are at risk for drug–nutrient, food–drug, and drug–drug interactions. Anorexia of aging also is a major public health problem.

- Arthritis is a prevalent chronic health problem in this age group. Weight management is a key element of arthritis treatment.

- Chronic constipation is a common complaint among older adults. Fluids, fiber, and regular exercise can reduce the likelihood of constipation.

- Both poor oral and visual health can compromise the ability of older adults to consume a nutritionally adequate diet.

- Osteoporosis is a major health problem that can be addressed through adequate calcium, vitamin D, regular weight-bearing exercise, and medication, if needed.

- Adults can maintain independence while aging but may require special assistance to obtain and prepare food. Community resources can help respond to the needs of older adults and those of their caretakers and family.

## Study Questions

1. Which vitamins and minerals are most likely to be deficient in a child's diet?

2. Describe the hunger and malnutrition that occur in U.S. households. What federal programs help to address these problems?

3. Identify several chronic nutrition problems that can affect children. How can these problems be avoided?

4. What are typical nutritional concerns for adolescents?

5. What are some consequences of decreased immunity among older adults?

6. Compared with a younger adult, does a person older than 65 need more, less, or about the same amount of protein?

7. Why are older adults at risk of vitamin D deficiency?

8. Discuss minerals that may need special attention in assessment of an older adult's nutrition status.

9. What problems might older adults encounter with dietary supplements?

10. What is the role of physical activity in osteoporosis prevention? What nutritional factors are important?

## Try This

### Eat Like a Kid

Children, especially toddlers, tend to be exploratory, and take in the sensory nature of food—the textures, smells, and tastes. In fact, you were probably once this way. The purpose of this exercise is to eat a meal like a kid and gain an appreciation of food's textures and taste. Make some mashed potatoes, macaroni and cheese, buttered peas, or spaghetti (favorite "kid food") and eat it with your fingers. Explore your food and play with it. Try mixing foods. How does this experience make you feel?

### Aging Simulation

The purpose of this exercise is to simulate what it can be like to age and experience age-related declines in health. Have you ever thought of how difficult it is to be an older person with health problems and do routine tasks? Invite a few friends over and do the following, one per person for each activity:

- Put gloves on to simulate the difficulty of losing sensitivity in your hands.
- Use cotton balls in your ears to decrease your hearing ability.
- Apply some petroleum jelly to a pair of glasses or sunglasses to give yourself poor vision.

Now try a simple activity. Make a salad, or put a CD in your CD player and listen to it. After completing the activity, switch disabilities with your friends so everyone has experienced each of the limitations. What is it like to do these everyday activities with your impairment?

## What About Bobbie?

Let's pretend that Bobbie is in her sixties and has just read a newspaper article about how older people may have low intakes of vitamins E and $B_6$, magnesium, calcium, and iron. How do you think her diet compares to the needs of a 65-year-old woman? (You may want to review her one-day intake in the "Food Choices: Nutrients and Nourishment" chapter.) Although her calorie intake is probably much higher than that of most women in their sixties, let's look at her intake of these vitamins and minerals.

Bobbie was close to her RDA or AI for vitamin $B_6$, magnesium, and zinc, but her intake was lower for vitamin E and calcium. Because Bobbie's fat intake was ample, this low value for vitamin E probably reflects a lack of complete data for the vitamin E content of foods. As is true of many women in their sixties who have inadequate calcium intake, this increases Bobbie's risk of osteoporosis.

### Vitamin E

| | |
|---|---|
| RDA | 15 mg |
| Bobbie's intake | 9 mg |

### Vitamin $B_6$

| | |
|---|---|
| RDA | 1.5 mg |
| Bobbie's intake | 2.0 mg |

### Magnesium

| | |
|---|---|
| RDA | 320 mg |
| Bobbie's intake | 310 mg |

### Calcium

| | |
|---|---|
| RDA | 1,200 mg |
| Bobbie's intake | 710 mg |

### Zinc

| | |
|---|---|
| RDA | 8 mg |
| Bobbie's intake | 12 mg |

## References

1  Institute of Medicine, Food and Nutrition Board. *Dietary Reference Intakes for Energy, Carbohydrate, Fiber, Fat, Fatty Acids, Cholesterol, Protein, and Amino Acids.* Washington, DC: National Academies Press; 2002.

2  Kleinman RE, ed. *Pediatric Nutrition Handbook.* 6th ed. Elk Grove Village, IL: American Academy of Pediatrics; 2008; and Nicklas T, Johnson R, Academy of Nutrition and Dietetics. Position of the American Dietetic Association: nutrition guidance for healthy children ages 2 to 11 years. *J Am Diet Assoc.* 2008;108:1038–1047.

3  Kleinman RE, ed. Op. cit.

4  Nicklas T, Johnson R, Academy of Nutrition and Dietetics. Op. cit.

5  Neelon SE, Briley ME, Academy of Nutrition and Dietetics. Position of the American Dietetic Association: benchmarks for nutrition in child care. *J Am Diet Assoc.* 2011;111:607–615.

6  Pearson N, Biddle SJ. Sedentary behavior and dietary intake in children, adolescents, and adults: a systematic review. *Am J Prev Med.* 2011;41(2):178–188.

7  Kelly B, Halford JCG, Boyland EJ, et al. Television food advertising to children: a global perspective. *Am J Pub Health.* 2011;100(9):1730–1736.

8  Batada A, Seitz M, Wootan M. Nine out of 10 food advertisements shown during Saturday morning children's television programming are for foods high in fat, sodium, or added sugars, or low in nutrients. *J Am Diet Assoc.* 2008;108(4):673–678.

9  Boyland EJ, Harrold JA, Kirkham TC, et al. Food commercials increase preference for energy-dense foods, particularly in children who watch more television. *Pediatrics.* 2011;128(1):e93–e100.

10    Miller SA, Taveras EM, Rifas-Shiman SL, Gillman MW. Association between television viewing and poor diet quality in young children. *Int J Pediatr Obes*. 2008;3(3):168–176.

11    World Food Programme. Hunger stats. http://www.wfp.org/hunger/stats. Accessed 8/4/11.

12    Let's move! Child nutrition reauthorization Healthy Hunger-Free Kids Act of 2010 fact sheet. http://www.whitehouse.gov/sites/default/files/Child_Nutrition_Fact_Sheet_12_10_10.pdf. Accessed 8/4/11; and Nord M, Coleman-Jensen A, Andrews M, Carlson S. *Household Food Security in the United States, 2009*. ERR-108. US Department of Agriculture, Economic Research Service; November 2010.

13    Let's move! Child nutrition reauthorization Healthy Hunger-Free Kids Act of 2010 fact sheet. Op. cit.

14    Ibid.

15    American Psychiatric Association. *Diagnostic and Statistical Manual of Mental Disorders*. 4th ed. (DSM-IV). Washington, DC: American Psychiatric Association; 2000.

16    Kim Y, Chang H. Correlation between attention deficit hyperactivity disorder and sugar consumption, quality of diet, and dietary behavior in school children. *Nutr Res Pract*. 2011;5(3):236–245.

17    Stevens LJ, Kuczek T, Burgess JR, Hurt E, Arnold LE. Dietary sensitivities and ADHD symptoms: thirty-five years of research. *Clin Pediatr* (Phila). 2011;50(4):279–293; and McCann D, Barrett A, Cooper A, et al. Food additives and hyperactive behaviour in 3-year-old and 8/9-year-old children in the community: a randomised, double-blinded, placebo-controlled trial. *Lancet*. 2007;370:1560–1567.

18    Pelsser LM, Frankena K, Toorman J, et al. Effects of a restricted elimination diet on the behaviour of children with attention-deficit hyperactivity disorder (INCA study): a randomised controlled trial. *Lancet*. 2011;377: 494–503.

19    Ogden CL, Carroll MD, Curtin LR, Lamb MM, Flegal KM. Prevalence of high body mass index in US children and adolescents, 2007–2008. *JAMA*. 2010;303:242–249.

20    Gable S, Britt-Rankin J, Krull JL. Ecological predictors and developmental outcomes of persistent childhood overweight. CCR-42. US Department of Agriculture, Economic Research Service; 2008.

21    Let's Move! http://www.letsmove.gov. Accessed 8/4/11.

22    Ibid.

23    Daniels SR, Greer FR, Committee on Nutrition. Lipid screening and cardiovascular health in childhood. *Pediatrics*. 2008;122:198–208.

24    *Healthy People 2020*. Environmental health. http://www.healthypeople.gov/2020/topicsobjectives2020/overview.aspx?topicid=12. Accessed 8/4/11.

25    Wengrovitz AM, Brown MJ, Advisory Committee on Childhood Lead Poisoning. Recommendations for blood lead screening of Medicaid-eligible children aged 1–5 years: an updated approach to targeting a group at high risk. *MMWR*. 2009;58(RR09):1–11.

26    Centers for Disease Control and Prevention. Lead. http://www.cdc.gov/lead. Accessed 8/4/11.

27    Craig WJ, Mangels AR, Academy of Nutrition and Dietetics. Position of the American Dietetic Association: vegetarian diets. *J Am Diet Assoc*. 2009; 109(7):1266–1282.

28    Wagner CL, Greer FR, Section on Breastfeeding and Committee on Nutrition. Prevention of rickets and vitamin D deficiency in infants, children, and adolescents. *Pediatrics*. 2008;122(5):1142–1152.

29    American Association of Pediatrics. Children's health topics. Vitamin D. http://www.aap.org/healthtopics/vitamind.cfm. Accessed 8/4/11.

30    Kleinman RE, ed. Op. cit.

31    Institute of Medicine, Food and Nutrition Board. *Dietary Reference Intakes for Calcium and Vitamin D*. Washington, DC: National Academies Press; 2011.

32    Park S, Sappenfield WM, Huang Y, Sherry B, Bensyl DM. The impact of the availability of school vending machines on eating behavior during lunch: the Youth Physical Activity and Nutrition Survey. *J Am Diet Assoc*. 2010;110(10):1532–1536.

33    Minaker LM, Storey KE, Raine KD, et al. Associations between the perceived presence of vending machines and food and beverage logos in schools and adolescents' diet and weight status. *Public Health Nutr*. 2011;14(8):1350–1356; and Fox MK, Dodd AH, Wilson A, Gleason PM. Association between school food environment and practices and body mass index of US public school children. *J Am Diet Assoc*. 2009;109(suppl 2):S108–S117.

34    Centers for Disease Control and Prevention. Overweight and obesity. A growing problem. Updated 4/21/11. http://www.cdc.gov/obesity/childhood/problem.html. Accessed 8/5/11.

35    Reedy J, Krebs-Smith SM. Dietary sources of energy, solid fats, and added sugars among children and adolescents in the United States. *J Am Diet Assoc*. 2010;110:1477–1484; and Centers for Disease Control and Prevention. Beverage consumption among high school students—United States, 2010. *MMWR*. 2011;60(23):778–780.

36    Let's move! Child nutrition reauthorization Healthy Hunger-Free Kids Act of 2010 fact sheet. Op. cit.

37    Pasch KE, Lytle LA, Samuelson AC, Farbakhsh K, Kubik MY, Patnode CD. Are school vending machines loaded with calories and fat? An assessment of 106 middle and high schools. *J Sch Health*. 2011;81(4):212–218.

38    Fox MK, Gordon A, Nogales R, Wilson A. Availability and consumption of competitive foods in US public schools. *J Am Diet Assoc*. 2009;109(suppl 2):S57–S66.

39    Rovner AJ, Nansel TR, Wang J, Iannotti RJ. Food sold in school vending machines is associated with overall student dietary intake. *J Adolesc Health*. 2011;48(1):13–19.

40    American Academy of Pediatrics Committee on Nutrition and the Council on Sports Medicine. Clinical report—sports drinks and energy drinks for children and adolescents: are they appropriate? *Pediatrics*. 2011;127:1182–1189.

41    Centers for Disease Control and Prevention. Beverage consumption among high school students. Op. cit.

42    Ibid.

43    Danby FW. Nutrition and acne. *Clin Dermatol*. 2010;28(6):598–604; and Spencer EH, Ferdowsian HR, Barnard ND. Diet and acne: a review of the evidence. *Int J Dermatol*. 2009;48:339–347.

44    Marcason W. Milk consumption and acne—is there a link? *J Am Diet Assoc*. 2010;110(1):152.

45    Berra B, Rizzo AM. Glycemic index, glycemic load: new evidence for a link with acne. *J Am Coll Nutr*. 2009;28(suppl):450S–454S.

46    Nader PR, Bradley RH, Houts RM, et al. Moderate-to-vigorous physical activity from ages 9 to 15 years. *JAMA*. 2008;300:295–305.

47    Centers for Disease Control and Prevention. Overweight and obesity. The basics about childhood obesity. Updated 5/26/11. http://www.cdc.gov/obesity/childhood/basics.htm. Accessed 8/5/11.

48    Ibid.

49    Centers for Disease Control and Prevention. Overweight and obesity. A growing problem. Op. cit.

50    Watson LC, Kwon J, Nichols D, Rew M. Evaluation of the nutrition knowledge, attitudes, and food consumption behaviors of high school students before and after completion of a nutrition course. *Fam Consumer Sci Res J*. 2009;37(4):523–534.

51    Johnston LD, O'Malley PM, Bachman JG, Schulenberg JE. *Monitoring the Future. National results on adolescent drug use: overview of key findings, 2010*. Ann Arbor: Institute for Social Research, The University of Michigan; 2011. http://www.monitoringthefuture.org/pubs/monographs/mtf-overview2010.pdf. Accessed 8/5/11.

52    Ibid.

53    Centers for Disease Control and Prevention. Alcohol quick stats: binge drinking. http://www.cdc.gov/alcohol/quickstats/binge_drinking.htm. Accessed 8/5/11.

54    Department of Health and Human Services, Administration on Aging. A profile of older Americans: 2010. http://www.aoa.gov/aoaroot/aging_statistics/Profile/2010/2.aspx. Accessed 8/7/11.

55    Department of Health and Human Services, Administration on Aging. Projected population by single year of age, sex, race, and Hispanic origin for the United States: July 1, 2000 to July 1, 2050. 8/14/08. http://www.aoa.gov/AoARoot/Aging_Statistics/Minority_Aging/index.aspx. Accessed 7/30/11.

56    Federal Interagency Forum on Aging Related Statistics. Older Americans 2010. Key indicators of well-being. 2010. http://www.agingstats.gov/agingstatsdotnet/Main_Site/Data/2010_Documents/Docs/OA_2010.pdf. Accessed 8/7/11.

57    Bernstein MA, Luggen AS, eds. *Nutrition for the Older Adult*. Burlington, MA: Jones & Bartlett Learning; 2010.

58  Fiatarone-Singh MA, Bernstein MA. Exercise for the older adult: nutritional implications. In: Bernstein MA, Luggen AS, eds. Op. cit.

59  Ibid.

60  Salem GJ, Skinner JS, Chodzko-Zajko WJ, et al. Exercise and physical activity for older adults. *Med Sci Sports Exer*. 2009;41(7):1510–1530.

61  US Department of Health and Human Services. *2008 Physical Activity Guidelines for Americans*. ODPHP Publication No. U0036. Washington, DC: US Department of Health and Human Services; 2008.

62  Chodzko-Zajki W, Proctor D, Fiatarone-Singh M, et al. American College of Sports Medicine position stand. Exercise and physical activity for older adults. *Med Sci Sport Exerc*. 2009;41(7):1510–1530.

63  Larson Duyff R. Academy of Nutrition and Dietetics. *Complete Food and Nutrition Guide*. 3rd ed. Hoboken, NJ: John Wiley and Sons; 2006.

64  Moskovitz DN, Saltzman J, Kim YI. The aging gut. In: Chernoff R, ed. *Geriatric Nutrition: The Health Professional's Handbook*. 3rd ed. Burlington, MA: Jones & Bartlett Learning; 2006.

65  Paddon-Jones D, Rasmussen BB. Dietary protein recommendations and the prevention of sarcopenia. *Curr Opin Clin Nutr Metab Care*. 2009;12(1):86–90.

66  Institute of Medicine, Food and Nutrition Board. *Dietary Reference Intakes for Water, Potassium, Sodium, Chloride, and Sulfate*. Washington, DC: National Academies Press; 2004.

67  Ibid.

68  National Institutes of Health, Office of Dietary Supplements. Dietary supplement fact sheet. Vitamin D. http://ods.od.nih.gov/factsheets/vitamind/#en61. Accessed 8/7/11.

69  Ibid.

70  Institute of Medicine, Food and Nutrition Board. 2011. Op. cit.

71  Dangour AD, Breeze E, Clarke R, et al. Plasma homocysteine, but not folate or vitamin $B_{12}$, predicts mortality in older adults in the United Kingdom. *J Nutr*. 2008;138:1121–1128.

72  Haan MN, Miller JW, Aiello AE, et al. Homocysteine, B vitamins, and the incidence of dementia and cognitive impairment: results from the Sacramento Area Latino Study on Aging. *Am J Clin Nutr*. 2007;85(2):511–517.

73  Allen LH. How common is vitamin $B_{12}$ deficiency? *Am J Clin Nutr*. 2009;89(2):693S–696S.

74  Evans JR. Antioxidant vitamin and mineral supplements for slowing the progression of age-related macular degeneration. *Cochrane Database Syst Rev*. 2006 Apr 19;(2):CD000254.

75  Evans JR, Henshaw K. Antioxidant vitamin and mineral supplements for preventing age-related macular degeneration. *Cochrane Database Syst Rev*. 2008 Jan 23;(1):CD000253.

76  Devore E, Kang J, Stampfer M, Grodstein F. Total antioxidant capacity of diet in relation to cognitive function. *Am J Clin Nutr*. 2010;92:1157–1164.

77  Institute of Medicine, Food and Nutrition Board. 2011. Op. cit.

78  Ibid.

79  Nahin R, Pecha M, Welmerink D, et al. Concomitant use of prescription drugs and dietary supplements in ambulatory elderly people. *J Am Geriatric Soc*. 2009;57(7):1197–1205.

80  Buhr G, Bales CW. Nutritional supplements for older adults: review and recommendations—part I. *J Nutr Elder*. 2009;28(1):5–29.

81  Chapman IM. The anorexia of aging. *Clin Geriatr Med*. 2007;23(4):735–756.

82  National Institute of Arthritis and Musculoskeletal and Skin Diseases. Handout on health: osteoarthritis. Revised 7/10. http://www.niams.nih.gov/Health_Info/Osteoarthritis/default.asp. Accessed 8/8/11.

83  Sarubin Fragakis A, Thomson CA. *The Health Professional's Guide to Popular Dietary Supplements*. 3rd ed. Chicago: Academy of Nutrition and Dietetics; 2006.

84  National Eye Institute. The AREDS formulation and age-related macular degeneration. Are these high levels of antioxidants and zinc right for you? http://www.nei.nih.gov/amd/summary.asp. Accessed 8/8/11.

85  Devore E, Kang J, Stampfer M, Grodstein F. Op. cit.

86  Academy of Nutrition and Dietetics. Evidence Analysis Library. Nutrition across the spectrum of aging. Evidence Analysis project. Aging programs. http://www.adaevidencelibrary.com/topic.cfm?cat=4072. Accessed 8/30/11.

87  Kim K, Frongillo EA. Participation in food assistance programs modifies the relation of food insecurity with weight and depression in older adults. *J Nutr*. 2007;137:1005–1010.

# CHAPTER 14

# Food Safety and Technology: Microbial Threats and Genetic Engineering

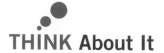

## THINK About It

1   Do you worry about getting sick from the food you eat?

2   To what extent do you rely on organically grown food to avoid pesticides?

3   What food safety measures, such as thawing meat in the refrigerator, do you practice at home?

4   Would genetically modified rice be welcome at your dinner table?

Visit **go.jblearning.com/inseldisco4e**

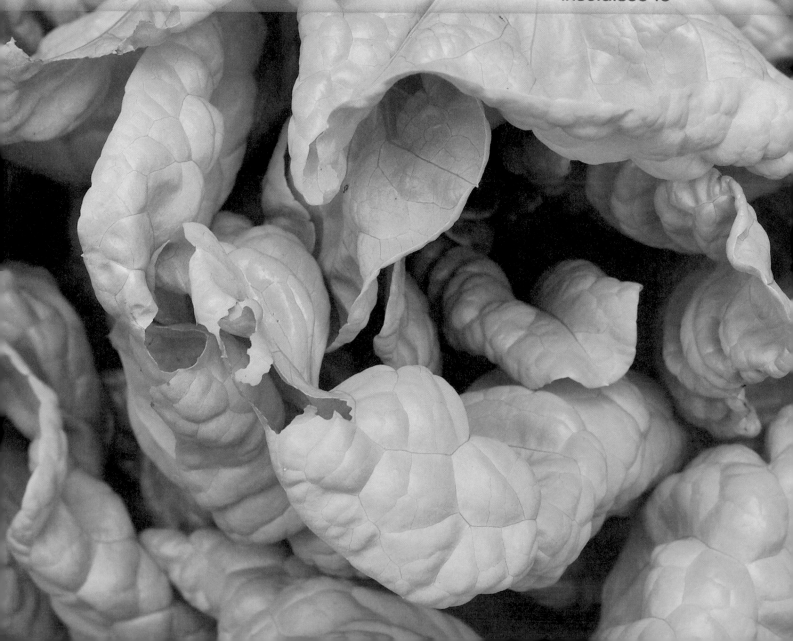

The newspaper headline screams, "Poorly Cooked Hamburger Meat Proves Fatal." You read further and discover that a child's death has been traced to bacteria thriving in undercooked hamburger meat. Additionally, several adults have become ill from the same source. This worries you. You hate well-done meat. You especially like your hamburgers blood red and your steaks rare. "Well," you ponder, "maybe I'll move my preferences up a notch to pink hamburgers and medium-rare steaks." Have you made the right choice? Or, should you investigate this issue further?

Although once confined mainly to cookbooks and textbooks, today food safety advice shows up in many places—the popular press, the classroom, even the *Dietary Guidelines for Americans, 2010*. What has prompted such enthusiasm? Recent headlines tell part of the story. In the 1990s, microbial contamination of such foods as hamburger, apple juice, eggs, raw sprouts, and frozen berries seriously sickened thousands and killed many, especially those most susceptible: young children, people with compromised immune systems, and seniors.

Consumers are voicing concerns about other food safety issues as well, including fears about excessive pesticide residues in plant foods, antibiotics and hormones in animals used for food, and hidden food allergens (e.g., nuts, milk, eggs) in prepared foods. Increasingly, consumers are checking prepared foods for ingredients to which they are allergic (e.g., caseinates as milk protein) and questioning preparation methods to avoid an allergen that may be an unintentional food additive (e.g., peanut material found in a milk chocolate candy might be residue left on machinery from earlier processing of peanut butter cups). Other, less frequently discussed food hazards include physical contamination with glass fragments and other sharp objects, heavy metals, and naturally occurring toxins in seafood and some agricultural products. (See **Figure 14.1**.)

## Food Safety

This chapter reviews major food safety hazards and touches on controversial issues such as the merits of organic foods, the use of food irradiation, and the production of genetically modified foods.

## Harmful Substances in Foods

In the United States and Canada most foodborne diseases are caused by microorganisms and can be prevented by preparers cleaning hands and surfaces, cooking foods sufficiently, and refrigerating foods promptly.

### Pathogens

In North America, most food safety experts agree that the chief cause of **foodborne illness** is pathogenic (disease-causing) microorganisms, including bacteria, viruses, and parasites. (See Table 14.1 for a list of common foodborne microbes and the serious illnesses they cause.) Researchers at the Centers for Disease Control and Prevention (CDC) estimate that each year approximately 48 million Americans (that's one in six) become sick, 128,000 require hospitalization, and 3,000 die from foodborne illnesses.[1] Foodborne illnesses are estimated to cost the United States $152 billion annually.[2] These figures take into account the estimated number of unrecognized and unreported food-caused illnesses. Such illnesses can range from relatively mild stomach upset to severe symptoms that can be fatal.

THINK About It 1

*Quick* Bite

**A Morbid Margin Note**
Every day more than 208,000 Americans get sick from something they ate. Fourteen of them die.

**foodborne illness** A sickness caused by food contaminated with microorganisms, chemicals, or other substances hazardous to human health.

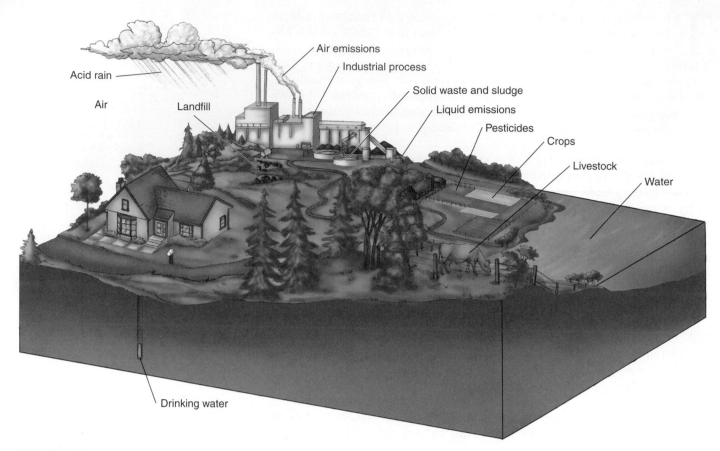

**Figure 14.1** **Heavy metals and other contaminants can be found in foods.** Industrial plants and automobiles release heavy metals and other contaminants into the air. Rainfall carries these contaminants to the soil. Plants for food crops and animal feed absorb contaminants from the soil. Runoff can pick up contaminants from pesticides, fertilizers, and animal manure. This pollutes surface water (lakes and streams), groundwater, and coastal water. Polluted water contaminates seafood and other fish that people eat.

**Table 14.1** ## Common Foodborne Pathogens and Illnesses

| Organism *Bacteria* | Sources | Diseases and Symptoms |
|---|---|---|
| *Campylobacter jejuni* | Raw poultry and meat and unpasteurized milk | Campylobacteriosis<br>*Onset:* usually 2 to 5 days after eating<br>*Symptoms:* diarrhea, stomach cramps, fever, bloody stools; lasts 7 to 10 days |
| *Clostridium botulinum* (illness is caused by a toxin produced by this organism) | Improperly canned foods, such as corn, green beans, soups, beets, asparagus, mushrooms, tuna, and liver pate; also, luncheon meats, ham, sausage, garlic in oil, lobster, and smoked and salted fish | Botulism<br>*Onset:* 18 to 36 hours after eating<br>*Symptoms:* nerve dysfunction, such as double vision, inability to swallow, speech difficulty, and progressive paralysis of respiratory system; can lead to death |
| *Escherichia coli* O157:H7 | Raw or undercooked meat, raw vegetables, unpasteurized milk, minimally processed ciders and juices, contaminated water | *E. coli* infection<br>*Onset:* 2 to 5 days after eating<br>*Symptoms:* watery and bloody diarrhea, severe stomach cramps, dehydration, colitis, neurological symptoms, stroke, and hemolytic uremic syndrome (HUS), a particularly serious disease in young children that can cause kidney failure and death |

| Table 14.1 | **Common Foodborne Pathogens and Illnesses** *(Continued)* |
|---|---|

| Organism | Sources | Diseases and Symptoms |
|---|---|---|
| *Listeria monocytogenes* | Soft cheeses, unpasteurized milk, hot dogs, luncheon meats, cold cuts, other deli-style meat and poultry<br>*Note:* resists salt, heat, nitrites, and acidity better than most microorganisms | Listeriosis<br>*Onset:* from 7 to 21 days after eating, but symptoms have been reported 9 to 48 hours after eating<br>*Symptoms:* fever, headache, nausea, and vomiting; primarily affects pregnant women and their fetuses, newborns, older adults, and people with cancer and compromised immune systems; can cause death in fetuses and babies |
| *Salmonella* | Raw or undercooked meats, poultry, eggs; raw milk and other dairy products; seafood; fresh produce, including raw sprouts; coconut; pasta; chocolate; foods containing raw eggs | Salmonellosis<br>*Onset:* 1 to 3 days after eating<br>*Symptoms:* nausea, abdominal cramps, diarrhea, fever, and headache |
| *Shigella* | Undercooked liquid or moist food that has been handled by an infected person | Shigellosis (bacillary dysentery)<br>*Onset:* 12 to 50 hours after eating<br>*Symptoms:* stomach cramps; diarrhea; fever; sometimes vomiting; and blood, pus, and mucus in stools |
| *Staphylococcus aureus* (illness is caused by a toxin produced by this organism) | Meat and poultry; egg products; tuna, potato, and macaroni salads; cream filled pastries and other foods left unrefrigerated for long periods<br>*Note: S. aureus* is frequently found in cuts on skin and in nasal passages | Staphylococcal food poisoning<br>*Onset:* 1 to 6 hours after eating<br>*Symptoms:* diarrhea, vomiting, nausea, stomach pain, and cramps; lasts 1 to 2 days |
| *Vibrio vulnificus* | Raw seafood, especially raw oysters | Vibrio infection<br>*Onset:* 1 to 7 days<br>*Symptoms:* chills, fever, nausea and vomiting, and possibly death, especially in people with underlying health problems |
| **Viruses**<br>Hepatitis A | Raw shellfish from polluted water, food handled by an infected person | Hepatitis A<br>*Onset:* average about 1 month after exposure<br>*Symptoms:* at first, malaise, loss of appetite, nausea, vomiting, and fever; after 3 to 10 days, jaundice and darkened urine; severe cases can result in liver damage and death |
| Noroviruses (Norwalk-like virus) | Raw shellfish from polluted water; salads, sandwiches, and other ready-to-eat foods handled by an infected person; noroviruses are highly contagious and spread rapidly from person to person due to the ease of transmission | Gastroenteritis<br>*Onset:* 1 to 3 days<br>*Symptoms:* nausea, vomiting, diarrhea, stomach pain, headache, and low-grade fever |
| **Protozoa**<br>*Anisakis* | Raw fish | Anisakiasis<br>*Onset:* 12 to 24 hours<br>*Symptoms:* abdominal pain; can be severe |
| *Cryptosporidium* | Food that comes in contact with sewage; contaminated water; foods handled by a person who did not wash hands after using the toilet | Cryptosporidiosis<br>*Onset:* 1 to 12 days<br>*Symptoms:* profuse watery stools, stomach pain, loss of appetite, vomiting, and low-grade fever |
| *Giardia lamblia* | Consumption of contaminated water, contamination of food by an infected person | Giardiasis<br>*Onset:* 1 to 3 days<br>*Symptoms:* diarrhea, abdominal cramps, nausea |
| *Toxoplasma gondii* | Raw or undercooked meat and, under certain conditions, unwashed fruits and vegetables; also, cats shed cysts in their feces during acute infection—organism may be transmitted to humans, if feces are handled | Toxoplasmosis<br>*Onset:* 10 to 13 days<br>*Symptoms:* fever, headache, rash, sore muscles diarrhea; can kill a fetus or cause severe defects, such as mental retardation |

## *Quick* Bite

### Is It Stomach Flu or Food Poisoning?

Both flu and food poisoning can produce similar symptoms—miserable vomiting, abdominal cramping, and diarrhea. Although we often do not know the exact cause, stomach flu tends to occur in the winter months and is preceded by other symptoms, such as sore throat. Food poisoning tends to occur in summer months, and symptoms usually appear suddenly without warning. Symptoms may not begin until 12 to 72 hours after eating tainted food. If many people who ate the same food get sick around the same time, it's probably food poisoning.

**botulism** An often fatal type of food poisoning caused by a toxin released from *Clostridium botulinum*, a bacterium that can grow in improperly canned low-acid foods.

***Salmonella*** Rod-shaped bacteria responsible for many foodborne illnesses.

***Escherichia coli (E. coli)*** Bacteria that are the most common cause of urinary tract infections. Because they release toxins, some types of *E. coli* can rapidly cause shock and death.

## *Quick* Bite

### Sticky *Salmonella*

One in four Americans suffer a foodborne illness each year. In 2009, people were reported sickened in 46 states and more than 3,200 products were recalled, costing the food industry over $1 billion. What made more than 700 people sick? Not the most likely foods, such as undercooked chicken and hamburgers but rather *Salmonella*-contaminated peanut butter and foods with peanut products.

Development of foodborne illness results from the interaction of three factors: the pathogen, the host, and the environment in which they exist and interact.[3] Foodborne illnesses can result directly from infection with a pathogen or from toxins produced by a pathogenic microorganism. For example, the bacterium *Staphylococcus aureus*, a common bacterium found on the skin of many healthy people, creates havoc with the gastrointestinal tract by producing a toxin. When food containing *S. aureus* stands unrefrigerated, the bacteria begin multiplying. After several hours, the expanding bacterial population can produce enough nasty toxin to cause nausea, vomiting, and abdominal cramps. Staphylococcal food poisoning is common and causes approximately 250,000 illnesses each year.[4] Fortunately, the illness usually dissipates after a day or so of vomiting and feeling miserable, with no further harmful effects. Another toxin-producing bacterium, *Clostridium botulinum*, causes the rare, but deadly, illness **botulism**. Improperly canned foods, as well as garlic in oil preparations, are sources of botulism. Honey can be contaminated with *C. botulinum*, but the acid in adult stomachs kills the bacteria. Infants produce insufficient amounts of stomach acid to kill *C. botulinum*, so even small amounts of contaminated honey can be fatal.

*Salmonella* bacteria cause more than 1 million cases of foodborne illness and almost 400 deaths each year, according to CDC estimates.[5] *Salmonella* bacteria are prevalent on poultry and in eggs as well as in a wide variety of other foods. Choosing eggs cooked "over easy" is potentially disastrous because inadequate cooking can leave you vulnerable to the misery of salmonellosis. (See the FYI feature "Safe Food Practices" for more information on how to protect yourself from foodborne illness.)

*Escherichia coli (E. coli)* are a diverse group of bacteria. Although most varieties are harmless, others can make you sick. Some types cause diarrhea, whereas others cause more serious illnesses, even death. Many foods, including eggs, dairy products, meat and poultry, seafood, fresh produce, unpasteurized juices, and cereal grains, can harbor these disease-causing bacteria.

Because bacteria and other infectious organisms are pervasive in the environment, the contamination of food can occur anywhere from the farm to your plate. Many organisms capable of causing foodborne illness in humans are naturally present in food-producing animals and their environment. For example, *Salmonella enteritidis* bacteria enter eggs directly from the egg-laying hen, and *E. coli* are normally present in the intestines of cattle. Microorganisms natural to the marine environment, but toxic to humans, can contaminate seafood. (See the FYI feature "Seafood Safety.")

Exposure to animal manure or sewage runoff can contaminate crops. Sewage runoff into rivers and streams also can contaminate fish that live there. In the food-processing stage, contamination can occur from dirty equipment, rodent droppings, improper food storage, and infectious employees who fail to wash their hands adequately or take proper precautions when handling food. Poor food safety practices in retail facilities and at home also can contaminate food.

Patterns of foodborne illness have changed dramatically over the last several decades as our food production has become more centralized. When food animals and produce were grown, prepared, and eaten on the family farm, the consequences of errors in food handling were generally limited to a single family. Now, much of the food we eat is mass-produced at central locations and distributed widely to restaurant chains and supermarkets. Although most food poisoning cases arise from poor food handling in homes and restaurants, contamination at a processing plant can make hundreds or even thousands of people ill. This can have nationwide implications and, therefore, receives intense national media attention.

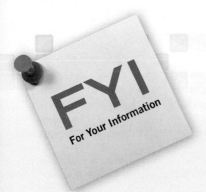

# Safe Food Practices

Because bacteria grow rapidly between 40°F and 140°F (4°C–60°C), most food should be kept out of this temperature range, known as the Danger Zone. Cold temperatures keep bacteria from multiplying; the fewer bacteria, the less the risk of illness. Proper cooking (or other heat treatment such as pasteurization) kills the bacteria. These principles serve as the basis for many of the following recommended food-handling practices.

## Buying Food

- Buy from reputable dealers and grocers who keep their selling areas and facilities clean and sanitary and maintain food at the appropriate temperature—for example, holding dairy foods, eggs, meats, seafood, and certain produce such as cut melons and raw sprouts at refrigerator temperatures.
- Don't buy foods in cans with dents or bulges. Avoid torn, crushed, or open food packages. Also, avoid buying packages that are above the frost line in the store's freezer. If the package cover is transparent, look for frost or ice crystals, signs that the product has been stored for a long time or thawed and refrozen.

## Storing Food

- Separate raw, cooked, and ready-to-eat foods while shopping, preparing, or storing.
- Refrigerate perishable items as quickly as possible after purchase. The refrigerator temperature should be 40°F or colder. Check it periodically with a thermometer to make sure the correct temperature is being maintained.
- Keep eggs in their original carton and store them in the refrigerator itself, not on the door, where the temperature is warmer.
- If raw meat, poultry products, or fresh seafood will be used within two days, store them in the coldest part of the refrigerator, usually under the freezer compartment or in a special "meat keeper." Store the packages loosely to allow air to circulate freely around each package, and be sure to wrap them tightly so raw juices can't leak out and contaminate other foods.
- If raw meat, poultry, and seafood will not be used within two days, store them in the freezer, which should have a temperature of 0°F. Check this temperature periodically, too, and adjust as needed.

- Read label directions for storing other foods; for example, mayonnaise and ketchup need to be refrigerated after they have been opened.
- Store potatoes and onions in a cool dark place but not under the sink because leakage from pipes can contaminate and damage them. Keep them away from household cleaning products and other chemicals as well.

## Preparing Food

- Wash hands thoroughly with warm, soapy water for at least 20 seconds before beginning food preparation and every time you handle raw foods, including fresh produce.
- Defrost meat, poultry, and seafood products in the refrigerator, microwave oven, or in a water-tight plastic bag submerged in cold water (the water must be changed every 30 minutes). Never defrost at room temperature—an ideal temperature for bacteria to grow and multiply.
- Marinate foods in the refrigerator. Discard the marinade after use because it contains raw juices, which may harbor bacteria; make a separate batch for basting food while cooking.
- Always use a clean cutting board. Wash cutting boards with hot water, soap, and a scrub brush. Then sanitize them in an automatic dishwasher or by rinsing with a solution of 5 milliliters (1 teaspoon) chlorine bleach to about 1 liter (1 quart) of water. If possible, use one cutting board for fresh produce and a separate one for raw meat, poultry, and seafood. Once cutting boards become excessively worn or develop hard-to-clean grooves, you should replace them.
- Before opening canned foods, wash the top of the can to prevent dirt from coming in contact with the food.
- Wash fresh fruits and vegetables thoroughly with cold water. It is not necessary to wash or rinse meat or poultry.

- Avoid eating dough or batter containing raw eggs because of the risk of *Salmonella enteritidis*, a bacterium that can live in eggs.

## Cooking Food

- Cook foods to the USDA Recommended Safe Minimum Internal Temperatures: 145°F for whole meats with a three-minute "rest period," 160°F for ground meats, and 165°F for all poultry.[1]
- The only safe way to know whether food is "done" is to use a food thermometer. According to USDA, one of every four hamburgers turns brown before reaching a safe internal temperature.
- During the three-minute "rest period" after meat is removed from the heat source, the internal temperature remains constant or continues to rise, which destroys pathogens.
- Never place cooked food on a plate that previously held raw meat, poultry, or seafood.
- When microwaving foods, rotate the dish and stir its contents several times to ensure even cooking. Follow recommended standing times, then check meat, poultry, and seafood products with a thermometer to make sure they have reached the correct internal temperature.
- Cook eggs until the white is firm and the yolk begins to harden.

## Serving Food

- Keep hot foods at 140°F or higher and cold foods at 40°F or lower.
- Refrigerate or freeze leftovers and perishables within two hours or sooner.
- Date leftovers so they can be used within a safe time—generally, three to five days in the refrigerator.

1    US Department of Agriculture, Food Safety and Inspection Service. USDA revises recommended cooking temperature for all whole cuts of meat, including pork, to 145°F. *Constituent Update*. 2011;13(21).

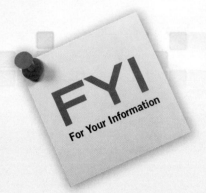

# Seafood Safety

Seafood can be a delicious and heart-healthy part of our diets. However, as with all food, contamination can have serious consequences. Seafood is one of the most rapidly perishable foods, so proper refrigeration and rapid processing and transport to the consumer are essential. Although certain types of microbial contaminants and toxins are unique to seafood, properly handled and cooked seafood is as safe to eat as most other foods. To kill seafood parasites, cook the fish or freeze it for at least 72 hours.

Eating raw seafood is risky business. Despite the popularity of such dishes as sashimi, sushi, and raw oysters, uncooked fish, no matter how carefully prepared, poses a risk for infection. People with liver disease, diabetes, cancer, or other diseases that impair immune function should be especially careful to stay away from

raw seafood. Pregnant women also should avoid uncooked seafood; some physicians recommend that pregnant women avoid seafood altogether. The rest of us should think twice before enjoying those raw oysters and sashimi and, at the very least, should make sure they are fresh and from a reliable source before letting those slippery delicacies pass our lips.

Seafood-related illness falls into several categories. Sources of infection include bacteria, viruses, and parasites. Toxins occur naturally in some fish, and human pollution may contaminate seafood. The following are several examples of seafood-caused illness:

- Raw or undercooked shellfish such as oysters, clams, and mussels may be contaminated with bacteria such as *Salmonella*, *Vibrio* species, and *Staphylococcus aureus*. Hepatitis A (caused by a virus) and gastroenteritis are other illnesses that can be contracted by eating uncooked shellfish from polluted waters.
- Fish such as mahi-mahi, tuna, and bluefish that have begun to spoil can cause scombroid poisoning. A toxin in these decomposing fish causes flushing, itching, and headache. Cooking does not destroy the toxin, so

the best prevention is proper refrigeration and rapid use of fresh fish.
- Some tropical fish, such as red snapper and barracuda, may contain ciguatera toxin, which can cause gastrointestinal and neurological problems in humans. Larger warm-water fish are most often implicated in this illness. The toxin is actually produced by tiny plants that are eaten by small fish. When larger fish consume many small fish, the toxin can accumulate. The flesh of these large fish may contain enough of the toxin to make humans very ill. Heating or freezing does not destroy this toxin.
- *Anisakis* is a parasite found in raw fish. After a person eats an infected fish, the larvae of this roundworm can invade the human stomach, causing severe abdominal pain. Cooking or freezing the fish for at least 72 hours can kill this parasite.
- Red tide is a well-known phenomenon in which huge numbers of tiny toxic organisms called dinoflagellates infest seawater. Shellfish in the area become poisonous as a result. Respiratory paralysis and death are possible effects of eating shellfish from red tide areas.

- Pollution is a serious problem, especially near population centers where industrial wastes and human sewage flow into the water. Heavy metals such as mercury can accumulate in larger fish (e.g., sharks, swordfish) that have been exposed to mercury in their environment for long periods. The *Dietary Guidelines for Americans, 2010* advise pregnant and breastfeeding women to limit white (albacore) tuna to 6 ounces per week and to completely avoid eating tilefish, shark, swordfish, and king mackerel.[1]
- Dioxin and polychlorinated biphenols (PCBs) also can accumulate in fish living in polluted water. Commercial seafood companies tend to avoid contaminated areas, but local fishers who frequently catch and eat fish from these waters may be at some risk.

1  US Department of Health and Human Services and US Department of Agriculture. *Dietary Guidelines for Americans, 2010*. Executive Summary. 2010. http://www.cnpp.usda.gov/Publications/DietaryGuidelines/2010/PolicyDoc/ExecSumm.pdf. Accessed 6/7/11.

## Table A  Understanding Seafood Safety

| Condition | Explanation |
| --- | --- |
| Scombroid poisoning | Scombroid poisoning is a type of food intoxication caused by the consumption of scombroid and scombroid-like marine fish species that have begun to spoil with the growth of particular types of food bacteria. Fish most commonly involved are members of the Scombridae family (tunas and mackerels) and a few nonscombroid relatives (bluefish, mahi-mahi, and amberjacks). The suspect toxin is an elevated level of histamine generated by bacterial degradation of substances in the muscle protein. |
| *Anisakis* | *Anisakis simplex* (herring worm) and *Pseudoterranova* (*Phocanema, Terranova*) *decipiens* (cod or seal worm) are anisakid nematodes (roundworms) that have been implicated in human infections caused by the consumption of raw or undercooked seafood. Anisakiasis is the term generally used to refer to the acute disease in humans. |
| Red tide | When temperature, salinity, and nutrients reach certain levels, algae grow very fast or "bloom" and accumulate into dense, visible patches near the surface of the water. Red tide is a common name for such a phenomenon where certain species of phytoplankton contain reddish pigments and "bloom" such that the water appears to be colored red. The term red tide is a misnomer because the reddish color is not associated with tides. A small number of species produce potent neurotoxins that can cause illness and even death. |
| Polychlorinated biphenols (PCBs) | A group of toxic, persistent chemicals used as insulation for electrical transformers and capacitors and as lubricants in gas pipeline systems. PCBs are a serious health problem because of their persistence in the environment, accumulation in the body, and potential for a long-term negative effect on health. In the United States, their manufacture was stopped in 1976. |

## Prions and Mad Cow Disease

**Bovine spongiform encephalopathy (BSE)**, also known as **mad cow disease**, is a chronic degenerative disease that affects the central nervous system of cattle. Once thought to infect only cows, scientists have found that BSE can cause a rare, but fatal, brain-wasting disease in humans.

Researchers believe that **prions**—proteins found in the cells of humans and other mammals—are responsible for BSE. When mammals eat tissues contaminated with abnormal prions, they can develop BSE. Cooking and irradiation do not kill or deactivate abnormal prions.

The skull, brain, eyes, vertebral column, and spinal cord of cows at least 30 months of age are most likely to harbor abnormal prions. The tonsils and a portion of the small intestine of all cattle also may contain the agent. To protect the safety of meat, milk, and dairy products, Canadian and U.S. agencies prohibit these cow parts in the human food supply. Government agencies also regulate and provide guidance to manufacturers who produce cow-derived foods, such as gelatin and some dietary supplements.

**Key Concepts** *Foodborne pathogens are a major cause of illness in the United States and Canada. Pathogenic (disease-causing) agents include bacteria, viruses, parasites, and prions. Contamination of food can occur at many points along the food processing chain from farm to table.*

## Chemical Contamination

To avoid foods exposed to chemicals, more and more people are turning to **organic foods**. (See the "Organic Alternatives" section in this chapter.) Yet food safety experts consider contamination by pathogenic microorganisms to create much greater risk to public health than contamination by chemicals. Chemical contaminants include pesticides, drugs, pollutants, and natural toxins.

## Pesticides

**Pesticides** play an important role in food production by controlling plant diseases, weeds, insects, and other pests. Pesticides protect crops and ensure a substantial yield, thus assuring consumers of a wide variety of foods at affordable prices. Without these chemicals, many argue that crop production would fall and prices for food would rise.

Every year, the U.S. Food and Drug Administration (FDA) collects thousands of domestic and imported food samples and analyzes them for pesticide residues.[6] During the period from 2004–2006, the FDA found no illegal residues in more than 98 percent of domestic or more than 94 percent of imported samples. When a violation occurred, it usually involved the use of a pesticide on crops for which it was not approved, rather than an excessive level. Results for the past 15 years have been fairly consistent.[7]

The FDA also samples and analyzes domestic and imported animal feeds for pesticide residues. This monitoring focuses on feeds for livestock and poultry—animals that become or produce foods for human consumption. Despite these reassuring results, concerns about pesticides in food persist. Processing methods can either reduce or concentrate pesticide residues in foods. (See **Figure 14.2**.) Infants and young children are particularly susceptible to the hazards of pesticides. Their small size and rapid growth make them especially vulnerable to pesticide residues, which can accumulate in their bodies over their lifetimes. Enacted in 1996, the Food Quality Protection Act includes landmark protections for the young. For the first time, manufacturers had to show that pesticide levels are safe for infants and children. In addition, when determining a safe level for a pesticide in a food, the Environmental Protection Agency (EPA) must account for the cumulative effect of exposures to similar pesticides and toxic chemicals.[8]

*Quick* **Bite**

**How Many *Salmonella* Does It Take?**
In 1994, 224,000 people in 41 states came down with *Salmonella* food poisoning from eating contaminated ice cream. The amazing part? The ice cream contained only about six *Salmonella* bacteria per serving.

**bovine spongiform encephalopathy (BSE)** A chronic degenerative disease, widely referred to as *mad cow disease*, that affects the central nervous system of cattle.

**mad cow disease** See *bovine spongiform encephalopathy (BSE)*.

**prions** Short for *proteinaceous infectious particle*. Self-reproducing protein particles that can cause disease.

**organic foods** Foods that originate from farms or handling operations that meet the standards set by the USDA National Organic Program. The methods of organic food production eschew modern synthetic pesticides and chemical fertilizers—organic foods do not contain genetically modified organisms and are not processed using irradiation, industrial solvents, or chemical food additives.

**pesticides** Chemicals used to control and kill insects, diseases, weeds, fungi, and other pests on plants, vegetables, fruits, and animals.

*Quick* **Bite**

**A Not So Dirty Dozen**
The Environmental Working Group (EWG), an environmental advocacy organization, publishes an annual list of the "Dirty Dozen"—fruits and vegetables suspected of having the greatest potential for contamination with pesticide residues. According to UC Davis researchers, however, the "findings conclusively demonstrate that consumer exposures to the 10 most frequently detected pesticides on EWG's 'Dirty Dozen' commodity list are at negligible levels and that the EWG methodology is insufficient to allow any meaningful rankings among commodities."

**integrated pest management (IPM)** Economically sound pest control techniques that minimize pesticide use, enhance environmental stewardship, and promote sustainable systems.

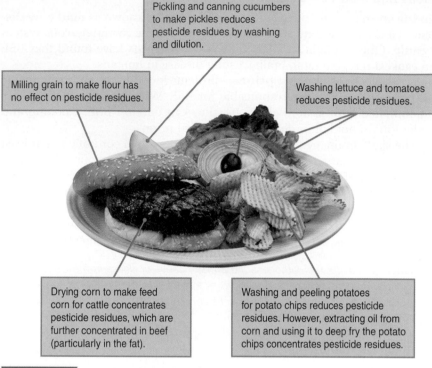

Pickling and canning cucumbers to make pickles reduces pesticide residues by washing and dilution.

Milling grain to make flour has no effect on pesticide residues.

Washing lettuce and tomatoes reduces pesticide residues.

Drying corn to make feed corn for cattle concentrates pesticide residues, which are further concentrated in beef (particularly in the fat).

Washing and peeling potatoes for potato chips reduces pesticide residues. However, extracting oil from corn and using it to deep fry the potato chips concentrates pesticide residues.

**Figure 14.2** **Pesticide pathways to dinner.** Food processing and preparation methods can either reduce or concentrate pesticide residues in foods.

1. **Legal control**
State and federal guidelines are designed to limit the spread of pests.

2. **Biological control**
Beneficial organisms, such as predators, parasites, and viruses, are released into the environment to suppress pest organisms.

3. **Cultural control**
Rotation, sanitation, and other good farming techniques are employed to help reduce pest populations.

4. **Physical control**
Barriers, traps, and the location and timing of planting are all used to control pest infestations.

5. **Genetic control**
Resistant plant strains are developed to reduce the impact of pests.

6. **Chemical control**
Conventional pesticides, biopesticides, pheromones, and other chemicals are used to prevent or suppress pest outbreaks. The chemical controls are specific to a pest species and are ideally short-lived in the environment. In addition, the chemicals are used at their lowest effective rate and may be alternated to help prevent the development of pest resistance.

**Figure 14.3** **Integrated pest management.** Integrated pest management is a sustainable approach that combines prevention, avoidance, monitoring, and suppression strategies in a way that minimizes economic, health, and environmental risks. It minimizes pesticide use and promotes economically sound practices.

Excessive use of synthetic pesticides, herbicides, and fertilizers contributes substantially to the pollution of soil and water. Overuse can be particularly hazardous to farm workers, whose exposure to these chemicals typically is much higher than consumers'. Overuse also threatens wildlife. Today, many farmers use **integrated pest management (IPM)** to reduce pesticide use. (See **Figure 14.3**.) IPM methods include crop rotation, use of natural rather than synthetic pesticides, and planting nonfood crops nearby that lure pests away from food crops. Releasing sterile fruit flies into orchards also allows reductions in pesticide use. Because fruit flies produce no offspring when they mate with sterile partners, the overall fruit fly population drops.

## Organic Alternatives

Organic foods are grown or produced without synthetic pesticides and without synthetic fertilizers. In the United States, the growth of the organic food industry can be seen in the expanding number of retailers offering a variety of organic foods and the widespread introduction of new organic products.[9] In 2010, sales of organic foods exceeded $26 billion and that number continues to grow.[10] Growth of the industry reflects, in part, America's distrust of technology and a desire to return to a simpler, more "natural" way of food production.

The Organic Foods Production Act and the National Organic Program (NOP) are intended to assure U.S. consumers that the organic foods they purchase are produced, processed, and certified to consistent national standards. The labeling requirements of this program apply to raw meats, fresh produce, and processed foods that contain organic ingredients. Foods that are sold, labeled, or represented as organic must be produced and processed in accordance with the NOP standards.[11] Table 14.2 outlines the requirements for labeling a food product as being organic.

| Table 14.2 | **Labeling Requirements for Organic Food** |
|---|---|

Labeling requirements are based on the percentage of a product's ingredients that are organic.

*Foods Labeled "100 Percent Organic" and "Organic"*

- Products labeled "100 percent organic" must contain only organically produced ingredients (excluding water and salt).
- Products labeled "organic" must consist of at least 95 percent organically produced ingredients (excluding water and salt). Any remaining ingredients must consist of nonagricultural substances approved on the National List maintained by the USDA National Organic Program or nonorganically produced agricultural products included on the National List at 205.606 that are not commercially available in organic form.
- Products that meet the requirements may display these terms and the percentage of organic content on their principal display panel.
- The USDA seal and the seal or mark of certifying agents may appear on product packages and in advertisements.
- Foods labeled "100 percent organic" and "organic" cannot be produced using excluded methods, sewage sludge, or ionizing radiation.

*Processed Products Labeled "Made with Organic (Specified Ingredients)"*

- Products that contain at least 70 percent organic ingredients can use the phrase "made with (specified) organic ingredients" and list up to three of the organic ingredients or food groups on the principal display panel. For example, soup made with at least 70 percent organic ingredients and only organic vegetables may be labeled either "soup made with organic peas, potatoes, and carrots" or "soup made with organic vegetables."
- Nonagricultural ingredients used in the remaining 30 percent of the products must be approved on the National List maintained by the USDA National Organic Program. For example, citric acid and sodium bicarbonate appear on this list.
- Foods labeled "made with (specified) organic ingredients" cannot be produced using excluded methods, sewage sludge, or ionizing radiation.
- The percentage of organic content and the certifying agent's seal or mark may be used on the package. However, the USDA seal cannot be used anywhere on the package.

*Processed Products That Contain Less Than 70 Percent Organic Ingredients*

- These products cannot use the term *organic* anywhere on the primary display panel. However, they may identify the specific ingredients that are organically produced on the ingredients statement on the information panel.

*Other Labeling Provisions*

- Any product labeled as organic must identify each organically produced ingredient in the ingredient statement on the information panel.
- The name of the certifying agent of the final product must be displayed on the information panel.
- There are no restrictions on the use of other truthful labeling claims, such as "no drugs or growth hormones used," "free range," or "sustainably harvested." However, claims on meat and poultry are subject to USDA–FSIS approval.

Source: USDA, National Organic Program. Organic labeling and marketing information. Washington, DC; April 2008. http://www.ams.usda.gov/AMSv1.0/getfile?dDocName=STELDEV3004446. Accessed 6/7/11.

Under the NOP, farm and processing operations that grow and process organic foods must be certified by the USDA. The certification process includes an on-site inspection to verify that the applicant's operation complies with strict national organic standards. Certifying agents may collect and test soil, water, waste, plant and animal tissues, and processed products. A certified operation may label its products or ingredients as organic and may use the "USDA Organic" seal (see **Figure 14.4**).

Even though there is no scientific evidence that genetic engineering and irradiation of foods present unacceptable risks, public opposition to these practices led the NOP to prohibit use of these technologies with organic foods. Although irradiation and genetic engineering have been approved for use in agriculture and may offer certain benefits for the environment and human health, consumers strongly oppose their use in organically grown foods.

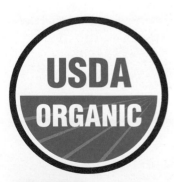

| Figure 14.4 | **The USDA Organic seal.** |
|---|---|

Source: Courtesy of the USDA.

Because of consumer opposition, foods produced with these techniques are prohibited from carrying the organic label.[12]

Organic farming has its drawbacks. The use of manure as a natural fertilizer raises food safety concerns. The organic producer must manage animal and plant waste materials so they do not contribute to contamination of crops, soil, or water. Manure runoff can pollute nearby lakes and streams. Some critics charge that organic farming is "elitist" and that synthetic fertilizers and pesticides are necessary to meet the food needs of an expanding world population. They also point out that complete freedom from pesticides cannot be guaranteed, no matter how carefully a food is produced, because pesticide residues may still exist in soil, water, and air.

**THINK**
**About It**
**2**

Organic foods are not pesticide-free foods. Organic farmers can use natural and approved synthetic pesticides to control weeds and insects.[13] In fact, a review of results from the USDA Pesticide Data Program found that 23 percent of organic food samples tested were positive for pesticide residues.[14] Microbial contaminants that cause foodborne illness can be found in organic as well as conventional foods. Consumers must handle all food appropriately, whether organically or conventionally grown.

### Animal Drugs

Current agricultural practice depends heavily on the use of drugs in food animals and food-producing animals raised specifically to provide meat, milk, and eggs. Producers use drugs to maintain animal health and well-being, as well as to increase production. Keeping animals in good health reduces the chance that disease will spread from animals to humans, and healthy animals can use nutrients for growth and production rather than to fight infection. But there is a possibility that drugs used in animals could enter human food and possibly increase the risk of ill health in humans.

Many researchers fear that overuse of animal antibiotics will contribute to the emergence of antibiotic-resistant microorganisms that could threaten human health. Another potential problem, though with less widespread effects, is that humans with drug allergies could have reactions to drug residues in food-producing animals. Some people worry that the widespread use of hormones may impair animal health or the quality of the food obtained from treated animals.

There are five major classes of drugs used in animals raised for food:[15]

1. Topical antiseptics, bactericides, and fungicides used to treat skin or hoof infections, cuts, and abrasions
2. Ionophores, which are feed additives that alter stomach microorganisms to more efficiently digest feeds and to help protect against some parasites
3. Hormone and hormonelike production enhancers (anabolic hormones for meat production and bovine somatotropin for increased milk production in dairy cows)
4. Antiparasitics
5. Antibiotics used to prevent infections, treat disease, and promote growth

The FDA is responsible for ensuring that drugs approved for use in animals are safe not only for the animals but also for humans who eat food produced from the animals. In addition, the FDA enforces regulations to ensure that drugs are used properly in cows, chickens, and seafood. However, FDA surveillance is not perfect; government investigations have revealed that a few U.S. veterinarians and farmers illegally use animal drugs that are known to be dangerous to humans.

## Pollutants

**Pollutants** from animal manure and other wastes, factories, human sewage, and other runoff can contaminate food-production areas. For example, some scientists theorize that dioxin contamination of foods may cause human cancer. **Dioxins** are chemical compounds created in the manufacture, combustion, and chlorine bleaching of pulp and paper and in other industrial processes.[16] Dioxins can accumulate in the food chain and are potent animal carcinogens. Freshwater fish from inland waters highly contaminated with dioxins can contain significant amounts of these toxins, and regional advisories should be consulted prior to consumption.[17] The commercial fishing industry avoids areas of known dioxin pollution. Dioxins in tiny amounts are found in food packages, paper plates, and coffee filters made of bleached paper. Because the quantity of this toxic chemical is minimal, however, the FDA has concluded that use of these products poses no significant risk to human health.

## Natural Toxins

Other chemical contamination of food can occur from **natural toxins**. Examples include

- **Aflatoxins**, found in contaminated food or animal feed. Aflatoxins are produced by certain strains of *Aspergillus* fungi under certain conditions of temperature and humidity. The most pronounced contamination has been found in tree nuts, peanuts, and other oilseeds, such as corn and cottonseed. Aflatoxins have been implicated as a factor in the development of liver cancer, particularly in parts of the world where food and water are frequently contaminated with this fungus.
- **Ciguatera** and other marine toxins. These toxins can accumulate in seafood (mainly in large tropical fish) and, when ingested, cause serious problems, including paralysis, amnesia, and nerve toxicity. Commercial fishers avoid waters known to harbor ciguatera toxin. Ciguatera poisoning sometimes occurs when these fish are caught as part of recreational fishing. Cooking does not destroy these toxins.
- **Methyl mercury**. Mercury occurs naturally in the environment and is produced by human activities. It is soluble in water, where bacteria can cause chemical changes that transform mercury to methyl mercury, a more toxic form. Fish absorb methyl mercury from water passing over their gills and by eating other contaminated aquatic species. Larger predatory fish can consume many contaminated smaller fish, thereby accumulating higher levels of methyl mercury. (See **Figure 14.5**.) Because shark, swordfish, king mackerel, and tilefish contain high levels of mercury, the FDA and EPA recommend that women who may become pregnant, pregnant women, nursing mothers, and young children avoid eating these fish.[18] In addition, the *Dietary Guidelines for Americans, 2010* recommends that women who are pregnant or breastfeeding also limit white (albacore) tuna to 6 ounces per week because it is higher in methyl mercury.[19]
- **Poisonous mushrooms**. These plants produce toxic substances that can cause stomach upset, dizziness, hallucinations, and other neurological symptoms. The more lethal mushroom species can cause liver and kidney failure, coma, and death.
- **Solanine**, a toxic substance in raw potato skins. Solanine develops in the greenish layer of improperly stored potatoes. It can be removed by thoroughly peeling the potato.

*Quick* Bite

**Well-Traveled Dioxin**
In Nunavut, Canada's newest province, the breast milk of native Inuits has twice the average concentration of dioxin as does the milk of women in southern Quebec. Native Inuits primarily eat fatty animals high on the food chain. These animals accumulate dioxin, but where did the dioxin originate? Not Canada. Carried by the wind, most comes from industrial combustion in the eastern and midwestern United States and some originates as far away as Mexico.

**pollutants** Gaseous, chemical, or organic waste that contaminates air, soil, or water.

**dioxins** Chemical compounds created in the manufacture, combustion, and chlorine bleaching of pulp and paper and in other industrial processes.

**natural toxins** Poisons that are produced by or naturally occur in plants or microorganisms.

**aflatoxins** Carcinogenic and toxic factors produced by food molds.

**ciguatera** A toxin found in more than 300 species of Caribbean and South Pacific fish. It is a nonbacterial source of food poisoning.

**methyl mercury** A toxic compound that results from the chemical transformation of mercury by bacteria. In trace amounts, mercury is water-soluble and contaminates many bodies of water.

**poisonous mushrooms** Mushrooms that contain toxins that can cause stomach upset, dizziness, hallucinations, and other neurological symptoms.

**solanine** A potentially toxic alkaloid that is present with chlorophyll in the green areas on potato skins.

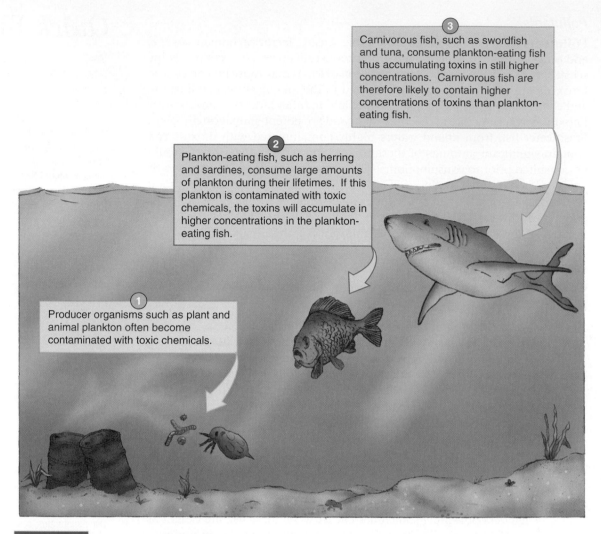

**Figure 14.5**   **Toxins in the food chain.** As toxins travel up the food chain, they become concentrated in larger fish.

A variety of compounds in herbs and spices also can be toxic. However, foodborne illness caused by these and other natural toxins is relatively rare compared with illness from pathogenic microorganisms.

### Other Food Contaminants

In the United States, about 2 percent of adults and 5 percent of infants and young children (nearly 11 million people) have food allergies. Eight major food groups—milk, eggs, fish, shellfish, tree nuts, peanuts, wheat, and soybeans—account for 90 percent of allergic reactions. Whenever these foods (or ingredients derived from them) are present in a food product, food labels must identify them.[20] (See **Figure 14.6.**) In an allergic person, these foods can cause a variety of reactions, including gastrointestinal problems, skin irritation, breathing difficulty, shock, and even death.

Contaminants such as glass, metal, and other objects may be introduced unintentionally during food production. Improper use of cleaning agents in food-contact areas can add these undesirable substances to food. Insects, dirt, and other undesirable items, although generally not a health hazard, also can find their way into food.

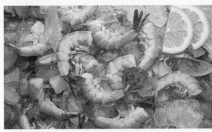
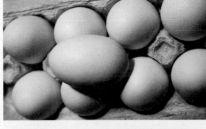
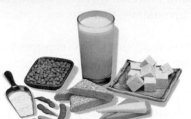
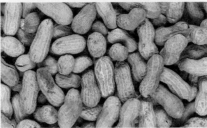

| Figure 14.6 | **Foods that commonly cause allergic reactions.** In sensitive people, an allergic reaction to food can be life threatening. |

**Key Concepts** *Chemical contaminants in foods include pesticides, natural toxins, and contamination related to pollution. Although organic foods are grown without synthetic pesticides or fertilizers, they still can contain chemical contaminants. Other potential food hazards are allergens and nonfood contaminants.*

## Keeping Food Safe

Having safe foods to eat requires the efforts of a great many people along the way from the farm to your plate. Imagine yourself enjoying a piece of broiled chicken. Consider that harmful contamination of that chicken could have occurred at the farm, in the processing plant, or during transportation to the supermarket. Once at the supermarket, the chicken might have been under-refrigerated or kept too long before being sold. After buying the chicken, you might have left it in a warm car or kept it in a refrigerator that was not cold enough. Your kitchen hygiene might not have been the best; and, finally, you could have undercooked the chicken. Considering the many opportunities for contamination, it is truly amazing that most of the time our food does not make us sick.

Keeping foods free from contamination is a job that falls to many parties. It is the responsibility not only of government officials at the national, state, and local levels but also of everyone who comes in contact with food—the producer, the manufacturer, the retailer, and, ultimately, the consumer.

### Government Agencies

The basis of modern food law is the Federal Food, Drug, and Cosmetic (FD&C) Act of 1938, which gives the Food and Drug Administration authority over food and food ingredients and defines requirements for truthful labeling of ingredients.

The FDA Food Safety Modernization Act (FSMA) was signed into law on January 4, 2011, with the goal of reforming the food safety system in the United States. The primary objective of FSMA is to ensure the U.S. food supply is safe by enabling the FDA to focus more on preventing food safety problems rather than primarily reacting to problems after they occur. Under the new law, the FDA has greater authority to enforce compliance with prevention-

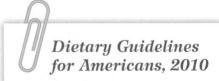

*Dietary Guidelines for Americans, 2010*

**Key Recommendations**
- Follow food safety recommendations when preparing and eating foods to reduce the risk of foodborne illnesses.

**Key Recommendations for Specific Population Groups**
- *Women who are pregnant or breastfeeding.* Due to their high methyl mercury content, limit white (albacore) tuna to 6 ounces per week and do not eat the following four types of fish: tilefish, shark, swordfish, and king mackerel.

**critical control points (CCPs)** Operational steps or procedures in a process, production method, or recipe at which control can be applied to prevent, reduce, or eliminate a food safety hazard.

***Food Code*** A reference published periodically by the Food and Drug Administration for restaurants, grocery stores, institutional food services, vending operations, and other retailers on how to store, prepare, and serve food to prevent foodborne illness.

and risk-based food safety standards and to better respond to and contain problems when they do occur. The law also enables the FDA to better ensure the safety of imported foods and to build an integrated national food safety system in partnership with state and local authorities.[21] At the federal level, six agencies (see **Figure 14.7**) share responsibility for food safety:

1. The Food and Drug Administration (FDA) enforces laws governing the safety of domestic and imported food, except meat and poultry.
2. The Centers for Disease Control and Prevention (CDC) monitors outbreaks of foodborne diseases, investigates their causes, and determines proper prevention.
3. The USDA Food Safety and Inspection Service (FSIS) enforces laws governing the safety of domestic and imported meat and poultry products.
4. The USDA Cooperative State Research, Education, and Extension Service (CSREES) develops research and education programs on food safety for farmers and consumers.
5. The USDA Agricultural Research Service (ARS) conducts research to extend knowledge of various agricultural practices, including those involving animal and crop safety.
6. The Environmental Protection Agency (EPA) regulates public drinking water and approves pesticides and other chemicals used in the environment.

State and local health and agricultural departments oversee food safety in their jurisdictions, often in conjunction with federal agencies.

### Hazard Analysis Critical Control Point

Hazard Analysis Critical Control Point (HACCP) is a food industry program that focuses on preventing contamination by identifying areas in food production and retail where contamination could occur. HACCP also is an important line of defense against intentional contamination by bioterrorists. (See the FYI feature "At War with Bioterrorism.")

Companies and retailers analyze their food-production processes and determine **critical control points (CCPs)**—points at which hazards could occur. They then determine measures that they can institute at these points to prevent, control, or eliminate the hazards.[22] (See Table 14.3.) Critical control points can occur anywhere in a food's production—from its raw state through processing and shipping to purchase by the consumer. Preventive measures can include proper cooking, chilling, and sanitizing, as well as preventing cross-contamination and improving employee hygiene.

The USDA requires HACCP for the food products it regulates—meat and poultry. The FDA, which regulates all other foods, requires HACCP in the seafood and low-acid canned-food industries and for the juice industry.[23] Also, the FDA has incorporated HACCP principles into its ***Food Code***, a reference for restaurants, grocery stores, institutional food services, vending operations, and other retailers on how to store, prepare, and serve food to prevent foodborne illness.[24] The FDA updates and publishes the *Food Code* periodically as a model for states to adopt and use to regulate retail food establishments in their jurisdictions.

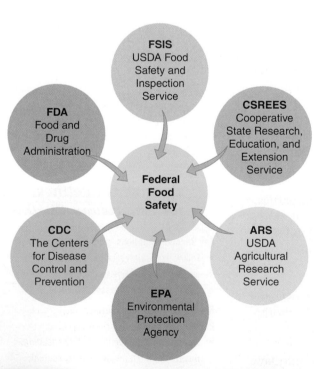

**Figure 14.7    Government agencies that help protect our food supply.** Although the FDA has primary responsibility for the safety of much of our food supply, many government agencies provide oversight.

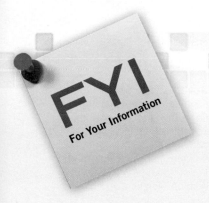

# At War with Bioterrorism

Late one afternoon, restaurant owner Dave Lutgens first felt nauseated and then experienced mild stomach cramps. By evening he was dizzy and disoriented. Suffering from diarrhea, he had to crawl to reach the toilet. Weak and dehydrated, he was wracked with chills, fever, and vomiting. Two days later his wife became ill with the same symptoms. By the end of the week, 13 employees were sick as well as dozens of customers. The culprit was *Salmonella typhimurium*, a rod-shaped bacteria responsible for many foodborne illnesses. But this was not a simple case of food poisoning. Occurring in 1984, this was a criminal assault on the small Oregon town of Dalles. The Rajaneesh religious cult attempted to sway local election results by poisoning people to keep them away from the polls. The cult deliberately perpetrated this terrifying food experience by contaminating a number of self-service salad bars and coffee creamers with home-grown *Salmonella*. Ten restaurants were affected, and more than 700 people fell ill from the biological attack.

Biocriminals also have struck in Canada. In 1970, four students in Montreal, Quebec, were admitted to the hospital after eating eggs inoculated with a parasitic nematode, *Ascaris suum*. They had signs of a parasitic infection and suffered from asthma and other lung problems. In 2000, 27 people suffered food poisoning after drinking coffee from a single vending machine at Lavalle University in Quebec City. The coffee had been laced with arsenic. In 2003, arsenic-laced coffee also poisoned more than a dozen people after a church service in New Sweden, Maine. One person died. After September 11, 2001, food bioterrorism received a surge of attention in the United States in an effort to protect against a large-scale terrorist attack on the nation's food or water supply.[1]

Food and water poisonings can be initiated by any of these three agents:[2]

1. *Bioterrorism and biowarfare:* Terrorist acts by state-sponsored organizations or hate groups. Few such events have occurred to date.
2. *Biocrime:* Intent to harm for personal gain or revenge. A few dozen events have occurred during recent decades.
3. *Biomisfortune:* Naturally occurring foodborne disease. Virtually all foodborne disease falls into this category, which is a daily concern for public health agencies everywhere.

Bioterrorist attacks can range from making false statements or accusations to actively inflicting injury on people, animals, or crops. Threats can be as devastating as actual destruction. Just claiming that a product has been intentionally contaminated can be sufficient to trigger an expensive recall and harmful adverse publicity. Product tampering, whether a hoax or real, can provide notoriety to the perpetrator, who is attempting to terrorize people and businesses.

Our food supply is an obvious route for the delivery of chemical and biological agents. Food production and distribution is a complex system not protected easily from the deliberate introduction of toxic agents. The attacks on the World Trade Center and Pentagon and the anthrax assaults have increased the concern and vigilance of the United States and Canadian governments, which are acutely aware that public food and water supplies are among the most vulnerable avenues for terrorist attacks.

At ports of entry, food inspection facilities, and research labs and buildings, government personnel are at a heightened state of alert. To prevent the entry of animal or plant pests and diseases, they are carrying out intensified product and cargo inspections of travelers and baggage. Food safety inspectors have been given a mandate to be alert to any irregularities at food-processing facilities. Within processing facilities, specific plans for security should be developed. Such plans can be based on HACCP principles.[3]

The FDA has adopted five broad strategies to counter bioterrorism:[4]

1. *Awareness:* Increasing awareness through collecting, analyzing, and spreading information and knowledge
2. *Prevention:* Identifying specific threats or attacks that involve biological, chemical, radiological, or nuclear agents
3. *Preparedness:* Developing and making available medical countermeasures, such as drugs, devices, and vaccines
4. *Response:* Ensuring rapid and coordinated response to any terrorist attacks
5. *Recovery:* Ensuring rapid and coordinated treatment for any illness that may result from a terrorist attack

The Public Health Security and Bioterrorism Preparedness and Response Act of 2002 (sometimes called the Bioterrorism Act) mandated that the FDA take numerous steps to protect the safety and security of the U.S. food supply. Since then, the FDA has developed additional food safety regulations, increased domestic and foreign surveillance, and continued to work toward reducing threats and vulnerabilities.[5]

What can consumers do to protect themselves from food contamination? We must be the final judges of the safety of the food we buy. At a minimum, we should:

1. Make sure the food package or can is intact before opening it. If it has been damaged or dented or opened prior to purchase, call it to the attention of the appropriate person.
2. Be alert to abnormal color, taste, and appearance of a food item. If you have any doubt, don't eat it.
3. If the food appears to be tampered with, report it immediately.
4. Follow safe food-handling practices.

1   Position of the American Dietetic Association: food and water safety. *J Am Diet Assoc.* 2009;109:1449–1460.

2   Sobel J. Epidemiologic preparedness and response to terrorist events involving the nation's food supply. Paper presented at Centers for Disease Control and Prevention Health Preparedness Conference; February 2005.

3   Bledsoe GE, Rasco BA. Addressing the risk of bioterrorism in food production. *Food Technol.* 2002;56(2):43–47.

4   Meadows M. The FDA and the fight against terrorism. *FDA Consumer.* January–February 2004. http://www.nti.org/e_research/source_docs/us/commission_reports/10.pdf. Accessed 6/7/11.

5   US Food and Drug Administration. Building a stronger defense against bioterrorism. Updated 6/7/11. http://www.fda.gov/ForConsumers/ConsumerUpdates/ucm048251.htm. Accessed 6/7/11.

**Table 14.3    Hazard Analysis and Critical Control Point (HACCP)**

| | |
|---|---|
| Step 1: Analyze hazards. | Identify the potential hazards associated with a food. The hazard could be biological (e.g., a microbe), chemical (e.g., mercury), or physical (e.g., ground glass or metal). |
| Step 2: Identify critical control points (CCPs). | Identify points in a food's production path—from its raw state through processing and shipping to consumption—where a potential hazard can be controlled or eliminated. Examples of CCPs are cooking, chilling, handling, cleaning, and storage. |
| Step 3: Establish preventive measures with critical limits for each control point. | An example is setting the minimum cooking temperature and time to ensure safety for a particular food (the temperature and time are critical limits). |
| Step 4: Establish procedures to monitor the control points. | Such procedures might include determining how and by whom cooking time and temperature should be monitored. |
| Step 5: Establish corrective actions to be taken when a critical limit has not been met. | For example, reprocessing or disposing of food if the minimum cooking temperature is not met. |
| Step 6: Establish effective record keeping to document the HACCP system. | For example, recording hazards and their control methods, the monitoring of safety requirements, and action taken to correct potential problems. |
| Step 7: Establish procedures to verify that the system is working consistently. | For example, testing time-recording and temperature-recording devised to verify that a cooking unit is working properly. |

**Note:** The HACCP method focuses on preventing hazards, relies heavily on scientific principles, permits efficient government oversight, and places greater responsibility on the food operations to ensure food safety.

**Source:** Data from US Food and Drug Administration. Hazard Analysis and Critical Control Point principles and application guidelines. Updated 6/18/09. http://www.fda.gov/Food/FoodSafety/HazardAnalysisCriticalControlPointsHACCP/HACCPPrinciplesApplicationGuidelines/default.htm. Accessed 6/7/11.

**Key Concepts** *Food safety is the responsibility of many agencies at the federal and state levels. The use of the Hazard Analysis Critical Control Point system allows government and industry to identify possible sites of food contamination and correct problems before they occur.*

### The Consumer's Role in Food Safety

Food safety advice to consumers used to consist of a simple message: "Keep hot foods hot and cold foods cold." (See **Figure 14.8**.) Now food safety experts urge consumers to follow the following four rules (see **Figure 14.9**):[25]

1. *Clean.* Wash hands and surfaces often. Clean fruits and vegetables. Meat and poultry should *not* be washed or rinsed.
2. *Separate.* Don't cross-contaminate. When shopping, preparing, or storing food, separate raw, cooked, and ready-to-eat foods.
3. *Cook.* Cook to proper temperatures. Avoid unpasteurized milk and juices, raw sprouts, raw or partially cooked eggs, and raw or undercooked meat and poultry.
4. *Refrigerate promptly.* Defrost foods properly and quickly refrigerate perishable foods.

Once a consumer takes possession of a food, food safety becomes his or her responsibility. Unfortunately, studies show that many consumers fail to follow safe food practices in the home. Current public health efforts focus on teaching consumers—from young children to older Americans—safe food practices in the home. (See the FYI feature "Safe Food Practices.")

Some food-handling practices are so important that the federal government requires specific instructions or warnings on labels of certain foods. Following outbreaks of illness from *E. coli* O157:H7 in contaminated hamburger in 1993, the USDA mandated instructions on labels of raw meat and poultry to encourage consumers to follow recommendations for safe handling and cooking of these products.

Labels of unpasteurized or otherwise untreated packaged juice products carry a warning statement about the product's possible danger to children,

THINK
About It

3

*Quick* Bite

**College Students Dissatisfied with Food Choices**
Only 28 percent of college students surveyed were satisfied with the healthful food offerings at their schools, according to consumer researchers. Nearly two-thirds said they eat at on-campus dining facilities, and almost half want more options to omit or substitute ingredients.

older adults, and people with weakened immune systems. The warning states that the product has not been pasteurized and therefore may contain harmful bacteria that can cause serious illness in these high-risk groups. This requirement was made after a number of people became seriously ill from drinking unpasteurized apple juice that was contaminated with *E. coli*.

Fresh eggs must be handled carefully, and even eggs with clean, uncracked shells may occasionally contain *Salmonella* that can cause an intestinal infection. The FDA requires the following safe handling statement on egg cartons:[26]

*SAFE HANDLING INSTRUCTIONS: To prevent illness from bacteria, keep eggs refrigerated, cook eggs until yolks are firm, and cook foods containing eggs thoroughly.*

Food manufacturers may voluntarily place other safe handling instructions on the label, such as those for proper cooking and storage of the item. Consumers should always follow these instructions.

## Who's at Increased Risk for Foodborne Illness?

Although everyone should follow safe food practices, infants and young children, pregnant women, older adults, and those who are immunocompromised or have certain chronic conditions must be especially careful about following safe food practices. In particular, they should not eat or drink raw (unpasteurized) milk or any products made from raw milk. They also should not eat raw or partially cooked eggs or foods containing raw eggs, raw or undercooked meat and poultry, raw or undercooked fish or shellfish, unpasteurized juices, and raw sprouts.

People who are at risk include individuals with the following conditions:

- Immune disorders, such as HIV infection
- Cancer
- Diabetes
- Long-term steroid use, such as for asthma or arthritis
- Liver disease
- Hemochromatosis, an iron storage disorder that affects the liver
- Stomach problems, including the effects of previous stomach surgery and low stomach acid (e.g., from chronic antacid use)

Because these conditions are more common in older adults, seniors have an increased risk of foodborne illness. Young children do not have fully developed immune systems, so they are particularly vulnerable to serious illness from foodborne disease. Also, pregnant women and their fetuses are at special risk from the bacterium *Listeria monocytogenes* and the parasite *Toxoplasma gondii*. Both of these microorganisms can harm—even kill—fetuses and young babies.

## A Final Word on Food Safety

A totally risk-free system of food production is an unreasonable and unattainable goal. The United States and Canada enjoy a reputation as having food supplies that are among the safest in the world. We expect our food to be clean, fresh, and not contaminated with debris, chemicals, or organisms that cause sickness or discomfort. To make sure it stays that way, food safety

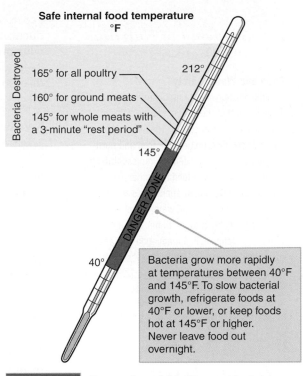

**Safe internal food temperature °F**

Bacteria Destroyed

165° for all poultry

160° for ground meats

145° for whole meats with a 3-minute "rest period"

212°

145°

DANGER ZONE

40°

Bacteria grow more rapidly at temperatures between 40°F and 145°F. To slow bacterial growth, refrigerate foods at 40°F or lower, or keep foods hot at 145°F or higher. Never leave food out overnight.

**Figure 14.8**  **Temperature guide.** To prevent bacterial growth, keep hot food hot and cold food cold.

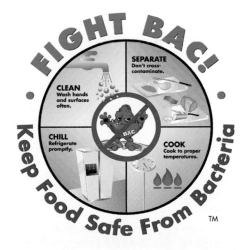

**FIGHT BAC!**
**Keep Food Safe From Bacteria** ™

**CLEAN** Wash hands and surfaces often.

**SEPARATE** Don't cross-contaminate.

**CHILL** Refrigerate promptly.

**COOK** Cook to proper temperatures.

**Clean:**  Wash hands and surfaces often
**Separate:**  Don't cross-contaminate
**Cook:**  Cook to proper temperatures
**Chill:**  Refrigerate properly

**Figure 14.9**  **Keeping harmful bacteria at bay.** Although our food supply generally is safe, food safety practices in the home are the weakest link in the food chain from farm to kitchen table. Make sure to follow the four basic practices: clean, separate, cook, and chill.

**Source:** Courtesy of Partnership for Food Safety Education, www.fightbac.org.

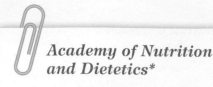

## Academy of Nutrition and Dietetics*

**Food and Water Safety**

It is the position of the American Dietetic Association that the public has the right to a safe food and water supply. The Association supports collaboration among food and nutrition professionals, academics, representatives of the agriculture and food industries, and appropriate government agencies to ensure the safety of the food and water supply by providing education to the public and industry, promoting technological innovation and applications, and supporting further research.

**Source:** Reproduced from Albrecht JA, Nagy-Nero D. Position of the Academy of Nutrition and Dietetics: food and water safety. *J Am Diet Assoc.* 2009;109:1449–1460.

\* Formerly the American Dietetic Association

## *Quick* Bite

### How Good Are Your Food Safety Habits?

Do Americans practice food safety in their own kitchens? Apparently not. A study conducted by the FDA and the CDC showed that one-half of people surveyed ate undercooked eggs in the past year. Twenty percent of people ate undercooked hamburger, and 25 percent of men and 14 percent of women failed to wash their hands with soap after handling raw meat.

**pasteurization** A process for destroying pathogenic bacteria by heating liquid foods to a prescribed temperature for a specified time.

**preservatives** Chemicals or other agents that slow the decomposition of a food.

## *Quick* Bite

### Where Do *E. coli* Hang Out?

Ground beef is the most common source of *E. coli* bacteria, but *E. coli* also has been found on apples and lettuce.

experts are continually trying to ensure that every participant in the food production chain—from the farmer who produces the food to the manufacturer who processes it to the retailer who sells it and to the consumer who buys it—undertakes measures to help reduce and perhaps even eliminate foodborne disease. That's one reason food safety advice today is turning up in so many places—to ensure that everyone gets the word on food safety.

**Key Concepts** *Consumers play a huge role in food safety. They can avoid foodborne illness by following a few simple food-handling and preparation rules: keep hands and food preparation areas clean; avoid cross-contamination of foods; cook foods adequately; refrigerate foods promptly. People who have weak or less-developed immune systems are at higher risk for foodborne illnesses.*

## Food Technology

Technology is having an increasingly greater impact on the food we eat. Our use of preservatives, other preservation techniques, and genetic engineering have implications for our food supply in the years to come and have triggered debates about their risks and benefits.

## Food Preservation

In our modern society, few people grow their own vegetables, fruits, and grains, or keep livestock as a source of meat and milk. Rather, we shop for our food, typically at a large, full-service supermarket. Because we don't consume our food at the point of harvest or slaughter, we use food preservation methods to help maintain the quality of the foods we purchase. Among food preservation methods are the addition of chemical preservatives, canning or freezing, **pasteurization**, and irradiation.

## Preservatives

**Preservatives** are added to foods to prevent spoilage and increase shelf life. The most common antimicrobial agents are salt and sugar. Other preservatives, such as potassium sorbate and sodium propionate, extend the shelf life of baked goods and many other products. Antioxidants are a type of preservative that prevents the changes in color and flavor caused by exposure to air. Common antioxidants include vitamins C and E, sulfites, and BHA and BHT.

### Preparation for Preservation

Some preservation techniques, such as salting and fermenting, date to ancient times and are still practiced along with their modern counterparts—freezing, canning, pasteurization, and the like (see **Figure 14.10**). Salting, drying, or fermenting foods creates an environment in which bacteria cannot multiply and, therefore, cannot cause food spoilage. Canned foods are heated quickly to a temperature that kills microbes and then are sealed airtight to prevent both contamination and oxidative damage. Freezing temperatures not only keep bacteria from multiplying but also prevent normal enzymatic changes in food that would cause spoilage. Pasteurization of milk or other beverages uses a very high temperature for a very short time to kill bacteria but minimizes changes that would result from longer heating. The food industry and the North American public readily accept these food preservation methods. One of the most modern preservation techniques—irradiation—is also the most controversial, in part because of our fear of anything that has to do with radiation.

## Irradiation

Before it received official approval, food **irradiation** underwent more than 40 years of scientific research and testing—more than any other food technology.[27] During irradiation, foods are exposed to a measured dose of radiation to reduce or eliminate pathogenic bacteria, including *E. coli* O157:H7, *Salmonella*, and *Campylobacter*, the chief causes of foodborne illness today. Irradiation also can destroy insects and parasites, reduce spoilage, and inhibit sprouting and delay ripening of certain fruits and vegetables. Irradiated strawberries, for example, stay unspoiled for up to three weeks versus three to five days for untreated berries. Irradiation also is effective in raw poultry and meat, where it can reduce levels of many pathogens significantly. Although some people fear irradiation will make the food radioactive, this concern is unfounded. The energy used to irradiate foods passes through the food and leaves no residue—in the same way that microwaves pass through food. Despite its benefits, use of irradiation remains rare in North America.

Because food manufacturers fear consumer rejection, they have been reluctant to use irradiation on their products. Some consumers and advocacy groups protest its use because they are concerned that irradiation may compromise a food's nutritional value and change its texture, taste, or appearance. However, food irradiation may cause less nutritive loss than conventional methods of food preservation.[28] At appropriate doses, irradiation of food does not significantly change its flavor, texture, or appearance.[29] Many organizations, including the Academy of Nutrition and Dietetics, the American Medical Association, and the World Health Organization, endorse irradiation as a means of providing the public with a safer food supply.

The FDA has approved irradiation for:

- Spices and dry vegetable seasoning to decontaminate and control insects and microorganisms
- Dry or dehydrated enzyme preparations to control insects and microorganisms
- Fruits and vegetables to inhibit maturation
- Poultry and red meat to control spoilage and pathogenic microorganisms
- All the foods above, to control insects, mites, and other arthropod pests

The FDA requires labels of irradiated foods to state that the product was "treated with irradiation" or "treated by irradiation" and display the international symbol for irradiation, the radura. (See **Figure 14.11**.)

Some experts believe the time is right for food irradiation to become more widespread. News stories about deaths related to foodborne illness have made the public more aware of the need for protection against contamination of food. As more consumers become aware of the benefits of irradiation, the demand for irradiated foods is expected to increase.

## Bacteriophages

The Food and Drug Administration has approved a mixture of viruses as a food additive to protect people from bacterial infections. The viruses used in the additive are called **bacteriophages** ("bacteria eaters"). A bacteriophage is any virus that infects bacteria.

Bacteriophages are common in soil, water, and our bodies. In the human gut and oral cavity, bacteriophages are normal

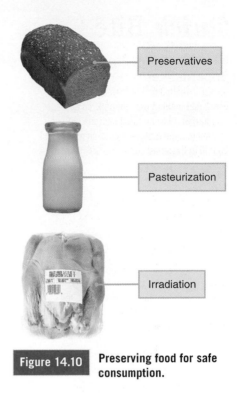

Preservatives

Pasteurization

Irradiation

**Figure 14.10** **Preserving food for safe consumption.**

**irradiation** A food preservation technique in which foods are exposed to measured doses of radiation to reduce or eliminate pathogens and kill insects, reduce spoilage, and, in certain fruits and vegetables, inhibit sprouting and delay ripening.

**bacteriophage** A virus that infects bacteria.

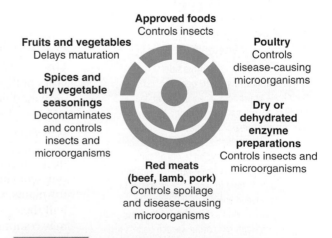

**Approved foods**
Controls insects

**Fruits and vegetables**
Delays maturation

**Poultry**
Controls disease-causing microorganisms

**Spices and dry vegetable seasonings**
Decontaminates and controls insects and microorganisms

**Dry or dehydrated enzyme preparations**
Controls insects and microorganisms

**Red meats (beef, lamb, pork)**
Controls spoilage and disease-causing microorganisms

**Figure 14.11** **FDA approved uses of irradiation.** Irradiation can retard spoilage and reduce risk of foodborne illness.

# *Quick* Bite

**Bacteria at the Supermarket**
Bacteria abound on the surface of supermarket meat. A piece of pork, on average, may harbor a few hundred bacteria per cubic centimeter, and a piece of chicken may have 10,000 in the same area.

**genetically modified (GM) foods** Foods produced using plant or animal ingredients that have been modified using gene technology.

**biotechnology** The set of laboratory techniques and processes used to modify the genome of plants or animals to create desirable new characteristics. Genetic engineering in the broad sense.

# *Quick* Bite

**Wood vs. Plastic: The Cutting Controversy**
Which type of cutting board is safer to use while cutting meat: wood or plastic? Both have drawbacks. A wood cutting board tends to absorb bacteria, sucking them down into the wood fibers. This may be safer than a plastic board, which keeps bacteria on the surface, in an easy position to rub off onto food and other objects. However, with use, wooden cutting boards tend to keep more on the surface than new wooden boards, acting more like plastic boards. What's the solution? Keep cutting boards clean by heating wooden boards in the microwave or putting plastic boards in the dishwasher.

and beneficial microbial inhabitants. Bacteriophages infect only bacteria and do not bother mammalian or plant cells.

The additive can be sprayed onto ready-to-eat meat and poultry products to protect consumers from the potentially life-threatening bacterium *Listeria monocytogenes*. The approved bacteriophage mixture targets *Listeria* and will thrive only when *Listeria* are present.

Under the Federal Meat Inspection Act and the Poultry Products Inspection Act, both administered by the USDA, the use of the bacteriophage preparation must be declared on labeling as an ingredient. Consumers will see "bacteriophage preparation" on the label of meat or poultry products that have been treated with the additive.[30]

**Key Concepts** *Various processing methods help protect us from contamination of food by pathogens. Drying, salting, canning, freezing, and pasteurizing are methods that consumers accept. Irradiation is a process in which foods are exposed to a measured dose of radiation to reduce or eliminate pathogenic bacteria. The FDA has approved spraying ready-to-eat meats and poultry products with bacteriophages, viruses that infect bacteria. Although government and professional organizations deem irradiation a safe procedure, consumers are still wary.*

# Genetically Modified Foods

**Genetically modified (GM) foods** have arrived, and most of us are already dining on them. When you prepare a dinner of broccoli and tofu, some of the soybeans used to make the tofu probably came from plants genetically modified to resist herbicide sprays or insect pests or both. And, although your broccoli is currently "natural," you can be sure that in a lab somewhere genetically modified broccoli seeds are sprouting, perhaps with enhanced nutrient or other phytochemical levels. If you are eating tenderloin tonight, the steak probably came from a steer fed on genetically modified corn that had its DNA altered by the addition of foreign genes to allow the plant to resist insect pests and herbicides.

Should you be indignant that these new foods are showing up on your table without any indication on the label, or should you be grateful that these high-tech methods are keeping crop yields high and food costs low? An informed answer to this question requires some understanding of how genetic engineering works, how new crops and foods are regulated, and how gene modification of crops and animals differs from the classical methods of agricultural breeding that have been practiced for thousands of years.

## A Short Course in Plant Genetics

How do GM food plants differ from those developed through traditional cross-pollination and hybridization? The answer, surprisingly, is that most crop modifications achieved by DNA manipulation and associated techniques of **biotechnology** also could be achieved with classical techniques, but the time scale and expense are very different. (See **Figure 14.12**.)

The classical techniques for breeding a plant with new characteristics have been practiced for hundreds of years. They involve crossing two plants with different characteristics, then growing the resulting hybrid seeds and looking for plants with the desired combination of characteristics. Hybrid plants get half their genes from one parent and half from the other. Though the hybrid may combine favorable qualities from both parents, a lot of undesirable genetic baggage must be sorted out after formation of such a hybrid. It usually takes dozens of additional crosses, and many years, to separate the desirable genes from the undesirable, and the process has a large element of chance. Due to

CROP DEVELOPMENT

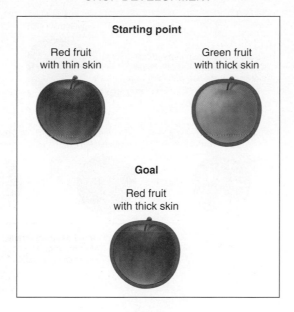

GENETIC ENGINEERING

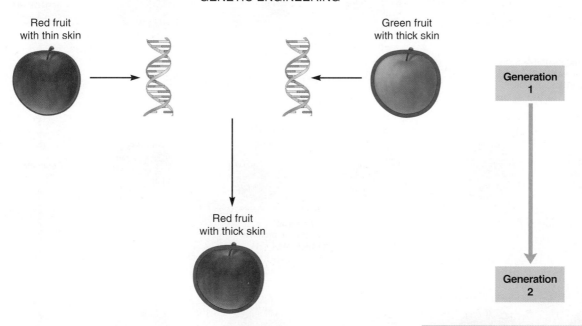

Scientists can use genetic engineering to combine certain traits in a single generation.

**Figure 14.12** **Genetic engineering and traditional breeding.** Genetic engineering can fast-track crop development that can take years with traditional breeding practices.

*(Continues)*

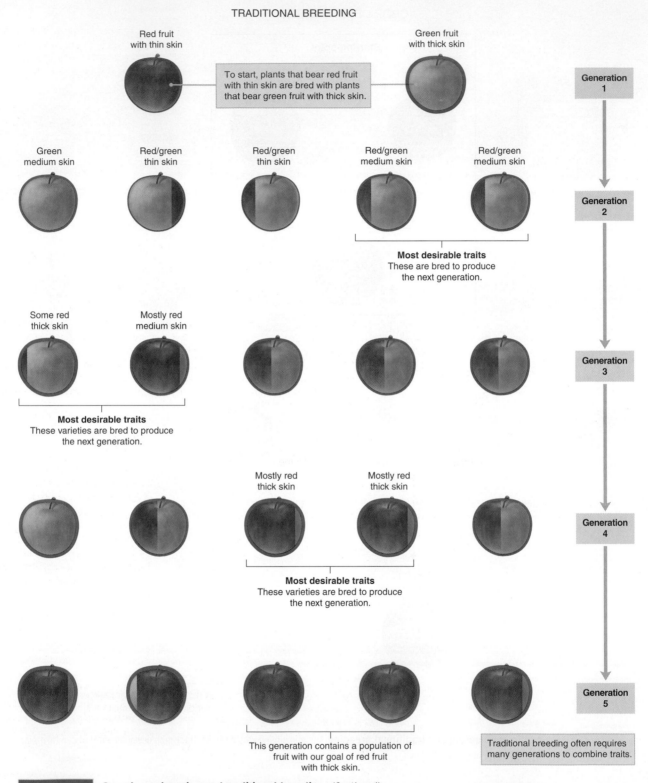

**Figure 14.12**  **Genetic engineering and traditional breeding.** *(Continued)*

human intervention, today virtually every crop plant species differs greatly from its original, wild form.

**Genetic engineering**, in contrast, allows scientists to transform a plant one gene at a time, using well-established methods for manipulating DNA sequences and integrating them into the plant **genome** (its set of genes). Because many plant genes have already been identified, and complete DNA sequences of many plant genomes will be available soon, we can anticipate that the genetic engineering of plants will become increasingly powerful and precise. Designing a new GM plant should come to resemble a manufacturing process rather than the tedious guessing game of classical genetics. In some cases, a gene can be selected and introduced into plant cells, and new GM seeds can be prepared within a year or two. When we consider that it took

> **genetic engineering** Manipulation of the genome of an organism by artificial means for the purpose of modifying existing traits or adding new genetic traits.
>
> **genome** The total genetic information of an organism, stored in the DNA of its chromosomes.

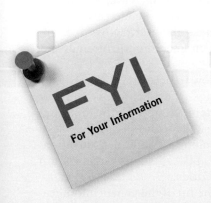

# Are Nutrigenomics in Your Future?

Nutritional genomics, or *nutrigenomics*, is the study of how different foods can interact with particular genes to alter a person's risk of developing diseases such as type 2 diabetes, obesity, heart disease, and cancer.

Many of these diseases are especially common among minority populations. African American men, for example, have a 60 percent greater chance of being diagnosed with prostate cancer than do Caucasian men.[1] Half of all adult Pima Indians in the United States have type 2 diabetes, compared with 6.5 percent of adult Americans of Caucasian descent. Genetics, diet, economic and social conditions, culture, and behavior may all contribute to these differences.[2]

Thanks to human genomics research, we now know that all people share the vast majority of human genetic information. Indeed, any two individuals share 99.9 percent of their DNA sequence—or about 1 difference in every 1,000 base pairs. Similarly, racial and ethnic groups share most genetic variations. The small differences that do exist are responsible for diverse human characteristics such as hair and skin colors; height and weight potential; and other "gene-based" variations, such as susceptibility to disease. The incidence of disease or patterns of progression differ among different groups. Risk factors for common diseases such as obesity, coronary heart disease, diabetes, prostate cancer, and birth defects must take into account both genetic and environmental/behavioral/social factors. The science of nutrigenomics studies how genes, diet, and disease interact to create health disparities for certain human populations that evolved from different geographic regions.

Although diet can be a serious risk factor for a number of diseases, the exact effect of different food components may depend on a person's genetic makeup. Thus, it is not a question of whether your genes are good or bad but rather how they interact with your environment. A single-letter change in DNA in people from Scandinavia 10,000 years ago, for example, allows most Caucasian adults today to drink cow's milk without getting sick due to lactose intolerance.[3]

The nutrigenomics effort seeks to identify genes controlled by nutrients and other naturally occurring chemicals in food and to study how some of these genes can tip the balance between health and disease. Nutrients alter molecular processes such as DNA structure, gene expression, and metabolism, which, in turn, may alter disease initiation, development, or progression. Individual genetic variations can influence how nutrients are assimilated, metabolized, stored, and excreted by the body. Nutritional genomics will enable individuals to better manage their health and well-being by precisely matching their diets to their unique genetic makeup.

The conceptual basis for this new branch of genomic research can best be summarized by the following "Five Tenets of Nutrigenomics":[4]

1. Under certain circumstances and in some individuals, diet can be a serious risk factor for a number of diseases.
2. Common dietary chemicals can act on the human genome, either directly or indirectly, to alter gene expression or structure.
3. The degree to which diet influences the balance between healthy and disease states may depend on an individual's particular genetic makeup.
4. Some diet-regulated genes (and their normal, common variants) are likely to play a role in the onset, incidence, progression, and/or severity of chronic diseases.
5. Dietary intervention based on knowledge of nutritional requirements, nutritional status, and genotype (i.e., "intelligent nutrition")

can be used to prevent, mitigate, or cure chronic disease.

Just as pharmacogenomics has inspired the concepts of "personalized medicine" and "designer drugs," the new field of nutrigenomics is opening the way for "personalized nutrition."[5] In other words, by understanding our nutritional needs, our nutritional status, and our genotype, nutrigenomics should enable people to better manage their health and well-being by precisely matching their diets with their unique genetic makeup. Stay tuned!

1. University of California–Davis. New center will probe links between diet, genes, and disease. Press release. 1/21/03. http://www.news.ucdavis.edu/search/news_detail.lasso?id=6238. Accessed 11/14/11.
2. Ibid.
3. Enattah NS, et al. Identification of a variant associated with adult-type hypolactasia. *Nat Genet.* 2002;30(2):233–237.
4. National Institute on Minority Health and Health Disparities, Center of Excellence for Nutritional Genomics. What is nutrigenomics, and how does it relate to me? University of California–Davis. http://nutrigenomics.ucdavis.edu. Accessed 10/28/08.
5. McCarthy JJ, Hilfiker R. The use of single-nucleotide polymorphism maps in pharmacogenomics. *Nat Biotechnol.* 2000;18(5):505–508.

centuries of selection and breeding to transform the weedy wild maize plant of pre-Columbian Mexico into our modern varieties of corn, the scale and speed of the gene revolution in agriculture are astounding.

## Genetically Modified Foods: An Unstoppable Experiment?

The United States accounts for nearly two-thirds of all biotechnology crops planted globally. GM food crops grown by U.S. farmers include corn, cotton, soybeans, canola, squash, and papaya. (See **Figure 14.13**.) About 85 percent of the U.S. soybean crop and over 75 percent of the cotton crop are genetically modified.[31] Other major producers of GM crops are Argentina, which plants primarily biotech soybeans; Canada, whose principal biotech crop is canola; Brazil, which recently approved the planting of GM soybeans; China, where the acreage of GM cotton continues to increase; and South Africa, where cotton is also the principle biotech crop. The increased yields and lower costs associated with GM crops make them attractive to farmers. There is now strong, perhaps unstoppable, momentum to continue and expand GM crop plantings.

European countries, however, have been slow to accept GM crops. They are concerned about possible ecological damage from such crops and fear potential unintended consequences of genetic "tampering" with the food supply. Although some U.S. consumer groups voice similar concerns, agribusiness, the Academy of Nutrition and Dietetics, the American Medical Association, the National Academy of Science, and the Food and Agriculture Organization have been supportive of the trend toward GM foods.[32]

The GM crops mentioned earlier are just the tip of the genetic-modification iceberg; hundreds more are under development in university laboratories and in the labs of giant agribusinesses. Research in plant biotechnology

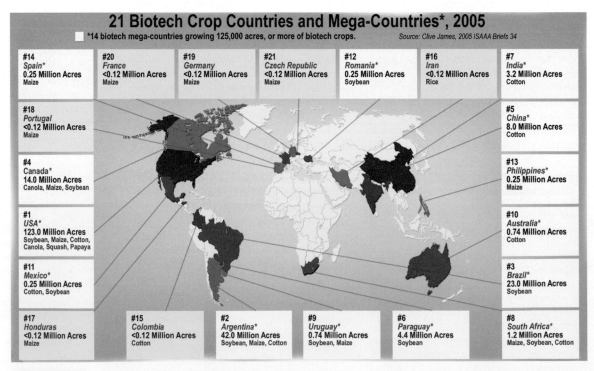

**Figure 14.13**   **Major GM crop producing countries.** The United States and other Western Hemisphere nations are the world's leading producers of genetically modified crops.

**Source:** Courtesy of International Service for the Acquisition Applications (ISAAA); Brief 34: 2005.

has focused primarily on characteristics that improve resistance to pests, reduce the need for pesticides, and increase the ability of the plant to survive adverse growing conditions such as drought, soil salinity, and cold. Many of these goals would be achievable with classical selection techniques, but, with genetic engineering, they move from laboratory to table in decades rather than centuries.

If only plant genes were involved in GM food production, there would be much less controversy. However, *any* gene, including genes from bacteria and animals, can be introduced into a plant genome. Some people find this frightening, and an imaginative term, *Frankenfoods*, has been coined to express the "unnatural" nature of some GM products. But how unnatural is the exchange of DNA between species? It may be reassuring to realize that organisms have been swapping DNA for eons, with no help from humans. Foreign DNA can be carried from one species to another by a variety of viruses, for example. Nature has already performed millions of "gene modifications" on its own, and exchange of DNA is an established part of the evolutionary process. Now that we can do our own experiments with DNA manipulation, we hope the benefits will be increased.

## Benefits of Genetic Engineering

Whatever the risks, no one can argue with the success of these GM techniques. For instance, a bacterial gene was used to create insect-resistant varieties of corn, potatoes, and soybeans. This gene, the **Bt gene**, was taken from the soil bacterium *Bacillus thuringiensis*. When inserted into a plant genome, the Bt gene directs the production of a protein in the plant that makes the plant toxic to insects. Such crops have been extremely successful and produce high yields without use of insecticides.

Bt-modified crops, which are now grown in the United States over an area larger than Rhode Island, are a boon to both the economy and the environment. Because chemical insecticides are not necessary, many benign insects are spared, and insect **biodiversity** is preserved. Similarly, other plants can be genetically modified to resist the effects of common herbicides. Chemical sprays that are lethal to most plant life have no effect on these GM plants. The crop plant grows larger in the absence of weeds, and the farmer gets a better yield with less effort and expense.

The economic benefits of GM foods are clearly substantial. Increased yields of important food plants can help feed increasing populations without the need for putting more land under the plow or increasing the use of toxic insecticides. In the coming century, this may be the difference between starvation and adequate nutrition in many developing countries.

It is easy to imagine how manipulation of plant amino acids and plant oils could yield superior foods, which not only would be able to satisfy calorie requirements but also would address protein and vitamin needs. A strain of rice, genetically modified to be rich in beta-carotene, known as Golden Rice, could benefit the more than 1 million children in developing countries who die or are weakened by vitamin A deficiency.[33] In developed countries, where heart disease and cancer loom as greater risks than malnutrition, the ability to adjust the saturation level of plant lipids or to boost beneficial phytochemicals would be of great value to public health. But do these undoubted benefits outweigh the risks?

THINK
About It
4

## Risks

What are the specific risks of GM foods? Many consumers are concerned about whether these new foods are safe to eat. The answer to this concern is

**Bt gene** *Bacillus thuringiensis* (Bt) is a bacterium that produces a protein called the Bt toxin. One of the bacterium's genes, the Bt gene, carries the information for the Bt toxin. Inserting a copy of the Bt gene into plants enables them to produce Bt toxin protein and resist some insect pests. The Bt protein is not toxic to humans.

**biodiversity** The countless species of plants, animals, and insects that exist on the earth. An undisturbed tropical forest is an example of the biodiversity of a healthy ecosystem.

a fairly unequivocal yes. When a new protein or other substance is introduced into a food, the FDA requires substantial testing to demonstrate its safety. With GM foods, the principal risk appears to be the possibility of introducing a new allergen into a GM food.[34] To be cautious, the FDA has focused on allergy issues. Under the law and the FDA's biotech food policy, companies must tell consumers on the food label when a product includes a gene from a food that commonly causes an allergic reaction.

Of greater concern, and more difficult to predict, are environmental effects, though no ecological disasters have occurred thus far. For example, what if the Bt-containing plants lead to the development of insects resistant to Bt-modified plants and to other insecticides? Another concern is the development of herbicide-resistant weeds, or "superweeds." When herbicide-resistant crops are planted in proximity to related wild plants, pollen may drift from food plant to weed, and the resistant genes might be passed to the weedy cousins of the GM plants. In the presence of herbicide, this might lead to the rapid selection of herbicide-resistant weeds. A final concern is that the herbicide-resistant food plants may become so successful that they are planted over a vast acreage in developing countries and sprayed with excessive amounts of herbicides. In the worst scenario, this could lead to a loss of many species of unmodified plants as well as the insect and animal communities that depend on them. Many scientists feel that the loss of biodiversity is one of the greatest threats to the planet today. Because of the complexity and interdependence of the biosphere, this is perhaps the greatest unknown and the greatest danger of unmonitored use of GM crops. Table 14.4 summarizes current concerns and scientific research areas.

## Regulation

The FDA regulates foods and food safety, and it oversees genetically modified foods as well as conventional foods. For foods derived from new varieties of plants, the FDA takes the position that whether modified by traditional breeding or genetic engineering, testing for safe human consumption is the legal responsibility of the producer or manufacturer of the foods. Crops such as Bt-modified soybeans do not require special testing, labeling, or FDA

---

**Table 14.4** **GM Concerns and Current Research**

*1. GM Crops Will Hurt Innocent Creatures*
Will crops engineered to contain insecticides harm nondestructive species important to biodiversity? Although laboratory studies show that genetic modifications to plants can harm nontarget insects, such as monarch butterflies, field studies suggest the risk is small.

*2. GM Crops Will Lead to the Emergence of Superweeds*
Will genetic modifications that give crops the ability to kill insect pests or withstand certain herbicides migrate to weeds? Almost every crop has weedy relatives somewhere in the world. Despite anecdotal reports, studies have not found superweeds. Yet to avoid pollen spreading from modified genes to weeds, scientists warn that GM crops should not be grown near weedy relatives.

*3. GM Crops Will Have Sudden Failures*
Will target insect pests become tolerant to insecticides in GM plants and will weeds become immune to herbicides sprayed on herbicide-resistant GM crops? Could these threats become unstoppable? Although there are no documented GM crop failures, scientists believe they are likely. Are current prevention measures adequate? Critics and proponents disagree.

approval. Although the plant expresses the Bt protein, the beans do not contain it. Except for some foreign DNA sequences, the beans are identical to unmodified soybeans. However, when a new substance is added to a food, FDA review and approval are necessary. Thus, if a new substance is produced or introduced into a food by genetic means, it must be tested as though it were a food additive.

Some consumer groups are pushing for mandatory labeling of GM foods. They believe consumers have the right to know whether a food is bioengineered. Other groups desire labeling so they can adhere to cultural or religious beliefs that may ban certain animal foods. Because the FDA believes the way a food is developed or produced is irrelevant information, current FDA policy does not require labeling of GM foods.

The FDA does require that food labels disclose any significant difference between the bioengineered food and its conventional counterpart. Such differences would include changes in nutritional properties, the presence of an allergen that consumers would not expect in the food, or any property that would require special handling, storage, cooking, or preservation.

Similar to U.S regulations, Health Canada requires special labeling for genetically modified foods when there is a potential for allergic reactions, and a different name must be used for a GM food that is different in composition or nutritional value. Voluntary positive ("does contain") and voluntary negative ("does not contain") labeling is permitted, provided the statements are factual and not misleading or deceptive.[35]

Many groups (government agencies, such as the FDA; professional organizations, such as the Academy of Nutrition and Dietetics; and consumer advocacy groups) are monitoring developments in biotechnology. Websites for these organizations can be a source of policy statements and breaking news in this area. Regardless of our views on genetic manipulation of food plants, research and development will continue.

**Key Concepts** *Genetic engineering allows scientists to transform a plant one gene at a time, using well-established methods for manipulating DNA sequences. The goals of genetic modification of foods are higher yields, lower costs, increased amounts of critical nutrients, and a healthier mix of plant oils. Because of the complexity and interdependence of the biosphere, loss of genetic biodiversity is perhaps the greatest unknown and the greatest danger of unmonitored GM crops.*

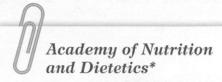

### *Academy of Nutrition and Dietetics\**

**Agricultural and Food Biotechnology**

It is the position of the American Dietetic Association that agricultural and food biotechnology techniques can enhance the quality, safety, nutritional value, and variety of food available for human consumption and increase the efficiency of food production, food processing, food distribution, and environmental and waste management. The Academy of Nutrition and Dietetics encourages the government, food manufacturers, food commodity groups, and qualified food and nutrition professionals to work together to inform consumers about this new technology and encourage availability of these products in the marketplace.

**Source:** Reproduced from Bruhn C, Earl R. Position of the Academy of Nutrition and Dietetics: agricultural and food biotechnology. *J Am Diet Assoc.* 2006;106(2):285–293.

\* Formerly the American Dietetic Association

# Learning Portfolio

## Key Terms

## Study Points

- Foodborne illness is extremely common; it affects millions of Americans each year. Estimates of the frequency of foodborne illness are difficult because the vast majority of foodborne illnesses go unreported.

- The incidence of foodborne illness may be on the rise in the United States and Canada. Many factors are responsible, including the increased centralization of food preparation, food imports, an increasing population of especially susceptible individuals (such as the elderly and those with weakened immune systems), and failure of consumers and retail establishments to follow appropriate food safety measures.

- Microorganisms cause most foodborne diseases in the United States and Canada. Most of these illnesses are preventable.

- *Staphylococcus aureus* is one of the most common causes of foodborne illness. Onset of illness is rapid, typically occurring between 30 minutes and a few hours after consuming the contaminated food.

- Common symptoms of foodborne illness are diarrhea, nausea, abdominal cramps, and sometimes fever. The severity of the illness depends on the type of organism and the amount of contaminant eaten.

- Ensuring a safe food supply is a farm-to-table continuum involving producers, manufacturers, retailers, and consumers.

- Pesticides, animal drugs, natural toxins, and pollutants are the major forms of chemical food contamination.

- The government monitors imported and domestic foods for pesticide residues by testing food samples for both amounts and types of pesticides. Efforts are under way to reduce the allowable amounts of certain pesticides in order to avoid harm to infants and children.

- The FDA evaluates drugs used in food-producing animals for safety in both animals and humans. Overuse of animal antibiotics could contribute to the emergence of antibiotic-resistant microorganisms that could threaten human health.

- The government and the food industry use the Hazard Analysis Critical Control Point system to prevent food contamination.

- Consumers must take responsibility for food safety in their homes. Cleaning hands and surfaces, avoiding cross-contamination, cooking foods adequately, and refrigerating foods promptly are important steps that prevent foodborne illness.

- Food preservation techniques inhibit growth of microorganisms. Canning, drying, freezing, fermentation, and pasteurization are common methods.

- Although the FDA has approved food irradiation for numerous uses, it is rarely used, mostly because of consumer fears. Food irradiation does not make foods radioactive. It can kill insects and most microorganisms. Appropriate doses of radiation extend the shelf life of many foods.

- Genetically modified (GM) foods are most likely already on your table. Soybeans, corn, and potatoes are some of the GM foods being commercially produced. Concerns about GM foods include worries about decreasing biodiversity and the development of herbicide-resistant weeds.

## Study Questions

1. What are the two main ways that pathogenic bacteria can cause foodborne illness?

2. Why shouldn't your 97-year-old great-grandmother drink homemade eggnog made from raw eggs?

3. How can you limit your intake of pesticides, according to the Consumers Union?

4. List four naturally occurring toxins.

5. What does "HACCP" stand for, and what is its purpose?

6. What are some ways to keep food safe at home?

7. List the most common food preservation techniques.

8. What are scientists' two major concerns about GM crops?

# Try This

## Bacterial Detective

What sources of bacteria do you encounter in your everyday activities? Here's an experiment to find out.

### First, you'll need ...

Cotton swabs
Six or more Petri dishes with agar

If you are unable to obtain a set of agar-filled Petri dishes from your school or local health department, you can make your own culture medium. Here's how:

- Add 2 teaspoons of unflavored gelatin (1 packet) and 2 teaspoons of sugar to 2/3 cup of water.
- Bring the solution to a boil and stir for one minute until everything is dissolved. Pour ¼-inch of the solution into each Petri dish or other suitable container.

### Then, using separate Petri dishes,

1. Pluck a hair and lay it in one Petri dish, labeled "Hair."

2. Sneeze or cough into another Petri dish, labeled "Cough."

3. Run a cotton swab around a nostril and carefully zigzag it across the agar in another Petri dish, labeled "Nose."

4. Run a cotton swab across a dampened kitchen sink sponge and carefully zigzag it across the agar in another Petri dish, labeled "Sponge."

5. Run a cotton swab around a clean kitchen countertop and carefully zigzag it across the agar in another Petri dish, labeled "Countertop."

6. Use the same procedure to collect additional samples from any other area in which bacteria may be present.

7. Store the Petri dishes in a warm environment, at a constant temperature around 80°F. Check your specimens periodically. Within a week, you should see something growing!

What do you observe? Which Petri dishes show the most growth? Which show the least? Does this change your ideas about cleaning habits?

## Organic Foods

Organic foods are increasing in popularity. Are organic foods widely available in your neighborhood? What types of organic produce can you find? Go to either a natural food store or the local grocery store and look at the array of organic produce. Compare the prices of organic produce and nonorganic produce. Do you think the cost differences outweigh possible benefits? Compare the look of the organic and nonorganic produce. Do you see any differences? What other organic products can you find?

# References

1   Centers for Disease Control and Prevention. Foodborne disease. Food safety at CDC. Questions and answers about foodborne disease. How many cases of foodborne disease are there in the United States? http://www.cdc.gov/foodsafety/facts.html#howmanycases. Accessed 6/2/11.

2   Institute of Food Technologists. Foodborne illness costs US 152 B annually. 3/10. http://www.ift.org/food-technology/daily-news/2010/march/10/foodborne-illness-costs-us-152-b-annually.aspx. Accessed 6/2/11.

3   Ibid.

4   Centers for Disease Control and Prevention. Questions and answers about foodborne illness (sometimes called "food poisoning"). What are the most common foodborne diseases? http://www.cdc.gov/foodsafety/facts.html#mostcommon. Accessed 6/2/11.

5   Ibid.

6   US Food and Drug Administration. Residue monitoring reports. FDA pesticide program residue monitoring: 1993–2008. 2010. http://www.fda.gov/Food/FoodSafety/FoodContaminantsAdulteration/Pesticides/ResidueMonitoringReports/default.htm. Accessed 6/2/11.

7   Ibid.

8   US Environmental Protection Agency. Pesticide program. Assessing health risks from pesticides. 2007. http://www.epa.gov/opp00001/factsheets/riskassess.htm. Accessed 6/2/11.

9   Dimitri C, Oberholtzer L, US Department of Agriculture. A report from the Economic Research Service. Marketing US organic foods: recent trends from farms to consumers. Economic Information Bulletin No. 58. 9/09. http://www.ers.usda.gov/publications/eib58/eib58.pdf. Accessed 6/2/11.

10  Organic Trade Association. U.S. organic industry valued at nearly $29 billion in 2010. Greenfield, MA: Organic Trade Association; April 2011. http://www.ota.com/index.html. Accessed 6/2/11.

11  US Department of Agriculture. National Organic Program, organic labeling and marketing information. Agricultural Marketing Service. 4/08. http://www.ams.usda.gov/AMSv1.0/getfile?dDocName=STELDEV3004446&acct=nopgeninfo. Accessed 6/2/11.

12  US Department of Agriculture. National Organic Program, organic production and handling standards. Agricultural Marketing Service. 4/08. http://www.ams.usda.gov/AMSv1.0/getfile?dDocName=STELDEV3004445. Accessed 6/2/11.

13  Ibid.

14  Winter CK, Katz JM. Dietary exposure to pesticide residues from commodities alleged to contain the highest contamination levels. J Toxicol. 2011;2011:589674.

15  Committee on Drug Use in Food Animals, Panel on Animal Health, Food Safety, and Public Health, National Research Council. The Use of Drugs in Food Animals. Washington, DC: National Academies Press; 1999.

16  Food and Agriculture Organization. Fact sheet. Dioxins in the food chain: prevention and control of contamination. 4/06. http://www.fao.org/ag/agn/agns/files/Dioxin_fact%20sheet.pdf. Accessed 6/3/11.

17  Mozaffarian D, Rimm EB. Fish intake, contaminants, and human health: evaluating the risks and the benefits. JAMA. 2006;296(15):1885–1899.

18  Environmental Protection Agency, US Department of Health and Human Services. EPA–FDA Joint Federal Advisory for Mercury in Fish. What you

need to know about mercury in fish and shellfish. 3/04. http://water.epa.gov/scitech/swguidance/fishshellfish/outreach/advice_index.cfm. Accessed 6/3/11.

19  US Department of Health and Human Services, US Department of Agriculture. *Dietary Guidelines for Americans, 2010.* 7th ed. Washington, DC: US Government. Printing Office; December 2010.

20  US Food and Drug Administration. Food allergens. What you need to know. 2011. http://www.fda.gov/food/resourcesforyou/Consumers/ucm079311.htm. Accessed 6/3/11.

21  US Department of Health and Human Services. FDA Food Safety Modernization Act. http://www.fda.gov/Food/FoodSafety/FSMA/default.htm. Accessed 11/15/11.

22  US Department of Health and Human Services, US Food and Drug Administration. Hazard Analysis and Critical Control Point principles and application guidelines. 6/09. http://www.fda.gov/Food/FoodSafety/HazardAnalysisCriticalControlPointsHACCP/HACCPPrinciplesApplicationGuidelines/default.htm. Accessed 6/3/11.

23  US Department of Health and Human Services, US Food and Drug Administration. Hazard Analysis and Critical Control Point (HAACP). Updated 4/27/11. http://www.fda.gov/food/foodsafety/hazardanalysiscriticalcontrolpointshaccp/default.htm. Accessed 6/3/11.

24  US Department of Health and Human Services, US Food and Drug Administration. *Food Code.* 11/18/09. http://www.fda.gov/Food/FoodSafety/RetailFoodProtection/FoodCode/default.htm. Accessed 6/3/11.

25  Partnership for Food Safety Education. Fight Bac! Four simple steps to food safety. http://www.fightbac.org. Accessed 6/3/11; and US Department of Health and Human Services, US Department of Agriculture. Op. cit.

26  Food labeling, safe handling statements, labeling of shell eggs; refrigeration of shell eggs held for retail distribution, final rule. *Federal Register.* 2000;65:76091–76114.

27  Environmental Protection Agency. Radiation protection. History of food irradiation. Updated 3/24/11. http://www.epa.gov/radiation/sources/food_history.html. Accessed 6/6/11.

28  Iowa State University Extension Service. Consumer questions about food irradiation. Updated 6/9/10. http://www.extension.iastate.edu/foodsafety/irradiation/index.cfm?articleID=25&parent=3. Accessed 6/6/11.

29  Centers for Disease Control and Prevention. Food irradiation. Updated 10/11/05. http://www.cdc.gov/ncidod/dbmd/diseaseinfo/foodirradiation.htm#howaffect. Accessed 6/6/11.

30  Bren L. Bacteria-eating virus approved as food additive. *FDA Consumer.* January–February 2007.

31  US Department of Agriculture. Biotechnology. Frequently asked questions about biotechnology. http://www.usda.gov/wps/portal/usda/usdahome?contentid=BiotechnologyFAQs.xml&navid=AGRICULTURE. Accessed 6/7/11.

32  Position of the American Dietetic Association: agriculture and food biotechnology. *J Am Diet Assoc.* 2006;106(2):285–293.

33  Tang G, Qin J, Dolnikowski GG, et al. Golden Rice is an effective source of vitamin A. *Am J Clin Nutr.* 2009;89(6):1776–1783.

34  Selgrade MK, Bowmann CC, Ladies GS, et al. Safety assessment of biotechnology products for potential risk of food allergy: implications of new research. *Toxicol Sci.* 2009;110(1):31–39.

35  Health Canada. The regulation of genetically modified foods. Updated 11/25/05. http://www.hc-sc.gc.ca/sr-sr/pubs/biotech/reg_gen_mod-eng.php. Accessed 6/7/11.

# CHAPTER 15

# World View of Nutrition: The Faces of Global Malnutrition

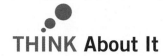

**THINK About It**

1 Have you ever experienced hunger without being able to satisfy it within a day?

2 Have you seen evidence of hunger or malnutrition in your community?

3 What can you do to help eliminate hunger in North America?

4 How do you feel about the United States sending food to impoverished nations?

**Visit go.jblearning.com/inseldisco4e**

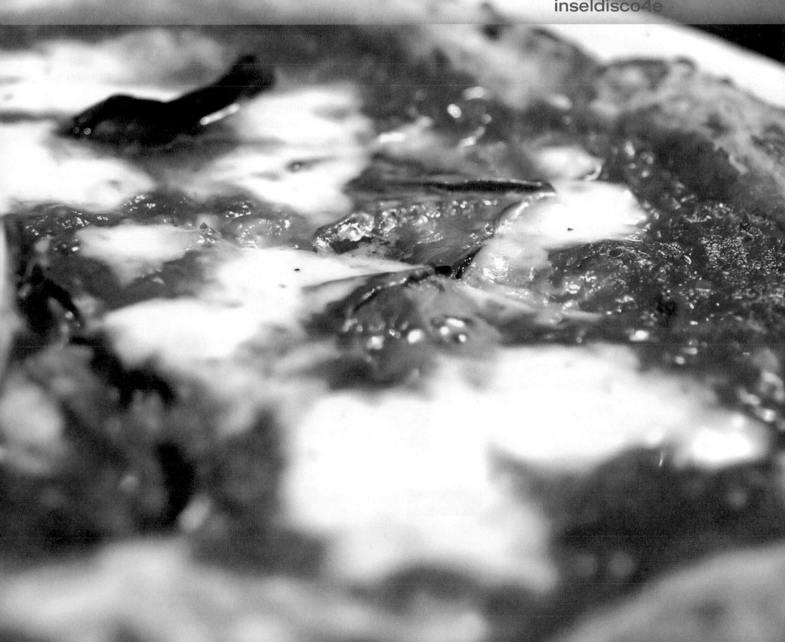

E ach day on your way to class, you pass a soup kitchen. You look at the long line of men and women waiting to get their meals and wonder what brought them to this point. You wonder how many similar soup lines exist in your community and how many people need food assistance but can't get it. If **hunger** exists in our rich country, what about people living in poor countries?

In 2010, 925 million people worldwide did not have enough to eat. This figure includes 19 million people in developed countries,[1] although most of the world's hungry live in developing countries (see **Figure 15.1**). The majority of undernourished people live in Asia and the Asian Pacific (578 million people); the region with the highest proportion of undernutrition is sub-Saharan Africa (239 million people).[2] Worldwide, more than half the deaths of children younger than 5 years are caused directly or indirectly by **malnutrition**, which kills more than 10 million children per year.[3]

In this chapter, we look at hunger and malnutrition. By *hunger*, we don't mean that mildly empty feeling one gets before mealtime. We mean the inability, day after day, to satisfy basic nutrition needs, the gnawing emptiness that creates a constant focus on eating and how to obtain food. In contrast to the hunger dieters feel from cutting calories, this deprivation is involuntary and unwanted.

Technically speaking, *malnutrition* can be any kind of unhealthy nutritional status, including the result of imbalance and excess—obesity or toxicity from oversupplementation, for example. And although we touch on obesity as an emerging issue, even in developing countries, in this chapter *malnutrition* generally refers to undernutrition resulting from hunger.

Along the spectrum of malnutrition and hunger is the less extreme condition of **food insecurity**, the ongoing worry about having enough to eat. At the opposite end of the spectrum is **food security**, access to nutritionally adequate and safe food. Most people in the industrialized world are food-secure. Overabundance and obesity are the primary problems in these popu-

**hunger** The internal, physiological drive to find and consume food. Unlike appetite, which may not entail hunger, hunger often is experienced as an awareness of a lack of food, often manifesting as an uneasy or painful sensation, but one may be unaware of his or her own hunger. A recurrent and involuntary lack of access to food may produce malnutrition over time.

**malnutrition** Failure to achieve nutrient requirements, which can impair physical and/ or mental health. It may result from consuming too little food or from a shortage or imbalance of key nutrients.

**food insecurity** (1) Limited or uncertain availability of nutritionally adequate and safe foods or (2) limited or uncertain ability to acquire acceptable foods in socially acceptable ways.

**food security** Access to enough food for an active, healthy life, including (1) the ready availability of nutritionally adequate and safe foods and (2) an assured ability to acquire acceptable foods in socially acceptable ways.

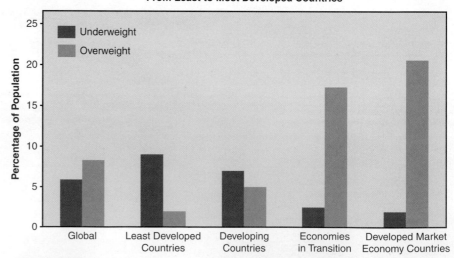

**From Least to Most Developed Countries**

Figure 15.1 | **Global nutrition transition and obesity.** As poor countries become more prosperous, they acquire some of the problems, including obesity, along with the benefits of becoming a more developed nation. In the developing world, a number of changes in diet, physical activity, health and nutrition, collectively known as the "nutrition transition," lead to increased rates of obesity.

**Source:** Courtesy of the Food and Agriculture Organization of the United Nations using data from WHO.

lations, but malnutrition is a serious problem among certain groups, such as the homeless and urban poor.

## Malnutrition in the United States

Malnutrition and hunger are serious problems not only in developing countries but also in the United States and other industrialized countries. Among those who suffer the worst malnutrition are the homeless, children, older adults, the working poor, and the rural poor.

### The Face of American Malnutrition

In the food-rich United States, food insecurity remains a problem.[4] (See **Figure 15.2**.) It is characterized by anxiety about having enough to eat and about running out of food and having no money to purchase more. Some people actually go hungry in the United States: During 2009, 50.2 million people, including 17.2 million children, lived in one of the 17.4 million U.S. households experiencing food insecurity.[5]

Households that are struggling to meet basic food needs tend to follow a typical pattern as their plight worsens. First, adults worry about having enough food. Then, they stretch resources and juggle other necessities, with more of the budget going for fixed expenses than for food. The quality and variety of the diet decline. Next, the adults eat less and less often. And finally, as food becomes more limited, the children also eat less. Families cope with food insecurity in various ways. When there is not enough food, common strategies include eating less varied diets and participating in local and federal emergency relief and food assistance programs.[6]

THINK
About It
1

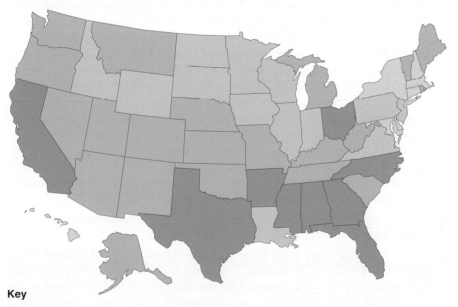

**Key**

■ Food insecurity below national average
■ Food insecurity near national average
■ Food insecurity above national average

**Figure 15.2**    **Prevalence of food insecurity.** State-to-state differences in food insecurity reflect both differences in the makeup of state populations, such as the income, employment, age, education, and family structure of their residents, as well as differences in state characteristics, such as economic conditions, the accessibility and use of food assistance programs, and tax policies.

**Source:** Nord M, Coleman-Jensen A, Andrews M, Carlson S. *Household Food Security in the United States, 2009.* USDA; November 2010. Economic Research Service. Report No. 108. http://www.ers.usda.gov/Publications/ERR108/ERR108.pdf. Accessed 7/23/11.

## Quick Bite

### Food Recovery and Gleaning

Each year more than 96 billion pounds of food produced in this country go to waste. Programs throughout the country are rescuing much of this wholesome food and distributing it to people in need. "Gleaning" is harvesting excess food from farms, orchards, and packing houses. Perishable items also are salvaged from wholesale and retail markets; fresh foods that are wholesome but will spoil before they can be sold are given to local food pantries and meal providers. Canned goods and other staples are collected from groceries, distributors, food processors, and individual homes. Even surplus food from restaurants, caterers, and other food services is collected by some charities for local food programs.

| Table 15.1 | Poverty Guidelines: Income Levels Defined as Poverty for a Given Household Size |
|---|---|

| Persons in Family | 48 Contiguous States and Washington, DC | Alaska | Hawaii |
|---|---|---|---|
| 1 | $10,890 | $13,600 | $12,540 |
| 2 | 14,710 | 18,380 | 16,930 |
| 3 | 18,530 | 23,160 | 21,320 |
| 4 | 22,350 | 27,940 | 25,710 |
| 5 | 26,170 | 32,720 | 30,100 |
| 6 | 29,990 | 37,500 | 34,490 |
| 7 | 33,810 | 42,280 | 38,880 |
| 8 | 37,630 | 47,060 | 43,270 |
| For each additional person, add: | 3,820 | 4,780 | 4,390 |

**Note:** Despite the limits to the use of household income as a proxy for estimating food insecurity, poverty remains an intuitively reasonable indicator. Keep in mind that, in addition to food, income must cover housing, clothing, transportation, medical care, and other essentials.

**Source:** Reproduced from US Department of Health and Human Services, Office of the Secretary. Annual update of the HHS poverty guidelines. *Federal Register.* 2011;76(13):3637–3638.

Surprisingly, obesity is more prevalent among low-income, food-insecure groups than among those with higher incomes. Households with little money often rely on cheaper, high-calorie foods to stave off hunger. Families try to maximize caloric intake for each dollar spent, which can lead to overconsumption of calories and a less healthful diet. Historically, obesity has hit low-income Americans the hardest. Their limited financial resources and worsening food insecurity shift food purchases to cheaper, easier, high-energy options that can contribute to obesity.[7] Those who live in a state of food insecurity consume significantly fewer healthful foods and micronutrients. Although such suboptimal diets usually do not lead to overt deficiency diseases, more subtle effects are serious and costly, showing up years later as chronic illness or more immediately as reduced immune function. More illness, more medicines, more doctor visits and hospital stays, more missed days and poorer performance at school and work, poor pregnancy outcomes, delayed growth and development—suboptimal nutrition contributes to them all.

## Prevalence and Distribution

How much hunger and food insecurity exist in the United States? Until recently, it was difficult to measure. Estimates were based on the percentage of the population living in poverty, with the assumption that they were at risk of undernutrition. Such estimates are somewhat flawed because being at risk does not necessarily mean that people are poorly nourished. Many people with limited financial resources manage to eat well. However, under certain circumstances, such as loss of a job, people who live well above the poverty line (see Table 15.1) may be food-insecure.

The U.S. Department of Agriculture (USDA) tracks hunger with an annual **Food Security Supplement Survey**, which asks about food availability and hunger in the household. (See Table 15.2.) In a recent survey, food insecurity was strongly associated with poverty and was interlinked with economic

**Food Security Supplement Survey** A federally funded survey that measures the prevalence and severity of food insecurity and hunger.

**THINK**
**About It**
**2**

and social factors. Food insecurity and hunger were highest in households headed by single women with children and in Hispanic and African American households.[8] Geographically, food insecurity is more common in large cities and rural areas and, regionally, is more prevalent in the South. (See **Figure 15.3**.) To combat food insecurity and hunger effectively, nutrition programs must be accompanied by social and economic efforts.

## The Working Poor

Employment does not guarantee that families always have enough to eat. Often the pay is too little to lift households out of poverty, and work-related expenses, such as transportation or child care, further deplete family budgets. Food insecurity can be as common among the working poor as the unemployed. Low-paid workers may be unaware that they still qualify for food-assistance programs. However, their work hours may preclude program participation.

Migrant farm workers may have access to plenty of fresh produce but are poorly paid and may not have the money to buy other foods. Farm workers and undocumented workers (illegal aliens) may not qualify for government programs to help the poor or may not sign up for fear of deportation.

### Food Deserts

People in remote rural areas may live far from food resources and lack access to transportation. Areas that lack access to affordable healthy foods such as low-fat milk products, whole grains, fruits, and vegetables are termed *food deserts*.[9] Approximately 6,501 food deserts exist in the United States.[10]

### The Isolated

Some people become isolated despite living in populated cities. Even though they live in a crowded neighborhood or apartment building, they are alone and are physically or mentally unable to obtain adequate food.

### Older Adults

The infirmities of age, along with feelings of vulnerability, keep some older adults homebound and lonely, conditions hardly conducive to a healthy appetite. Physical ailments may make cooking and eating difficult, while actu-

---

**Table 15.2**  **Sample Questions from the Food Security Questionnaire**

*Light Food Insecurity*
"We worried whether our food would run out before we got money to buy more." Was that often, sometimes, or never true for you in the last 12 months?
"The food that we bought just didn't last and we didn't have money to get more." Was that often, sometimes, or never true for you in the last 12 months?

*Moderate Food Insecurity*
In the last 12 months did you or other adults in the household ever cut the size of your meals or skip meals because there wasn't enough money for food?
In the last 12 months, were you ever hungry but didn't eat because you couldn't afford enough food?

*Severe Food Insecurity*
In the last 12 months did you or other adults in the household ever not eat for a whole day because there wasn't enough money for food?
(For households with children) In the last 12 months did any children ever not eat for a whole day because there wasn't enough money for food?

**Source:** Reproduced from Nord M, Coleman-Jensen A, Andrews M, Carlson S. *Household Food Security in the United States, 2009.* USDA; November 2010. Economic Research Service. Report No. 108. http://www.ers.usda.gov/Publications/ERR108/ERR108.pdf. Accessed 7/23/11.

---

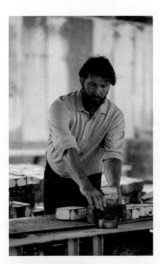
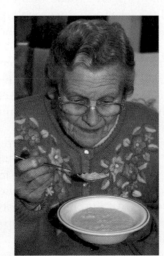
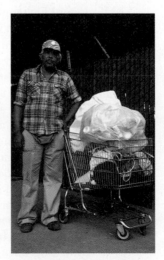
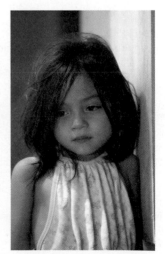

**Figure 15.3**    **Americans at risk.** Americans most at risk for hunger include working poor, older adults, homeless people, and children.

## Quick Bite

**A Dire Doubling in Less Than Three Decades**
In less than three decades (from 1998 to 2025), the number of people with obesity-related diabetes is expected to double. Three-quarters of this growth is projected to occur in developing countries.

**Food Research and Action Center (FRAC)** Founded in 1970 as a public interest law firm, FRAC is a nonprofit child advocacy group that works to improve public policies to eradicate hunger and undernutrition in the United States.

**Table 15.3** **USDA Food and Nutrition Service Food Assistance Programs**

Supplemental Nutrition Assistance Program (SNAP)
Women, Infants, and Children (WIC) Program
- Farmers' Market Nutrition Program
- Senior Farmers' Market Nutrition Program
School meals
- National School Lunch Program (NSLP)
- School Breakfast Program (SBP)
- Fresh Fruit and Vegetable Program
- Special Milk Program
- Team Nutrition
Summer Food Service Program (SFSP)
Child and Adult Food Care Program (CACFP)
Food assistance for disaster relief
Food distribution
- Schools/Child Nutrition Commodity Program
- Food Distribution Program on Indian Reservations (FDPIR)
- Nutrition Services Incentive Program
- The Emergency Food Assistance Program (TEFAP)

**Source:** Data from USDA Food and Nutrition Service. Nutrition assistance programs. http://www.fns.usda.gov/fns. Accessed 7/23/11.

ally increasing nutrient needs. Older adults often have small incomes, with little prospect for improvement. Like others with limited resources, they cut food purchases to pay for other necessities. Although food assistance may be available, pride or shame may keep an older person from participating in such programs.

### The Homeless or Inadequately Housed

The homeless rely on soup kitchens and other public programs for much of their food. Some resort to handouts and even forage through garbage. Many are mentally ill or substance abusers. The addict often has little interest in eating and may sell available food to buy more drugs. Many other people live in welfare hotels, single-room-occupancy facilities, or rooming houses without storage or cooking facilities. Budget-stretching strategies such as buying food in bulk and carefully using leftovers are out of the question for these people; as the monthly budget dwindles, they often rely on fast-food meals and then soup kitchens.

### Children

Perhaps no group is more vulnerable to hunger than the young. Growth and development are delayed in poorly nourished children. They get sick more often. It is harder for them to concentrate in school. Children are captives of their family circumstances; poverty and lack of nutritious food in the household are beyond a child's control. In the United States, roughly 21.3 percent of households with children and adolescents (ages 18 and under) were food-insecure at some time during 2009.[11]

## Attacking Hunger in America

Government efforts to fight hunger began during the Great Depression of the 1930s. From that modest beginning, federal efforts have grown to include at least 14 programs that address hunger. (See Table 15.3.) The School Lunch Program was created in 1946, after many young men failed the physical requirements for military service in World War II because of poor nutrition. The Food Stamp Program (now called the Supplemental Nutrition Assistance Program [SNAP]), begun on a small scale years earlier, was greatly expanded in the early 1970s following an exposé on hunger in Appalachia and the Mississippi Delta and the television documentary "Hunger in America." The federal government initiated the Special Supplemental Nutrition Program for Women, Infants, and Children (WIC) in the 1970s in response to concerns about maternal and child health. Other government programs have since been added to meet the special needs of the young, the elderly, the disadvantaged, and the disabled. The **Food Research and Action Center (FRAC)** is a national nonprofit advocacy group that fights hunger and undernutrition at the national, state, and local levels.

Nonprofit community agencies, charities, religious organizations, and similar groups create a large network of food pantries, soup kitchens, and services for home-delivered meals. (See the FYI feature "Hungry and Homeless.") Most federal government programs for direct distribution of food or meals operate at the local level through these networks. Both laypeople and professionals, such as dietitians, work in these programs, either as volunteers or as staff, to fight hunger and malnutrition.

Food assistance programs have greatly reduced the prevalence of hunger but not of food insecurity, which requires social and economic change. The following are among the federal government's most far-reaching programs against hunger.

THINK
About It

3

## The Supplemental Nutrition Assistance Program

On October 1, 2008, the Food Stamp Program was renamed the Supplemental Nutrition Assistance Program (SNAP). SNAP is the main food security program in the United States. Recipients can use benefits to purchase food but not nonfood items such as paper goods, pet food, and alcohol. The benefit amount varies according to household size and income level.

Actually, the term *food stamp* is becoming a misnomer. Almost half the people who receive benefits use **Electronic Benefits Transfer (EBT)** cards. (See **Figure 15.4**.) The card resembles and functions like a debit card. Each month the household's benefit amount is credited to the card, which is then used at participating retailers and farmers' markets.

> **Electronic Benefits Transfer (EBT)** Electronic delivery of government benefits by a single plastic card that allows access to food benefits at point-of-sale locations.

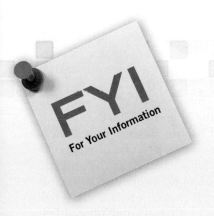

# Hungry and Homeless

A shabbily dressed man slowly pushes a shopping cart along the sidewalk. It is laden with bottles and cans that he can redeem for cash. In front of a supermarket, a woman and child clutch a sign scrawled with the words "Hungry. Please help." On a street corner, a man confronts every passing car with a sign that says "Will work for food." When confronted by a homeless person, do you feel uncomfortable? Do you turn away? Or, do you try to help?

The U.S. Conference of Mayors' Task Force on Hunger and Homelessness reports that between 2009 and 2010, among the people who requested emergency food assistance, 56 percent were persons in families, 30 percent were employed, 19 percent were older adults, and 17 percent were homeless.[1]

Who are the homeless? Roughly, 24 percent of homeless adults are severely mentally ill, 20 percent are physically disabled, 19 percent are employed, 14 percent are victims of domestic violence, 14 percent are veterans, and 3 percent are HIV positive.[2]

Hunger in the homeless is caused by a number of interrelated factors, including low-paying jobs, unemployment and related problems, high housing costs, substance abuse, poverty or lack of income, and food stamp cuts. Family members—children and their parents—most frequently request emergency food assistance. Among households with children, unemployment is the primary cause for homelessness, followed by lack of affordable housing, poverty, low-paying jobs, and domestic violence. Lack of affordable housing is the leading cause of homelessness for unaccompanied individuals, followed by mental illness and lack of needed psychological services, substance abuse and lack of needed medical services, and poverty.[3]

Complex challenges face the homeless, who may sleep in the streets or in emergency shelters. The homeless get food from many sources—shelters, drop-in centers, fast-food restaurants, and garbage bins. Approximately 4.8 million households (including 8.8 million adults and 4.5 million children) obtained food from pantries at least once in 2008.[4] Soup kitchens are a primary source of meals, yet navigating this system to obtain adequate food can be a formidable and time-consuming task. Almost 70 percent of food-insecure households did not use a food pantry despite knowing that they were available in their community.[5] Also, although homeless people often are eligible for food stamps, they are extremely limited in their ability to store and prepare food, and few restaurants are authorized to accept SNAP benefits.

A major public health concern for homeless people is not only whether they are getting enough to eat but also the nutritional quality of their diet. This concern is complicated by the special needs of infants, children, and women, especially pregnant women. The diet of food-insecure people, especially children, often is nutritionally inadequate for numerous key nutrients and low in fruit and vegetable intake. Poor diets put the homeless at an increased risk for illness and chronic conditions. Pregnant women, children, and people with compromised health status are particularly vulnerable.

Homeless families and individuals rely on emergency food assistance facilities not only during emergencies but also for extended periods. Unfortunately, these facilities are strained beyond their capacities. Due to limited space, emergency shelters must turn away families with children experiencing homelessness and unaccompanied individuals. During 2009–2010, an average of 27 percent of homeless persons in need of food assistance did not receive it.

Some shelters have resorted to rationing to extend their food resources to a greater number of people. Because of a lack of resources, over half may be forced to turn people away. Addressing hunger is a top priority. Once access to food is secure, obtaining a nutritionally adequate diet and dealing with health issues become reasonable goals.

1. US Conference of Mayors. *A Status Report on Hunger and Homelessness in America's Cities. A 27-City Survey.* 12/10. http://www.usmayors.org/pressreleases/uploads/2010HungerHomelessnessReportfinalDec212010.pdf. Accessed 7/23/11.

2. Ibid.

3. Ibid.

4. Position of the American Dietetic Association: food insecurity in the United States. *J Am Diet Assoc.* 2010;110:1368–1377.

5. Ibid.

6. Ibid.

7. Ibid.

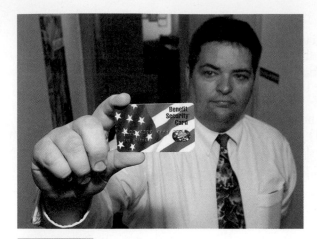

**Figure 15.4** **Electronic Benefits Transfer card.** Electronic Benefits Transfer (EBT) is an electronic system that allows recipients to authorize transfer of their government benefits from a federal account to a retailer account to pay for products received.

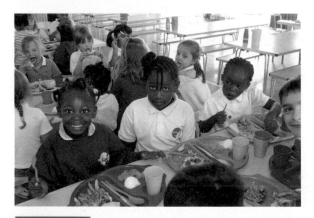

**Figure 15.5** **National School Lunch Program.**

**Child and Adult Care Food Program** A federally funded program that reimburses approved family child-care providers for USDA-approved foods served to preschool children; also provides funds for meals and snacks served at after-school programs for school-age children and to adult day care centers serving chronically impaired adults or people over age 60.

**Feeding America** The largest charitable hunger-relief organization in the United States. Its mission is to feed America's hungry through a nationwide network of member food banks and to engage the country in the fight to end hunger.

## Special Supplemental Nutrition Program for Women, Infants, and Children

The WIC program provides food to pregnant and breastfeeding women, infants, and preschoolers. More than 9 million women and children receive WIC benefits each month.[12] To be eligible for WIC services, the participant must be at nutritional risk and the household's income must be less than the federal definition of poverty level. For a family of four in fiscal year 2010, the eligibility cut-off point is an annual income of no more than $40,793.[13]

Nutrition assessment and nutrition education are important components of the WIC program. In most states, participants receive coupons, "checks," or EBT cards for specific categories of healthful foods, and they use them at participating grocery stores. Unlike SNAP benefits, the amount of the WIC benefit varies with nutritional need, not income.

## National School Lunch Program

The National School Lunch Program ensures that children in primary and secondary schools receive at least one healthful meal every school day (supplemented in many areas by the School Breakfast Program). For a family of four for the 2011–2012 school year, the child's meals are free if the household income is less than $29,055; the allotment for meals is reduced if the household income exceeds $29,055 but is less than $41,348.[14] School lunches must comply with the *Dietary Guidelines for Americans, 2010* and provide one-third or more of dietary requirements for key nutrients. The program operates in more than 101,000 public and nonprofit private schools and residential child-care institutions. It provides nutritionally balanced, low-cost or free lunches to more than 31 million children each school day.[15] (See **Figure 15.5**.)

## Child and Adult Care Food Program

The **Child and Adult Care Food Program** provides funds for children's meals and snacks at nonprofit licensed child-care centers, day care homes, after-school programs, and similar settings. Nutritious meals for older adults or disabled people are also funded at nonprofit facilities such as adult day care centers and recreation centers.

## Feeding America

**Feeding America**, formerly known as *America's Second Harvest*, is the largest charitable hunger-relief organization in the United States. This network of more than 200 member food banks and food-rescue organizations secures and distributes more than 3 billion pounds of donated food and groceries throughout the United States. Each year, Feeding America provides food assistance to more than 37 million hungry people, including 14 million children and 3 million seniors.[16]

Feeding America focuses on nutritious products such as fresh produce, seafood, meat, cereal, rice, and pasta. The organization also works to effect changes in public attitudes and laws that assist Americans who are hungry or at risk of being hungry. Feeding America works to educate the general public and keep them informed about hunger in America.

**Key Concepts** *Although overt malnutrition in the United States is uncommon, more than 17.4 million American households experience food insecurity at some time during the* *year. Food insecurity and hunger are interlinked with poverty. Groups at risk include the working poor, the isolated, the homeless, children, and older adults. A large network of individual volunteers, nonprofit agencies, and charities, together with major government programs such as SNAP, WIC, and School Lunch, have done much to reduce hunger. However, food insecurity, which continues among an unacceptably large number of people, must be overcome by social and economic improvements. Feeding America is the largest charitable hunger-relief organization in the United States.*

### Malnutrition in the Developing World

"Proper nutrition and health are fundamental human rights," according to the **World Health Organization (WHO)**. "Nutrition is a cornerstone that affects and defines the health of all people, rich and poor. It paves the way for us to grow, develop, work, play, resist infection and aspire to realization of our fullest potential as individuals and societies. Conversely, malnutrition makes us all more vulnerable to disease and premature death."[17]

Hunger is a global problem. (See **Figure 15.6**.) "The number and the proportion of undernourished people have declined, but they remain unacceptably high. Undernourishment remains higher than before the food and economic crises, making it ever more difficult to achieve international hunger targets," says the **Food and Agriculture Organization (FAO)** of the United Nations.[18]

"The world food system is in trouble and the hot spots of food risks will be where high food prices combine with shocks from weather or political crises. These are recipes for disaster," says Joachim von Braun, the Director General of the International Food Policy Research Institute.[19]

> THINK
> About It
> **4**

### The World Food Equation

Income growth, climate change, high energy prices, globalization, and urbanization are transforming food consumption. Soaring food prices are hitting the world's most vulnerable—those who must spend a substantial part of their income on food. Today, the world consumes more than it produces, and the cost of food has been rising steadily, reversing a downward trend of more than four decades. Food stocks are at a low, and the food supply is vulnerable to unpredictable factors, such as adverse weather. During a disaster, food prices rise rapidly while family incomes decline, thus producing an economic mismatch that is the root cause of most famines.[20]

### Global Economic Boom

Some developing countries are undergoing rapid economic expansion. People in emerging economies, such as China, India, Brazil, and at least 10 African countries, have become more prosperous and are changing their diets. Since 1990, China has nearly doubled its consumption of meat, fish, and dairy products. Because it takes 7 pounds of grain to produce 1 pound of meat, this shift removes grain from the global marketplace. In just the past few years, China has changed from being one of the largest corn exporters to importing corn.[21]

### Oil Prices and Biofuels

Record oil prices have driven up costs along the entire food production chain—from fertilizer to diesel oil for tilling, planting, and harvesting to storage and shipping. High oil prices also make food stocks a more attractive alternative fuel. Production of biodiesel and other biofuels is pressuring the global markets for wheat, corn, sugar, oil-containing seeds, cassava, palm oil, and other crops.

---

**World Health Organization (WHO)** A global organization that directs and coordinates international health work. Its goal is the attainment by all peoples of the highest possible level of health, defined as a state of complete physical, mental, and social well-being and not merely the absence of disease or infirmity.

**Food and Agriculture Organization (FAO)** The largest autonomous UN agency; the FAO works to alleviate poverty and hunger by promoting agricultural development, improved nutrition, and the pursuit of food security.

---

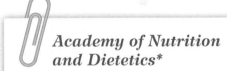

*Academy of Nutrition and Dietetics**

**Addressing World Hunger, Malnutrition, and Food Insecurity**

It is the position of the American Dietetic Association that access to adequate amounts of safe, nutritious, and culturally appropriate food at all times is a fundamental human right. Hunger continues to be a worldwide problem of staggering proportions. The Association supports programs and encourages practices that combat hunger and malnutrition, produce food security, promote self-sufficiency, and are environmentally and economically sustainable.

**Source:** Reproduced from Struble MB, Aomari LL. Position of the Academy of Nutrition and Dietetics: addressing world hunger, malnutrition, and food insecurity. *J Am Diet Assoc.* 2003;103(8):1046–1057.

* Formerly the American Dietetic Association

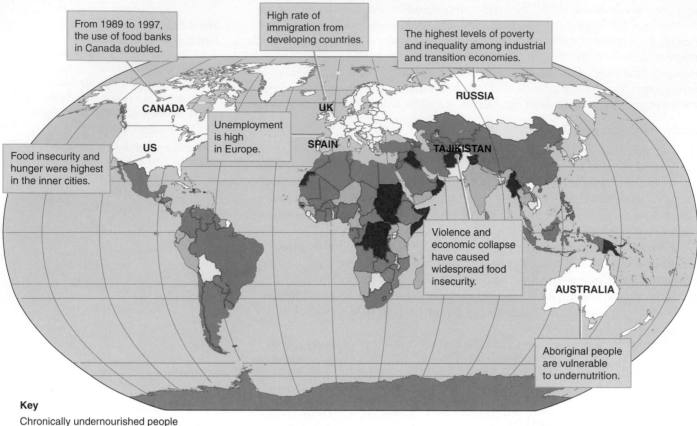

From 1989 to 1997, the use of food banks in Canada doubled.

High rate of immigration from developing countries.

The highest levels of poverty and inequality among industrial and transition economies.

CANADA

RUSSIA

UK

US

Unemployment is high in Europe.

SPAIN

TAJIKISTAN

Food insecurity and hunger were highest in the inner cities.

Violence and economic collapse have caused widespread food insecurity.

AUSTRALIA

Aboriginal people are vulnerable to undernutrition.

**Key**
Chronically undernourished people

- ■ Less than 5%
- ■ 5–10%
- ■ 10–20%
- ■ 20–30%
- ■ 30–40%
- ■ 40% and above
- □ Comparable data not available

**Figure 15.6** **Global hunger.** Although the proportion of the world's population that is chronically undernourished has been decreasing over the last few decades, undernutrition is still widespread, particularly in certain regions. Furthermore, projections to the year 2010 suggest that there will be little change in the absolute number of chronically undernourished people.

**Source:** Food and Agriculture Organization of the United Nations. Hunger: Interactive world hunger map. http://www.fao.org/hunger/en. Accessed 7/27/11.

### Global Climate Change and Severe Weather Events

As a consequence of climate change, farmers will face growing unpredictability and variability in water supplies and increasing frequency of droughts and floods. However, these impacts will vary tremendously from place to place. According to experts with the FAO, "The livelihoods of rural communities and the food security of a predominantly urban population are at risk from water-related impacts linked primarily to climate variability. The rural poor, who are the most vulnerable, are likely to be disproportionately affected."[22]

Water is fundamental to the stability of global food production. Reliable access to water increases agricultural yields, and a lack of sustainable water management places global food security at risk. In developing countries, drought is the single most common natural cause of severe food shortages. Floods are another major cause of food emergencies. To the extent that climate change increases rainfall variability and the frequency of extreme weather events, it will threaten food security.

### The Fight Against Global Hunger

International relief agencies and government programs help combat food shortages and hunger. Some U.S. agencies involved in the fight against global

*Quick* Bite

**Where Were You Born?**
Your survival was greatly influenced by the location of your birth. Angola has the highest infant mortality rate (195 deaths per 1,000 live births), according to estimates for year 2000. Other countries with high infant mortality rates include Sierra Leone (148 per 1,000), Afghanistan (149 per 1,000), and Liberia (134 per 1,000). At the other end of the spectrum is Finland (4 per 1,000). Canada (5 per 1,000) has a lower infant mortality rate than the United States (7 per 1,000).

hunger are the USDA; the U.S. State Department, through its Agency for International Development; and the Centers for Disease Control and Prevention (CDC), through the Center for Communicable Diseases. These agencies offer both short-term emergency efforts and long-term programs for repair and rebuilding.

Long-term solutions to hunger are tremendously complex; they require economic, political, and social change as well as improvements in nutrition, food production, and environmental safeguards. As you study the critical nutrient deficiencies in the developing world, you will see that poverty, infection, poor sanitation, and social upheaval interact with nutrient shortages to bring about these deficiencies.

## Social and Economic Factors

Poverty, overpopulation, and migration to overcrowded cities are closely interrelated causes of hunger. (See **Figure 15.7**.) Each of those situations compounds the effects of the others as they steadily drive a population toward malnutrition.

### Poverty

Poverty, hunger, and malnutrition stalk one another in a vicious circle, compromising health and wreaking havoc on the development of entire countries and regions. A large percentage of the global population—especially those in developing countries—bear this triple burden.

Poverty is the most important underlying reason for chronic hunger.[23] Obviously, poverty limits access to food. It limits purchase of farming supplies to grow food, boats and equipment to fish, and storage equipment to prevent spoilage. It limits access to medical care. It compromises efforts at sanitation. It discourages education and the chance for personal advancement.

For nations, poverty means paralyzed economic development and too few jobs; inadequate investments in infrastructure and basic housing; and too few resources to train doctors, nutritionists, nurses, and other healthcare workers.

### Population Growth

Population growth in many regions is outstripping gains in food production, education, employment, health care, and economic progress. The burgeoning numbers stress limited environmental resources, contributing to environmental degradation and pollution. In rural areas where farmland is limited, each small parcel of family land is subdivided with each generation, until there is too little land to support each family.

You might think that poverty would pressure parents to limit family size, but, ironically, poverty and sickness do just the reverse. Where child mortality rates are high, having many babies is a guarantee some children will survive. In countries that have no economic safeguards for disability, unemployment, or old age, parents consider their children a source of security and support in times of need. Many other factors contribute to large families, from ignorance of birth control methods to the attitude that big families reflect the father's masculinity. Some political and religious groups also encourage high birth rates and fast population growth as a way to achieve political or military

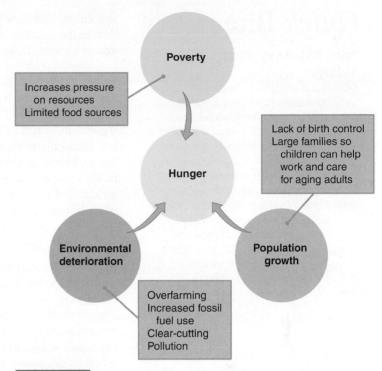

| Figure 15.7 | **Major problems causing hunger.** Poverty, population growth, and environmental degradation interact to intensify hunger problems. |

## Quick Bite

**World Food Summit Goals: Can We Meet the Challenge?**

The World Food Summit has pledged to halve the number of undernourished people by 2015. Although the proportion of malnourished people has declined, the number of hungry people has remained virtually unchanged since 1990–1992. To meet the summit's 2015 goal, the world must reduce the number of hungry people by 31 million annually—10 times the reduction achieved since 1990–1992.

*Quick* Bite

**Food Supply vs. Food Safety**
Sometimes obtaining food is more important than safety. Food from street vendors is important in the diets of many urban populations, particularly the socially disadvantaged. Health authorities responsible for food safety should balance their risk management with issues of food availability and hunger. Rigorous application of codes and regulations suited to larger and permanent food-service establishments may cause the disappearance of the street vendors, with consequent aggravation of hunger and malnutrition. WHO encourages the development of regulations that empower vendors to take greater responsibility for the preparation of safe food.

*Quick* Bite

**Rehydration Therapy for Diarrhea**
Simple and inexpensive packets of carbohydrate and salts diluted with sterile water replace lost fluids and electrolytes. These packets are saving thousands of people each year.

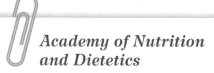

*Academy of Nutrition and Dietetics*

**Nutrition Intervention and Human Immunodeficiency Virus Infection**
It is the position of the Academy of Nutrition and Dietetics that efforts to optimize nutritional status through individualized medical nutrition therapy, assurance of food and nutrition security, and nutrition education are essential to the total system of health care available to people with human immunodeficiency virus (HIV) infection throughout the continuum of care.

**Source:** Reproduced from Fields-Gardner C, et al. Position of the American Dietetic Association and Dietitians of Canada: nutrition intervention in the care of persons with human immunodeficiency virus infection. *J Am Diet Assoc.* 2004;104(9):1425-1441.

dominance. To slow population growth, socioeconomic and cultural changes that make smaller family size acceptable, even desirable, must accompany access to birth control.

### Urbanization

Urbanization is a worldwide trend. As rural lands become too crowded or exhausted farmland no longer supports good crops, rural people migrate to the city in hopes of jobs and a better life. Unfortunately, in fast-growing cities, social disorder, sanitary conditions, and living standards may be much worse. Hunting, fishing, foraging, and gardening—sources of accessible food in the rural setting—are seldom an option in the city. Breastfeeding becomes impractical for many mothers who could nurse their babies while doing farm work but cannot do so with jobs in the city.

## Infection and Disease

Infection interacts with malnutrition, each making its victim more vulnerable to the other, each making the other worse, in a downward spiral. Nutrient deficiencies lower resistance to infections. In turn, the fever of infection speeds depletion of calories and nutrients. Other symptoms (e.g., loss of appetite, weakness, nausea, mouth lesions) limit ability to eat. Infectious diarrhea is especially dangerous, quickly wasting what few nutrients are consumed; infants and young children can die quickly from loss of electrolytes. Programs that prevent or control infection (e.g., immunizations, improvements in hygiene and sanitation, safe water supplies, access to medicine and medical care) all indirectly improve nutrition status.

Infection with the human immunodeficiency virus (HIV) provides a dramatic demonstration of the interaction between malnutrition and infection. (See the FYI feature "AIDS and Malnutrition.") Transmission of the virus from mother to fetus is greater when the mother is deficient in vitamin A. Among those who are afflicted, the infection progresses fastest in people who are poorly nourished. Severe loss of weight and muscle are hallmarks of the advanced disease, acquired immune deficiency syndrome (AIDS). Globally, AIDS is the fourth leading cause of death. More than 33 million people are living with HIV, partly because infected people are living longer than before, and AIDS-related deaths have declined in recent years.[24] Ninety-seven percent of people living with HIV/AIDS live in low- and middle-income countries, and an estimated 67 percent of all people living with HIV worldwide live in sub-Saharan Africa, where it is the leading cause of death. Other areas experiencing severe epidemics include Eastern Europe, Latin America, Asia, and Central Asia. In 2009, approximately 370,000 children were newly infected with HIV, bringing the total number of children living with HIV to 2.1 million. About half of all new adult HIV infections occur among people aged 15 to 24 years.[25]

## Political Disruptions

Social upheavals and natural disasters such as floods and drought can leave famine in their wake. The resulting displacement of populations and inequitable food distribution usually lead to hunger and malnutrition.

### War

Whereas poverty is the underlying cause of chronic mild to moderate malnutrition, war and its aftermath cause severe malnutrition and famine. War diverts limited financial resources from development efforts to expenditures for fighting and destruction. Men and women no longer farm, fish, or bring home a paycheck—they are in the army. Households become fatherless and sometimes motherless, often permanently. Crops and croplands are destroyed, along with irrigation systems, food-processing facilities, and transportation infrastructure, which may have taken decades to develop.

### Refugees

Masses of refugees—many very young, old, infirm, and already weakened by chronic hunger—find themselves without the basic elements of sustenance. The resulting famine has become an all too common sight on the evening news. International relief agencies have learned to respond to these emergencies quickly and with great determination, but logistic difficulties (e.g., mobilizing manpower, obtaining foods, transporting supplies, setting up feeding stations) may slow relief until it is too late for the sickest or weakest. Some refugee groups are inaccessible, hidden, or intentionally kept hungry as part of a political plan; emergency food may never reach many of them.

### Sanctions

International sanctions and embargoes create food shortages, both directly and indirectly, by limiting access to agricultural supplies, fuel, and food-processing supplies. Some people argue that shortages created by embargoes hurt powerless people rather than government officials; others say that such actions are preferable to war.

*Quick* **Bite**

**Accidental Solution**
Sometimes a solution to undernutrition is not planned. On October 9, 1998, the *Wall Street Journal* carried the headline, "In Guatemala, Organic Farms Sprout on Civil War Turf." During the country's 35-year civil war, local farmers abandoned their land. As the farmlands reverted to jungle and pesticide levels diminished, wild spices thrived. With the trend for "organic" spices, coffee, and natural dyes, the premium prices commanded by these new crops could be significant for the farmers' incomes.

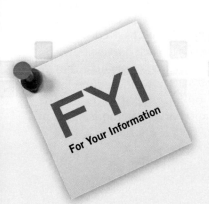

## AIDS and Malnutrition

Like other infections, HIV interacts with malnutrition in a vicious, devastating cycle. Left untreated, HIV infection progresses to acquired immunodeficiency syndrome (AIDS). The virus attacks by destroying its victim's immune system. When a person is unable to fight infections and malignancies, disease quickly depletes marginal nutrient stores, speeding the way to severe malnutrition and death. But malnutrition and HIV interact on several other levels, as well:[1]

- Poor nutrition contributes to declining immune function, HIV progression, and further deterioration in health.
- HIV is transmitted to infants in breast milk; but in impoverished regions substitutions for breast milk typically increase infantile diarrhea, malnutrition, and death.
- AIDS leaves mothers too weak to feed and care for their children. Eventually AIDS turns children into orphans.
- AIDS disables parents so they cannot work to support and feed their families.
- Among those who are afflicted, the infection progresses faster in people who are poorly nourished.
- Weight loss and muscle wasting in an infected person are associated with faster progression of HIV disease and AIDS.

- Infections that accompany AIDS cause fever and diarrhea, making malnutrition worse. Nausea and loss of appetite also contribute to malnutrition.
- Severe protein-energy malnutrition (PEM) is characteristic of untreated AIDS and frequently the ultimate cause of death.
- Adequate dietary intake and nutrient absorption are essential to achieving the maximum benefit of antiretroviral treatment for HIV/AIDS.

More than 34 million people worldwide were living with HIV in 2010.[2] Sub-Saharan Africa, Southeast and Central Asia, Latin America, and Eastern Europe continue to be areas with a high prevalence of HIV. Without treatment or a cure, these people are doomed to death, usually within 10 years of the initial infection. The fate of severe

PEM in millions of people appears unavoidable. If we do not arrest the continued transmission of HIV, the number of PEM victims will climb even higher.

1   UNAIDS Joint United Nations Programme on HIV/AIDS. HIV, food security, and nutrition. Policy Brief. 5/08. http://www.unaids.org/en/media/unaids/contentassets/dataimport/pub/manual/2008/jc1515_policy_brief_nutrition_en.pdf. Accessed 7/27/11.

2   UNAIDS Joint United Nations Programme on HIV/AIDS. Homepage. http://www.unaids.org/en. Accessed 7/27/11.

## *Quick* Bite

**Emergency Management**
Imagine a civil war in a developing country that displaces tens of thousands of people. What are the most important measures for preventing sickness and death among these refugees? Protection from violence heads the list, closely followed by adequate food rations, clean water and sanitation, diarrheal disease control, measles immunization, and maternal and child health care.

## *Quick* Bite

**Know Thine Enemy**
Crops have a critical role in feeding the world's burgeoning population. "Responsible biotechnology is not the enemy; starvation is," says former President Jimmy Carter.

## Agriculture and Environment: A Tricky Balance

Advances in agriculture increase food supplies and reduce food costs. Because the economies of most developing countries are based on agriculture, improvements boost rural incomes and buying power, increase demand for agricultural labor, stimulate commerce among small vendors and food processors, and ultimately help a nation's economy.

Dramatic gains in agricultural productivity took place in the 1960s and 1970s with the development of new seed varieties, especially rice and corn. The seeds greatly increased crop yields. Expectations were so strong that these seeds would finally solve the world's food shortage that their development and use was dubbed the "Green Revolution." Despite its successes, the Green Revolution had limitations. The seeds required irrigation and heavy use of pesticides and fertilizers, which poor farmers could not afford. (See the FYI feature "Tough Choices.") The farming techniques were sometimes hard on the environment. Gains from the Green Revolution have now about reached their limit and, if current trends continue, threaten to be lost to the population explosion.

Proponents of agricultural biotechnology see it as another step along the continuum of plant-breeding techniques and a promising tool to increase crop production. Some uses of biotechnology are well accepted—for example, diagnostic kits that identify plants and insects by DNA and tissue culture for plant reproduction, a technique already in widespread commercial use. More controversial is the modification of plant genetic material. The technology has the potential to improve plants' resistance to disease, tolerance to adverse conditions, yield, and nutritional quality.

At the other end of the technology spectrum is a renewed appreciation and conservation of traditional seed varieties, those selected over the generations by local farmers because they do well in local conditions. In developing countries, farmers typically save some of these seeds at each harvest to use in the next planting season. The seeds grow well in the regions where they've evolved, whereas imported seeds, no matter how carefully bred, often fail.

In addition to seed selection, strategies to optimize agriculture include irrigation, soil preparation, improved planting and harvest methods, erosion

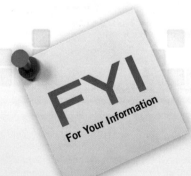

# Tough Choices

Imagine you live in a poor village of a developing country. How would you make these choices?

- You've learned you must boil your drinking water to prevent diarrhea. But that means cutting young trees for firewood. You recently planted those trees to stop erosion. What do you do?
- You've recently given birth to your fourth child. Your husband was injured in an accident and is unable to work. But, you can work at a nearby factory and use your pay to buy food and clothes for the older

children. How would you feed the new baby?
- Your small herd of goats provides milk for your young children. You like the goats because they can survive in the rough, hilly countryside, but the goats are overgrazing the grasses on the hillside. What can you do?
- Insects have destroyed your crop. In the past, you burned fields after harvest to control insects, but you've learned that

"slash and burn" is bad for the land. You've thought about using a chemical pesticide, but it is too expensive. You could clear the jungle for another growing field. Do you have other choices? What should you do?
- You can grow either vegetables to feed your family or a "cash crop" to sell for export. The cash crop would help pay for medicine and other necessities. Which should you grow?

prevention, fertilization, pest control, and flood control. The methods should be affordable, suitable for the level of local development, and protective of the environment. For example, where there is an abundant supply of willing farm laborers and gasoline is expensive, using heavy-duty farm machinery makes little sense. Other examples include mulching to conserve water and control weeds, and using manure (after composting to kill pathogens) to reduce the need for fertilizer.

### Environmental Degradation

Environmental degradation is a growing concern in both the developing and the industrialized world. In developing countries, there is pressure for more land to support rapidly expanding populations. In industrialized countries, there is pressure from the affluent for more land, more houses, larger properties, more recreation areas, and so on. Residents of the industrialized world consume vast amounts of resources (e.g., water, fuel, wood, paper, textiles, food) without a thought and often without making the small effort to conserve or recycle. Residents of the developing world consume much less per person, but the impact of their numbers is greater.

Environmental degradation has nutritional consequences because it threatens food production. Urbanization and the expansion of cities reduce acreage available for farming. The pressure to supply food to growing populations leads to clear-cutting marginal land, eventually eroding hilly terrain or quickly exhausting fragile rain forest soils. Overdependence on irrigation can drain water, eventually creating deserts. The destruction of vast areas of natural ground cover can lead to global climate changes. Overuse of pesticides and fertilizers pollutes waterways, destroying fish and seafood.

**Key Concepts** *Despite gains in eradicating malnutrition, almost all undernourished people in the world live in developing countries. Factors that allow hunger to continue include rising food prices, poverty, poor sanitation, urbanization, and inefficient food distribution. Infection, especially AIDS, rapid population growth, wars, and environmental degradation threaten to reverse hard-won gains.*

## Malnutrition: Its Nature, Its Victims, and Its Eradication

Most diseases of nutritional deficiency exist throughout the developing world but seldom in isolation. Typically, the malnourished person has two or more coexisting deficiencies, each increasing the severity of the other. Keep the potential for this deadly synergy in mind as we discuss some major categories of malnutrition.

### Protein-Energy Malnutrition

Lack of protein and also energy can have devastating consequences, especially on the young. In kwashiorkor, the body and face swell with excess fluid, the hair turns wispy and red, and a terrible rash develops; without treatment, the person dies. Marasmus paints an even more dramatic picture of sunken eyes, shriveled limbs, and a clearly visible outline of the skeleton; it is as deadly as kwashiorkor.

Protein-energy malnutrition (PEM) is by far the most lethal form of malnutrition, and children are its most visible victims.[26] Their fast growth creates high nutrient demands, leaving them especially vulnerable to inappropriate food distribution in the family, inappropriate infant and child feeding practices, and interactions of infection with malnutrition. PEM typically develops after a child is weaned from the breast. Men in the household may have priority for nutritious food. In big families, the young child must also compete for food with many siblings.

## *Quick* Bite

In the developing world, breastfeeding is almost always essential to an infant's survival. Inappropriate bottle-feeding puts a baby at grave risk. Relative to income, formula is usually very expensive and often is diluted to make it "stretch." Contaminated water and lack of other hygienic requirements for bottle preparation cause diarrhea. The combination of diarrhea and nutritional deficiency from watered-down formula often is fatal.

A tremendous educational effort, including promotion of breastfeeding, has reduced the global prevalence and severity of infant and childhood PEM. Severe PEM typified by kwashiorkor or marasmus has become more sporadic, occurring mainly as a result of war or natural disaster. However, mild to moderate PEM continues to pose a grave problem in the developing world, putting children at risk of delayed growth, impaired psychological development, and the deadly interactions of disease and malnutrition.

### Iodine Deficiency Disorders

Iodine deficiency is the world's most common cause of preventable brain damage and a main cause of impaired cognitive development in children.[27] Its impairment of intellectual ability and work performance is potentially so widespread that **iodine deficiency disorders (IDDs)** can actually slow a nation's social and economic development.

Iodine deficiency is most devastating during pregnancy, causing spontaneous abortions, stillbirths, and birth defects, including cretinism, a disease of mental retardation that is often severe. Deafness and spastic paralysis are likely to accompany the retardation. In regions of Africa, dwarfism also occurs where diets rich in goitrogen-containing vegetables (e.g., cassava, cabbage) make the deficiency worse. Moreover, iodine deficiency is damaging at all ages, limiting mental development in infants and children and producing apathy and marginal mental function in adults.

Iodine deficiency disorders are endemic throughout much of the developing world where the soil is low in iodine. These areas typically are mountainous or far from the oceans. They often are isolated and impoverished. Fifty-four countries are still iodine-deficient.[28] The WHO estimates that 31.5 percent (266 million) of school-age children have insufficient iodine intake.[29] (See **Figure 15.8.**)

Disturbing though these figures are, great strides have been made in IDD prevention, mainly through iodizing salt. More than two-thirds of households throughout the world now use iodized salt,[30] and, in countries with salt iodization programs in place for five years or more, the improvement in iodine status has been dramatic. The cost is merely 5 cents per person per year.

### Vitamin A Deficiency

Vitamin A deficiency is the leading cause of preventable blindness in children. It also increases the risk of disease and death from severe infections. In pregnant women, vitamin A deficiency causes night blindness and may increase the risk of maternal mortality.

Vitamin A deficiency is a public health problem in more than half of all countries, especially those in Africa and Southeast Asia, hitting young children and pregnant women in low-income countries hardest. The nutrient is crucial for maternal and child survival, and supplying adequate vitamin A in high-risk areas can significantly reduce mortality. Conversely, its absence causes a needlessly high risk of disease and death. An estimated 250 million preschool children are vitamin A–deficient. Of the estimated 250,000 to 500,000 children who become blind every year from vitamin A deficiency, one-half will die within 12 months of losing their sight.[31]

**iodine deficiency disorders (IDD)** A wide range of disorders due to iodine deficiency that affect growth and development.

Vitamin A deficiency often coexists with marginal PEM. The vitamin deficiency predisposes infants and children to diarrheal diseases, which, in turn, worsen the child's nutritional status, leading to severe PEM. Common childhood infections, most notably measles, are much more serious in vitamin A–deficient children, with a much greater risk of death or permanent damage from complications.

In communities where vitamin A deficiency exists, pregnant and breast-feeding women often experience night blindness, an early symptom of deficiency. Maternal death, poor pregnancy outcome, and failure to lactate are all increased with vitamin A deficiency. Vitamin A levels in the breast milk of these women are likely to be low as well, putting their infants at later risk of deficiency.

Many countries are taking a multipronged approach to vitamin A deficiency that includes promotion of breastfeeding, fortification of foods, supplementation, and nutrition education. Foods such as eggs, dairy foods, and liver are promoted as important for women and children; educational programs also encourage growing and eating fruits and vegetables high in beta-carotene. However, dietary change can be difficult and slow. The best sources of vitamin A often are the most expensive or inaccessible. For absorption and conversion to vitamin A, beta-carotene requires dietary fat—another expensive item in many areas—and other factors not completely understood. Meanwhile, periodic single, large-dose vitamin A supplements, often given in tandem with maternal–child immunizations, are proving an effective short-term measure.

Biotechnology may have a significant impact on vitamin A deficiency. Through genetic engineering, scientists have developed a new strain of rice that is rich in beta-carotene. When these rice plants are crossed with locally grown strains of rice, they become suited to a particular region's climate and growing conditions. If local farmers and consumers accept such crops, bioengineered rice may play a critical role in feeding the world's burgeoning population and alleviating widespread vitamin A deficiency.[32]

### Iron-Deficiency Anemia

Iron deficiency is the most common nutritional disorder in the world. The numbers are staggering: 2 billion people—over 30 percent of the world's population—are anemic, mainly due to iron deficiency. In resource-poor areas, the condition frequently is worsened by infectious diseases, including malaria, HIV/AIDS, and hookworm infestation.[33] Although iron deficiency occurs in all age groups, fast growth in young children and reproductive blood loss in women make them especially vulnerable to low-iron diets. Anemia impairs childhood development, work capacity, learning capacity, and resistance to disease.[34] Anemia during pregnancy increases illness and death rates for mother and baby. For all groups of people, anemia can cause profound fatigue, and severe anemia causes death.

The anemias of the developing world demonstrate the interaction of multiple nutrient deficiencies, which, in turn, interact with infection, sanitation, and poverty. Supplying iron alone is seldom enough to correct the problem. Iron-deficient diets are typically high in starch and cereal grains. During digestion, cereals may bind with the very limited iron the diet provides, preventing its absorption. Other blood-building nutrients, such as vitamins $B_6$ and $B_{12}$ and folate, are in short supply as well.

Anemia-producing parasites are common in areas of iron deficiency, aggravating the effects of poor diet. Blood cells are destroyed by malarial infections. Intestinal malabsorption and intestinal bleeding are caused by hookworm, which is prevalent where human waste contaminates the fields

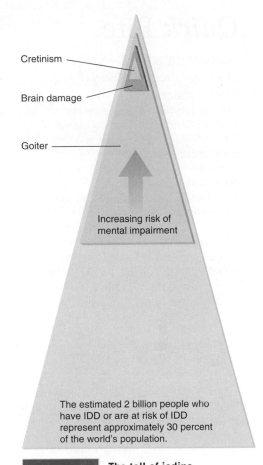

Cretinism

Brain damage

Goiter

Increasing risk of mental impairment

The estimated 2 billion people who have IDD or are at risk of IDD represent approximately 30 percent of the world's population.

**Figure 15.8** **The toll of iodine deficiency.** Iodine deficiency remains the single greatest cause of preventable brain damage and mental retardation worldwide.

## *Quick* Bite

**The Importance of Rice**
Rice is the principal food crop for one-half of the world's population.

## *Quick* Bite

### Overweight and Malnourished: It Knows No Boundaries

Take a 14-year-old African-American boy living in Baltimore. While watching hours of television or playing video games, he is like many Americans: he eats too much junk food. He knows he is obese. What he doesn't know is that his body is starving for *omega*-3 fatty acids and other essential nutrients like vitamins and minerals required for good development and health.

Now take a 14-year-old boy from Nigeria. He has poor, uneducated parents and has to share a small bowl of rice and legumes with his three siblings every day. He walks several miles to school daily, often in intense heat. He is emaciated and frequently endures pangs of hunger. For Nigerian children like this, malnutrition usually starts before they are born due to poor prenatal care.

They are an ocean apart, yet both boys suffer from malnutrition, ranging from undernutrition with resulting short stature and below normal weight for the Nigerian to overconsumption of high-fat foods with little or no exercise leading to obesity for the American. Research tells us that both these forms of malnutrition weaken a person's defenses against various infections and make one more prone to diseases, including measles, malaria, tuberculosis, respiratory and diarrheal diseases, HIV/AIDS, and some cancers.

**Source:** Courtesy of Dr. Cyril O. Enwonwu, Professor of Biochemistry, University of Maryland. First published in *The Baltimore Sun*.

where people walk barefoot, and by other parasites, acquired when human waste contaminates the water that people drink or in which people bathe.

People debilitated by anemia may be too weak to build outhouses, too poor to buy shoes or fuel to boil water, or too apathetic to clear standing water where malaria-carrying mosquitoes breed. Moreover, they often do not understand the connection between sanitation, infection, and malnutrition. Added to this mix are excessive blood loss from repeated pregnancies, inherited blood disorders such as sickle cell disease, and chronic bacterial or viral infections such as HIV.

Timely treatment can restore personal health and raise national productivity levels by as much as 20 percent.[35] The WHO has developed a comprehensive package of public health measures based on a three-pronged approach:

1. *Increase iron intake.* Dietary diversification, including iron-rich foods and enhancement of iron absorption, food fortification, and iron supplementation.
2. *Control infection.* Immunization and control programs for malaria and parasitic worm diseases.
3. *Improve nutritional status.* Prevention and control of other nutritional deficiencies, such as vitamin $B_{12}$, folate, and vitamin A.

### Deficiencies of Other Micronutrients

Deficiencies of zinc and calcium often coexist with other deficiencies, contributing to illness and death during periods of growth and threatening immune function and skeletal health in people who survive to old age.

Selenium deficiency, although limited to only a few countries, has serious consequences. It occurs where the soil is selenium-poor, in distinct regional patterns in China and Russia. In China, where the deficiency is most severe, it predisposes individuals to the fatal Keshan disease, in which heart muscle is destroyed. Keshan disease affects mainly women and children. The condition can be prevented by selenium supplementation or by fortification, as in programs undertaken in New Zealand, where soil is also low in selenium.

The classical deficiency diseases beriberi, pellagra, and scurvy still occur among the world's poorest and most underprivileged people. Most often, however, these diseases strike the victims of war and political strife—the refugees. Diets based on milled cereals and starchy roots, all poor thiamin sources, predispose refugee populations to beriberi. People who rely on corn-based diets low in niacin and tryptophan are susceptible to pellagra. The disruption of refugee life can easily tip the balance from marginal deficiency to overt deficiency disease.

### Overweight and Obesity

Obesity is a growing health problem worldwide and is increasingly being recognized as a form of malnutrition.[36] Obesity has reached epidemic proportions globally, with more than 1 billion adults overweight—at least 300 million of them clinically obese. It is a major contributor to the global burden of chronic disease and disability.[37] In developing countries, obesity often exists right alongside undernutrition. Obesity exists in areas of economic advancement and in urban areas. Its prevalence is rising rapidly in Latin America and the Caribbean, but obesity still is relatively uncommon in Asia and Africa.

Societal changes and the worldwide nutrition transition are driving the obesity epidemic. Economic growth, modernization, urbanization, and globalization of food markets are just some of the forces thought to underlie the epidemic.

As incomes rise and populations become more urban, diets high in complex carbohydrates give way to more varied diets with a higher proportion of fats, saturated fats, and sugars. Calorie-dense foods that have few other nutrients often are cheap, satisfying, convenient, and heavily promoted; some are foreign brands that have become affordable status symbols. In poor communities, cultural attitudes toward overweight may be more accepting and even admiring.

At the same time, large shifts toward less physically demanding work have been observed worldwide. Moves toward less physical activity are also found in the increasing use of automated transport, technology in the home, and more passive leisure pursuits. The reductions in energy expenditure can be dramatic.

If an individual is overweight, can we assume that the person is well nourished? Not necessarily. A new trend in developed countries is the presence of malnutrition with obesity. With too little physical activity, obese individuals may be eating too many calories of poor-nutrient foods and not enough nutritious foods such as vegetables and fruit. The availability of an overabundance of inexpensive, poor food choices in combination with lack of accessible opportunities for physical activity are just some of the factors contributing to the obesogenic environment in which many people are currently living.[38]

**Key Concepts** *The most critical nutritional deficiencies in today's developing world are deficiencies of protein, calories, iodine, vitamin A, and iron. There have been gains in reducing the severity and prevalence of protein-energy malnutrition through breastfeeding promotion, nutrition education, and improvements in food supplies. Fortification and supplementation programs are effectively attacking iodine and vitamin A deficiencies but have had less success overcoming iron deficiency. All the underlying causes of malnutrition must be addressed to reduce and eliminate these and other deficiencies.*

# Learning Portfolio

## Key Terms

## Study Points

- Hunger and malnutrition continue to be problems in both industrialized and developing countries.

- Although most people in the United States are food-secure, malnutrition is a serious problem among the working poor, the rural poor, the homeless, older adults, and children.

- Many federal programs address hunger in the United States. Among them are the Supplemental Nutrition Assistance Program (SNAP); the Special Supplemental Nutrition Program for Women, Infants, and Children (WIC); the National School Lunch and Breakfast Programs; and the Child and Adult Care Food Program. Feeding America is the largest charitable hunger-relief organization in the United States.

- Progress against global hunger and malnutrition is slow and uneven. It is estimated that more than 900 million people in the developing world do not have enough to eat.

- Social and economic factors, infection, disease, political disruptions, natural disasters, and inequitable food distribution all contribute to hunger in the developing world.

- Advances in agricultural practices have increased food supplies and reduced food costs in the developing world; however, the increase in production has led to environmental degradation as a result of urbanization, clear-cutting, overirrigation, and soil erosion.

- Protein-energy malnutrition (PEM) refers to physical conditions, such as kwashiorkor and marasmus, that result from not having enough to eat.

- Infants and children are most likely to suffer from PEM. However, nutrition education efforts, including promotion of breastfeeding, have reduced the severity and prevalence of PEM.

- Iodine deficiency is the largest cause of preventable brain damage and impaired cognitive development in the developing world. It can cause damage to people of all ages.

- Great strides have been made in preventing iodine deficiency disorders (IDD) through salt iodization programs. More than two-thirds of households in IDD-affected countries now use iodized salt.

- Vitamin A deficiency is the leading cause of preventable childhood blindness. It also makes its victims more vulnerable to infection, diarrheal diseases, and PEM.

- Pregnant and breastfeeding women with vitamin A deficiency are at increased risk of death, poor pregnancy outcomes, and lactation failure.

- Many countries are taking a multipronged approach to vitamin A deficiency that includes promotion of breastfeeding, fortification of foods, supplementation, and nutrition education.

- The best sources of vitamin A often are expensive and inaccessible to people in developing countries. Scientists have developed new bioengineered strains of rice that are rich in beta-carotene and that may play a critical role in alleviating widespread vitamin A deficiency.

- The anemias of the developing world demonstrate the interaction of multiple nutrient deficiencies, which, in turn, interact with infection, poor sanitation, and poverty.

- Food fortification and iron supplementation for women and children are the mainstays of anemia prevention and treatment, along with efforts to overcome poverty and improve sanitation.

- The classical deficiency diseases beriberi and pellagra still occur among the world's poorest and most underprivileged people.

- In some developing countries, obesity exists right alongside undernutrition.

## Study Questions

1. What is the difference between food insecurity and hunger?

2. What is food security?

3. What groups are most at risk for food insecurity in the United States?

4. List some organizations and programs that fight hunger and food insecurity in the United States.

5. List four causes of malnutrition worldwide.

6. List four common nutritional deficiencies worldwide.

7. What populations are at increased risk of nutritional deficiencies, and why?

# Try This

## Try Giving Up Your Stove and Refrigerator

A homeless person has no kitchen facilities to store or prepare food. For one day, eat a balanced diet without resorting to cooking or using your refrigerator. Some foods you could eat include the following:

Breads, bagels, tortillas, rolls

Cereals

Crackers

Milk—canned, evaporated, or aseptically packaged

Cheese—hard cheeses keep well

Pudding cups (single-serve, nonrefrigerated type)

Tuna/chicken—canned

Sardines, salmon—canned

Nuts, peanut butter

Beans—canned

Fruits and vegetables—fresh, canned, dried fruits

How satisfying did you find this eating pattern? What did you miss most? What would it be like to eat this way for an extended time?

## Community Food Programs

The purpose of this exercise is to see how you can contribute to decreasing or eliminating food insecurity in your community. Look in the phone book (under "Food Programs" and "Human Services") to see what programs are available. Consider volunteering at your local food bank or another community program to help feed people who do not have the means to feed themselves.

# References

1   Food and Agriculture Organization of the United Nations. Hunger. http://www.fao.org/hunger/en. Accessed 7/23/11.

2   Ibid.

3   Bryce J, Boschi-Pinto C, Shibuya K, Black R. WHO estimates of the causes of death in children. *Lancet.* 2005;365(9465):1147–1152.

4   Position of the American Dietetic Association: food insecurity and hunger in the United States. *J Am Diet Assoc.* 2010;110(9):1368–1377.

5   USDA Economic Research Service. Food security in the United States: key statistics and graphics. http://www.ers.usda.gov/Briefing/FoodSecurity/stats_graphs.htm#how_many. Accessed 7/22/11.

6   Position of the American Dietetic Association. Op. cit.

7   Finkelstein EA, Strombotne KL. The economics of obesity. *Am J Clin Nutr.* 2010;91(5):1520S–1524S.

8   USDA Economic Research Service. Op. cit.

9   Centers for Disease Control and Prevention. Food deserts. http://www.cdc.gov/features/fooddeserts. Accessed 7/23/11.

10  USDA food desert locator. http://www.ers.usda.gov/data/fooddesert/fooddesert.html. Accessed 7/23/11.

11  USDA Economic Research Service. Op. cit.

12  Special Supplemental Nutrition Program for Women, Infants And Children (WIC) data as of August 1, 2011. http://www.fns.usda.gov/pd/37WIC_Monthly.htm. Accessed 8/15/11.

13  USDA Food and Nutrition Service. WIC income eligibility guidelines 2009–2010. http://www.fns.usda.gov/wic/howtoapply/incomeguidelines09-10.htm. Accessed 8/15/11.

14  US Department of Agriculture. Child nutrition programs—income eligibility guidelines *Federal Register.* 2011;76(58). http://www.fns.usda.gov/cnd/governance/notices/iegs/IEGs11-12.pdf. Accessed 7/23/11.

15  USDA Food and Nutrition Service. National School Lunch Program. 9/10. http://www.fns.usda.gov/cnd/lunch. Accessed 7/23/11.

16  Feeding America. About us. http://feedingamerica.org. Accessed 7/23/11.

17  Brundtland GH. *Nutrition, Health, and Human Rights.* Geneva, Switzerland: World Health Organization, 2003. http://www.who.int/director-general/speeches/1999/english/19990412_nutrition.html. Accessed 7/23/11.

18  Food and Agriculture Organization of the United Nations. The state of food insecurity in the world. http://www.fao.org/publications/sofi/en. Accessed 7/23/11.

19  von Braun J. *The World Food Situation.* Washington, DC: International Food Policy Research Institute; December 2007. http://www.ifpri.org/pubs/fpr/pr18.asp. Accessed 7/23/11.

20  Sheeran J. The New Face of Hunger. Keynote address. 4/18/08. Center for Strategic and International Studies. Washington, DC.

21  Ibid.

22  Turral H, Burke J, Faurès J-M. *Climate Change, Water, and Food Security.* Rome: Food and Agriculture Organization of the United Nations; 2011.

23  Hunger Notes. 2011 world hunger and poverty facts and statistics. http://www.worldhunger.org/articles/Learn/world%20hunger%20facts%202002.htm. Accessed 7/23/11.

24  Joint United Nations Programme on HIV/AIDS (UNAIDS). http://www.unaids.org/en. Accessed 7/27/11; and Joint United Nations Programme on HIV/AIDS (UNAIDS), World Health Organization. AIDS epidemic update. 2009. http://www.who.int/hiv/pub/epidemiology/epidemic/en/index.html. Accessed 7/23/11.

25  Joint United Nations Programme on HIV/AIDS (UNAIDS). HIV/AIDS. http://www.usaid.gov/our_work/global_health/aids/News/aidsfaq.html#world. Accessed 7/23/11.

26  World Health Organization. Protein-energy malnutrition. http://www.wpro.who.int/health_topics/protein_energy. Accessed 7/23/11.

27  World Health Organization. Micronutrient deficiencies: iodine deficiency disorders. http://www.who.int/nutrition/topics/idd/en. Accessed 7/23/11.

28  Ibid.

29  de Benoist B, McLean E, Andersson M, Rogers L. Iodine deficiency in 2007: global progress since 2003. *Food Nutr Bull.* 2008;29(3).

30  World Health Organization. Micronutrient deficiencies: iodine deficiency disorders. Op. cit.

31  World Health Organization. Micronutrient deficiencies: vitamin A deficiency. 2009. http://www.who.int/nutrition/topics/vad/en/index.html. Accessed 7/23/11.

32  Tang G, Qin J, Dolnikowski GG, Russell RM, Grusak MA. Golden Rice is an effective source of vitamin A. *Am J Clin Nutr.* 2009;89(6):1776–1783.

33  World Health Organization. Micronutrient deficiencies: iron deficiency anaemia. http://www.who.int/nutrition/topics/ida/en/index.html. Accessed 7/23/11.

34  Ibid.

35  Ibid.

36  Hunger Notes. Op. cit.

37  World Health Organization. *Global Strategy on Diet Physical Activity and Health. Obesity and Overweight.* Geneva, Switzerland: World Health Organization. http://www.who.int/hpr/NPH/docs/gs_obesity.pdf. Accessed 7/23/11.

38  US Department of Agriculture and US Department of Health and Human Services. *Dietary Guidelines for Americans, 2010.* 7th ed. Washington, DC: US Government Printing Office; 2010.

# Appendix 1 — *Nutrition and Health for Canadians*

► **Canadian Guidelines for Nutrition**

► **Nutrient Intake Recommendations for Canadians**

► ***Canada's Food Guide to Healthy Eating***

► ***Canada's Food Guide***

► ***Canadian Physical Activity Guidelines***

► **Nutrition Labeling for Canadians**

► **Canadian Diabetes Association's Meal Planning Guide**

## Canadian Guidelines for Nutrition

For more than 60 years, the Canadian government has worked to promote healthy and nutritious eating habits. In 1987, Health and Welfare Canada began a major review of the system for guiding Canadians on their food choices. To perform the review, the government appointed two advisory committees—the Scientific Review Committee and the Communications and Implementation Committee.

After examining research evidence available on nutrition and public health, the Scientific Review Committee issued a report in 1990 called *Nutrition Recommendations.* The report included both updated Recommended Nutrient Intakes (RNI) and a scientific description of a healthy dietary pattern that would deliver adequate nutrients for health and reduce the risk of nutrition-related chronic diseases.

Meanwhile, the Communications and Implementation Committee translated these scientific findings into understandable guidelines and outlined implementation strategies in a report called *Action Towards Healthy Eating: Technical Report* (1990). This report suggested that Canada develop a "total diet approach" towards healthy eating. A total diet approach would give consumers a better idea of eating patterns associated with reducing the risk of developing chronic diseases.

In 1990, the government issued *Nutrition Recommendations: A Call for Action*, a summary report produced jointly by the Scientific Review Committee and the Communications and Implementation Committee.

## A Revised Food Guide

In accordance with the recommendations of its two advisory groups, the Health Department undertook to revise *Canada's Food Guide*. In 1992, the agency launched *Canada's Food Guide to Healthy Eating* and an explanatory document called *Using the Food Guide*. It promoted dietary diversity, a reduction in total fat intake, and an active lifestyle and offered consumers a pattern for establishing healthy eating habits in their daily selection of foods.

Moreover, the guide introduced a number of new concepts. A range of servings from the four food groups accommodated the wide range of energy needs for different ages, body sizes, activity levels, genders, and conditions such as pregnancy and nursing. The wide range of servings in grain products, vegetables, and fruits was designed to give consumers a better idea of the type of diet that would help reduce the risk of developing nutrition-related chronic diseases.

The guide also introduced a category of "other" foods such as sweets, fats such as butter, and drinks like coffee, that, though part of the diets of many Canadians, would traditionally not have been mentioned in a food guide. The guide recommended moderation in the consumption of these foods and acknowledged their role, along with the wide range of servings in grains, vegetables, and fruits, as a "total diet approach" to healthy eating.

## A Work in Progress

Some groups and organizations challenged specific aspects of the government's *Nutrition Recommendations.* In a typically Canadian twist, the government responded to challengers by including them in the development process. When the Canadian Pediatric Society, for example, queried the dietary recommendations on fat consumption in children, the Society was invited to join Health Canada in researching the issue. The result was *Nutrition Recommendations Update: Dietary Fat and Children* (1993), which adjusted the recommendation of appropriate levels of dietary fat for growing children. In 1995, Health Canada issued *Canada's Food Guide to Healthy Eating: Focus on Preschoolers* as a background paper for educators and communicators.

A thorough review of the 1992 *Food Guide* began in 2002. Many strengths as well as some challenges in understanding and using the information from the 1992 *Food Guide* were identified. An assessment of the nutritional adequacy of the 1992 *Food Guide* using Dietary Reference Intakes was undertaken. The assessment also sought to address changes in the food supply and patterns of food use. Extensive stakeholder consultation was also carried out. Health Canada worked with three advisory groups, an external *Food Guide* Advisory Committee, an Interdepartmental Working Group, and the Expert Advisory Committee on Dietary Reference Intakes throughout the revision process. In 2007, Health Canada released *Eating Well with Canada's Food Guide*, which is available in 10 languages. In addition, *A Food Guide for First Nations, Inuit, and Métis*, which recognizes the cultural, spiritual, and physical importance of traditional aboriginal foods, was also released in 2007.

Health Canada has positioned nutrition in a broader health context, which includes physical activity and a positive outlook on life. One result of this comprehensive approach was the Vitality Leaders Kit (1994), intended to help community leaders promote healthy eating, active living, and positive self-image and body image in an integrated way. *Canada's Physical Activity Guide* was released in 1998, followed by the *Guide for Older Adults* and the *Guides for Children and Youth.* In 2011, the Public Health Agency of Canada released new physical activity guidelines. Canadians are now encouraged to refer to Get Active Tip Sheets for the latest information on physical activity.

## Looking Ahead

The job of keeping Canada's nutrition policy and consumer guidelines up-to-date is an ongoing task. New scientific research on nutrition and health continually uncovers new relationships and connections between them. Consumer tastes in foods vary in response to prevailing fashions and shifting demographics. Global trade also influences the food choices that appear on the Canadian dinner table.

The science underlying nutrition recommendations knows no borders. An increasingly complex knowledge base on nutrients, food and health, global trade, and international agreements requires international efforts. Scientists from Canada and the United States worked with the National Academy of Sciences to develop the Dietary Reference Intakes (DRIs), recommended nutrient intake levels for healthy people in the United States and Canada.

To keep abreast of the latest developments in Canada's nutrition policies, visit the Food and Nutrition area of the Health Canada website at: http://www.hc-sc.gc.ca/fn-an/index-eng.php.

## Nutrient Intake Recommendations for Canadians

Health Canada has reviewed and made recommendations on nutrient requirements on a periodic basis since 1938. Known as the Recommended Nutrient Intakes, or RNI, these values were last published in 1990 as part of *Nutrition Recommendations: The Report of the Scientific Review Committee.* Since that time, there have been advances in science and by 1994, it was clear that it was time to initiate another review of the scientific data.

At the same time, the Food and Nutrition Board of the National Academy of Sciences was beginning a consultation process on the review of the Recommended Dietary Allowances, the nutrient recommendations used in the United States. Health Canada considered that participating in the U.S. review would offer several advantages to Canada. These were as follows:

- The science underlying nutrient requirements knows no borders and scientists everywhere are utilizing the same knowledge produced from studies conducted all over the world.
- The knowledge base on nutrients, foods, and health is increasing rapidly in scope and complexity. This increases the need for specialized expertise. Participating in the U.S. review permits Canada to expand the base of scientific expertise that could be utilized.
- International trade considerations, including NAFTA, suggest that the harmonization of the science base underlying nutrition policy will facilitate harmonization of such trade-related matters as nutrition labeling and food composition.

Canadian and American scientists establish Dietary Reference Intakes (DRIs) through a review process overseen by the Food and Nutrition Board of the Institute of Medicine, National Academy of Sciences. DRIs have replaced the RNIs and are found printed inside the covers of this text.

The National Academy of Sciences is an American private nonprofit society of distinguished scholars engaged in scientific and engineering research, dedicated to the advancement of science and technology and to their use for the general welfare. The Academy has a mandate that requires it to advise the U.S. federal government on scientific and technical matters.

The Food and Nutrition Board (FNB) is a unit of the Institute of Medicine, part of the National Academy of Sciences. The Board is a multidisciplinary group of biomedical scientists with expertise in various aspects of nutrition, food sciences, biochemistry, medicine, public health, epidemiology, food toxicology, and food safety. The major focus of the FNB is to evaluate emerging knowledge of nutrient requirements and relationships between diet and the reduction of risk of common chronic diseases and to relate this knowledge to strategies for promoting health and preventing disease.

## Canada's Food Guide

Scientists have known for some time that adequate nutrition is essential for proper growth and development. More recently, healthy eating has been accepted as a significant factor in reducing the risk of developing nutrition-related problems, including heart disease, cancer, obesity, hypertension (high blood pressure), osteoporosis, anemia, dental decay, and some bowel disorders.

### What "Reducing Risk" Means

Reducing risk means lowering the chances of developing a disease. It does not guarantee the prevention of a disease. Since the development of disease involves several factors, risk reduction usually involves several different strategies or approaches. Healthy eating is just one positive action that may help to avoid a potential problem.

### Healthy Eating with *Canada's Food Guide*

The revised *Food Guide* was designed to meet the body's needs for vitamins, minerals, and other nutrients; to reduce the risk of obesity, type 2 diabetes, heart disease, and certain types of cancer and osteoporosis; and to enhance the overall health and vitality of Canadians over the age of 2. The *Food Guide* outlines the recommended number of servings from the different food groups based on age and gender. **Figure 1.1** shows the current *Food Guide*.

## Canadian Physical Activity Guidelines

High levels of physical inactivity are a serious threat to public health in Canada. Nearly two-thirds of Canadians are not active enough to achieve optimal health benefits. These Canadians are at risk for heart disease, obesity, high blood pressure, adult-onset diabetes, osteoporosis, stroke, depression, and colon cancer. Although physical activity levels increased during the 1980s and early 1990s, the progress has stalled. Health Canada estimates that physical inactivity results in at least 21,000 premature deaths annually.

The *Canadian Physical Activity Guidelines*, produced by the Canadian Society for Exercise Physiology, provides a standard set of Canadian guidelines for physical activity. It provides information to help Canadians understand how to achieve health benefits by being physically active. The guide complements the popular *Canada's Food Guide to Healthy Eating* and provides concrete examples of how to incorporate physical activity into daily life.

The guide recommends an adult 18–64 years should accumulate 105 minutes of physical activity each week to stay healthy or improve your health. Moderate to vigorous physical activity should occur in bouts of 10 minutes or more. **Figure 1.2** shows the complete Physical Activity Guide, which provides physical activity recommendations for all ages.

Federal, provincial, and territorial governments are working to reduce the number of inactive Canadians. Canada's *Physical Activity Guidelines* are a major step toward building the knowledge and awareness necessary for all Canadians to become more active. These guidelines now include physical activity recommendations for children 5–11 years; youths 12–17 years; adults 18–64 years; and older adults 65 and older.

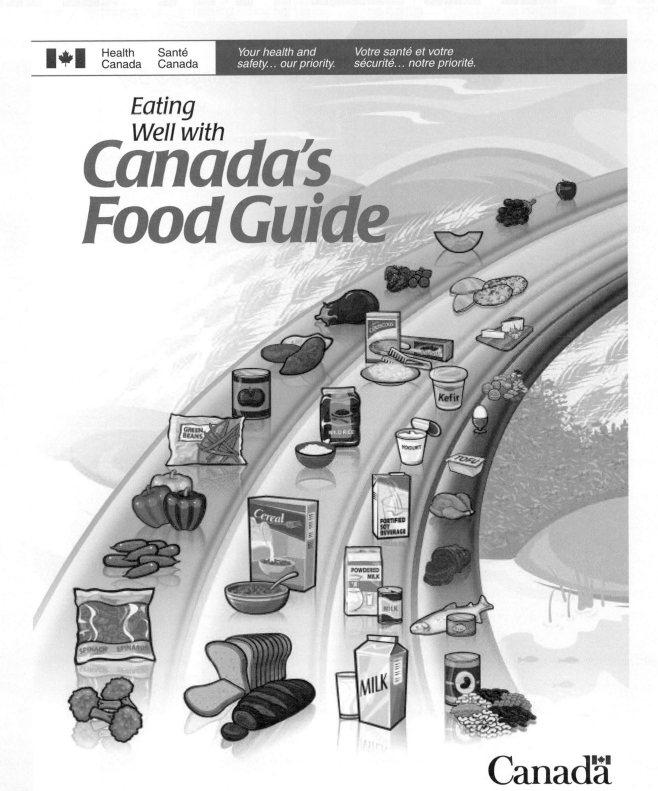

# Recommended Number of *Food Guide Servings* per Day

| | Children | | | Teens | | Adults | | | |
|---|---|---|---|---|---|---|---|---|---|
| Age in Years | 2-3 | 4-8 | 9-13 | 14-18 | | 19-50 | | 51+ | |
| Sex | Girls and Boys | | | Females | Males | Females | Males | Females | Males |
| **Vegetables and Fruit** | 4 | 5 | 6 | 7 | 8 | 7-8 | 8-10 | 7 | 7 |
| **Grain Products** | 3 | 4 | 6 | 6 | 7 | 6-7 | 8 | 6 | 7 |
| **Milk and Alternatives** | 2 | 2 | 3-4 | 3-4 | 3-4 | 2 | 2 | 3 | 3 |
| **Meat and Alternatives** | 1 | 1 | 1-2 | 2 | 3 | 2 | 3 | 2 | 3 |

The chart above shows how many Food Guide Servings you need from each of the four food groups every day.

Having the amount and type of food recommended and following the tips in *Canada's Food Guide* will help:

• Meet your needs for vitamins, minerals and other nutrients.
• Reduce your risk of obesity, type 2 diabetes, heart disease, certain types of cancer and osteoporosis.
• Contribute to your overall health and vitality.

## What is One Food Guide Serving?
### Look at the examples below.

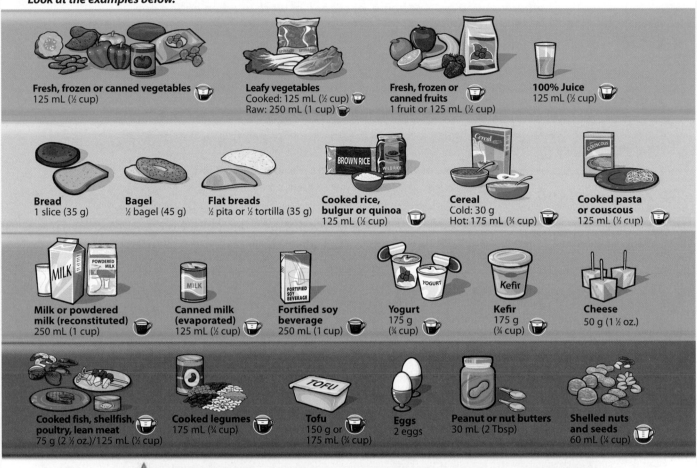

**Fresh, frozen or canned vegetables**
125 mL (½ cup)

**Leafy vegetables**
Cooked: 125 mL (½ cup)
Raw: 250 mL (1 cup)

**Fresh, frozen or canned fruits**
1 fruit or 125 mL (½ cup)

**100% Juice**
125 mL (½ cup)

**Bread**
1 slice (35 g)

**Bagel**
½ bagel (45 g)

**Flat breads**
½ pita or ½ tortilla (35 g)

**Cooked rice, bulgur or quinoa**
125 mL (½ cup)

**Cereal**
Cold: 30 g
Hot: 175 mL (¾ cup)

**Cooked pasta or couscous**
125 mL (½ cup)

**Milk or powdered milk (reconstituted)**
250 mL (1 cup)

**Canned milk (evaporated)**
125 mL (½ cup)

**Fortified soy beverage**
250 mL (1 cup)

**Yogurt**
175 g
(¾ cup)

**Kefir**
175 g
(¾ cup)

**Cheese**
50 g (1 ½ oz.)

**Cooked fish, shellfish, poultry, lean meat**
75 g (2 ½ oz.)/125 mL (½ cup)

**Cooked legumes**
175 mL (¾ cup)

**Tofu**
150 g or
175 mL (¾ cup)

**Eggs**
2 eggs

**Peanut or nut butters**
30 mL (2 Tbsp)

**Shelled nuts and seeds**
60 mL (¼ cup)

### Oils and Fats

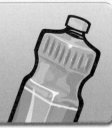

- Include a small amount – 30 to 45 mL (2 to 3 Tbsp) – of unsaturated fat each day. This includes oil used for cooking, salad dressings, margarine and mayonnaise.
- Use vegetable oils such as canola, olive and soybean.
- Choose soft margarines that are low in saturated and trans fats.
- Limit butter, hard margarine, lard and shortening.

## *Make each Food Guide Serving count...*
*wherever you are – at home, at school, at work or when eating out!*

▸ **Eat at least one dark green and one orange vegetable each day.**
  - Go for dark green vegetables such as broccoli, romaine lettuce and spinach.
  - Go for orange vegetables such as carrots, sweet potatoes and winter squash.

▸ **Choose vegetables and fruit prepared with little or no added fat, sugar or salt.**
  - Enjoy vegetables steamed, baked or stir-fried instead of deep-fried.

▸ **Have vegetables and fruit more often than juice.**

▸ **Make at least half of your grain products whole grain each day.**
  - Eat a variety of whole grains such as barley, brown rice, oats, quinoa and wild rice.
  - Enjoy whole grain breads, oatmeal or whole wheat pasta.

▸ **Choose grain products that are lower in fat, sugar or salt.**
  - Compare the Nutrition Facts table on labels to make wise choices.
  - Enjoy the true taste of grain products. When adding sauces or spreads, use small amounts.

▸ **Drink skim, 1%, or 2% milk each day.**
  - Have 500 mL (2 cups) of milk every day for adequate vitamin D.
  - Drink fortified soy beverages if you do not drink milk.

▸ **Select lower fat milk alternatives.**
  - Compare the Nutrition Facts table on yogurts or cheeses to make wise choices.

▸ **Have meat alternatives such as beans, lentils and tofu often.**

▸ **Eat at least two Food Guide Servings of fish each week.***
  - Choose fish such as char, herring, mackerel, salmon, sardines and trout.

▸ **Select lean meat and alternatives prepared with little or no added fat or salt.**
  - Trim the visible fat from meats. Remove the skin on poultry.
  - Use cooking methods such as roasting, baking or poaching that require little or no added fat.
  - If you eat luncheon meats, sausages or prepackaged meats, choose those lower in salt (sodium) and fat.

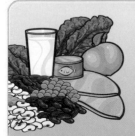

*Enjoy a variety of foods from the four food groups.*

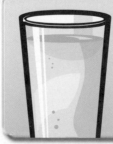

**Satisfy your thirst with water!**

Drink water regularly. It's a calorie-free way to quench your thirst. Drink more water in hot weather or when you are very active.

\* Health Canada provides advice for limiting exposure to mercury from certain types of fish. Refer to www.healthcanada.gc.ca for the latest information.

## *Advice for different ages and stages...*

### Children

Following *Canada's Food Guide* helps children grow and thrive.

Young children have small appetites and need calories for growth and development.

- Serve small nutritious meals and snacks each day.

- Do not restrict nutritious foods because of their fat content. Offer a variety of foods from the four food groups.

- Most of all... be a good role model.

### Women of childbearing age

All women who could become pregnant and those who are pregnant or breastfeeding need a multivitamin containing **folic acid** every day. Pregnant women need to ensure that their multivitamin also contains **iron**. A health care professional can help you find the multivitamin that's right for you.

Pregnant and breastfeeding women need more calories. Include an extra 2 to 3 Food Guide Servings each day.

**Here are two examples:**
- Have fruit and yogurt for a snack, or

- Have an extra slice of toast at breakfast and an extra glass of milk at supper.

### Men and women over 50

The need for **vitamin D** increases after the age of 50.

In addition to following *Canada's Food Guide*, everyone over the age of 50 should take a daily vitamin D supplement of 10 μg (400 IU).

## How do I count Food Guide Servings in a meal?

### Here is an example:

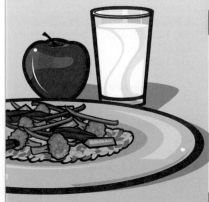

| Vegetable and beef stir-fry with rice, a glass of milk and an apple for dessert | | |
|---|---|---|
| 250 mL (1 cup) mixed broccoli, carrot and sweet red pepper | = | 2 **Vegetables and Fruit** Food Guide Servings |
| 75 g (2 ½ oz.) lean beef | = | 1 **Meat and Alternatives** Food Guide Serving |
| 250 mL (1 cup) brown rice | = | 2 **Grain Products** Food Guide Servings |
| 5 mL (1 tsp) canola oil | = | part of your **Oils and Fats** intake for the day |
| 250 mL (1 cup) 1% milk | = | 1 **Milk and Alternatives** Food Guide Serving |
| 1 apple | = | 1 **Vegetables and Fruit** Food Guide Serving |

# Eat well and be active today and every day!

## The benefits of eating well and being active include:

- Better overall health.
- Lower risk of disease.
- A healthy body weight.
- Feeling and looking better.
- More energy.
- Stronger muscles and bones.

## Be active

To be active every day is a step towards better health and a healthy body weight.

*Canada's Physical Activity Guide* recommends building 30 to 60 minutes of moderate physical activity into daily life for adults and at least 90 minutes a day for children and youth. You don't have to do it all at once. Add it up in periods of at least 10 minutes at a time for adults and five minutes at a time for children and youth.

**Start slowly and build up.**

## Eat well

Another important step towards better health and a healthy body weight is to follow *Canada's Food Guide* by:

- Eating the recommended amount and type of food each day.

- Limiting foods and beverages high in calories, fat, sugar or salt (sodium) such as cakes and pastries, chocolate and candies, cookies and granola bars, doughnuts and muffins, ice cream and frozen desserts, french fries, potato chips, nachos and other salty snacks, alcohol, fruit flavoured drinks, soft drinks, sports and energy drinks, and sweetened hot or cold drinks.

## Read the label

- Compare the Nutrition Facts table on food labels to choose products that contain less fat, saturated fat, trans fat, sugar and sodium.

- Keep in mind that the calories and nutrients listed are for the amount of food found at the top of the Nutrition Facts table.

## Limit trans fat

When a Nutrition Facts table is not available, ask for nutrition information to choose foods lower in trans and saturated fats.

### Nutrition Facts
Per 0 mL (0 g)

| Amount | % Daily Value |
|---|---|
| **Calories** 0 | |
| **Fat** 0 g | 0 % |
| Saturates 0 g | 0 % |
| + Trans 0 g | |
| **Cholesterol** 0 mg | |
| **Sodium** 0 mg | 0 % |
| **Carbohydrate** 0 g | 0 % |
| Fibre 0 g | 0 % |
| Sugars 0 g | |
| **Protein** 0 g | |

| | | | |
|---|---|---|---|
| Vitamin A | 0 % | Vitamin C | 0 % |
| Calcium | 0 % | Iron | 0 % |

## Take a step today...

- ✓ Have breakfast every day. It may help control your hunger later in the day.
- ✓ Walk wherever you can – get off the bus early, use the stairs.
- ✓ Benefit from eating vegetables and fruit at all meals and as snacks.
- ✓ Spend less time being inactive such as watching TV or playing computer games.
- ✓ Request nutrition information about menu items when eating out to help you make healthier choices.
- ✓ Enjoy eating with family and friends!
- ✓ Take time to eat and savour every bite!

*For more information, interactive tools, or additional copies visit Canada's Food Guide on-line at:* **www.healthcanada.gc.ca/foodguide**

*or contact:*

Publications
Health Canada
Ottawa, Ontario K1A 0K9
**E-Mail:** publications@hc-sc.gc.ca
**Tel.:** 1-866-225-0709
**Fax:** (613) 941-5366
**TTY:** 1-800-267-1245

Également disponible en français sous le titre : Bien manger avec le Guide alimentaire canadien

This publication can be made available on request on diskette, large print, audio-cassette and braille.

# Canadian Physical Activity Guidelines

**FOR CHILDREN - 5 – 11 YEARS**

## Guidelines

 For health benefits, children aged 5-11 years should accumulate at least 60 minutes of moderate- to vigorous-intensity physical activity daily. This should include:

 Vigorous-intensity activities at least 3 days per week.

 Activities that strengthen muscle and bone at least 3 days per week.

 More daily physical activity provides greater health benefits.

### Let's Talk Intensity!

Moderate-intensity physical activities will cause children to sweat a little and to breathe harder. Activities like:

- Bike riding
- Playground activities

Vigorous-intensity physical activities will cause children to sweat and be 'out of breath'. Activities like:

- Running
- Swimming

### Being active for at least **60 minutes** daily can help children:

- Improve their health
- Do better in school
- Improve their fitness
- Grow stronger
- Have fun playing with friends
- Feel happier
- Maintain a healthy body weight
- Improve their self-confidence
- Learn new skills

### Parents and caregivers can help to plan their child's daily activity. Kids can:

- ☑ Play tag – or freeze-tag!
- ☑ Go to the playground after school.
- ☑ Walk, bike, rollerblade or skateboard to school.

- ☑ Play an active game at recess.
- ☑ Go sledding in the park on the weekend.
- ☑ Go "puddle hopping" on a rainy day.

*60 minutes a day. You can help your child get there!*

 PARTICIPACTION

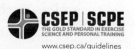 CSEP | SCPE
THE GOLD STANDARD IN EXERCISE
SCIENCE AND PERSONAL TRAINING
www.csep.ca/guidelines

**Figure 1.2A** *Canadian Physical Activity Guidelines for Children: 5–11 Years.*

**Source:** Canadian Physical Activity Guidelines, © 2011. Used with permission from the Canadian Society for Exercise Physiology, www.csep.ca/guidelines.

# Canadian Physical Activity Guidelines

**FOR YOUTH - 12 – 17 YEARS**

## Guidelines

 For health benefits, youth aged 12-17 years should accumulate at least 60 minutes of moderate- to vigorous-intensity physical activity daily. This should include:

 Vigorous-intensity activities at least 3 days per week.

 Activities that strengthen muscle and bone at least 3 days per week.

 More daily physical activity provides greater health benefits.

### Let's Talk Intensity!

Moderate-intensity physical activities will cause teens to sweat a little and to breathe harder. Activities like:

- Skating
- Bike riding

Vigorous-intensity physical activities will cause teens to sweat and be 'out of breath'. Activities like:

- Running
- Rollerblading

### Being active for at least **60 minutes** daily can help teens:

- Improve their health
- Do better in school
- Improve their fitness
- Grow stronger
- Have fun playing with friends
- Feel happier
- Maintain a healthy body weight
- Improve their self-confidence
- Learn new skills

### Parents and caregivers can help to plan their teen's daily activity. Teens can:

- ☑ Walk, bike, rollerblade or skateboard to school.
- ☑ Go to a gym on the weekend.
- ☑ Do a fitness class after school.

- ☑ Get the neighbours together for a game of pick-up basketball, or hockey after dinner.
- ☑ Play a sport such as basketball, hockey, soccer, martial arts, swimming, tennis, golf, skiing, snowboarding…

*Now is the time. 60 minutes a day can make a difference.*

 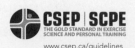

www.csep.ca/guidelines

**Figure 1.2B**  *Canadian Physical Activity Guidelines for Youth:* 12–17 Years.

Source: Canadian Physical Activity Guidelines, © 2011. Used with permission from the Canadian Society for Exercise Physiology, www.csep.ca/guidelines.

# Canadian Physical Activity Guidelines

## FOR ADULTS - 18 – 64 YEARS

## Guidelines

 To achieve health benefits, adults aged 18-64 years should accumulate at least 150 minutes of moderate- to vigorous-intensity aerobic physical activity per week, in bouts of 10 minutes or more.

 It is also beneficial to add muscle and bone strengthening activities using major muscle groups, at least 2 days per week.

 More physical activity provides greater health benefits.

### Let's Talk Intensity!

Moderate-intensity physical activities will cause adults to sweat a little and to breathe harder. Activities like:

- Brisk walking
- Bike riding

Vigorous-intensity physical activities will cause adults to sweat and be 'out of breath'. Activities like:

- Jogging
- Cross-country skiing

### Being active for at least **150 minutes** per week can help reduce the risk of:

- Premature death
- Heart disease
- Stroke
- High blood pressure
- Certain types of cancer
- Type 2 diabetes
- Osteoporosis
- Overweight and obesity

And can lead to improved:

- Fitness
- Strength
- Mental health (morale and self–esteem)

### Pick a time. Pick a place. Make a plan and move more!

- ☑ Join a weekday community running or walking group.
- ☑ Go for a brisk walk around the block after dinner.
- ☑ Take a dance class after work.
- ☑ Bike or walk to work every day.

- ☑ Rake the lawn, and then offer to do the same for a neighbour.
- ☑ Train for and participate in a run or walk for charity!
- ☑ Take up a favourite sport again or try a new sport.
- ☑ Be active with the family on the weekend!

*Now is the time. Walk, run, or wheel, and embrace life.*

 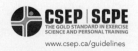

**Figure 1.2C** *Canadian Physical Activity Guidelines for Adults:* 18–64 Years.

Source: Canadian Physical Activity Guidelines, © 2011. Used with permission from the Canadian Society for Exercise Physiology, www.csep.ca/guidelines.

# Canadian Physical Activity Guidelines

## FOR OLDER ADULTS - 65 YEARS & OLDER

## Guidelines

 To achieve health benefits, and improve functional abilities, adults aged 65 years and older should accumulate at least 150 minutes of moderate- to vigorous-intensity aerobic physical activity per week, in bouts of 10 minutes or more.

 It is also beneficial to add muscle and bone strengthening activities using major muscle groups, at least 2 days per week.

 Those with poor mobility should perform physical activities to enhance balance and prevent falls.

 More physical activity provides greater health benefits.

### Let's Talk Intensity!

Moderate-intensity physical activities will cause older adults to sweat a little and to breathe harder. Activities like:

- Brisk walking
- Bicycling

Vigorous-intensity physical activities will cause older adults to sweat and be 'out of breath'. Activities like:

- Cross-country skiing
- Swimming

### Being active for at least **150 minutes** per week can help reduce the risk of:

- Chronic disease (such as high blood pressure and heart disease) and,
- Premature death

And also help to:
- Maintain functional independence
- Maintain mobility
- Improve fitness
- Improve or maintain body weight
- Maintain bone health and,
- Maintain mental health and feel better

### Pick a time. Pick a place. Make a plan and move more!

- ☑ Join a community urban poling or mall walking group.
- ☑ Go for a brisk walk around the block after lunch.
- ☑ Take a dance class in the afternoon.
- ☑ Train for and participate in a run or walk for charity!

- ☑ Take up a favourite sport again.
- ☑ Be active with the family! Plan to have "active reunions".
- ☑ Go for a nature hike on the weekend.
- ☑ Take the dog for a walk after dinner.

***Now is the time. Walk, run, or wheel, and embrace life.***

 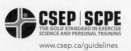

**Figure 1.2D**    *Canadian Physical Activity Guidelines for Older Adults:* 65 Years and Older.

Source: Canadian Physical Activity Guidelines, © 2011. Used with permission from the Canadian Society for Exercise Physiology, www.csep.ca/guidelines.

## The Nutrition Facts Box

The Nutrition Facts box allows consumers to make informed choices.

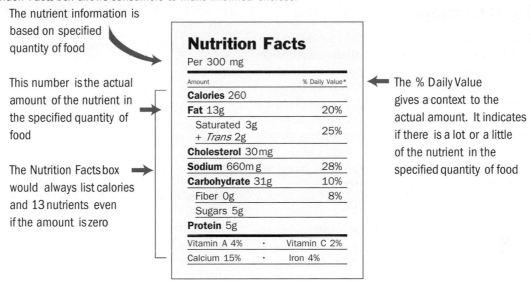

The nutrient information is based on specified quantity of food

This number is the actual amount of the nutrient in the specified quantity of food

The Nutrition Facts box would always list calories and 13 nutrients even if the amount is zero

**Nutrition Facts**

Per 300 mg

| Amount | % Daily Value* |
|---|---|
| **Calories** 260 | |
| **Fat** 13g | 20% |
| Saturated 3g + *Trans* 2g | 25% |
| **Cholesterol** 30mg | |
| **Sodium** 660mg | 28% |
| **Carbohydrate** 31g | 10% |
| Fiber 0g | 8% |
| Sugars 5g | |
| **Protein** 5g | |

| | |
|---|---|
| Vitamin A 4% | Vitamin C 2% |
| Calcium 15% | Iron 4% |

The % Daily Value gives a context to the actual amount. It indicates if there is a lot or a little of the nutrient in the specified quantity of food

| Figure 1.3 | **How to read a food label.** |
|---|---|

## Nutrition Labeling for Canadians

The nutrition label is one of the most useful tools in selecting foods for healthy eating (**Figure 1.3**). The *Food Guide* outlines a pattern of healthy eating; the nutrition label supports the *Food Guide* by helping consumers to choose foods according to healthy eating messages.

Consumers can use labels to compare products and make choices on the basis of nutrient content. For example, consumers can choose a lower-fat product based on the fat content given on the labels.

Consumers also can use label information to evaluate products in relation to healthy eating. For instance, the *Nutrition Recommendations* advise Canadians to get 30 percent or less of their day's energy (kilocalories/kilojoules) from fat. This translates into a range of fat, in grams, that can be used as a benchmark against which individual foods and meals can be evaluated. The *Food Guide* covers a range of energy needs from 1,800 to 3,200 kilocalories (7,500 to 13,400 kilojoules) per day. A fat intake of 30 percent or less of a day's calories means a fat intake between 60 and 105 grams of fat.

## Label Claims

A claim on a food label highlights a nutritional feature of a product. It is known to influence consumers' buying habits. Manufacturers often position label claims in a bold, banner-format on the front panel of a package or on the side panel along with the nutrition label. Because a label claim must be backed up by detailed facts relating to the claim, the consumer should look for the nutrition label for more information.

### Nutrient Content Claims

A nutrient content claim describes the amount of a nutrient in a food. A food whose label carries the claim *high fibre* must contain 4 grams or more of fiber per reference amount and serving of stated size. A "sodium-free" food must contain less than 5 milligrams of sodium per reference amount and serving of stated size.

### Diet-Related Health Claims

Optional health claims highlight the characteristics of a diet that reduces the chance of developing a disease such as cancer or heart disease. They also tell how the food fits into the diet.

| Characteristic of the Diet: | Reduced Risk of: |
|---|---|
| Low in sodium and high in potassium | High blood pressure |
| Adequate in calcium and vitamin D | Osteoporosis |
| Low in saturates and trans fats | Heart disease |
| Rich in fruits and vegetables | Some types of cancer |

For the latest information, visit the Nutrition Labeling area of the Health Canada website at http://www.inspection.gc.ca/english/fssa/lebeti/nutrition-pagee.shtml.

## Canadian Diabetes Association's Meal Planning Guide

The Canadian Diabetes Association (CDA) works to promote the health of Canadians through diabetes research, education, service, and advocacy. In response to the introduction of new medications and new methods for the management of diabetes, the CDA has revised its meal planning guide. Like the Exchange Lists, the CDA meal planning guide was designed to make it easier for people with diabetes to eat the right amount of food for their insulin supply. The system is based on two concepts: Most foods are eaten by people with diabetes in measured amounts, and foods within each of the system's eight food groups can be interchanged.

The new guide, *Beyond the Basics: Meal Planning for Diabetes Prevention and Management,* has several features. First, food items have been modified to reflect current thinking on heart health, glycemic index, and carbohydrate counting. A wider range of multicultural foods have also been added. Portion sizes have been adjusted to be more similar to *Canada's Food Guide,* and to the Quebec and U.S. meal planning systems. The guide also used color coding to help consumers: green for "choose more often" or "everyday" foods and amber for "choose less often" or "special occasion foods." The listed portions of all carbohydrate-rich foods now contain 15 grams of available carbohydrate (total carbohydrate minus fiber and half of any sugar alcohols).

*Beyond the Basics* classifies foods into eight food groups:

- Grains & Starches
- Fruits
- Milk & Alternatives
- Other Choices
- Vegetables
- Meat & Alternatives
- Fats
- Extras

Within each group, food items are listed along with portions to show how much of one food is interchangeable with another food in the same group. In the past, symbols for the meal planning guide food groups were used on food labels, but this has been phased out with the new food labeling regulations. However, the CDA partnered with Dietitians of Canada to develop *Healthy Eating Is In Store for You*™, an educational program to help Canadians interpret the nutrition label. For more information visit the CDA site: http://www.diabetes.ca/diabetes-and-you/nutrition/healthy-eating.

# Appendix 2 *ATP Produced from Macronutrients*

| Pathway | ATP formed by pathway | ATP formed by electron transport chain |
|---|---|---|
| **Glycolysis (1 glucose)** | | |
| Net 2 ATP (4 produced – 2 used) | 2 | |
| 2 NADH[a] | | 3 to 5 |
| | | |
| **Pyruvate to Acetyl CoA (2 pyruvate)** | | |
| First pyruvate → Acetyl CoA | | |
| 1 NADH | | 2.5 |
| Second pyruvate → Acetyl CoA | | |
| 1 NADH | | 2.5 |
| | | |
| **Citric Acid Cycle (twice)** | | |
| First acetyl CoA → Citric acid cycle | | |
| 1 GTP (ATP) | 1 | |
| 1 FADH$_2$ | | 1.5 |
| 3 NADH | | 7.5 |
| Second acetyl CoA → Citric acid cycle | | |
| 1 GTP (ATP) | 1 | |
| 1 FADH$_2$ | | 1.5 |
| 3 NADH | | 7.5 |
| Subtotal | 4 | 26 to 28 |
| | | **Total = 30 to 32** |

**Figure 2.1** **The complete breakdown of glucose.** These metabolic pathways and molecules move energy from glucose to ATP. Complete breakdown of one glucose molecule yields 30 to 32 ATP.

**Note:** [a] Each NADH molecule formed in the cytosol by glycolysis will produce either 2.5 or 1.5 ATP molecules in the electron transport chain. NADH formed by the citric acid cycle will produce 2.5 ATP molecules in the electron transport chain.

| Pathway | ATP yield |
|---|---|
| **Beta Oxidation (stearic acid C18:0)** | |
| 8 NADH | 20 |
| 8 FADH$_2$ | 12 |
| **Citric Acid Cycle (9 acetyl CoA)** | |
| | |
| 1 GTP x 9 = 9 GTP | 9 |
| 1 FADH$_2$ x 9 = 9 FADH$_2$ | 13.5 |
| 3 NADH x 9 = 27 NADH | 67.5 |
| Subtotal | 122 |
| ATP needed to start beta-oxidation | −2 |
| **Net Yield** | **120** |

**The Grand Total:**
120 ATP molecules from one molecule of stearic acid

**Figure 2.2** **The complete breakdown of stearic acid.** The complete breakdown of one 18-carbon fatty acid yields about four times as much ATP as the complete breakdown of 1 glucose molecule.

| Pathway | ATP yield |
|---|---|
| **Alanine to Pyruvate** | 0 |
| **Pyruvate to Acetyl CoA** | |
| 1 NADH | 2.5 |
| **Citric Acid Cycle** | |
| 1 GTP (ATP) | 1 |
| 1 $FADH_2$ | 1.5 |
| 3 NADH | 7.5 |
| **Total** | **12.5** |

**Figure 2.3**   **The complete breakdown of alanine.** The complete breakdown of the amino acid alanine yields about one-third the ATP of the complete breakdown of 1 glucose molecule.

| Pathway | ATP yield |
|---|---|
| **Methionine to Succinyl CoA**[a] | 0 |
| **Citric Acid Cycle (partial)** | |
| 1 GTP (ATP) | 1 |
| 1 $FADH_2$ | 1.5 |
| 1 NADH | 2.5 |
| **Total** | **5** |

**Figure 2.4**   **The complete breakdown of methionine.** The complete breakdown of the amino acid methionine yields about one-sixth the ATP of 1 glucose molecule.

**Note:** [a] Succinyl CoA is an intermediate of the citric acid cycle.

# Answers to Study Questions

## Chapter 1

1. Any three of the following: taste, smell, texture, appearance
3. Carbohydrates, lipids (fats and oils), proteins, vitamins, minerals, and water
5. Macrominerals are found in and used by the body in the largest amounts. Microminerals are found in and used by the body in smaller amounts.
7. An epidemiological study observes and compares how disease rates vary among different population groups and identifies conditions related to diseases or conditions within the populations. This enables researchers to identify associations between factors within the population and the particular disease being studied.
9. A placebo is an imitation treatment that looks the same as the experimental treatment (such as a sugar pill) but has no effect. The placebo is important for reducing bias because subjects do not know if they are receiving the intervention and are less inclined to alter their responses or reported symptoms based on what they think should happen.

## Chapter 2

1. Undernutrition is poor health resulting from the depletion of nutrients due to inadequate nutrient intake over time. It is most often associated with poverty, alcoholism, and some types of eating disorders.

    The most common type of overnutrition in the United States is due to the regular consumption of excess calories, fats, saturated fats, and cholesterol.
3. Grains: 6 ounce-equivalents; half should be whole grains

    Vegetable group: 2½ cups

    Fruits: 2 cups

    Milk: 3 cups

    Meat and beans: 5½ ounce-equivalents
5. The Estimated Average Requirement (EAR) is the nutrient intake level that is estimated to meet the needs of 50 percent of the individuals in a life-stage and gender group.

    The Recommended Dietary Allowance (RDA) is the daily intake level that meets the needs of most (97 to 98 percent) people in a life-stage and gender group.

An Adequate Intake (AI) level is set when an RDA has yet to be established due to a lack of knowledge and need for more scientific research.

The Tolerable Upper Intake Level (UL) is the maximum daily intake level that is unlikely to pose health risks to almost all of the individuals in a life-stage and gender category.

7. Calories

    Calories from fat

    Total fat

    Saturated fat

    Trans fat

    Cholesterol

    Sodium

    Total carbohydrate

    Dietary fiber

    Sugars

    Protein

    Calcium, iron, vitamins A and C (all as a % Daily Value)
9. Nutrient content claims describe the level of a nutrient or dietary substance in the product using terms such as *good source*, *high*, or *free*.

    A health claim is any statement that associates a food or a substance in a food with a disease or health-related condition.

    A structure/function claim describes a benefit related to a nutrient-deficiency disease or describes the role of a nutrient or dietary ingredient intended to affect a structure or function in humans; for example, *calcium helps build strong bones*.

## Chapter 3

1. Phytochemicals are plant chemicals, including pigments and antioxidants. They help plants resist bacteria and fungi, the destructive effects of free radicals, and high levels of UV sunlight. When we eat plants that contain phytochemicals, we receive many of the same protections.
3. Food additives may improve a food's nutritional value, maintain its palatability and consistency, provide leavening, control acidity or alkalinity, enhance flavor, or prevent spoilage.
5. DSHEA defines a dietary supplement as any product intended to supplement the diet, and it

requires the word *supplement* to be clearly printed on the label.

7. • Check the label for the USP-Verified mark, which indicates that the manufacturer followed standards established by the U.S. Pharmacopeia.
   • Remember that just because something is natural does not mean it is safe.
   • Consider purchasing a supplement from one of the large, nationally known manufacturers because they generally have tighter quality controls.
9. The traditional macrobiotic diet is a vegetarian diet that gets progressively more restrictive, with the "highest level" consisting of little more than brown rice and water. The diet has since evolved to a simpler one-level regimen based on whole-grain cereals and vegetables, a small amount of fish and no other animal products, and no fruit.

# Chapter 4

1. Mouth, esophagus, stomach, small intestine, large intestine, and rectum.
3. Hydrochloric acid produced by cells that line the stomach lowers the pH of the stomach contents to about 2. Mucus, also produced by stomach lining cells, protects these cells from the acid environment.
5. Vascular system (blood circulatory system) and lymphatic system

# Chapter 5

1. A monosaccharide is a single sugar unit (e.g., glucose, fructose, and galactose). A disaccharide (e.g., maltose, sucrose, and lactose) is a molecule of two single sugar units. A polysaccharide (e.g., starch and fiber) is a long chain of sugar units.
3. Both starch and fiber are long chains of glucose molecules, but we are unable to digest the bonds between the glucose units in fiber. Therefore, fiber moves through the small intestine undigested while starch is broken down into glucose and absorbed.
5. Plant foods are our main dietary sources of carbohydrates. Grains, legumes, and vegetables provide starches and fibers. Fruits provide sugars and fibers. Milk and other dairy products provide sugar in the form of lactose. Sweets and soft drinks contain carbohydrates in the form of sugars.
7. An excessive amount of added sugar probably translates into an excessive amount of calories, and overconsumption of calories leads to weight gain. Overweight and obesity are, in turn, associated with

increased risk of chronic disease. Excess sugar intake also increases risk for dental caries.

## Spotlight on Alcohol

1. Most beer is up to 5 percent alcohol (some exceed 6 percent), wine is 8–14 percent alcohol, and liquor is typically 35–45 percent alcohol.
3. The liver
5. Ethnicity
   Age
   Gender
   Body size and composition
7. Harmful effects of alcohol:
   Addiction
   Accidents and violence
   Birth defects
   Emotional and social problems
   Cardiomyopathy
   Brain effects (acute and long term)
   Liver disease
   Gastritis
   Pancreatitis
   Cancer
   Anemia
   Osteoporosis
   Peripheral neuropathy
   Helpful effects of alcohol:
   Raises protective HDL cholesterol levels
   May inhibit formation of blood clots
   Stress relief and relaxation
   Protection against heart disease

# Chapter 6

1. If all the bonds between the carbon atoms in a fatty acid chain are single bonds, then the fatty acid is called a saturated fatty acid. A fatty acid with one double bond in the fatty acid chain is a monounsaturated fatty acid (MUFA); one with two or more double bonds is a polyunsaturated fatty acid (PUFA).
3. Linoleic acid and alpha-linolenic acid
5. 1. Energy source (9 kilocalories per gram)
   2. Energy reserve (triglycerides in fat cells)
   3. Insulation and protection (visceral and subcutaneous fat)
   4. Carrier of fat-soluble compounds
   5. Contribute sensory qualities to foods
7. Only foods from animal sources contain cholesterol. Organ meats such as brain and liver contain very

high levels of cholesterol. Other sources are egg yolks, meats, and dairy products.

9. Total fat: 20–35 percent of kilocalories
   Saturated fat: less than 10 percent of kilocalories
   Cholesterol: less than 300 milligrams per day

# Chapter 7

1. Indispensable amino acids cannot be made in the body and must be obtained from the diet.

   Dispensable amino acids can be manufactured in the body when enough nitrogen, carbon, hydrogen, and oxygen are available.

   Conditionally indispensable amino acids are amino acids that your body makes under normal circumstances, but, when one has certain deficiencies and disorders, the body can no longer produce them, and they must be obtained from the diet.

3. Antibodies are blood proteins that attack and inactivate bacteria and viruses that can cause infection. Each protein antibody has a specific shape that allows it to attack and destroy a specific foreign invader.

5. Although the protein in one plant food may lack certain amino acids, the protein in another plant food may be a complementary protein that completes the amino acid pattern. So, the protein in one plant food can provide the essential amino acid(s) that the other plant food is missing.

   1. Beans and rice
   2. Peanut butter on bread
   3. Pasta with beans

7. Vegetarian diets:
   - Contain less fat, saturated fat, and cholesterol
   - Contain vegetables and fruits high in antioxidants and that contain dietary fiber and phytochemicals

   Vegetarians:
   - Have lower blood cholesterol levels
   - Are less likely to develop heart disease
   - Have lower weight
   - Are less likely to have high blood pressure
   - Have lower rates of cancer

## Spotlight on Metabolism

1. ATP is the energy form usable by all cells, so it is called the universal energy currency.

3. Glycolysis; anaerobic
   Pyruvate to acetyl CoA; aerobic
   Citric acid cycle; aerobic
   Electron transport chain; aerobic

5. An amino acid is considered either glucogenic or ketogenic, based on whether its carbon skeleton can be made into glucose or acetyl CoA. If an amino acid's carbon skeleton can be converted to pyruvate or a citric acid cycle intermediate, it can follow gluconeogenic pathways to glucose. Such amino acids are glucogenic. If a carbon skeleton is converted to acetyl CoA, it cannot be made into glucose. It can, however, be made into a ketone body, so these amino acids are ketogenic.

7. Energy is stored as glycogen in the liver and muscle tissues and as triglyceride in the adipose tissue. The largest store of energy is the adipose tissue.

# Chapter 8

1. Energy balance is the relationship between your energy intake and energy output. You are in energy equilibrium when your energy or caloric intake equals the amount of energy or calories you expend. People who maintain their weight over time are in energy equilibrium whether or not they are aware of their intake or expenditure. Positive energy balance (intake > output) results in weight gain while negative energy balance (intake < output) results in weight loss.

3. • Resting Energy Expenditure: The energy expended while the body is at rest, which includes basic physiological functions such as heartbeat, muscle contraction, respiration, and so on.
   • Thermic Effect of Food: The energy expended to digest, metabolize, and store ingested macronutrients.
   • Physical Activity: The increase in metabolic rate caused by any movement of skeletal muscles.

5. Underweight        $< 18.5 \text{ kg/m}^2$
   Overweight         25 to 29.9 $\text{kg/m}^2$
   Obese              $\geq 30 \text{ kg/m}^2$
   These standards are the same for men and women.

7. Excess fat accumulation is associated with increased fat cell size, called hypertrophic obesity. In hypertrophic obesity, fat cells become larger than normal as they fill with fat. When the capacity of these cells reaches its maximum, the body generates more fat cells. Hyperplastic obesity is characterized not only by increased fat cell size but also increased cell number.

9. A balanced diet of moderate caloric intake
   Adequate exercise
   Cognitive-behavioral strategies for changing habits and behavior patterns

Attention to balancing self-acceptance and the desire for change

11. The term *underweight* is defined as a BMI of less than 18.5 kg/m². The *Dietary Guidelines for Americans* defines underweight as a BMI lower than 19 kg/m².

# Chapter 9

1. Fat-soluble vitamins first travel in the lymphatic system (inside chylomicrons) before entering the bloodstream.

   Water-soluble vitamins are absorbed directly into the bloodstream.

   Most fat-soluble vitamins are not readily excreted and are stored in the liver and adipose tissue.

   Most water-soluble vitamins are readily excreted and stored in limited quantities.

3. Vitamin D is called the "sunshine vitamin" because UV sunlight hitting the skin makes vitamin D from cholesterol. Like all hormones, vitamin D is made in one part of the body and acts elsewhere in the body.

5. Blood clotting

7. Thiamin functions in energy metabolism as the coenzyme thiamin pyrophosphate (TPP). TPP helps in the breakdown of glucose, synthesis of RNA and DNA, and synthesis of neurotransmitters.

   Riboflavin functions in energy metabolism as coenzymes that participate in reactions that break down glucose, fatty acids, and amino acids for energy.

   Niacin coenzymes function in 200 metabolic pathways including pathways in energy metabolism and fatty acid synthesis.

   Vitamin $B_6$ functions in amino acid metabolism and in the synthesis of hemoglobin and neurotransmitters.

   Folate is essential to the synthesis of DNA, and good folate status prevents some birth defects. Folate also helps lower homocysteine levels.

   Vitamin $B_{12}$ activates folate and maintains the myelin sheath that protects nerve fibers and supports red blood cell synthesis.

   Pantothenic acid functions in energy metabolism as part of coenzyme A.

   Biotin acts as a coenzyme critical to energy and amino acid metabolism, as well as in fatty acid synthesis.

   Vitamin C is important in collagen synthesis, assists with absorption of iron, and is an antioxidant.

9. The only water-soluble vitamins with demonstrated toxicity are niacin, vitamin $B_6$, and vitamin C.

Excessive amounts of niacin can cause "niacin flush," nausea, headache, and blurred vision. Over time, liver damage can result. Excessive amounts of vitamin $B_6$ can cause irreversible nerve damage, and excessive doses of vitamin C can cause abdominal cramps and diarrhea.

# Chapter 10

1. Water is needed to transport nutrients and wastes, provide shock absorption and lubrication, facilitate chemical reactions, and regulate body temperature.

3. Calcium is important for blood clotting, nerve function, muscle contractions, and cell metabolism. When dietary intakes do not meet calcium needs, calcium is withdrawn from the bone to compensate, thus making the bone weaker and increasing risk for the development of osteoporosis.

5. The initial stage of iron deficiency is depletion of iron stores. In the second stage of iron deficiency, there is a decrease in functional or transport iron. The third and most severe stage of iron deficiency is anemia.

7. Goiter is an enlarged thyroid gland. Both iodine deficiency and iodine toxicity can cause goiter.

9. Chromium appears to enhance the effects of insulin and helps move glucose into cells. Good sources of chromium are brewer's yeast, processed meats, whole grains, green beans, and broccoli.

# Chapter 11

1. ATP–CP energy system
   Lactic acid energy system
   Oxygen energy system

   The ATP–CP energy system is used during the first few seconds to one minute of exercise. The lactic acid energy system is used in short-duration activities and at the end of endurance activities. The oxygen energy system is used during longer-duration activities.

3. It is recommended that athletes consume 60 percent of their calories from carbohydrates. Fat intake should be less than 30 percent of calories, with the remainder of energy intake coming from protein.

5. The adult nonathlete's RDA for protein is 0.8 grams per kilogram of body weight per day. This is less than the recommended intake for endurance athletes, which is 1.2 to 1.4 grams per kilogram of body weight per day. The protein recommendation for strength athletes is 1.6 to 1.7 grams of protein per kilogram of body weight per day.

7. Sports anemia is a condition of low hemoglobin concentration in the blood that results from an

increase in fluid (plasma) volume. Endurance training temporarily increases plasma volume. Because sports anemia is a result of increased plasma volume, it is not considered a true anemia like those caused by lack of iron, folate, or vitamin $B_{12}$.

9. Disordered eating
   Amenorrhea
   Premature osteoporosis

## Spotlight on Eating Disorders

1. Anorexia nervosa:
   - Body weight < 85% of expected weight (or BMI ≤ 17.5 kg/m²)
   - Intense fear of weight gain
   - Inaccurate perception of own body size, weight, or shape
   - Amenorrhea (in females after menarche)

   Bulimia nervosa:
   - Recurrent binge eating (at least two times per week for three months)
   - Recurrent purging, excessive exercise, or fasting (at least two times per week for three months)
   - Excessive concern about body weight or shape
   - Absence of anorexia nervosa

   Binge-eating disorder:
   - Recurrent binge eating (at least two times per week for six months)
   - Marked distress with at least three of the following:
     - Eating very rapidly
     - Eating until uncomfortably full
     - Eating when not hungry
     - Eating alone
     - Feeling disgusted or guilty after a binge
   - No recurrent purging, no excessive exercising, and no fasting
   - Absence of anorexia nervosa

3. Treatment usually involves a combination of hospitalization, psychotherapy, and pharmacotherapy. The first goal of treatment is to stabilize the patient's medical condition. Research suggests that with intensive therapy, most patients can achieve normal weight. However, they may struggle all their lives with a moderate to severe preoccupation with food and body weight, poor social relationships, and depression. The earlier the patient begins treatment, the better the prognosis.

5. During a binge, individuals with bulimia typically consume massive quantities of highly palatable "forbidden" foods, such as pastry, ice cream, and candy. This gorging takes place over a relatively short time span—say, an hour or two. Binges may contain up to 10,000 kilocalories. Afterward, feeling physically ill from overindulgence, sufferers use a variety of purging techniques, such as:
   - Self-induced vomiting
   - Excessive quantities of laxatives
   - Strict fasting
   - Heightened exercise

## Chapter 12

1. In the first stage of fetal growth, called the blastogenic stage, the fertilized egg rapidly divides and begins to differentiate. During the embryonic stage, the major organ systems form. The fetal stage is the longest stage of development, and during this stage the fetus grows dramatically in size.

3. Calories: increased by 340 kilocalories per day during the second trimester and by 450 kilocalories in the third trimester
   Protein: increased from 0.8 grams per kilogram per day to 1.1 grams per kilogram per day during pregnancy
   Folate: increased by 200 micrograms per day (from 400 to 600 micrograms per day)
   Iron: increased by 9 milligrams per day (from 18 to 27 milligrams per day)

5. Infants who are breastfed have a lower incidence of respiratory, gastrointestinal, and ear infections. Infants also have lower incidence of allergies, diarrhea, and bacterial meningitis. Breastmilk stimulates development of the infant's immune system. Breastfeeding stimulates uterine contractions following delivery. This helps to control blood loss and returns the uterus to its normal size more quickly. Breastfeeding may reduce a woman's risk for ovarian and breast cancer, and for osteoporosis.

7. Babies need approximately 0.7 liters of water each day in the first six months of life and 0.8 liters per day from age 7 months to 1 year. Breastfed and formula-fed infants do not need supplemental water; the breast milk and properly mixed formula provide enough water for adequate hydration until significant amounts of solid foods have been added to the diet.

9. According to the American Academy of Pediatrics, solid foods (anything other than breast milk or infant formula) are not needed before the age of 6 months. Then new foods should be introduced one at a time to check for any allergies or intolerances. Most parents begin with infant rice cereal, mixed to a thin consistency with water, breast milk, or infant formula. After the infant is eating cereal several times

a day, strained fruits and vegetables are introduced one at a time.

## Chapter 13

1. Iron, possibly zinc, vitamin D, and vitamin E (if parents follow a low-fat diet).
3. Chronic nutrition problems that can affect children include obesity, lead toxicity, and early onset of indicators of heart disease. Infants and toddlers should not be given low-fat, high-fiber diets; when children reach the age of 3, dietary changes consistent with the *Dietary Guidelines for Americans* can gradually be made. Making sure children have regular physical activity and limiting sedentary activity such as television viewing are important factors in reducing obesity and chronic disease risk.
5. Decreased immune function can result in increased risk of respiratory infections, urinary tract infections, pressure sores, and foodborne illness.
7. Older people have less ability to produce active vitamin D from sun exposure; they typically are exposed to less sunlight; and they often do not consume enough dairy products, which are good sources of vitamin D.
9. Some nutrients in large amounts can be toxic.

    Supplements can affect the absorption of other nutrients or interfere with the absorption and metabolism of prescription medication.

    Excessive use of vitamin supplements can result in hypervitaminosis (high levels of vitamins in the blood).

    Supplements may contain more vitamin A than is needed in an elder's diet, which may lead to liver dysfunction, bone and joint pain, headaches, and other problems.

    Large amounts of vitamin C can increase the likelihood of kidney stones and gastric bleeding.

## Chapter 14

1. Some types of pathogenic bacteria can directly infect a person who consumes contaminated food. Other bacteria may produce a toxin that can cause foodborne illness.

3. The following suggestions by the Consumers Union will help you limit your intake of pesticides: wash and peel produce, and eat a wide variety of fruits and vegetables.
5. HACCP stands for Hazard Analysis and Critical Control Point. It is a process used by both the government and industry to prevent food contamination by identifying areas in food production where contamination can occur.
7. • Salting
   • Fermenting
   • Canning
   • Freezing
   • Pasteurization
   • Irradiation

## Chapter 15

1. Food insecurity is the worry that one does not have the resources to obtain adequate food. Hunger is the physical sensation of unease or pain caused by a lack of food. Food insecurity can exist with or without hunger.
3. Working poor
   People in rural, isolated areas
   Elders
   Homeless
   Children
5. Any four of the following:
   • Poverty
   • Population growth
   • Urbanization
   • Infection and disease
   • War
   • Political sanctions
   • Natural disasters
   • Inequitable food distribution
7. Children, women, the elderly, and refugees are at increased risk of malnutrition due to lack of education and employment, sex discrimination, and dependency on others.

# Glossary

**ABC model of behavior** A behavioral model that includes the external and internal events that precede and follow the behavior. The "A" stands for antecedents, the events that precede the behavior ("B"), which is followed by consequences ("C") that positively or negatively reinforce the behavior.

**absorption** The movement of substances into or across tissues; in particular, the passage of nutrients and other substances into the walls of the gastrointestinal tract and then into the bloodstream.

**Acceptable Macronutrient Distribution Ranges (AMDRs)** Range of intakes for a particular energy source that are associated with reduced risk of chronic disease while providing adequate intakes of essential nutrients.

**acesulfame K [ay-see-SUL-fame]** An artificial sweetener that is 200 times sweeter than common table sugar (sucrose). Because it is not digested and absorbed by the body, acesulfame contributes no calories to the diet and yields no energy when consumed.

**acetaldehyde** A toxic intermediate compound formed by the action of the alcohol dehydrogenase enzyme during the metabolism of alcohol.

**acetyl CoA** A key intermediate product in the metabolic breakdown of carbohydrates, fatty acids, and amino acids. It consists of a two-carbon acetate group linked to coenzyme A, which is derived from pantothenic acid.

**acidosis** An abnormally low blood pH (below about 7.35) due to increased acidity.

**acne** An inflammatory skin eruption that usually occurs in or near the sebaceous glands of the face, neck, shoulders, and upper back.

**acrolein** A pungent decomposition product of fats, generated from dehydrating the glycerol component of fats; responsible for the coughing attacks caused by the fumes released by burning fat. This toxic water-soluble liquid vaporizes easily and is highly flammable.

**active transport** The movement of substances into or out of cells against a concentration gradient. Active transport requires energy (ATP) and involves carrier (transport) proteins in the cell membrane.

**additives** Substances added to food to perform various functions, such as adding color or flavor, replacing sugar or fat, improving nutritional content, or improving texture or shelf life.

**adenosine diphosphate (ADP) [ah-DEN-oh-seen di-FOS-fate]** A molecule composed of adenosine and two phosphate groups.

**adenosine triphosphate (ATP) [ah-DEN-oh-seen try-FOS-fate]** A high-energy compound composed of adenosine and three phosphate groups. ATP is the main direct fuel that cells use to synthesize molecules, contract muscles, transport substances, and perform other tasks. Breaking down ATP to adenosine diphosphate (ADP) releases energy, and forming ATP from ADP captures energy.

**Adequate Intake (AI)** The nutrient intake that appears to sustain a defined nutritional state or some other indicator of health (e.g., growth rate, normal circulating nutrient values) in a specific population or subgroup. AI is used when there is insufficient scientific evidence to establish an EAR.

**adipocytes** Fat cells.

**adipose tissue** Body fat tissue.

**adolescence** The period between onset of puberty and adulthood.

**aerobic [air-ROW-bic]** Referring to the presence of or need for oxygen. The complete breakdown of glucose, fatty acids, and amino acids to carbon dioxide and water occurs only via aerobic metabolism. The citric acid cycle and electron transport chain are aerobic pathways.

**aerobic endurance** The ability of skeletal muscle to obtain a sufficient supply of oxygen from the heart and lungs to maintain muscular activity for a prolonged time.

**aflatoxins** Carcinogenic and toxic factors produced by food molds.

**albumin** A protein that circulates in the blood and helps transport many minerals and some drugs.

**alcohol** Common name for ethanol or ethyl alcohol. As a general term, it refers to any organic compound with one or more hydroxyl (–OH) groups.

**alcohol dehydrogenase (ADH)** The enzyme that catalyzes the oxidation of ethanol and other alcohols.

**alcohol poisoning** An overdose of alcohol. The body is overwhelmed by the amount of alcohol in the system and cannot metabolize it fast enough.

**aldehyde dehydrogenase (ALDH)** The enzyme that catalyzes the conversion of acetaldehyde to acetate, which forms acetyl CoA.

**aldosterone [al-DOS-ter-own]** A hormone secreted from the adrenal glands that acts on the kidneys to regulate electrolyte and water balance. It raises blood pressure by promoting retention of sodium (and thus water) and excretion of potassium.

**alkalosis** An abnormally high blood pH (above about 7.45) due to increased alkalinity.

**alpha (α) bonds** Chemical bonds linking monosaccharides, which can be broken by human intestinal enzymes, releasing the individual monosaccharides. Starch, maltose, and sucrose contain alpha bonds.

**alpha-linolenic acid [al-fah-lin-oh-LEN-ik]** An essential *omega*-3 fatty acid that contains 18 carbon atoms and 3 carbon–carbon double bonds (18:3).

**Alzheimer's disease (AD)** A presenile dementia characterized by accumulation of plaques in certain regions of the brain and degeneration of a certain class of neurons.

**amenorrhea [A-men-or-Ee-a]** Absence or abnormal stoppage of menses in a female; commonly indicated by the absence of three to six consecutive menstrual cycles.

**amino acid pool** The amino acids in body tissues and fluids that are available for new protein synthesis.

**amino acids** Organic compounds that function as the building blocks of protein.

**amniotic fluid** The fluid that surrounds the fetus; contained in the amniotic sac inside the uterus.

**amylopectin [am-ih-low-PEK-tin]** A branched-chain polysaccharide composed of glucose units.

**amylose [AM-ih-los]** A straight-chain polysaccharide composed of glucose units.

**anabolic steroids** Several compounds derived from testosterone or prepared synthetically. They promote body growth and masculinization and oppose the effects of estrogen.

**anabolism [an-A-bol-iz-um]** Any metabolic process whereby cells build complex substances from simple, smaller units.

**anaerobic [AN-ah-ROW-bic]** Referring to the absence of oxygen or the ability of a process to occur in the absence of oxygen. Glycolysis is an anaerobic pathway.

**android obesity [AN-droyd]** Excess storage of fat located primarily in the abdominal area.

**anemia** Abnormally low concentration of hemoglobin in the bloodstream; can be caused by impaired synthesis of red blood cells, increased destruction of red blood cells, or significant loss of blood.

**anencephaly** A type of neural tube birth defect in which part or all of the brain is missing.

**angular stomatitis** Inflammation and cracking at the corners of the mouth; a symptom of riboflavin deficiency.

**anions** Ions that carry a negative charge.

**anorexia athletica** Eating disorder associated with competitive participation in athletic activity.

**anorexia nervosa [an-or-EX-ee-uh ner-VOH-sah]** An eating disorder marked by prolonged decrease of appetite and refusal to eat, leading to self-starvation and excessive weight loss. It results in part from a distorted body image and intense fear of becoming fat, often linked to social pressures.

**anorexia of aging** Loss of appetite and wasting associated with old age.

**antibodies [AN-tih-bod-eez]** Infection-fighting protein molecules in blood or secretory fluids that tag, neutralize, and help destroy pathogenic microorganisms (e.g., bacteria, viruses) or toxins.

**antidiuretic hormone (ADH)** A hormone secreted by the pituitary gland that increases blood pressure and prevents fluid excretion by the kidneys. Also called vasopressin.

**antioxidant** A substance that combines with or otherwise neutralizes a free radical, thus preventing oxidative damage to cells and tissues.

**appetite** A psychological desire to eat that is related to the pleasant sensations often associated with food.

**ariboflavinosis** Riboflavin deficiency.

**aspartame [AH-spar-tame]** An artificial sweetener composed of two amino acids. It is 200 times sweeter than sucrose and sold by the trade name NutraSweet.

**atherosclerosis** A type of "hardening of the arteries" in which cholesterol and other substances in the blood build up in the walls of arteries. As the process continues, the arteries to the heart may narrow, cutting down the flow of oxygen-rich blood and nutrients to the heart.

**ATP–CP energy system** A simple and immediate anaerobic energy system that maintains ATP levels. Creatine phosphate is broken down, releasing energy and a phosphate group, which is used to form ATP.

**autonomic nervous system (ANS)** The part of the central nervous system that regulates the automatic responses of the body; consists of the sympathetic and parasympathetic systems.

**avidin** A protein in raw egg whites that binds biotin, preventing its absorption. Avidin is denatured by heat.

**bacteriophage** A virus that infects bacteria.

**beriberi** Thiamin-deficiency disease. Symptoms include muscle weakness, loss of appetite, nerve degeneration, and edema in some cases.

**beta ($\beta$) bonds** Chemical bonds linking monosaccharides, which sometimes can be broken by human intestinal enzymes. Lactose contains digestible beta bonds, and cellulose contains nondigestible beta bonds.

**beta-glucans** Functional fiber, consisting of branched polysaccharide chains of glucose, that helps lower blood cholesterol levels. Found in barley and oats.

**beta-oxidation** The breakdown of a fatty acid into numerous molecules of the two-carbon compound acetyl coenzyme A (acetyl CoA).

**bile** An alkaline, yellow-green fluid that is produced in the liver and stored in the gallbladder. Bile emulsifies dietary fats, aiding fat digestion and absorption.

**binge** Consumption of a very large amount of food in a brief time (e.g., two hours) accompanied by a loss of control over how much and what is eaten.

**binge drinking** Consuming excessive amounts of alcohol in short periods of time.

**binge eaters** Individuals who routinely consume a very large amount of food in a brief period of time (e.g., two hours) and lose control over how much and what is eaten.

**binge-eating disorder** An eating disorder marked by repeated episodes of binge eating and a feeling of loss of control. The diagnosis is based on a person's having an average of at least two binge-eating episodes per week for six months.

**bioavailability** A measure of the extent to which a nutrient becomes available to the body after ingestion and thus is available to the tissues.

**biodiversity** The countless species of plants, animals, and insects that exist on the earth. An undisturbed tropical forest is an example of the biodiversity of a healthy ecosystem.

**bioelectrical impedance analysis (BIA)** Technique to estimate amounts of total body water, lean tissue mass, and total body fat. It uses the resistance of tissue to the flow of an alternating electric current.

**bioflavonoids** Naturally occurring plant chemicals, especially from citrus fruits, that reduce the permeability and fragility of capillaries.

**biosynthesis** Chemical reactions in which complex biomolecules, especially carbohydrates, lipids, and proteins, are formed from simple molecules.

**biotechnology** The set of laboratory techniques and processes used to modify the genome of plants or animals to create desirable new characteristics. Genetic engineering in the broad sense.

**blastogenic stage** The first stage of embryonic gestation during which tissue proliferation by rapid cell division begins.

**bleaching process** A complex light-stimulated reaction in which rod cells lose color as rhodopsin is split into vitamin A (retinal) and opsin.

**BodPod** A device used to measure the density of the body based on the volume of air displaced as a person sits in a sealed chamber of known volume.

**body composition** The chemical or anatomical composition of the body. Commonly defined as the proportions of fat, muscle, bone, and other tissues in the body.

**body dysmorphic disorder (BDD)** An eating disorder in which a distressing and impairing preoccupation with an imagined or slight defect in appearance is the primary symptom.

**body fat distribution** The pattern of fat distribution on the body.

**body image** A person's mental concept of his or her physical appearance, constructed from many different influences.

**body mass index (BMI)** Body weight (in kilograms) divided by the square of height (in meters), expressed in units of kg/m$^2$.

**bolus [BOH-lus]** A chewed, moistened lump of food that is ready to be swallowed.

**botulism** An often fatal type of food poisoning caused by a toxin released from *Clostridium botulinum*, a bacterium that can grow in improperly canned low-acid foods.

**bovine spongiform encephalopathy (BSE)** A chronic degenerative disease, widely referred to as *mad cow disease*, that affects the central nervous system of cattle.

**bran** The layers of protective coating around the grain kernel that are rich in dietary fiber and nutrients.

**Bt gene** *Bacillus thuringiensis* (Bt) is a bacterium that produces a protein called the Bt toxin. One of the bacterium's genes, the Bt gene, carries the information for the Bt toxin. Inserting a copy of the Bt gene into plants enables them to produce Bt toxin protein and resist some insect pests. The Bt protein is not toxic to humans.

**buffers** Compounds that can take up and release hydrogen ions to keep the pH of a solution constant. The buffering action of proteins and bicarbonate in the bloodstream plays a major role in maintaining the blood pH at 7.35 to 7.45.

**built environment** Any human-formed, developed, or structured areas, including the urban environment that consists of buildings, roads, fixtures, parks, and all other human developments that form its physical character.

**bulimia nervosa [bull-EEM-ee-uh]** An eating disorder marked by consumption of large amounts of food at one time (binge eating) followed by a behavior such as self-induced vomiting, use of laxatives, excessive exercise, fasting, or other practices to avoid weight gain.

**calcitonin** A hormone secreted by the thyroid gland in response to elevated blood calcium. It stimulates calcium deposition in bone and calcium excretion by the kidneys, thus reducing blood calcium.

**calcitriol** See *25-hydroxyvitamin D [25(OH)D]*.

**calmodulin** A calcium-binding protein that regulates a variety of cellular activities, such as cell division and proliferation.

**calorie** The general term for energy in food and used synonymously with the term *energy*. Often used instead of *kilocalorie* on food labels, in diet books, and in other sources of nutrition information.

**cancer** A term for diseases in which abnormal cells divide without control. Cancer cells can invade nearby tissues and can spread through the bloodstream and lymphatic system to other parts of the body.

**carbohydrate loading** Changes in dietary carbohydrate intake and exercise regimen before competition to maximize glycogen stores in the muscles. It is appropriate for endurance events lasting 60 to 90 consecutive minutes or longer. Also known as *glycogen loading*.

**carbohydrates** Compounds, including sugars, starches, and dietary fibers, that usually have the general chemical formula $(CH_2O)_n$, where $n$ represents the number of $CH_2O$ units in the molecule. Carbohydrates are a major source of energy for body functions.

**carcinogens [kar-SIN-o-jins]** Any substances that cause cancer.

**cardiac output** The amount of blood expelled by the heart.

**cardiovascular disease (CVD)** General term for all disorders affecting the heart and blood vessels.

**carnitine [CAR-nih-teen]** A compound that transports fatty acids from the cytosol into the mitochondria, where they undergo beta-oxidation.

**carotenoids** A group of yellow, orange, and red pigments in plants. Some of these compounds are precursors of vitamin A.

**case control studies** Investigations that use a group of people with a particular condition rather than a randomly selected population. These cases are compared with a control group of people who do not have the condition.

**catabolism [ca-TA-bol-iz-um]** Any metabolic process whereby cells break down complex substances into simpler, smaller ones.

**catalyze** To speed up a chemical reaction.

**cations** Ions that carry a positive charge.

**cecum** The blind pouch at the beginning of the large intestine into which the ileum opens from one side and which is continuous with the colon.

**celiac disease [SEA-lee-ak]** A disease that involves an inability to digest gluten, a protein found in wheat, rye, and barley. If untreated, it causes flattening of the villi in the intestine, leading to severe malabsorption of nutrients. Symptoms include diarrhea, fatty stools, swollen belly, and extreme fatigue.

**cells** The basic structural units of all living tissues. Cells have two major parts—the nucleus and the cytoplasm.

**cellulose [SELL-you-los]** A straight-chain polysaccharide composed of hundreds of glucose units linked by beta bonds. It is nondigestible by humans and a component of dietary fiber.

**central nervous system (CNS)** The brain and the spinal cord. The central nervous system transmits signals that control muscular actions and glandular secretions along the entire GI tract.

**ceruloplasmin** A copper-dependent enzyme that enables iron to bind to transferrin. Also known as *ferroxidase I*.

**chain length** The number of carbons that a fatty acid contains. Foods contain fatty acids with chain lengths of 4 to 24 carbons, and most have an even number of carbons.

**cheilosis** Inflammation and cracking of the lips; a symptom of riboflavin deficiency.

**chemical energy** Energy contained in the bonds between atoms of a molecule.

**Child and Adult Care Food Program** A federally funded program that reimburses approved family child-care providers for USDA-approved foods served to preschool children; also provides funds for meals and snacks served at after-school programs for school-age children and to adult day care centers serving chronically impaired adults or people over age 60.

**childhood** The period of life from age 1 to the onset of puberty.

**chitin** A long-chain structural polysaccharide of slightly modified glucose. Found in the hard exterior skeletons of insects, crustaceans, and other invertebrates; also occurs in the cell walls of fungi.

**chitosan** Polysaccharide derived from chitin.

**cholesterol [ko-LES-te-rol]** A waxy lipid (sterol) whose chemical structure contains multiple hydrocarbon rings.

**choline** A nitrogen-containing compound that is part of phosphatidyl-choline, a phospholipid. Choline also is part of the neurotransmitter acetylcholine. The body can synthesize choline from the amino acid methionine.

**chylomicron [kye-lo-MY-kron]** A large lipoprotein formed in intestinal cells following the absorption of dietary fats. A chylomicron has a central core of triglycerides and cholesterol surrounded by phospholipids and proteins.

**chyme [KIME]** A mass of partially digested food and digestive juices moving from the stomach into the small intestine.

**ciguatera** A toxin found in more than 300 species of Caribbean and South Pacific fish. It is a nonbacterial source of food poisoning.

**ciliary action** Wavelike motion of small hairlike projections on some cells.

**circular muscle** Layers of smooth muscle that surround organs, including the stomach and the small intestine.

**circulation** Movement of substances through the vessels of the cardiovascular or lymphatic system.

**cis fatty acid** An unsaturated fatty acid with a bent carbon chain. Most naturally occurring unsaturated fatty acids are *cis* fatty acids.

**citric acid cycle** The aerobic metabolic pathway in mitochondria that breaks down acetyl CoA to yield two molecules of carbon dioxide, one molecule of GTP, and pairs of high-energy electrons. It transfers the electrons to three molecules of $NAD^+$ (yielding three NADH) and one molecule of FAD (yielding one $FADH_2$). Also known as the *Krebs cycle* and the *tricarboxylic acid cycle*.

**clinical trials** Studies that collect large amounts of data to evaluate the effectiveness of a treatment.

**coenzyme A** A cofactor derived from the vitamin pantothenic acid.

**coenzymes** Organic compounds, often derived from B vitamins, that combine with inactive enzymes to form active enzymes.

**cofactors** Compounds required for an enzyme to be active. Cofactors include coenzymes and metal ions such as iron, copper, and magnesium.

**colic** Periodic inconsolable crying in an otherwise healthy infant that appears to result from abdominal cramping and discomfort.

**collagen** The most abundant fibrous protein in the body. Collagen is the major constituent of connective tissue, forms the foundation for bones and teeth, and helps maintain the structure of blood vessels and other tissues.

**colon** The portion of the large intestine extending from the cecum to the rectum. It is made up of four parts: the ascending, transverse, descending, and sigmoid colons.

**color additive** Any dye, pigment, or other substance that can impart color when added or applied to a food, drug, or cosmetic or to the human body.

**colostrum** A thick yellow fluid secreted by the breast during pregnancy and the first days after delivery.

**complementary and alternative medicine (CAM)** A broad range of healing philosophies, approaches, and therapies that include treatments and health care practices not taught widely in medical schools, not generally used in hospitals, and not usually reimbursed by medical insurance companies.

**complementary foods** Any foods or liquids other than breast milk or infant formula fed to an infant.

**complementary proteins** Two or more incomplete food proteins whose assortment of amino acids make up for, or complement, each other so the combination provides sufficient amounts of all the indispensable amino acids.

**complete proteins** Proteins that supply all of the indispensable amino acids in the proportions the body needs. Also known as *high-quality proteins*.

**complex carbohydrates** Chains of more than two monosaccharides. May be oligosaccharides or polysaccharides.

**compulsive overeating** See *binge-eating disorder*.

**concentration gradients** Differences between the solute concentrations of two solutions.

**conditionally indispensable amino acids** Amino acids that are normally made in the body (dispensable) but become indispensable under certain circumstances, such as during critical illness. Also called *conditionally essential amino acids*.

**cone cells** Cells in the retina that are sensitive to bright light and translate it into color images.

**congeners** Biologically active compounds in alcoholic beverages that include nonalcoholic ingredients as well as other alcohols such as methanol. Congeners contribute to the distinctive taste and smell of the beverage and may increase intoxicating effects and subsequent hangover.

**conjugated linoleic acid (CLA)** A polyunsaturated fatty acid in which the position of the double bonds has moved so that a single bond alternates with two double bonds.

**connective tissues** Tissues composed primarily of fibrous proteins, such as collagen, and that contain few cells. Their primary function is to bind together and support various body structures.

**constipation** Infrequent and difficult bowel movements, followed by a sensation of incomplete evacuation.

**control group** A set of people used as a standard of comparison to the experimental group. The people in the control group have characteristics similar to those in the experimental group and are selected at random.

**cornea** The transparent outer surface of the eye.

**correlations** Connections co-occurring more frequently than can be explained by chance or coincidence but without a proven cause.

**C-reactive protein (CRP)** A protein released by the body in response to acute injury, infection, or other inflammatory stimuli. CRP is associated with future cardiovascular events.

**creatine** An important nitrogenous compound found in meats and fish and synthesized in the body from amino acids (glycine, arginine, and methionine).

**creatine phosphate** An energy-rich compound that supplies energy and a phosphate group for the formation of ATP. Also called *phosphocreatine*.

**cretinism** A congenital condition often caused by severe iodine deficiency during gestation; characterized by arrested physical and mental development.

**critical control points (CCPs)** Operational steps or procedures in a process, production method, or recipe at which control can be applied to prevent, reduce, or eliminate a food safety hazard.

**critical period of development** Time during which the environment has the greatest impact on the developing embryo.

**cystic fibrosis** An inherited disorder that causes widespread dysfunction of the exocrine glands, resulting in chronic lung disease, abnormally high levels of electrolytes (e.g., sodium, potassium, chloride) in sweat, and deficiency of pancreatic enzymes needed for digestion.

**cytoplasm** The material of the cell, excluding the cell nucleus and cell membranes. The cytoplasm includes the semifluid cytosol, the organelles, and other particles.

**cytosol** The semifluid inside the cell membrane, excluding organelles. The cytosol is the site of glycolysis and fatty acid synthesis.

**Daily Values (DVs)** A single set of nutrient intake standards developed by the Food and Drug Administration to represent the needs of the "typical" consumer; used as standards for expressing nutrient content on food labels.

**dark adaptation** The process that increases the rhodopsin concentration in your eyes, allowing them to detect images in the dark better.

**deamination** The removal of the amino group ($-NH_2$) from an amino acid.

**Delaney Clause** The part of the 1960 Color Additives Amendment to the Federal Food, Drug, and Cosmetic Act that bars the FDA from approving any additives shown in laboratory tests to cause cancer.

**denaturation** A change in the three-dimensional structure of a protein resulting in an unfolded polypeptide chain that cannot fulfill the protein's function. Treatment with heat, acid, alkali, or extreme agitation can denature most proteins.

**diarrhea** Watery stools due to reduced absorption of water.

**dietary fiber** Carbohydrates and lignins that are naturally in plants and are nondigestible; that is, they are not digested and absorbed in the human small intestine.

**dietary folate equivalents (DFE)** A measure of folate intake used to account for the high bioavailability of folic acid taken as a supplement compared with the lower bioavailability of the folate found in foods.

***Dietary Guidelines for Americans*** The *Guidelines* are the foundation of federal nutrition policy and is jointly developed by the U.S. Department of Agriculture (USDA) and the Department of Health and Human Services (DHHS). These science-based guidelines are intended to reduce the number of Americans who develop chronic diseases such as hypertension, diabetes, cardiovascular disease, obesity, and alcoholism.

**Dietary Reference Intakes (DRIs)** A framework of dietary standards that include Estimated Average Requirement (EAR), Recommended Dietary Allowance (RDA), Adequate Intake (AI), and Tolerable Upper Intake Level (UL).

**dietary standards** Set of values for recommended intake of nutrients.

**Dietary Supplement Health and Education Act (DSHEA)** Legislation that regulates dietary supplements.

**dietary supplements** Products taken by mouth in tablet, capsule, powder, gelcap, or other nonfood form that contain one or more of the following: vitamins, minerals, amino acids, herbs, enzymes, metabolites, or concentrates.

**digestion** The process of transforming the foods we eat into units for absorption.

**digestive secretions** Substances released at different places in the GI tract to speed the breakdown of ingested carbohydrates, fats, and proteins.

**diglyceride** A molecule of glycerol combined with two fatty acids.

**dioxins** Chemical compounds created in the manufacture, combustion, and chlorine bleaching of pulp and paper and in other industrial processes.

**dipeptide** Two amino acids joined by a peptide bond.

**direct additives** Substances added to foods for a specific purpose.

**disaccharides [dye-SACK-uh-rides]** Carbohydrates composed of two monosaccharide units chemically linked. They include sucrose (common table sugar), lactose (milk sugar), and maltose.

**disordered eating** An abnormal change in eating pattern related to an illness, a stressful event, or a desire to improve one's health or appearance. If it persists it may lead to an eating disorder.

**dispensable (nonessential) amino acids** Amino acids the body can make if supplied with adequate nitrogen. Dispensable amino acids do not need to be supplied in the diet.

**diuresis** The formation and secretion of urine.

**diuretics [dye-u-RET-iks]** Drugs or other substances that promote the formation and release of urine. Diuretics are given to reduce body fluid volume in treating such disorders as high blood pressure, congestive heart disease, and edema. Both alcohol and caffeine act as diuretics.

**diverticulitis [dy-vur-tik-yoo-LY-tis]** A condition that occurs when small pouches in the colon (diverticula) become infected or irritated. Also called *left-sided appendicitis*.

**diverticulosis [dy-vur-tik-yoo-LOH-sis]** A condition that occurs when small pouches (diverticula) push outward through weak spots in the colon.

**double-blind study** A research study set up so neither the subjects nor the investigators know which study group is receiving the placebo and which is receiving the active substance.

**duodenum [doo-oh-DEE-num]** The portion of the small intestine closest to the stomach. The duodenum is 25 to 30 cm (10 to 12 in.) long and wider than the remainder of the small intestine.

**eating disorders** A spectrum of abnormal eating patterns that eventually may endanger a person's health or increase the risk for other diseases. Generally, psychological factors play a key role.

*Eating Well with Canada's Food Guide* Recommendations to help Canadians select foods to meet energy and nutrient needs while reducing the risk of chronic disease. The *Food Guide* is based on the *Nutrition Recommendations for Canadians* and Canada's Guidelines for Healthy Eating and is a key nutrition education tool for Canadians aged 2 to 3 years and older.

**eclampsia** The occurrence of seizures in a pregnant woman that are unrelated to brain conditions.

**edema** Swelling caused by the buildup of fluid between cells.

**eicosanoids** A class of hormonelike substances formed in the body from long-chain essential fatty acids.

**electrolytes [ih-LEK-tro-lites]** Substances that separate into charged particles (ions) when dissolved in water or other solvents and thus become capable of conducting an electrical current. The terms *electrolyte* and *ion* often are used interchangeably.

**Electronic Benefits Transfer (EBT)** Electronic delivery of government benefits by a single plastic card that allows access to food benefits at point-of-sale locations.

**electron transport chain** An organized series of protein carrier molecules located in mitochondrial membranes. As high-energy electrons delivered by NADH and $FADH_2$ traverse the electron transport chain to oxygen, it produces ATP and water.

**elimination** The removal of undigested food from the body.

**embryonic stage** The developmental stage between the time of implantation (about two weeks after fertilization) through the seventh or eighth week; the stage of major organ system differentiation and development of main external features.

**emetics** Agents that induce vomiting.

**emulsifiers** Agents that blend fatty and watery liquids by promoting the breakup of fat into small particles and stabilizing their suspension in a watery solution.

**endosperm** The middle portion of a grain kernel; high in starch to provide food for the growing plant embryo.

**enemas** Infusions of fluid into the rectum, usually for cleansing or other therapeutic purposes.

**energy** The capacity to do work. The energy in food is chemical energy, which the body converts to mechanical, electrical, or heat energy.

**energy balance** The balance in the body between amounts of energy consumed and expended.

**energy equilibrium** A balance of energy intake and output that results in little or no change in weight over time.

**energy intake** The caloric or energy content of food provided by the sources of dietary energy: carbohydrate (4 kcal/g), protein (4 kcal/g), fat (9 kcal/g), and alcohol (7 kcal/g).

**energy output** The use of calories or energy for basic body functions, physical activity, and processing of consumed foods.

**enrich** To add vitamins and minerals lost or diminished during food processing, particularly the addition of thiamin, riboflavin, niacin, folic acid, and iron to grain products.

**enteric nervous system** A network of nerves located in the gastrointestinal wall.

**enterohepatic circulation [EN-ter-oh-heh-PAT-ik]** Recycling of certain compounds between the small intestine and the liver.

**enzymes [EN-zimes]** Proteins in the body that speed up the rate of chemical reactions but are not altered in the process.

**epinephrine** A hormone released in response to stress or sudden danger, epinephrine raises blood glucose levels to ready the body for "fight or flight." Also called *adrenaline*.

**epiphyses** The heads of the long bones that are separated from the shaft of the bone until the bone stops growing.

**epithelial cells** The millions of cells that line and protect the external and internal surfaces of the body. Epithelial cells form epithelial tissues such as skin and mucous membranes.

**epithelial tissues** Closely packed layers of epithelial cells that cover the body and line its cavities.

**ergogenic aids** Substances that can enhance athletic performance.

*Escherichia coli (E. coli)* Bacteria that are the most common cause of urinary tract infections. Because they release toxins, some types of *E. coli* can rapidly cause shock and death.

**esophageal sphincter** The opening between the esophagus and the stomach that relaxes and opens to allow the bolus to travel into the stomach, and then closes behind it. Acts as a barrier to prevent the reflux of gastric contents. Also called the *cardiac sphincter*.

**esophagitis** Inflammation of the esophagus.

**esophagus [ee-SOFF-uh-gus]** The food pipe that extends from the pharynx to the stomach.

**essential fatty acids (EFAs)** Fatty acids that the body needs but cannot synthesize and must obtain from the diet.

**essential nutrients** Substances that must be obtained in the diet because the body either cannot make them or cannot make adequate amounts of them.

**Estimated Average Requirement (EAR)** The intake value that meets the estimated nutrient needs of 50 percent of individuals in a specific life-stage and gender group.

**Estimated Energy Requirement (EER)** Dietary energy intake that is predicted to maintain energy balance in a healthy adult of a defined age, gender, weight, height, and level of physical activity consistent with good health.

**ethanol** Chemical name for drinking alcohol. Also known as ethyl alcohol.

**ethyl alcohol** See *ethanol*.

**experimental group** A set of people being studied to evaluate the effect of an event, substance, or technique.

**Exchange Lists** Lists of foods that in specified portions provide equivalent amounts of carbohydrate, fat, protein, and energy. Any food in an Exchange List can be substituted for any other without markedly affecting macronutrient intake.

**excretion** The process of separating and removing waste products of metabolism.

**extracellular fluid** The fluid located outside of cells. It is composed largely of the liquid portion (plasma) of the blood and the fluid between cells in tissues (interstitial fluid), with fluid in the GI tract, eyes, joints, and spinal cord contributing a small amount. It constitutes about one-third of body water.

**extreme obesity** Obesity characterized by body weight exceeding 100 percent of normal; a condition so severe it often requires surgery.

**extrusion reflex** A young infant's response when a spoon is put in its mouth; the tongue is thrust forward, indicating that the baby is not ready for spoon feeding.

**facilitated diffusion** A process by which carrier (transport) proteins in the cell membrane transport substances into or out of cells down a concentration gradient.

**FAD** Flavin adenine dinucleotide (FAD), a coenzyme derived from the B vitamin riboflavin, becomes $FADH_2$ as it accepts a pair of high-energy electrons for transport in cells.

**failure to thrive (FTT)** Abnormally low gains in length (height) and weight during infancy and childhood; may result from physical problems or poor feeding, but many affected children have no apparent disease or defect.

**fasting hypoglycemia** A type of hypoglycemia that occurs because the body produces too much insulin even when no food is eaten.

**fast-twitch (FT) fibers** Muscle fibers that can develop high tension rapidly. These fibers can fatigue quickly but are well suited to explosive movements in sprinting, jumping, and weight lifting.

**fat replacers** Compounds that imitate the functional and sensory properties of fats but contain less available energy than fats.

**fatty acids** Compounds containing a long hydrocarbon chain with a carboxyl group (–COOH) at one end and a methyl group ($–CH_3$) at the other end.

**fatty liver** Accumulation of fat in the liver, a sign of increased fatty acid synthesis.

**Feeding America** The largest charitable hunger-relief organization in the United States. Its mission is to feed America's hungry through a nationwide network of member food banks and to engage the country in the fight to end hunger.

**fermentation** The anaerobic conversion of various carbohydrates to carbon dioxide and an alcohol or organic acid.

**ferritin** A major storage form of iron.

**fetal alcohol syndrome** A set of physical and mental abnormalities observed in infants born to women who abuse alcohol during pregnancy. Affected infants exhibit poor growth, characteristic abnormal facial features, limited hand–eye coordination, and mental retardation.

**fetal stage** The period of rapid growth from the end of the embryonic stage until birth.

**fibrin** A stringy, insoluble protein that is the final product of the blood-clotting process.

**flatulence** The presence of excessive amounts of air or other gases in the stomach or intestines.

**flatus** Lower intestinal gas that is expelled through the rectum.

**flavor** The collective experience that describes both taste and smell.

**fluorosis** Mottled discoloration and pitting of tooth enamel caused by prolonged ingestion of excess fluoride that is characterized in children by discoloration and pitting of the teeth.

**Food and Agriculture Organization (FAO)** The largest autonomous UN agency; the FAO works to alleviate poverty and hunger by promoting agricultural development, improved nutrition, and the pursuit of food security.

**Food and Nutrition Board** A board within the Institute of Medicine of the National Academy of Sciences. It is responsible for assembling the group of nutrition scientists who review available scientific data to determine appropriate intake levels of the known essential nutrients.

**foodborne illness** A sickness caused by food contaminated with micro-organisms, chemicals, or other substances hazardous to human health.

***Food Code*** A reference published periodically by the Food and Drug Administration for restaurants, grocery stores, institutional food services, vending operations, and other retailers on how to store, prepare, and serve food to prevent foodborne illness.

**food groups** Categories of similar foods, such as fruits or vegetables.

**food insecurity** (1) Limited or uncertain availability of nutritionally adequate and safe foods or (2) limited or uncertain ability to acquire acceptable foods in socially acceptable ways.

**food label** Labels required by law on virtually all packaged foods and having five requirements: (1) a statement of identity; (2) the net contents (by weight, volume, or measure) of the package; (3) the name and address of the manufacturer, packer, or distributor; (4) a list of ingredients; and (5) nutrition information.

**Food Research and Action Center (FRAC)** Founded in 1970 as a public interest law firm, FRAC is a nonprofit child advocacy group that works to improve public policies to eradicate hunger and undernutrition in the United States.

**food security** Access to enough food for an active, healthy life, including (1) the ready availability of nutritionally adequate and safe foods and (2) an assured ability to acquire acceptable foods in socially acceptable ways.

**Food Security Supplement Survey** A federally funded survey that measures the prevalence and severity of food insecurity and hunger.

**fortify** Refers to the addition of vitamins or minerals that were not originally present in a good.

**free radicals** Short-lived, highly reactive chemicals often derived from oxygen-containing compounds, which can have detrimental effects on cells, especially DNA and cell membranes.

**French paradox** The phenomenon observed in the French, who have a lower incidence of heart disease than people whose diets contain comparable amounts of fat. Part of the difference has been attributed to the regular and moderate drinking of red wine.

**fructose [FROOK-tose]** A common monosaccharide naturally present in honey and many fruits. Also called *levulose* or *fruit sugar*.

**full-term baby** A baby delivered during the normal period of human gestation, between 38 and 41 weeks.

**functional dyspepsia** Chronic pain in the upper abdomen not due to any obvious physical cause.

**functional fiber** Isolated nondigestible carbohydrates, including some manufactured carbohydrates, that have beneficial effects in humans.

**functional food** A food that may provide a health benefit beyond basic nutrition.

**galactose [gah-LAK-tose]** A monosaccharide that has a structure similar to glucose; usually joined with other monosaccharides.

**gallbladder** A pear-shaped sac that stores and concentrates bile from the liver.

**galvanized** Describes iron or steel with a thin layer of zinc plated onto it to protect against corrosion.

**gastric lipase** An enzyme in the stomach that primarily breaks down butterfat.

**gastrin [GAS-trin]** A hormone released from the walls of the stomach and duodenum that stimulates gastric secretions and motility.

**gastritis** Inflammation of the stomach.

**gastroesophageal reflux** A backflow of stomach contents into the esophagus, accompanied by a burning pain because of the acidity of the gastric juices.

**gastroesophageal reflux disease (GERD)** Tissue damage to the esophagus due to the reflux of gastric contents.

**gastrointestinal (GI) tract [GAS-troh-in-TES-tin-al]** The connected series of organs and structures used for digestion of food and absorption of nutrients; also called the alimentary canal or the digestive tract.

**Generally Recognized as Safe (GRAS)** Refers to substances that are "generally recognized as safe" for consumption and can be added to foods by manufacturers without establishing their safety by rigorous experimental studies. Congress established the GRAS list in 1958.

**genetically modified (GM) foods** Foods produced using plant or animal ingredients that have been modified using gene technology.

**genetic engineering** Manipulation of the genome of an organism by artificial means for the purpose of modifying existing traits or adding new genetic traits.

**genome** The total genetic information of an organism, stored in the DNA of its chromosomes.

**geophagia** Ingestion of clay or dirt.

**germ** The innermost part of a grain that can grow into a new plant. Germ is rich in protein, oils, vitamins, and minerals.

**gestational diabetes** A condition that results in high blood glucose levels during pregnancy.

**ghrelin** A hormone produced by the stomach that stimulates feeding by increasing release of neuropeptide Y.

**glossitis** Inflammation of the tongue; a symptom of riboflavin deficiency.

**glucagon [GLOO-kuh-gon]** Produced by the pancreas, this hormone promotes the breakdown of liver glycogen to glucose and, thus, increases blood glucose levels.

**glucogenic** A term describing an amino acid whose carbon skeleton can be used in gluconeogenesis to form glucose.

**gluconeogenesis [gloo-ko-nee-oh-JEN-uh-sis]** Synthesis of glucose within the body from noncarbohydrate precursors such as amino acids, lactic acid, and glycerol. Fatty acids cannot be converted to glucose.

**glucose [GLOO-kose]** A common monosaccharide that is a component of disaccharides (sucrose, lactose, and maltose) and various complex carbohydrates; present in the blood. Also known as *dextrose*.

**glutathione peroxidase** A selenium-containing enzyme that reduces toxic hydrogen peroxide formed within cells; works with vitamin E to reduce free radical damage.

**glycerol [GLISS-er-ol]** The backbone of mono-, di-, and triglycerides; alone, it is a thick, smooth liquid.

**glycogen [GLY-ko-jen]** A very large, highly branched polysaccharide composed of multiple glucose units. Sometimes called *animal starch*, glycogen is the primary storage form of glucose in animals.

**glycogenesis** The formation of glycogen from glucose.

**glycogen loading** See *carbohydrate loading*.

**glycolysis [gligh-COLL-ih-sis]** The anaerobic pathway that breaks down a glucose molecule into two molecules of pyruvate and yields two molecules of ATP and two molecules of NADH. Glycolysis occurs in the cytosol of a cell.

**goiter** A chronic enlargement of the thyroid gland, visible as a swelling at the front of the neck; usually associated with iodine deficiency.

**goitrogens** Compounds that interfere with iodine absorption and can induce goiter.

**growth charts** Charts that plot the weight, length, and head circumference of infants and children as they grow.

**GTP (guanosine triphosphate)** A high-energy compound, similar to ATP but with three phosphate groups linked to guanosine instead of adenosine.

**gums** Dietary fibers, which contain galactose and other monosaccharides, found between plant cell walls.

**gynoid obesity** Excess storage of fat located primarily in the buttocks and thighs. Also called *gynecoid obesity*.

**hangover** The collection of symptoms experienced by someone who has consumed a large quantity of alcohol. Symptoms can include pounding headache, fatigue, muscle aches, nausea, stomach pain, heightened sensitivity to light and sound, dizziness, and possibly depression, anxiety, and irritability.

**head circumference** Measurement of the largest part of the infant's head (just above the eyebrows and ears); used to determine brain growth.

**health claim** Any statement that associates a food or a substance in a food with a disease or health-related condition. The FDA authorizes health claims.

**heartburn** Burning pain behind the breastbone area caused by acidic stomach contents backing up into the esophagus.

**heat capacity** The amount of energy required to raise the temperature of a substance 1°C.

**heme** A chemical complex with a central iron atom that forms the oxygen-binding part of hemoglobin and myoglobin.

**heme iron** The iron found in the hemoglobin and myoglobin of animal foods.

**hemicelluloses [hem-ih-SELL-you-los-es]** A group of large polysaccharides in dietary fiber that are fermented more easily than cellulose.

**hemochromatosis** A hereditary disorder in which excessive absorption of iron results in abnormal iron deposits in the liver and other tissues.

**hemoglobin [HEEM-oh-glow-bin]** The oxygen-carrying protein in red blood cells that consists of four heme groups and four globin polypeptide chains. The presence of hemoglobin gives blood its red color.

**hemosiderin** An insoluble form of storage iron.

**herbal therapy (phytotherapy)** The therapeutic use of herbs and other plants to promote health and treat disease. Also called *phytotherapy*.

**high-density lipoproteins (HDL)** The blood lipoproteins that contain high levels of protein and low levels of triglycerides. Synthesized primarily in the liver and small intestine, HDL picks up cholesterol released from dying cells and other sources and transfers it to other lipoproteins. HDL cholesterol sometimes is called "good cholesterol."

**hormones** Chemical messengers that are secreted into the blood by one tissue and act on cells in another part of the body.

**hunger** The internal, physiological drive to find and consume food. Unlike appetite, hunger is often experienced as a negative sensation, often manifesting as an uneasy or painful sensation; the recurrent and involuntary lack of access to food that may produce malnutrition over time.

**husk** The inedible covering of grain; also known as the *chaff*.

**hydrochloric acid (gastric acid)** A very strong acid of chloride and hydrogen atoms made by stomach glands and secreted into the stomach. Also called *gastric acid*.

**hydrogenation [high-dro-jen-AY-shun]** A chemical reaction in which hydrogen atoms are added to a fat; hydrogenation produces more saturated fatty acids and converts some unsaturated fatty acids from a *cis* form to a *trans* form.

**hydrolysis** A reaction that breaks apart a compound through the addition of water.

**hydrostatic weighing** See *underwater weighing*.

**hydroxyapatite** A crystalline mineral compound of calcium and phosphorus that makes up bone.

**hyperactivity** A maladaptive and abnormal increase in activity that is inconsistent with developmental levels. Includes frequent fidgeting, inappropriate running, excessive talking, and difficulty in engaging in quiet activities.

**hypercellular obesity** Obesity due to an above-average number of fat cells.

**hypercholesterolemia** High blood cholesterol (total cholesterol).

**hyperglycemia [HIGH-per-gly-SEE-me-uh]** Abnormal high concentration of glucose in the blood.

**hyperplastic obesity (hyperplasia)** Obesity due to an increase in both the size and number of fat cells.

**hypertension** Condition in which resting blood pressure persistently exceeds 140 mm Hg systolic or 90 mm Hg diastolic.

**hyperthermia** A much higher than normal body temperature.

**hypertrophic obesity** Obesity due to an increase in the size of fat cells.

**hypervitaminosis** High levels of vitamins in the blood, usually a result of excess supplement intake.

**hypoglycemia [HIGH-po-gly-SEE-mee-uh]** Abnormally low concentration of glucose in the blood; any blood glucose value below 40 to 50 mg/dL of blood.

**hypogonadism** Decreased functional activity of the gonads (ovaries or testes) with retardation of growth and sexual development.

**hypothalamus [high-po-THAL-ah-mus]** A region of the brain involved in regulating hunger and satiety, respiration, body temperature, water balance, and other body functions.

**hypotheses** Scientists' "educated guesses" to explain phenomena.

**hypothyroidism** The result of a lowered level of circulating thyroid hormone, with slowing of mental and physical functions.

**ileum [ILL-ee-um]** The terminal segment of the small intestine (about 150 cm [5 ft] long), which opens into the large intestine.

**immune response** A coordinated set of steps, including production of antibodies, that the immune system takes in response to an antigen.

**incomplete proteins** Proteins that lack one or more indispensable amino acids. Also called *low-quality proteins*.

**indirect additives** Substances that become part of the food in trace amounts due to its packaging, storage, or other handling.

**indispensable (essential) amino acids** Amino acids the body cannot make at all or cannot make in sufficient quantities to meet the body's needs. Indispensable amino acids must be supplied in the diet.

**infancy** The period between birth and 12 months of age.

**infantile anorexia** Severe feeding difficulties that begin with the introduction of solid foods to infants. Symptoms include persistent food refusal for more than one month, malnutrition, parental concern about the child's poor food intake, and significant caregiver–infant conflict during feeding.

**inorganic** Any substance that does not contain carbon, excepting certain simple carbon compounds such as carbon dioxide and monoxide. Common examples include table salt (sodium chloride) and baking soda (sodium bicarbonate).

**insensible water loss** The continual loss of body water by evaporation from the respiratory tract and diffusion through the skin.

**insulin [IN-suh-lin]** Produced by the pancreas, this hormone stimulates the uptake of blood glucose into cells, the formation of glycogen in the liver, and various other processes.

**insulin resistance** State in which enough insulin is produced but cells do not respond to the action of insulin. Also called *insulin insensitivity*.

**integrated pest management (IPM)** Economically sound pest control techniques that minimize pesticide use, enhance environmental stewardship, and promote sustainable systems.

**intermediate-density lipoproteins (IDL)** The lipoproteins formed when lipoprotein lipase strips some of the triglycerides from VLDL.

**International Units (IU)** An outdated system to measure vitamin activity, this measurement does not consider differences in bioavailability.

**interstitial fluid [in-ter-STISH-ul]** The fluid between cells in tissues, usually high in sodium and chloride. Also called *intercellular fluid*.

**intervention studies** See clinical trials.

**intracellular fluid** The fluid in the body's cells. It usually is high in potassium and phosphate and low in sodium and chloride. It constitutes about two-thirds of total body water.

**intravascular fluid** The fluid portion (plasma) of the blood contained in arteries, veins, and capillaries. It accounts for about 15 percent of the extracellular fluid.

**intrinsic factor** A protein released from cells in the stomach wall that binds to and aids in the absorption of vitamin $B_{12}$.

**iodine deficiency disorders (IDD)** A wide range of disorders due to iodine deficiency that affect growth and development.

**iodopsin** Color-sensitive pigment molecules in cone cells that consist of opsinlike proteins combined with retinal.

**ions** Atoms or groups of atoms with an electrical charge resulting from the loss or gain of one or more electrons.

**iron overload** Toxicity from excess iron.

**irradiation** A food preservation technique in which foods are exposed to measured doses of radiation to reduce or eliminate pathogens and kill insects, reduce spoilage, and, in certain fruits and vegetables, inhibit sprouting and delay ripening.

**irritable bowel syndrome (IBS)** A disruptive state of intestinal motility with no known cause.

**isoflavones** Plant chemicals that include genistein and daidzein and may have positive effects against cancer and heart disease. Also called *phytoestrogens*.

**jejunum [je-JOON-um]** The middle section of the small intestine (about 120 cm [4 ft] long), lying between the duodenum and ileum.

**keratin** A water-insoluble fibrous protein that is the primary constituent of hair, nails, and the outer layer of the skin.

**Keshan disease** Selenium-deficiency disease that impairs the structure and function of the heart.

**ketoacidosis** Acidification of the blood caused by a buildup of ketone bodies. It is primarily a consequence of uncontrolled type 1 diabetes mellitus and can be life threatening.

**ketogenesis** The process in which excess acetyl CoA from fatty acid oxidation is converted into ketone bodies.

**ketogenic** A term describing an amino acid broken down to acetyl CoA (which can be converted into ketone bodies).

**ketone bodies** Molecules formed when insufficient carbohydrate is available to completely metabolize fat. Formation of ketone bodies is promoted by a low glucose level and high acetyl CoA level within cells. Acetone, acetoacetate, and beta-hydroxybutyrate are ketone bodies. Beta-hydroxybutyrate is sometimes improperly called a ketone.

**ketones [KEE-tonez]** Organic compounds that contain a chemical group consisting of C=O (a carbon–oxygen double bond) bound to two hydrocarbons. Pyruvate and fructose are examples of ketones. Acetone and acetoacetate are both ketones and ketone bodies. Although beta-hydroxybutyrate is not a ketone, it is a ketone body.

**ketosis [kee-TOE-sis]** Abnormally high concentration of ketone bodies in body tissues and fluids.

**kilocalories (kcal) [KILL-oh-kal-oh-rees]** Units used to measure energy. Food energy is measured in kilocalories (1,000 calories = 1 kilocalorie).

**Krebs cycle** See *citric acid cycle*.

**kwashiorkor** A type of malnutrition that occurs primarily in young children who have an infectious disease and whose diets supply marginal amounts of energy and very little protein. Common symptoms include poor growth, edema, apathy, weakness, and susceptibility to infections.

**lactate** A three-carbon compound that is produced when insufficient oxygen is present in cells to break down pyruvate to acetyl CoA. Often called *lactic acid*.

**lactation** The process of synthesizing and secreting breast milk.

**lactation consultants** Health professionals trained to specialize in education about and promotion of breastfeeding; may be certified as an International Board Certified Lactation Consultant (IBCLC).

**lacteal** A small lymphatic vessel in the interior of each intestinal villus that picks up fat-soluble compounds from intestinal cells.

**lactic acid energy system** Anaerobic energy system; using glycolysis, the process rapidly produces energy (ATP) and lactate. Also called *anaerobic glycolysis*.

**lactose [LAK-tose]** A disaccharide composed of glucose and galactose; also called *milk sugar* because it is the major sugar in milk and dairy products.

**lanugo [lah-NEW-go]** Soft, downy hair that covers a normal fetus from the fifth month but is shed almost entirely by the time of birth. It also appears on semistarved individuals who have lost much of their body fat, serving as insulation normally provided by body fat.

**large intestine** The tube (about 150 cm [5 ft] long) extending from the ileum of the small intestine to the anus. The large intestine includes the appendix, cecum, colon, rectum, and anal canal.

**laxatives** Substances that promote evacuation of the bowel by increasing the bulk of the feces, lubricating the intestinal wall, or softening the stool.

**lean body mass** The portion of the body exclusive of stored fat, including muscle, bone, connective tissue, organs, and water.

**lecithin** In the body, a phospholipid with the nitrogen-containing component choline. In foods, lecithin is a blend of phospholipids with different nitrogen-containing components.

**legumes** A family of plants with edible seed pods, such as peas, beans, lentils and soybeans; also called *pulses*.

**leptin** A hormone produced by adipose cells that signals the amount of body fat content and influences food intake.

**let-down reflex** The release of milk from the breast tissue in response to the stimulus of the hormone oxytocin. The major stimulus for oxytocin release is the infant suckling at the breast.

**lignins [LIG-nins]** Insoluble fibers composed of multiring alcohol units that constitute the only noncarbohydrate component of dietary fiber.

**lingual lipase** A fat-splitting enzyme secreted by cells at the base of the tongue.

**linoleic acid [lin-oh-LAY-ik]** An essential *omega*-6 fatty acid that contains 18 carbon atoms and 2 carbon–carbon double bonds (18:2); a thin liquid at room temperature.

**lipids** A group of fat-soluble compounds that includes triglycerides, sterols, and phospholipids.

**lipogenesis [lye-poh-JEN-eh-sis]** Synthesis of fatty acids from acetyl CoA derived from the metabolism of fats, alcohol, and some amino acids.

**lipoprotein** A complex that transports lipids in the lymph and blood. Lipoproteins consist of a central core of triglycerides and cholesterol surrounded by a shell composed of proteins, cholesterol, and phospholipids. The various types of lipoproteins differ in size, composition, and density.

**lipoprotein a [Lp(a)]** A substance that consists of an LDL "bad cholesterol" part plus a protein (apoprotein a) whose exact function is currently unknown.

**lipoprotein lipase** The major enzyme responsible for the breakdown of lipoproteins and triglycerides in the blood.

**liver** The largest glandular organ in the body, it produces and secretes bile, detoxifies harmful substances, and helps metabolize carbohydrates, lipids, proteins, and micronutrients.

**longitudinal muscle** Muscle fibers aligned lengthwise.

**Lou Gehrig's disease** A syndrome marked by muscular weakness and atrophy due to a degeneration of motor neurons of the spinal cord. Technically known as *amyotrophic lateral sclerosis (ALS)*.

**low-birth-weight infant** A newborn who weighs less than 2,500 grams (5.5 pounds) as a result of either premature birth or inadequate growth in utero.

**low-density lipoproteins (LDL)** The cholesterol-rich lipoproteins that result from the breakdown and removal of triglycerides from intermediate-density lipoprotein. LDL cholesterol sometimes is called "bad cholesterol."

**lumen** Cavity or hollow channel in any organ or structure of the body.

**lycopene** One of a family of plant chemicals, the carotenoids. Others in this big family include alpha-carotene and beta-carotene.

**lymph** Fluid that travels through the lymphatic system, made up of large fat particles and fluid drained from the areas between the cells.

**lymphatic system** A system of small vessels, ducts, valves, and organized tissue (e.g., lymph nodes) through which lymph moves from its origin in the tissues toward the heart.

**lymphocytes** White blood cells that are primarily responsible for immune responses. Present in the blood and lymph.

**macrobiotic diet** A highly restrictive dietary approach applied as a therapy for risk factors or chronic disease in general.

**macrominerals** Major minerals required in the diet and present in the body in large amounts compared with trace minerals.

**macronutrients** Nutrients, such as carbohydrate, fat, or protein, that are needed in relatively large amounts in the diet.

**macrophages** Large immune system cells that function as patrol cells and engulf and kill foreign invaders.

**macular degeneration** Progressive deterioration of the macula, an area in the center of the retina, that eventually leads to loss of central vision.

**mad cow disease** See *bovine spongiform encephalopathy (BSE)*.

**major minerals** Major minerals are required in the diet and are present in the body in large amounts compared with trace minerals.

**malabsorption syndromes** Conditions that result in imperfect, inadequate, or otherwise disordered gastrointestinal absorption.

**malnutrition** Failure to achieve nutrient requirements, which can impair physical and/or mental health. It may result from consuming too little food or from a shortage or imbalance of key nutrients.

**maltose [MALL-tose]** A disaccharide composed of two glucose molecules; sometimes called *malt sugar*. Maltose seldom occurs naturally in foods but is formed whenever long molecules of starch break down.

**marasmus** A type of malnutrition resulting from chronic inadequate consumption of protein and energy that is characterized by wasting of muscle, fat, and other body tissue.

**Meals on Wheels** A voluntary, nonprofit organization established to provide nutritious meals to homebound people (regardless of age) so they may maintain their independence and quality of life.

**megadoses** Doses of a nutrient that are 10 or more times the recommended amount.

**megaloblastic anemia** Excess amounts of megaloblasts (immature red blood cells) in the blood caused by deficiency of folate or vitamin $B_{12}$.

**menadione** A medicinal form of vitamin K. Also known as *vitamin $K_3$*.

**menaquinones** The form of vitamin K that comes from animal sources or is produced by intestinal bacteria. Also known as *vitamin $K_2$*.

**menarche** First menstrual period.

**Menkes' syndrome** A genetic disorder that results in copper deficiency.

**metabolic fitness** The absence of all metabolic and biochemical risk factors associated with obesity.

**metabolic pathway** A series of chemical reactions that either break down a large compound into smaller units (catabolism) or synthesize more complex molecules from smaller ones (anabolism).

**metabolic syndrome** A cluster of at least three of the following risk factors for heart disease: hypertriglyceridemia (high blood triglycerides), low HDL cholesterol, hyperglycemia (high blood glucose), hypertension (high blood pressure), and excess abdominal fat.

**metabolism** All chemical reactions within organisms that enable them to maintain life. The two main categories of metabolism are catabolism and anabolism.

**metabolites** Substances produced during metabolism.

**methanol** The simplest alcohol. Also known as methyl alcohol and wood alcohol.

**methyl alcohol** See *methanol*.

**methyl mercury** A toxic compound that results from the chemical transformation of mercury by bacteria. In trace amounts, mercury is water-soluble and contaminates many bodies of water.

**micelles** Tiny emulsified fat packets. They are composed of emulsifier molecules (phospholipids) oriented with their fat-soluble part facing inward and their water-soluble part facing outward toward the surrounding aqueous environment.

**microcytic hypochromic anemia** Anemia characterized by small, pale red blood cells that lack adequate hemoglobin to carry oxygen; can be caused by deficiency of iron or vitamin $B_6$.

**microencephaly** A type of neural tube birth defect in which the brain is abnormally small.

**microminerals** See *trace minerals*.

**micronutrients** Nutrients, such as vitamins and minerals, that are needed in relatively small amounts in the diet.

**microsomal ethanol-oxidizing system (MEOS)** An energy-requiring enzyme system in the liver that normally metabolizes drugs and other foreign substances. When the blood alcohol level is high, alcohol dehydrogenase cannot metabolize it fast enough, and the excess alcohol is metabolized by the MEOS.

**microvilli** Minute, hairlike projections that extend from the surface of absorptive cells facing the intestinal lumen.

**mineralization** The addition of minerals, such as calcium and phosphate, to bones and teeth.

**minerals** Inorganic compounds needed for growth and for regulation of body processes.

**mitochondria (mitochondrion)** The sites of aerobic production of ATP, where most of the energy from carbohydrate, protein, and fat is captured. Called the "power plants" of the cell, the mitochondria are where the citric acid cycle and electron transport chain are located. A human cell contains about 2,000 mitochondria.

**mitochondrial membrane** The mitochondria are enclosed by a double shell separated by an intermembrane space. The outer membrane acts as a barrier and gatekeeper, selectively allowing some molecules to pass through while blocking others. The inner membrane is where the electron transport chain is located.

**monoglyceride** A molecule of glycerol combined with one fatty acid.

**monosaccharides** Single sugar units. The common monosaccharides are glucose, fructose, and galactose.

**monounsaturated fatty acid** A fatty acid in which the carbon chain contains one double bond.

**morbid obesity** See *extreme obesity*.

**morning sickness** A persistent or recurring nausea that often occurs during early pregnancy, frequently—but not always—in the morning.

**motor proteins** Proteins that use energy and convert it into some form of mechanical work. Motor proteins are active in processes such as cell division, muscle contraction, and sperm movement.

**mucilages** Gelatinous soluble fibers containing galactose, mannose, and other monosaccharides; found in seaweed.

**mucosa [myu-KO-sa]** The innermost layer of a cavity. The inner layer of the gastrointestinal tract (the intestinal wall). It is composed of epithelial cells and glands.

**mucus** A slippery substance secreted in the GI tract (and other body linings) that protects cells from irritants.

**multilevel marketing** A system of selling in which each salesperson recruits assistants who then recruit others to help them. The person at each level collects a commission on sales made by the later recruits.

**multiple sclerosis** A progressive disease that destroys the myelin sheath surrounding nerve fibers of the brain and spinal cord.

**muscle fibers** Individual muscle cells.

**myelin sheath** The protective coating that surrounds nerve fibers.

**myoglobin** The oxygen-transporting protein of muscle that resembles blood hemoglobin in function.

**NAD⁺** Nicotinamide adenine dinucleotide ($NAD^+$), a coenzyme derived from the B vitamin niacin, becomes NADH as it accepts a pair of high-energy electrons for transport in cells.

**National Center for Complementary and Alternative Medicine (NCCAM)** An NIH organization established to stimulate, develop, and support objective scientific research on complementary and alternative medicine for the benefit of the public.

**National Institutes of Health (NIH)** A Department of Health and Human Services agency composed of 27 separate institutes and centers with a mission to advance knowledge and improve human health.

**National School Lunch Program** A USDA program that provides nutritious lunches and the opportunity to practice skills learned in classroom nutrition education; enacted in 1946 to provide U.S. children with at least one healthful meal every school day.

**natural killer cells** Nonspecific lymphocytes that spontaneously attack and kill cancer cells and cells infected by microorganisms. They are "natural" killers because they do not need to recognize a specific antigen in order to attack and kill.

**natural toxins** Poisons that are produced by or naturally occur in plants or microorganisms.

**negative energy balance** Energy intake is lower than energy expenditure, resulting in a depletion of body energy stores and weight loss.

**negative nitrogen balance** Nitrogen intake is less than the sum of all sources of nitrogen excretion.

**negative self-talk** Mental or verbal statements made to one's self that reinforce negative or destructive self-perceptions.

**neonate** An infant from birth to 28 days.

**neophobia** A dislike for anything new or unfamiliar.

**neotame** An artificial sweetener similar to aspartame, but one that is sweeter and does not require a warning label for people with phenylketonuria.

**neural tube defects (NTD)** Birth defects resulting from failure of the neural tube to develop properly during early fetal development.

**neuropeptide Y (NPY)** A neurotransmitter widely distributed throughout the brain and peripheral nervous tissue. NPY activity has been linked to eating behavior, depression, anxiety, and cardiovascular function.

**neurotransmitters** Substances released at the end of a stimulated nerve cell that diffuse across a small gap and bind to another nerve cell or muscle cell, stimulating or inhibiting it.

**niacin equivalents (NE)** A measure that includes preformed dietary niacin as well as niacin derived from tryptophan; 60 milligrams of tryptophan yield about 1 milligram of niacin.

**night blindness** The inability of the eyes to adjust to dim light or to regain vision quickly after exposure to a flash of bright light.

**night-eating syndrome (NES)** An eating disorder in which a habitual pattern of interrupting sleep to eat is the primary symptom.

**nitrogen balance** Nitrogen intake minus the sum of all sources of nitrogen excretion.

**nitrogen equilibrium** Nitrogen intake equals the sum of all sources of nitrogen excretion; nitrogen balance equals zero.

**nonessential fatty acids** Fatty acids that your body can make when they are needed. It is not necessary to consume them in the diet.

**nonexercise activity thermogenesis (NEAT)** The output of energy associated with fidgeting, maintenance of posture, and other minimal physical exertions.

**non-heme iron** The iron in plants and animal foods that is not part of hemoglobin or myoglobin.

**normal weight** BMI at or above $18.5 \text{ kg/m}^2$ and less than $25 \text{ kg/m}^2$.

**nucleic acids** A family of more than 25,000 molecules found in chromosomes, nucleoli, mitochondria, and the cytoplasm of cells.

**nucleus** The primary site of genetic information in the cell, enclosed in a double-layered membrane.

**nutrient density** A description of the healthfulness of foods. Foods high in nutrient density are those that provide substantial amounts of vitamins and minerals and relatively few calories; foods low in nutrient density are those that supply calories but relatively small amounts of vitamins and minerals (or none at all).

**nutrients** Any substances in food that the body can use to obtain energy, synthesize tissues, or regulate functions.

**nutrigenomics** The study of how nutrition interacts with specific genes to influence a person's health.

**nutrition** The science of foods and their components (nutrients and other substances), including the relationships to health and disease (actions, interactions, and balances); processes within the body (ingestion, digestion, absorption, transport, functions, and disposal of end products); and the social, economic, cultural, and psychological implications of eating.

**Nutrition Labeling and Education Act (NLEA)** An amendment to the Food, Drug, and Cosmetic of 1938. The NLEA made major changes to the content and scope of the nutrition label and to other elements of the food labels. Final regulations were published in 1993 and went into effect in 1994.

**nutritive sweeteners** Substances that make foods sweet and can be absorbed and yield energy in the body.

**obesity** Excessive accumulation of body fat leading to a body weight in relation to height that is substantially greater than some accepted standard. A BMI at or above $30 \text{ kg/m}^2$.

**obesogenic environment** Circumstances in which a person lives, works, and plays in a way that promotes the overconsumption of calories and discourages physical activity and calorie expenditure.

**obsessive-compulsive disorder** A disorder in which a person attempts to relieve anxiety by ritualistic behavior and continuous repetition of certain acts.

**Older Americans Act Nutrition Program** A federally funded program (formerly known as the *Elderly Nutrition Program*) that provides older adults with nutritionally sound meals through meals-on-wheels programs or in senior citizen centers and similar congregate settings.

**olestra** A fat replacer made from a sucrose backbone with six to eight fatty acids attached. The fatty acid arrangement prevents breakdown by the digestive enzyme lipase, so the fatty acids are not absorbed. Olestra can withstand heat and is stable at frying temperatures. Its trade name is Olean.

**oligopeptide** Four to 10 amino acids joined by peptide bonds.

**oligosaccharides** Short carbohydrate chains composed of 3 to 10 sugar molecules.

***omega*-3 fatty acid** An essential fatty acid; alpha-linolenic acid is the major type.

***omega*-6 fatty acid** An essential fatty acid; linoleic acid is the primary type.

**opsin** A protein that combines with retinal to form rhodopsin in rod cells.

**orexin** A class of hormones in the brain that may affect human food consumption.

**organelles** Various membrane-bound structures that form part of the cytoplasm. Organelles perform specialized metabolic functions.

**organic** In chemistry, any compound that contains carbon, except carbon oxides (e.g., carbon dioxide) and sulfides and metal carbonates (e.g., potassium carbonate). The term *organic* also is used to denote crops that are grown without synthetic fertilizers or chemicals.

**organic foods** Foods that originate from farms or handling operations that meet the standards set by the USDA National Organic Program. The methods of organic food production eschew modern synthetic pesticides and chemical fertilizers—organic foods do not contain genetically modified organisms and are not processed using irradiation, industrial solvents, or chemical food additives.

**orthomolecular medicine** The preventive or therapeutic use of high-dose vitamins to treat disease.

**osmosis** The movement of a solvent, such as water, through a semipermeable membrane from the dilute to the concentrated side until the concentrations on both sides of the membrane are equal.

**osteoblasts** Bone cells that synthesize and excrete the extracellular matrix that forms the structure of bone.

**osteoclasts** Bone cells that break down bone structure and release calcium and phosphate into the blood.

**osteomalacia** A disease in adults that results from vitamin D deficiency; it is marked by softening of the bones, leading to bending of the spine, bowing of the legs, and increased risk for fractures.

**osteoporosis** A bone disease characterized by a decrease in bone mineral density and the appearance of small holes in bones due to loss of minerals.

**overweight** BMI at or above 25 $kg/m^2$ and less than 30 $kg/m^2$.

**oxalate (oxalic acid)** An organic acid in some leafy green vegetables, such as spinach, that binds to calcium to form calcium oxalate, an insoluble compound the body cannot absorb.

**oxaloacetate** A four-carbon intermediate compound in the citric acid cycle. Acetyl CoA combines with free oxaloacetate in the mitochondria, forming citric acid and beginning the cycle.

**oxidation** Oxygen attaches to the double bonds of unsaturated fatty acids. Oxidation causes fats to become rancid.

**oxygen energy system** A complex energy system that requires oxygen. To release ATP, it completes the breakdown of carbohydrate and fatty acids via the citric acid cycle and electron transport chain.

**oxytocin** A pituitary hormone that stimulates the release of milk from the breast.

**palatable** Pleasant tasting.

**pancreas** An organ that secretes enzymes that affect the digestion and absorption of nutrients and that releases hormones, such as insulin, which regulate metabolism as well as the way nutrients are used in the body.

**pancreatic amylase** Starch-digesting enzyme secreted by the pancreas.

**parathyroid hormone (PTH)** A hormone secreted by the parathyroid glands in response to low blood calcium. It stimulates calcium release from bone and calcium absorption by the intestines, while decreasing calcium excretion by the kidneys. It acts in conjunction with 25(OH)D to raise blood calcium. Also called parathormone.

**passive diffusion** The movement of substances into or out of cells without the expenditure of energy or the involvement of transport proteins in the cell membrane. Also called *simple diffusion*.

**pasteurization** A process for destroying pathogenic bacteria by heating liquid foods to a prescribed temperature for a specified time.

**pathogenic** Capable of causing disease.

**pectins** A type of dietary fiber found in fruits.

**peer review** An appraisal of research against accepted standards by professionals in the field.

**pepsin** A protein-digesting enzyme produced by the stomach.

**pepsinogen** The inactive form of the enzyme pepsin.

**peptide bond** The bond between two amino acids formed when a carboxyl (–COOH) group of one amino acid joins an amino (–$NH_2$) group of another amino acid, releasing water in the process.

**perceived exertion** The subjective experience of how difficult an effort is.

**peristalsis [per-ih-STAHL-sis]** The wavelike, rhythmic muscular contractions of the GI tract that propel its contents down the tract.

**pernicious anemia** A form of anemia that results from an autoimmune disorder that damages cells lining the stomach and inhibits vitamin $B_{12}$ absorption; causes vitamin $B_{12}$ deficiency.

**pesticides** Chemicals used to control and kill insects, diseases, weeds, fungi, and other pests on plants, vegetables, fruits, and animals.

**pH** A measurement of the hydrogen ion concentration, or acidity, of a solution.

**phenylketonuria (PKU)** An inherited disorder that causes a lack of the enzyme that metabolizes phenylalanine.

**phosphate group** A chemical group that contains phosphate (–$PO_4$) attached to a larger molecule. Attaching a phosphate group, along with two fatty acids, to a glycerol backbone forms a phospholipid.

**phosphocreatine** See *creatine phosphate*.

**phospholipids** Compounds that consist of a glycerol molecule bonded to two fatty acid molecules and a phosphate group with a nitrogen-containing component. Phospholipids have both water-soluble and fat-soluble regions, which makes them good emulsifiers.

**photosynthesis** The process by which green plants use light energy from the sun to produce carbohydrates from carbon dioxide and water.

**phylloquinone** The form of vitamin K that comes from plant sources. Also known as *vitamin $K_1$*.

**phytate (phytic acid)** A phosphorus-containing compound in the outer husks of cereal grains that binds with minerals and inhibits their absorption.

**phytochemicals** Substances in plants that may possess health-protective effects, even though they are not essential for life.

**phytoestrogens** Plant compounds that have weak estrogen activity in the body.

**phytosterols** Sterols found in plants. Phytosterols are poorly absorbed by humans and reduce intestinal absorption of cholesterol. They recently have been introduced as a cholesterol-lowering food ingredient.

**placebo** An inactive substance that is outwardly indistinguishable from the active substance whose effects are being studied.

**placebo effect** A physical or emotional change that is not due to properties of an administered substance. The change reflects participants' expectations.

**placenta** The organ formed during pregnancy that produces hormones for the maintenance of pregnancy and across which oxygen and nutrients are transferred from mother to infant; it also allows waste materials to be transferred from infant to mother.

**plasma** The fluid portion of the blood that contains blood cells and other components.

**poisonous mushrooms** Mushrooms that contain toxins that can cause stomach upset, dizziness, hallucinations, and other neurological symptoms.

**pollutants** Gaseous, chemical, or organic waste that contaminates air, soil, or water.

**polysaccharides** Long carbohydrate chains composed of more than 10 sugar molecules. Polysaccharides can be straight or branched.

**polyols** See *sugar alcohols*.

**polypeptide** More than 10 amino acids joined by peptide bonds.

**polyphenols** Organic compounds that may produce bitterness in coffee and tea.

**polyunsaturated fatty acid** A fatty acid in which the carbon chain contains two or more double bonds.

**positive energy balance** Energy intake exceeds energy expenditure, resulting in an increase in body energy stores and weight gain.

**positive nitrogen balance** Nitrogen intake exceeds the sum of all sources of nitrogen excretion.

**positive self-talk** Constructive mental or verbal statements made to one's self to change a belief or behavior.

**post-traumatic stress disorder (PTSD)** An anxiety disorder characterized by an emotional response to a traumatic event or situation involving severe external stress.

**precursor** A substance that is converted into another active substance. Enzyme precursors also are called *proenzymes*.

**pre-diabetes** Blood glucose levels higher than normal but not high enough to warrant a diagnosis of diabetes.

**preeclampsia** A condition of late pregnancy characterized by maternal hypertension, edema, and proteinuria.

**pregorexia** A term used to describe pregnant women who reduce calories and exercise in excess in an effort to control pregnancy weight gain.

**prematurity** Birth before 37 weeks of gestation.

**preservatives** Chemicals or other agents that slow the decomposition of a food.

**preterm delivery** A delivery that occurs before the 37th week of gestation.

**prions** Short for *proteinaceous infectious particle*. Self-reproducing protein particles that can cause disease.

**prior-sanctioned substance** All substances that the FDA or the U.S. Department of Agriculture (USDA) had determined were safe for use in specific foods before passage of the 1958 Food Additives amendment are designated as prior-sanctioned substances. These substances are exempt from the food additive regulation process.

**proenzymes** Inactive precursors of enzymes.

**prolactin** A pituitary hormone that stimulates the production of milk in breast tissue.

**proteases [PRO-tea-aces]** Enzymes that break down protein into peptides and amino acids.

**protein digestibility-corrected amino acid score (PDCAAS)** A measure of protein quality that takes into account the amino acid composition of the food and the digestibility of the protein.

**protein-energy malnutrition (PEM)** A condition resulting from long-term inadequate intakes of protein and energy that can lead to wasting of body tissues and increased susceptibility to infection.

**protein hydrolysates** Proteins that have been treated with enzymes to break them down into amino acids and shorter peptides.

**proteins** Large, complex compounds consisting of many amino acids connected in varying sequences and forming unique shapes.

**protein turnover** The constant breakdown and synthesis of proteins in the body.

**provitamin A** Carotenoid precursors of vitamin A in foods of plant origin, primarily deeply colored fruits and vegetables.

**provitamins** Inactive forms of vitamins that the body can convert into active usable forms. Also referred to as vitamin precursors.

**psyllium** The dried husk of the psyllium seed.

**puberty** The period of life during which the secondary sex characteristics develop and the ability to reproduce is attained.

**purge** Emptying of the GI tract by self-induced vomiting and/or misuse of laxatives, diuretics, or enemas.

**pyloric sphincter** A circular muscle that forms the opening between the duodenum and the stomach. It regulates the passage of food into the small intestine.

**pyruvate** The three-carbon compound that results from glycolysis. Cells also can make glucose from pyruvate, but this process requires energy and several enzymes not involved in glycolysis. Pyruvate also can be derived from glycerol and some amino acids.

**reactive hypoglycemia** A type of hypoglycemia that occurs about one hour after eating carbohydrate-rich food. The body overreacts and produces too much insulin in response to food, rapidly decreasing blood glucose.

**rectum** The muscular final segment of the intestine, extending from the sigmoid colon to the anus.

**refined sweeteners** Substances composed of monosaccharides and disaccharides that have been extracted and processed from other foods.

**resistant starch** A starch that is not digested.

**resting energy expenditure (REE)** The minimum energy needed to maintain basic physiological functions (e.g., heartbeat, muscle function, respiration). The resting metabolic rate (RMR) extrapolated to 24 hours.

**resting metabolic rate (RMR)** A clinical measure of resting energy expenditure performed three to four hours after eating or performing significant physical activity.

**restrained eaters** Individuals who routinely avoid food as long as possible, and then gorge on food.

**retina** A paper-thin tissue that lines the back of the eye and contains cells called rods and cones.

**retinal** The aldehyde form of vitamin A; one of the retinoids; the active form of vitamin A in the retina; interconvertible with retinol.

**retinoic acid** The acid form of vitamin A; one of the retinoids; formed from retinal but not interconvertible; helps growth, cell differentiation, and the immune system; does not have a role in vision or reproduction.

**retinoids** Compounds in foods that have chemical structures similar to vitamin A. Retinoids include the active forms of vitamin A (retinol, retinal, and retinoic acid) and the main storage forms of retinol (retinyl esters).

**retinol** The alcohol form of vitamin A; one of the retinoids; the main physiologically active form of vitamin A; interconvertible with retinal.

**retinol activity equivalent (RAE)** A unit of measurement of the vitamin A content of a food. One RAE equals 1 microgram of retinol.

**rhodopsin** Found in rod cells, this light-sensitive pigment molecule consists of a protein called opsin combined with retinal.

**rickets** A bone disease in children that results from vitamin D deficiency.

**rod cells** Light-sensitive cells in the retina that react to dim light and transmit black-and-white images.

**saccharin [SAK-ah-ren]** An artificial sweetener that tastes about 300 to 700 times sweeter than sucrose. Neither digested nor absorbed, saccharin contributes no calories to the diet.

**salivary amylase [AM-ih-lace]** An enzyme that catalyzes the hydrolysis of amylose, a starch. Also called *ptyalin*.

**salivary glands** Glands in the mouth that release saliva.

*Salmonella* Rod-shaped bacteria responsible for many foodborne illnesses.

**salts** Compounds that result when the hydrogen of an acid is replaced with a metal or a group that acts like a metal.

**satiation** Feeling of satisfaction and fullness that terminates a meal.

**satiety** The effects of a food or meal that delay subsequent intake. Feeling of satisfaction and fullness following eating that quells the desire for food.

**saturated fatty acid** A fatty acid completely filled by hydrogen, with all carbons in the chain linked by single bonds.

**School Breakfast Program** A USDA program that assists schools in providing a nutritious morning meal to children nationwide.

**seborrheic dermatitis** Disease of the oil-producing glands of the skin; a symptom of riboflavin deficiency.

**segmentation** Periodic muscle contractions at intervals along the GI tract that alternate forward and backward movement of the contents, thereby breaking apart chunks of the food mass and mixing in digestive juices.

**simple carbohydrates** Monosaccharides and disaccharides; simple carbohydrates. Sugars composed of a single sugar molecule (a monosaccharide) or two joined sugar molecules (a disaccharide).

**skeletal muscles** Muscles composed of bundles of parallel, striated muscle fibers under voluntary control. Also called *voluntary muscle* or *striated muscle*.

**skinfold measurements** A method to estimate body fat by measuring the thickness of a fold of skin and subcutaneous fat.

**sleep apnea** Periods of absence of breathing during sleep.

**slow-twitch (ST) fibers** Muscle fibers that develop tension more slowly and to a lesser extent than fast-twitch muscle fibers. ST fibers have high oxidative capacities and are slower to fatigue than fast-twitch fibers.

**small intestine** The tube (approximately 3 meters [10 ft] long) where the digestion of protein, fat, and carbohydrate is completed and where the majority of nutrients are absorbed. The small intestine is divided into three parts: the duodenum, the jejunum, and the ileum.

**soda loading** Consumption of bicarbonate (baking soda) to raise blood pH. The intent is to increase the capacity to buffer acids, thus delaying fatigue. Also known as *bicarbonate loading*.

**solanine** A potentially toxic alkaloid that is present with chlorophyll in the green areas on potato skins.

**Special Supplemental Nutrition Program for Women, Infants, and Children (WIC)** A USDA program that provides federal grants to states for supplemental foods, healthcare referrals, and nutrition education for low-income pregnant, breastfeeding, and nonbreastfeeding postpartum women and/or infants and children at nutritional risk.

**sphincters [SFINGK-ters]** Circular bands of muscle fibers that surround the entrance or exit of a hollow body structure (e.g., the stomach) and act as valves to control the flow of material.

**spina bifida** A type of neural tube birth defect.

**sports anemia** A lowered concentration of hemoglobin in the blood due to dilution. The increased plasma volume that dilutes the hemoglobin is a normal consequence of aerobic training.

**squalene** A cholesterol precursor found in whale liver and plants.

**standard drink** One serving of alcohol (about 15 grams) is equal to 12 ounces of beer, 4 to 5 ounces of wine, or 1.5 ounces of liquor.

**starch** The major storage form of carbohydrate in plants; starch is composed of long chains of glucose molecules in a straight (amylose) or branching (amylopectin) arrangement.

**stem cells** Formative cells whose daughter cells may differentiate into other cell types.

**sterols** A category of lipids that includes cholesterol. Sterols are hydrocarbons with several rings in their structures.

**stevia** See *stevioside*.

**stevioside** A dietary supplement, not approved for use as a sweetener, that is extracted and refined from *Stevia rebaudiana* leaves.

**stomach** The enlarged, muscular, saclike portion of the digestive tract between the esophagus and the small intestine, with a capacity of about 1 quart.

**structure/function claims** These statements may claim a benefit related to a nutrient-deficiency disease (e.g., *vitamin C prevents scurvy*) or describe the role of a nutrient or dietary ingredient intended to affect a structure or function in humans (e.g., *calcium helps build strong bones*).

**subcutaneous fat** Fat stores under the skin.

**sucralose** An artificial sweetener made from sucrose. Sucralose is nonnutritive and about 600 times sweeter than sugar.

**sucrose [SOO-crose]** A disaccharide composed of one molecule of glucose and one molecule of fructose joined together. Also known as *table sugar*.

**sugar alcohols** Compounds formed from monosaccharides; commonly used as nutritive sweeteners. Also called *polyols*.

**Summer Food Service Program** A USDA program that helps children in lower-income families to continue receiving nutritious meals during long school vacations when they do not have access to school lunch or breakfast.

**Supplementary Nutrition Assistance Program (SNAP)** A USDA program that helps single people and families with little or no income to buy food. Formerly known as the *Food Stamp Program*.

**Supplement Facts panel** Content label that must appear on all dietary supplements.

**tagatose** An artificial sweetener derived from lactose that has the same sweetness as sucrose with only half of the calories.

**taste threshold** The minimum amount of flavor that must be present for a taste to be detected.

**teratogen** Any substance that causes birth defects.

**thermic effect of food (TEF)** The energy used to digest, absorb, and metabolize energy-yielding foodstuffs. It constitutes about 10 percent of total energy expenditure but is influenced by various factors.

**thiamin pyrophosphate (TPP)** A coenzyme of which the vitamin thiamin is a part. It plays a key role in removing carboxyl groups in chemical reactions and helps drive the reaction that forms acetyl CoA from pyruvate during metabolism.

**thyroid-stimulating hormone (TSH)** Hormone secreted from the pituitary gland at the base of the brain; regulates synthesis of thyroid hormones.

**tocopherol** The chemical name for vitamin E. There are four tocopherols (alpha, beta, gamma, and delta), but only alpha-tocopherol is active in the body.

**tocotrienol** Four compounds (alpha, beta, gamma, and delta) chemically related to tocopherols. The tocotrienols and tocopherols are collectively known as vitamin E.

**toddler** A child between 12 and 36 months of age.

**Tolerable Upper Intake Levels (ULs)** The maximum levels of daily nutrient intakes that are unlikely to pose health risks to almost all of the individuals in the group for whom they are designed.

**total energy expenditure (TEE)** The total of the resting energy expenditure (REE), energy used in physical activity, and energy used in processing food (TEF); usually expressed in kilocalories per day.

**total fiber** The sum of dietary fiber and functional fiber.

**trace minerals** Trace minerals are present in the body and required in the diet in relatively small amounts compared with major minerals; also known as *microminerals*.

***trans* fatty acid** An unsaturated fatty acid with a straighter chain than a *cis* fatty acid, usually as a result of hydrogenation; *trans* fatty acids are more solid than *cis* fatty acids.

**transferrin** A protein synthesized in the liver that transports iron in the blood to the red blood cells for use in heme synthesis.

**trehalose** A disaccharide of two glucose molecules but with a linkage different from maltose. Used as a food additive and sweetener.

**tricarboxylic acid (TCA) cycle** See *citric acid cycle*.

**triglycerides** Fats composed of three fatty acid chains linked to a glycerol molecule.

**trimesters** Three equal time periods of pregnancy, each lasting approximately 13 to 14 weeks.

**tripeptide** Three amino acids joined by peptide bonds.

**tryptophan** An amino acid that serves as a niacin precursor in the body. In the body, 60 milligrams of tryptophan yield about one milligram of niacin, or 1 niacin equivalent (NE).

**25-hydroxyvitamin D [25(OH)D]** The active form of vitamin D. It is an important regulator of blood calcium levels.

**type 1 diabetes** Diabetes that occurs when the body's immune system attacks beta cells in the pancreas, causing them to lose their ability to make insulin.

**type 2 diabetes** Diabetes that occurs when target cells (e.g., fat and muscle cells) lose the ability to respond normally to insulin.

**ulcer** A craterlike lesion that occurs in the lining of the stomach or duodenum; also called a *peptic ulcer* to distinguish it from a skin ulcer.

**umami [ooh-MA-mee]** A Japanese term that describes a delicious meaty or savory sensation. Chemically, this taste detects the presence of glutamate.

**underwater weighing** Determining body density by measuring the volume of water displaced when the body is fully submerged in a specialized water tank. Also called *hydrostatic weighing*.

**underweight** BMI less than 18.5 $kg/m^2$.

**unsaturated fatty acid** A fatty acid in which the carbon chain contains one or more double bonds.

**urea** The main nitrogen-containing waste product in mammals. Formed in liver cells from ammonia and carbon dioxide, urea is carried via the bloodstream to the kidneys, where it is excreted in the urine.

**urinary tract infection (UTI)** An infection of one or more structures in the urinary tract; usually caused by bacteria.

**U.S. Department of Agriculture (USDA)** The government agency that monitors the production of eggs, poultry, and meat for adherence to standards of quality and wholesomeness. The USDA also provides public nutrition education, performs nutrition research, and administers the WIC program.

**U.S. Pharmacopeia (USP)** Established in 1820, the USP is a nonprofit health care organization that sets quality standards for a range of health care products.

**vascular system** A network of veins and arteries through which the blood carries nutrients. Also called the *blood circulatory system*.

**very-low-calorie diets (VLCD)** Diets supplying 400 to 800 kilocalories per day, which include adequate high-quality protein, little or no fat, and little carbohydrate.

**very-low-density lipoproteins (VLDL)** The triglyceride-rich lipoproteins formed in the liver. VLDL enters the bloodstream and is gradually acted upon by lipoprotein lipase, releasing triglyceride to body cells.

**villi** Small fingerlike projections that blanket the folds in the lining of the small intestine. Singular is *villus*.

**visceral fat** Fat stores that cushion body organs.

**vitamin precursors** See *provitamins*.

**vitamins** Organic compounds necessary for reproduction, growth, and maintenance of the body. Vitamins are required in miniscule amounts.

**waist circumference** The waist measurement, as a marker of abdominal fat content, can be used to indicate health risks.

**wasting** The breakdown of body tissue, such as muscle and organ, for use as a protein source when the diet lacks protein.

**weight cycling** Repeated periods of gaining and losing weight. Also called *yo-yo dieting*.

**weight management** The adoption of healthful and sustainable eating and exercise behaviors that reduce disease risk and improve well-being.

**Wilson's disease** Genetic disorder of increased copper absorption, which leads to toxic levels in the liver and heart.

**wood alcohol** Common name for methanol.

**World Health Organization (WHO)** A global organization that directs and coordinates international health work. Its goal is the attainment by all peoples of the highest possible level of health, defined as a state of complete physical, mental, and social well-being and not merely the absence of disease or infirmity.

**xerophthalmia** A condition caused by vitamin A deficiency that dries the cornea and mucous membranes of the eye.

# Index